MATERNAL, FETAL, AND NEONATAL PHYSIOLOGY

A CLINICAL PERSPECTIVE

Susan Tucker Blackburn, Ph.D., R.N.,C., F.A.A.N.

Professor, Department of Parent and Child Nursing
School of Nursing, University of Washington
Seattle, Washington

Donna Lee Loper, M.S., R.N., C.N.S.

Neonatal Clinical Nurse Specialist and Nursery Clinical Coordinator
San Francisco General Hospital and Medical Center
San Francisco, California

W.B. SAUNDERS COMPANY
A Division of Harcourt Brace & Company

Philadelphia London Toronto Montreal Sydney Tokyo

W.B. SAUNDERS COMPANY
A Division of
Harcourt Brace & Company

The Curtis Center
Independence Square West
Philadelphia, Pennsylvania 19106

Library of Congress Cataloging-in-Publication Data

Blackburn, Susan, Ph.D.

Maternal, fetal, and neonatal physiology: a clinical perspective / Susan
Tucker Blackburn, Donna Lee Loper.

    p.   cm.

ISBN 0–7216–2936–9

1. Pregnancy.   2. Fetus—Physiology.   3. Infants (Newborn)—
Physiology.   I. Loper, Donna Lee.   II. Title. [DNLM:
1. Fetus—physiology.   2. Infant, Newborn—physiology.
3. Pregnancy—physiology.   WQ 205 B628m] RG558.B58
1992

612.6'3—dc20

DNLM/DLC   91–6872

Editor: Thomas Eoyang
Designer: Dorothy Chattin
Production Manager: Ken Neimeister
Manuscript Editor: Arlene Friday
Illustration Coordinator: Peg Shaw
Indexer: Kathleen Cole

Maternal, Fetal, and Neonatal Physiology   ISBN 0–7216–2936–9

Last digit is the print number: 9   8   7   6   5

Contributor and Reviewers

Contributor

Karen Ann Thomas, Ph.D., R.N.
Assistant Professor
Department of Parent and Child Nursing
University of Washington
Seattle, Washington

Reviewers

Mary K. Barger, M.P.H., R.N., C.N.M.
UCSF/UCSD Intercampus Graduate Studies
   in Nurse-Midwifery
La Jolla, California

Jane L. Berry, M.S.N., R.N.,C.
Hospital of the University of Pennsylvania
Philadelphia, Pennsylvania

Mary L. Dickey, M.S.N., R.N., C.N.A.
North Bay Medical Center
Fairfield, California

**Rosmarie A. Fuller, M.S.N., R.N.,
I.B.C.L.C.**
Anna Jaques Hospital
Newburyport, Massachusetts

Mary F. Haire, M.S.N., R.N.
Copper Basin Medical Center
Copperhill, Tennessee

Diane Holditch-Davis, Ph.D., R.N.
University of North Carolina at Chapel Hill
Chapel Hill, North Carolina

Maribeth Inturrisi, M.S., R.N.
The Medical Center of the University of
   California at San Francisco
San Francisco, California

Tracy B. Karp, M.S., R.N.C., N.N.P.
Primary Children's Medical Center
Salt Lake City, Utah

Kathryn A. Lee, R.N., Ph.D.
University of California, San Francisco
San Francisco, California

Cynthia A. Levy, M.S.N., R.N.,C.
St. Louis Children's Hospital
St. Louis, Missouri

Mary Beth Malloy, M.S.N., R.N.
Loyola University Medical Center
Maywood, Illinois

Barbara Medoff-Cooper, Ph.D., F.A.A.N.
University of Pennsylvania
Philadelphia, Pennsylvania

Sally B. Olds, M.S.N., R.N.,C.
Beth-El College of Nursing
Colorado Springs, Colorado

**Rosanne Perez-Woods, Ed.D., R.N.,
C.P.N.P., F.A.A.N.**
Loyola University of Chicago
Chicago, Illinois

Deborah Woolley Perlis, Ph.D., C.N.M.
University of Colorado School of Nursing
Denver, Colorado

**Kathrine L. Peters, M.N., R.N.,
Ph.D. Candidate**
University of Washington
Seattle, Washington

Preface

Accurate assessment and clinical care appropriate to the developmental and maturational stage of the mother, fetus, and neonate depend on a thorough understanding of normal physiologic processes and the ability of the caregiver to understand the impact of pathologic deviations on these processes. Information on normal perinatal physiology and its clinical implications can be found in various sources, including journal articles, general physiology texts, core nursing texts, and medical references. In our experience of teaching students and acting as preceptors for clinical staff, we found that the material in these sources was fragmented, too basic in level, focused on one phase of the perinatal period without integration within the maternal-fetal-neonatal unit, too medically oriented, or lacked the clinical applications relevant to patient care and thus did not adequately meet the needs of nurses in specialty and advanced clinical practice.

We attempted to create, therefore, a single text that brought together detailed information on the physiologic changes that occur throughout the perinatal period, with emphasis on the mother, fetus, and neonate and the interrelationships between them. The purpose of this book is not to provide a manual of specific assessment and intervention strategies or to focus on pathophysiology, but rather to provide the practitioner with information on normal physiologic adaptations and developmental physiology that provides the scientific basis and rationale underlying assessment and management of the low- and high-risk pregnant woman, fetus, and neonate. Since the focus of this book is on physiologic adaptations, psychological aspects of perinatal care are not addressed. These aspects are certainly important but are not within the realm of this text.

This textbook provides detailed descriptions of the physiologic processes associated with the perinatal client: mother, fetus, or neonate. The major focus is on the normal physiologic adaptations of the pregnant woman during the antepartum, intrapartum, and postpartum periods; anatomic and functional development of the fetus; transition and adaptation of the infant at birth; and developmental physiology of the neonate (term and preterm), including a summary of maturation of each body system during infancy and childhood. We also examine the clinical implications of these physiologic adaptations as they relate to the pregnant woman, the maternal-fetal unit, and the neonate. Each chapter relates the impact of normal physiologic adaptations to clinical assessment and interventions with low- and high-risk women and neonates with selected health problems. Of special interest to those seeking quick access to clinical information are the tabular recommendations for clinical practice that index content describing the scientific basis and rationale underlying each recommendation.

Given the growing recognition that advanced practice nursing is based on a sound physiologic as well as a sound nursing theoretical base, we hope that this book will be seen as a useful foundation reference for specialty and advanced practice nurses in both primary and acute settings, as well as for graduate programs in maternal, perinatal, and neonatal nursing, and nurse midwifery. As the collaborative perspective on perinatal care gains power, this book may also hold appeal for other health care professionals involved in obstetrics and neonatology, including physicians, physical and occupational therapists, respiratory therapists, and nutritionists.

SUSAN TUCKER BLACKBURN
DONNA LEE LOPER

Acknowledgments

We would like to acknowledge the many individuals whose help and support were critical in making this book a reality. These include former and current students, nursing staff, and faculty colleagues who stimulated us to expand our knowledge of perinatal physiology and to examine the scientific basis for nursing interventions with pregnant women and neonates. We would also like to thank these individuals for their support and help during the development of this book. The women, neonates, and their families whom we have cared for during our years in perinatal nursing and from whom we have learned a great deal also stimulated us to write this book. We deeply appreciate the efforts of the reviewers listed on page iii, whose constructive comments and suggestions helped in refining the content and in making this book more useful for the intended audience. Warm appreciation and heartfelt thanks go to Karen Thomas, friend and colleague, for her contribution of the fetal and neonatal content in Chapter 12, "The Neuromuscular and Sensory Systems." A special acknowledgment also goes to our editor, Thomas Eoyang, who supported this project from its conception and provided helpful feedback and guidance over the past few years.

Finally, we would like to thank our families for their support, guidance, and encouragement in all our endeavors.

Contents

UNIT I
REPRODUCTIVE AND DEVELOPMENTAL PROCESSES 1

CHAPTER 1   Biologic and Physiologic Basis for
Reproduction 3

Basic Genetic Mechanisms and Principles   3
Causes and Transmission of Genetic Diseases   6
Embryonic and Fetal Development of the Reproductive System   10
Fetal Endocrinology   18
Common Anomalies   20
Gametogenesis   23
Reproductive Processes   24
Clinical Implications   29

CHAPTER 2   The Prenatal Period and Placental
Physiology 36

Overview of Pregnancy   37
Conception   40
Clinical Implications Related to Conception   45
Embryonic and Fetal Development   49
Clinical Implications Related to Embryonic and Fetal
    Development   60
The Placenta and Placental Physiology   63
Umbilical Cord   81
Amnion and Chorion   82
Amniotic Fluid   83
Clinical Implications Related to Placental Physiology   84
Multiple Pregnancy   95

CHAPTER 3   Parturition and Uterine Physiology 109

The Uterus   109
The Myometrium   111
Physiology of Parturition   113
Clinical Implications for the Pregnant Woman and Her Fetus   122

CHAPTER 4   The Postpartum Period and Lactation
Physiology 136

Involution of the Reproductive Organs   137
Endocrine Changes   139
Physiology of Lactation   141

UNIT II
ADAPTATIONS IN MAJOR BODY SYSTEMS IN THE PREGNANT WOMAN, FETUS, AND NEONATE 157

CHAPTER 5   The Hematologic and Hemostatic Systems ... **159**
Maternal Physiologic Adaptations   160
Clinical Implications for the Pregnant Woman and Her Fetus   171
Development of the Hematologic System in the Fetus   176
Neonatal Physiology   179
Clinical Implications for Neonatal Care   186
Maturational Changes During Infancy and Childhood   195

CHAPTER 6   Cardiovascular System **201**
Maternal Physiologic Adaptations   202
Clinical Implications for the Pregnant Woman and Her Fetus   212
Development of the Cardiovascular System in the Fetus   228
Neonatal Physiology   240
Clinical Implications for Neonatal Care   246
Maturational Changes During Infancy and Childhood   253

CHAPTER 7   The Respiratory System **262**
Maternal Physiologic Adaptations   263
Clinical Implications for the Pregnant Woman and Her Fetus   270
Development of the Respiratory System in the Fetus   276
Neonatal Physiology   289
Clinical Implications for Neonatal Care   309
Maturational Changes During Infancy and Childhood   324

CHAPTER 8   The Renal System and Fluid and Electrolyte Homeostasis **336**
Maternal Physiologic Adaptations   337
Clinical Implications for the Pregnant Woman and Her Fetus   346
Development of the Renal System in the Fetus   354
Neonatal Physiology   358
Clinical Implications for Neonatal Care   365
Maturational Changes During Infancy and Childhood   371

CHAPTER 9   The Gastrointestinal and Hepatic Systems and Perinatal Nutrition **379**
Maternal Physiologic Adaptations   380
Clinical Implications for the Pregnant Woman and Her Fetus   389
Development of the Gastrointestinal and Hepatic Systems in the Fetus   397
Neonatal Physiology   408
Clinical Implications for Neonatal Care   417
Maturational Changes During Infancy and Childhood   429

CHAPTER 10   The Immune System and Host Defense Mechanisms **439**
Maternal Physiologic Adaptations   440
Clinical Implications for the Pregnant Woman and Her Fetus   446
Development of Host Defense Mechanisms in the Fetus   464

Neonatal Physiology   467
Clinical Implications for Neonatal Care   474
Maturational Changes During Infancy and Childhood   482

CHAPTER 11   The Integumentary System **491**
Maternal Physiologic Processes   492
Clinical Implications for the Pregnant Woman and Her Fetus   498
Development of the Integumentary System in the Fetus   499
Transitional Events   507
Neonatal Physiology   508
Clinical Implications for Neonatal Care   511
Maturational Changes During Infancy and Childhood   516

CHAPTER 12   The Neuromuscular and Sensory Systems ... **522**
Maternal Physiologic Adaptations   523
Clinical Implications for the Pregnant Woman and Her Fetus   528
Development of the Neuromuscular and Sensory Systems in the
    Fetus   538
Neonatal Physiology   551
Clinical Implications for Neonatal Care   565
Maturational Changes During Infancy and Childhood   575

UNIT III
ADAPTATIONS IN METABOLIC PROCESSES IN THE
PREGNANT WOMAN, FETUS, AND NEONATE 581

CHAPTER 13   Carbohydrate, Fat, and Protein
Metabolism **583**
Maternal Physiologic Adaptations   584
Clinical Implications for the Pregnant Woman and Her Fetus   591
Fetal Development of Carbohydrate, Fat, and Protein
    Metabolism   598
Neonatal Physiology   603
Clinical Implications for Neonatal Care   606
Maturational Changes During Infancy and Childhood   609

CHAPTER 14   Calcium and Phosphorus Metabolism **614**
Maternal Physiologic Adaptations   614
Clinical Implications for the Pregnant Woman and Her Fetus   618
Development of Calcium and Phosphorus Metabolism in the
    Fetus   621
Neonatal Physiology   623
Clinical Implications for Neonatal Care   626
Maturational Changes During Infancy and Childhood   631

CHAPTER 15   Bilirubin Metabolism **636**
Maternal Physiologic Adaptations   636
Clinical Implications for the Pregnant Woman and Her Fetus   637
Development of Bilirubin Metabolism in the Fetus   638
Neonatal Physiology   639
Clinical Implications for Neonatal Care   644
Maturational Changes During Infancy and Childhood   654

CHAPTER 16   Thyroid Function **660**

Maternal Physiologic Adaptations   660
Clinical Implications for the Pregnant Woman and Her Fetus   663
Development of Thyroid Function in the Fetus   667
Neonatal Physiology   668
Clinical Implications for Neonatal Care   670
Maturational Changes During Infancy and Childhood   672

CHAPTER 17   Thermoregulation **677**

Maternal Physiologic Adaptations   677
Clinical Implications for the Pregnant Woman and Her Fetus   678
Neonatal Physiology   679
Clinical Implications for Neonatal Care   684
Maturational Changes During Infancy and Childhood   693

Index **699**

Reproductive and Developmental Processes

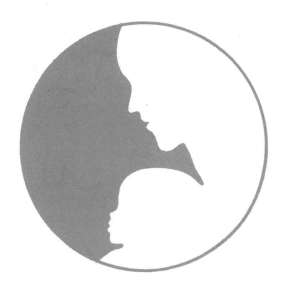

CHAPTER 1

Biologic and Physiologic Basis for Reproduction

Basic Genetic Mechanisms and Principles
    Chromosomes and Genes
    DNA Structure and Function
    DNA Replication
    Cell Division
        Mitosis
        Meiosis
Causes and Transmission of Genetic Diseases
Embryonic and Fetal Development of the
    Reproductive System
    Development of the Gonads
    Development of the Genital Ducts
    Development of the External Genitalia

Fetal Endocrinology
Common Anomalies
Gametogenesis
    Spermatogenesis
    Oogenesis
    Abnormal Gamete Development
Reproductive Processes
    Female
    Male
Clinical Implications
    Infertility
    Contraception

The biologic and physiologic basis for reproduction includes the embryonic development of the reproductive system from fertilization to puberty, including the process of gametogenesis. The ability to reproduce is modified throughout the life span and is influenced by deoxyribonucleic acid (DNA) and chromosomal structure and function. Therefore, these areas are also included in this chapter.

BASIC GENETIC MECHANISMS AND PRINCIPLES

Chromosomes and Genes

There are between 50,000 and 100,000 genes in an individual's total gene pool (genome).

These genes direct protein synthesis while regulating the rate at which protein is synthesized. This means that genes are important in determining and maintaining structural integrity and cell function and in regulating biochemical and immunologic processes.[31]

Chromosomes are composed of DNA, proteins, and some ribonucleic acid (RNA). This entire structure is known as chromatin. Genes have a specific location on the chromosome, called a locus. Autosomal genes are located on the autosomes (chromosomes common to both sexes), which are homologous (a pair of chromosomes with identical gene arrangements). In the male, there exists a pair of nonhomologous chromosomes, which are the X and Y sex chromosomes.

3

One copy of a gene normally occupies any given locus. In somatic cells, the chromosomes are paired so that there are two copies of each gene (alleles). These corresponding genes at a given locus on homologous chromosomes govern the same trait but not necessarily in the same way. If gene pairs are identical, they are homozygous; if different, the pair is said to be heterozygous. In the heterozygous state, one of the alleles may be expressed over the other. This allele is considered dominant, meaning that only one member of a pair of homologous chromosomes is responsible for the trait. On the other hand, recessive traits can be expressed only when the allele responsible for that trait is present on both chromosomes or when the dominant allele is not present (as with X-linked genes). Codominance occurs when both alleles are expressed, as is the case in the AB blood group.

Although the full complement of genes is present in somatic cells, genes are selectively switched on and off in cells. Therefore, all genes are not active at the same time. This activation process is important during development and is influenced by age, cell type, and function.

A genotype refers to either the genetic makeup of a particular gene pair or the total genetic pool for an individual. The observable expression of a specific trait is referred to as the phenotype. A trait may be a biochemical property, an anatomic structure, a cell or organ function, or a mental characteristic. Therefore, traits are derived from the action of the gene and not from the gene itself.[9, 31, 67]

The way in which a particular trait is transmitted to offspring is referred to as the mode of inheritance. Autosomal dominant traits are the result of a dominant allele at a particular locus on an autosome. When a characteristic is the result of a recessive allele, the mode of inheritance is known as autosomal recessive. Polygenic traits are governed by the additive effect of two or more alleles at different loci.[9] The traits expressed by autosomal genes usually occur with the same frequency in males as in females.

The latter is not true of sex-linked traits. These traits occur with higher frequency in males than in females. This is because the genes located on the X chromosome are present in only one copy in males. Therefore, the genes that are on that chromosome are expressed and are considered hemizygous.[9, 51]

DNA Structure and Function

The transmission of hereditary information from one cell to another is the function of DNA. DNA contains the instructions for the synthesis of proteins that then determine the structure and function of that cell. The nucleus holds the DNA, and protein assembly occurs within the cytoplasm. The transfer of information from the nucleus to the site of synthesis is the role of RNA, which is synthesized on the surface of DNA.

Both DNA and RNA are nucleic acids made up of a nitrogenous purine or pyrimidine base, a five-carbon sugar, and a phosphate group. Together these substrates form a nucleotide that is linked in a linear sequence by phosphodiester bonds. DNA is composed of two antiparallel complementary chains of opposite polarity. These strands form a double helix in which the sides are the phosphate and sugar groups and the crossbars are complementary bases held by hydrogen bonds. Only complementary bases form stable bonds; therefore adenine (A) always pairs with thymine (T), and guanine (G) always pairs with cytosine (C). Thus, the sequence of the bases on one strand determines the sequence of bases on the other. The passage of information from DNA to RNA is called transcription; the assemblage of the proper sequence on amino acids is translation (Table 1–1).

In RNA, uracil (U) pairs with adenine because thymine is not present. There are three major types of RNA: (1) messenger RNA (mRNA), (2) ribosomal RNA (rRNA), and (3) transfer RNA (tRNA). Messenger RNA receives information from the DNA, serving as the template for protein synthesis. Transfer RNA maneuvers the amino acids to mRNA and positions them correctly during protein synthesis. One of the structural components at the protein assemblage site is rRNA.

Gene structure is relatively simple. The sequence of bases along the polynucleotide provides the code that specifies the sequence of amino acids. Each of the 20 amino acids is designated by a specific sequence of three bases. A gene is a single protein, which is a series of codes. The four bases can be arranged in 64 triplet combinations, of which 61 are used to specify the 20 amino acids.

TABLE 1–1
Sequence of Events in Transcription and Translation

TRANSCRIPTION
1. The two strands of the DNA double helix separate in the region of the gene to be transcribed.
2. Free nucleotides base pair with the nucleotide bases in DNA.
3. The nucleotide triphosphates paired with one strand of DNA are linked together by DNA-dependent RNA polymerase to form mRNA containing a sequence of bases complementary to the DNA base sequence.

TRANSLATION
4. mRNA passes from the nucleus to the cytoplasm where one end of the mRNA binds to a ribosome.
5. Free amino acids combine with their corresponding tRNAs in the presence of specific aminoacyl-tRNA synthetase enzymes in the cytoplasm.
6. Amino acid–tRNA complexes bind to sites on the ribosome and the three base anticodons in tRNA pair with the corresponding codons in mRNA.
7. Each amino acid is then transferred from its tRNA to the growing peptide chain, which is attached to the adjacent tRNA.
8. The tRNA freed of its amino acid is released from the ribosome.
9. A new amino acid–tRNA complex is attached to the vacated site on the ribosome.
10. mRNA moves one codon step along the ribosome.
11. Steps 6 to 10 are repeated over and over.
12. The completed protein chain is released from the ribosome when the termination codon in mRNA is reached.

From Vander, A.J., et al. (1980). *Human physiology, the mechanisms of body function* (3rd ed., p. 60). New York: McGraw-Hill.

The other three codes are termination codes, which designate the end of a gene.

DNA Replication

When a cell divides, the accurate replication of the genetic material stored within the DNA of the parent cell is essential. In principle, the replication process is very similar to mRNA synthesis on the surface of DNA. During DNA replication the strands uncoil, relax, and separate, the exposed bases pairing with complementary free nucleotides. DNA polymerase links the nucleotides together, the result being two identical molecules of DNA. Once the two have been formed they pass on an identical set to each daughter cell.

Cell Division

Genetic material is passed on to daughter cells in two ways. For somatic cells it is through mitosis, and for germ cells it is via meiosis. Although we understand the stages of cell division, currently there is little known about the molecular events that occur or how the process is initiated or regulated.[67]

Mitosis

Mitosis is the process by which growth of the organism occurs and cells repair and replace themselves. This process maintains the diploid chromosome number of 46 and forms two daughter cells that are exact replicas of the parent, unless mutation occurs.

The period between the end of one cell division and the beginning of the next is known as interphase. Cells spend most of their time in interphase, as division takes approximately an hour. DNA replication does occur during this phase, however, lasting 10 to 12 hours.

Just prior to cell division the duplicated DNA threads, known as chromatin, change from a loose, relaxed mass and become condensed and tightly coiled, forming rod-shaped structures called chromosomes. This condensing process facilitates the transfer of DNA to the daughter cells. This change is the first sign of cell division.

As the cell enters prophase the chromosomes are double, each consisting of two sister threads (chromatids). The two chromatids are joined at a single point called the centromere. Late in prophase the nuclear membrane begins to disintegrate. The centrioles (two small cylindrical bodies) separate and move to opposite sides of the cell. A number of microtubules can be seen; these are the spindle fibers, and they extend from one side of the cell to the other, between the centrioles.

During metaphase the chromatids line up on the metaphase plate in the center of the cell. Other spindle fibers now extend from the centrioles and are attached to the centromere region of the chromosome. The centromeres divide in the next phase (anaphase), and the single-stranded chromosomes are pulled to opposite poles.

As the chromosomes reach their respective poles they begin to uncoil and elongate. The cell begins to constrict along a plane perpendicular to the spindle apparatus, creating a division in the cell membrane. This constriction continues, creating two cells. At the end of this phase (telophase), the nucleolus and nuclear membrane re-form and the spindle fibers disappear. Division is complete, and the two daughter cells move into interphase (Fig. 1–1).

Meiosis

Meiosis is the process of germ cell division that is designed to reduce the number of chromosomes from diploid (2n) to haploid (n). In this process there are two sequential divisions. The first meiotic division is a reduction division; the second is an equational one. The result of meiosis is daughter cells that have 23 chromosomes: one chromosome from each pair of autosomes and one sex chromosome. Fusion of sperm and ovum restores the cell to the diploid number of chromosomes.

The first meiotic division consists of four phases (prophase, metaphase, anaphase, and telophase). Prophase is longer and more complex, being divided into five stages. In the first stage (leptotene) the chromosomes are thread-like but already duplicated. Although consisting of two chromatids, the chromosome appears as a single strand. The nuclear membrane is intact. As the cell moves into the zygotene stage, homologous chromosomes pair up (synapsis) and in a zipper-like fashion become bivalents. The chromosomes shorten and condense during the pachytene stage.

The two chromatids in each chromosome are distinct and can be seen clearly during this stage. The four chromatids of the homologous chromosomes are grouped together in a tetrad. Crossover and exchange of genetic material (recombination) can occur at this time. The sites of exchange are called chiasmata. The pairs of chromatids separate from each other during the diplotene stage. Once this separation is completed the nuclear membrane dissolves (diakinesis stage). The chromosomes are maximally condensed, chiasmata are terminated, and normal disjunction occurs.

Between diakinesis and metaphase I the nucleolus disappears and spindle fibers form. In metaphase the chromosomes line up on the metaphase plate. Homologous chromosomes are paired and attached to spindle fibers at the centromere. The centrioles are at opposite poles. In anaphase I the centromeres are not divided and the chromatids are pulled to opposite poles. The bivalents are separated, and one half of each homologous chromosome goes to each pole.

In telophase I the nuclear membranes re-form and cell division can be seen. One duplicated member of each chromosome pair is in each daughter cell as the parent cell finishes dividing.

In the second meiotic division no DNA replication occurs. The duplicated chromosomes in each daughter cell line up along the metaphase plate, centrioles are again polarized, and spindle fibers are in place. As the cell moves from metaphase II to anaphase II, the centromeres divide and the chromatids separate and move to opposite poles. In telophase II the nuclear membrane re-forms and cell division occurs at the end of the stage. The end result is four haploid cells, with one half of each chromosome pair in each cell (Fig. 1–1).

CAUSES AND TRANSMISSION OF GENETIC DISEASES

Genetic diseases are the result of a detrimental change in the number or composition of individual genes or in the entire chromosome. These changes are heritable because of DNA replication. New changes in a single gene are called point mutations and are estimated to occur approximately five times per newly created genome. Many of these changes do not affect the structural genes and are not deleterious; instead, genetic variation is introduced into the species.[59]

Heritable disorders caused by such changes are called mendelian diseases, because mutations are then governed by the mendelian principles of inheritance (Table 1–2). Genetic diseases resulting from the mutation of a single allele are called dominant; those that cause mutation of a gene pair are called recessive. Cytogenetic or chromosomal diseases result when a large number of genes are damaged. Individuals born with chromosomal defects often demonstrate physical and mental handicaps.[9, 49, 59]

Besides these physical and mental effects, genetic mutations may result in inherited biochemical disorders characterized by defective or deficient cellular functioning. The consequences of this alteration are dependent upon the type of molecule affected, type of defect, usual metabolic reaction, usual site of action, remaining residual activity, gene interactions, and milieu of the body as well as the degree of adaptation that is possible.[9, p.65]

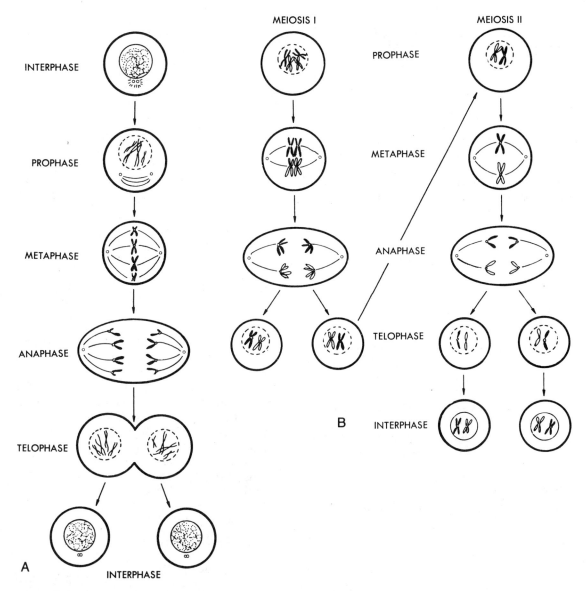

FIGURE 1–1. Comparison of the stages of mitosis *(A)* and meiosis *(B)*. (From Whaley, L.F. (1974). *Understanding inherited disorders* (pp. 11, 12). St. Louis: CV Mosby.)

Most of the inherited biochemical disorders and sex-linked disorders are single gene mutations, whereas major chromosome errors are of two basic types: a change in number, or a change in structure.

Changes in Chromosome Number

Deviations from euploidy (the correct number of chromosomes) are of two types. Polyploidy refers to an exact multiple of the haploid (23) set of chromosomes. Aneuploidy is the term applied to all the situations in which there is not an exact multiple. Monosomy is a subset of the latter, in which one member of a pair of chromosomes is missing. Trisomy refers to the presence of an extra chromosome.

Changes in Chromosome Structure

Variations in this area are widespread. Some have very little effect, while others are devastating. There are four major alterations in chromosome structure: (1) deletions, (2) du-

TABLE 1–2
Mendelian Principles of Inheritance

PRINCIPLE OF DOMINANCE
In the competition of two genes at the same locus on paired chromosomes, one gene may mask or conceal the other. The individual manifests the dominant gene's characteristic. The concealed trait is termed recessive.

PRINCIPLE OF SEGREGATION
During meiosis paired chromosomes are separated to form two gametes. Therefore, the genes remain unchanged and are transferred from one generation to the next.

PRINCIPLE OF INDEPENDENT ASSORTMENT
When displayed traits have alleles at two or more loci, each is distributed within the gametes randomly, independent of each other.

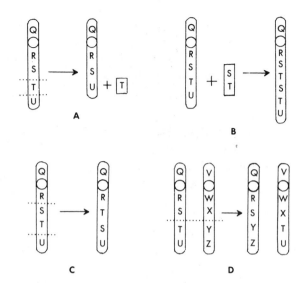

FIGURE 1–2. Major types of aberrations in chromosome and structure. *A,* Deletion; *B,* duplication; *C,* inversion; and *D,* translocation. (From Whaley, L.F. (1974). *Understanding inherited disorders* (p. 74). St. Louis: CV Mosby.)

plications, (3) inversions, and (4) translocations (Fig. 1–2).

Deletion

Deletions, the loss of part of a chromosome, can occur anywhere on the chromosome. Terminal deletions are those occurring on the ends. Interstitial deletions occur along the body of the chromosome with the ends reattaching. If the broken piece is without a centromere, the piece will be lost during cell division. Occasionally, broken fragments may be incorporated into another chromosome.

Duplication

This is a situation in which extra copies of genes are created or obtained during crossing-over. The results of this duplication may or may not be visible.

Inversion

Inversions result from two breaks and the subsequent 180-degree rotation of the broken segment. This results in a sequence change and rearrangement of genes in reverse order. Chromosome pairing cannot occur during meiosis when inversions exist, resulting in an increased incidence of spontaneous abortions. This may explain some cases of infertility.

Translocation

Translocations occur after breaks have happened. Genetic material is transferred to another chromosome. In reciprocal translocation no genetic material is lost, because two chromosomes exchange pieces (balanced translocation). If material is gained or lost, that is considered an unbalanced translocation. Children with balanced translocations appear normal; those with unbalanced translocations may have multiple anomalies.

There are several other forms of structural change, and the reader is referred to a basic genetics text for further discussions in this area.

Sex-Linked Inheritance

Genes on the X chromosome are identified as X-linked, whereas those on the Y chromosomes are Y-linked. There are many such X-linked genes; however, there is limited evidence for Y-linked genes except for those of maleness.[49] Males can transmit X-linked genes to their daughters but not to their sons, and sons can receive X-linked genes only from their mothers. Female offspring can be either homozygous or heterozygous for X-linked genes because of their dual X chromosomes. Males, on the other hand, are hemizygous for X-linked genes, because they have only one X chromosome.

X-Linked Recessive Inheritance

In males, an X-linked recessive gene is always expressed, because there is no corresponding gene on the Y chromosome to be dominant. In females, recessive genes of this nature are usually expressed only when the allele is present in the homozygous form. Occasionally a female may demonstrate the trait secondary to the random inactivation of one of the X chromosomes in each cell. The degree to which this individual expresses the trait depends on the proportion of cells in which the dominant gene has been inactivated. The larger the proportion the greater the likelihood that the X-linked trait will be visible (Table 1–3).

X-Linked Dominant Inheritance

In this situation, the trait will be demonstrated in both males and females. Who will be affected and to what degree depend on the genotype of the parents. All the daughters of an affected father will receive the X chromosome with the dominant gene and will express the disease. However, none of the sons of this father will be affected.

When the mother is heterozygous, the chances are that half the offspring will be affected. If the mother is homozygous, all the children will be affected, regardless of the father's status. If the father is also affected, the daughters will be homozygous for the disease. In situations in which the father does not exhibit the trait and the mother is heterozygous, the probability is that all their daughters and half their sons will be affected (Table 1–4).

Y-Linked Inheritance

Since only males have Y chromosomes and there is no corresponding allele on the X

TABLE 1–3
Major Characteristics of X-Linked Recessive Inheritance Disorders

The mutant gene is on the X chromosome.
One copy of the mutant gene is needed for phenotypic effect in males.
Two copies of the mutant gene are usually needed for phenotypic effect in females.
Males are more frequently affected than females.
Unequal X inactivation can lead to manifesting heterozygote in female carriers.
Transmission is often through heterozygous (carrier) females.
All daughters of affected males are carriers.
All sons of affected males are normal.
There is no male-to-male transmission.
There are some fresh gene mutations.

Adapted from Cohen, F.L. (1984). *Clinical genetics in nursing practice* (p. 84). Philadelphia: JB Lippincott.

TABLE 1–4
Major Characteristics of X-Linked Dominant Inheritance Disorders

The mutant gene is located on the X chromosome.
One copy of the mutant gene is needed for phenotypic manifestation.
X inactivation modifies the gene effect in females.
Often lethal in males and so may see transmission only in female line.
Affected families show excess of female offspring.
Affected male transmits gene to all his daughters and none of his sons.
Affected males have affected mothers (unless it is a new mutation).
There is no male-to-male transmission.
There is no carrier state.
Disorders are relatively uncommon.

Adapted from Cohen, F.L. (1984). *Clinical genetics in nursing practice* (p. 85). Philadelphia: JB Lippincott.

chromosome, these traits occur only in males. If a Y-linked trait is present, it will be expressed. There is no dominance or recessiveness. When a father with a Y-linked chromosome transfers genetic material, all the sons will be affected and none of the daughters.

Autosomal Inheritance

The inheritance of these traits is dependent upon the differences between alleles of a particular locus on an autosomal pair. In this situation, it makes no difference which parent carries the genotype, because the autosomes are the same in both sexes.

Autosomal Dominant Inheritance

In autosomal dominant disorders, the disease is expressed in the heterozygote state and the probability of transmitting it to the offspring is 50% with each pregnancy. Although rarely encountered in humans, the homozygous version of an autosomal dominant disorder is lethal. The vast majority of these diseases cannot be identified through laboratory examination. Consequently, careful history taking and physical examination must be done.[31] Whenever the gene is present it is expressed in the phenotype and can be traced through a number of generations. Expression of these genes rarely skips a generation, and a person not affected will not transmit the gene. Therefore, the affected individual will have an affected parent, unles the condition is the result of fresh mutation.[70]

Other characteristics include a wide variation in expression in those individuals affected. Penetrance may also not be complete. Penetrance refers to whether or not there is phenotypic recognition of the mutant gene. If a gene is fully penetrant, the trait it controls is always manifested in the individual. If it is not fully penetrant, the disease may appear to skip a generation; that is, a particular genotype produces a particular trait in some individuals but not in others.

It is not uncommon for an autosomal dominant characteristic to appear for the first time as a fresh mutation. These types of mutations are also seen in sex-linked recessive disorders. Increased paternal age may contribute to these disorders (Table 1–5).[9, 49]

Autosomal Recessive Inheritance

A trait governed by a recessive allele is expressed only when the homozygous condition exists.[9] When both parents exhibit the trait, all their children are affected. If an affected person marries a homozygous unaffected individual, their children will be heterozygous for the trait and will not manifest the disease, but they will be carriers. If two carriers marry, then the probability (for each pregnancy) is about 25% that the child will manifest the disease, 50% that the child will be a carrier, and 25% that the child will neither have the disease nor be a carrier. When an affected person marries a carrier, the probability is about 50% that a child will have the disease and 50% that the child will be a

TABLE 1–5
Major Characteristics of Autosomal Dominant Inheritance Disorders

The mutant gene is on an autosome.
One copy of the mutant gene is needed for effects to be evident.
Males and females are affected in equal numbers.
There is no sex difference in clinical manifestations.
Vertical family history through several generations may be seen.
There is wide variability of expression.
Penetrance may be incomplete.
There is an increased paternal age effect.
Fresh gene mutation is frequent.
Later age of onset is frequent.
Male-to-male transmission is possible.
Normal offspring of an affected person have normal children.
The least negative effect is on reproductive fitness.
Structural protein defect is often involved.
Few are able to be detected biochemically.
Disorder tends to be less severe than the recessive disorders.

Adapted from Cohen, F.L. (1984). *Clinical genetics in nursing practice* (p. 80). Philadelphia: JB Lippincott.

TABLE 1–6
Major Characteristics of Autosomal Recessive Inheritance Disorders

The mutant gene is located on an autosome.
Two copies of the mutant gene are needed for phenotypic manifestations.
Males and females are affected in equal numbers.
There is usually no sex difference in clinical manifestations.
Affected individual receives one mutant gene from each parent.
Family history is usually negative, especially for vertical transmission (in more than one generation).
Other affected individuals in family in same generation (horizontal transmission) may be seen.
Consanguinity is often present.
Fresh gene mutation is rare.
Age of disease onset is early newborn, infancy, and early childhood.
The greatest negative effect is on reproductive fitness.
Often involve enzyme defect or deficiency.
Disease course is usually severe.
Disease is often amenable to prenatal diagnosis.
Biochemical carrier detection assay is often available.

Adapted from Cohen, F.L. (1984). *Clinical genetics in nursing practice* (p. 77). Philadelphia: JB Lippincott.

carrier. Usually an affected child is the offspring of two heterozygotes who are themselves normal. Consanguineous marriages increase the probability of this (Table 1–6).[49]

EMBRYONIC AND FETAL DEVELOPMENT OF THE REPRODUCTIVE SYSTEM

Embryonic and fetal development of the reproductive system involves the formation of the gonads, genital ducts, and external genitalia from undifferentiated primordial structures within the embryo that are adapted to meet the functional need of the two sexes. For the male, the gonads differentiate into the testes, and the duct system becomes the efferent ductules of the testes, the duct of the epididymis, ductus deferens, seminal vesicles, and most of the urethra. The external genitalia become specialized to form the penis and scrotum (Fig. 1–3). For the female, the gonads differentiate into the ovaries, and the duct system becomes the uterine (fallopian) tubes, uterus, and vagina. The external genitalia are the vulva (Fig. 1–4). The development of these systems is complex, being strikingly different as well as mutually exclusive.[23]

This developmental process begins at fertilization with the determination of genetic sex, passing through three other stages prior to birth. These include differentiation of go-

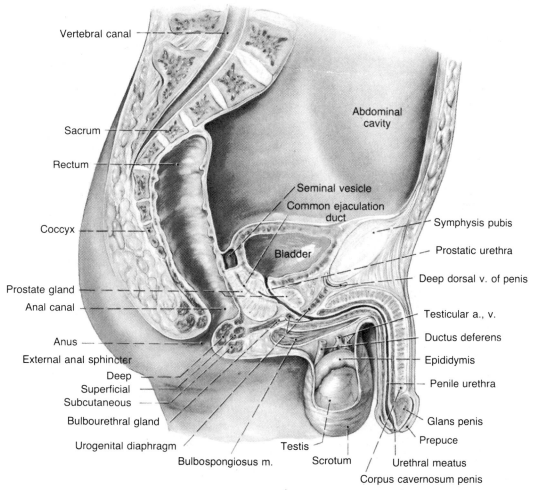

FIGURE 1–3. Male reproductive system. (From Jacob, S.W. & Francone, C.A. (1989). *Elements of anatomy and physiology* (2nd ed., p. 281). Philadelphia: WB Saunders.)

nadal sex, somatic sex, and neuroendocrine sex. After birth sexual differentiation continues with the development of social sex, psychological sex, and secondary sex characteristics.[54] These stages determine the final sexual characteristics and behavior of the individual.[45]

Genetic sex is determined at the time of fertilization and consists of genic sex as defined by the genes. Chromosomal sex is defined by the sex chromosome complement. Gonadal sex is defined by the structure and function of the gonads; somatic sex involves all other genital organs; and neuroendocrine sex is established by the cyclic or continuous production of gonadotropin-releasing hormones.[54]

Prenatally the reproductive system develops from analogous undifferentiated structures in both sexes. The basic pattern is the female phenotype; the male system develops only when the Y chromosome, testosterone, and other organizing substances are present. This is true of the external genitalia as well. Prenatal sexual development occurs in three different areas: the gonads, the genital ducts, and the external genitalia.

Development of the Gonads

The gonads in the human consist of the ovaries in the female and the testes in the male. These structures are derived from three cellular sources: (1) primordial germ cells, (2) underlying mesenchyme, and (3) coelomic epithelium. The primordial germ cells, large spherical primitive sex cells, are visible in the 4th week of gestation.[62] Origi-

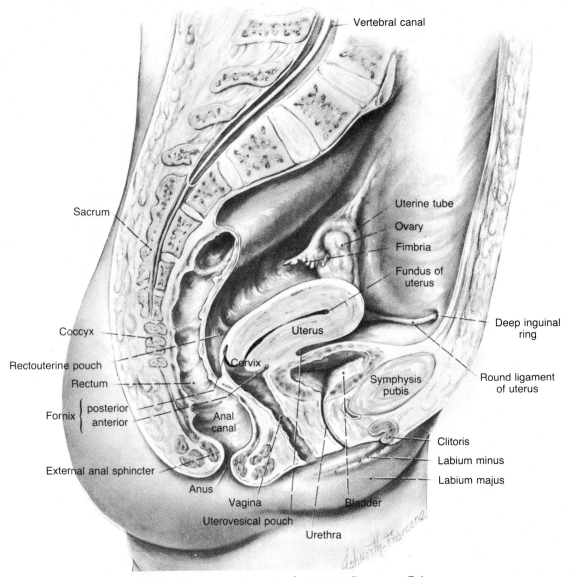

FIGURE 1–4.   Female reproductive system. (From Jacob, S.W. & Francone, C.A. (1989). *Elements of anatomy and physiology* (2nd ed., p. 287). Philadelphia: WB Saunders.)

nating among the endodermal cells of the wall of the yolk sac, near the origin of the allantois, the primordial germ cells migrate by ameboid movements along the dorsal mesentery of the hindgut to the gonadal ridge. Meiotic division continues during this migration. These cells are then incorporated into the mesenchyme and the primary sex cords during the 6th week of gestation and are destined to become the oogonia or spermatogonia.[46]

The mechanism for attraction between the gonadal tissue and the primordial germ cells is unknown. Apparently, there are cell sur-

face components that are responsible for guiding the migration and identifying the final stopping place.[54]

Indifferent Stage

During the 5th week of gestation, a thickening of the coelomic epithelium on the medial side of the mesonephros can be seen; this becomes the gonadal ridge.[23, 46] The surface cells proliferate to form a solid cord of cells that grow downward with finger-like projections into the mesenchyme.[1, 23, 46] These are the primary sex cords. It is during this time that the gonads separate from the mesonephros.[23]

The gonads at the end of 6 weeks remain sexually indistinguishable. Two layers can be identified within the gonads, the cortex (coelomic epithelium) and the medulla (mesenchyme). In the XX embryo, the cortex differentiates into the ovary and the medulla essentially regresses. In the XY embryo, however, the medulla differentiates into the testes and the cortex regresses (Fig. 1–5).

Development of the Testes

The Y chromosome has a strong testis-determining effect on the medulla of the indifferent gonad.[46] The primary sex cords condense and extend even farther into the medulla. Here they branch, canalize, and anastomose to form a network of tubules, the rete testis. These cords are separated from the surface epithelium by a dense layer of connective tissue, the tunica albuginea. Septa grow from the tunica into the medulla to divide the testis into approximately 250 wedge-shaped lobules.[23] Each lobule contains approximately one to three seminiferous tubules, interstitial cells, and supporting cells.

Canalization of the seminiferous cords results in formation of the walls of the tubules by Sertoli (supporting) cells and spermatogenic (germinal) epithelium, which is derived from the primary germ cells.[23, 46] The Sertoli cells multiply during growth of the cords until they constitute the majority of the epithelium during fetal life and provide nutrients for the maturing spermatids in adult life.[46, 54] It is the Sertoli cells that produce the antimüllerian hormone that results in the degeneration of the paramesonephric ducts.[32] These cells may also inhibit spermatogonia meiosis in the fetal testis.[33, 69]

The process of cellular reorganization is the first step in male differentiation and is most likely controlled by the sex-determining genes associated with the Y chromosome. Wachtel and associates suggest that the H-Y (histocompatibility-Y) antigen gene found on the Y chromosome is the regulator of gonadal differentiation.[68] Those cells having the Y chromosome would join with each other through the H-Y antigen and its receptor. This would lead to an increased synthesis of H-Y antigen, resulting in the development of the testicular cords and interstitium from the blastema.[54]

The mesenchyme contributes masses of interstitial cells (Leydig cells), which proliferate between the tubules. These cells produce testosterone and are functional almost immediately. The Leydig cells are highly active in the 3rd, 4th, and 5th gestational months.[23, 55] The rise in testosterone parallels the increase in Leydig cells.[50] After 18 weeks, the number of Leydig cells and testosterone levels decrease (Fig. 1–5).[37]

It is testosterone that induces the masculinization of the external genitalia. In addition, the Leydig cells produce genital duct inducer and suppressor substances that initiate the development of the mesonephric ducts and suppress the development of the paramesonephric ducts.[46] Once initiated, testosterone synthesis does appear to be regulated by human chorionic gonadotropin (hCG), however.[29]

The testicles start to descend into the inguinal canal during the 6th month, entering the scrotal swellings shortly before birth.[54] Gonadotropin stimulation as well as the Leydig cells seems to regulate this descent.[20]

Development of the Ovaries

In XX embryos gonadal development occurs more slowly, the ovary being identifiable at 10 weeks.[46] The primary sex cords do develop and extend into the medulla of the developing ovary but are not prominent and later degenerate. By the 12th week, the medulla is mainly connective tissue with scattered groups of cells that represent the prospective rete ovarii.[54] The rete ovarii appears to be derived from migrating mesonephric cells, which may later give rise to the follicular cells.[7]

During the 4th month, secondary sex cords (cortical cords) are thought to grow into the gonad from the germinal epithelium (surface epithelium).[1, 46] As the cortical cords enlarge, the primordial germ cells are incorporated into them. At around 16 weeks the cords begin to break up into clusters, resulting in surrounding of the primitive ova (oogonia) by a single layer of flattened follicular cells derived from the cortical cords.[46] This complex is termed the primordial follicle and will later develop into the primary follicle once the oocyte is formed and a single or multiple layer of low columnar follicular cells surrounds the oocyte.[1, 23, 46]

The surface epithelium becomes separated from the follicles, which lie in the cortex, by a thin fibrous capsule, the tunica albuginea.

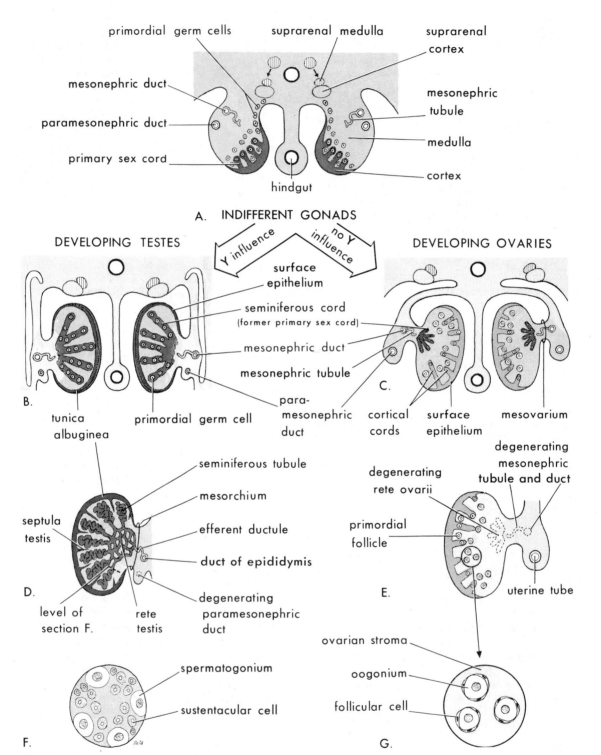

FIGURE 1–5.   *See legend on opposite page*

The ovary, like the testis, separates from the regressing mesonephros, becoming suspended by its own mesentery (mesovarium) (Fig. 1–5).[46]

Female gonadal differentiation is probably regulated by a gene located on the X chromosome.[2, 22] This gene is somehow linked to the testis-organizing gene so that the ovary's gene acts only if the testis gene is not active.[54] For primary ovarian differentiation only one X chromosome need be present; however, in 45,X individuals the ovary degenerates before birth.[23, 46, 54]

Androgen conversion into estrogen has been demonstrated from the fetal age of 8 weeks, although serum increases are not encountered. This may indicate that estrogens act locally, stimulating follicle development.[14, 15, 54]

Development of the Genital Ducts

Both the male and the female embryos have two pairs of genital ducts, the mesonephric (wolffian) duct and the paramesonephric (müllerian) duct. The mesonephric duct originates as part of the urinary system and during the 6th week is incorporated into the developing gonad. The paramesonephric ducts develop alongside the mesonephric ducts in both sexes but reach complete development only in the female.[23] The female ducts differentiate autonomously without external regulatory factors, whereas the male system is regulated by testicular androgens and müllerian-inhibiting hormone.[54]

Indifferent Stage

The mesonephric ducts drain the mesonephric kidneys and develop into the ductus deferens, the epididymides, and the ejaculatory ducts in the male when the second kidney tubules degenerate. In the female, the mesonephric ducts almost completely degenerate.

The paramesonephric ducts develop bilaterally alongside the mesonephric ducts. The paramesonephric ducts run caudally parallel to the mesonephric ducts, then cross in front of them, fusing to form a Y-shaped canal.[46]

Male Genital Duct Development

Under the influence of androgens and the nonsteroid suppressor/inducer substance, the mesonephric duct is incorporated into the genital system (Fig. 1–6). It is the suppressor substance that inhibits the development of the paramesonephric ducts in the male.[40, 54]

The majority of the mesonephric tubules disappear, except those that are in the region of the testes. These 5 to 12 mesonephric tubules lose their glomeruli and join with the rete testis.[23] This creates a communication between the gonads and the mesonephric duct. At this point they are called the efferent ductules; they greatly elongate and become convoluted, making up the majority of the caput epididymidis. The mesonephric duct becomes the ductus epididymidis in this region. Below this area, the mesonephric duct incorporates muscle tissue and becomes the ductus deferens (vas deferens).

The epididymides are narrow, tightly coiled tubes approximately 5 to 6 meters in

---

FIGURE 1–5. Schematic sections illustrating differentiation of the indifferent gonads into testes or ovaries. *A,* Six weeks, showing the indifferent gonads composed of an outer cortex and an inner medulla. *B,* Seven weeks, showing testes developing under the influence of a Y chromosome. Note that the primary sex cords have become seminiferous cords. *C,* Twelve weeks, showing ovaries beginning to develop in the absence of a Y chromosome. Cortical cords have extended from the surface epithelium, displacing the primary sex cords centrally into the mesovarium, where they form the rudimentary rete ovarii. *D,* Testis at 20 weeks, showing the rete testis and the seminiferous tubules derived from the seminiferous cords. An efferent ductule has developed from a mesonephric tubule, and the mesonephric duct has become the duct of the epididymis. *E,* Ovary at 20 weeks, showing the primordial follicles formed from the cortical cords. *F,* Section of a seminiferous tubule from a 20-week fetus. Note that no lumen is present at this stage and that the seminiferous epithelium is composed of two kinds of cell. *G,* Section from the ovarian cortex of a 20-week fetus, showing three primordial follicles containing oogonia. (From Moore, K.L. (1988). *The developing human* (4th ed., p. 264). Philadelphia: WB Saunders.)

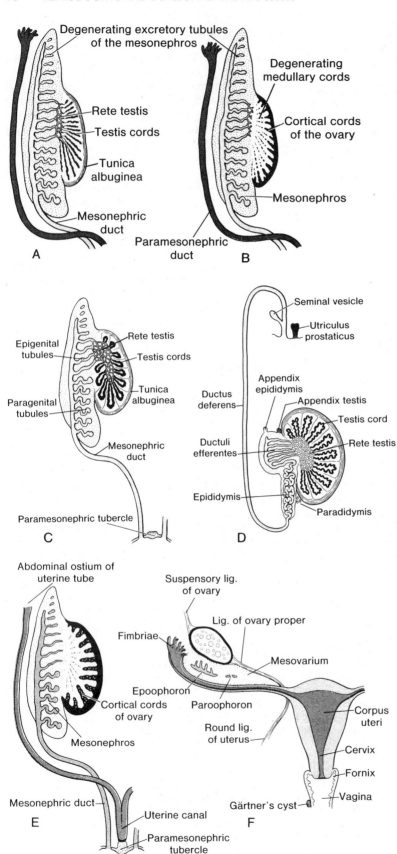

FIGURE 1–6. Differentiation and development of the genital ducts. Diagram of the genital ducts in the 6th week of development in the male (A) and in the female (B). The mesonephric and paramesonephric ducts are present in both. Note the excretory tubules of the mesonephros and their relationship to the developing gonad in both sexes. C, Diagram of the genital ducts in the male in the 4th month of development. Cranial and caudal (paragenital tubules) segments of the mesonephric system regress. D, The genital duct after descent of the testis. Note the horseshoe-shaped testis cords, the rete testis, and the ductuli efferentes entering the ductus deferens. The paradidymis is formed by the remnants of the paragenital mesonephric tubules. The paramesonephric duct has degenerated except for the appendix testis and the utriculus prostaticus. E, Schematic drawing of the genital ducts in the female at the end of the 2nd month of development. Note the paramesonephric or müllerian tubercle and formation of the uterine canal. F, The genital ducts after descent of the ovary. The only parts remaining of the mesonephric system are the epoophoron, paroophoron, and Gartner's cyst. Note the suspensory ligament of the ovary, the ligament of the ovary proper, and the round ligament of the uterus. (From Langman, J. (1981). *Medical embryology* (4th ed., pp. 249, 251, 252). Baltimore/London: Williams & Wilkins.)

length, which run along the top and side of each testis. These structures serve as a reservoir for maturing spermatozoa and contribute to semen production.

The vas deferens is the excretory duct for the testes. It runs from the epididymis through the inguinal canal into the abdominal cavity behind the bladder, where it joins the seminal vesicle duct emptying into the ejaculatory duct and urethra.

A lateral outgrowth from the lower end of the mesonephric duct gives rise to a seminal vesicle. The area of the mesonephric duct between the duct of the gland and the urethra becomes the ejaculatory duct. The urethra makes up the remainder of the male genital duct system (see Fig. 1–3).[46]

Experimental evidence indicates that fetal testosterone is the inducing factor for the development of the mesonephric duct.[34, 60] Lacking sufficient exposure to testosterone, the mesonephric duct degenerates by the end of the 4th month.[54]

Female Genital Duct Development

In the female embryo, the mesonephric ducts regress and the paramesonephric ducts develop (Fig. 1–6). Female sexual development is not dependent upon the presence of ovaries.[46] The paramesonephric duct becomes the oviduct, uterus, and proximal vagina in the female, degenerating by the end of the 2nd month in the male.[56]

The cranial unfused portions of the paramesonephric ducts develop into the fallopian tubes; the caudal portion fuses to form the uterovaginal primordium. The latter gives rise to the epithelium and glands of the uterus and to the vaginal wall. The endometrial lining and the myometrium are derived from the surrounding mesenchymal tissue.

The uterus is mainly an abdominal organ in the newborn infant, and the cervix is relatively large. These characteristics change with growth and development. The uterus is divided into two parts, the corpus (body) and the cervix, with the corpus consisting of the fundus, main body, and isthmus.

The cervix is the lower portion of the uterus that projects into the vagina and posteriorly toward the sacrum. It is composed primarily of connective tissue along with some smooth muscle (about 10%) and elastic fibers. The cervix is also divided into three sections: the internal os, opening into the isthmus; the cervical canal; and the external os, opening into the vagina.

The vaginal epithelium is derived from the endoderm of the urogenital sinus, and the fibromuscular wall of the vagina develops from the uterovaginal primordium. Initially the vagina is a solid cord (the vaginal plate); the vaginal lumen is formed as the central cells of the plate break down.

The fallopian tubes are a pair of tubes that extend along the edge of the broad ligament and open into the cornua of the uterus on each side. They function as a repository for the ovulated ovum and as the conduit along which the ovum travels between the ovary and uterus.

The broad ligaments are formed from the peritoneal folds that occur during fusion of the paramesonephric ducts. The broad, wing-like folds extend from the lateral portions of the uterus to the pelvic wall. The folds of the broad ligaments are continuous with the peritoneum and divide the pelvis into anterior and posterior portions. Between the layers of the broad ligament the mesenchyme proliferates to form loose connective tissue and smooth muscle. This complex of tissue provides support and attachment for the uterus, fallopian tubes, and ovaries (see Fig. 1–4).

Development of the External Genitalia

The early development of the external genitalia is similar in both the male and the female embryos. Distinguishing characteristics can be seen during the 9th week of gestation, with definitive characteristics being fully formed by the 12th week.[46]

Indifferent Stage

The external genitalia are bipolar in the early stages. Early in the 4th week at the cranial end of the cloacal membrane a swelling can be identified; this is the genital tubercle. Labioscrotal swellings and urogenital folds soon develop alongside the cloacal membrane. The genital tubercle elongates at this time and is the same length in both sexes.

The urorectal septum fuses with the cloacal membrane, dividing the membrane into a dorsal anal membrane and a ventral urogenital membrane. These membranes rupture around the 8th week, forming the anus and urogenital orifice. The urethral groove, which is continuous with the urogenital orifice, forms on the ventral surface of the genital tubercle at this time (Fig. 1–7).[46]

Male External Genitalia

The androgens produced by the fetal testes induce the masculinization of the external genitalia of the male embryo. The genital tubercle continues to elongate, forming the penis and pulling the urogenital folds forward. This results in the development of the lateral walls of the urethral groove by the urogenital folds. The posterior-to-anterior fusion of the urogenital folds as they come in contact results in the development of the spongy urethra and the progressive movement of the urethral orifice toward the glans of the penis. The opening, however, remains on the undersurface of the phallus.

Backward growth of a plate of ectodermal tissue from the tip of the phallus to the urethra forms the terminal part of the urethra. Once canalized, the urinary and reproductive systems will have achieved an open system. This, along with the descent of the testes into the genital swellings (scrotum), completes the development of the external genitalia (Fig. 1–7).[1]

After the penile urethra has formed, the connective tissue surrounding the urethra becomes condensed to form the corpus cavernosum urethrae, in which numerous wide and convoluted blood vessels having many arteriovenous anastomoses develop.[23] The labioscrotal swellings also grow toward each other and fuse to form the scrotum. Tisssue swelling occurs in order to dilate the inguinal canal and scrotum in preparation for the descent of the testes in the 7th or 8th month of gestation.[1]

Descent of the testes is moderated by many forces, including the enlargement of the pelvis, trunk growth, and the testes' remaining relatively stationary, as well as the influence of gonadotropins and androgens.[46] At about 32 weeks, the testes will actually enter the scrotum. Once passage is complete, the inguinal canal contracts around the spermatic cord. The spermatic cord consists of the vas deferens, blood vessels, and nerves.

In most situations (97% of cases), the testes will have descended bilaterally prior to delivery. During the first 3 months following delivery, the majority of undescended testes will descend without intervention.[46]

Female External Genitalia

Without androgens, feminization of the neutral external genitalia occurs. Initially the genital tubercle grows rapidly; however, it gradually slows, becoming the relatively small clitoris. The clitoris develops like the penis, except that the urogenital folds do not fuse. Both the urethra and the vagina open into the common vestibule, which is widely open after the disappearance of the urogenital membrane. The opening is flanked by the urethral folds and the genital swellings, which become the labia minora and majora, respectively (Fig. 1–7).

FETAL ENDOCRINOLOGY

Large quantities of steroids are produced by the products of conception (placenta and fetus). Some of these substances are dependent upon the viability and well-being of the fetus and placenta, whereas others do not require the fetus to be viable for production to continue. In the latter situation, progesterone continues to be produced at levels that are unchanged.

Early in development steroid-producing cells appear. They can be seen first in the trophoblastic tissue of the placenta; however, the syncytiotrophoblast lacks several of the key enzymes necessary for steroid metabolism. Therefore, the placenta is an incomplete steroidogenic tissue and must receive precursors from exogenous sources (i.e., the fetus or maternal system) (see Chapter 2). The reproductive system of the fetus is dependent upon the functioning of several glands: the pituitary gland, the adrenal gland, and the gonads.

Pituitary

The pituitary gland plays a major role in regulating the principal steroid-secreting glands (adrenal gland and gonads) via a negative feedback mechanism. In general, most of the fetal pituitary hormones are apparent by the 10th week of pregnancy. The plasma concentration of these hormones rises for the first 20 weeks of gestation. At this time, the negative feedback loop comes into operation and the production and release of pituitary hormones become more finely regulated.[26] Two gonadotropins, luteinizing hormone (LH) and follicle-stimulating hormone (FSH),

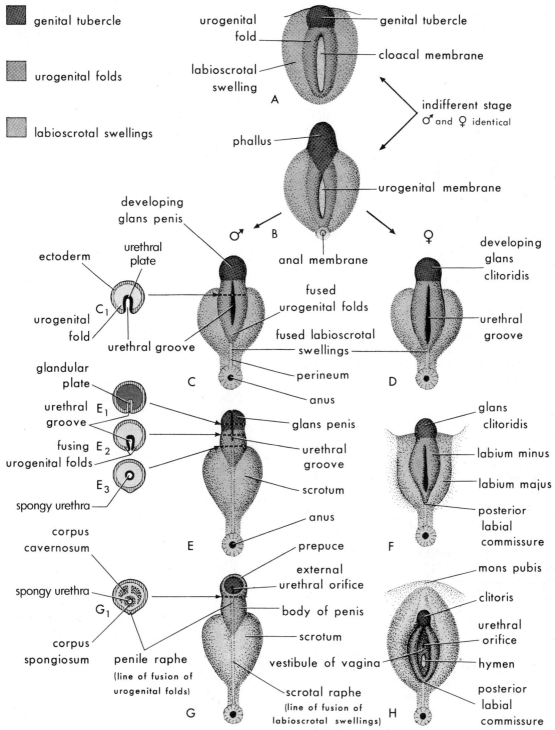

FIGURE 1–7. Differentiation and development of the external genitalia. *A* and *B,* Diagrams illustrating development of the external genitalia during the indifferent stage (4 to 7 weeks). *C, E,* and *G,* Stages in the development of the male external genitalia at about 9, 11, and 12 weeks, respectively. To the left are schematic transverse sections (C_1, E_1 to E_3, G_1) through the developing penis, illustrating formation of the spongy urethra. *D, F,* and *H,* Stages in the development of female external genitalia at 9, 11, and 12 weeks, respectively. (From Moore, K. L. (1988). *The developing human* (4th ed., p. 272). Philadelphia: WB Saunders.)

appear in the fetal pituitary gland at 9 to 10 weeks' gestation. They reach their peaks at about 20 to 22 weeks' gestation. The concentration of LH is higher than that of FSH, and females have higher levels than males.[17, 30]

Follicle-stimulating hormone promotes development of follicles in females; it stimulates growth of seminiferous tubules and initiates spermatogenesis in males. Luteinizing hormone increases the synthesis and secretion of testosterone in the male embryo and stimulates steroid synthesis in all ovarian cells. In the female, LH also induces ovulation in an FSH-primed follicle.

Releasing hormones are synthesized in the hypothalamus and secreted into the portal system, which connects the hypothalamus with the anterior pituitary gland. These releasing hormones stimulate the anterior pituitary to synthesize or release adrenocorticotropic hormone (ACTH), detectable in the fetal pituitary by 8 weeks.[26] ACTH is then liberated into the systemic circulation to act on the adrenal cortex, potentiating growth of the fetal zone in the adrenal gland.

Adrenal

The human fetal adrenal gland develops a fetal zone of considerable size during gestation, being as large as the mid-gestation kidney. Involution occurs during the first year of life.[28] The adrenals are responsible for biosynthesis and secretion of glucocorticoids and for the production of adrenal androgens by the adult zone of the fetal cortex. The inner fetal zone produces primarily dehydroepiandrosterone (DHA) and its sulfate (DHA-S), which serve as precursors of estrone or estradiol-17β in the placenta. Estriol is formed in the placenta from 16-hydroxydehydroepiandrosterone, derived primarily from the fetus (see Chapter 2).

The adrenal's large size allows the fetus to secrete up to 200 mg of adrenal androgens daily, predominantly DHA-S, as compared with the adult, who secretes only 20 to 30 mg of DHA-S.[26] The placenta lacks 16- and 17-hydroxylase activity; therefore placental estrogen production is dependent upon an external source of DHA-S. The fetus supplies 90% of the DHA-S to the placenta after 16-hydroxylation by the fetal liver.[26]

Owing to the fetal adrenal's inability to convert pregnenolone to progesterone, progesterone must come from some exogenous source. Once this becomes available, the fetal zone preferentially converts progesterone to corticosteroids.[4] The placenta utilizes maternal precursors for progesterone synthesis. Progesterone is then transported to the fetus, which uses it to produce corticosteroids (e.g., DHA-S) that the placenta uses to produce estrogen. This demonstrates the intimate interrelationship between the maternal, placental, and fetal systems. If abnormal development leads to absence of the fetal hypophysis, the fetal zone of the adrenal gland will not be formed and DHA-S will not be produced.

Gonads

At about the time the adrenal gland can be identified (6 weeks), the Leydig cells can be found within the testes. The increased activity in these cells coincides with maximal human chorionic gonadotropin (hCG) production in the placenta. An interrelationship between the rise in hCG and testosterone has been suggested by Kaplan and Grumbach.[36]

Androgen-sensitive cells have a receptor within the cell that binds testosterone so that it can be transported to the nucleus. The testes appear to secrete testosterone starting at 7 to 8 weeks of gestation, promoting maturation of the spermatogenic tubules and virilization of the male embryo. Testosterone stimulates mesonephric duct, urogenital sinus, urogenital tubercle, and urogenital swelling differentiation. All but the mesonephric duct require testosterone as a prehormone that must be reduced by the cell to dihydrotestosterone before it can bind to the receptor site.

Many of the anomalies encountered in the reproductive system are related to deviations from normal interactions and patterns of development. They often produce a sterile individual, with abnormal phenotypic characteristics. Fewer than 1% of humans are born with errors of sex differentiation; this includes errors at the chromosomal, gonadal, and phenotypic levels.[61]

COMMON ANOMALIES

The anomalies encountered in the reproductive systems may be secondary to any of three major factors: (1) genetic makeup, (2) endocrine and hormonal environment, and (3) mechanical events. Each may lead to alterations in development and reproductive ability. Because the embryo is bipotential, when genetic or hormonal factors alter development the embryo may develop various degrees of intermediate sex (intersexuality or hermaphroditism). True hermaphrodites have both ovarian and testicular tissue, whereas pseudohermaphrodites have either one or the other but have incongruence between chromosomal sex and gonadal sex. The former is extremely rare, and pseudohermaphroditism occurs only once in 25,000 births.[45, 46] Table 1–7 provides a classification of intersexuality. Mechanical congenital

TABLE 1–7
Classification of Intersexuality

DISORDERS OF GONADAL DEVELOPMENT
Klinefelter's syndrome
Gonadal dysgenesis
    Turner's syndrome
    Mosaicism
    Structural abnormality of the second X chromosome
    Normal karyotype (pure gonadal dysgenesis)
True hermaphroditism
Male pseudohermaphroditism
    Primary gonadal defect
    Y chromosomal defect
DISORDERS OF FETAL ENDOCRINOLOGY
Female pseudohermaphroditism with partial virilization
    Congenital adrenal hyperplasia
        21-Hydroxylase deficiency without salt wasting
        21-Hydroxylase deficiency with salt wasting
        11β-Hydroxylase deficiency (hypertensive)
        3β-ol Dehydrogenase deficiency
    Nonadrenal female pseudohermaphroditism
        Maternal androgenization
            Exogenous androgen
            Virilizing tumors
        Idiopathic
Male pseudohermaphroditism with partial failure of virilization
    Abnormalities of müllerian-inhibiting factor synthesis or action
    Defects in testosterone action
        Complete androgen-binding protein deficiency (complete testicular feminization)
        Partial defects of androgen cytosol receptors (incomplete testicular feminization; familial incomplete male pseudohermaphroditism type I)
        5α-Reductase deficiency (familial incomplete male pseudohermaphroditism type II)
    Testosterone biosynthesis defect
        Pregnenolone synthesis defect (lipid adrenal hyperplasia)
        3β-Hydroxysteroid dehydrogenase deficiency
        17α-Hydroxylase deficiency
        17,20-Desmolase deficiency
        17β-Hydroxysteroid dehydrogenase deficiency

From Mishell, D. R. & Goebelsmann, U. (1991). Disorders of sexual differentiation. In D. R. Mishell, V. Davajan, & R. A. Lobo (Eds.), *Infertility, contraception & reproductive endocrinology* (3rd ed., p. 322). Boston: Blackwell Scientific Publishers.

anomalies are somewhat more common and are related to developmental arrests, interference, or failures that result in changes in normal morphologic patterns.

Gonadal Agenesis

Absence of one or both gonads is a rare disorder. If agenesis is unilateral, absence of the renal system on the affected side is common.[54] Failure or defective development of nephrogenic mesenchyme is probably the cause, although the etiology of such failure is not known.

Hermaphroditism

Hermaphrodites are extremely rare; chromosomal constitution may be either 46,XX, 46,XY, or mosaic XX/XY. These individuals have both ovaries and testes either as separate organs or as a single ovotestis. Usually the gonadal tissue is not functional, but in some individuals oogenesis and spermiogenesis may occur simultaneously. The external genitalia are ambiguous, but the rest of the physical appearance may be either male or female. This abnormality seems to be the result of an error in sexual determination and lack of dominance of the cortex or medulla of the genital ridge.[23, 45, 46]

Possible causes include translocation of testicular differentiation genes to the X chromosome, a mutant gene, or undetected XY cells in the gonad. The presence of uterus and fallopian tubes indicates defective functioning of the müllerian-inhibiting hormone. In those individuals who are mosaic 46,XX/XY, the etiology involves the union of two zygotes of different genetic sex. The two cell lines develop normally, limits being set by their topographic distribution during ontogeny.[54]

Male Pseudohermaphroditism

These male infants have more or less dysgenetic testes with an XY constitution. There is incomplete differentiation of the external genitalia secondary to testicular dysgenesis and insufficient testosterone production. This abnormality may be associated with ambisexual internal genitalia, owing to inadequate inducer/suppressor substance production.[23, 46, 58]

Causes may include a deficiency in the 5α-reductase enzyme necessary to convert testosterone to dihydrotestosterone so that external virilization can occur. In testicular feminization syndrome there is an inability to bind androgens in target tissues, while in other situations transmission of androgens from the receptor to the nucleus is blocked.[23, 24, 46]

Externally the genitalia will be either ambiguous or feminine. Internal structures will also vary. These male infants have varying degrees of phallic and paramesonephric duct development, even though their chromosomes are 46,XY. When differentiation occurs, males with 5α-reductase deficiencies have testosterone and its derivatives in the external genitalia tissue but not in the developing mesonephric duct. It would seem that testosterone appears in the mesonephric ducts after the period of tissue sensitivity has passed.[24, 46]

Males with the X-linked gene for testicular feminization (genotype 46,XY) have normally differentiated testes; however, these children look like normal females. The vagina ends in a blind pouch, and the uterus and fallopian tubes are nonexistent or rudimentary.[46] The testes are usually intraabdominal or inguinal, or they may descend into the labia majora. There are high levels of circulating testosterone with elevated levels of gonadotropins. Unfortunately, testosterone receptor sites will not bind or incorporate testosterone into the cells at the labioscrotal and urogenital folds.[24]

Moore suggests that these "females" represent an extreme form of male pseudohermaphroditism.[46] They have female genitalia, and at puberty there is normal development of secondary sex characteristics; menstruation does not occur, however. The psychosexual orientation of these children is female, and they should be raised as such.[46]

Female Pseudohermaphroditism

The chromosome composition of these female infants is 46,XX, but there is congenital virilization of the external genitalia. This is usually termed adrenogenital syndrome, meaning hyperfunction of the adrenal cortices associated with ambiguous genitalia. The most common cause is an excessive production of androgens, which may be due to maternal disease (e.g., adrenal tumor) but is more likely to be of fetal origin. Lack of 21-hydroxylase (an enzyme involved in steroid metabolism) is frequently the cause.

Most often there are clitoral hypertrophy, partial fusion of the labia majora, and a persistent urogenital sinus. The infants who are afflicted with this syndrome do have functioning ovaries, fallopian tubes, uterus, and cervix. The mesonephric duct does not develop. Often there are other metabolic disorders that require complex care.[24]

Hypospadias

Hypospadias (urethral orifice on the ventral surface of the penis) may be a variety of pseudohermaphroditism especially if the penis is very abnormal. The more severe the degree of hypospadias the higher the possibility of testicular dysgenesis and of cryptorchidism.[23] This defect occurs once in every 300 live births and is probably due to inadequate androgen production resulting in urogenital fold fusion failure and incomplete spongy urethra formation.[46] There are four types of hypospadias, with 80% being either glandular or penile. The other 20% are penoscrotal or perineal. Variations in this defect are due to the timing and degree of hormonal failure.[46]

Epispadias

Epispadias is a relatively rare congenital anomaly, occurring once in every 30,000 live births. It is a dorsal surface urethral opening often associated with exstrophy of the bladder. It may be glandular or penile and is probably due to caudal development of the genital tubercle, resulting in the urogenital sinus' being on the dorsal surface once the membrane has ruptured.[46]

Turner's Syndrome

One of the most common sex chromosome abnormalities is Turner's syndrome. Of all aborted fetuses it is estimated that 0.8–1% are the result of this chromosomal aberration. Occurring once in every 4000 to 5000 live births, the absence or deletion of an X chromosome results in either 46/XO with an abnormally structured chromosome or a 45/XO setup. Mosaics with XX/XO often have functioning ovaries. In most other cases, however, there is ovarian dysgenesis associated with other somatic abnormalities.[23]

Uterovaginal Malformation

Fusion defects of the paramesonephric ducts result in varying degrees of structural duplication. Complete fusion failure leads to the development of two complete genital tracts in which the vagina is divided in two by a septum, with a separate cervix and uterine body associated with each half (didelphia). If one of the paramesonephric ducts fails to develop entirely, the result will be uterus unicornis. Various other anomalies may also result, including a single vagina with double cervices, a single vagina and cervix associated with a uterus subdivided into halves, or a single uterus that is incompletely separated by a septum (bicornate, unicornous, vagina simplex). Any of these anomalies may result in infertility.[1, 46]

GAMETOGENESIS

Once anatomic structures are laid down and endocrine cycles are in place, the development and release of sperm and ova become the primary directive of the gonads. This process is known as gametogenesis and begins in prenatal life.

Gametogenesis is the process by which the primordial germ cell develops into mature gametes. These processes are known as spermatogenesis and oogenesis in the male and female, respectively.

Spermatogenesis

Sperm development consists of spermiogenesis and spermatogenesis. Spermatogenesis is the reduction of chromosomes from 46 to 23 (diploid to haploid), whereas spermiogenesis is the maturation process of the primitive spermatogonium into the highly specialized sperm cell.

Spermatogenesis begins at puberty with the release of androgen. Once begun the process is continuous. In fetal life, the spermatogonia are located inside the seminiferous tubules. At puberty, the lining cells release androgen, which initiates mitotic division of the spermatogonia. As the size of the spermatogonia increases, the cells become designated as primary spermatocytes (46 chromosomes).

Through meiotic division (the first maturational division) the primary spermatocytes reduce their chromosome count to half (haploid) and are now two secondary spermatocytes. The second maturational division is without chromosomal duplication and results in the formation of four spermatids. Division stops here.

The spermatids undergo spermiogenesis, which is the transformation process from ordinary cell structure to sperm cell with head, acrosome, neck, body, and tail. From the initial growth phase of the spermatogonia to the final product, the process takes approximately 64 to 74 days. Once completed, the sperm are set free in the seminiferous tubules and transported via the fluid to the epididymis and ductus deferens, where they are stored.

At ejaculation, somewhere between 300 million and 500 million sperm are released in 2 to 5 ml of seminal fluid. Of these, 75 to 80% are normal. The sperm are transported to the ampulla of the fallopian tube via peristalsis of the organs (penis, uterus, fallopian tubes) as well as by self-motility. Depending on the alkalinity of the surrounding fluid (vaginal and uterine), sperm are able to traverse 2 to 3 mm per minute in the female reproductive tract.

Sperm viability, as it relates to the ability to fertilize, lasts 24 to 48 hours after ejaculation. Viability is enhanced by the pH of the semen, which is 7.5 to 8.0. The alkalinity affords the sperm protection from the acid environment of the vaginal tract.

Ninety seconds after ejaculation (during penile/vaginal intercourse) the sperm enters the cervical mucosa. At mid-cycle the mucus is thinned out, being 99% water. The rest of the time it is only 89% water and is a barrier to sperm entry.

Of the 300 million to 500 million discharged, only 300 to 1000 sperm will actually make it into the vicinity of the ovum. This occurs approximately 1 hour after ejaculation. The ovum apparently secretes some type of chemotactic substance that guides the sperm in the right direction. The sperm receives energy from fructose found in the semen, which is metabolized by the mitochondria in the neck of the sperm.

The role of sperm in fertilization is threefold: (1) to supply the paternal complement of chromosomes, (2) to reach and penetrate the egg, and (3) to activate the egg into further cell division. The sperm's unique design allows the latter two events to occur.

Oogenesis

Oogenesis is the process of ovum development, which unlike spermatogenesis begins in fetal life. During early fetal life proliferation of the oogonia is rapid. By 20 weeks' gestation there are between 5 million and 7 million ova. These cells continue to enlarge, becoming primary oocytes. By birth a layer of follicular cells surrounds the primary oocytes, and they are designated primordial follicles. The first maturational (meiotic) division has started but stops part way through. These cells are then dormant until puberty.

At birth there are approximately 2 million ova left within the ovaries, since many have degenerated via a process known as atresia. This process continues, so that at puberty only 300,000 to 400,000 ova remain.

During puberty FSH and LH are released, causing an increase in the size of the oocyte as well as formation of the zona pellucida. Prior to ovulation the first meiotic division is completed, resulting in an unequal division of the cytoplasm and yielding one secondary oocyte and one polar body. The polar body degenerates.

Once the first meiotic division is completed, the secondary oocyte begins the second maturational division. It too is arrested part way through, to be completed once the ovum has been penetrated by the sperm. If penetration does occur, division is completed and the cytoplasm is once again unequally divided, yielding one mature oocyte and another polar body that also disintegrates.

For each menstrual cycle, 1000 oocytes will undergo maturational changes. Usually only one is released and the others degenerate. This roughly translates into each woman's having 400 cycles in her lifetime. Menopause is the time when few if any ova are left and the ovary is structurally as well as functionally changed.

The viability of the oocyte is very short, probably less than 24 hours. Aging and structural changes begin before 24 hours have passed. The role of the ovum in fertilization is also threefold: (1) to contribute all the nutrition for the zygote until implantation, (2) to reject all but one sperm, and (3) to provide the maternal chromosome complement.

Abnormal Gamete Development

Abnormal gamete development is the result of either chromosomal or morphologic abnormalities. The impact of maternal or paternal age at the time of conception can be seen in fresh gene mutations. The older the parents the greater the likelihood that they will generate germ cells that harbor gene mutations that can be passed on to the embryo. The likelihood of chromosomal abnormalities increases after the age of 35.[46, 66]

Nondisjunction is an error in meiotic division in which homologous chromosomes fail to separate and move to opposite poles of the cell. As a result, one gamete will have 24 chromosomes and the other will have only 22. Once fertilization occurs, the gamete with 24 chromosomes forms a zygote with 47 chromosomes. This chromosomal pattern is termed trisomy.

In the alternative situation, a 45-chromosome zygote is formed from the joining of a 22- and a 23-chromosome gamete. This situation is known as monosomy, since there is one chromosome missing.

Beyond chromosomal abnormalities, gametes may experience alterations in morphology. This is much less common in oocytes than in sperm. Although some oocytes may have two or more nuclei, they probably never mature.

In each ejaculate up to 20% of the sperm are grossly abnormal, having either two heads or two tails. Their ability to fertilize the ovum is probably limited owing to decreased or abnormal motility and inability to pass through the cervical mucus, thereby terminating their access to the ovum. An increase in the percentage of abnormal sperm can have an impact on fertility.[10, 46]

REPRODUCTIVE PROCESSES

Female

Endocrinology

The hormones of reproduction in the female are released by the hypothalamus, anterior pituitary, and ovaries. The cyclic release of these hormones in the female is associated with the menstrual cycle, which is discussed later.

HYPOTHALAMIC HORMONES

Gonadotropin-releasing hormone or factor (GnRH) is a peptide hormone produced by the hypothalamic neurons. GnRH acts on the anterior pituitary to stimulate release of LH and FSH. GnRH has also been called luteinizing hormone releasing hormone (LHRH) and luteinizing hormone releasing factor (LRF).

PITUITARY GONADOTROPINS

The anterior pituitary secretes three gonadotropins: LH, FSH, and prolactin. LH and FSH are glycoprotein hormones that act synergistically and sequentially to regulate the ovarian cycle by stimulating maturation of an ovarian follicle and regulating secretion of the ovarian hormones.

FSH acts on the ovarian granulosa cells along with estrogen to stimulate both follicular growth and formation of LH receptors on the granulosa cells. The appearance of LH receptors stimulates production of progesterone by the follicle. FSH secretion is cyclic, peaking at mid-cycle at the same time but at lower levels than the LH surge.

LH stimulates the theca cells of the ovary to synthesize androgens, which are converted to estrogens by the granulosa cells. The increase in estrogen inhibits maturation of other follicles. LH and FSH act synergistically to complete follicular maturation and ovulation, with a large LH surge at mid-cycle (12 to 36 hours prior to ovulation). The secretion of FSH and LH is influenced by the feedback effects of estrogens and, to a lesser extent, progesterone on the hypothalamic-pituitary-ovarian axis.

The anterior pituitary also secretes prolactin. Prolactin may enhance follicle maturation and function of the corpus luteum. Prolactin has important roles in initiating and maintaining lactation and in development of the mammary ducts during pregnancy. Elevated levels of prolactin in the nonpregnant woman may lead to infertility, since prolactin decreases the responsiveness of the anterior pituitary gland to GnRH and of the ovarian follicles to LH and FSH.

OVARIAN HORMONES

The ovaries produce four hormones: estrogens, progesterone, androgens, and folliculostatin. The estrogens, progesterone, and androgens are steroid hormones. Folliculostatin is a protein hormone.[18, 19, 52, 57, 67]

The principal estrogens produced by the ovaries are estrone (E_1) and estradiol-17β (E_2). Estradiol is secreted by the granulosa cells of the follicle from androgens produced by the theca cells surrounding the follicle. Estrogen levels peak immediately prior to the LH surge and ovulation. Estrogens stimulate development of primary and secondary sex characteristics in the female, influence changes associated with the endometrial cycle, stimulate contractions in the fallopian tubes, and influence the hypothalamic-pituitary-ovarian axis via feedback loops. During pregnancy significant amounts of estrogens are synthesized by the placenta.[18]

Progesterone is mainly produced by the corpus luteum during the luteal phase following ovulation. It stimulates development of the endometrium (in preparation for implantation) and alters the structure of the cervical mucus to prevent sperm entry. Progesterone also acts on the hypothalamus to increase basal body temperature. Circulating levels peak 7 to 8 days after the LH surge. If pregnancy does not occur, the corpus luteum regresses and progesterone levels fall.

The ovaries also produce androgens, which serve as precursors for estrogen synthesis, and folliculostatin. Folliculostatin, which is produced by the granulosa cells, is thought to provide negative feedback to regulate FSH secretion.

Puberty

In girls, changes during puberty include alterations in the reproductive organs, onset of menstruation, and development of secondary sex characteristics. The onset of the first menstrual period is called menarche. Puberty usually occurs about 2 years earlier in girls than in boys.

The mechanisms that trigger puberty and menarche are still unclear. The physical changes are in response to an increased production of gonadotropins and ovarian hormones, which begins gradually about 2 years prior to the onset of puberty.[35]

Prior to the first menstrual period there are changes in the organs of reproduction and somatic growth. A somatic growth spurt usually occurs between ages 9 and 14. The first change in the reproductive organs is the appearance of glandular breast tissue (breast bud) between 8 and 13 years of age, often accompanied by the appearance of hair on the mons pubis.

Changes during puberty in girls, in addition to menarche, include development of the breast and labia majora and labia minora; increase in size and length of the vagina, uterus, and fallopian tubes; increase in vaginal secretions and decreased vaginal pH; development of pubic and axillary hair; widening of the pelvis; and deposition of fat in the breasts, hips, and buttocks.[13, 41]

The age at which menstruation begins in the United States is usually between 11 and

14 years. The age of menstrual onset is influenced by nutritional status, weight, general health and genetic background, exercise, and environmental factors. Menarche usually occurs about 2 years after the appearance of the breast bud and generally occurs after a height growth spurt. The initial menstrual periods are irregular and anovulatory and lack a secretory phase.[13, 35]

Menstrual Cycle

The menstrual cycle is a reflection of the cyclic release of hormones along the hypothalamic-pituitary-ovarian axis. The release of these hormones results in characteristic changes in ovarian hormone production, follicular development, and ovulation known as the ovarian cycle. The changes along this hormonal axis and within the ovary induce cyclic structural and functioning changes within other parts of the reproductive system, including the endometrium of the uterus (endometrial cycle), cervical mucus, and vagina.

OVARIAN CYCLE

The ovarian cycle consists of three phases: follicular, ovulatory, and luteal.[19, 35, 57, 67] The follicular or preovulatory phase begins with initiation of menstruation and continues until immediately prior to ovulation. During this phase one of the graafian follicles within the ovary matures. Mature ovarian graafian follicles consist of a primary oocyte, granulosa cells, zona pellucida membrane, and theca cells. During each menstrual cycle one follicle completes the maturational process and is ovulated (Fig. 1–8).

The process of follicle maturation takes about 12 to 14 days, but this can be variable. Maturation of the follicle begins under the influence of LH and FSH with an increase in size and accumulation of fluid creating a large fluid-filled sac. Estrogen production increases concomitantly. The rate of estrogen secretion increases rapidly beginning about 1 week prior to ovulation, peaking 24 hours prior to the LH surge. By the end of the follicular phase the follicle bulges on the surface of the ovary.

The ovulatory phase extends from the estrogen peak to ovulation. The oocyte completes its first meiotic division 36 to 48 hours prior to ovulation, becoming a secondary oocyte. The mid-cycle LH surge, accompanied by a smaller increase in FSH, occurs

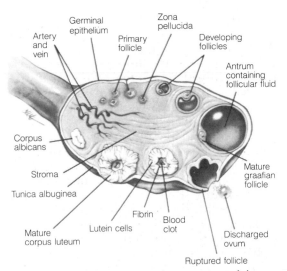

FIGURE 1–8. The ovary and maturation of the ovarian follicle. (From Olds, S.A., London, M.L., & Ladewig, P.A. (1989). *Maternal-newborn nursing: A family-centered approach* (p. 138). Menlo Park, CA: Addison-Wesley.)

12 to 36 hours before ovulation. Prior to the LH surge, estrogen levels decrease and progesterone levels begin to rise.

Ovulation begins with small avascular spots (stigma) that appear on the ovarian surface over the protruding follicle. The stigma forms a vesicle, which ruptures, extruding the secondary oocyte surrounded by the zona pellucida along with the follicular fluid and cells.

After ovulation the walls of the follicle collapse inward. LH causes the remaining tissues to become vascularized and undergo morphologic and metabolic changes to form the corpus luteum, which secretes progesterone and some estrogen. Progesterone levels continue to increase, peaking 7 to 8 days post ovulation. The luteal phase lasts 14 days and ends with the onset of menstruation. If conception does not occur, the corpus luteum regresses, progesterone levels fall, and menstruation begins.

ENDOMETRIAL CYCLE

The changing patterns of gonadotropic and ovarian hormones stimulate changes within the endometrium of the uterus. The endometrial cycle is divided into three phases: proliferative, secretory, and menstrual.[35, 52, 57]

The proliferative phase of the endometrial cycle overlaps the follicular phase of the ovarian cycle, beginning post menstruation and ending with ovulation. After menstruation the endometrium is very thin. During the proliferative phase the endometrium thickens from 1 mm to between 3 and 5 mm, owing to epithelial cell lengthening. The endometrium becomes more vascularized, and endometrial glands proliferate. All these changes are under the influence of estrogen secreted by the maturing follicle. The length of this phase is variable.

The secretory phase corresponds to the luteal phase of the ovarian cycle, extending from ovulation to the onset of menstruation. This phase is usually 14 days long (range, 12 to 16 days) and is primarily under the influence of progesterone from the corpus luteum. During the secretory phase the endometrium and its stroma continue to thicken. Blood vessels proliferate, dilate, and become coiled. The endometrial glands continue to hypertrophy and begin to secrete a fluid rich in glycogen. If conception does not occur, regression of the corpus luteum and fall in progesterone and estrogen levels lead to degenerative changes in the endometrium.

During the menstrual phase the endometrium undergoes vasospasm, ischemic necrosis, and sloughing of the endometrial tissue. After the initial vasospasm the blood vessels dilate, resulting in menstrual flow. This phase is also variable in length, lasting 3 to 6 days. The onset of menstruation is considered to be day 1 of the menstrual cycle. The correlation of the ovarian and endometrial cycles for an "ideal" 28-day cycle is illustrated in Figure 1–9.

Characteristic changes in the vaginal epithelial cells and in the quantity, viscosity, elasticity, and cellular pattern of cervical mucus are evident during the menstrual cycle. During the proliferative phase the cervical mucus is scant and viscous and demonstrates minimal spinnbarkeit and ferning. Spinnbarkeit describes the elasticity of mucus or the ability of the mucus to form along thin threads. Ferning is an arborization pattern caused by increased sodium chloride content that is seen in dried mucus around the time of ovulation. Under the influence of estrogen, immediately prior to ovulation, the cervical mucus becomes thin, clear, watery, and elastic (maximum spinnbarkeit) and develops a ferning pattern. Changes in the vaginal epithelial cells also occur with ovulation as these cells become larger, flatter, and cornified.[21, 57]

Climacteric

The female climacteric is the period of life characterized by the cessation of menstruation and decrease in ovarian hormones. The climacteric may last for many years. During this time there is decreased production of estrogen, with an increased production of gonadotropic hormones in an attempt to stimulate the now unresponsive ovary to produce estrogen. The exact stimulus for the climacteric is not well understood, although it is related to the disappearance of oocytes and follicles which are responsive to gonadotropins. Since production of the ovarian hormones (particularly estrogen) is dependent on cyclic follicular maturation, the levels of estrogen decrease and the cyclic balance of ovarian and endometrial cycles is disrupted.[35]

The major alterations during the climacteric are menstrual, vasomotor, musculoskeletal, cardiovascular, and reproductive and are primarily due to decreased estrogen. Menopause, or the cessation of regular menstruation for 6 months or more, may occur gradually or abruptly between 45 and 50 years of age in 50% of women, before age 45 in 25%, and after age 50 in 25%.[35] In general, the period prior to menopause is associated with marked alterations in the length and frequency of menstrual cycles.

Other changes in the reproductive system include atrophy of the vagina, uterus, cervix, vulva, pelvic floor, and breasts. Vaginal atrophy is associated with alteration in the vaginal mucosa, irritation, increased risk of vaginal infections, and painful intercourse.

The climacteric is characterized by vasomotor instability with generalized cutaneous vasodilation or vasoconstriction. These vasomotor changes are accompanied by a feeling of warmth (hot flashes), flushing of the skin, and sweating, or feelings of chill and cold extremities. Musculoskeletal changes include decreased muscle length, tone, and strength; osteoporosis; reduction in bone density; decrease in height; and reduction in skeletal strength, with an increased risk of fractures. There is a decrease in skin elasticity. Cardiovascular alterations include increased arteriosclerosis and coronary artery disease. The type and intensity of alterations in body systems and physiologic function during the climacteric vary significantly from woman to woman.[21, 35]

Since most of the changes associated with

PHASE	MENSTRUAL	EARLY FOLLICULAR	ADVANCED FOLLICULAR	OVULATION	EARLY LUTEAL	ADVANCED LUTEAL	PREMEN-STRUAL
Days	1–3 to 5	4 to 6–8	9 to 12–16	12–16	15–19	20–25	26–32
Ovary	Involution of corpus luteum	Growth and maturation of graafian follicle		Ovulation	Active corpus luteum		Involution of corpus luteum
Estrogen	Diminution	Progressive increase		High concentration	Secondary rise		Decreasing
Progesterone	———————— Absent ————————			Appearing	——— Rising ———		Decreasing
Endometrium	Menstrual desquamation and involution	Reorganization and proliferation	Further growth and watery secretion	—	Active secretion and glandular dilatation	Accumulation of secretion and edema	Regressive
Pituitary secretion							
FSH	Fairly constant until just before ovulation			Moderate increase just before	——— Rapid decrease to previous levels ———		
LH	——————— Same as above ———————			Marked increase just before	——————— Same as above ———————		

FIGURE 1–9. Correlation of the ovarian and endometrial cycles (ideal 28-day cycle). (From Pritchard, J.A. & MacDonald, P.C. (1980). *Williams obstetrics* (16th ed., p. 84). New York: Appleton-Century-Crofts, Courtesy of Appleton-Century-Crofts, Publishing Division of Prentice-Hall, Inc., Englewood Cliffs, NJ.)

the climacteric are related to the decrease in estrogen, treatment by estrogen replacement may be used. Estrogen replacement therapy is controversial, with many advantages as well as risks. The major disadvantage associated with this therapy is the increased risk for endometrial and breast cancer.[35]

Male

Endocrinology

The hormones of the male reproductive system are released by the hypothalamus, anterior pituitary, and testes. Release is both systemic and local, being continuous or acyclic after puberty. Slight diurnal changes in plasma testosterone levels occur. The release of male reproductive hormones is controlled by a negative feedback loop along the hypothalamic-pituitary-testicular axis.

Testosterone is an androgen produced by the Leydig cells of the testes. Initial production of testosterone early in embryonic development is responsible for development of the male reproductive organs and external genitalia. Production becomes active again at puberty. Testosterone is necessary for spermatogenesis, development of male secondary sex characteristics, bone growth, growth and development of male reproductive organs, sexual drive, and potency.[21, 57, 67] The testes also produce small amounts of other androgens.

The hypothalamus regulates the testicular environment by secreting gonadotropin-releasing hormone (GnRH), which is moderated further by norepinephrine, serotonin, endorphin, melatonin, and dopamine. GnRH secretion occurs once every 70 to 90 minutes. The pulsatile pattern is required for the production and release of LH and FSH by the anterior pituitary.[8]

Both LH and FSH act directly on the testes, stimulating spermatogenesis and testosterone production. Both hormones have a high affinity for their respective receptors. Once bound, they activate the protein kinase cascade via cyclic adenosine monophosphate (cAMP).[65]

LH stimulates the Leydig cells to initiate steroidogenesis by synthesizing androgens from cholesterol precursors. Along with androgen production, LH is responsible for triggering spermatogenesis.

The effects of FSH complement those of LH. FSH binds to receptor sites in the Sertoli cells, stimulating the production of proteins that in turn affect spermatogenesis. FSH is also responsible for facilitating mitosis in the spermatogonia and initiating meiosis in the spermatocyte. Last, FSH seems to be necessary for the maturation of the spermatid. Normal levels of FSH are necessary to maintain normal sperm quality.[6, 38, 39, 42]

Testicular testosterone is thought to act directly on the germ cells and Sertoli cells.

Through diffusion and active transport testosterone supports the germinal epithelium and regulates spermatogenesis.

Puberty

Reproductive capability in men begins with spermarche. Unlike menarche, which occurs toward the end of puberty, spermarche begins early in puberty, preceding the peak growth spurt, occurring on an average at 13½ years of age.[6] Puberty takes about 4 years to complete, beginning somewhere between 11 and 16 years of age. During this time there are growth and development of the reproductive organs, rapid physical growth, and development of secondary sex characteristics.[41, 67]

The specific stimulus or mechanism for initiating puberty is not known. There is an increase in the release of pituitary gonadotropins, which stimulates the production of androgens, particularly testosterone. It is the synthesis of testosterone and other androgens that results in the changes in the reproductive system and somatic tissue.

The major changes include the enlargement of the testes and penis; development of pubic, axillary, facial, and body hair; rapid skeletal growth; hypertrophy of the larynx, with subsequent deepening of the voice; increased activity of the sweat and sebaceous glands; and muscular hypertrophy.[41] Along with this, the seminiferous tubules begin sperm production. The earliest observable changes are the enlargement of the testes and scrotum resulting from growth of the seminiferous tubules. Ejaculation generally can occur about a year after the growth of the penis.

Sperm Production

Sperm production takes place within the complex endocrine environment described previously. The development of mature germ cells in the seminiferous tubules involves three stages: (1) mitosis—spermatogonial multiplication, (2) meiosis—production of haploid cells, and (3) spermiogenesis—maturation of spermatids to mature spermatozoa. The androgens and proteins produced locally modulate the stage of spermatogenesis seen within the tubule.[6, 63]

The seminiferous tubule can be divided into two zones. The basal compartment is the outer layer (zone 1) of the tubule, and the adluminal compartment is the inner luminal layer. The basal compartment is composed of stem cells (termed spermatogonia) that are renewed through mitosis. Some of these continue to proliferate and serve as stem cells, whereas others separate from the basal membrane and begin to migrate toward the lumen. These cells are known as preleptotene spermatocytes. As migration progresses the cells undergo further morphologic changes, becoming primary spermatocytes. The first and second meiotic divisions occur with further differentiation in the adluminal zone, resulting in the formation of secondary spermatocytes and spermatids.

The luminal spermatids continue to mature (spermiogenesis). This transformation is a complex sequence of changes within the cell organelles, resulting in the development of the unique sperm characteristics.

The sperm are then moved down the tubules by contraction and fluid secretion by the Sertoli cells. The evolution process takes approximately 70 ± 4 days.[72] Little is known about the mechanisms that govern the time this takes, but the germ cells must progress through the process at a predetermined rate or they degenerate.[28]

At the time of their release into the tubules, the spermatozoa are still morphologically immature and lack motility. While traversing the epididymis (which takes 14 to 21 days) they continue to differentiate. It is in the proximal epididymis that forward motility is achieved.[6]

Climacteric

Males do not experience a cessation in reproductive ability in the same manner that females experience menopause. There is a gradual decline in testosterone production and in spermatogenesis in the thirties and forties. Reproductive ability is usually not compromised, however. In later life, atrophy of the external genitalia occurs. Concomitantly there are involution of the testes and degenerative changes in the Leydig cells, thereby diminishing the production of testosterone. The age at which these events occur is variable among individual men, and some do not experience them at all.[21, 67]

CLINICAL IMPLICATIONS

The ability to control the reproductive process and determine the timing of pregnancy is the desire of many couples. Therefore, contraception is discussed in this section, as are problems related to fertility.

Infertility

Infertility has been defined as a situation in which "conception does not occur after one year of sexual exposure in a couple trying to achieve pregnancy."[12, p.38] Primary infertility is the term used when there has been no previous conception, whereas secondary infertility designates infertility following previous conceptive ability. The actual incidence of infertility is unknown; however, it is estimated that 10 to 15% of all married couples experience infertility.[48]

There are numerous causes for infertility, including those related to ovulation; structural problems; sperm abnormalities; metabolic, endocrine, and immunologic factors; and subclinical genital infections.[12] These are summarized in Table 1–8.

Proper steroid secretion by the ovary is essential in controlling the hypothalamic and pituitary function. Any disruption in the central nervous system, hypothalamus, or pituitary and ovarian unit and its coordinated synchronized interactions can result in ovarian insufficiency. This condition is incompatible with reproduction because ovulation is either absent or markedly impaired.[5] Pharmacologic intervention with steroid preparations is the current therapy for this type of failure.

The major cause of tuboperitoneal damage is pelvic inflammatory disease, whereas obstruction of the fallopian tubes is often the result of adhesions secondary to endometri-

osis. Surgical intervention may reestablish patency and enhance conception.[43]

Male factors are responsible for 30 to 40% of the cases of infertility. Men who have azoospermia, complete sperm immobility, or total teratospermia are clearly infertile. The probability of pregnancy is high if the ejaculate always contains more than 20 million sperm/ml, with 50% showing good forward motility, and 60% being normal in morphology. There are very few treatments known to increase fertility in men who do not achieve these values. Table 1–9 provides a list of the classification and causes of semen abnormalities.

In the male there are numerous factors that affect the sperm's capacity to fertilize. These include the consistency and volume of the seminal fluid, motility, viability, and morphology. The seminal plasma serves as a vehicle and a diluent for spermatozoa. It also buffers the sperm cells from the hostile vaginal environment while providing the energy source for survival. The plasma volume and chemical composition are dependent upon testosterone. Therefore, alterations in viscosity impair sperm transport, and increased or decreased volume or a change in pH indicates the abnormal functioning of the contributing organs.[16]

It is unclear what the normal range for sperm count should be. Biweekly sampling has demonstrated fluctuations in count from 5 million to 170 million/ml. Men with sperm counts of greater than 250 million/ml seem to be infertile for unknown reasons. There is probably no definite lower concentration limit below which all men are infertile; however, less than 20 million/ml is considered a low normal count and seems to reduce the likelihood of fertilization.[16, 28]

Few sperm are required for fertilization, but they must be motile. Assessment of this is based on the percentage of motile sperm; greater than 50% is considered normal.[16] Progressive (forward) movement is also assessed and rated as poor, good, or excellent. A loss of motility in 10 to 20% of sperm over 3 hours is considered to be normal.[16, 28]

Sperm have a unique topography, and there is a clear correlation between sperm morphology and capacity to fertilize. Usually there are a variety of defects seen rather than a single consistent abnormality. When 40 to 60% of the sperm are normal, fertility does not seem to be affected. The morphology of the abnormal sperm may help to provide a clue to the possible causes.[16, 28]

TABLE 1–8
Factors Accounting for Infertility

FACTOR	PERCENTAGE AFFECTED
Failure of ovulation	10–15
Endometriosis, pelvic adhesions, tubal disease	30–40
Male factors	30–40
Abnormal sperm (inability to penetrate cervical mucus)	10–15
Metabolic, endocrine, and immunologic factors or subclinical genital infections	5
Unable to diagnose	10

Compiled from Davajan, V. & Mishell, D.R. (1986). Evaluation of the infertile couple. In D.R. Mishell & V. Davajan (Eds.), *Infertility, contraception & reproductive endocrinology* (2nd ed.). Oradell, NJ: Medical Economics Books.

Infertility is an ever-increasing problem as couples delay conception into their thirties. New diagnostic techniques and treatment modalities are being developed based on the increasing understanding we have of the processes involved in reproduction (see Chapter 2).

Contraception

Reversible contraception is the temporary blocking of fertility. Sterilization should be considered a permanent method of prevention regardless of the new surgical techniques being designed to attempt reversal and reestablish fertility. All the contraceptive methods have advantages and disadvantages. These need to be thoroughly explained to couples, although this is usually discussed with the woman because the only temporary contraceptive developed for the man is the condom (Table 1–10).

As of 1982, approximately 68% of the married couples in the United States practiced some form of birth control.[47] Sterilization (when all females between the ages of 5 and 44 years are considered) is the most common method of fertility control in the United States; oral contraceptives are the most popular of the nonsurgical modalities. Vasectomy has become increasingly popular since 1965, with an estimated 250,000 men each year undergoing the procedure.

Contraceptive method effectiveness refers to the theoretical effectiveness of the method when used correctly. Use effectiveness, the rate of effectiveness in actual application, is influenced by the instruction provided, the motivation to use, and amount of experience with the technique. Generally, those methods used at the time of coitus have a much lower use effectiveness than method effectiveness. Contraceptive failure is more likely to occur with couples wanting to delay a pregnancy than with those wanting to prevent any further pregnancies or any pregnancy at all. Contraceptive failure has been correlated with age, socioeconomic status, and level of education. Failure rates decline with increasing use (experience) and with increasing age.

TABLE 1–9
Etiology of Semen Abnormalities

FINDING	CAUSE
Abnormal Count	
Azoospermia	Klinefelter's syndrome or other genetic disorders
	Sertoli-cell–only syndrome
	Seminiferous tubule of Leydig cell failure
	Hypogonadotropic hypogonadism
	Ductal obstruction, including Young's syndrome
	Varicocele
	Exogenous factors
Oligozoospermia	Genetic disorder
	Endocrinopathies, including androgen receptor defects
	Varicocele and other anatomic disorders
	Maturation arrest
	Hypospermatogenesis
	Exogenous factors
Abnormal Volume	
No ejaculate	Ductal obstruction
	Retrograde ejaculation
	Ejaculatory failure
	Hypogonadism
Low volume	Obstruction of the ejaculatory ducts
	Absence of seminal vesicles and vas deferens
	Partial retrograde ejaculation
	Infection
High volume	Unknown factors
Abnormal Motility	Immunologic factors
	Infection
	Varicocele
	Defects in sperm structure
	Metabolic or anatomic abnormalities of sperm
	Poor liquefaction of semen
Abnormal Viscosity	Cause unknown
Abnormal Morphology	Varicocele
	Stress
	Infection
	Exogenous factors
	Unknown factors
Extraneous Cells	Infection or inflammation
	Shedding of immature sperm

From Bernstein, G. S. (1991). Male factor in infertility. In D. R. Mishell, V. Davajan, & R. A. Lobo (Eds.), *Infertility, contraception & reproductive endocrinology* (3rd ed., p. 629). Boston: Blackwell Scientific Publishers.

TABLE 1–10
Available Contraceptives for Couples in the U.S.

Abstinence from and alternatives to sexual intercourse
Condoms
Combined birth control pills
Progestin-only or mini-pill
Morning-after pills or IUD insertion
IUDs that are medicated with copper
IUDs that elaborate progesterone
Diaphragms
Cervical caps
Spermicidal sponges and suppositories
Contraceptive foam
Natural family planning methods
Tubal ligation and hysterectomy
Vasectomy
Therapeutic abortion
Levonorgestrel implants

Adapted from Hatcher, R.A., et al. (1986). *Contraceptive technology 1986–1987* (13th ed., p. 295). New York: Irvington Publishers.

The lowest failure rates have been found in women who wished to prevent a pregnancy, had the highest income, and were over 30 years of age.[3, 27, 44, 47, 48]

Barrier Methods

These methods include spermicides, diaphragm, cervical cap, cervical sponge, and condom. They are designed to prevent the sperm from crossing the cervical mucosa. Spermicides must be used with each act of intercourse. They contain a spermicidal ingredient (usually nonoxynol 9) that is designed to kill or immobilize sperm on contact. Effectiveness of this method is comparable to that of the diaphragm; the latter is an actual physical barrier imposed across the vagina to cover the cervix. Diaphragm effectiveness is dependent upon the fit and the ability to place the barrier appropriately. Teaching with return demonstrations is necessary in order to ensure the latter. The more experienced the individual is with the method the more effective the contraception. Diaphragms must be prescribed and fitted by a physician or nurse practitioner and should be used in conjunction with a spermicide.[11, 53]

The condom is currently the only temporary method of birth control for the male. It is a widely used contraceptive not only in the United States but also throughout the world. Males who are motivated and consistently use the condom exactly as directed with each act of coitus have a theoretical failure rate of 2 pregnancies/100 women/year. The actual rate is closer to 10 per year. There is currently a resurgence in condom use in the United States. This is probably because of the protection it provides against sexually transmitted diseases, e.g., human immunodeficiency virus (HIV).[25, 44, 64]

Oral Contraceptives

Oral contraceptives (OC) come in three major forms: fixed-dose combination, combination phasic, and daily gestagen (progestin). The most frequently used are the combination formulations, which are the most effective in preventing pregnancy by inhibiting the mid-cycle gonadotropin surge and preventing ovulation. They also alter the cervical mucus, making it more viscous, thereby slowing or inhibiting sperm penetration. Along with

this, they alter uterine motility, which affects ova and sperm transport and reduces the endometrial production of glycogen, altering the energy store available to a blastocyst in the uterine cavity.[44, 53]

The daily gestagen-only preparations do not stop ovulation consistently. Their mechanisms of contraception are related more to the other physiologic changes. Because of these inconsistencies, the pregnancy rate is higher (i.e., 2.5%/year compared with 2%). These pills may be prescribed for women for whom estrogen is contraindicated.[25, 44] The reader is referred to contraception texts for discussion of conditions that are contraindications to OC use and of the many side effects associated with estrogen and progestin use.[25, 44]

Intrauterine Devices

One of the main benefits of intrauterine devices (IUDs) is that a single act provides long-term contraception. Along with this there are fewer systemic side effects. All IUDs have similar use and method failure rates, and pregnancy seems to be related more to the skill of the individual inserting the device. High fundal placement is desirable. After the first year the accidental pregnancy rate drops steadily, approaching that for oral contraceptives. The incidence of adverse effects (bleeding and pain) usually decreases with duration of use as well.[25, 44]

The mechanism of action for IUDs is spermicidal. The local inflammatory reaction caused by the foreign substance within the uterus results in an increase in leukocytes. As the leukocytes break down, toxic by-products are released, creating a noxious environment for either sperm or blastocyst (although sperm reaching the oviducts is an infrequent event). Beyond this, the endometrium appears to become less receptive to the embryo and implantation does not occur. The addition of copper to the IUD increases the inflammatory reaction, making pregnancy less likely.[3, 25, 44]

The inflammatory response usually resolves quickly with removal of the IUD, and the resumption of fertility is not delayed. The rates of subsequent pregnancy are equal to those in women who discontinue use of barrier methods.[44]

Contraceptive Implants

Recent research has looked at long-term reversible and irreversible contraception utilizing implants. Recently, subdermal implants made up of Silastic rods containing levonorgestrel (LNG) have become available to women desiring long-term contraception. The synthetic steroid is released at a steady rate for 5 years or longer, causing systemic changes that result in ovulation inhibition (in about 50% of ovulatory cycles) and thickened cervical mucus, which reduces sperm penetration.

There are currently two versions of this contraceptive method. Norplant consists of six hollow rods 3 cm in length that release LNG at a rate of 40 µg/day. This provides a pregnancy protection rate that is similar to that of sterilization. The second version (Norplant–2) consists of two solid implants. Both are placed under the skin of the upper arm with the patient under local anesthesia and are considered to be effective for 3 to 5 years. The rods can be removed at any time, and fertility is rapidly restored.

Further research into alternative methods of contraception continues, with much focus on a contraceptive vaccine that can be administered to men. As more knowledge about reproduction and the endocrine control of the different stages is acquired, options for controlling the process will become available for both males and females.

TABLE 1–11
Clinical Implications for the Mother and Neonate Related to Chromosomes and Reproductive Biology

Parents with a familial history of chromosomal or genetic abnormalities should receive genetics counseling with an explanation of how chromosomes can be altered during gametogenesis or division (pp. 6–10).

Couples who do not achieve pregnancy at the end of 1 year of consistent sexual exposure should obtain fertility counseling and a fertility work-up (pp. 29–30).

Contraceptive alternatives need to be explored with women and men; selection should be based on motivation, lifestyle, and advantages for use (pp. 31–33).

Neonates born with abnormal genitalia require a complete endocrine evaluation, ultrasonography of internal structures, and chromosomal assessment (pp. 10–11, 20–23).

Psychosocial orientation should be discussed with parents of an infant with ambiguous genitalia (pp. 20–23).

Page numbers in parentheses following each implication refer to the pages where the rationale for the intervention is discussed.

SUMMARY

This chapter has attempted to provide an overview of the physiologic mechanisms of gametogenesis and demonstrate the complexities of these processes. Our knowledge remains limited but continues to expand as further research is conducted. The more we understand about reproductive endocrinology and the actual mechanisms of reproduction and genetic transfer, the more we can hope for ways to improve perinatal outcome. Clinical implications for the mother and neonate can be found in Table 1–11.

REFERENCES

1. Beck, F., Moffat, D.B., & Davies, D.P. (1985). *Human embryology* (2nd ed.). Oxford: Blackwell/Year Book Medical Publishers.
2. Boczkowski, K. (1971). Sex determination and gonadal differentiation in man. A unifying concept of normal and abnormal sex development. *Clin Genet, 2,* 379.
3. Bounds, W. (1984). Male and female barrier contraceptive methods. In M. Filshie & J. Guillebaud (Eds.), *Contraception: Science and practice.* London: Butterworths.
4. Branchaud, C.L., et al. (1985). Functional zonation of the midgestation human fetal adrenal cortex: Fetal versus definitive zone use of progesterone for cortisol synthesis. *Am J Obstet Gynecol, 151,* 271.
5. Breckwoldt, M., et al. (1986). Classification and diagnosis of ovarian insufficiency. In V. Insler & B. Lunenfeld (Eds.), *Infertility: Male and female.* New York: Churchill Livingstone.
6. Buster, J.E. & Saurer, M.V. (1989). Endocrinology of conception. In S.A. Brody & K. Ueland (Eds.), *Endocrine disorders in pregnancy.* Norwalk, CT: Appleton & Lange.
7. Byskov, A.G. (1978). The anatomy and ultrastructure of the rete system in the fetal mouse ovary. *Biol Reprod, 19,* 720.
8. Carmel, P.W., et al. (1976). Pituitary stalk portal blood collection in rhesus monkeys: Evidence for pulsatile release of gonadotropin-releasing hormone (GnRH). *Endocrinology, 99,* 243.
9. Cohen, F.L. (1984). *Clinical genetics in nursing practice.* Philadelphia: JB Lippincott.
10. Cormack, D.H. (1984). *Introduction to histology.* Philadelphia: JB Lippincott.
11. Craig, S. & Hepburn, S. (1985). The effectiveness of barrier methods of contraception with and without spermicide. *Contraception, 25,* 132.
12. Davajan, V. & Mishell, D.R. (1986). Evaluation of the infertile couple. In D.R. Mishell & V. Davajan (Eds.), *Infertility, contraception & reproductive endocrinology* (2nd ed.). Oradell, NJ: Medical Economics Books.
13. Fordney, D.S. (1980). Adolescence. In S.L. Romney, et al. (Eds.), *Gynecology & Obstetrics: The Healthy Care of Women* (2nd ed.). New York: McGraw-Hill.
14. George, F.W. & Wilson, J.D. (1978). Conversion of androgen to estrogen by the human fetal ovary. *Clin Endocrinol Metab, 47,* 550.

15. George, F.W., et al. (1978). Estrogen content of the embryonic rabbit ovary. *Nature* (London), *274*, 172.

16. Glezerman, M. & Vartoov, B. (1986). Semen analysis. In V. Insler & B. Lunenfeld (Eds.), *Infertility: Male and female*. New York: Churchill Livingstone.

17. Gluckman, P.D., Grumback, M.M., & Kaplan, S.L. (1981). The neuroendocrine regulation and function of growth hormone and prolactin in the mammalian fetus. *Endocr Rev, 2*, 363.

18. Gondos, B. & Hobel, C.V. (1973). Interstitial cells in the human fetal ovary. *Endocrinology, 93*, 736.

19. Greenhill, J.P. & Friedman, E.A. (1974). *Biological principles and modern practice of obstetrics*. Philadelphia: WB Saunders.

20. Hadziselimovic, F. & Girard, J. (1977). Pathogenesis of cryptorchidism. *Horm Res, 8*, 76.

21. Hafez, E.S.E. (1980). *Human reproduction: conception and contraception* (2nd ed.). Hagerstown, MD: Harper & Row.

22. Hamerton, J.L. (1968). Significance of sex chromosome derived heterochromatin in mammals. *Nature, 219*, 910.

23. Hamilton, W.J., Boyd, J.D., & Mossman, H.W. (1976). *Human embryology: Prenatal development of form and function* (4th ed.). London: Macmillan.

24. Haseltine, F.P. (1983). Sex differentiation: Current concepts. In J.B. Warshaw (Ed.), *The biological basis of reproductive and developmental medicine*. New York: Elsevier Biomedical.

25. Hatcher, R.A., et al. (1986). *Contraceptive technology 1986 –1987* (13th ed.). New York: Irvington.

26. Heinrichs, W.L. & Gibbons, W.E. (1989). Endocrinology of pregnancy. In S.A. Brody & K. Ueland (Eds.), *Endocrine disorders in pregnancy*. New York: Appleton & Lange.

27. Hendershot. G.E., et al. (1982). Infertility and age: An unresolved issue. *Fam Plann Perspect, 14*, 287.

28. Hudson, B., et al. (1985). Virility and fertility. In R.P. Shearman (Ed.), *Clinical reproductive endocrinology*. Edinburgh: Churchill Livingstone.

29. Huhtaniemi, I. (1977). Studies on steroidogenesis and its regulation in human fetal adrenal and testis. *Steroid Biochem, 8*, 491.

30. Jaffe, R.B. (1986). Endocrine physiology of the fetus and fetoplacental unit. In S.S.C. Yen & R.B. Jaffe (Eds.), *Reproductive endocrinology: Physiology, pathophysiology and clinical management*. Philadelphia: WB Saunders.

31. Jones, O.W. (1989). Basic genetics and patterns of inheritance. In R.K. Creasy & R. Resnik (Eds.), *Maternal-fetal medicine: Principles and practice* (2nd ed.). Philadelphia: WB Saunders.

32. Josso, N., et al. (1977). The antimullerian hormone. *Recent Prog Horm Res, 33*, 117.

33. Jost, A., et al. (1974). Sertoli cells and early testicular differentiation. In R.E. Mancini & L. Martini (Eds.). *Male fertility and sterility*. London: Academic Press.

34. Jost, A., et al. (1973). Studies on sex differentiation in mammals. *Recent Prog Horm Res, 29*, 1.

35. Judd, H.L. & Meldrum, D.R. (1981). Physiology and pathophysiology of menstruation and menopause. In S.L. Romney, et al. (Eds.), *Gynecology and obstetrics, health care of women* (2nd ed.). New York: McGraw-Hill.

36. Kaplan, S.L. & Grumbach, M.M. (1978). Pituitary and placental gonadotropins and sex steroids in the human fetus and subhuman primate fetus. *Clin Endocrinol Metab, 7*, 487.

37. Kaplan, S.L., et al. (1976). The ontogenesis of pituitary hormones and hypothalamic factors in the human fetus: Maturation of central nervous system regulation of anterior pituitary function. *Recent Prog Horm Res, 32*, 161.

38. Kruegger, P.M., et al. (1974). New evidence for the role of Sertoli cell and spermatogonia in the feedback control of FSH secretion in male rats. *Endocrinology, 95*, 955.

39. Lacroix, M., et al. (1977). Secretion of plasminogen activator by Sertoli cell enriched cultures. *Mol Cell Endocrinol, 9*, 227.

40. Langman, J. (1981). *Medical embryology* (4th ed.). Baltimore: Williams & Wilkins.

41. Lowery, G.H. (1977). *Growth and development of children* (7th ed.). Chicago: Year Book Medical Publishers.

42. Matsumoto, A.M., et al. (1986). Chronic human chorionic gonadotropin administration in normal men: Evidence that follicle-stimulating hormone is necessary for the maintenance of quantitatively normal spermatogenesis in man. *J Clin Endocrinol Metab, 62*, 1184.

43. McComb, P., et al. (1986). Investigation of tubo-peritoneal causes of female infertility. In V. Insler & B. Lunenfeld (Eds.), *Infertility: Male and female*. New York: Churchill Livingstone.

44. Mishell, D.R. (1986). Contraceptive use and effectiveness. In D.R. Mishell & V. Davajan (Eds.), *Infertility, contraception & reproductive endocrinology* (2nd ed.). Oradell, NJ: Medical Economics Books.

45. Mishell, D.R. & Goebelsmann, U. (1986). Disorders of sexual differentiation. In D.R. Mishell & V. Davajan (Eds.), *Infertility, contraception & reproductive endocrinology* (2nd ed.). Oradell, NJ: Medical Economics Books.

46. Moore, K.L. (1986). *The developing human: Clinically oriented embryology* (3rd ed.). Philadelphia: WB Saunders.

47. Mosher, W.D. (1983). *Vital and health statistics*, Series 23. Data from the National Survey of Family Growth, No. 7, DHHS Publication PHS 81.

48. Mosher, W.D. (1983). Infertility trends among U.S. couples: 1965–1976. *Fam Plann Perspect, 12*, 22.

49. Muir, B. (1983). *Essentials of genetics for nurses*. New York: John Wiley.

50. Niemi, M., et al. (1965). Histochemistry and fine structure of the interstitial tissue in the human foetal testis. In G.E.W. Wolstenholme & M. O'Connor (Eds.), *Ciba Foundation colloquia on endocrinology: Endocrinology of the testis* (Vol 16). London: J & A Churchill.

51. Ohno, S. (1967). *Sex chromosomes and sex-linked genes*. New York: Springer-Verlag.

52. Page, E.W., et al (1981). *Human reproduction* (3rd ed.). Philadelphia: WB Saunders.

53. Peel, J. & Potts, M. (1970). *Textbook of contraceptive practice*. London: Cambridge University Press.

54. Pelliniemi, L. & Dym, M. (1980). The fetal gonad and sexual differentiation. In D. Tulchinsky & K. Ryan (Eds.), *Maternal-fetal endocrinology*. Philadelphia: WB Saunders.

55. Pelliniemi, L.J. & Niei, M. (1969). Fine structure of the human foetal testis. I. The interstitial tissue. *Z Zellforsch, 99*, 507.

56. Pinkerton, J.H.M., et al. (1961). Development of the human ovary—A study using histochemical technics. *Obstet Gynecol, 18*, 152.

57. Prichard, J.A. & MacDonald, P.C. (1980). *Williams*

obstetrics (16th ed.). New York: Appleton-Century-Crofts.

58. Sarto, G.E. & Opitz, J.M. (1973). The XY gonadal agenesis syndrome. *J Med Genet, 10*, 288.

59. Short, E.M. (1988). Genetic disorders. In G.N. Burrow & T.F. Ferris (Eds.), *Medical complications during pregnancy* (3rd ed.). Philadelphia: WB Saunders.

60. Siiteri, P.K. & Wilson, J.D. (1974). Testosterone formation and metabolism during male sexual differentiation in the human embryo. *J Clin Endocrinol Metab, 38*, 113.

61. Simpson, J.L. (1978). *Disorders of sexual differentiation: Etiology and clincial delineation.* New York: Academic Press.

62. Spiegelman, M. & Bennett, D. (1973). A light- and electron-microscopic study of primordial germ cells in the early mouse embryo. *J Embryol Exp Morphol, 30*, 97.

63. Steinberger, E. (1970). Hormonal control of mammalian spermatogenesis. *Physiol Rev, 51*, 1.

64. Strokes, B. (1980). Men and family planning. *Worldwatch Paper, 41*, 92.

65. Swerdloff, R.S. & Bhasin, S. (1984). Male reproductive physiology. In J. Aimen (Ed.), *Infertility: Diagnosis and management.* New York: Springer-Verlag.

66. Thompson, M.W. (1986). *Medical genetics* (4th ed.). Philadelphia: WB Saunders.

67. Vander, A.J., et al. (1980). *Human physiology, the mechanisms of body function* (3rd ed.). New York: McGraw-Hill.

68. Wachtel, S.S., et al. (1975). Possible role for H-Y antigen in the primary determination of sex. *Nature, 257*, 235.

69. Wartenberg, H. (1978). Human testicular development and the role of the mesonephros in the origin of a dual Sertoli cell system. *Andrologia, 10*, 1.

70. Whaley, L.F. (1974). *Understanding inherited disorders.* St. Louis: CV Mosby.

CHAPTER 2

The Prenatal Period and Placental Physiology

Overview Of Pregnancy
First Trimester
Second Trimester
Third Trimester
Conception
Ovarian Function
Sperm Transport
Fertilization
Cleavage and Zygote Transport
Clinical Implications Related to Conception
Donor Artificial Insemination
In Vitro Fertilization
Gamete Intrafallopian Transfer
Spontaneous Abortion and Recurrent Pregnancy
Loss
Embryonic And Fetal Development
Principles of Morphogenesis
Overview of Embryonic Development
Overview of Fetal Development
The Intrauterine Environment
**Clinical Implications Related to Embryonic and
Fetal Development**
Critical Periods of Development
Principles of Teratogenesis
The Placenta and Placental Physiology
Placental Development
Placental Structure
Placental Circulation
Placental Function

Umbilical Cord
Amnion and Chorion
Amniotic Fluid
Amniotic Fluid Volume and Turnover
Amniotic Fluid Production and Disposition
Composition of Amniotic Fluid
**Clinical Implications Related to Placental
Physiology**
Transfer of Substances Across the Placenta
Perinatal Pharmacology
Alterations in the Appearance of the Placenta
and Membranes
Placental Function and Postdate Gestation
Assessment of Fetal Status and Placental
Function
Alterations in Amniotic Fluid Volume
Abnormalities of the Cord and Placenta
Multiple Pregnancy
Monozygotic Twins
Dizygotic Twins
Placental Abnormalities in Multiple Gestation

The prenatal period encompasses the period from conception to birth. During this period the pregnant woman experiences major physiologic and psychological changes that support maternal adaptations and fetal growth and development as well as prepare the mother for the birth process and transition to parenthood. Simultaneously the embryo and fetus are developing from a single cell to a complex organism. Supporting this development are the placenta, fetal membranes (amnion and chorion), and amniotic fluid. These structures protect and nourish the embryo and fetus and are essential for the infant's survival, growth, and development. Alterations in maternal physiology, endocrine function, embryonic and fetal development, or placental function and structure can lead to maternal disorders and fetal death, malformations, poor growth, or preterm birth. Assessment of placental size and function and amniotic fluid volume and composition is useful in evaluating fetal growth and health status during gestation. This chapter describes events that result in conception and provides an overview of pregnancy, related endocrinology, and development of the embryo, fetus, and placenta. Specific clinical implications related to normal and abnormal aspects of the development and functional status are discussed.

OVERVIEW OF PREGNANCY

The duration of pregnancy averages 266 days (38 weeks) post ovulation, or 280 days (40 weeks) after the first day of the last menstrual period. This equals 10 lunar months, or just over 9 calendar months. During these months, the almost solid uterus, with a cavity of 10 ml or less, develops into a large thin-walled organ. The total volume of the contents of the uterus is 5 L or more at term, 500 to 1000 times the original capacity.[224]

Most of the changes encountered during pregnancy are progressive and can be attributed to either hormonal responses or physical alterations secondary to fetal size. The preimplantation endocrine system controls the reproductive cycles in males and females. In the woman, this system is controlled by the cyclic release of pituitary gonadotropins and secretion of estrogen and progesterone by the ovary (see Chapter 1).

The pregnancy-specific or postimplantation endocrine system controls the integrity and duration of gestation. These processes include prolongation of the corpus luteum by human chorionic gonadotropin (hCG); production of estrogen, progesterone, and human placental lactogen (hPL) by the placenta; and release of oxytocin (by the posterior pituitary), prolactin (by the anterior pituitary), and relaxin (by the ovary, uterus, and placenta). Changes in specific organ systems and metabolic processes during pregnancy and clinical implications are described in detail in Units II and III. This section presents an overview of physiologic changes during each trimester of pregnancy. Concomitant with these adaptations and equally significant are psychological adaptations. These adaptations are not discussed since the focus of this text is on physiologic changes.

First Trimester

During the first trimester the woman experiences the first signs and symptoms of pregnancy. The first sign of pregnancy is usually cessation of menses. The average cycle length is 28 days, with a range of 15 to 45 days (see Chapter 1). The first missed period is suggestive of pregnancy; by the time the second period is missed, pregnancy becomes probable. Brief or scant bleeding may occur during pregnancy, most commonly in the first trimester around the time of implantation.

Breast tenderness and tingling, especially around the nipple area, may occur beginning at 4 to 6 weeks. Increased breast size and vascularity are usually evident by the end of the 2nd month and are due to growth of the secretory duct system. Colostrum leakage may occur by 3 months. Enlargement of the sebaceous glands around the nipple (Montgomery's glands) may also be apparent.

Nausea with or without vomiting may occur any time of the day or night. This symptom usually begins about 6 weeks after the onset of the last menstrual period and continues for 6 to 12 weeks or longer in some women. An increase in frequency of urination during the first trimester is related to the pressure exerted on the bladder by the growing uterus. This pressure subsides by about 12 weeks, as the uterus rises and enters the abdominal cavity. Excessive fatigue is often experienced and may last throughout the first 12 weeks. The cause of this fatigue is unknown, but it may be a response to hormonal shifts. Hormonal changes are also thought to be responsible for the dyspnea experienced during this period.

Physical signs associated with pregnancy include Goodell's sign (softening of the cervix and vagina with increased leukorrheal discharge), Hegar's sign (softening and increased compressibility of the lower uterine segment), and Chadwick's sign (bluish-purple discoloration of the vaginal mucosa, cervix, and vulva) by 8 weeks. Although a presumptive sign of pregnancy, Chadwick's sign is only useful in primiparous women.

By 8 to 10 weeks, fetal heart tones can be auscultated by Doppler ultrasonography. Real-time ultrasound can pick up fetal heart movements about 2 weeks earlier. Maternal cardiovascular changes are also occurring, with cardiac volume as well as cardiac output already beginning to increase. These changes contribute to increased renal plasma flow and glomerular filtration.[224] Weight gain during these 3 months is usually small.

Second Trimester

This trimester is characterized by marked maternal changes as the fetus' presence becomes more evident. The uterus, which started as a pear-shaped organ, is now ovoid, as length increases over width. With this growth, the uterus moves into the abdominal cavity and begins to displace the intestines. The tension and stretching of the broad ligament may lead to low, sharp painful sensations. Normally contractions during the second trimester are irregular and usually painless.

The increasing vascularity of the vagina and pelvic viscera may result in increased sensitivity and heightened arousal and sexual interest. Mucorrhea is not uncommon as a result of the hyperactivity of the vaginal glandular tissues. This change may increase the pleasure experienced during sexual intercourse. Spontaneous orgasm and multiple orgasm may occur owing to the increased congestion.

Leukorrhea often occurs, with thick, white, acidotic (pH, 3.5 to 6.0) discharge that may contribute to inhibition of pathogenic colonization of the vagina.[96] Perineal structures also enlarge as a result of the vasocongestion, increased vascularity, hypertrophy of the perineal body, and fat deposition that began during the first trimester.

The breasts become increasingly more nodular. Colostrum can be easily expressed now. The nipples are larger and more deeply pigmented. The areolae have also broadened. Increased skin pigmentation occurs elsewhere as well. The line from the symphysis to the pubis (linea alba) may darken very distinctly and is referred to as the linea nigra. Darkening of the skin over the forehead and cheeks (chloasma gravidarum) can also result from the hormonal changes. Deeper pigmentation changes seem to occur in women with darker complexions. Most pigmentation changes resolve following delivery.

Other cutaneous changes include the appearance of spider nevi and capillary hemangiomas. The former usually resolve, while the latter may shrink but often do not completely disappear after delivery. The breakdown of underlying connective tissue may result in reddish, irregular stretch marks on the abdomen, buttocks, thighs, or breasts. Although little can be done to prevent the formation of stretch marks, they may fade with time.

Increased estrogen levels may result in hyperemic, soft, swollen gums that bleed easily. Increased salivation also may occur. Good oral and dental care is important. Elevated progesterone levels decrease the motility of the gastrointestinal tract. By the end of the second trimester esophageal regurgitation may lead to heartburn. Fluid retention and constipation also may occur as pregnancy progresses.

Maternal blood volume rises significantly during these months and hematocrit and hemoglobin levels fall. Blood pressure decreases slightly, whereas the heart rate increases by 10 to 20 beats per minute. Cardiac output increases slowly from the first trimester. Some women present with a grade II systolic murmur.[224] Glomerular filtration rates increase over the second and third trimesters. Bladder tone is decreased, and the ureters have lost tone and are more tortuous, increasing the risk of urinary tract infection.

Protein and carbohydrate needs increase markedly, contributing to the weight gain during this phase. Fetal movement (quickening) is first perceived by the mother at 16 to 20 weeks (earlier in successive pregnancies). These movements become perceptible to a hand on the mother's abdomen toward the end of this period. By 20 weeks, the uterus will be at the level of the umbilicus (Fig. 2–1).[96]

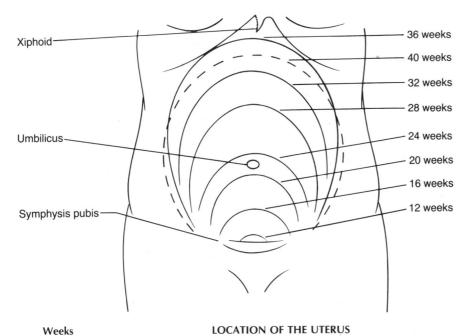

Weeks	LOCATION OF THE UTERUS
1–2	The uterus is a pelvic organ for the first 3 months of pregnancy, palpable on vaginal examination.
12th	The uterus fills the pelvic cavity. The fundus is felt level with or just above the upper margin of the symphysis pubis. The uterus is the size of a small grapefruit and feels globular and firm.
16th	The fundus is halfway between the symphysis pubis and the umbilicus and is ovoid in shape.
20th	The fundus is about 1–2 fingerbreadths below the umbilicus.
24th	The fundus is 1–2 fingerbreadths above the umbilicus and may rotate to the right; it feels less firm.
28th	The fundus is halfway between the umbilicus and the xiphoid, about 3 fingerbreadths above the umbilicus.
32nd	The fundus is ¾ the distance between the umbilicus and the xiphoid, or about 3 fingerbreadths below the xiphoid.
36th	The fundus is at or just below the xiphoid.
40th	The fundus drops several fingerbreadths, particularly in primigravidae.

FIGURE 2–1. Approximate height of the fundus during pregnancy. (Adapted from Carr, K.C. (1976). *Perinatal nurse clinician program. Maternal-fetal pathway syllabus*. Seattle: University of Washington.)

Third Trimester

Once again fatigue, dyspnea, and increased urinary frequency are experienced. Fatigue and dyspnea are related to the increased weight and pressure exerted by the greatly enlarged uterus. Thoracic breathing predominates. Increased urinary frequency is due to pressure of the presenting part against the bladder.

The uterine wall is thin (1.5 cm or less). The myometrium softens and is easily indented. The fetus can be easily palpated through the uterine wall, and fetal movements are quite visible. The uterus reaches almost to the liver, and broad ligament pain may become more intense as tension is increased. Uterine contractions become more regular and uncomfortable and are easily detected and palpable at 38 to 40 weeks.

The heart is displaced slightly to the left now owing to the increased pressure from the enlarged uterus. Blood pressure rises slightly, and cardiac output remains unchanged. Blood volume peaks at about 32 weeks. Dependent edema frequently occurs as blood return from the lower extremities is reduced. Increasing pelvic congestion, relaxation of the smooth muscle in the veins, and the increased pressure of the growing fetus lead to varicosities of the perineum and rectum. Constipation and obesity may lead to development of engorged blood vessels.[96, 224]

The intestines and stomach are displaced

by the growing uterus. The upper portion of the stomach may herniate, increasing the hiatus of the diaphragm. This produces heartburn and decreases the stomach's holding capacity. Renal blood flow is decreased. The bladder is pulled up and out of the true pelvis by the growing uterus. This stretches the urethra and increases the susceptibility to urinary tract infection.

The increased elasticity of connective and collagen tissue leads to relaxation and hypermobility of the pelvic joints. Separation of the symphysis pubis results in instability of the sacroiliac joint. The center of gravity has shifted lower with development of a progressive lordosis in order to compensate for the anterior shift of the uterus. Balance is maintained by an enhanced cervicodorsal curvature leading to difficulty in walking and the characteristic waddling gait. Stress on the ligaments and muscles of the middle and lower back and spine may lead to discomfort and back pain.[224]

Most women tolerate these changes without difficulty; however, many become tired of pregnancy late in gestation. The process of conception and the changes related to pregnancy are truly remarkable events. The coming together of all factors brings about the appropriate and necessary environment for the nurturance and development of the next generation.

CONCEPTION

In order for conception to occur, a precise set of sequential events must take place. The probability of a viable conception per menstrual cycle is only 0.3 at best.[57, 74, 211, 212] The process of conception and fetal survival is selective, as evidenced by implantation failures and the approximately 50% anomaly rate encountered in spontaneously aborted fetuses.[153] The menstrual and endometrial cycles necessary for conception and early support of the fertilized ovum are described in Chapter 1. This section will examine ovarian function, ovulation, sperm transport, fertilization, and cleavage and zygote transport.

Ovarian Function

The ovary combines two important functions: gametogenesis and steroid hormone synthesis. Integration of ovarian steroid synthesis, follicle maturation, ovulation, and corpus luteum function is essential for fertilization and implantation. Estrogen and progesterone have significant effects on tubal and uterine motility, endometrial proliferation, and the properties of the cervical mucus.[97]

The close proximity of the germ cells and steroid-producing cells in the ovary allows the ovary to control follicle maturation, ovulation, and corpus luteum formation, function, and regression. The hypothalamus and anterior pituitary regulate these morphologic changes through secretion of gonadotropin-releasing hormone (GnRH) and gonadotropins. Follicle stimulating hormone (FSH) and luteinizing hormone (LH) act synergistically. FSH is primarily responsible for stimulating follicular development; LH affects biosynthesis of steroids in the ovary (see Chapter 1).

The three hormones produced by the ovary in significant quantities are (1) estradiol (produced by the granulosa cells), (2) androstenedione (synthesized by the ovarian stroma and theca cells), and (3) progesterone (produced by the corpus luteum).[97] As the follicle grows and matures, the number of granulosa cells increases, as does production and secretion of estradiol. Local concentrations and balance between estrogen and androgen are probably important in determining whether a follicle matures or undergoes atresia.[123, 228, 234]

Estradiol has several activities that prepare the follicle for ovulation. Estradiol produced in the ovary induces formation of additional granulosa cell FSH receptors and stimulates further growth and replication of the granulosa cells. Development of these cells results in further increases in concentrations of estradiol in the antral fluid and in the serum. Induction of FSH and duplication of granulosa cells promote further follicular development. A cohort of developing follicles selectively undergoes rapid development with a single (dominant) follicle within the cohort maturing at a faster rate.

Follicle Maturation

Follicle maturation begins with the primary oocyte in the diplotene stage of its first meiotic division (see Chapter 1). This division was initiated in fetal life and the oocyte has remained dormant until now. Granulosa (follicular) cells surrounding the oocyte may secrete a substance ("oocyte maturation inhibitor") to keep this process arrested. The primordial follicles are covered by a single layer of granulosa cells. In order to become a primary follicle, several layers of granulosa cells must develop. This initial development can proceed without FSH stimulation.[179] Further development requires both gonadotropin and ovarian hormone stimulation. Follicle maturation takes about 14 days and is illustrated in Figure 2–2.

While the primary follicle is in the preantral stage, the oocyte enlarges and becomes surrounded by the zona pellucida, which is a thick, amorphous glycoprotein coating. The granulosa cells continue to duplicate and multiply, forming several layers around the oocyte. Theca cells develop from the surrounding stroma, forming several connective tissue layers (theca folliculi) that subsequently differentiate into the theca interna (similar to steroid-producing cells) and the theca externa (primarily connective tissue) (Fig. 2–2).

FSH interacts with receptors on the granulosa cells to stimulate both aromatization of the androgens produced in theca cells and production of estradiol. FSH also stimulates the granulosa cells to produce estradiol, creating a cyclic process of granulosa cell formation, FSH receptor formation, and further estradiol production. These processes favor maturation of the follicle to the preovulatory state. FSH stimulates LH receptor development on the granulosa cells, and the mid-cycle surge of LH provides enough hormone to react with these receptors. This interaction halts granulosa cell proliferation and initiates progesterone production.

As the oocyte increases in size and granulosa cells proliferate, fluid produced by the these cells accumulates, producing a space (antrum). The antral cavity enlarges and at mid-cycle is easily detected by ultrasonography. The oocyte is pushed to the side and surrounded by a mound of follicular cells (cumulus oophorus). The dominant follicle produces large quantities of estradiol, which enhance development of its granulosa cells and increase the number of FSH receptors so that further development can continue. At the same time, levels of circulating FSH are decreased through a feedback loop, which then stops the development of the other follicles within the cohort. The theca cells have become vascularized, allowing the dominant follicle increased access to the dwindling supply of FSH.

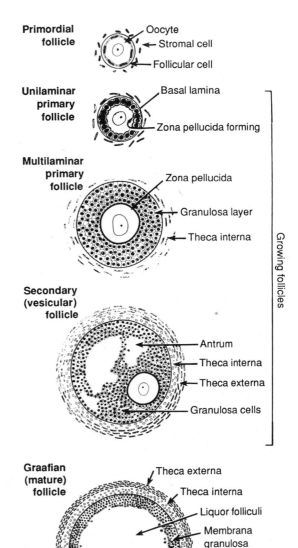

FIGURE 2–2. Follicle maturation. (From Junqueira, L.C., Carneiro, J., & Kelley, R.O. (1989). *Basic histology* (6th ed., p. 441). Norwalk, CT: Appleton & Lange.)

The oocyte completes its first meiotic division 36 to 48 hours prior to ovulation, forming the secondary oocyte (23 chromosomes plus most of the cell cytoplasm) and first polar body. The small polar body is nonfunctional and degenerates (see Chapter 1).

Ovulation

The fully developed preovulatory follicle is approximately 20 mm in diameter. There are multiple layers of granulosa cells lining the antral side of the basement membrane, and a cumulus of granulosa cells surrounds the oocyte. The oocyte is covered by the zona pellucida. The theca cells surrounding the follicle are fully vascularized. The follicle produces large amounts of estradiol; the level peaks about 24 hours prior to ovulation.[105]

LH levels are also rising, which increases production of progesterone by the dominant follicle through interaction of LH with LH receptors on granulosa cells. The rise in progesterone occurs 12 to 24 hours prior to ovulation and elicits a rapid and marked surge in LH secretion, paralleling the mid-cycle FSH peak.[172] This LH peak is essential for ovulation. The mid-cycle surge of LH initiates ovulation by stimulating prostaglandin (PGF and PGE) synthesis and initiating completion of the first meiotic division of the oocyte. The surge also causes a decrease in estradiol production. A rise in prostaglandin and production of proteolytic enzymes are also necessary for follicular rupture.

Ovulation begins with a protrusion or bulge on the ovarian wall. A small avascular spot (stigma) develops, forms a vesicle, and ruptures, extruding the secondary oocyte, follicular fluid, and cells. Rupture does not seem to be related to increased intrafollicular pressure but is thought to be caused by action of proteases such as collagenase and plasmin, which cause dissolution of connective tissues.[104] The oocyte is surrounded by the zona pellucida and corona radiata (radially arranged granulosa cells). The second meiotic division begins with ovulation, then stops and is not completed until fertilization. The oocyte is swept by the fimbriae into the fallopian tube. Muscular contraction of the tube and, primarily, beating of the cilia move the ovum along the tube to the ampulla (site of fertilization). If unfertilized, the ovum usually dies within 24 hours.[104]

Corpus Luteum

After ovulation the follicular walls and theca collapse inward and become vascularized. The granulosa cells undergo a luteinizing process to form the corpus luteum, which secretes progesterone and a small amount of estrogen (by theca cells). The luteinization process begins prior to ovulation and is dependent upon adequate levels of LH. Following ovulation this process continues in the theca interna and the remains of the granulosa cells. These cells grow rapidly for 2 to 3 days, followed by a vascularization stage. Secretion of estrogen and progesterone by the corpus luteum peaks 8 days after ovulation. The accumulation of lipids during this time makes the corpus luteum bright orange-yellow. If fertilization has taken place, implantation occurs during the latter part of this week. The implanted trophoblast secretes human chorionic gonadotropin (hCG), a luteotropin that stimulates the corpus luteum to continue to function and may alter the metabolism of the uterus to prevent the release of substances that result in luteal regression. If implantation does not occur, hCG is not produced, the corpus luteum begins to regress, and involution begins. The decline in steroids results in menstruation.

The corpus luteum is not essential for pregnancy maintenance once the placenta has developed the capacity to secrete estrogens and progesterone. The corpus luteum is probably essential for continuation of the pregnancy for the first 6 to 7 weeks.[226] From 6 to 10 weeks there is a transition period in which both the placenta and corpus luteum are producing hormones; by 7 weeks the placenta is capable of producing sufficient progesterone to maintain pregnancy.[46, 226] At 6 to 8 weeks, there is a dip in progesterone levels indicating a decline in corpus luteum functioning. This is followed by a secondary rise in progesterone (presumably due to placental takeover) without a rise in the metabolite 17α-hydroxyprogesterone (secreted by corpus luteum). Around 32 weeks there is a more gradual rise in this metabolite indicating placental utilization of fetal precursors.[46]

Sperm Transport

Spermatozoa have not completely differentiated when they are released into the lumen of the seminiferous tubules. They are nonmotile and incapable of fertilization. Sperm are moved down the seminiferous tubules and through the epididymis and vas deferens by the pressure of additional sperm forming behind them, seminal fluid, and peristaltic action. Maturation of the sperm occurs during their 9- to 14-day passage through the epididymis. Sperm are stored in the vas deferens and epididymis prior to ejaculation.

Ejaculation occurs through the urethra with contraction of the ampulla and the ejaculatory duct upon orgasm.

The volume of ejaculate ranges from 2 to 5 ml and contains 50 million to 100 million sperm/ml. Men with less than 20 million sperm/ml are likely to be sterile.[255] Some spermatozoa are immature, senescent, and abnormal, and generally only the normal and strongest sperm are able to complete the journey within the female reproductive tract to the upper end of the fallopian tube. Sperm become motile in the semen. Semen provides fructose for energy and an alkaline pH for protection against the acid environment of the vagina and dilutes the sperm to improve motility. The seminal fluid may also enhance motility by dilution of an epididymal inhibitory factor.[110]

The neck and midpiece of the spermatozoa contain a pair of centrioles, the base of the tail apparatus, and the mitochondrial sheath. The mitochondria are arranged in a tight helical spiral around the anterior portion of the flagellum (tail). Mitochondria supply the adenosine triphosphate (ATP) required for independent motility. Sperm must reach the ovum within an allotted time or exhaust their energy supply and die. Sperm survival in the uterus is relatively short, since phagocytosis by leukocytes begins within a few hours. Most sperm do not survive for more than 24–48 hours.[110]

Once deposited at the external cervical os, a percentage of the ejaculated sperm will cross the cervical mucus facilitated by a decrease in mucus viscosity at mid-cycle, allowing for more rapid migration. Within minutes the sperm enter the uterine cavity although some get caught in cervical crypts and endometrial glands. Sperm can reach the upper end of the fallopian tube (site of fertilization) as soon as 5 minutes after ejaculation, and most arrive in the ampulla within 1 to 6 hours. A gentle pumping action of the uterus may facilitate sperm transport. Uterine motility may be stimulated by prostaglandins in seminal fluid that cause smooth muscle contraction.[83, 110]

The sperm appear to be responsive to some chemical released by the ovum. This chemotactic substance diffuses outward in all directions, with the highest concentration at the surface of the ovum.[110] Thus sperm must respond to small changes in chemical concentrations within the female genital tract to "find" the ovum.

Fertilization

The process of fertilization takes 24 hours and begins with contact between the sperm and secondary oocyte and ends with fusion of the nuclei of the sperm and the ovum. Fertilization usually occurs in the upper third of the fallopian tube, usually in the ampulla. Prior to fertilization the sperm must undergo two final maturational changes: capacitation and the acrosome reaction. Capacitation involves removal of the glycoprotein coat and seminal plasma proteins from the plasma membrane over the acrosome (head of the sperm), which allows the acrosomal reaction to occur. Capacitation takes about 7 hours and usually occurs in the tubes but may begin while the sperm is still in the uterus. This process is stimulated by chemicals in the female genital tract and follicular fluid.[104, 191]

Of the millions of sperm in the ejaculate, only a few thousand enter the fallopian tubes, with only a few hundred reaching the vicinity of the ovum. Although it only takes one sperm to penetrate the ovum, it appears that several hundred are necessary to effect passage of the spermatozoa through the corona radiata to the ovum. The number of spermatozoa that are ejaculated does not appear to influence the number of sperm that enter the fallopian tubes unless very low counts occur.[83, 110]

In order for successful penetration of the corona radiata and zona pellucida to be accomplished, the acrosome reaction must occur with release of enzymes through small holes in the acrosomal membrane. These enzymes include hyaluronidase (for penetration of the corona radiata); a trypsin-like substance (for digestion of the zona pellucida); and sperm lysin, or zona lysin (for penetration of the zona pellucida).[191] Once a sperm has passed through the zona pellucida a zonal reaction occurs with physicochemical alterations in the zona pellucida that make it impenetrable to other sperm. The mechanisms behind this remain unclear.

The sperm head attaches to the surface of the oocyte, and their plasma membranes fuse. The head and tail of the sperm enter the oocyte, leaving the outer plasma membrane of the sperm attached to the outer membrane of the oocyte (Fig. 2–3). The mechanism by which penetration of the oocyte's membrane is accomplished is unknown. Cortical granules have been identified in the membrane in animal models immediately

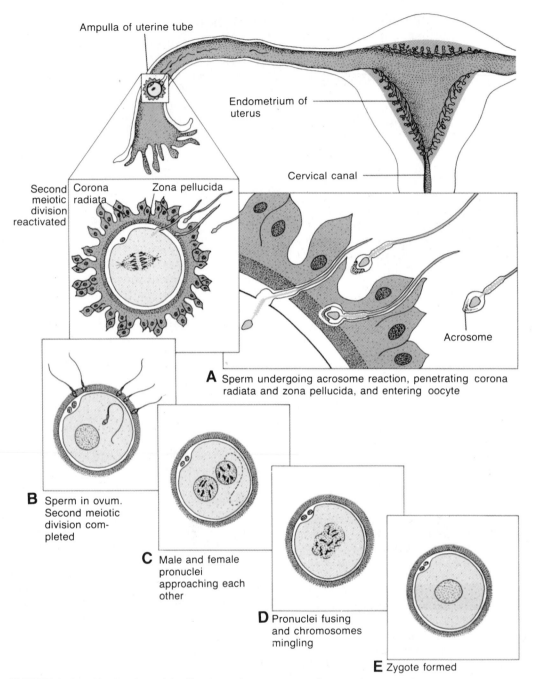

FIGURE 2–3. Mechanism of fertilization. The sequence of events begins with contact between a sperm and a secondary oocyte in the ampulla of the fallopian tube and ends with formation of a zygote. (From Moore, K.L. (1988). *Essentials of human embryology* (p. 3). Philadelphia: BC Decker.)

after ovulation. Granules remain evident until the membrane is penetrated. The contents of the granules are exuded by exocytosis into the space around the membrane and may prevent other sperm from entering the ovum.[19]

The oocyte reacts to sperm penetration by completing the second meiotic division of the ovum and extrusion of the second polar body into the perivitelline space. The nucleus enlarges and is called the female pronucleus. The oocyte is now mature and metabolically active. After entering the cytoplasm of the oocyte, the tail of the sperm degenerates and the head enlarges to form the male pronucleus. Each pronucleus has 23 chromosomes (22 autosomes and 1 sex chromosome). Sex of the offspring is determined by the male, depending on whether the sperm that enters the ovum contains an X or a Y chromosome.

The female and male pronuclei approach each other, their membranes disintegrate, and the nuclei fuse (Fig. 2–3). Chromatin strands intermingle, and the diploid number (46) of chromosomes is restored. The zygote (from the Greek meaning "yoked together") is complete, and mitotic division (cleavage) begins. The zygote measures 0.2 mm in diameter and carries the genetic material necessary to create a unique human being. Fertilization results in species variation, with half of the chromosomes coming from the mother and half from the father, mixing the genes each parent originally received from their parents.[19, 191]

Cleavage and Zygote Transport

Cleavage involves a series of rapid mitotic cell divisions that begins with the first mitotic division of the zygote and ends with formation of the blastocyst. The zygote divides into two daughter cells (blastomeres) about 30 hours after fertilization; each of these cells divides into two smaller cells, which also divide, and so forth (Fig. 2–4). The dividing cells are contained by the zona pellucida and become progressively smaller with each subsequent division, with no change in the total mass of the zygote. Cell division occurs about every 12 hours. By 3 to 4 days the zygote has divided into 8 to 16 blastomeres and is a solid cluster of cells called the morula.[46]

The zygote remains in the ampulla for the first 24 hours, then is propelled down the fallopian tube by ciliary action over the next few days. The zygote reaches the uterine cavity 3 to 4 days after fertilization (about 90 hours or 5 days after follicle rupture). As fluid from the uterine cavity (which provides nutrients for the organism) enters the morula, the blastocyst is formed. The blastocyst consists of four distinct components: (1) zona pellucida, a thick glycoprotein membrane that is beginning to stretch and thin; (2) trophoblast, a one-cell-thick outer layer of flattened cells that will form the placenta; (3) inner cell mass, a one- or two-cell-thick crescent-shaped cluster of cells that will form the embryo; and (4) fluid-filled blastocyst cavity.[191, 230] The zona pellucida protects the zygote from adhering to the mucosa of the fallopian tube and from recognition and rejection by the maternal immune system.[107] The blastocyst floats free in the uterine cavity from 90 to 150 hours after ovulation, then begins to implant (Fig. 2–5).

CLINICAL IMPLICATIONS RELATED TO CONCEPTION

Issues surrounding conception relate to the ability of couples to conceive and maintain pregnancies until the fetus can survive outside the uterus. Infertility (see Chapter 1) is the principal symptom of conception failure. Failure to conceive can result from disorders of ovulation, spermatogenesis, and gamete transport. Recent years have brought increased knowledge of these factors, with development of technologies such as artificial insemination, therapeutic donor insemination, ovulation induction, microsurgery, laser surgery, in vitro fertilization (IVF), gamete intrafallopian transfer (GIFT), zygote intrafallopian transfer (ZIFT), cryopreservation, frozen embryo transfer (FET), donation of eggs or preembryos, and surrogate mothering for couples having difficulty achieving conception. Three of the more common procedures (artificial insemination, IVF, and GIFT) are discussed in this section.

Donor Artificial Insemination

Artificial insemination with donor sperm has been used to treat infertility since the nineteenth century.[77] Currently, somewhere between 6000 and 10,000 couples or individuals avail themselves of this technique in order to achieve pregnancy. This therapy may be employed when azoospermia, oligospermia, decreased sperm motility, or other sperm abnormalities are present. When vasectomy is nonreversible or genetic disorders are possible, artificial insemination may be an option. Single women who desire a child may also opt to use this method in order to conceive.

Candidates for insemination must ovulate regularly or respond to ovulation-inducing drug therapy. Basal body temperatures are utilized to monitor ovulation and to time insemination attempts appropriately. Serial serum progesterone levels, cervical mucus

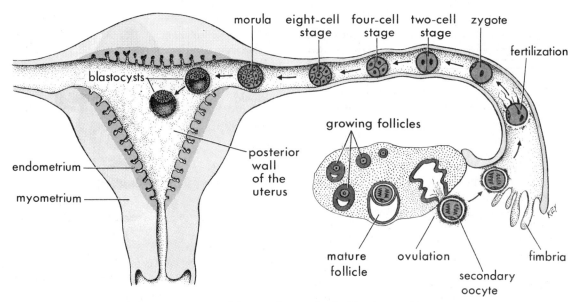

FIGURE 2–4.   Diagrammatic summary of the ovarian cycle, fertilization and human development during the 1st week. (From Moore, K.L. (1988). *The developing human* (4th ed., p. 35). Philadelphia: WB Saunders.)

changes, serial ultrasound, or the presence of luteinizing hormone in urine or blood may also be utilized in determining the right time for insemination. The techniques currently used include deposition of sperm into the upper vagina at the cervical os, or inside the cervical canal, or directly into the uterus.[87]

The donor is matched to the couple phenotypically and by blood type. Reported success rates are 5 to 20% per month with 70 to 90% of couples conceiving within 6 months.[18] Fresh or frozen semen is inserted one to two times per mid-cycle. Test samples are screened for infection prior to insemination. Fresh semen is rarely used, because of concern over sexually transmitted diseases and HIV infection.[176] Pregnancy outcomes are better than those in normal conception cycles even though cryopreservation impairs fertility to some extent.[229]

In Vitro Fertilization

In vitro fertilization literally means fertilization that takes place outside the body in test tubes or in a petri dish. The first infant conceived in this manner was a baby girl born in England in 1978.[87] Since that time, thousands of infants have been born utilizing this technique.[46] Originally in vitro fertilization (IVF) was developed for women with blocked or absent fallopian tubes. This continues to be the main reason for use of IVF, although

other indications include endometriosis unresponsive to conventional therapy, low sperm counts, immunologic disorders unresponsive to therapy, hostile cervical mucus or sperm antibodies, control of sex-linked disorders, and idiopathic infertility.[87] Women who are over 40 years of age have decreased success rates and increased spontaneous abortion rates.

The procedure is done in four stages: ovulation induction and monitoring, follicular aspiration, fertilization, and embryo transfer. The goal of ovulation induction is recruitment of a large number of follicles to increase the number of embryos that can be transferred and thus the percentage of successful pregnancies per IVF cycle.[253] Drugs given on day 2 or 3 of the menstrual cycle to induce maturation of more than one follicle include clomiphene citrate, FSH, GnRH, bromocriptine, menotropins (Pergonal or human menopausal gonadotropin), and hCG. The maturing ova are monitored by serial serum estradiol, ultrasound, and cervical mucus changes. Estradiol measurements are included because adequate ovary visualization may be difficult. Once adequate follicular size is achieved or preovulatory estradiol levels are appropriate, follicular aspiration can occur.[68, 246]

The woman is given hCG to enhance the final stages of follicular maturation and to control timing of ovulation, which occurs

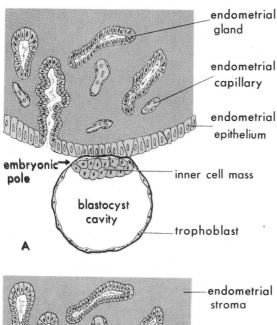

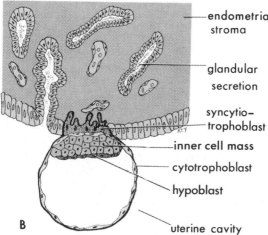

FIGURE 2–5. Early implantation of the blastocyst. *A,* Day 6; the trophoblast is attached to the endometrial epithelium at the embryonic pole of the blastocyst. *B,* Day 7; the syncytiotrophoblast has penetrated the epithelium and has started to invade the endometrial stroma (framework of connective tissue). (From Moore, K.L. (1988). *The developing human* (4th ed., p. 34). Philadelphia: WB Saunders.)

within 36 to 37 hours. Therefore oocytes are collected immediately prior to this time (usually 34 to 35 hours after the hCG injection). Collection is done by either laparoscopy or ultrasound-directed aspiration.

After follicle aspiration and processing of the semen sample from the father, the ova are identified, placed in a special nutrient culture medium and incubated at body temperature for 6 to 8 hours. Capacitated sperm are then mixed with the ova, and the mixture is incubated for 48 to 72 hours to allow for fertilization and adequate early cell divi-

sion.[46, 87] Approximately 50,000 to 200,000 sperm are needed, and at least 100,000 sperm per oocyte are preferred. If oligospermia exists, success rates can be increased if 500,000 sperm/ml are utilized for insemination purposes.[66]

Embryo transfer generally occurs when the zygote has reached a 2- to 8-cell stage (after 35 to 60 hours), with timing varying between different centers. The zygotes are injected via a catheter into the cervix. Up to four zygotes are transferred to increase the likelihood of pregnancy.[253] Bed rest is recommended following transfer. Progesterone by injection is begun on the day of transfer and is continued daily for 2 weeks to support the corpus luteum.[213] A serum β-hCG assay is done at 2 weeks to determine if implantation has occurred. Progesterone supplements are continued for up to 10 weeks if implantation has taken place. Unused zygotes may be frozen and stored.

Success rates of 10 to 35% are reported.[73,75,161] The risk of multiple pregnancy is increased owing to use of superovulatory agents and the transfer of multiple preembryos. The incidence of congenital anomalies does not appear to be higher. The cesarean section rate is higher in many centers, which has been attributed to the "premium" nature of these babies (i.e., the effort and expense the parents have invested in conceiving this infant) and malpresentation with multiple gestations. The higher rate of preterm labor that has also been reported is most likely due to the occurrence of multiple gestations.[46]

The emotional, physical, and financial stress is high in these families. At any phase in the cycle the process may need to be stopped, resulting in frustration and disappointment. The need for blood draws, ultrasound, and injections can require the woman to spend many hours in the clinic, which contributes to the stress. Each attempt at in vitro fertilization can cost as much as $8,000 (averaging $4,000 to $5,000), which many health insurance carriers do not pay; and the chance of an unsuccessful outcome is greater than the chance of a successful pregnancy.[87]

Gamete Intrafallopian Transfer

Gamete intrafallopian transfer (GIFT) was developed in 1984 and is the process of transferring eggs and sperm directly into the fallopian tube via a fine catheter.[13] This therapy was developed for use in infertile couples when there was doubt that the gametes would be able to reach the fallopian tubes or when male factor or idiopathic infertility existed.[46, 87] The woman must have at least one healthy patent fallopian tube in order to qualify for this treatment modality.

The three stages of this therapy include induction, oocyte retrieval, and gamete transfer to fallopian tubes. Ovarian induction is the same as in IVF. Oocyte retrieval is by laparotomy or transvaginally using ultrasonographic techniques. The ova are mixed with capacitated sperm, and the mixture is transferred to the fallopian tubes. During retrieval the four best eggs are found, and two are transferred to each tube. Fertilization takes place within the natural environment and successive events progress normally. Reported success rate vary from 15 to 40%.[14, 55] The cost is less than with IVF since embryo incubation is not needed, making GIFT a viable alternative to couples who meet the requirements.

Spontaneous Abortion and Recurrent Pregnancy Loss

Along with techniques designed to help infertile couples achieve conception, there are newer modalities and therapies that help fertile couples maintain pregnancy. For 1 in 200 to 400 couples pregnancy is achieved but not maintained.[18, 229] The definition of abortion is termination of pregnancy prior to 22 weeks' gestation or when the fetal weight is less than 500 g.[128] The true incidence of abortion is approximately 50% owing to the high loss rate that occurs in the early weeks following conception. The majority of these abortions are caused by chromosomal aberrations in the sperm or egg. When only spontaneous abortions (4 to 20 weeks) are considered, however, the rate is between 6.5 and 21% with the majority of authors agreeing on a 10 to 17% rate.[128] Sensitive assays for hCG suggest that 15 to 20% of pregnancies are lost between implantation and 6 weeks.[536] Early abortions are usually due to some type of fetal abnormality, while late pregnancy losses are associated with abnormal fetal development and maternal complications. Anomalies are more common in products of conception than in viable births, and are usually associated with chromosomal abnormalities.[37, 257]

Habitual (recurrent) abortion is characterized as three or more consecutive abortions conceived with the same partner. Primary habitual aborters are those women who have never carried a pregnancy beyond 16 weeks; secondary aborters have carried one or more pregnancies beyond 16 weeks. The habitual abortion rate is 0.3 to 0.5%.[128] Clinical studies have demonstrated that the risk of abortion after three consecutive abortions is 30 to 55%, depending on the cause.[220, 232, 274] The chance of a live birth following three abortions without a previous live birth is 40 to 50%. These odds improve to 70% if the couple has had at least one previous normal pregnancy.[178]

The reason for spontaneous abortion and habitual abortion varies. Possible causes include anatomic, genetic, endocrine, infectious, metabolic, male, immunologic, and systemic disease factors. About 15 to 56% of women with a history of habitual abortion present with one or more abnormalities, but in many cases the cause is not known. This can be extremely devastating to couples whose hopes rise with each pregnancy.

Approximately 12 to 15% of habitual abortions are related to uterine malformations. The most frequent cause of recurrent abortion is a septate uterus, with a 70 to 80% successful pregnancy rate after surgical repair.[273] Cervical abnormalities related to congenital factors or traumatic events may result in cervical incompetence and increased abortion rates. The rate of second trimester abortions increases after portio amputation or conization of the cervix (depending on the size of the cone).[128]

Genetic abnormalities are common causes of spontaneous abortion. Between 8 and 13% of couples with recurrent early losses have some genetic abnormality. The most frequent cause is a translocation (44%), with mosaicism, deletions, and inversions constituting the majority of other causes.[128, 236, 263, 273] Balanced translocations were found in 23 to 37% of couples with a history of abortion and fetal malformation (versus a usual rate of 0.4%).[47] Karyotyping should be considered for individuals with such a history, although this procedure does not uncover single gene defects or abnormalities of meiosis in sperm cells.

If the parents' karyotypes are abnormal, nothing can be done to lessen the chance of recurrent abortion. Known genetic abnormalities are associated with only a 32%

chance of achieving a successful pregnancy with a normal child.[178] Karyotyping of the aborted products of conception may also be possible. Aneuploidy and euploidy are associated with a high likelihood of subsequent abortions. Aneuploidy is often related to aging of the ovum or sperm. Treatment includes accurately timed or donor insemination.[255]

Endocrine abnormalities include inadequate secretory endometrium, low serum progesterone levels, and a luteal phase less than 11 days. Low progesterone levels may also be a sign of impending abortion. In 23 to 35% of women who experienced recurrent pregnancy failure, decreased serum progesterone levels during the luteal phase and an inadequate corpus luteum were reported. Treatment of endocrine abnormalities with progesterone yields a 90% chance of achieving a successful pregnancy.[178] Usually progesterone vaginal suppositories are used from a few days after ovulation until the placenta assumes hormone production.

Many infectious agents have been implicated in recurrent abortions; however, causal relationship has not been established. For example, women with recurrent abortions have a higher incidence of positive T-mycoplasma cultures and improved pregnancy rates after antimicrobial therapy.[125, 144, 257]

Oligozoospermia and teratozoospermia are found more often in men whose partners abort early.[15] The male factor is not confirmed in habitual abortions and needs further investigation.

Maternal systemic disorders such as diabetes and thyroid dysfunction have been sporadically reported as a cause of repeated abortion; however, current evidence does not support these disorders as factors in habitual abortion.[135] Some women with a history of habitual abortion have been found to have a subclinical autoimmune disease that is associated with fetal growth retardation and death during the second trimester.[220] Habitual abortion may be the result of an allograft reaction probably related to HLA (human lymphocyte antigens). The fetus has antigens from both parents. In an allograft reaction, the maternal immune system response to antigens on placental or fetal tissues is abnormal. In this situation, the mother's body does not recognize the presence of shared fetal antigens and therefore does not produce enhancing antibodies or suppressor cells necessary to maintain the pregnancy (see Chapter 10).[128, 178]

EMBRYONIC AND FETAL DEVELOPMENT

The infant develops progressively from the single cell fertilized egg to a highly complex multicellular organism. The genetic constitution of the individual is established at the time of fertilization. During development of the embryo and fetus genetic information is unfolded to control morphologic development. Alterations in the genetic information or morphologic development can modify structure and function of cells and organs and result in congenital defects. This section provides an overview of embryonic and fetal development including discussion of basic principles of morphogenesis and implications for the pathogenesis of developmental defects. Principles of genetics are discussed in Chapter 1; development of specific body systems is described in Units II and III.

Principles of Morphogenesis

Embryonic development combines growth, differentiation, and organization of cellular components at all levels. As development progresses, differential synthesis is established, resulting in cellular differentiation. Growth is the process of creating more of a substance that is already present through increase in cell size and number. In contrast, differentiation is the creation of new types of substances, cells, tissues, and organs that were not previously present. Organization is the process by which these elements are coordinated into functional integrated units. Morphogenesis is the production of a special form, shape, or structure of a cell or group of cells and occurs by the precise organization of cell populations into distinct organs.[106]

The human embryo's progression through stages of development is shared by many other creatures (phylogenetic recapitulation). As a result animal models can be useful in understanding developmental processes and deviations in humans. Development and maturation generally proceed in a cephalocaudal direction. Morphogenesis is accomplished by a variety of mechanisms.

Cell Differentiation

Initially all cells are similar and unspecialized. All cells must pass through two phases in order to become specialized. In the first phase (determination) the cell becomes restricted in its developmental capabilities and loses the ability to develop in alternative ways. Cell determination occurs for the first time in the blastocyst, with formation of the inner cell mass (which forms the embryo) and trophoblast (which becomes the placenta). In the second phase (differentiation) cells develop distinctive morphologic and functional characteristics. Differentiation seems to be regulated by interactions between cell populations.[30]

Induction

Induction is the process by which cells in one part of the embryo influence cells around them to develop in a specific way. Induction requires two types of tissue: (1) inductors, or cells that stimulate reactions in surrounding cells (probably via release of chemical or protein substances called evocators), and (2) induced tissue, which is made up of cells that have the capacity or competence to respond to the evocators. At some point inductors and inducers lose their ability to perform these actions.[111]

Secondary induction is a chain of developmental events and is a common way many parts of the embryo are formed. For example, in the nervous system the notochord is a primary inductor or organizer for brain development. The forebrain reacts to secondary inductors in the mesoderm to form the optic cup, which then induces adjacent ectoderm to form the eye lens. The eye lens then induces epidermis around it to form the corneal epithelium. If any of these steps is interfered with, the next stage in development may not occur or occur abnormally. If these alterations occur early in the developmental sequence, complete organ agenesis may result.[30, 111]

Differential Cell Proliferation

Differential cell proliferation results from localized differences in rates of cell division. These differences may lead to a buildup of cells in certain areas or result in a phenomenon called invagination in which cells growing more slowly than those around them appear to be "sinking" into tissues. In reality one set of cells is actually overtaking the other cells in growth. This phenomenon can be seen during the development of the neural groove, the oral cavity, and the nostrils. The rate of cell proliferation seems to be modulated by interactions at the surface of the cells or by systemic and local trophic factors that stimulate proliferation during organogenesis. A period of rapid cell proliferation often precedes differentiation.[30] Proliferation inhibition by teratogenic agents may cause defects. Growth inhibition can also be caused by lack of space (when space runs out, tissues stop proliferating). For example, with a diaphragmatic hernia the intestinal contents are in the thoracic cavity and inhibit lung development.[30, 111]

Programmed Cell Death

Cell death is a precisely timed event, possibly under genetic control, that occurs in many of the embryonic tissues as part of normal development. The process involves the release of lysosomal hydrolytic enzymes that dissolve cells, thereby altering the tissues. This mechanism is responsible for lumen formation in solid tubes (trachea and parts of the gut) and the disappearance of the webbing between the fingers and toes. If enzyme release is inhibited, syndactyly, some forms of bowel atresia, or imperforate anus may result. If enzyme activity is increased, micromelia (shortened limbs) may result.[29, 30]

Cell Size and Shape Changes

Cell size and shape changes occur with elongation or narrowing and swelling or shrinkage. Elongation or narrowing is accomplished by the coordinated activities of cell microfilaments and microtubules. Microtubules contain tubulin, a substance that alters its length when polymerized (i.e., joined together to form a molecule of higher molecular weight). Certain chemicals (including some found in microorganisms) inhibit tubulin polymerization and normal microfilament action. Changes in osmotic balance or interference in transport of elements across the membranes results in swelling or shrinkage of cells.[30, 111]

Cell Migration

During development some cells move around in a fashion similar to that of an ameba. This process is dependent on microtubular and microfilament elongation and contraction. Migration involves the elongation of the leading edge of the cell, followed by adhesion of the cell to a new contact point. Contraction of the cell towards the new adhesion site results in movement of the cell. Alterations or interference with the enzyme system may limit cell migration and result in a defect. Hirschsprung's disease (absence of intestinal ganglion cells) results from failure of neural crest cells to migrate. From 3 to 6 months' gestation there is normally migration of millions of cells within the central nervous system from their point of origin in the periventricular area to their eventual loci in the cerebrum and cerebellum. Alterations in this migration can result in defects in CNS organization and function.[30, 111, 235]

Cell Recognition and Adhesion

This mechanism involves the adhesion of certain cells, such as the neural folds, which meet and fuse to form the neural tube. The recognition and adhesion process involves interaction of specific substrates such as glycoproteins, or cell surface enzymes, on one cell with complementary substrates or enzymes on the membrane of another cell. A similar mechanism is seen with adhesion during cell migration. Interference with cellular membrane substrates may prevent adhesion. This mechanism may be responsible for cleft palate or neural tube defects.[30, 235]

Folding of the Embryo

The embryo begins as a straight line of cells. As new cells form, the embryo is forced to conform to available space. To adapt to the confined space, the embryo folds (curves) in both transverse and longitudinal planes. Folding in the transverse plane causes the embryo to become cylindrical in shape; longitudinal folding results in the head and tail folds. Structures within the embryo also undergo folding to conform to the space available to them. Examples are seen in the heart and intestines.[191, 235]

Differential Maturity

Various tissues and organs are at different stages of maturity throughout development. For example, the gut and bladder are essentially structurally complete at birth, whereas the long bones and lung alveoli do not reach maturity for years after birth. Therefore various organs are more or less vulnerable to insults and toxic agents at different stages of development.

Overview of Embryonic Development[191]

Preembryonic development occurs from the time of conception and zygote formation until 2 weeks' gestation. By the time of implantation the inner cell mass consists of 12 to 15 cells. At about 7 days the first of three germ cell layers that give rise to the embryo, the hypoblast or primitive endoderm, appears. During the 2nd week, the bilaminar embryo develops as the inner cell mass differentiates to form the epiblast along the inner part of the amniotic cavity.

The developing organism appears as a flat disc with a connecting stalk that will become the umbilical cord. During this week cytotrophoblast cells form an exocoelomic membrane around the inner wall of the blastocyst cavity to form the primitive yolk sac (Fig. 2–6). Connective tissue (extraembryonic mesoderm) fills in the space between the cytotrophoblast cells and the exocoelomic membrane. Near the end of the 2nd week, cavities appear in the extraembryonic mesoderm and fuse to form the extraembryonic coelom. A secondary yolk sac (Fig. 2–6) develops from the primary sac (which gradually disintegrates). This yolk sac provides for early nutrition of the embryo and is eventually incorporated into the primitive gut. An endodermal cell thickening (prochordal plate) appears at one end of the disc and is the future site of the mouth and cranial region.[191]

The embryonic period lasts from 2 weeks postfertilization until the end of the 8th week. This period is the time of organogenesis. Table 2–1 and Fig. 2–7 summarize major stages in development of specific organ systems. Development of specific organ systems is described in detail in Unit II. This section provides on overview of major events during embryogenesis.

The 3rd week coincides with the first missed menstrual period. During the 3rd week, growth becomes more rapid, with development of the mesoderm and establishment of the trilaminar embryo; formation of the neural tube (CNS), somites (bones and

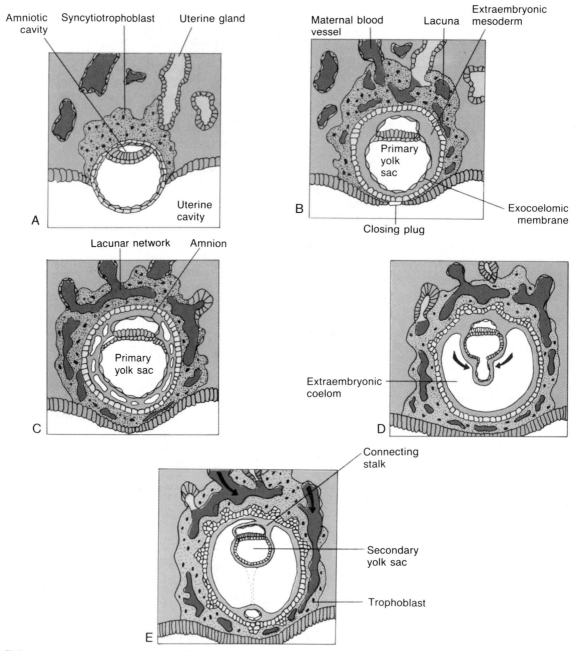

FIGURE 2–6. Formation of the yolk sac and lacunar network. *A,* 8 days; *B,* 10 days; *C,* 12 days; *D* and *E,* 2nd week. (From Moore, K.L. (1988). *Essentials of human embryology* (pp. 11, 13). Philadelphia: BC Decker.)

other supporting structures), and coelom (body cavities); and development of a primitive cardiovascular system.[191]

The primitive streak (thick band of epiblast cells) appears at 15 days in the midline of the dorsal aspect of the embryonic disc. Cells in the primitive streak migrate between the endoderm and ectoderm to form the mesoderm; the epiblast layer becomes the ectoderm, establishing the trilaminar embryo. Cells from the mesoderm later migrate out into the embryonic body to become mesenchyme and form supporting tissues.[191]

The ectoderm layer will eventually form

TABLE 2–1
Timetable of Human Development

AGE (Days)	SIZE (mm)	GENERAL BODY FORM	AGE (Days)	SIZE (mm)	RESPIRATORY SYSTEM
1	0.100	Zygote	27	3.3	Lung primordia appear
5	0.125	Blastocyst	35	5.0	Primary and lobar bronchi formed
18	1.5	Neural plate	49	20.0	Segmental bronchi develop
26	3.0	Closure of anterior neuropore Arms buds appear	180	230.0	Alveolar ducts form
28	3.5	Closure of posterior neuropore Leg buds appear			
35	6.0	Tail regression			
38	8.0	Hand plate Umbilical hernia			
56	25.0	Facial clefts closed Eyelids formed			
70	45.0	Intestines return to abdomen Eyelids fused			
196	240.0	Eyelids open			

AGE	SIZE	NERVOUS SYSTEM	AGE	SIZE	GENITOURINARY SYSTEM
18	1.5	Neural plate and groove develop	24	2.5	Pronephros primordium
24	3.0	Optic vesicles appear	28	4.0	Differentiation of mesonephros and mesonephric ducts
26	3.0	Anterior neuropore closed	35	6.0	Primordium of kidney pelvis and differentiation of metanephros Bulging of genital ridge
27	3.3	Posterior neuropore closed Ventral horn cells appear	42	13.0	Division of cloaca Separation of bladder and urachus Primordium of gonad present External genitalia indifferent
31	4.3	Anterior and posterior nerve roots appear	49	20.0	Müllerian duct primordium Degeneration of wolffian duct in female Gonadal tissue differentiating
35	5.0	Five cerebral vesicles Choroid plexuses appear Dorsal root ganglia present	56	26.0	Body of uterus and cervix complete Testis and ovary distinct
42	13.0	Primordium of cerebellum evident	100	125.0	Primary follicles evident in ovaries
56	25.0	Differentiation of cerebral cortex Meninges distinct			
150	225.0	Five fissures in cerebral cortex Spinal cord ends at L_3			
180	230.0	Myelinization increases			

Table continued on following page

TABLE 2–1
Timetable of Human Development *Continued*

AGE	SIZE	CARDIOVASCULAR SYSTEM	AGE	SIZE	SENSE ORGANS
18	1.5	Cardiogenic plate present	24	3.0	Optic vesicle present Auditory placode visible
23	3.0	Primitive vascular system Heart tubes fuse First aortic arch appears	28	3.5	Lens primordium evident Otocyst cut off Olfactory placode present
30	4.5	Septum primum develops Aortic arches present	35	5.0	Lens vesicle separated Olfactory pits present
38	8.0	Septum secundum and interentricular septum appear Absorption of bulbus cordis	42	13.0	Hyaloid artery identifiable Retinal pigmentation present Pinnae forming
42	13.0	Ductus venosus visible Division of truncus arteriosus	49	20.0	Lens solid Eyelids appear Semicircular canals present Cochlear duct
49	20.0	Interatrial septum complete Interventricular septum complete Superior vena cava appears Inferior vena cava appears Pulmonary vein absorption	70	45.0	Eyelids fused
56	25.0	Sinus venosus absorbed Definitive plan of main blood vessels	196	240.0	Eyelids open

AGE	SIZE	DIGESTIVE SYSTEM	AGE	SIZE	SKELETAL SYSTEM
22	2.8	Formation of foregut and hindgut	22	2.0	Appearance of somites
25	3.0	Liver bud appears Rupture of buccopharyngeal membrane	28	4.0	Primordia of upper and lower limbs
28	4.0	Primordium of stomach visible Dorsal pancreas evident Cloaca present	35	5.0	Appearance of myotomes in limbs
35	5.0	Atrophy of tailgut Primordium of ventral pancreas and spleen evident	42	13.0	Subdivision of limbs occurs Finger rays in hand plate evident Cartilaginous models appear
38	8.0	Herniation of intestines Division of cloaca	49	20.0	Primary centers of ossification begin to appear
49	20.0	Rectum and bladder separated Anal membrane ruptured Duodenum occluded Lumen in gallbladder Pancreas fused	56	26.0	Palatal processes grow medially Digits of upper and lower limbs clearly separated
56	25.0	Duodenum recanalized	63	35.0	Fusion of palate completed
63	50.0	Intestines return to abdomen			

the central and peripheral nervous systems, epidermis, hair, nails, inner ear, epithelium of the sensory organs, nasal cavity and mouth, salivary glands, and mucous membranes. The middle mesoderm layer develops into the dermis, muscle, connective tissue, skeleton (tendon, bones, cartilage), circulatory and lymphatic systems, kidneys, gonads, and the lining of the pericardial, pleural, and peritoneal cavities. The endoderm forms the epithelium of the digestive, respiratory, and urinary tracts as well as the thyroid and parathyroid.[191]

Development is in a cranial to caudal direction, with the embryo initially being a pear shaped disc with a broad cephalic end and a narrow caudal end. The primitive streak elongates cranially to form a midline rod of cells or notochord. The notochord extends to the prochordal plate, where the endoderm and ectoderm fuse into the oropharyngeal membrane. Other cells from the primitive streak migrate around the notochord and prochordal plate to form a cardiogenic area where the heart will develop. At the caudal end the endoderm and ectoderm fuse into the cloacal membrane.

The ectoderm over the notochord thickens to form the neural plate, which will eventually form the neural tube, which gives rise to the brain and spinal cord. The mesoderm on either side of the notochord thicken to form two long columns that divide into paired cuboidal bodies (somites). Somites give rise to the skeleton and its associated musculature and much of the dermis. Somite development is used to distinguish the stage of development. The foregut and body cavities begin to develop. Mesoderm cells aggregate in the cardiogenic area at 18 to 19 days to form two endocardial tubes, which fuse by 19 to 20 days. Primitive blood cells and vessels develop in the yolk sac, chorion, and embryo, and by 21 days' gestation they link with heart tubes to form a primitive cardiovascular system.

The 4th week is a time of body building. The embryo becomes cylindrical and begins to assume a C-shape owing to transverse and longitudinal folding. The neural tube fuses during days 21 to 28. The cranial area enlarges and develops cephalic and cervical flexure, with the head oriented in the characteristic flexed position. The heart is prominent and begins beating at 22 days. Small swellings become visible on the lateral body walls at 26 (arm buds) and 28 (leg buds) days.

The branchial arches (from which the face, mandible, and pharynx will develop) become visible; however, facial structures are not distinct and human likeness is not clear yet. The embryo is now 2 to 5 cm long.[191]

As the embryonic period moves into the 5th week, the form develops a human-like appearance. Head growth is rapid owing to brain development. The embryo further flexes into the characteristic C-shape and the facial area comes into close approximation with the heart prominence. The forelimbs begin to develop, and paddle-shaped hand plates with digital ridges are visible. The heart chambers are forming, and five distinct areas in the brain are visible. The cranial nerves are present. Retinal pigment and the external ear begin to appear.

Limb differentiation continues in the 6th week; short webbed fingers develop, and toe rays form. The face is much more distinct, the jaws are visible, and the nares and upper lip are present. Heart development is almost complete, and circulation is well established. The liver is prominent and producing blood cells. The intestines enter the proximal portion of the umbilical cord.

The last 2 weeks of the embryonic period are a time of facial, organ system, and neuromuscular development. The head is rounded and more erect although still disproportionately large. The eyes are open, and the eyelids are developing. The eyelids fuse by the end of the 8th week and do not open again until week 25. The mouth, tongue, and palate are complete. The external ear is distinct, although it is still low on the head. The regions of the limbs are distinct, and elbow and wrist flexion are possible. Fingers are longer and the toes are differentiated. The feet have moved to the midline. The forearms gradually rise above the shoulder level, and the hands often cover the lower face. The abdomen is less protuberant, and the body is covered by thin skin.[191]

Neuromuscular development leads to movement, which can be seen on ultrasound although not felt. The gastrointestinal and genitourinary systems have separated, and the kidneys have achieved their basic structure. Although the internal genitalia have differentiated, the external genitalia have not. The rectal passage is complete, and the anal membrane is perforated, resulting in an open digestive system.

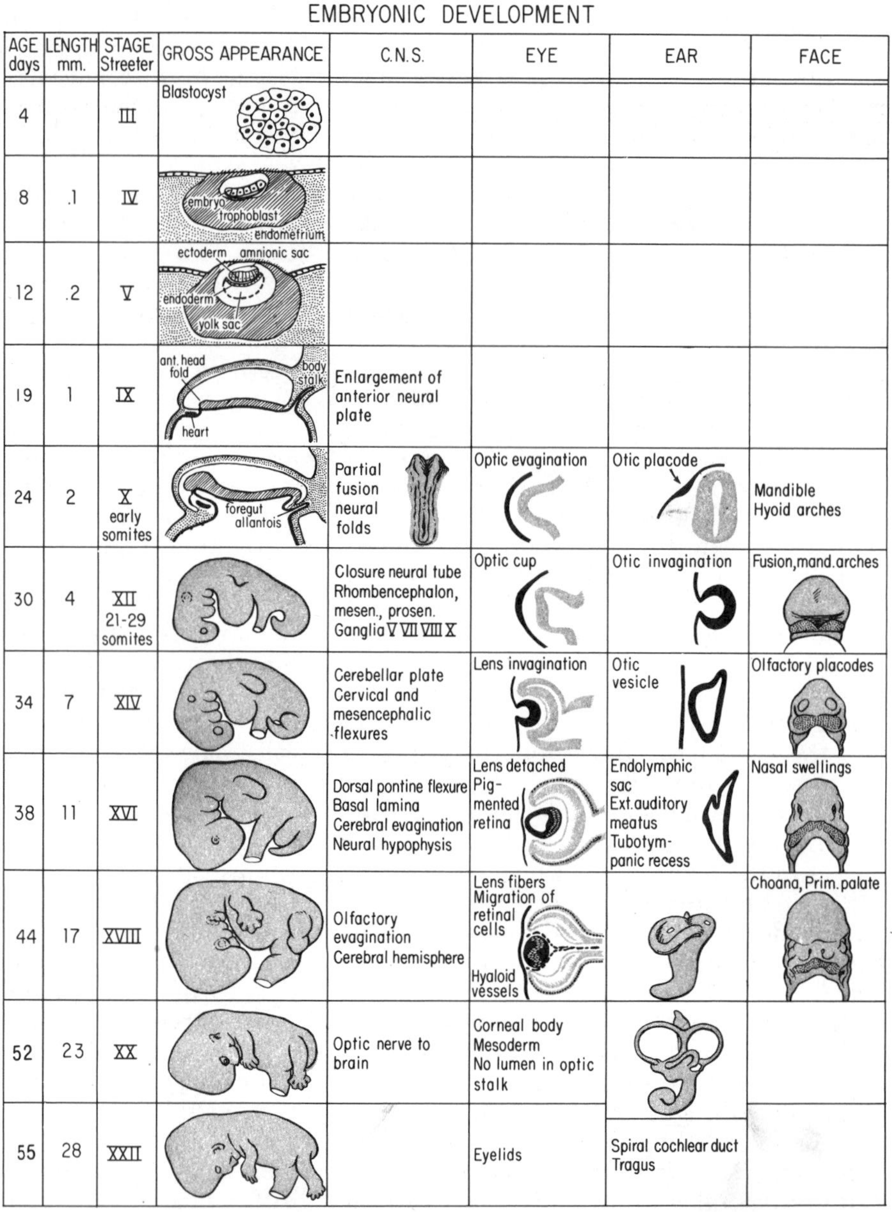

EMBRYONIC DEVELOPMENT

AGE days	LENGTH mm.	STAGE Streeter	GROSS APPEARANCE	C.N.S.	EYE	EAR	FACE
4		III	Blastocyst				
8	.1	IV	embryo, trophoblast, endometrium				
12	.2	V	ectoderm, amnionic sac, endoderm, yolk sac				
19	1	IX	ant. head fold, body stalk, heart	Enlargement of anterior neural plate			
24	2	X early somites	foregut, allantois	Partial fusion neural folds	Optic evagination	Otic placode	Mandible Hyoid arches
30	4	XII 21-29 somites		Closure neural tube Rhombencephalon, mesen., prosen. Ganglia V VII VIII X	Optic cup	Otic invagination	Fusion, mand. arches
34	7	XIV		Cerebellar plate Cervical and mesencephalic flexures	Lens invagination	Otic vesicle	Olfactory placodes
38	11	XVI		Dorsal pontine flexure Basal lamina Cerebral evagination Neural hypophysis	Lens detached Pigmented retina	Endolymphic sac Ext. auditory meatus Tubotympanic recess	Nasal swellings
44	17	XVIII		Olfactory evagination Cerebral hemisphere	Lens fibers Migration of retinal cells Hyaloid vessels		Choana, Prim. palate
52	23	XX		Optic nerve to brain	Corneal body Mesoderm No lumen in optic stalk		
55	28	XXII			Eyelids	Spiral cochlear duct Tragus	

FIGURE 2–7. Timetable of human embryonic and fetal development. (From Smith, D.W. (1988). *Recognizable patterns of human malformation* (4th ed., end plates). Philadelphia: WB Saunders.)

Overview of Fetal Development[191]

The fetal period extends from the end of the 8th week of gestation until term. All major systems and external features are established or have begun to develop. During the early fetal period (9 to 20 weeks) there is further differentiation of body structures with a gradual increase in functional ability. By 6 months the fetus has achieved 60% of its eventual length and 20% of its weight. During the late fetal period (20 weeks to term) further maturation of organ and body systems occurs along with a marked increase in weight. Organization is a prominent feature of this period.

During weeks 9 through 12 the embryo is 5 to 8 cm long and weighs 8 to 14 g. The head is half the body length. The body length doubles during these 3 weeks. Head growth slows down, the neck lengthens, and the chin is lifted off the chest. The face is broad with widely set eyes, fused lids, and low set ears. Teeth begin forming under the gums, and

EXTREMITIES	HEART	GUT, ABDOMEN	LUNG	UROGENITAL	OTHER
					Early blastocyst with inner cell mass and cavitation (58 cells) lying free within the uterine cavity.
					Implantation Trophoblast invasion Embryonic disc with endoblast and ectoblast
		Yolk sac			Early amnion sac Extraembryonic mesoblast, angioblast Chorionic gonadotropin
	Merging mesoblast anterior to pre-chordal plate	Stomatodeum Cloaca		Allantois	Primitive streak Hensen's node Notochord Prechordal plate Blood cells in yolk sac
	Single heart tube Propulsion 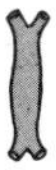	Foregut		Mesonephric ridge	Yolk sac larger than amnion sac
Arm bud 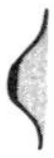	Ventric. outpouching Gelatinous reticulum 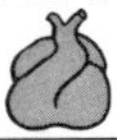	Rupture stomatodeum Evagination of thyroid, liver, and dorsal pancreas.	Lung bud 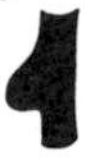	Mesonephric duct enters cloaca	Rathke's pouch Migration of myotomes from somites
Leg bud 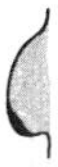	Auric. outpouching Septum primum 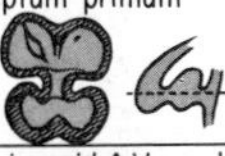	Pharyngeal pouches yield parathyroids, lat. thyroid, thymus Stomach broadens	Bronchi 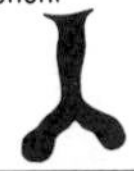	Ureteral evag. Urorect. sept. Germ cells Gonadal ridge Coelom, Epithelium 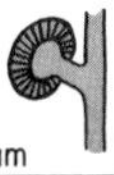	
Hand plate, Mesench. condens. Innervation 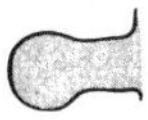	Fusion mid. A-V canal Muscular vent. sept. 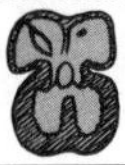	Intestinal loop into yolk stalk Cecum Gallbladder Hepatic ducts Spleen	Main lobes 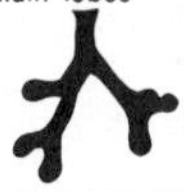	Paramesonephric duct Gonad ingrowth of coelomic epith. 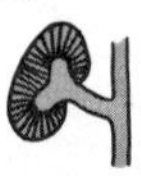	Adrenal cortex (from coelomic epithelium) invaded by sympathetic cells = medulla Jugular lymph sacs
Finger rays, Elbow 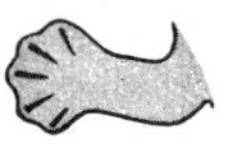	Aorta Pulmonary artery Valves Membrane ventricular septum	Duodenal lumen obliterated Cecum rotates right Appendix	Tracheal cartil. 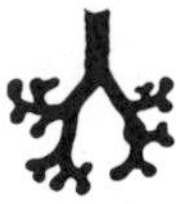	Fusion urorect. sept. Open urogen. memb., anus Epith. cords in testicle 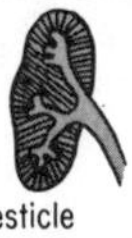	Early muscle
Clearing, central cartil. 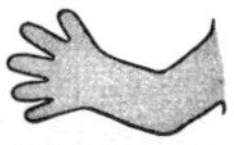	Septum secundum 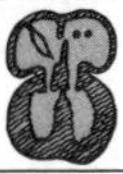			S-shaped-vesicles in in nephron blastema connect with collecting tubules from calyces	Superficial vascular plexus low on cranium
Shell, Tubular bone 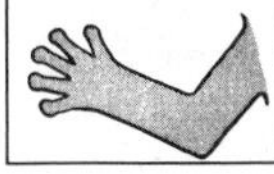				A few large glomeruli Short secretory tubules Tunica albuginea Testicle, interstitial cells	Superficial vascular plexus at vertex

FIGURE 2–7 *Continued*

the palate fuses. Fingernails become apparent, and the arms reach their final relative length.

Micturition and swallowing of amniotic fluid begin. The esophageal lumen forms, and the intestines reenter the abdominal cavity and assume their fixed positions. The bone marrow begins blood formation. The external genitalia differentiate, and by 12 weeks sexual determination is possible visually.

From 13 to 16 weeks rapid growth continues. The length of the embryo almost doubles during these weeks. The embryo weighs 20 g by the end of the 16th week. The eyes and ears have achieved more normal positions, giving the face a distinctively human look. Fetal skin is extremely thin, and lanugo is present. There is increased muscle and bone development, which along with establishment of neuromuscular connections results in increased fetal movements. Skeletal ossification continues and can be seen on x-ray film by 16 weeks. Brown fat deposition and meconium formation begin.

Growth slows slightly during the next month (17 to 20 weeks) and the legs reach their final relative positions. During this pe-

FETAL DEVELOPMENT

AGE weeks	LENGTH cm. C-R	LENGTH cm. Tot.	WT. gm.	GROSS APPEARANCE	CNS	EYE, EAR	FACE, MOUTH	CARDIO-VASCULAR	LUNG
7½	2.8			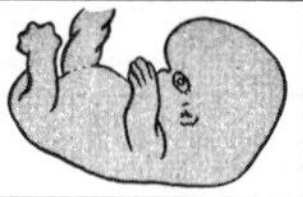	Cerebral hemisphere 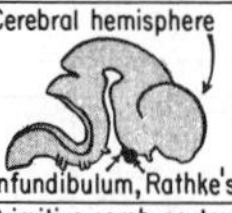 / Infundibulum, Rathke's	Lens nearing final shape	Palatal swellings 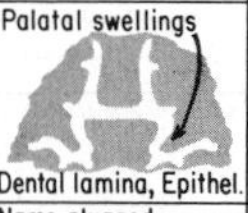 / Dental lamina, Epithel.	Pulmonary vein into left atrium	
8	3.7			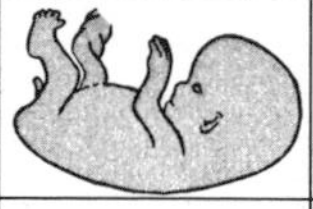	Primitive cereb. cortex 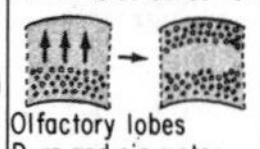 / Olfactory lobes / Dura and pia mater.	Eyelid / Ear canals	Nares plugged / Rathke's pouch detach. 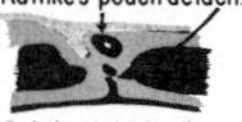 / Sublingual gland	A-V bundle / Sinus venosus absorbed into right auricle	Pleuroperitoneal canals close 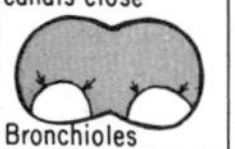 / Bronchioles
10	6.0				Spinal cord histology 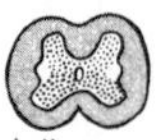 / Cerebellum	Iris / Ciliary body / Eyelids fuse / Lacrimal glands / Spiral gland different	Lips, Nasal cartilage / Palate 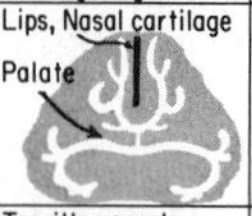		Laryngeal cavity reopened
12	8.8			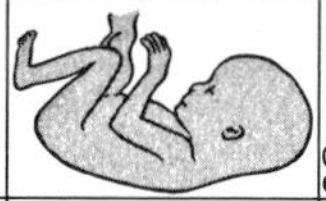	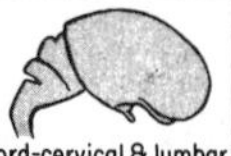 Cord-cervical & lumbar enlarged, Cauda equina	Retina layered / Eye axis forward / Scala tympani	Tonsillar crypts / Cheeks 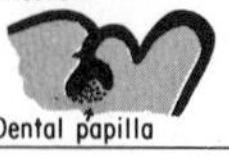 / Dental papilla	Accessory coats, blood vessels	Elastic fibers
16	14				Corpora quadrigemina / Cerebellum prominent / Myelination begins	Scala vestibuli 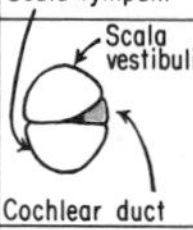 / Cochlear duct	Palate complete / Enamel and dentine	Cardiac muscle condensed	Segmentation of bronchi complete
20				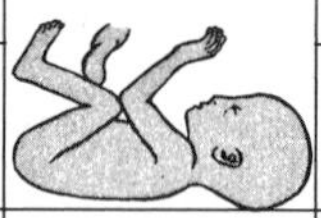		Inner ear ossified	Ossification of nose		Decrease in mesenchyme / Capillaries penetrate linings of tubules
24	32		800		Typical layers in cerebral cortex / Cauda equina at first sacral level		Nares reopen / Calcification of tooth primordia		Change from cuboidal to flattened epithelium / Alveoli
28	38.5		1100	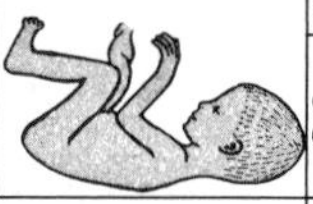	Cerebral fissures and convolutions	Eyelids reopen / Retinal layers complete / Perceive light			Vascular components adequate for respiration
32	43.5		1600	Accumulation of fat		Auricular cartilage	Taste sense		Number of alveoli still incomplete
36	47.5		2600						
38	50		3200		Cauda equina, at L-3 / Myelination within brain	Lacrimal duct canalized	Rudimentary frontal maxillary sinuses	Closure of: foramen ovale ductus arteriosus umbilical vessels ductus venosus	
First postnatal year +				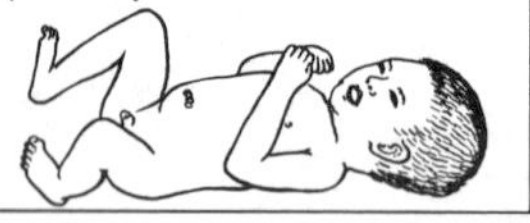	Continuing organization of axonal networks / Cerebrocortical function, motor coordination / Myelination continues until 2-3 years	Iris pigmented, 5 months / Mastoid air cells / Coordinate vision, 3-5 months / Maximal vision by 5 years	Salivary gland ducts become canalized / Teeth begin to erupt 5-7 months / Relatively rapid growth of mandible and nose	Relative hypertrophy left ventricle	Continue adding new alveoli

FIGURE 2–7 *Continued*

riod quickening is felt by the first-time mother (earlier with successive pregnancies). Fetal heart tones are now audible with a stethoscope. Myelinization of the spinal cord begins. Head hair, eyelashes, and eyebrows can be seen. The sebaceous glands are active, resulting in vernix caseosa deposition. Lung development continues as bronchial branching is completed and terminal air sacs begin to develop. The pulmonary capillary bed is forming in preparation for gas exchange. By 20 weeks the fetus weighs about 300 g and is 25 cm long.

After 20 weeks weight increases substantially. By 24 to 25 weeks the fetus weighs 650 to 780 g and is 30 cm long. The body is better proportioned. The skin is translucent, and subcutaneous fat has yet to be laid down. Fingerprint and footprint ridges are formed, and the eye is structurally complete.

During weeks 25 to 28 the gas exchange ability of the lungs improves so that extrauterine life can be sustained. Subcutaneous fat begins to form, and head hair and lanugo are well developed. The eyes open as the lids unfuse. CNS development allows initiation of

GUT	UROGENITAL	SKELETAL MUSCLE	SKELETON	SKIN	BLOOD, THYMUS LYMPH	ENDOCRINE
Pancreas, dorsal and ventral fusion	Renal vesicles 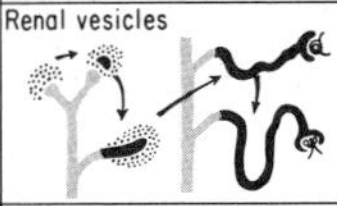	Differentiation toward final shape	Cartilaginous models of bones Chondrocranium Tail regression	Mammary gland 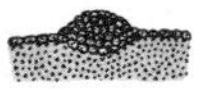		Parathyroid associated with thyroid Sympathetic neuroblasts invade adrenal
Liver relatively large Intestinal villi	Müllerian ducts fusing 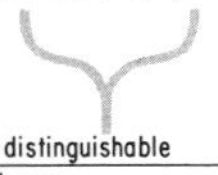 Ovary distinguishable	Muscles well represented Movement	Ossification center 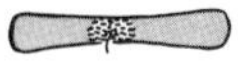 Sternum 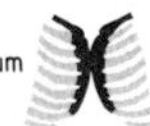	Basal layer 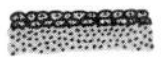	Bone marrow Thymus halves unite Lymphoblasts around the lymph sacs	Thyroid follicles
Gut withdrawal from cord Pancreatic alveoli Anal canal	Testosterone Renal excretion Bladder sac Müllerian tube into urogenital sinus Vaginal sacs, prostate	Perineal muscles	Joints 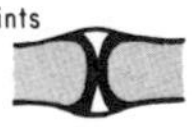	Hair follicles 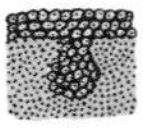 Melanocytes	Enucleated R.B.C.'s Thymus yields reticulum and corpuscles Thoracic duct Lymph nodes; axillary iliac	Adrenalin Noradrenalin
Gut muscle layers Pancreatic islets Bile	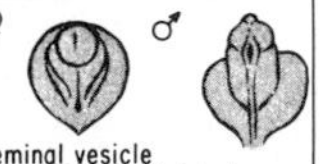 ♀ ♂ Seminal vesicle Regression, genital ducts		Tail degenerated Notochord degenerated	Corium, 3 layers Scalp, body hair Sebaceous glands Nails beginning	Blood principally from bone marrow Thymus-medullary and lymphoid	Testicle-Leydig cells Thyroid-colloid in follicle Anterior pituitary acidophilic granules Ovary-prim. follicles
Omentum fusing with transverse colon Mesoduodenum, asc. & desc. colon attach to body wall. Meconium. Gastric, intest. glands	Typical kidney Mesonephros involuting Uterus and vagina Primary follicles	In-utero movement can be detected	Distinct bones	Dermal ridges hands Sweat glands Keratinization		Anterior pituitary-basophilic granules
	No further collecting tubules			Venix caseosa Nail plates Mammary budding	Blood formation decreasing in liver	
						Testes-decrease in Leydig cells
						Testes descend
	Urine osmolarity continues to be relatively low			Eccrine sweat Lanugo hair prominent Nails to fingertips		
			Only a few secondary epiphyseal centers ossified in knee		Hemoglobin 17-18 gm Leukocytosis	
			Ossification of 2nd epiph. centers-hamate, capitate, proximal humerus, femur New ossif. 2nd epiph. centers till 10-12 yrs. Ossif. of epiphyses till 16-18 yrs.	New hair, gradual loss of lanugo hair	Transient (6 wk) erythroid hypoplasia Hemoglobin 11-12 gm 7S gamma globulin produced by 6 wks. Lymph nodes develop cortex, medulla	Transient estrinization Adrenal-regression of fetal zone Gonadotropin with feminization of ♀ 9-12 yr. (onset); masc. of ♂ 10-14 yr. (onset)

FIGURE 2–7 *Continued*

rhythmic breathing movements and partial temperature control. The testes begin to descend into the scrotum.

From 29 weeks to term fat and muscle tissue are laid down and skin thickness increases. Although the bones are fully formed, ossification is not complete. Vernix caseosa and lanugo begin to disappear as term gestation is approached and growth slows. The testes descend into the scrotum. The infant fills the uterine cavity and the extremities are flexed against the body. Myelinization progresses, and sleep-wake cycles are established. By 38 to 40 weeks fetal size averages 3000 to 3800 g and 45 to 50 cm.

The Intrauterine Environment

The uterine environment provides the ideal stimulation for the development and refining of the organ systems so that transition to and interaction with the extrauterine environment are possible. The amniotic fluid provides the space for the developing fetus to grow and protection from the external environment. Amniotic fluid cushions against external pressure, allowing pressure to the uterus to be transmitted from one side to the other with minimal exertion on the fetus. The weightless space allows for the symmetric development of the face and body. Adequate volume facilitates normal lung development and, until late gestation, exercise and neuromuscular development. The amniotic sac and uterine wall give the fetus something to push against during "practice" activities.

The maternal body provides the fetus with a darkened environment, which may become grayer as the uterus grows and stretches. Auditory stimuli are rich and include the sound of the maternal heart beat, peristalsis, and blood flow through the placenta. Most of these sounds are patterned and rhythmic. Extrauterine sounds, such as voices and music, are transmitted in a muted form to the fetus. The maternal system maintains a warm thermal environment. Kinesthetic and vestibular stimulation are provided by maternal movement and changes in position. Other less well defined patterns of stimulus that have a powerful impact on the activity and responses of the fetus and neonate include maternal biorhythms and diurnal, circadian, and sleep-wake cycles (see Chapter 12).

Exposure of the fetus to these stimuli and events provides appropriate experiences that enhance neurologic organization and establishment of synaptic connections. These activities are critical for successful transition to extrauterine life and establishing physiologic and social relationships necessary to assure survival.

CLINICAL IMPLICATIONS RELATED TO EMBRYONIC AND FETAL DEVELOPMENT

Growth and development in the uterus is usually a peaceful yet richly stimulating experience. Early on, the infant develops morphologic characteristics upon which functional and neurobehavioral characteristics develop later in gestation and after birth. Embryonic and fetal development can be altered by a variety of internal and external events and teratogens, which result in structural and functional defects. Fetal defects can result from malformation, deformation, or disruption. A malformation is an embryonic

alteration in morphogenesis (e.g., renal agenesis). Causes of human malformations are listed in Table 2–2. Deformation defects are the abnormal form, shape, or position of a body part arising from extrinsic mechanical forces (e.g., clubfoot due to fetal restraint), whereas a disruption is caused by an external force that alters a previously normal tissue (e.g., amputation of a fetal part by an amniotic band).[135, 188, 256] This section examines critical periods of development and events that can disrupt the usual course of development.

Critical Periods of Development

In 1921 Stockard documented critical moments in development during which congenital malformations were more likely to develop.[256a] The most likely period for structural defects to occur is during organogenesis, since exposure of the embryo to a teratogenic agent either during or before a critical stage in development of that organ can lead to malformation.[191, 274]

The time of greatest susceptibility during development is defined as the time when the highest incidence of defects occur (usually gross anatomic defects). Other defects, especially functional defects, have peaks in sensitivity at different times during development. These periods of sensitivity vary depending on the timing and duration of the period of cell proliferation (e.g., brain growth and development extend into early childhood and thus are vulnerable for a longer period of time).[191, 279]

Prior to conception damage can occur to the chromosomes of one or both parents, or they may have inherited defective genes from their parents. Alterations in spermatogenesis,

TABLE 2–2
Causes of Human Malformations

CAUSE		%
Known genetic transmission		20
Chromosomal anomalies		5
Environmental factors		10
Irradiation	<1%	
Infections (viral)	2–3%	
Maternal disorders	1–2%	
Drugs and chemicals	4–5%	
Multifactorial/unknown		65
Total		100

From Iams, J.D. & Rayburn, W.F. (1980). Drug use during pregnancy: Part 2, Drug effects on the fetus. *Perinatal Press, 4,* 131.

in seminal fluid or sperm transport in the male, or in oogenesis or the environment of the vagina, cervix, or uterus of the female may also alter development.

The preembryonic stage (up to 14 days) is a time of little morphologic differentiation. During the first part of this period the zygote is protected by the zona pellucida. Exposure to teratogens during this period usually has an all-or-nothing effect, i.e., either the damage is so severe that the zygote is aborted or there are no apparent effects. Teratogens or environmental disturbances may interfere with implantation of the blastocyst or cause death and early abortion. However, most congenital anomalies probably do not arise during this period, probably owing to the lack of differentiation. Most cells within the inner cell mass are not yet programmed to become specific structures. Thus, damage to a few cells does not alter development if the preembryo is able to produce sufficient cells to restore the volume.[279] If the teratogen is potent or the dosage is high, the effect is death or possibly mitotic dysjunction during cleavage, with chromosomal alterations that subsequently cause malformation syndromes rather than local defects. If only a few cells are damaged, development continues although the schedule programmed by genetic material may be delayed.[279]

The period of organogenesis (15 to 60 days after conception) is a period of extreme sensitivity to teratogens and the period when most congenital malformations develop. Insults early in this period (15 to 30 days) are likely to result in death if the embryo is damaged. Early events in organ formation are generally most sensitive to extraneous forces, although in some systems (e.g., the sensory organs) critical periods occur during relatively late stages. The more specialized the metabolic requirements of a group of cells, the more sensitive they are to deprivation and damage; therefore, they are more likely to experience malformation.[279]

From 11 weeks to term the fetus becomes increasingly resistant to damage from toxic agents. The ability to produce major structural deviations is reduced as organ systems become organized (see Fig. 2–7). Once the definitive form and relationships within a system are established, gross anatomic defects are no longer possible. However, the functional role of the organ system can still be altered.[191, 279] Histogenesis of most systems continues postnatally until complete maturation of that system is achieved. Therefore, defects can occur at the microscopic level, or functional abilities can be altered, resulting in physiologic defects and delayed growth. Insults during late fetal life and early infancy can lead to dysfunction such as brain damage or deafness, prematurity, growth retardation, stillbirth, infant death, or malignancy.

Principles of Teratogenesis

A teratogen is any substance, organism, physical agent, or deficiency state present during gestation that is capable of inducing abnormal postnatal structure or function (biochemical, physiologic, or behavioral) by interfering with normal embryonic and fetal development.[67] Six general principles that govern the action of teratogens have been identified:[67, 70, 278, 279]

1. *Susceptibility to a teratogenic agent is dependent upon the genotype of the embryo and the manner in which the agent interacts with environmental factors.* The genetic makeup of the developing embryo is the environmental programmer to which the teratogenic agent is introduced. This programming means that the genes and extrinsic factors interact in varying degrees with varied responses in different individuals and species. Since individual sensitivity is dependent upon the biochemical and morphologic makeup of that particular individual, data from animal models and sometimes even from studies on other individuals cannot always be applied.

2. *Susceptibility to teratogenic agents is dependent on the timing of the exposure and the developmental stage of the embryo.* A basic precept of biology is that the more immature an organism is the more susceptible that organism is to change. This suggests that there is a critical period where teratogenic events have the greatest impact. As discussed above, the period of greatest susceptibility is during the first trimester, when cell differentiation and organogenesis are occurring. Structural and functional maturation continue after birth, and therefore many systems remain susceptible to alterations in later development.

Malformations resulting from incomplete morphogenesis within an organ usually have their origin prior to the time organ structure is complete. The exact time at which a specific defect occurs cannot be determined; it can be said only that a defect occurred at some time *prior* to a particular point. For example, anencephaly must occur prior to closure of the anterior neural tube (25 to 26 days); meningomyelocele prior to closure of the posterior neural tube (27 to 28 days); cleft palate prior to fusion of the maxillary palatal shelves (10 weeks); cleft lip prior to closure of the lip (38 days); tracheoesophageal fistula prior to separation of the foregut into the trachea and primitive esophagus (30 days); ventricular septal defect prior to closure of the ventricular septum (6 weeks); diaphragmatic hernia prior to closure of the pleuroperitoneal canal (6 weeks); and omphalocele prior to or during return of the gut to the abdomen (10 to 10.5 weeks).[191]

3. *Teratogenic agents act in specific ways on cells or tissues to cause pathogenesis.* Unfavorable factors within the environment are able to trigger changes in developing cells that alters their subsequent development. These changes are not specific to the type of causative factor, and initial changes may result in a variety of alterations within the embryo. These early changes may not be discernible because they occur subcellularly at the molecular level. Pathogenesis is the visible sign of cellular damage and may occur from cell necrosis or by secondary interference with cellular interactions, i.e., induction, adhesion, and migration; reduced biosynthesis of macromolecules; or accumulation of foreign materials, fluids, or blood.

4. *The final manifestations of abnormal development are death, malformation, growth retardation, and functional disorders.* For the early embryo a teratogenic event will most likely result in death. Once organogenesis begins, teratogenic events lead to malformation in the organs or organ systems. The insult might also make the embryo more susceptible to death or general cell necrosis resulting in a reduced cell mass and slower overall rate of growth. Functional defects may be induced throughout infancy and childhood.

5. *Access to the embryo by environmental teratogens depends on the nature of the agent.* There are several routes by which agents reach the embryo or fetus. One route is an indirect method in which influencing agents such as ultrasound, ionizing radiation, and microwaves pass directly through maternal tissue without modification. Chemical agents or their metabolites reach developing tissues directly via transmission across the placenta. Whether they reach toxic or teratogenic concentrations depends on maternal dosage, rate

of absorption, and maternal homeostatic capabilities as well as physical properties of the agent and the placenta. Pathogenic organisms may also reach the fetus by ascending the vaginal canal and cervix.

6. *As the dosage increases, manifestations of deviant development increase.* There appears to be a threshold at which embryotoxicity occurs and damage is initiated. When the threshold of effect is exceeded, cell damage or death exceeds restoration. Different types of embryotoxicity exist for different thresholds. A given teratogenic effect may be induced by a variety of agents. For example, a specific defect may result from infection, drugs, genetic alteration, an environmental toxin, or a combination of these factors.[67, 70, 278, 279]

The proposed mechanisms of teratogenesis include

1. *Gene mutation.* Mutation is the basis of heritable developmental defects and is the result of a change in the sequence of nucleotides. If the change appears in the germinal cell line, it is likely to be heritable. A mutation in a somatic cell will be passed to daughter cells but cannot be transferred to the next generation.

2. *Chromosome breaks and nondisjunction.* These alterations lead to excesses, deficiencies, or rearrangements of chromosomes, chromatids, or their parts and can be transmitted to offspring.

3. *Mitotic interference.* Interference with mitosis can result from inhibition of DNA synthesis, prevention of spindle formation, or failure of chromosome separation.

4. *Altered nucleic acid integrity or function.* These alterations occur secondary to biochemical changes that interfere with nucleic acid replication, transcription, natural base incorporation, or RNA translation and protein synthesis. Since processes such as protein synthesis are essential for survival of the embryo, interference usually results in death rather than malformation.

5. *Lack of precursors, substrates, or coenzymes needed for biosynthesis.* These deficiencies result in slowed or altered growth and differentiation and occur because of dietary deficiencies, placental transfer failure, maternal absorption failure, or the presence of specific analogues or antagonists.

6. *Altered energy sources.* As a result of interference with energy pathways (glucose sources, glycolysis, citric acid cycle, terminal electron transport systems), the energy needs

of the rapidly proliferating and synthesizing tissues of the embryo are not met.

7. *Enzyme inhibitions.* Inhibition of critical enzymes interferes with cell functioning, cellular repair, differentiation, and growth.

8. *Osmolar imbalance.* These imbalances lead to pathogenesis by causing edema which impinges upon the embryo.

9. *Altered membrane characteristics.* These changes can result in abnormal membrane permeability and lead to osmolar imbalances and edema.[278, 279]

The ultimate result of any of these mechanisms is an organ with too few functioning cells. The cells needed for normal differentiation are lacking, thus disturbing development.[67] Table 2–3 explains the successive stages in the pathogenesis of a developmental defect.

THE PLACENTA AND PLACENTAL PHYSIOLOGY

The human placenta is a hemochorial villous organ that is essential for transfer of nutrients and gases from the mother to the fetus and for removal of fetal waste products. Alterations in placental development and function markedly influence fetal growth and development and the ability of the infant to survive in intrauterine and extrauterine environments.

Placental Development

Implantation

Implantation begins at about 150 hours after ovulation and involves three distinct processes:

1. loss of the zona pellucida ("hatching" of the blastocyst) 4 to 5 days after fertilization, followed by rapid proliferation of the trophoblast to form the trophoblast cell mass;
2. adherence of the blastocyst to the endometrial surface, which occurs in the early luteal phase of the menstrual cycle;
3. erosion of the epithelium of the endometrial surface, with burrowing of the blastocyst beneath the surface.[42, 86, 142]

By 5 to 6 days after fertilization (7 to 9 days after follicle rupture) the blastocyst rests on and adheres to the endometrium. The endometrium remains receptive to implantation for only a few days.[73] The mechanism by which the site of implantation is selected is unknown. The site is usually near a small capillary.[112] Prostaglandin metabolism increases with localized changes seen at the eventual site of the implantation beginning up to 24 hours prior to adherence of the

TABLE 2–3
Successive Stages in the Pathogenesis of a Developmental Defect

MECHANISMS	PATHOGENESIS	COMMON PATHWAYS	FINAL DEFECT
Initial types of changes in developing cells or tissues after teratogenic insult: Mutation (gene) Chromosomal breaks, nondisjunction, etc. Mitotic interference Altered nucleic acid integrity or function Lack of normal precursors, substrates, etc. Altered energy sources Changed membrane characteristics Osmolar imbalance Enzyme inhibition	Ultimately manifested as one or more types of abnormal embryogenesis: Excessive or reduced cell death Failed cell interactions Reduced biosynthesis Impeded morphogenetic movement Mechanical disruption of tissues	Too few cells or cell products to effect localized morphogenesis or functional maturation Other imbalances in growth and differentiation	

Beginning with the initial types of changes in developing cells or tissues (the mechanisms) and continuing to the final defect: One or more mechanisms are initiated by the teratogenic cause from the environment. This leads to changes in the developmental system which become manifested as abnormal embryogenesis. This in turn leads into pathways that are often characterized by too few cells or cell products to effect normal morphogenesis or functional maturation. The suggestion that this is a single or common pathway for all developmental defects is conjecture.

From Wilson, J.G. (1977). Current status of teratology: General principles and mechanisms derived from animal studies. In J.G. Wilson & F.C. Fraser (Eds.), *Handbook of teratology: General principles and etiology* (p. 55). New York: Plenum Press.

blastocyst to the endometrium.[46, 112] These changes may be influenced by signals from uterine proteins or enzymes mediated by ovarian steroid hormones.[46, 112, 113] The place of attachment is usually on the anterior or posterior wall of the upper part of the uterus but can occur at a variety of other intrauterine and extrauterine sites.

The blastocyst orients itself so that the embryonic pole containing the embryo-forming inner cell mass contacts the endometrial surface first. By day 6 or 7 trophoblast cells have begun to invade the endometrium. Finger-like projections of trophoblast cells protrude between the cells of the endometrial epithelium into the endometrial stroma.[86]

On the 7th day after fertilization, the trophoblast begins to differentiate into two layers: the inner cytotrophoblast and the outer syncytiotrophoblast layer.[86] The mononuclear cytotrophoblast is a mitotically active layer that forms new syncytial cells, the chorionic villi, and the amnion. The syncytiotrophoblast is a thick multinuclear mass, without distinct cell boundaries, which puts out finger-like projections that invade the endometrial epithelium, engulfing uterine cells (see Fig. 2–5).[16] Slight bleeding may occur during this process, which may be mistaken for a scanty, short menstrual period.

The trophoblast produces human chorionic gonadotropin (hCG), which maintains the corpus luteum during early pregnancy. The trophoblast is also thought to produce Schwangerschaftsprotein 1 (SP1), which appears to have an immunosuppressive function.[7] SP1 (also call PAPP-A, or pregnancy-associated plasma protein-A) and hCG appear in maternal blood 6 to 14 days after ovulation. These substances induce the histologic, hormonal, and immunologic changes necessary for implantation and continuation of the pregnancy and may be mechanisms through which the fetus' presence is signaled to the mother.[7]

Many ova that are fertilized never implant. Moore indicates that one third to one half of all zygotes never become blastocysts.[191] Hertig estimates that 70 to 75% of blastocysts implant and 51% of these survive to the 2nd week.[117] Sixteen percent of this latter group are later spontaneously aborted. Implantation can be electively inhibited by administration of low dose estrogen for several days following sexual intercourse ("morning-after" pill).[137] Estrogen preparations such as diethylstilbestrol act by altering the normal balance of estrogen and progesterone during the secretory phase of the endometrial cycle (see Chapter 1) making the endometrial lining unsuitable for implantation. Estrogen may also accelerate passage of the zygote along the fallopian tube so that it arrives in the uterus before the secretory phase of the endometrial cycle is established.[191]

Implantation is complete by 10 days after fertilization.[86] At 10 days the blastocyst lies beneath the endometrial surface and is covered by a blood clot and cellular debris. By 12 days the endometrial epithelium has regenerated in this area.[142] Although visualization of the gestational sac by ultrasound has been reported as early as 11 days after conception (25 days after the onset of the last menstrual period), visualization is more common at 5 to 6 weeks.[169]

ECTOPIC PREGNANCY

Extrauterine implantation results in an ectopic pregnancy and occurs in 1 in 80 to 250 pregnancies.[214] The incidence of ectopic pregnancy has tripled since 1970. It accounts for 10 to 11% of maternal mortality in the United States and is the most common cause of death in the first 20 weeks of pregnancy.[69, 130, 226] The increased incidence is thought to be due to the prevalence of sexually transmitted and pelvic inflammatory disease and possibly to the use of intrauterine devices.[130] The most common site for an ectopic pregnancy is the fallopian tubes. This probably results from delay in transport of the zygote from the site of fertilization to the uterine cavity. The delay is often due to tubal adhesions or mucosal damage from pelvic inflammatory disease (PID).[191] PID and salpingitis disrupt and damage the tubal mucosa, decreasing the number of cilia, which are essential for timely movement of the zygote along the tube. Alterations in the concentrations of progesterone, estrogen, and prostaglandins may also delay ovum transport.[56, 107, 130] If transport is delayed, the blastocyst emerges from the zona pellucida while in the fallopian tube and adheres to and implants in tubal mucosa.

Endometrium and Decidua

The uterine endometrial lining consists of an epithelial layer that contains ciliated and mucus secreting cells.[205] These cells penetrate into the endometrial stroma and may enter the underlying myometrium. The endometrium is divided into three functional zones. The deepest basalis layer lies adjacent to the myometrium. This layer responds to progesterone stimulus with secretory activity and provides the base for endometrial regeneration after menstrual sloughing. The two superficial layers of endometrium are the outer compacta and the middle spongiosa, which contains glands and blood vessels.

Early nutrition of the blastocyst is from digestion of substances in endometrial tissue and the capillaries that diffuse into the inner cell mass. Under stimulation of progesterone and estrogen the epithelium and stromal cells become progressively hypertrophic and develop subnuclear vacuoles rich in glycogen and lipids.[60, 142] These endometrial changes during pregnancy are known as the decidual reaction, and the altered endometrial lining is known as the decidua. In addition to its role in early nutrition of the embryo, the decidua may also protect the endometrium and myometrium from uncontrolled invasion by the trophoblast cell mass.[142]

The decidua is divided into three sections (Fig. 2–8). The decidua capsularis, just above the area of trophoblastic proliferation, initially covers the growing embryo. With development of the chorion, the decidua capsularis gradually disappears. The portion of the decidua on which the blastocyst rests forms a soft, spongy vascular bed known as the decidua basalis, site of the future placenta. The remaining portion is known as the decidua parietalis (or decidua vera).

With embryonic growth, the decidua basalis is progressively compressed. The glands and blood vessels become distorted and assume oblique and horizontal courses. The decidua basalis forms the maternal portion of the placenta and the stratum in which separation of the placenta will occur at delivery.[191, 224] As the embryo fills the lumen of the uterus, the decidua capsularis disappears. Eventually the chorion laeve and decidua parietalis meet and fuse, obliterating the uterine cavity (Fig. 2–8).[142]

Placentation

As the syncytiotrophoblast proliferates and invades the endometrial stroma, the blastocyst slowly sinks into the endometrium. The syncytiotrophoblast is thought to lack transplantation antigens and therefore is not rejected by the mother.[148, 191, 214] Erosion of maternal endometrial capillaries by the syncytiotrophoblast leads to development of intersyncytial spaces or lacunae (see Fig. 2–6) beginning 8 days after conception. At this stage the trophoblast has a sponge-like appearance. The lacunae fill with a nutritive substance containing maternal blood and glandular fluid that diffuses through the trophoblast to the embryo. Individual lacunae fuse into lacunar networks which will later develop into the intervillous spaces. Maternal blood flows into the lacunae via "controlled seepage"; there are no direct arterial openings into the lacunae.[142, 281] Endometrial capillaries around the implanted embryo become congested and dilated, forming sinusoids. As the trophoblast erodes these sinusoids, maternal blood seeps into the lacunar networks to form a primitive uteroplacental circulation 17 days after conception.[276]

DEVELOPMENT OF THE AMNIOTIC CAVITY

The amniotic cavity appears during the 2nd week as the blastocyst is burrowing into the endometrium. Small spaces appear between the inner cell mass and cytotrophoblast. By 8 days these spaces coalesce to form a narrow amniotic cavity that gradually enlarges to completely surround the fetus (Fig. 2–9).

The amniotic cavity develops a thin epithelial roof or lining. This lining is the amnion, which arises from amnioblasts (amniogenic cells) from the cytotrophoblast. The floor of the amniotic cavity is formed from the embryonic epiblast germ layer. Initially a small amount of fluid may be secreted by the amniotic epithelial cells, but the major early source of amniotic fluid is probably maternal serum. With advancing gestation, the epithelial cells of the amnion become more cuboidal or columnar and are covered with microvilli.[191]

DEVELOPMENT OF VILLI

Initially the lacunae are separated by trabecular columns of syncytial trophoblast (primary villous stems), which provide the framework for development of the villi. Chorionic villi begin to appear toward the end of the 2nd week as proliferation of the inner cytotrophoblast layer produces columns of cells or finger-like processes known as primary chorionic villi. A mesenchymal core grows within these columns. Blood vessels within the villi will later arise from this mesenchymal core.[63, 142]

As the columns of cytotrophoblast cells

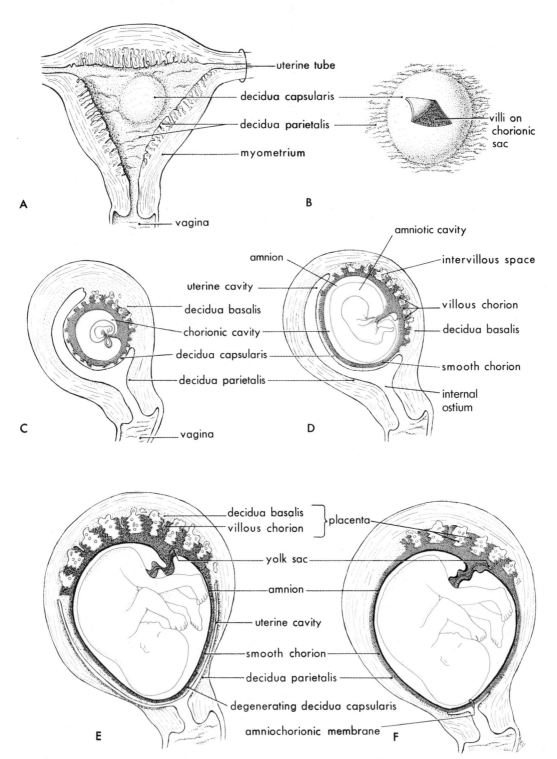

FIGURE 2–8. Changes in the decidual layers with growth of the embryo and fetus. *A,* Drawing of a frontal section of the uterus showing the elevation of the decidua capsularis caused by the expanding chorionic sac of a 4-week embryo, implanted in the endometrium on the posterior wall. *B,* Enlarged drawing of the implantation site. The chorionic villi have been exposed by cutting an opening in the decidua capsularis. *C* to *F,* Drawing of sagittal sections of the gravid uterus from the 5th to 22nd weeks, showing the changing relations of the fetal membranes to the decidua. In *F,* the amnion and chorion are fused with each other and the decidua parietalis, thereby obliterating the uterine cavity. Note in *D* to *F* that the chorionic villi persist only where the chorion is associated with the decidua basalis; here they form the villous chorion (fetal portion of the placenta). (From Moore, K.L. (1988). *The developing human.* (4th ed., p. 106). Philadelphia: WB Saunders.)

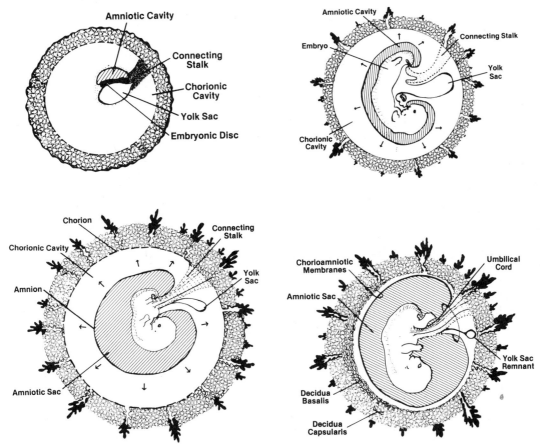

FIGURE 2–9. Formation of the amniotic cavity. (Reprinted from *The Human Placenta: Clinical Perspectives* by J. P. Lavery, p. 258, with permission of Aspen Publishers, Inc., © 1987.)

proliferate, they extend through the syncytiotrophoblast, expanding laterally to meet and fuse with adjoining cytotrophoblast columns. This forms the cytotrophoblastic shell and divides the syncytiotrophoblast into an inner layer and a peripheral layer. The peripheral layer degenerates and is replaced by fibrinoid material.[86, 142]

The cytotrophoblastic shell is the point of contact between the fetal tissue and maternal tissue and attaches the chorionic sac to the basal plate (Fig. 2–10). The basal plate is formed by the compact and spongy zones of the maternal decidua basalis, remnants of the trophoblast, and fibrinoid material. This shell is complete by 15 days after fertilization.[127] By the end of the 4th month the shell has regressed, with replacement of the cytotrophoblast cell columns by fibrinoid material (Rohr's layer) and formation of clumps (islands) of cytotrophoblast cells.[86] A layer of fibrinoid material (Nitabuch's layer) also de-

velops within the spongy zone of the decidua basalis. This is the level of placental separation at delivery (Fig. 2–11).[214]

Villi containing blood vessels arise by 18 to 21 days (Fig. 2–12).[7, 16] At 21 to 22 days a primitive fetoplacental circulation is established between blood in the villi, vessels forming in the embryo, primitive heart, and blood islands in the yolk sac. The villi that arise from the chorionic plate and attach to the maternal decidua basalis are known as anchoring or stem villi. Branch villi grow from the sides of stem villi and project into the intervillous space (Fig. 2–12). Branch villi, which constitute approximately 60% of the villi in the mature placenta, are the major area of exchange between maternal and fetal circulations.[60, 86]

Initially there are two divisions within the chorionic villi. The chorion laeve forms the chorion; the chorion frondosum forms the fetal portion of the placenta. At first villi

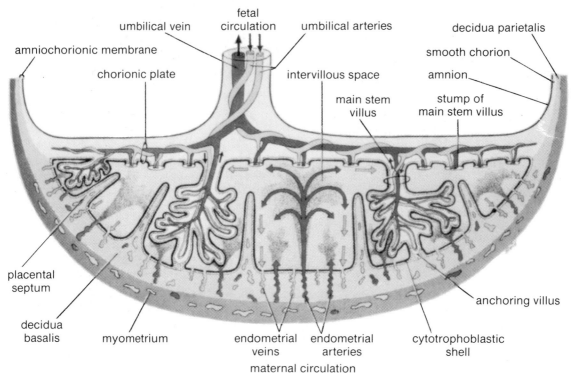

FIGURE 2–10. Placental structure and circulation at term. (From Moore, K.L. (1988). *The developing human* (4th ed., p. 109). Philadelphia: WB Saunders.)

cover the entire surface of the chorionic sac. Beginning at about 8 weeks, villi near the decidua capsularis become compressed, blood flow decreases, and the villi degenerate, leaving a bare avascular area (smooth chorion, or chorion laeve). Simultaneously, villi near the decidua basalis (villous chorion, or chorion frondosum) rapidly enlarge, increase in number and develop a mesenchymal core and blood vessels (see Fig. 2–8).

Anchoring villi grow more slowly than other portions of the placenta. As a result, during the 3rd month folds of the basal plate are pulled up into the intervillous spaces (see Fig. 2–11). These folds (known as the placental septa) do not extend to the chorionic plate and have no known morphologic or physiologic function.[86, 142, 276]

By 40 to 50 days after ovulation the trophoblast has invaded far enough into the endometrium to reach and erode maternal spiral arterioles. Invasion of the trophoblastic tissue ceases. Spurts of maternal arterial blood form localized hollows (intervillous spaces) around the villi within the chorion frondosum (see Fig. 2–11).[60, 224]

The mature placenta is established by 8 to 10 weeks after conception. The chorion laeve

fuses onto the decidua vera, forming the chorion or outer fetal membrane. The inner membrane, the amnion, is derived from the amniogenic cells (amnioblasts) of the cytotrophoblast. Although the amnion and chorion are often thought of as fusing, they do not actually grow together; rather, the amnion is passively pushed against the chorion.

Placental Growth

By 4 months the placenta has achieved its full thickness with no new lobules or stem villi added after 10 to 12 weeks.[175] Circumferential placental growth continues with further ramification of stem villi (via growth and extension of new trophoblast sprouts, followed by growth of the mesenchymal core and development of blood vessels), lengthening of existing villi, and increases in the size and number of placental capillaries.[60, 191, 224, 276] As a result, the surface area for placental exchange continues to increase until late in gestation. Trophoblast sprouts not used to form new villi may break off, enter maternal circulation, and lodge in the mother's lung capillaries.

After 30 weeks' gestation syncytial knots develop, pulling the syncytium and its nuclei

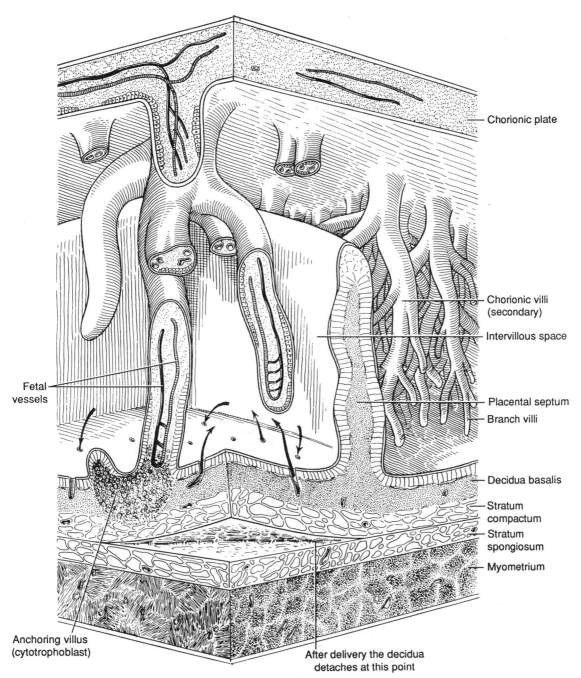

Chorionic plate

Chorionic villi
(secondary)

Intervillous space

Placental septum

Branch villi

Fetal
vessels

Decidua basalis

Stratum
compactum

Stratum
spongiosum

Myometrium

Anchoring villus
(cytotrophoblast)

After delivery the decidua
detaches at this point

FIGURE 2–11. Diagrammatic composition of placental tissues near term. Arrows indicate the blood flow from uteroplacental arteries to the intervillous space and back to the uteroplacental veins. (From Duplessis, G. D. T. and Haegel, P. (1971). *Embryologie.* New York: Masson. English edition by Springer-Verlag, 1972; Chapman and Hall, 1972; Masson, 1972.)

into "piles" several layers thick and leaving a thin attenuated anuclear membrane in the intervening areas.[276] These areas (known as the vasculosyncytial membrane) appear to, but do not actually, fuse with dilated fetal

capillaries and are thought to be specialized regions that facilitate placental gas exchange.[84, 86, 142, 276]

The rate of cellular proliferation deceases after 34 to 36 weeks, but cellular hypertrophy

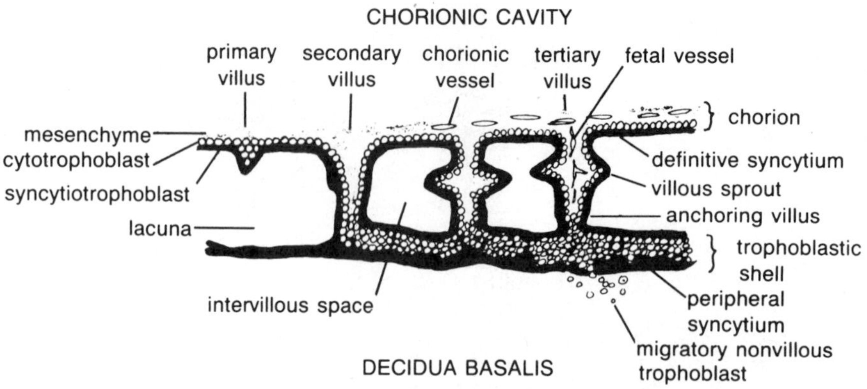

CHORIONIC CAVITY

FIGURE 2–12. Early development of the placenta progressing from 9 to 13 days (left side of figure) to 13 to 21 days (right side of figure). (Reprinted from *The Human Placenta: Clinical Perspectives* by J. P. Lavery, p. 28, with permission of Aspen Publishers, Inc., © 1987.)

continues to term.[39, 260] The placenta eventually occupies one third of the inner uterine surface. Until 15 to 16 weeks the placenta is larger than the fetus; the fetus then becomes larger than the placenta, so that by term the fetus is five to six times heavier than the placenta.[39, 121, 175, 217] The early growth of the placenta establishes a wide area of maternal blood flow (so the placenta is not dependent on relatively few blood vessels for perfusion) and adequate trophoblastic tissue for production of sufficient hCG to maintain the corpus luteum and thus the pregnancy. At term the placenta is a 500- to 600-g disc, 15 to 20 cm in diameter and 2 to 3 cm thick.[191]

Increases in villous surface area and thinning of placental tissue layers increase the functional efficiency of the placenta during pregnancy. During the first 2 months the relatively few villi are greater than 170 μm in diameter, vascularized by a small central fetal vessel and covered by two layers of trophoblast (syncytial outer layer and inner layer of cytotrophoblast) of uniform thickness. At this stage the villous stroma consists of a loose network of primitive mesenchymal tissue and many Hofbauer cells (tissue macrophage).[49, 86, 276, 281] From 8 to 30 weeks the number of villi increase and the average diameter decreases to about 70 μm. The stroma is then thinner and more compact and contains fibroblasts and collagen fibers with fewer Hofbauer cells.[86] By term, the placental villi are approximately 35 to 40 μm in diameter. The trophoblastic layer and stroma have thinned considerably, and few cytotrophoblast cells are seen.[217, 276]

The area-to-volume ratio of the placenta progressively increases. Surface area increases from 5 m² (28 weeks) to 11 m² (term), while the syncytium decreases in thickness from 10 mm² to 1.7 mm² late in gestation. The actual surface area is closer to 90 m² because of the presence of extensive microvilli on the surface of the syncytial trophoblast covering the villi.[60, 81, 224] Transfer efficiency of placental tissue increases sixfold. The trophoblast layer and connective tissue thin so that the capillaries lie closer to the syncytial trophoblast, decreasing the distance nutrients and waste products have to travel.[60]

Although villous growth continues to near term, the placenta also undergoes degenerative changes (increased syncytial knots, intervillous thrombi, fibrin deposits, infarcts, calcification). Abnormal growth of the placenta may also occur. Hypoplasia of the syncytial trophoblast can alter implantation and result in abortion, abruptio placentae, or poor development of terminal villi, increasing the risk of stillbirth or preterm delivery. Hyperplasia and reactivation of the syncytial growth layer, possibly due to suboptimal oxygenation, have been observed in women with hypertension and with prolonged pregnancy. Although the amount of cytotrophoblast decreases with gestation, the remaining tissue retains its proliferative capacity so the cytotrophoblast can be reactivated to replace damaged or destroyed syncytiotrophoblast.[86, 134] However, this hyperplasia may be followed by degenerative changes.[175, 224]

Separation of the Placenta

Placental separation and expulsion occur during the third stage of labor. The afterbirth consists of maternal and fetal tissues. Maternal tissues include the decidua basalis (maternal portion of the placenta), decidua parietalis, and any remaining decidua capsularis. Fetal tissues include the chorion frondosum (fetal portion of the placenta), chorion laeve, amnion and umbilical cord. Retained fragments of the placenta and membranes can lead to uterine atony, hemorrhage, or infection.

The sudden emptying of the uterus with delivery of the fetus rapidly reduces the surface area of the placental site to an area approximately 10 cm in diameter. This reduction in the base of support for the placenta leads to compression and shearing of the placenta from the uterine wall.[150] The usual site of placental separation is within the spongy layer of the decidua basalis. This layer has been described as being like the "... lines of perforation found between postal stamps."[150, p.155] The placenta may separate from the central area to the margins with inversion so that the fetal surface presents first (Schultze's mechanism), or from the margins toward the center with initial presentation of the maternal surface (Duncan's mechanism). Placentas implanted in the fundus of the uterus are more likely to separate via Schultze's mechanism; those implanted lower on the uterine wall usually separate by Duncan's mechanism (although these placentas may invert prior to expulsion).

Placental Structure

Although the placenta contains maternal and fetal components, it is primarily a fetal structure composed of extensively branching, closely packed fetal villi containing fetal blood vessels (see Fig. 2–11). Three types of villi can be identified: (1) stem or anchoring villi, which consist of multiple branches and function to stabilize the villous tree; (2) intermediate villi, located between the stem and terminal villi; and (3) terminal or branch villi, which are the areas of maternal-fetal exchange.[130, 140, 142] On the fetal side the placenta is covered by the chorionic plate, a thin membranous structure continuous with the fetal membranes. On the maternal side the outer layer of trophoblast cells fuse to the decidua basalis.

The fetal portion of the placenta is divided into 50 to 60 cotyledons or lobes, each arising as a primary stem villus supplied by primary branches of the umbilical vessels from the chorionic plate. Each cotyledon is divided into one to five subunits or lobules.[276] Lobules are globular structures with a central cylindrical space that is relatively empty.[86] This space is thought to arise because of preferential growth of villi in relation to entry of maternal spiral arteries into the intervillous spaces.[276] Beneath the chorionic plate the primary stem villi divide into secondary stem villi. These villi run parallel to the chorionic plate, dividing into tertiary stem villi, which project downward through the parenchyma of the placenta around the central space and anchor onto the basal plate (see Fig. 2–11).[63, 86, 276] Each primary stem villus may give rise to varying numbers of secondary stem villi and lobules.[86] The terminal villi branch off of the tertiary stem villi.

The placental septa divide the maternal surface of the placenta into an average of 15 to 20 lobes, each containing two or more main stem villi and their branches.[60, 175, 224] The term "cotyledon" is commonly used to describe these lobes. Fox suggests that, since the maternal lobes are just areas between placental septa with no physiologic or morphologic significance, cotyledon should really be used to describe portions of the villus tree that arise from a single primary stem villus.[86]

Maternal and fetal circulations are separated by several layers of tissue. These tissues are called the placental membrane or placental barrier. A substance, such as oxygen, moving from the maternal circulation to the fetal circulation must pass from maternal blood through five tissue layers in order to reach the fetal blood: (1) the microvillous membrane of the trophoblast; (2) the syncytiotrophoblast cells of the villus; (3) the basal membrane of the trophoblast; (4) the connective tissue mesoderm of the villus; and (5) the epithelium of the fetal blood vessel (Fig. 2–13). The layers of the placental barrier are modified as the cytotrophoblast ceases to form a continuous layer after about 12 weeks and is replaced by a fibrinoid layer.[175, 191, 193] The connective tissue mesoderm thins, and the fetal capillaries increase in number and size.

Placental Circulation

Adequate blood flow to and through the placenta from both fetal and maternal circulations is essential for adequate exchange of nutrients, gases, and waste products. However, nearly half of the combined maternal-fetal blood flow to the placenta is not involved

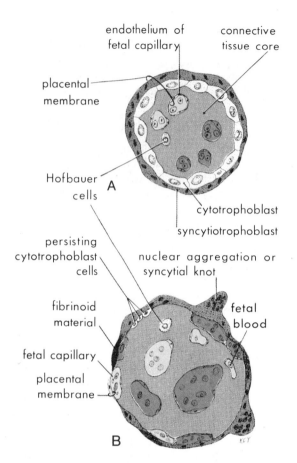

endothelium of fetal capillary

connective tissue core

placental membrane

Hofbauer cells

A

cytotrophoblast

syncytiotrophoblast

persisting cytotrophoblast cells

nuclear aggregation or syncytial knot

fibrinoid material

fetal blood

fetal capillary

placental membrane

B

FIGURE 2–13. The placental membrane or barrier. *A* and *B,* Drawings of sections through a chorionic villus at 10 weeks and at full term, respectively. (From Moore, K.L. (1988). *The developing human* (4th ed., p. 110). Philadelphia: WB Saunders.)

in maternal-fetal transfer owing to maternal and fetal shunts within the uteroplacental circulation (Fig. 2–14).[42] The fetal shunt is the portion of umbilical blood flow that does not supply an area of exchange between maternal and fetal blood. Approximately 17 to 25% of the total umbilical blood flow is used to supply the fetal membranes and placental tissue. Maternal shunt is the portion of uterine blood flow that does not supply the intervillous spaces. Approximately 20 to 27% of uterine arterial blood supplies the myometrium and cervix. At term the uterus extracts 30 to 35 ml O_2/min from maternal blood.[81]

Fetal-Placental Circulation

Deoxygenated blood from the fetus passes via the two umbilical arteries, which spiral around the umbilical vein, to the placenta. Each artery supplies half of the placenta. Prior to entering the placenta the two umbilical arteries are connected by several anastomosed vessels. These arteries tend to fuse close to the surface of the placenta.[86, 122] As the cord enters the placenta, the arteries divide and branch radially onto the chorionic plate before entering the villi. The chorionic vessels branch into 20 to 40 villous trunks or lobular arteries, which branch further into multiple smaller villous vessels, forming an extensive arteriovenous system within each villus. The veins converge back into the umbilical vein at the umbilical cord.

The rate of fetal blood flow in the placenta is about 500 ml/min.[86] Blood flow is dependent on fetal heart activity and regulated by the interaction of blood pressure, fetal right-to-left shunts, and systemic and pulmonary vascular resistance.[8, 81] Contraction of smooth muscle fibers in stem villi may help pump blood from the placenta back to the fetus.[129, 145] The placenta is a low resistance circuit in the fetal circulatory system (see Chapter 6) owing to minimal umbilical innervation.

Maternal Uteroplacental Circulation

Blood flows to the uterus via the uterine arteries, which are branches of the internal iliac and ovarian arteries from the abdominal aorta. The proportion of the maternal cardiac output supplying the uterus and intervillous space (IVS) increases during pregnancy peaking at 20 to 25% by term.[158] The increased blood flow is mediated by the low-resistance uteroplacental circuit, alterations in maternal cardiac output and systemic and peripheral vascular resistance (see Chapter 6) and hormonal and chemical influences.[114, 254, 272]

Maternal blood enters the IVS via uteroplacental arteries in the endometrium. By term, blood in these spaces is supplied by 100 to 200 maternal uteroplacental arteries and removed by 75 to 175 veins.[142] Blood flow in the IVS is pulsatile, entering this space through arterial inlets as a funnel shaped stream under the influence of the maternal blood pressure and flowing toward the chorionic plate or "roof" of the placenta (see Fig. 2–11).[60, 225] As the pressure dissipates, blood flows around the villi allowing exchange of materials between maternal and fetal circulation. Blood leaves the IVS via

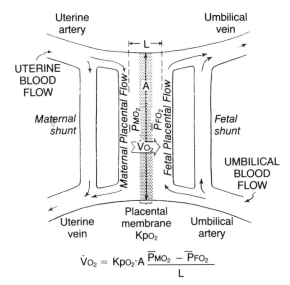

$$\dot{V}_{O_2} = K_{PO_2} \cdot A \frac{\overline{P}_{MO_2} - \overline{P}_{FO_2}}{L}$$

$\dot{V}_{O_2}$ = Rate of oxygen transfer
K_{PO_2} = Placental diffusion constant for oxygen
A = Placental surface area
$\overline{P}_{MO_2}$ = Average oxygen tension in maternal placental blood
$\overline{P}_{FO_2}$ = Average oxygen tension in fetal placental blood
L = Average transplacental diffusion distance for oxygen

FIGURE 2–14. Schematic diagram of placental circulation and physiologic shunts. (From Metcalfe, J., Bartels, H., & Moll, W. (1967). Gas exchange in the pregnant uterus. *Physiol Rev, 47,* 782.)

wide venous outlets into the uteroplacental veins and subchorial, interlobular, and marginal venous lakes.[81, 175, 276]

Maternal blood flowing into and through intervillous spaces moves through a series of pressure gradients. Pressure in the uteroplacental arteries is higher than that in the IVS, which is higher than maternal venous pressure during diastole. Overall the pressures within this system are low owing to anatomic changes in maternal uterine blood vessels. As a result, the maternal arterial blood pressure is not transmitted to the IVS, and pressure gradients from the arterial to venous sides are relatively small (i.e., pressure averages 25 mmHg in the uteroplacental arteries, 15 to 20 mmHg in the IVS, and 5 to 10 mmHg in the uterine veins).[9, 86, 225] Ramsey and Donner suggest that blood does not enter the intervillous space as a jet or spurt, as is often described, but rather "... much as water from an actively flowing brook penetrates a reed-filled marsh."[225]

The intervillous space in the mature placenta contains about 150 ml of blood, which is completely replenished three to four times a minute.[134, 175, 185] The rate of blood flow

within the maternal side of the placenta increases during pregnancy from 50 ml/min at 10 weeks to 500 to 600 ml/min by term.[17, 81, 224] Uterine contractions limit the entry of blood into the IVS but do not squeeze out a significant amount of blood. Thus oxygen transfer to the fetus is decreased during a normal contraction but does not cease since transfer continues from blood remaining in the IVS.

The arteries of the endometrium (decidua) and myometrium undergo marked physiologic changes during pregnancy that convert the uterine spiral arteries into uteroplacental arteries. These changes are mediated by nonvillous migratory cytotrophoblast (see Fig. 2–12). Two types of migratory cytotrophoblast have been described: endovascular and interstitial, or stromal.[80, 142]

Endovascular migratory cytotrophoblast cells invade the spiral arteries in the decidua and myometrium, replacing spiral artery endothelium and destroying muscular and elastic elements in medial tissue.[64, 86] Much of the arterial wall is replaced by fibrinoid material that arises from maternal fibrin and from proteins secreted by the cytotrophoblast. The endovascular cytotrophoblast migrates into the maternal tissue in two waves. During the initial wave at 6 to 10 weeks, spiral arteries in the decidua are altered; during the second wave, beginning at 14 to 16 weeks and lasting for 4 to 6 weeks, spiral arteries in the myometrium, and occasionally distal portions of the radial arteries, are altered.[142]

The interstitial, or stromal, migratory cytotrophoblast initially destroys the ends of decidual blood vessels. This promotes flow of maternal blood into the lacunae and IVS and prepares these arteries for the action of the endovascular cytotrophoblast. Later these cells migrate into the myometrium to prepare the spiral arteries for action of the second wave of endovascular cytotrophoblast.[33, 142]

Changes in the maternal arteries, particularly disruption of the muscular and elastic elements, enhance the capacity of the uteroplacental vessels to accommodate the increased blood volume needed to supply the placenta. These vessels are also functionally denervated owing to decreased neurotransmitter sites. As a result of these changes, the arteries are almost completely dilated and are no longer responsive to circulatory pressor agents or influences of the autonomic nervous system.[141, 242, 262, 272] Control of the uteroplacental circulation is at the level of the radial arteries and is mediated primarily by local influences.[80] These changes may be mediated by placental production of prostacyclin (PGI$_2$). Prostacyclin, the most potent vasodilator produced by the placenta, is thought to maintain vasodilation of these vessels, prevent platelet aggregation, and enhance cell disengagement (needed for disruption of elastic and muscular elements).[272]

The importance of these changes for fetal survival and growth can be appreciated by examining situations such as spontaneous abortion, pregnancy-induced hypertension, and intrauterine growth retardation in which invasion of the spiral arteries by migratory cytotrophoblast does not occur or is abnormal. Recurrent spontaneous abortion in some women may be due to absent or inadequate conversion of spiral ateries to uteroplacental arteries. Absence of changes in decidual arteries has been associated with late first trimester loss, and absence of myometrial artery changes with second trimester loss.[134]

Pregnancy-induced hypertension (PIH) is associated with alterations in the normal invasion of the spiral arteries by the cytotrophoblast (Fig. 2–15).[43, 89] This defect, which may have a genetic basis, may be the initial event in the development of PIH.[272] Generally the first cytotrophoblast wave proceeds normally, but there is failure of the second wave.[142, 230] Thus decidual spiral arteries undergo the usual physiologic changes, but the myometrial arteries do not. The uninvaded arterial segments may also develop atherosclerosis with necrosis and invasion of

the damaged wall by fibrin and other substances.[62] Alterations in the normal changes within the uterine arteries in women with PIH lead to (1) decreased perfusion of the IVS due to the retained muscular coat and inability of the vessels to dilate sufficiently to accommodate the increased blood flow and (2) hypertension in the uteroplacental arteries due to continued sensitivity of these vessels to circulatory pressor agents and the influences of the autonomic nervous system.[142]

PIH has been associated with alterations in production of placental prostacyclin (PGI$_2$) and thromboxane (TXA$_2$) (see Fig. 3–5). Prostacyclin is produced in many tissues and is a potent vasodilator and inhibitor of platelet aggregation and uterine contractility, which acts to promote increased uteroplacental blood flow during pregnancy. Conversely, TXA$_2$ is a potent vasoconstrictor that opposes the action of prostacyclin. Women with PIH have been reported to have an imbalance in levels of these mediators produced by the placenta with elevated TXA$_2$ and decreased prostacyclin (see Chapter 6), which may alter the usual changes in the uterine blood vessels.[272]

Underperfusion of the intervillous spaces may lead to occlusion of small arterioles within the villi. These changes can markedly alter fetal growth and health status and are similar to changes reported with some growth retarded fetuses. Failure of the normal cytotrophoblastic invasion of the decidua and myometrium and subsequent arterial changes occur in about half the mothers of infants with isolated growth retardation.[231, 245]

Placental Function

The placenta has four major activities: metabolic, endocrine, immunologic, and transport.

Placental Metabolism

Placental metabolic functions are particularly important early in pregnancy in providing nutrition and energy for the developing fetus and for the placenta itself. The placenta has a high metabolic rate. Rates of oxygen consumption and glucose utilization by the placenta approximate those of the brain.

The placenta is an active synthesizer of glycogen, fatty acids, cholesterol, and enzymes. The placenta produces protective and enhancement enzymes such as sulfatase, which enhances the excretion of fetal estro-

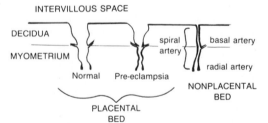

FIGURE 2–15.   Pattern of uteroplacental vascular changes in normal pregnancies and those complicated by pregnancy-induced hypertension (PIH). In normal pregnancy, physiologic vascular changes extend from the intervillous space to the radial arteries; in PIH these changes are limited to the decidua. Nonplacental spiral arteries and placental and nonplacental basal arteries are not involved in these vascular changes. (Reprinted from *The Human Placenta: Clinical Perspectives* by J. P. Lavery, p. 33, with permission of Aspen Publishers, Inc., © 1987.)

gen precursors, and insulinase, which increases the barrier to the transfer of insulin.[60, 81, 157] Relatively large amounts of ammonia and lactate are produced by the placenta and may be important in stimulating metabolic activity of the fetal liver. The impact of alterations in these metabolic processes on placental function and transport during pathologic states is not clear, but they decrease the capacity of the fetus to tolerate labor and transition to extrauterine life.

Placental Endocrinology

Placental endocrine activities are important in maintaining pregnancy and inducing metabolic adaptations in the mother and fetus. The placenta synthesizes polypeptide hormones (human chorionic gonadotropin and human placental lactogen) and steroid hormones (estrogens and progesterone) as well as mediators such as pregnancy-associated plasma proteins (PAPP), glycoproteins, and growth factors. Some hormones produced by the placenta are exclusively of placental origin; others are produced in collaboration with the fetoplacental and maternal units and have been used to evaluate fetal-placental well-being.

The four main hormones synthesized by the placenta are human chorionic gonadotropin, human placental lactogen, progesterone, and estrogens. The placenta also produces both pituitary-like and gonad-like peptide hormones (placental corticotropin, human chorionic thyrotropin, melanocyte stimulating hormone, and β-endorphins), hypothalamus-like releasing hormones (human chorionic somatostatin and corticotropin releasing hormones), and gut hormones (gastrin and vasoactive intestinal peptide).[114, 239, 249] The placenta, membranes, and fetus also synthesize a variety of peptide growth factors including epidermal growth factor (EGF), nerve growth factor (NGF), platelet-derived growth factor (PDGF), skeletal growth factor, and insulin-like growth factors I (somatomedin) and II.[159] Little is known regarding specific actions of these growth factors. They are thought to stimulate growth-related activities either directly or indirectly by influencing transplacental nutrient flux or acting as chemical mediators at the cellular level.[159, 192, 239]

HUMAN CHORIONIC GONADOTROPIN

Human chorionic gonadotropin (hCG) is a glycoprotein with alpha and beta subunits that is biologically similar to luteinizing hormone (LH). The major function of hCG is to maintain the corpus luteum during early pregnancy. It may also stimulate the fetal testes and adrenal gland to enhance testosterone and corticosteroid secretion, stimulate production of placental progesterone, and suppress maternal lymphocyte responses thereby preventing rejection of the placenta by the mother.[114, 206, 217]

Human chorionic gonadotropin is produced primarily by syncytiotrophoblast cells in the blastocyst and embryo, although small amounts may be produced by other trophoblast tissue.[107, 239] Although detection of hCG has been reported prior to implantation, generally hCG is not detectable in maternal serum until 8 to 10 days postconception or by the 9th day after the LH surge.[130] This timing correlates with formation of the lacunae and diffusion of hCG from the trophoblast into maternal blood. Significant serum concentrations of hCG can be detected about 12 days after follicle rupture in normal pregnancies. Concentrations of hCG in maternal serum double every 1.4 to 2 days (range, 1.3 to 3.3 days) until peak values are reached 60 to 90 days postconception (Fig. 2–16).[130]

Urine hCG can be detected 26 to 28 days after conception and is identified by isoimmunologic analysis. Home pregnancy tests of maternal urine are now usually positive as early as 1 day after the first missed period. These tests have a sensitivity of 80 to 90% and a specificity of 95%.[200] Concentrations of hCG decrease after 10 to 11 weeks and reach a plateau at low levels by 100 to 130 days. By 2 weeks after delivery hCG disappears. Persistently low levels may indicate an abnormal placenta or ectopic pregnancy; levels remain elevated in women with hydatidiform moles.[107, 224, 239]

HUMAN PLACENTAL LACTOGEN

Human placental lactogen (hPL), also called human chorionic somatomammotropin (hCS) or chorionic growth hormone, consists of a single polypeptide chain similar in structure to that of human growth hormone. It promotes fetal growth by altering maternal protein, carbohydrate, and fat metabolism (see Chapter 13). The primary role of hPL is regulating glucose availability for the fetus. It is an insulin antagonist that increases maternal metabolism and use of fat as an energy substrate and reduces glucose usage. As a

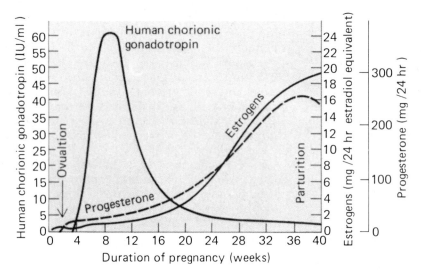

FIGURE 2–16. Patterns of excretion of human chorionic gonadotropin (hCG), progesterone, and estrogen during pregnancy. (From Guyton, A.C. (1987). *Human physiology and mechanisms of disease* (4th ed., p. 643). Philadelphia: WB Saunders.)

result more glucose is available for transport to the fetus.[114, 239]

Production of hPL by the syncytiotrophoblast begins 12 to 18 days after conception (5 to 10 days after implantation), rises during pregnancy, and levels off by 34 to 36 weeks at 1 to 2 g/day.[130, 224, 239, 266] Secretion of hPL is regulated by glucose; decreased serum glucose leads to increased hPL secretion and increased maternal lipolysis.[114] As early as 4 weeks postconception, hPL can be detected in maternal serum; little is found in maternal urine. It has a short half-life so maternal serum levels reflect the rate of production. Levels have been examined for use as a placental function test, but the feasibility of this has not yet been established.[33, 224, 266] Maternal serum hPL has been used in several European centers in diagnosing fetal growth retardation.[50]

STEROIDOGENESIS

Progesterone and the estrogens are steroid hormones whose synthesis increases rapidly during pregnancy (Fig. 2–16). Early in gestation the corpus luteum is the main synthesis site, but by 7 weeks the placental syncytial trophoblast has taken over as the major producer. Steroidogenesis during pregnancy is based on a complex set of interactions by separate organ systems. Each system lacks essential enzymes necessary for creation of the final hormone. Placental production of progesterone and estrogens is an example of a function that requires cooperative efforts of the mother, placenta, and fetus. The placenta lacks certain enzymes needed for pro-

duction of estriol; these enzymes are present in the fetal adrenal. The fetus is the major source of precursors for the estrogens, and the mother is the major source of precursors for the progesterone (Fig. 2–17). Placental progesterone also serves as a precursor for fetal synthesis of corticosteroids, testosterone, and androgens.[114, 141, 224]

Progesterone. Progesterone is produced by the corpus luteum (under the influence of hCG) during the first 5 weeks after fertilization. After that period progesterone is synthesized using cholesterol precursors from the mother. A fetus is not essential for placental progesterone production, which continues even after fetal death.[217] Progesterone production in late pregnancy is about 250 to 300 mg/day.[114] The active progesterone metabolites are 5α-reduced metabolite, 5α-pregnane-3,20-dione, and deoxycorticosterone (DOC). The fist two contribute to the altered response to the pressor action of angiotensin II during pregnancy. The role of DOC in pregnancy is unknown.[46]

During pregnancy progesterone acts to decrease myometrial activity and irritability, constrict myometrial vessels, decrease sensitivity of the maternal respiratory center to carbon dioxide, inhibit prolactin secretion, help suppress maternal immunologic responses to fetal antigens thereby preventing rejection of the fetus, relax smooth muscle in the gastrointestinal and urinary systems, increase basal body temperature, and increase sodium and chloride excretion.[224] β-Adrenergic agonists such as terbutaline and

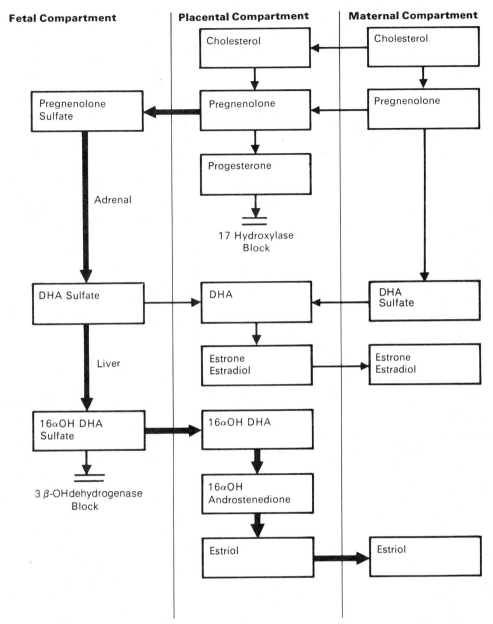

FIGURE 2–17. Steroid production by the maternal, fetal, and placental compartments. (From Speroff, L., Glass, R.H., & Kase, N. (1983). *Clinical gynecologic endocrinology and infertility* (3rd ed., p. 276). Baltimore: Williams & Wilkins.)

isoproterenol increase progesterone production.[239]

The most important role of progesterone in the fetus is to serve as the substrate pool for fetal adrenal gland production of glucocorticoids and mineralocorticoids. The fetal adrenal lacks enzymes in the 3β-hydroxysteroid dehydrogenase, δ4-5 isomerase system necessary for synthesis of some impor-

tant corticosteroids. Therefore, the fetus must utilize progesterone substrate from the placenta in order to accomplish this.[46]

Estrogens. The three major estrogens are estrone, estradiol, and estriol. During pregnancy production of estrogens increases markedly, particularly estriol. Estrone and estradiol production increases about 100 times; estriol about 1000 times.[114] During pregnancy estrogens act to enhance myometrial activity, promote myometrial vasodilation, increase sensitivity of the maternal respiratory center to carbon dioxide, soften fibers in the cervical collagen tissue, increase pituitary secretion of prolactin, increase serum binding proteins and fibrinogen, decrease plasma proteins, and increase the sensitivity of the uterus to progesterone in late pregnancy.[224]

Early in pregnancy estriol is derived from estrone and estradiol. Production of estrogens and particularly estriol is dependent on interaction of the maternal-fetal-placental unit. Approximately 90% of the precursors for estriol are derived from the fetus; 40% of the precursors for estrone and estradiol come from the mother and 60% from the fetus.[224] The primary source of estriol precursors (dehydroepiandrosterone sulfate [DHEAS]) is the fetal adrenal under stimulation by fetal adrenocorticotropic hormone (ACTH). DHEAS is hydroxylated in the fetal liver and further metabolized by the placenta to form estriol. Estriol is secreted by the placenta into maternal circulation and eventually excreted in maternal urine (Fig. 2–17). Maternal serum and urinary estriol levels rise rapidly during early pregnancy, more slowly between 24 and 32 weeks, and then increase rapidly again in the last 6 weeks. Although seldom used currently, estriol assays were one of the earlier methods of assessing fetal well-being and placental function for management of complicated pregnancies.[141, 224]

Placental Immunologic Function

The immunologic functions of the placenta include protection of the fetus from pathogens and prevention from rejection by the mother. The fetus differs in genetic makeup from the mother, yet is not rejected. Possible explanations for this phenomenon include reduced antigenicity of the trophoblast that is in direct contact with maternal blood, immunologic enhancement, and presence of blocking antibodies.[100, 206] The latter two mechanisms are discussed in Chapter 10. The fibrinoid glycoprotein coating of the trophoblast acts as an antigenic barrier and contains an alpha globulin of the IgG class. Electronegative properties make the coating capable of blocking stimulation of maternal lymphocytes by fetal antigens, decreasing cell-mediated responses. The coating is produced by maternal liver and appears within 48 hours after implantation.[82, 206] Prior to that time, the zona pellucida forms a barrier between maternal and fetal tissues.

The placenta also protects the fetus from pathogens. Many bacteria are too large to cross placenta, although most viruses and some bacteria are able to cross. The placenta also allows passage of maternal antibodies of the IgG class primarily via pinocytosis, although some may cross by diffusion. This may also be a disadvantage since both protective and potentially deleterious antibodies cross the placenta (see Chapter 10).[82, 185, 206]

Placental Transport

Placental transfer or transport involves movement of gases, nutrients, waste materials, drugs, and other substances across the placenta from maternal to fetal circulation or from fetal to maternal circulation (Fig. 2–18). Transport across the placenta increases during the course of gestation owing to changes in placental structure (decreased distance between maternal and fetal blood), increased fetal and maternal blood flow, and greater fetal demands. Transfer can be modified by maternal nutritional status, exercise, and disease such as diabetes mellitus (glucose transport increases owing to maternal hyperglycemia), hypertension (decreased nutrient transfer from reduced uteroplacental blood flow), and alcoholism (ethanol impairs placental uptake of amino acids and glucose).[103, 115, 134, 193, 259, 261] Transfer of specific substances across the placenta is summarized in Table 2–4; relative concentrations of selected materials in fetal and maternal plasma are listed in Table 2–5. The mechanisms by which substances are transferred across the placenta include simple (passive) diffusion, facilitated diffusion, active transport, pinocytosis, endocytosis, bulk flow, solvent drag, accidental capillary breaks, and independent movement. Although mechanisms by which most materials cross the placenta are known, there is still uncertainty about specific aspects of these mechanisms and changes during gestation.[192, 248]

SIMPLE DIFFUSION

Diffusion is movement of a substance from higher to lower concentration or electrochemical gradients (Fig. 2–19A). The quan-

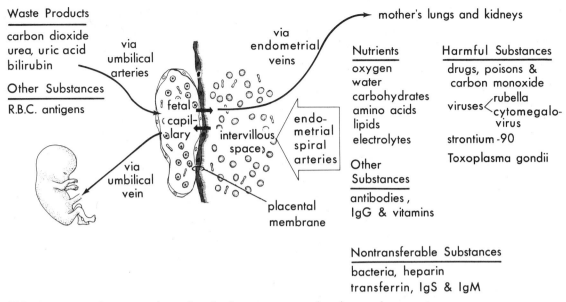

FIGURE 2–18.   Summary of transfer of substances across the placenta between the mother and fetus. (From Moore, K.L. (1988). *The developing human* (4th ed., p. 111). Philadelphia: WB Saunders.)

tity of a substance transferred is illustrated by the Fick diffusion equation:

$$Q/t = \frac{K\ A\ (C1\ -\ C2)}{L}$$

where Q/t is the quantity transferred/unit of time, K is the diffusion constant, A is the fetal surface area available for exchange, $C1$

$- C2$ is the concentration gradient across the placenta, and L is the thickness of the membrane across which the substance is to move.

Diffusion is the major mechanism of placental transfer. Simple diffusion is generally limited to smaller molecules that can pass through pores in the cell wall. Since the cell walls have a high lipid content, some lipid-soluble substances may cross directly through these lipid regions.[157, 175, 224] The cell walls can act as a barrier to some large non–lipid soluble substances such as muscle relaxants

TABLE 2–4
Mechanisms by Which Selected Substances are Transported Across the Placenta

MECHANISM	SUBSTANCE
Simple (passive) diffusion	Water, electrolytes, oxygen, carbon dioxide, urea, simple amines, creatinine, fatty acids, steroids, fat-soluble vitamins, narcotics, antibiotics, barbiturates, and anesthetics
Facilitated diffusion	Glucose, oxygen
Active transport	Amino acids, water-soluble vitamins, calcium, iron, iodine
Pinocytosis and endocytosis	Globulins, phospholipids, lipoproteins, antibodies, viruses
Bulk flow/solid drag	Water, electrolytes
Accidental capillary breaks	Intact blood cells
Independent movement	Maternal leukocytes, organisms such as *Treponema pallidum*

TABLE 2–5
Relative Concentrations of Nutrients and Other Substances in Maternal Versus Fetal Circulation

HIGHER IN FETUS	SIMILAR IN FETUS AND MOTHER	HIGHER IN MOTHER
Amino acids	Sodium	Total proteins
Total phosphorus	Chloride	Globulins
Lactate	Urea	Fibrinogen
Serum iron	Magnesium	Total lipids
Calcium		Phospholipids
Riboflavin		Fatty acids
Ascorbic acid		Glucose
		Cholesterol
		Vitamin A
		Vitamin E

Compiled from Longo, L. (1981). Nutrient transfer in the placenta. In *Placental transport* (pp. 15–20). Mead Johnson Symposium on Perinatal and Developmental Medicine, No. 18. Evansville, IN: Mead Johnson.

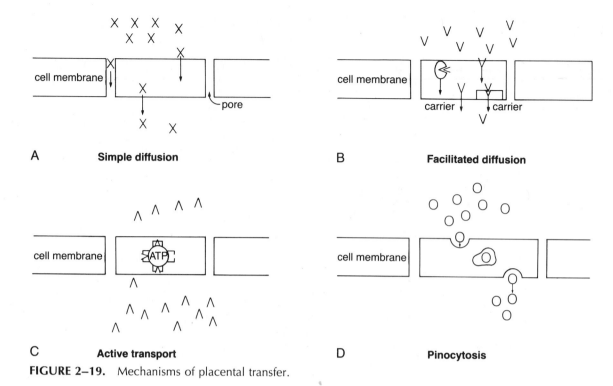

FIGURE 2–19. Mechanisms of placental transfer.

used with anesthesia. Table 2–4 lists substances that cross the placenta via simple diffusion.[81, 121, 157, 175, 193] Fat-soluble vitamins and cholesterol diffuse as lipoprotein complexes.[9] Compounds such as histamine, serotonin, angiotensin, and epinephrine diffuse readily, but significant concentrations may never reach the fetus owing to enzymatic deamination within the placenta.[157, 224] Free water crosses at a rate of 180 ml/sec, faster than any other known substance.[81]

Carbon dioxide is highly soluble in the placental membrane and diffuses readily. Oxygen diffuses with greater difficulty and therefore requires a considerable gradient of oxygen pressure on the either side of the membrane. The average gradient is about 20 mmHg for oxygen and 5 mmHg for carbon dioxide.[214] The oxygen gradient is higher because the placenta and myometrium also extract oxygen.[81] The rate of gas exchange across the placenta is limited by maternal and placental blood flow. The placenta consumes about 10 to 30% of the oxygen delivered to it.[9]

Although the placenta is similar to the lungs in terms of efficiency of gas exchange, the PO_2 levels of maternal and fetal blood leaving the placenta differ. These differences are due to the previously described vascular shunts in maternal and fetal circulations, nonuniform distribution of maternal and fetal blood flow, and differences in the positions of the maternal and fetal oxygen hemoglobin dissociation curves (see Chapter 7).[119, 120, 121, 160] When maternal blood flow exceeds fetal flow, the exchange of oxygen with fetal blood results in only minimal changes in maternal PO_2. Blood from these compartments contributes heavily to the PO_2 of mixed venous blood leaving the uterus. Conversely, oxygen exchange in areas in which fetal blood flow exceeds maternal flow depletes maternal reserves and equilibrates at a level similar to the fetal PO_2.[121] Placental gas exchange is discussed further in Chapter 7.

FACILITATED DIFFUSION

Facilitated diffusion involves transport via a protein carrier system to move substances across the placental membrane (Fig. 2–19*B*). Movement is from higher to lower concentration or electrochemical gradients. Glucose (fetal levels are 70 to 80% of maternal values) and possibly oxygen are transported from maternal to fetal circulation via facilitated diffusion. Placental glucose metabolism may partially account for differences in maternal and fetal glucose concentrations.[121] Glucose transport systems may become saturated at high concentrations.[4, 26, 27, 82]

ACTIVE TRANSPORT

Active transport utilizes energy-dependent carrier systems to move substances against concentration or electrochemical gradient (Fig. 2–19C). Amino acids, water-soluble vitamins, calcium, iron, and iodine cross the placenta via active transport (see Table 2–4).[54, 81, 121, 193] Active transport systems become saturated at high concentrations. Similar molecules may compete, reducing the movement of some substances across the placenta.[121]

Amino acids such as alanine, glutamine, threonine, and serine that are transported by multiple carrier systems are found in high concentrations in placental tissue.[193] The net movement of many amino acids is greater than that estimated for fetal growth needs, suggesting that the fetus also uses these substances for energy or the synthesis of other amino acids.[121, 193, 284] The amount of amino acids transported across the placenta increases markedly late in pregnancy owing to increased numbers of carriers. A carrier system for dipeptides has been identified, but most polypeptides and larger proteins that cross the placenta do so via pinocytosis or accidental capillary breaks.[92, 121] The only proteins transported in significant quantities are IgG (see Chapter 10) and retinol-binding protein.[73, 103, 113]

PINOCYTOSIS AND ENDOCYTOSIS

These mechanisms involve the engulfing of microdroplets of maternal plasma (pinocytosis) (Fig. 2–19D) or solid substances (endocytosis) by trophoblast cells. Substances in maternal plasma such as globulins, phospholipids, lipoproteins, and antibodies are transferred to the fetus or metabolized by the placenta. These mechanism are necessary to transfer molecules too large for diffusion or for which no carrier transport exists.

Maternal antibodies of the IgG class readily cross the placenta during the third trimester. Maternal IgA antibodies do not cross in significant amounts; IgM antibodies are not transferred. IgG antibodies from the mother can be protective (antibodies against diphtheria, measles, mumps) or potentially damaging (as occurs in Rh incompatibility or with maternal Graves' disease or myasthenia gravis) to the fetus (see Chapter 10).[185, 206]

BULK FLOW AND SOLVENT DRAG

Water crosses the placenta very rapidly. Bulk movement may occur with changes in hydrostatic or osmotic forces. Ions cross either by simple diffusion or by solvent drag as dissolved electrolytes are pulled across the placenta by the movement of water. This mechanism is useful in maintaining water and osmotic balances between maternal and fetal circulations.[81, 121, 175, 193]

Water movement varies within the placenta depending on the concentrations of various osmotically active substances and the hydrostatic pressure.[11, 121] Although large amounts of water move from mother to fetus, by the end of the placenta much of this water has moved back to the mother with a net flux to the fetus of 0.014 ml/min (or approximately 20 ml/day).[121]

ACCIDENTAL CAPILLARY BREAKS

Accidental capillary breaks and breaks in the villous covering permit passage of intact blood cells between maternal and fetal circulations. Small amounts (0.1 to 0.2 ml) of fetal cells can be found in maternal circulation intermittently during pregnancy. More extensive (>1 to 2 ml) fetomaternal hemorrhage may occur with placental separation and affect development of isoimmunization (see Chapter 10).[81, 175]

INDEPENDENT MOVEMENT

Maternal leukocytes or organisms such as *Treponema pallidum* may cross the placenta under their own power. Although many viruses can infect the fetus, the specific mechanisms through which they cross the placenta are unclear. Some viruses may be carried across via pinocytosis.[214]

UMBILICAL CORD

The umbilical cord contains two arteries and one vein surrounded by Wharton's jelly, a substance containing collagen, muscle, and mucopolysaccharide. The cord epithelium is formed by amnion. There are no other blood vessels nor neural tissue in the cord. The umbilical vessels are longer than the cord and tend to twist and spiral within the cord. The umbilical arteries contain four muscle layers: an inner circular layer, a longitudinal layer, and two helical layers. The helical layers function independently to coil both the arteries and the umbilical cord (usually in a counterclockwise direction).[122] Vasoresponsiveness to stimuli or drugs is thought to be myogenic.[151]

The cord is usually inserted into the center of the placenta but may be attached at any point. The cord arises from fusion of the connecting stalk with the yolk sac stalk and allantois at the end of the 4th week of gestation.[191] The umbilical vessels arise from the allantois and initially consist of four vessels. One of the two original umbilical veins invariably atrophies by 6 weeks after fertilization followed by dilation of the remaining (left) vessel.[122] Occasionally the right umbilical artery also regresses or does not form resulting in a two-vessel cord, which may be associated with other anomalies. The cord reaches its maximal length by 30 weeks and averages 55 cm (range, 30 to 90 cm) with a width of 1 to 2 cm.[214] Cord length is determined by intrauterine space and fetal activity.[184, 189]

The umbilical vessels constrict soon after delivery. Constriction of the umbilical arteries begins within 5 seconds of birth and is complete by 45 seconds; the umbilical vein begins to constrict within 15 seconds of delivery and is functionally closed by 3 to 4 minutes.[151] Placental transfusion and issues regarding timing of cord clamping are discussed in Chapter 5.

AMNION AND CHORION

The amnion and chorion are multilayered structures (Fig. 2–20) that begin to develop soon after fertilization and continue to grow until about 28 weeks' gestation. After this point further mitotic activity is rare, and enlargement takes place by stretching of the existing membranes.[151] Development of the amnion and chorion is described in the placental section.

The chorion or outer membrane contains blood vessels that atrophy as pregnancy advances, but no nerves. The four layers of the chorion (Fig. 2–20) are (1) the cellular layer (often absent at term); (2) the reticular layer (extends into the trophoblast, binding it to the underlying decidua); (3) the pseudobasement membrane; and (4) the trophoblast cells, which attach to and intermingle with cells of the decidua capsularis. The amnion consists of five layers (Fig. 2–20): (1) epithelial layer (with many microvilli and the site of significant fetal fluid exchange); (2) basement membrane; (3) compact layer (dense acellular layer that accounts for the strength of the amnion); (4) fibroblast layer (accounts for the thickness of amnion and permits distensibility); and (5) spongy layer (intermediate distensible layer between amnion and chorion containing a reticular network of collagen-like bundles and mucus).[38, 151] The amnion contains neither blood vessels nor nerves.

The amnion and chorion are not fused and up to 200 ml of amniotic fluid may accumulate in the intermembrane space.[243] The chorion is relatively fixed. The amnion is passively pushed against and moves over the chorion aided by mucus from the spongy

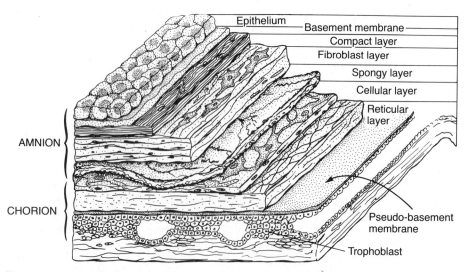

FIGURE 2–20. Layers of the human amnion and chorion. (Redrawn from Bourne, G.L. (1960). The microscopic anatomy of the human amnion and chorion. *Am J Obstet Gynecol, 79,* 1070.)

layer. As a result amnion can rupture, forming shreds of tissue (amniotic bands), while chorion remains intact. The amniotic bands may wrap around, constrict, or amputate fetal parts. The reason for rupture of the amnion is unknown but may be related to trauma.[138]

The fetal membranes are metabolically active, are involved in amniotic fluid turnover and may be important in initiation of labor (see Chapter 3). The amnion is a reservoir for storage of arachidonic acid, an essential prostaglandin precursor, and the chorion is a reservoir for progesterone.[151] The membranes and decidua are rich sources of enzymes such as phospholipase A_2 needed for formation of prostaglandins.[125] Cells of the amnion are involved in protein synthesis, protein and lipid secretion, and exchange of water, electrolytes, and other solutes. The amnion has a metabolic rate similar to that of the liver. The chorion contains renin and synthesizes prostaglandins.[2, 33, 99]

The ability of the membranes to stretch and resist rupture from increasing fetal size and amniotic fluid volume until the end of pregnancy is thought to be related to the collagen rich connective tissue layers of the amnion, which are 0.5 to 0.6 mm thick and have great tensile strength that is maintained throughout gestation.[213] Rupture of the membranes during labor or with delivery is primarily due to hyperdistention with pressure of the presenting part. Premature rupture of the membranes (rupture prior to the onset of uterine contractions) may be due to factors such as mechanical stress (polyhydramnios, multiple gestation), alterations in membranous collagen, or chorioamnionitis. In chorioamnionitis a variety of vaginal and cervical microorganisms have been demonstrated to produce proteases that alter membrane integrity and reduce the pressure needed for rupture.[98]

AMNIOTIC FLUID

Amniotic fluid provides space for symmetric fetal growth, maintains constant temperature and pressure, protects and cushions the fetus, allows free movement of the fetus, and distributes pressure from uterine contractions evenly over the fetus.[191, 224] Amniotic fluid antibacterial factors, such as transferrin (which binds iron needed by some bacteria and fungi for growth), fatty acids (which have a detergent effect on bacterial membrane), immunoglobulins (IgG and IgA), and lysozyme (which is bactericidal for gram-positive bacteria), help protect the fetus from infection (see Chapter 10).[149, 242]

Amniotic Fluid Volume and Turnover

The exact source and fate of amniotic fluid are unclear.[224] Amniotic fluid first appears as a droplet dorsal to the embryonic pole at about 3 weeks.[40, 191] There are approximately 7 ml of amniotic fluid by 8 weeks, 32 ml by 10 weeks, 200 ml by 16 weeks, and 400 ml by 25 weeks. The amount of fluid increases by 50 ml/week, peaks at 900 to 1000 ml by 34 weeks, and then decreases to term.[162, 191] In some women this decrease may begin as early as 28 to 30 weeks. Amounts of amniotic fluid at term vary widely, with a usual range of 500 to 1500 ml. The net volume turnover of amniotic fluid is about 95% per day.[41, 169] Turnover rate is independent of volume.[1, 33, 99]

Amniotic Fluid Production and Disposition

The cells of the amnion are separated by intracellular channels leading directly into the amniotic cavity that allow bulk flow of water and solutes. Transfer of water and most solutes across the amnion and chorion is governed by hydraulic, osmotic, and electrochemical forces. Water movement occurs as a result of a net imbalance between transmembrane hydrostatic pressure and effective osmotic pressure.[33, 99, 191] Some of the free water in amniotic fluid is thought to come from this transmembrane pathway. These pathways do not account for a significant portion of amniotic fluid production and turnover. Major sources for amniotic fluid production and exchange include

1. *Placenta and fetal membranes.* The fetal membranes are thought to be the second most important route of amniotic fluid clearance (after fetal swallowing) during the second half of gestation and account for an estimated 250 ml/day of amniotic fluid removal. Water crosses the membranes by either nondiffusional fast bulk flow or slower diffusional flow. The net transfer of water is

probably small except at the site of the placenta, where the chorioamniotic membrane is relatively close to maternal blood.[162]

2. *Uterine wall via sinusoidal vessels of the decidua.*

3. *Umbilical cord.* The cord arises from the same cell type as the amnion and is involved in fluid exchange after 4 weeks, with development of intracellular channels in cord membranes. The rate of water transfer between amniotic fluid and cord blood is approximately 40 to 50 ml/hour.[1, 2, 33, 99]

4. *Fetal skin.* Prior to complete keratinization of the fetal skin at 24 to 25 weeks (see Chapter 11), the skin is a site for transfer of water and solutes.[1, 2] Even after keratinization, large transcutaneous fluxes may continue.[41, 166] The significance of these fluxes in amniotic fluid homeostasis is uncertain.

5. *Fetal gastrointestinal tract.* Fetal swallowing is a major route for disposal of amniotic fluid. The fetus swallows approximately 7 ml/24 hours at 16 weeks, 16 ml/24 hours at 20 weeks, 120 ml/24 hours at 28 weeks and 200 to 600 ml/24 hours at term.[2, 3, 99, 162]

6. *Fetal respiratory tract.* The fetal lung secretes 200 to 400 ml of fluid/day. Tracheal fluid may contribute to amniotic fluid, although evidence concerning this is contradictory.[2, 4, 33, 41, 109, 162]

7. *Fetal renal/urinary tract.* Hypotonic urine is present in the bladder by 11 weeks. The fetus produces 3.5 ml of urine/hour at 25 weeks and 26 ml/hour, or 500 to 700 ml/day, at term. This latter value is similar to the amount of fluid swallowed by the term fetus. After 40 weeks fetal urine production declines.[2, 33, 99, 162, 280]

These pathways are summarized in Figure 2–21.

Amniotic fluid volume may also be influenced by other factors, including changes in tonicity of maternal serum and amniotic fluid prolactin, which seems to influence permeability of the amnion and chorion membranes.[2, 33] Although during the second half of pregnancy fetal urinary output and swallowing are considered to be the major factors regulating the amount of amniotic fluid, the interrelationships between amniotic fluid volume, fetal swallowing, and fetal urine output are unclear.[41]

Composition of Amniotic Fluid

Amniotic fluid is 98 to 99% water, with the remainder consisting of electrolytes, creati-nine, urea, bile pigments, renin, glucose, hormones, fetal cells, lanugo, and vernix caseosa. The composition of amniotic fluid changes with gestation. In early pregnancy amniotic fluid is similar to maternal and fetal serum with little particulate matter. During the second half of gestation amniotic fluid osmolality decreases to 92% of maternal serum values at term and is similar to dilute fetal urine with added phospholipids and other substances from the fetal lungs.[156, 240] Urea, creatinine, and uric acid concentrations increase as pregnancy progresses; whereas sodium and chloride levels decrease as fetal renal function matures.[1, 2, 99, 162, 271]

CLINICAL IMPLICATIONS RELATED TO PLACENTAL PHYSIOLOGY

An intact and adequately functioning placenta and amniotic fluid are critical for fetal survival and well-being. Without the placenta the fetus could not survive since it would have no alternatives for essential processes such as respiratory gas exchange and nutrition. This section discusses the roles of the placenta and amniotic fluid in low- and high-risk pregnancies, the implications for the fetus and neonate from placental dysfunction and alterations in amniotic fluid volume, and the bases for common cord and placental abnormalities.

Transfer of Substances Across the Placenta

Dancis suggested that in thinking of placental transfer, "Ask not whether a maternal nutrient crosses the placenta. Ask rather, how, how much, and how fast. Ask also as to fetal need."[59, p. 25] There are few compounds, endogenous or exogenous, that are unable to cross the placenta in detectable amounts given sufficient time and sensitivity of detection.[59] Placental transfer is influenced by the area of the placenta, physicochemical characteristics of the diffusing substance, concentration gradients, electrical potential differences, diffusing distance, degree of binding of a substance to hemoglobin or other blood proteins, permeability of the placental barrier, and the rates of maternal and fetal blood flow through the intervillous space and villi.[81, 121, 175, 193]

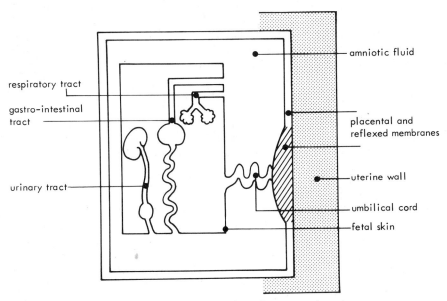

FIGURE 2–21. Pathways of amniotic fluid production and exchange. (From Wallenburg, H.C. (1977). The amniotic fluid I. Water and electrolyte homeostasis. *J Perinat Med*, *5*, 193.)

Diffusion of a substance across the placenta can be expressed as

$$\text{Diffusion} = \frac{\substack{\text{substance} \\ \text{characteristics}} \times \text{area} \times \substack{\text{concentration} \\ \text{gradient}}}{\text{distance}}$$

Increased surface area for exchange (as occurs with growth of the placenta along with the fetus), increased concentration gradient, and decreased diffusing distance each enhances transfer across the placenta. As the placenta matures, the distance between maternal and fetal blood decreases owing to thinning of the syncytial trophoblast and connective tissue and to increases in the size and number of capillaries in the villi. Transfer may be reduced with decreased surface area (small placenta, placental infarcts) or increased diffusing distance (placental edema, infection).

Physicochemical characteristics that influence movement across the placenta include lipid solubility, molecular weight, degree of ionization and protein binding. These characteristics can increase, decrease or prohibit movement of potentially harmful drugs and other substances from maternal to fetal circulation.[58, 81, 175, 224] Placental transfer may be increased or enhanced if a substance is lipid soluble (e.g., diazepam, lipoproteins) or unionized (e.g., phenobarbital), has a molecular weight less than 600 (e.g., propylthiouracil), or lacks significant binding to albumin (e.g.,

ampicillin).[189] Increased maternal to fetal concentration or electrochemical gradients also increase transfer. A substance may be prevented from crossing the placenta because it has a certain charge or molecular configuration (e.g., heparin) or certain size (e.g., bacteria, IgM), is altered or bound by enzymes within the placenta (e.g., amines, insulin), or is firmly bound to the maternal red blood cell or plasma protein (e.g., carbon monoxide).

The rate of maternal blood flow to and through the IVS and fetal blood flow to and through the villi influence placental transfer. Blood flow is the limiting factor in gas exchange across the placenta but also affects transfer of nutrients and waste products. During uterine contractions the entry of blood into the IVS is limited. Transfer of oxygen and other nutrients to the fetus may decrease but does not cease during contractions.[81, 86, 108, 116, 121, 193] The decrease in afferent blood flow during a contraction may be due to (1) compression and obliteration of the uteroplacental veins with increased IVS pressure, (2) occlusion of the uteroplacental arteries, or (3) increased intraluminal pressure within the uterus with alteration in the arteriovenous pressure gradients within the IVS.[6]

The fetus may become hypoxic and acidotic if contractions are hypertonic or if resting time between contractions is insufficient. If placental transfer is compromised by small placental size, infarcts, or edema, fetal distress may arise at lower levels of uterine activity. Since the quantity of oxygen reaching the fetus is primarily flow-limited, reduction of uteroplacental blood flow increases the risk of fetal hypoxia.

In addition to uterine contractions, factors that may alter uteroplacental blood flow include maternal position, anesthesia, nicotine and other drugs, emotional or physical stress, and degenerative changes within the placenta that are seen with hypertension, prolonged pregnancy, diabetes, or renal disease.[52, 158, 175, 193, 227] Maternal blood flow to and through the IVS can be altered by (1) changes in the systemic circulation (cardiac disease, small uterine artery); (2) changes in the number or size of the uteroplacental blood vessels (infection, degeneration); (3) compression of the uteroplacental blood vessels (tetanic or other abnormal contractions, polyhydramnios, multiple pregnancy); and (4) degenerative changes in the IVS associated with high-risk conditions such as maternal hypertension.[81]

Perinatal Pharmacology

Pharmacologic treatment during pregnancy is unique in that a drug taken by one person (pregnant woman) may significantly affect another (fetus).[59a] For many years it was believed that the placental barrier shielded the fetus. However the placenta provides little protection to the fetus from many drugs. The term "drug" is used generically in this section to refer to prescription and nonprescription pharmacologic agents, drugs of abuse, chemicals or additives in foods, and environmental agents such as pesticides, heavy metals, polychlorinated biphenyls (PCBs), herbicides, or other chemicals.[122a]

Factors that influence the effects of drugs in the fetus include individual drug characteristics, dosage and duration of use of the drug, genetic makeup of the mother and fetus (genetic susceptibility), timing in relation to stage of embryonic or fetal development, maternal physiology, and placental transfer. Placental transfer is affected by drug physicochemical characteristics (described in the previous section), blood flow, maturation, and metabolic activity. Once a drug reaches the fetal circulation the drug can (1) be metabolized by the fetal liver; (2)

bypass the fetal liver via the ductus venosus to enter specific fetal tissues or body compartments; (3) be eliminated by the fetal kidney into amniotic fluid (and perhaps be reswallowed in that fluid by the fetus); or (4) return to the maternal circulation via the umbilical arteries and placenta.[122a]

Drugs administered to the mother during pregnancy can affect the fetus in a variety of ways ranging from no effect to major structural or functional deficits. Drugs administered during labor affect the fetus primarily by exaggerating the degree of fetal asphyxia and influencing the rate and quality of infant recovery from birth, adaptation to extrauterine life, and neurobehavioral status. Factors influencing distribution of drugs and other substances within the fetus are summarized in Table 2–6. Effects of alterations in maternal physiology and of fetal and neonatal physiologic immaturity on pharmacokinetics in relation to specific body systems are discussed in Units II and III.

Alterations in the Appearance of the Placenta and Membranes

The appearance of the placenta (color, size, consistency) often provides clues to maternal or placental dysfunction or pathologic processes in the fetus. The color of the placenta is determined by fetal hemoglobin. The placenta is paler in immature infants and congested in infants of diabetic mothers. Pale placentas suggest fetal anemia. Edematous, pale and bulky placentas are seen with immune and nonimmune hydrops fetalis, twin-to-twin transfusion syndrome (donor twin), fetal congestive heart failure, and infection.[26, 131, 218, 276] These placentas may also contain more Hofbauer cells, an immature trophoblast layer, and other changes similar to those seen with hypoxia.

The placenta responds to hypoxia and ischemia with formation of excessive syncytial knots, proliferation of villous cytotrophoblast (Langhans) cells, fibrinoid necrosis of the villi, and thickening of the trophoblast basement membrane.[86, 276] The placentas from women with pregnancy-induced hypertension often have infarcts, hematomas, and characteristic histologic changes such as excessive proliferation of cytotrophoblast tissue within the villi and fibrin deposits.[138, 276] Infarctions are also seen in placentas of infants with intrauterine growth retardation whose

TABLE 2–6
Factors Influencing the Distribution of Drugs and Other Substances in the Fetus

FACTOR	POSSIBLE INFLUENCES
Type of drug	Factors that increase transfer include lipid solubility, low molecular weight (<600–650 daltons), un-ionized, and unbound.
Amount of drug	Transfer is increased by greater maternal-to-fetal gradient, especially for drugs transferred by diffusion.
Membrane permeability	Diffusion of substances increases with increasing gestation and greater placental efficiency.
	Some drugs have greater affinity for specific fetal tissues (e.g., tetracycline in teeth; warfarin in bones; dilantin in the fetal heart, since this is a highly lipid organ in the fetus, whereas in adults the CNS has a high lipid content owing to myelin sheaths; streptomycin in the otic nerve).
Fetal body water compartment	Drug distribution and dilution change as the total body water compartment decreases with increasing gestation; with an increased volume of distribution peak volumes of drugs are reduced, but excretion is delayed.
Fetal circulation	Maternal and fetal blood flow rates will influence transfer.
	Upon reaching the fetal circulation, drugs may be shunted by the ductus venosus past the liver (thus missing an opportunity for detoxification), with highest concentrations of these substances in blood going to the heart and upper body.
Serum protein binding	Protein binding of a drug in the maternal system limits the amount of free drug available for transfer to the fetus.
	Binding of drugs to macromolecules in the fetal circulation may increase the maternal-to-fetal transfer by maintaining a concentration gradient from the mother to fetus.
Receptor function	Functional ability of receptors on cell membranes increases with gestation, leading to increased specificity to respond to or exclude certain drugs.
Placental enzymes	Enzymes produced by the placenta, such as insulinase, may detoxify drugs and reduce tansfer to the fetus.
Gestational age	Many of the factors identified above are altered with advancing gestation and maturity of the fetus and placenta.
	The size and efficiency of the placental exchange area increase with increasing gestational age.
Fetal pH during labor	The fetal pH is usually 0.1 to 0.15 units below that of the mother; decrease in the fetal pH may increase the transfer of acidophilic agents from the mother to fetus.
	Hypoxia alters blood flow and thus drug distribution, metabolism and excretion; for example, with hypoxia, blood flow to the liver and kidneys may be reduced with preferential flow to the brain.
	Albumin binding of drugs may also be reduced, resulting in more free drug in the fetal circulation.

placentas are also small and in placentas from women with elevated hematocrits (>13 g/dl) in the second half of pregnancy.[204] In this latter group the infarctions may be due to increased blood viscosity and thrombosis. Placentas of women who smoke or who inhale second-hand smoke demonstrate hypertrophy with decreased diffusing distance and other changes consistent with chronic hypoxia.[198, 268]

Thrombi in the veins along the chorionic plate appear as yellow streaks on the surface of the placenta. These thrombi may embolize and are associated with velamentous insertion of the cord. Infarctions are often seen near the margins of the placenta; central infarctions are less common and more serious, since they may disrupt IVS circulation. Infarctions are areas of ischemic necrosis of primary villi resulting from obstruction of

IVS blood flow due to thrombi or marked impairment of blood flow in the spiral arteries.[276, 281] Initially these infarcted areas are red, later turning brown, gray, and then white with fibrin deposition and may be covered with necrotic decidua. Hematomas and thrombi may be seen in the IVS.[138, 276] Infarctions may be a way the fetus responds to villi that have inadequate maternal perfusion, that is, the flow of blood to the affected villus is reduced so blood normally flowing to that villus can be redistributed to areas where maternal circulation is adequate.[276]

Multiple plaques or nodules on the fetal surface of the placenta are found with amnion nodosum, squamous metaplasia (benign disorder), and infection.[276] With chorioamnionitis the placenta often has an opaque surface and may be foul smelling. Infection with *Candida albicans* is associated with white or yellow nodules on the placental surface.[138, 276]

Meconium staining of the membranes occurs in about 15% of pregnancies.[26] Since meconium is not discharged until after fetal gastrointestinal peptides such as motilin have reached critical levels (see Chapter 9), meconium passage is infrequent in preterm infants and common in postmature infants. Green membranes are not necessarily due to meconium, since accumulations of hemosiderin (as may occur with hemolysis and circumvallation) also stain the membranes green.[26] Green pigment can be found in amnionic macrophages an hour after meconium is discharged and in chorionic macrophage by 3 hours.[186] Other lesions of the amnion are associated with disorders such as gastroschisis and maternal lupus erythematosus.[10, 65, 163]

Placental Function and Postdate Gestation

The cause of postdate gestation is unknown but may relate to alterations in the hormonal regulation of labor onset (see Chapter 3). Postdate pregnancies (>42 weeks) are associated with changes in placental structure and function. Structural changes include increased syncytial degradation, fibrinoid deposits, fibrotic villi, villous necrosis with hemorrhage, and infarcts. Gas and nutrient transfer may be altered by fibrinoid degeneration of the decidual vessels and IVS, thickening of the vasculosyncytial membranes (important in gas exchange), and thrombosis and hyaline changes in the vessels of the stem villi.[42, 219, 262]

Alterations in placental function associated with postdate gestation develop over days to weeks. The placenta has adequate reserve in maternal and fetal shunts to compensate initially with decreased uteroplacental blood flow so that the fetus continues to receive the required 25 ml/min of oxygen.[42] With further degenerative changes these reserves become exhausted; nutritive, respiratory, and endocrine functions of the placenta are altered; and there is subsequent fetal growth retardation or hypoxia (with fetal distress, asphyxia, and meconium passage).[42, 53] Prolongation of pregnancy past 42 weeks requires close monitoring of placental function and fetal status.[72]

Assessment of Fetal Status and Placental Function

Assessment of placental function and analysis of the constituents of amniotic fluid are useful in evaluating the growth and health of the fetus and the ability of the fetus to withstand the stresses of labor and delivery. New techniques have improved monitoring of fetal and placental status with high risk pregnancies. Amniocentesis and more recently chorionic villus sampling allow for prenatal diagnosis of increasing numbers of chromosomal, genetic, and other congenital anomalies.

Evaluation of Placental Function

Techniques for evaluation of placental function consists of biochemical monitoring of the fetoplacental unit and antepartum fetal heart rate surveillance.

BIOCHEMICAL EVALUATION

The endocrine functions of the placenta and interactions of the maternal-fetal-placental unit have formed the basis for biochemical assessment of placental function and monitoring of fetal well-being. The placenta is an incomplete endocrine organ, i.e., production of hormones by the placenta during pregnancy depends on the availability of precursors from the mother or the fetus as well as the ability of the placenta to convert these precursors to active steroids (see Fig. 2–17). For many years measurement of maternal serum and urinary estriol was the most widely used of the endocrine-based tests of fetoplacental well-being.[141, 224] Serum and urinary estriol values may be diminished if there are problems with the fetus (pituitary, adrenal, or liver function), placenta (absent or insufficient enzymes, lesions, small size), or mother (gall bladder or liver disease, decreased renal function, or antibiotic use). Maternal antibiotics may interfere with estriol excretion by impairing hydrolytic activity of gut flora and reducing reabsorption of conjugate estriol from the gut for renal excretion.[141, 205, 224, 226]

Estriols can be evaluated using radioimmune or immunoreactive assays or glucometric analysis. Problems with estriol assessments include a wide range of normal values with an overlap between normal and abnormal values, high false positive rates (20 to 70%), day-to-day variations, and variations with maternal and fetal conditions unrelated to placental function.[12, 200] The reliability of estriol assessment is low, i.e., estriol assays have been reported to have a ± 10 to 15% diurnal and 20 to 30% day-to-day variation with repeat analysis of the same sample yielding up to a 40% difference in results.[200] As a result of these limitations and the development of other techniques (see below), estriol assessments currently have only very limited use in clinical management of pregnancies complicated by maternal diabetes, hypertension, or intrauterine growth retardation (IUGR).[12, 282] Estriol test results seem most useful when they are well within normal ranges and, if used at all, are used in conjunction with other assessments.

ANTEPARTUM FETAL HEART RATE SURVEILLANCE

Maternal estriol determinations and ultrasound are relatively poor predictors of fetal hypoxia.[215] Antepartum fetal heart rate (FHR) surveillance is used to evaluate uteroplacental insufficiency, a vague term often used to describe alterations in two components of placental function: nutrition and respiration.[12] Alterations in placental function due to impaired uterine or umbilical blood flow are thought to initially lead to disruption in nutrition (fetal growth retardation) and later to alterations in placental respiratory function (fetal hypoxia).[146, 216] If the fetus can compensate for the decreased placental blood flow and oxygen supply, heart rate variability will be normal. As changes in oxygenation become more severe, fetal compensatory mechanisms fail, leading to central asphyxia and heart rate alterations. Antepartum assessment of fetal heart rate is an indirect measurement of placental function in which actual or potential for fetal hypoxia, indicated by alterations in fetal heart rate patterns, is estimated using nonstress or contraction stress testing.

Nonstress testing (NST) uses external fetal monitoring to evaluate fetal heart rate responses to fetal activity. If the NST is nonreactive, a contraction stress test (CST) or oxytocin challenge test (OCT) is performed. A CST evaluates FHR response to uterine contractions, which may be induced by nipple stimulation or intravenous administration of oxytocin (OCT).[12, 215] Additional analysis of fetal status and chronic asphyxia may be accomplished using the fetal biophysical profile (FBP).[170] The FBP is a score based on evaluation of five parameters: fetal breathing movements, body movements, tone, amniotic fluid volume; and fetal heart rate reactivity. The first four parameters are measured by ultrasound, the last by NST.[169]

Amniotic Fluid Analysis

Cellular and biochemical components of amniotic fluid change with gestational age and are useful indicators of fetal maturity and well-being. Amniotic fluid samples are removed via amniocentesis, and the constituents are examined. Amniotic fluid contains cells from the amnion, fetal skin, buccal and bladder mucosa, and tracheal lining. Amniotic fluid cells can be examined early in pregnancy to determine fetal sex (important with sex-linked disorders) and to diagnose genetic and chromosomal disorders. Later, cellular and biochemical components of amniotic fluid can be used to evaluate fetal health and maturity (Table 2–7).

Genetic amniocentesis has traditionally been performed in most centers at 15 to 17 weeks (range, 14 to 20 weeks) (Fig. 2–22), since at this time amniotic fluid volume has reached 150 to 250 ml (so 20 to 30 ml can safely be removed), the uterus has reached the pelvic brim (so a transabdominal approach can be used), adequate fetal cells are available, diagnostic studies can be completed in time for a second trimester abortion (if that option is chosen by the parents), and the incidence of maternal and fetal complication (spotting, fluid leak, bleeding, infection, spontaneous abortion) is low (1 in 200).[217] Recent experiences in many centers with early amniocentesis at 9 to 14 weeks (Fig. 2–22) support the safety and reliability of this procedure.[78, 79] Amniotic fluid can be cultured for karyotype (to identify chromosomal abnormalities) or for biochemical assay (to identify specific inherited metabolic disorders); analyzed using DNA hybridization and restriction enzyme techniques (for detecting gene deletions that occur with disorders such as hemoglobinopathies); and analyzed for quantification of alpha-fetoprotein (screening for neural tube defects and other anomalies).[194, 264]

Chorionic Villus Sampling

Chorionic villus sampling (CVS) is an alternative to genetic amniocentesis that was first proposed about 20 years ago but was not

TABLE 2–7
Examples of Amniotic Fluid Values Used to Assess Fetal Status

VARIABLE MEASURED	RESULTS	IMPLICATIONS
Surfactants	Lecithin/sphingomyelin (L/S) ratio greater than or equal to 2:1 Phosphatidylglycerol (PG) and phosphatidylinositol (PI)*	Reduced incidence of respiratory distress syndrome Evidence of fetal lung maturity Reliability of these assessments may be reduced if samples are contaminated with blood or meconium or with the presence of polyhydramnios or maternal glucose intolerance
Bilirubin	Optical density of bilirubin (at 450 nm wavelength) of 0.01 at term	Altered with isoimmunization
Creatinine	2 mg/dl associated with a gestational age >37 weeks	Reflecting kidney development and fetal muscle mass May be altered with maternal renal disease, fetal anomalies, or dehydration
Cytology	20% or greater orange-staining cells	Presence of epithelial cells that contain or are coated with neutral lipids from fetal sebaceous glands (lipid-containing cells stain orange; other cells stain blue)

*See also Chapter 6.

practical until more recent improvement of ultrasound techniques.[217] CVS is generally performed 8 to 12 weeks after the last menstrual period (Fig. 2–22). Earlier, chorionic villi may not be well enough developed for adequate tissue sampling; later the chorion laeve is disappearing and the chorion frondosum is forming the definitive placenta.[34, 58, 200] A transcervical approach is used (be-cause the uterus is still in the pelvis) after the gestational sac and implantation site are located by ultrasound. Transabdominal approaches have also been used.

Living trophoblast tissue (15 to 30 mg) is aspirated from several sites on the chorion. This tissue can be analyzed for chromosome anomalies or with enzyme assay (for inborn errors of metabolism) or DNA analysis (he-

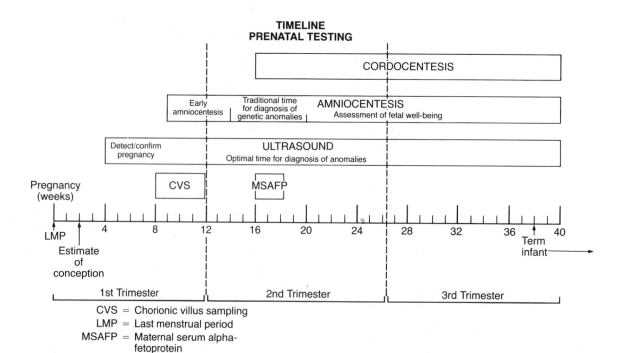

FIGURE 2–22. Timeline for prenatal testing. (Developed by Brock, K.A. (1990). University of Washington, Seattle.)

moglobinopathies).[200,250] Advantages of CVS include early diagnosis before the pregnancy is obvious to others and a decreased waiting period for results (<1 to 2 weeks versus 3 to 4 weeks with amniocentesis); disadvantages include a risk of spontaneous abortion, infection, bleeding and amniotic fluid leakage, uncertainty about long term effects on the infant, and inability to do alpha-fetoprotein assays for diagnosis of neural tube defects at this stage of gestation.[157, 214]

Umbilical Blood Sampling

Cordocentesis, or percutaneous umbilical blood sampling (PUBS), involves use of the umbilical cord to obtain fetal blood samples. Umbilical blood sampling has been used in the prenatal diagnosis of inherited blood disorders (hemoglobinopathies and coagulopathies), in detection of congenital infection, for rapid karyotyping of malformed fetuses, to assess fetal anemia (in Rh isoimmunization, thrombocytopenia), in evaluating acid-base status, and in fetal therapy (blood transfusion and injection of drugs such as digoxin).[58, 202] This technique is done using real-time ultrasound as early as 16 weeks after the last menstrual period (Fig. 2–22).[58] Complication rates of 0.5 to 1% have been reported.[58] Complications include infection, preterm labor, bleeding, thrombosis, and transient fetal arrhythmia.[71]

Alterations in Amniotic Fluid Volume

An understanding of the processes involved in the production of amniotic fluid and the pattern of fluid accumulation during pregnancy is necessary for assessing uterine growth and identifying women who need further evaluation. Alterations in production and removal of amniotic fluid can lead to polyhydramnios (hydramnios) or oligohydramnios.

Polyhydramnios

Polyhydramnios, or accumulation of more than 2 L of fluid in a single amniotic sac, can occur gradually during pregnancy or rapidly over a few days or weeks. Polyhydramnios is associated with maternal disease, multiple gestation, immune and nonimmune hydrops fetalis, Down syndrome and other chromo-

somal anomalies, and fetal gastrointestinal, cardiac, and neural tube anomalies.[40, 48] Essential polyhydramnios (i.e, due to no known cause) is thought to arise from an unexplained imbalance in water exchange between the fetus, mother, and amniotic fluid.[271]

Although multiple pregnancy frequently results in increased accumulation of amniotic fluid, in most cases this is not true polyhydramnios, since the fluid is distributed among several sacs, each sac containing usual amounts of fluid. An increased incidence of polyhydramnios has been reported in monozygotic monochorionic twins with arteriovenous anastomoses within their shared placenta and twin-to-twin transfusion syndrome. Development of polyhydramnios in these pregnancies may be the result of excessive urination, polycythemia, and transudation of fluids.[16, 197, 271] The elevated venous pressure and altered fluid dynamics seen with hydrops fetalis and some cardiovascular disorders may lead to excessive accumulation of amniotic fluid.[70] Polyhydramnios is more frequent in diabetic women, perhaps owing to fetal polyuria caused by fetal hyperglycemia or to alterations in osmotic gradients due to increased amniotic fluid glucose.[48]

Congenital anomalies are reported in 9 to 51% of pregnancies complicated by polyhydramnios.[48] Neural tube defects such as anencephaly and meningomyelocele may result in polyhydramnios owing to decreased fetal swallowing or transudation of fluid from the exposed meninges.[201, 222, 223, 238] Polyhydramnios associated with chromosomal anomalies may be related to reduced fetal swallowing and, in infants with Down syndrome, duodenal atresia. Although polyhydramnios is seen in most infants with esophageal or duodenal atresia (presumably owing to decreased fetal swallowing and decreased gut absorption), 2 to 10% of these pregnancies have normal amniotic fluid volume.[244, 271] The basis for this finding is unclear but suggests that amniotic fluid homeostasis is a very complex mechanism involving the interaction of many variables.

Oligohydramnios

Oligohydramnios (<500 ml at term or <50% of the usual accumulation of amniotic fluid at any stage of development) can occur at any time during gestation. Oligohydramnios is rarer than polyhydramnios and associated with amnion abnormalities, placental insufficiency, and fetal urinary anomalies.[33, 224] Oligohydramnios may lead to umbilical cord compression in labor and fetal distress.[154]

Inadequate amniotic fluid during labor can be due to premature rupture of the membranes, oligohydramnios, or early amniotomy.[143] A lack of adequate fluid removes the natural protective cushioning effect of this fluid and increases the risk of cord compression and variable fetal heart rate decelerations during contractions. These decelerations can sometimes be relieved by maternal position change and oxygen administration or by increasing amniotic fluid volume through intrauterine infusion of a saline solution (amnioinfusion).[91, 143]

Severe fetal renal anomalies (agenesis, dysplasia, or obstructive disorders) may lead to oligohydramnios because of decreased or no urine output. Bilateral renal agenesis in conjunction with pulmonary hypoplasia, musculoskeletal abnormalities, and a characteristic facies is known as Potter's syndrome and is associated with oligohydramnios. Several of the findings in Potter's syndrome may be deformation defects arising from lack of amniotic fluid.[135]

Movement produced by fetal muscular activity is an integral component of normal morphologic development. Mechanical forces can lead to defects either from intrinsic forces (such as fetal myoneuropathy, development of an organ in an abnormal and too small site, or alterations in the normal flow or volume of body fluids) or from external forces (such as a bicornate uterus, fibromas, or oligohydramnios) that interfere with fetal mobility.[188]

The constraints on fetal movement imposed by oligohydramnios can result in a cascade of developmental events resulting in fetal anomalies. These anomalies include congenital contracture (due to relative or complete immobilization of the joints in a confined space); lung hypoplasia (lack of room for development of the thorax and for the subsequent stretch or distention of lung tissue required for normal lung growth); shortened umbilical cord (length is related to fetal activity); dysmorphic facies including micrognathia, low set ears, small alae nasi, and hypertelorism (molding of the face by compressive forces); growth retardation (fetal motor activity seems important for normal development of muscle mass and weight gain); perhaps microgastria (lack of stretching and distention since the volume of amniotic fluid available for swallowing is reduced); and "loose" skin (stretched by the constrained fetus' attempts to move).[184, 187, 189, 190, 256] This sequence has been termed the fetal akinesia/hypokinesia deformation sequence (Fig. 2–23).[256]

Oligohydramnios is often associated with amnion nodosum. In this disorder yellow-gray nodules or plaques consisting of desquamated fetal epidermal cells, hair, and vernix are found in and on the amnion and on the placental surface (fetal side). This debris is probably pressed into the amnion by close approximation of the fetal skin and amnion in the presence of oligohydramnios.[271] Oligohydramnios may also occur with IUGR (owing to decreased urine flow rates) or with prolonged pregnancy.[3, 154]

Abnormalities of the Cord and Placenta

Abnormalities of the cord and placenta arise from alterations in implantation and placentation or from disorders of the trophoblast. Occasionally these abnormalities may have minimal effect on the fetus and the outcome of the pregnancy; more often, serious and sometimes fatal conditions develop so that the pregnancy cannot be maintained and is terminated early or fetal development and survival are threatened. At times maternal survival and reproductive function may also be compromised.

Abnormalities of Implantation and Separation

The major abnormalities of implantation and separation of the placenta are placenta previa, abruptio placentae, and placenta accreta. Placenta previa is implantation of the placenta over or near the internal cervical os so that it encroaches on a portion of the dilated cervix.[214] Placenta previa may be classified as total, partial, or marginal; low-lying placentas are sometimes included in this classification. Various theories have been proposed to explain the pathogenesis of placenta previa including defective vascularization of the endometrium, alteration of the normal ovum transport mechanism, and development of the placenta in the decidua capsularis.[224, 227]

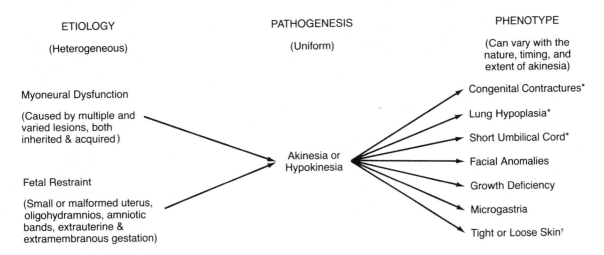

ETIOLOGY	PATHOGENESIS	PHENOTYPE
(Heterogeneous)	(Uniform)	(Can vary with the nature, timing, and extent of akinesia)

Myoneural Dysfunction

(Caused by multiple and varied lesions, both inherited & acquired)

Fetal Restraint

(Small or malformed uterus, oligohydramnios, amniotic bands, extrauterine & extramembranous gestation)

Akinesia or Hypokinesia

Congenital Contractures*

Lung Hypoplasia*

Short Umbilical Cord*

Facial Anomalies

Growth Deficiency

Microgastria

Tight or Loose Skin†

*This can lead to perinatal asphyxia and thus compound neurologic status.

†The skin tends to be tight and thin with myoneural dysfunction and loose with abundant folds in the case of fetal restraint.

FIGURE 2–23. The fetal akinesia/hypokinesia deformation sequence. (From Moessinger, A.C. (1989). Morphological consequences of depressed or impaired fetal activity. (From W.P. Smotherman & S.R. Robinson (Eds.), *Behavior of the fetus* (pp 163–173). Caldwell, NJ: Telford Press.)

If the blastocyst implants in endometrium that is poorly vascularized owing to atrophic or inflammatory changes, the placenta may develop a larger decidual surface area to compensate for an inadequate blood supply and grow downward into the lower uterine segment.[214, 224] If vascularization of the endometrium in the upper uterine segment is poor, the blastocyst may continue to descend, implanting by chance in healthier endometrium in the lower uterine segment. Altered transport of the blastocyst due to abnormal uterine motility, deviations in the size or shape of the uterine cavity, or fluid in the cavity can also result in displacement of the blastocyst to the lower uterus.[224] A scar from a previous cesarean section also predisposes to later placental previa.[203]

Normally the chorionic villi initially surround the entire embryo but later degenerate beneath the decidua capsularis forming the chorion laeve. By 4 months, the growing fetus fills the uterine cavity and the decidua capsularis fuses with the decidua vera (see Fig. 2–8). If chorionic villi near the lower uterus fail to degenerate as the decidua capsularis fuses with the decidua vera, these villi can become incorporated into the placenta and impinge on the lower uterine segment.[224,233]

Abruptio placentae is separation of a normally implanted placenta prior to the delivery of the fetus. Abruptio placentae is initiated by hemorrhage into the decidua basalis with formation of a hematoma that leads to separation and compression of the adjacent portion of the placenta. Hemorrhage may develop secondary to degenerative changes in the arteries supplying the intervillous space, with thrombosis, degeneration of the decidua, and vessel rupture with formation of a retroplacental hemorrhage.[214] The primary cause of placental abruption is unknown. Possible causes include maternal hypertension (secondary to essential hypertension, pregnancy-induced hypertension, chronic renal disease, or cocaine use), compression or occlusion of the inferior vena cava, circumvallate placenta, or trauma.[214] The incidence of abruptio placentae is markedly increased with maternal cocaine and crack use.[51] These drugs induce vasoconstriction of placental blood vessels and a sudden elevation in maternal blood pressure.

Placenta accreta is a general term used to describe any placental implantation in which there is abnormally firm adherence of the placenta to the uterine wall. As a result, there is partial or total absence of the decidua basalis and attachment of the placental villi to the fibrinoid (Nitabuch's) layer or to the myometrium. Occasionally the villi invade the myometrium (placenta increta) or penetrate through the myometrial wall (placenta percreta). Placenta accreta usually occurs when decidual formation is defective, such as with implantation over uterine scars or in the lower uterine segment. Placenta accreta is often associated with placenta previa and with significant morbidity including severe hemorrhage, uterine perforation, infection, and hysterectomy.[224]

Abnormalities of Placentation

The size and configuration of the placenta are influenced by the degree of vascularization of the decidua and the number and arrangement of the primitive villi that later comprise the fetal portion of the placenta.[224, 233] The major clinically significant abnormalities of placental configuration result in circumvallate, marginate, or succenturiate placentas.

With circumvallate placenta, the area of the chorionic plate is reduced. As chorionic villi invade the decidua, the fetal membranes fold back upon themselves, creating a dense, grayish-white raised ring encircling the central portion of the fetal surface. The fetal vessels forming the cord stop at this ring rather than covering the entire fetal surface of the placenta. The risk of abruptio placenta is increased with circumvallate placentas.[214] Marginate (or circumarginate) placenta also arises from a chorionic plate that is smaller than the basal plate. In these placentas the white ring composed of the fetal membranes coincides with the margin of the placenta, without the folding back of the membranes seen in circumvallate placentas.

The etiology of circumvallate and marginate placentas is uncertain, although partial or complete forms are seen in up to 25% of gestations.[276] Possible causes include subchorial infarcts, formation of insufficient chorion frondosum, and an abnormally deep implantation of the blastocyst causing part of the fetal surface to be covered by the decidua vera. These placentas are often asymptomatic, but complete forms have been linked to threatened abortion, preterm labor, painless vaginal bleeding after 20 weeks, placental insufficiency, and intrapartum and postpartum hemorrhage.[86, 217, 224, 233, 176]

Succenturiate placenta involves development of one or more smaller accessory lobes in the membranes that are attached to the main placenta by fetal vessels. This abnormality arises when a group of villi distant to the main placenta fail to degenerate, implan-

tation is superficial, or implantation occurs in a confined site (such as a bicornate uterus) so that attachment of the trophoblast also occurs on the opposing wall.[217] The accessory lobes may be retained, leading to postpartum hemorrhage or infection.[214, 233] These placentas are often associated with malrotation of the implanting blastocyst with velamentous insertion of the cord.[217]

Abnormalities of the Umbilical Cord

The umbilical cord may develop knots, loops, torsion or strictures. These alterations are associated with increased fetal mortality and morbidity.[86, 151] Excessively long cords (>100 cm) are more likely to develop knots, torsion, or prolapse. Abnormally short cords (<30 to 32 cm) are associated with asphyxia at birth owing to traction on the cord with fetal descent.[276] A single umbilical artery occurs in 1 in 200 newborns and probably arises from agenesis or degeneration of the missing vessel early in gestation. This anomaly is associated with a 15 to 20% incidence of fetal cardiovascular anomalies.[214]

Battledore placenta, or insertion of the cord at or near the margin of the placenta, may be clinically benign but has been linked to preterm labor, fetal distress, and bleeding in labor due to cord compression or vessel rupture. With velamentous insertion, the cord inserts into the membranes so that the vessels run between the amnion and chorion before entering into the placenta. These variations in insertion of the cord probably arise at the time of implantation.

Normally the blastocyst implants with the inner cell mass adjacent to the endometrium and the trophoblast that will form the placenta. The body stalk, which will become the cord, aligns with the center of the placenta. Rotation of the inner cell mass (and body stalk) gives rise to eccentric insertions of the cord. The degree of rotation will influence how far the umbilical cord will be from the center of the placenta (i.e., eccentric, marginal, or velamentous). Velamentous insertion may lead to rupture and fetal hemorrhage associated with a high fetal mortality, particularly with vasa praevia (when the fetal vessels are located along the lower uterine segment, crossing the internal cervical os, and presenting ahead of the fetus).[224, 276]

Gestational Trophoblastic Disease

Gestational trophoblastic disease includes hydatidiform mole and gestational trophoblastic tumors (derived from neoplastic hyperplastic changes).[181] Both forms of trophoblastic disease are associated with markedly elevated levels of hCG.[124, 251] Hydatidiform moles result from deterioration of the chorionic villi into a mass of clear vesicles. Histologically, hydatidiform mole is characterized by hyperplasia of the syncytiotrophoblast and the cytotrophoblast, edema of the avascular villous stroma, and cystic cavitations within the villous stroma. The villi become converted into molar cysts connected to each other by fibrous strands.[224] There may be no fetus (complete mole) or the remains of a degenerating fetus or amniotic sac (partial or incomplete mole). Rarely the fetus in an incomplete molar pregnancy survives to delivery.[181]

The karyotype of a complete mole is 46,XX and is thought to be derived from duplication of a haploid X-carrying (23,X) sperm. This mole is androgenic in origin, i.e., the ovum develops under the influence of a spermatozoon nucleus. The nucleus of the ovum is inactivated or lost prior to fertilization. A complete mole is associated with increased risk of choriocarcinoma.

In an incomplete mole the hydatidiform changes are focal, i.e., there is slowly progressive swelling of some villi (which are usually avascular), while other vascular villi develop with a functioning fetoplacental circulation.[224] The karyotype of this type of mole is usually triploid (69,XXX, 69,XXY, or 69,XYY). An incomplete mole results from fertilization of a normal haploid ovum (23,X) by two haploid sperm (dispermy) or a single diploid sperm.[181, 259] A third type involves heterozygous diploid fertilization of an empty ovum with two haploid sperm (46,XX or 46,XY). This form of mole is associated with an increased risk of gestational trophoblastic tumors.[181]

MULTIPLE PREGNANCY

The incidence of twins in the United States is 10 in 1000 deliveries, with other forms of multiple births seen less frequently.[126] The arrangement of membranes and placentas in twin and other multiple pregnancies is determined by the type twin and the stage of gestation at which twinning occurs. Multiple gestations can be detected by ultrasound as early as 6 to 8 weeks and reliably by 8 to 12 weeks. Approximately one-third of multiple gestations detected before 20 weeks result in birth of only one fetus owing to death of the other embryo(s) and reabsorption of the gestational sac or fetus.[169]

There are basically two types of twins, monozygotic (arising from division of a single ovum after fertilization) and dizygotic (simultaneous fertilization of two ova enclosed within a single follicle or theca, or ovulation of two ova from one or both ovaries that are then fertilized independently). Most (70%) twins are dizygotic. A third type has been proposed, with simultaneous fertilization of an ovum and its polar body by two sperm; but this is not well documented.[16, 147] This section focuses on twins, since higher order multiple pregnancies (triplets, quadruplets, etc.) can be monozygotic, dizygotic, or multizygotic, with attributes that are variations of findings characteristic of twins.

Twin zygosity cannot be determined solely on the number of placentas. Examinations to determine zygosity often require morphologic examination of the chorion, amnion, and yolk sac as well as evaluation of infant characteristics. Placentas and membranes of twins and other multiple births should always be saved and sent to pathology for accurate morphologic analysis.[21, 23]

Monozygotic (MZ) twins may have one or two placentas (which may be separate or fused). The placentas and membranes of MZ twins may be monochorionic-monoamnionic, monochorionic-diamnionic, or dichorionic-diamnionic (fused or separate). With higher order multiple births, placentas and membranes may also be multichorionic-multiamnionic. While dizygotic (DZ) twins always have two dichorionic-diamnionic placentas, the placentas may be fused and appear to be single. Fused placentas increase the risk of growth retardation in one or both infants, owing to competition for space, and abnormal cord insertions.[27] Potter calculated that about 80% of twins could be differentiated according to zygosity (i.e., as monozygotic or dizygotic) at or shortly after birth as follows (percentages are approximate): (1) 23% were monochorionic and therefore the infants monozygotic; (2) 30% were dichorionic with a male and female twin who therefore must be dizygotic; and (3) 27% were same sex twins but with different blood types and thus dizygotic.[221] The remaining 20% were same sex twins with similar blood types who were either MZ twins with dichorionic placentas (either separate or fused) or DZ twins of the same sex (with separate or fused placentas). Determination of the zygosity of these twins requires more intensive investigation such as tissue typing, enzymatic studies, dermatoglyphics, or DNA mapping.

Perinatal mortality is 3 to 11 times higher in twins than in singletons.[126] This risk is affected by zygosity and placental and membrane characteristics.[177, 209] For example, mortality is 2 to 3 times higher in monochorionic as in dichorionic (either DZ or MZ) twins.[22, 101, 177] Monochorionic twins tend to weigh less and are more frequently growth retarded in utero than are dichorionic twins.[76, 101] The incidence of congenital anomalies is higher in MZ twins than in DZ twins.[152, 195] Structural defects in MZ twins may arise from deformations due to limited intrauterine space, disruption of blood flow due to placental vascular anastomoses, or localized defects in early morphogenesis.[177, 241]

Monozygotic Twins

Monozygotic (MZ) twins occur in 3.5 to 4 in 1000 births.[147] The rate of MZ twinning is relatively constant worldwide and probably represents an accident in embryonic development. The etiology of this form of twins is unknown, although it has been proposed that MZ embryos arise from a delay in implantation secondary to adverse environmental conditions such as inadequate nutrition or oxygen deprivation.[25, 45, 165] MZ twinning can occur at three different stages of development: (1) during the early blastomere stage, (2) during formation of the inner cell mass, and (3) with development of the embryonic disc.[54] The stage of development determines the number of placentas and arrangement of membranes.

Separation of the ovum during the early blastomere stage usually occurs about 2 days after fertilization while the blastomere is in the 2- to 4-cell stage (Fig. 2–24). Since this is prior to differentiation of any cells, the two blastomeres will develop independently into morulae, blastocysts, and embryos, each with separate placentas, chorions, and amnions (dichorionic-diamnionic). These blastocysts will implant at separate sites. If these sites are close together the placentas may fuse. Membranes separating the embryos will contain the amnion-chorion of infant 1 and the chorion-amnion of infant 2 separated by their fused placentas.[16] This arrangement of infants, placentas, and membranes, which is identical to that of same sex DZ twins, requires blood typing, tissue typing, and other analyses to determine zygosity.

Separation and duplication of the inner cell mass during development of the blastocyst 4 to 7 days after fertilization give rise to the most common form of MZ twins (Fig. 2–24). The trophoblast layer that will become the placenta and chorion has already formed in the blastocyst prior to separation of the inner cell mass. The amnion and amniotic cavity, however, have not yet begun to form and will develop independently in each embryo. Thus this form of twinning is monochorionic-diamnionic with a single placenta. The membranes separating the embryos consist of two layers of amnion and one chorion. The placenta of these infants is larger than the placenta found with a single infant but smaller than two single placentas. These placentas have an increased frequency of abnormal configurations and cord attachments.[16]

Less frequently, twinning occurs owing to separation and duplication of the rudimentary embryonic disc with appearance of two embryonic nodes instead of one at 7 to 15 (possibly up to 17 days) after fertilization.[16, 54] Since the placenta, chorion, and amnion have all formed at this time, these twins are monochorionic-monoamnionic (Fig. 2–24). Monochorionic-monoamnionic infants account for only 1 to 2% of all MZ twins.[16] Perinatal mortality rate for this type of twins is 30 to 50% owing to twisting, knotting, and entanglement of the two umbilical cords within the single amniotic sac.[22, 86, 196] If this form of twinning occurs at 7 to 13½ days, two separate embryos are formed (Fig. 2–24).

Separation after 13½ days is usually incomplete, i.e., the embryonic disc divides but remains united at one or more points (fission theory), resulting in the formation of conjoined twins. Conjoined twins have also been suggested to arise after normal division of the embryonic disc into two cell masses that subsequently abut and join together (collision theory). Conjoined twins account for 1 in 2500 MZ twins.[16] The most common areas of fusion (either singularly or in combination) are the thorax, abdomen, and umbilical cord.

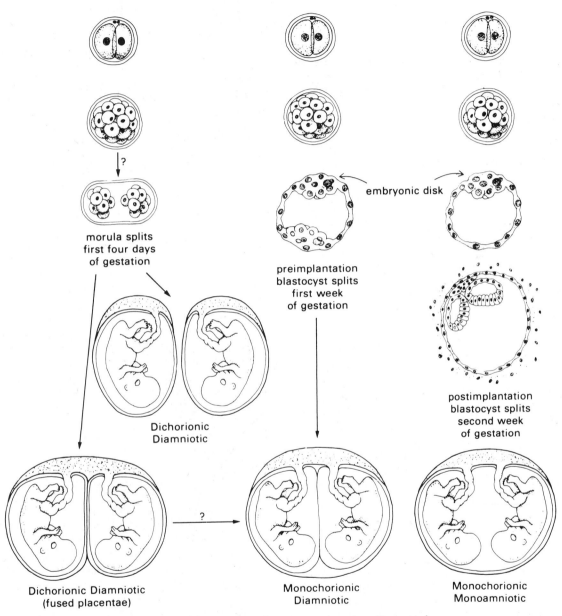

FIGURE 2–24. Development and placentation of monozygotic twins. (From Hafez, E.S.E. (Ed.). (1980). *Human reproduction: Conception and contraception* (2nd ed., p. 447). Hagerstown, MD: Harper & Row.)

Dizygotic Twins

The incidence of dizygotic (DZ) twins varies markedly among different racial groups ranging from 1 in 20 to 25 births in certain Nigerian tribal groups to 1 in 100 in Caucasian populations and 1 in 150 in Japanese women.[164] The incidence of DZ twinning is also influenced by a variety of endocrine, endogenous, exogenous, and iatrogenic (administration of gonadotropins for treatment of infertility) factors. DZ twinning has a strong maternal familial tendency. For example, the incidence of twins in female relatives of mothers of twins is 19% versus 10.7% among female relatives of fathers of twins.[16] Endocrine factors suggested in the etiology of DZ twins usually relate to increased levels of follicle-stimulating hormone (FSH) with overstimulation of the ovaries leading to release of more than one ovum.[208] Endogenous factors associated with an increased incidence of DZ twinning include increased parity, maternal age (peaking at 37 years), maternal height and weight (perhaps related to nutrition), and increased frequency of intercourse.[25, 44, 126, 133, 165, 207] Since DZ twins arise from separate ova, they have separate placentas, chorions and amnions (dichorionic-diamnionic), although their placentas may fuse if implanted close to each other (Fig. 2–25).

Placental Abnormalities in Multiple Gestations

Bardawil and colleagues categorize pathologic placental lesions associated with multiple gestation into four groups: (1) specific pathology directly due to the twinning process (conjoined twins, acardiac or amorphous fetuses, and vascular anastomoses); (2) pathologic lesions or conditions that arise as a consequence of group 1 lesions (entanglement of umbilical cords in monoamnionic twins, twin-to-twin transfusion, polyhydramnios, amnion nodosum, chimera in DZ twins); (3) lesions related to physical problems of accommodation due to decreased intrauterine space (circumvallate changes, velamentous or marginal cord insertion, vasa praevia); and (4) incidental lesions that can occur in any placenta and are not related to twinning per se.[16] Vascular lesions are described below, other lesions were discussed earlier in this chapter.

Vascular connections or anastomoses occur in 85 to 90% of the common placenta shared by monochorionic twins.[28, 258] Anastomoses in dichorionic fused placentas are rare (1 in 1000) but may account for chimerism in DZ twins. There have been no reports of vascular anastomoses in separate placentas.[16] Chimerism is uncommon but may complicate the determination of zygosity. The chimerous twin carries within its system genetically dissimilar blood or tissue from its fraternal twin. Movement of material from one twin to the other is thought to involve transfer of precursor blood cells or other immature cells through vascular communication during early stages of gestation when the fetal immune system is poorly developed. In chimerism, the recipient twin becomes tolerant of the foreign blood cells or tissue.[2, 16, 147, 265]

Placental vascular anastomoses can be arterial-arterial, venous-arterial, arterial-venous or venous-venous. The most common, artery-to-artery, are thought to be inconsequential.[16] Significant problems can arise with arterial-venous anastomoses. This type of anastomosis can lead to an imbalance in blood flow and development of fetal acardia and other anomalies or twin-to-twin transfusion. Arterial-venous anastomoses usually occur in a shared lobe supplied by an umbilical artery of one twin and drained by the umbilical vein of the other (Fig. 2–26).[276] Thus, a portion of the blood reentering the placenta from one fetus drains into the placental venous system of the second fetus (sometimes called the "third circulation"). The vascular flow is unidirectional and unless compensated by anastomoses in the opposite direction or other artery-to-artery anastomoses will result in a hydrodynamic imbalance.[16, 27]

Twin-to-twin transfusion syndrome which is seen in about 30% of MZ twins, may result from arterial-venous anastomoses.[20, 258] A difference in hemoglobin of 5 g/dl between infants is thought to indicate a significant transfusion.[210] The donor twin is smaller and anemic and may develop congestive heart failure; the larger, recipient twin is polycythemic and often hyperbilirubinemic and may develop hyperviscosity syndrome and disseminated intravascular coagulation.[35] Although vascular anastomoses are frequent and extensive in monochorionic-monoamnionic twins, especially in those with closely implanted umbilical cords, twin-to-twin transfusion syndrome is rare in this type of MZ twin. This finding may be because the anas-

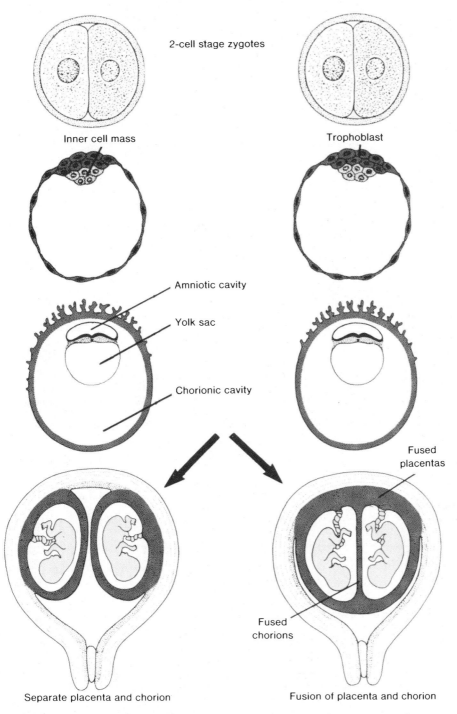

2-cell stage zygotes

Inner cell mass

Trophoblast

Amniotic cavity

Yolk sac

Chorionic cavity

Fused placentas

Fused chorions

Separate placenta and chorion

Fusion of placenta and chorion

FIGURE 2–25. Development and placentation of dizygotic twins. (From Sadler, T.W. (1985). *Langman's medical embryology* (5th ed., p. 104). Baltimore: Williams & Wilkins.)

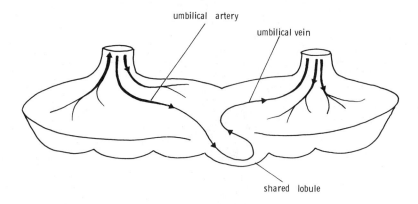

umbilical artery

umbilical vein

shared lobule

FIGURE 2–26. Vascular anastomoses in shared placental lobules with twin-to-twin transfusion. (From Wigglesworth, J.S. (1984). *Perinatal pathology* (p. 58). Philadelphia: WB Saunders.)

TABLE 2–8
Summary of Recommendations for Clinical Practice Related to the Prenatal Period and Placental Physiology

Counsel women regarding physical and physiologic changes during pregnancy (pp. 37–40, Chapters 5–17).
Provide counseling and health teaching to women and couples using alternative treatment modalities to conceive (pp. 45–48).
Recognize ethical issues related to reproductive technology (pp. 45–48).
Provide emotional support, counseling, and health teaching to couples with recurrent pregnancy loss (pp. 48–49).
Understand the basic processes involved in embryonic and fetal development (pp. 49–59, Table 2–1, Fig. 2–7).
Provide teaching to families regarding embryonic and fetal development at each stage of gestation (pp. 49–59).
Recognize critical periods of development and principles of teratogenesis (pp. 49–59, 60–63, Figure 2–7).
Recognize risks associated with fetal exposure to drugs and other environmental agents during pregnancy (pp. 60–63, Table 2–3).
Provide appropriate counseling and health teaching to promote optimal fetal development and health (pp. 49–50, 60–63, 84–86).
Provide counseling and health teaching to reduce exposure of the fetus to adverse environmental influences (pp. 60–63, Table 2–6).
Counsel women regarding use of drugs or exposure to other environmental agents during pregnancy (pp. 60–63, 86, Table 2–6).
Recognize and monitor women at risk for ectopic pregnancy (p. 64).
Understand the usual patterns of hCG production and counsel women regarding home pregnancy testing (pp. 64, 75, Figure 2–16).
Understand the basis for and counsel women regarding administration of low dose estrogen to prevent implantation (p. 64).
Provide health teaching regarding placental development and growth during gestation (pp. 63–70).
Recognize and monitor for factors that can alter placental growth and development or lead to pregnancy loss (pp. 69–70, 83–89).
Understand the dynamics of placental function throughout gestation and factors influencing transfer (pp. 74–81, 84–86).
Recognize and monitor for factors that can alter maternal-fetal-placental circulation (pp. 71–74).
Recognize the potential effects of maternal disorders on placental function and fetal development (pp. 70–74, 84–87).
Monitor fetal growth and development (pp. 61–63, 70–74, 84–86).
Monitor fetal growth and oxygenation in the woman with a postdate pregnancy (pp. 70, 88).
Assess maternal and fetal responses to compromised placental function (pp. 88–91).
Identify fetal risk situations during the ante- and intrapartum periods related to alterations in placental function (pp. 70–74, 83–88).
Understand endocrine functions of the placenta and interaction of the maternal-fetal-placental unit (pp. 75–78, 88–89, Figure 2–22).
Understand the rationale for fetal assessment tests (pp. 88–91).
Counsel women regarding the effects of estrogen and progesterone on body function and structure (pp. 76–78).
Recognize factors that may alter composition, production and removal of amniotic fluid (pp. 83–84, 91–92).
Monitor infants with a history of maternal polyhydramnios for congenital defects (p. 91).
Monitor infants with a history of maternal oligohydramnios for congenital anomalies and growth retardation (pp. 91–92).
Know implications of placental, umbilical cord, and trophoblastic disorders, and monitor at risk women and their infants (pp. 92–95).
Teach women who have experienced a multiple birth regarding the basis for development of monozygotic and dizygotic twins (or triplets, etc.) and implications of the arrangements of placentas and membranes (pp. 95–98).
Recognize and monitor for fetal and neonatal effects of placental abnormalities with monozygotic twins (p. 98).

Page numbers in parentheses following each intervention refer to the pages where the rationale for the intervention is discussed.

tomoses are so extensive there is no net hydrodynamic imbalance.[16, 28]

Placental vascular anastomoses can also be present between a living and a dead twin with subsequent passage of thromboplastic substances to the living twin. These substances can initiate intravascular coagulation, thrombosis, infarction, necrosis, alterations in organ function, and death.[177] Vascular abnormalities have been suggested as a cause for development of acardia or amorphous fetuses (shapeless mass of necrotic tissue and fibrin).[27, 241, 267] This anomaly likely arises in association with large artery-to-artery and vein-to-vein anastomoses. If pressure in the umbilical artery of the normal twin exceeds that in the artery of the other twin, circulation in the recipient twin may be reversed (i.e., blood flows to the twin via the umbilical arteries and returns to a large placental vein-to-vein anastomosis via the umbilical artery). The resultant low perfusion pressure, poor oxygenation, and circulatory reversal lead to development of multiple severe structural defects.[177] The abnormal twin continues to develop only if there is perfusion by the normal twin, who may subsequently develop cardiac hypertrophy, congestive heart failure, and hydrops fetalis.[177]

SUMMARY

The respiratory, nutritive, and endocrinologic functions of the placenta are critical for fetal growth and development and pregnancy outcome. A major component of nursing care for women with normal, at risk, and complicated pregnancies is providing appropriate counseling and health teaching to promote optimal fetal development and health and to prevent exposure of the fetus to adverse environmental influences. In order to accomplish this goal and to assess maternal and fetal responses to compromised placental function and identify fetal risk situations during the antepartum and intrapartum periods, the nurse must understand the factors influencing transfer of substances across the placenta. An understanding of endocrine functions and interactions of the maternal-fetal-placental unit provides a basis for assessing, monitoring, and teaching pregnant women undergoing various tests for clinical assessment of placental function and fetal well-being. Recommendations for nursing interventions are summarized in Table 2–8.

REFERENCES

1. Abramovich, D.R. (1979). Amniotic fluid. In R. Shearman (Ed.), *Human reproductive physiology*. Oxford: Blackwell.
2. Abramovich, D.R. (1981). Interrelation of fetus and amniotic fluid. *Obstet Gynecol Annu, 10*, 27.
3. Abramovich, D.R. et al. (1979). Fetal swallowing and voiding in relation to hydramnios. *Obstet Gynecol, 54*, 15.
4. Adams, F.H. et al. (1967). Control of flow of fetal lung fluid at the laryngeal outlet. *Respir Physiol, 2*, 202.
5. Adamson, E.G. (1983). Growth factors in development. In J.B. Warshaw (Ed.), *The biological basis of reproductive and developmental medicine* (pp. 307–336). New York: Elsevier Biomedical.
6. Adamsons, K. & Myres, R.E. (1975). Circulation in the intervillous space: Obstetrical considerations in fetal deprivation. In P. Gruenwald (Ed.), *The placenta and its maternal supply line* (pp. 158–177). Lancaster, England: Medical and Technical Publ.
7. Ahmed, A.G. & Klopper, A. (1983). Diagnosis of early pregnancy by assay of placental proteins. *Br J Obstet Gynaecol, 90*, 604.
8. Ahmed, A.G. & Klopper, A. (1985). Early fetal signals: Schwangerschaftsprotein 1 and human chorionic gonadotropin. In C.T. Jones & P.W. Nathanielsz (Eds.), *The physiological development of the fetus and newborn* (pp. 83–87). Orlando, FL: Academic Press.
9. Ahokas, R.A. & Anderson, G.D. (1987). The placenta as an organ of nutrition. In J.P. Lavery (Ed.), *The human placenta: Clinical perspectives* (pp. 207–220). Rockville, MD: Aspen.
10. Ariel, I.B. & Landing, B.H. (1985). A possibly distinctive vascular change of the amniotic epithelium associated with gastroschisis. *Pediatr Pathol, 2*, 283.
11. Armentrout, T. et al. (1977). Osmotic flow through the placental barrier of chronically prepared sheep. *Am J Physiol, 233*, H466.
12. Artal, R. & Brar, H.S. (1987). Tests of placental function. In J.P. Lavery (Ed.), *The human placenta: Clinical perspectives* (pp. 221–235). Rockville, MD: Aspen.
13. Asch, R.H. (1984). GIFT gamete intrafallopian transfer. Randolph, MA: Serono Symposia.
14. Asch, R.H. et al. (1986). Preliminary experiences with gamete intrafallopian transfer. *Fertil Steril, 40*, 53.
15. Bacz, A. (1987). The early pregnancy: A role of the male factor. *Eur J Obstet Gynecol Reprod Biol, 24*, 126.
16. Bardawil, W.A., Reddy, R.L., & Bardawil, L.W. (1988). Placental considerations in multiple pregnancy. *Clin Perinatol, 15*, 130.
17. Battaglia, F. (1982). New facts about fetal and placental metabolism. *Contemp Obstet Gynecol, 19*, 189.
18. Beck, W. (1982). Artificial insemination. *Postgrad Obstet Gynecol, 2*, 1.
19. Bedford, J.M. (1982). Fertilization. In C.R. Austin & R.V. Short (Eds.), *Reproduction in mammals: Germ cells and fertilization* (2nd ed.). Cambridge: Cambridge University Press.
20. Benirschke, K. (1958). Placental membranes in twins. *Obstet Gynecol Surv, 13*, 88.

21. Benirschke, K. (1961). Examination of the placenta. *Obstet Gynecol, 18*, 309.

22. Benirschke, K. (1961). Twin placenta in perinatal mortality. *NY State J Med, 61*, 1499.

23. Benirschke, K. (1961). Accurate recording of twin placentation. *Obstet Gynecol, 18*, 334.

24. Benirschke, K. (1970). Spontaneous chimerism in mammals: A critical review. *Curr Top Pathol, 51*, 1.

25. Benirschke, K. & Kim, C.K. (1973). Multiple pregnancy. *N Engl J Med, 288*, 1276.

26. Benirschke, K. (1987). Placental pathology. In A.A. Fanaroff & R.J. Martin (Eds.), *Neonatal-perinatal medicine—Diseases of the fetus and infant* (pp. 156–165). St. Louis: CV Mosby.

27. Benirschke, K. (1990). The placenta in twin gestation. *Clin Obstet Gynecol, 33*, 18.

28. Benirschke, K. & Driscoll, S.G. (1967). *The pathology of the human placenta*. New York: Springer-Verlag.

29. Bernfield, M.R. (1975). Developmental mechanisms of congenital anomalies. In *Biological and clinical aspects of malformations*. Mead Johnson Symposium on Perinatal and Developmental Medicine, No. 7. Evansville, IN: Mead Johnson.

30. Bernfield, M. (1983). Mechanisms of congenital malformations. In J.B. Warshaw (Ed.), *The biological basis of reproductive and developmental medicine*. New York: Elsevier Biomedical.

31. Bieber, F.R. & Driscoll, S.G. (1989). Evaluation of spontaneous abortion and of the malformed fetus. In G.B. Reed & A.E. Claireaux (Eds.), *Diseases of the fetus and newborn: Pathology, radiology, and genetics*. St. Louis: CV Mosby.

32. Bissonnette, J. (1981). Placenta transfer of carbohydrates. In *Placental Transport* (pp. 21–24), Mead Johnson Symposium on Perinatal and Developmental Medicine, No. 18. Evansville, IN: Mead Johnson.

33. Bolognese, R.J. & Roberts, N. (1982). Amniotic fluid. In R.J. Bolognese, R. H. Schwartz, & J. Schneider (Eds.), *Perinatal medicine* (pp. 184–211). Baltimore: Williams and Wilkins.

Blackmore, K.J. (1988). Prenatal diagnosis by CVS. *Obstet Gynecol Clin North Am, 15*, 179.

35. Blanchette, V. & Zipursky, A. (1987). Hematologic Problems In G.B. Avery (Ed.), *Neonatology* (pp. 638–688). Philadelphia: JB Lippincott.

36. Bleker, O.P. et al. (1975). Intervillous space during uterine contractions in human studies: An ultrasonic study. *Am J Obstet Gynecol, 123*, 697.

37. Boue, J., Boue, A., & Lazar, P. (1975). Retrospective and prospective epidemiological studies of 1500 karyotypes from spontaneous human abortions. *Teratology, 12*, 11.

38. Bourne, G.L. (1966). The anatomy of the amnion and chorion. *Proc Roy Soc Med, 59*, 1128.

39. Boyd, P.A. (1984). Quantitative structure of the human placenta from ten weeks of gestation until to term. *Early Hum Dev, 9*, 297.

40. Boylan, P. & Parisi, V (1986). An overview of hydramnios. *Semin Perinatol, 10*, 136.

41. Brace, R.A. (1986). Amniotic fluid volume and its relationship to fetal fluid balance: Review of experimental data. *Semin Perinatol, 10*, 103.

42. Brody, S.A. (1989). Endocrinology of postdate pregnancy. In S.A. Brody & K. Ueland (Eds.), *Endocrine disorders in pregnancy* (pp. 99–110). Norwalk, CT: Appleton & Lange.

43. Brosens, I., Robertson, W.B., & Dixon, G. (1972). The role of the spiral arteries in the pathogenesis of pre-eclampsia. *Obstet Gynecol Annu, 1*, 177.

44. Bulmer, M.G. (1959). The effect of parental age, parity and duration of marriage on the twinning rate. *Ann Hum Genet, 23*, 454.

45. Bulmer, M.G. (1970). *The biology of twinning in man*. Oxford: Clarendon Press.

46. Buster, J.E. & Sauer, M.V. (1989). Endocrinology of conception. In S.A. Brody & K. Ueland K (Eds.), *Endocrine disorders in pregnancy*. Norwalk, CT: Appleton & Lange.

47. Byrd, J.R., Askew, W.E., & McDonough, P.G. (1977). Cytogenetic findings in fifty-five couples with recurrent fetal wastage. *Fertil Steril, 28*, 519.

48. Cardwell, M.S. (1987). Polyhydramnios: A review. *Obstet Gynecol Surv, 42*, 612.

49. Castellucci, M., Zacchero, D., & Pescetto, G. (1980). A three-dimensional study of the normal human placental villous core. I. The Hofbauer cell. *Cell Tissue Res, 210*, 235.

50. Chard, T. (1987). What is happening to placental function tests. *Ann Clin Biochem, 24*, 435.

51. Chasnoff, I.J. et al. (1985). Cocaine use in pregnancy. *N Engl J Med, 313*, 666.

52. Clapp, J.F. (1982). The effects of maternal exercise during pregnancy on uterine blood flow and pregnancy outcome. In A.H. Moawad & M.D. Lindheimer (Eds.), *Uterine and placental blood flow* (pp. 177–183). New York: Masson Publishing.

53. Clifford, S.H. (1954). Postmaturity with placental dysfunction: Clinical syndrome and pathological findings. *J Pediatr, 44*, 1.

54. Corner, G.W. (1955). The observed embryology of human single-ovum twins and other multiple births. *Am J Obstet Gynecol, 70*, 933.

55. Corson, S.L. et al. (1986). Early experience with the GIFT procedure. *J Reprod Med, 31*, 219.

56. Critoph, F.N. & Dennis, K.J. (1978). Ciliary activity in the human oviduct. *Br J Obstet Gynaecol, 84*, 216.

57. Croxatto, H.B. et al. (1978). Studies on the duration of egg transport by the human oviduct II. Ovum location at various times following luteinizing hormone peak. *Am J Obstet Gynecol, 132*, 629.

58. Daffos, F. (1989). Access to the other patient. *Semin Perinatol, 13*, 252.

59. Dancis, J. (1981). Placental transport of amino acids, fats and minerals. In *Placental transport* (pp. 25–32). Mead Johnson Symposium on Perinatal and Developmental Medicine, No. 18. Evansville, IN: Mead Johnson.

59a. Dickason, E.J., Schult, M.O. &, Morris, E.M. (1978). *Maternal and infant drugs and nursing interventions*. New York: McGraw-Hill.

60. Enders, A.C. (1981). Anatomy of the placenta and its relationship to function. In *Placental transport* (pp. 3–7). Mead Johnson Symposium on Perinatal and Developmental Medicine, No. 18. Evansville, IN: Mead Johnson.

61. Dashi, M.J. (1986). Accuracy of consumer performed in-home tests for early pregnancy detection. *Am J Public Health, 76*, 512.

62. De Wolf, F., Robertson, W.B., & Brosens, I. (1975). The ultrastructure of acute atherosis in hypertensive pregnancy. *Am J Obstet Gynecol, 123*, 164.

63. Dempsey, E.W. (1972). The development of capillaries in the villi of early human placentas. *J Anat, 134*, 221.

64. DeWolf, F., DeWolf-Peeters, C., & Brosens, I. (1973). Ultrastructure of the spiral arteries in the

human placental bed at the end of normal pregnancy. *Am J Obstet Gynecol, 117*, 833.

65. DeWolf, F. et al. (1982). Decidual vasculopathy and extensive placental infarction in a patient with repeated thromboembolic accidents, recurrent fetal loss, and a lupus anticoagulant. *Am J Obstet Gynecol, 142*, 829.

66. Diamond, M.P. et al. (1985). Effect of the number of inseminating sperm and the follicular stimulation protocol of invitro fertilization of human oocytes in male factor and non-male factor couples. *Fertil Steril, 43*, 77.

67. Dicke, J.M. (1989). Teratology: Principles and practice. *Med Clin North Am, 73*, 567.

68. Dodson, M.G. et al. (1986). A detailed program review of in vitro fertilization with a discussion and comparison of alternative approaches. *Surg Gynecol Obstet, 162*, 89.

69. Dorfman, S.F. (1982). *Ectopic pregnancy surveillance.* Atlanta: Centers for Disease Control.

70. Doyle, D.K. (1986). Teratology: A primer. *Neonatal Network, 4*, 24.

71. Dunn, P.A., Weiner, S., & Ludomirski, A. (1989). Percutaneous umbilical blood sampling. *J Obstet Gynecol Neonatal Nurs, 17*, 308.

72. Eden, R.D. et al. (1982). Comparison of antepartum testing schemes for the management of the postdate pregnancy. *Am J Obstet Gynecol, 144*, 683.

73. Edwards, R.G. (1980). *Conception in the human female.* London: Academic Press.

74. Edwards, R.G. (1986). Causes of early embryonic loss in human pregnancy. *Hum Reprod, 1*, 185.

75. Eisenberg, E. & Wallach, E.E. (1984). In vitro fertilization and embryo transfer. *Postgrad Obstet Gynecol, 4*, 1.

76. Erkkola, R. et al. (1985). Growth discordancy in twin pregnancies: A risk factor not detected by measurements of biparietal diameter. *Obstet Gynecol, 66*, 203.

77. Ethics Committee of the American Fertility Society. (1986). Artificial insemination-donor. *Fertil Steril, 46*, 36s.

78. Evans, M.I. et al. (1988). Early genetic amniocentesis and chorionic villus sampling. *J Reprod Med, 33*, 450.

79. Evans, M.I., Johnson, M.P., & Drugan, A. (1990). Amniocentesis. In R.D. Eden & F.H. Boehm (Eds.), *Assessment and care of the fetus* (pp. 283–290). Norwalk, CT: Appleton & Lange.

80. Faber, J. (1969). Application of the theory of heat exchangers to the transfer of inert materials in the placenta. *Circ Res, 24*, 221.

81. Faber, J.J. & Thornburg, K.L. (1983). *Placental physiology.* New York: Raven Press.

82. Feldbush, T.L. & Lubaroff, D.M. (1977). Fundamental immunobiology. *Semin Perinatol, 1*, 113.

83. Fitzgerald, M.J.T. (1978). *Human embryology: A regional approach.* New York: Harper & Row.

84. Fox, H. (1967). The incidence and significance of vasculosyncytial membranes in the human placenta. *J Obstet Gynaecol Brit Comm, 74*, 28.

85. Fox, H. (1967). The significance of placental infarction in perinatal morbidity and mortality. *Biol Neonate, 11*, 87.

86. Fox, H. (1978). *Pathology of the placenta.* Philadelphia: WB Saunders.

87. Francis, G.R. & Nosek, J.A. (1988). Ethical considerations in contemporary reproductive technologies. *J Perinat Neonat Nurs, 1*, 37.

88. Freese, U.E. (1966). The fetal-maternal circulation of the placenta. I. Histomorphologic, plastoid injection, and X-ray cinematographic studies on human placentas. *Am J Obstet Gynecol, 94*, 354.

89. Frusca, T. et al. (1989). Histological features of uteroplacental vessels in normal and hypertensive patients in relation to birthweight. *Br J Obstet Gynaecol, 96*, 853.

90. Gaba, D.M. & Baden, J.M. (1985). Physiologic effects of drugs used in anesthesia. In J.M. Baden & J.B. Brodsky (Eds.), *The pregnant surgical patient* (p. 105). New York: Futura Publishing.

91. Galvan, B.J. et al. (1989). Using amnioinfusion for the relief of repetitive variable decelerations during labor. *J Obstet Gynecol Neonatal Nurs, 18*, 222.

92. Ganapathy, M.E. et al. (1985). Dipeptide transport in brush border membrane vesicles isolated from maternal term human placenta. *Am J Obstet Gynecol, 153*, 83.

93. Gitlin, D. & Gitlin, J. (1975). Fetal and neonatal development of human plasma proteins. In F.W. Putnam (Ed.), *The plasma proteins* (Vol 2, pp. 264–319). New York: Academic Press.

94. Gitlin, D. et al. (1964). The selectivity of the human placenta and the transfer of proteins from mother to fetus. *J Clin Invest, 43*, 1938.

95. Giudice, L.C. (1989). The endocrinology of recurrent spontaneous abortion. In S.A. Brody & K. Ueland (Eds.), *Endocrine disorders in pregnancy* (pp. 467–481). Norwalk, CT: Appleton & Lange.

96. Goddard, B. (1990). The role of the nurse in the prenatal period. In M.A. Auvenshine & M.G. Enriquez (Eds.), *Comprehensive maternity nursing: Perinatal and women's health.* Boston: Jones & Bartlett.

97. Goebelsmann, U. (1986). The menstrual cycle. In D.R. Mishell & V. Davajan (Eds.), *Infertility, contraception & reproductive endocrinology.* Oradell, NJ: Medical Economics Books.

98. Goldstein, I., Coppel, J.A., & Hobbins, J.C. (1989). Fetal behavior in preterm rupture of the membranes. *Clin Perinatol, 16*, 735.

99. Greenhill, J. & Friedman, E. (1974). Amniotic fluid. In J. Greenhill & E. Friedman (Eds.), *Biological principles and the modern practice of obstetrics* (pp. 75–83). Philadelphia: WB Saunders.

100. Gull, S.A. (1977). Maternal immune system during human gestation. *Semin Perinatol, 1*, 119.

101. Gruenwald, P. (1970). Environmental influences on twins apparent at birth. *Biol Neonate, 15*, 79.

102. Gruenwald, P. (1972). Expansion of placental site and maternal blood supply of primate placentas. *Anat Rec, 173*, 189.

103. Gruenwald, P. (1973). Lobular structure of hemochorial primate placentas. In P. Gruenwald (Ed.), *The placenta and its maternal supply line* (pp. 133–152). Lancaster, England: Medical and Technical Publishing.

104. Guyton, A.C. (1987). *Textbook of medical physiology* (7th ed.). Philadelphia: WB Saunders.

105. Hackeloer, B.J. et al. (1979). Correlation of ultrasonic and endocrinologic assessment of human follicular development. *Am J Obstet Gynecol, 135*, 12.

106. Hamilton, W.J., Boyd, J.D., & Mossman, H.W. (1972). *Human embryology* (4th ed.). Baltimore: Williams & Wilkins.

107. Hansen, R.P.S. (1984). Endocrine response in the fallopian tube. *Endocr Rev, 5*, 525.

108. Harbert, G.M. (1982). Effects of uterine contrac-

tions. In A.H. Moawad & M.D. Lindheimer (Eds.), *Uterine and placental blood flow* (pp. 193–199). New York: Masson Publishing.

109. Harding, R. et al. (1984). Composition and volume of fluid swallowed by fetal sheep. *Q J Exp Physiol, 69,* 487.

110. Harper, M.J.K. (1982). Sperm and egg transport. In C.R. Austin & R.V. Short (Eds.), *Reproduction in mammals: Germ cells and fertilization.* Cambridge: Cambridge University Press.

111. Harris, T. (1979). Fetal development and physiology. In A. Clark & D. Affonso (Eds.), *Childbearing: A nursing perspective* (pp. 234–236). Philadelphia: FA Davis.

112. Hayashi, R.H. (1987). Abnormalities of placental implanation. In J.P. Lavery (Ed.), *The human placenta: Clinical perspectives* (pp. 115–129). Rockville, MD: Aspen.

113. Heap, R., Flint, A., & Gadsby, J. (1979). Embryonic signals that establish pregnancy. *Br Med Bull, 35,* 129.

114. Heinrichs, W.L. & Gibbons, W.E. (1989). Endocrinology of pregnancy. In S.A. Brody & K. Ueland (Eds.), *Endocrine disorders in pregnancy* (pp. 65–80). Norwalk, CT: Appleton & Lange.

115. Henderson, G.I. et al. (1981). Inhibition of placental valine uptake after acute and chronic maternal ethanol consumption. *J Pharm Acol Exp Ther, 216,* 465.

116. Hendricks, C.H. (1958). The hemodynamics of a uterine contraction. *Am J Obstet Gynecol, 76,* 969.

117. Hertig, A.T. (1967). The overall problem in man. In K. Benirschke (Ed.), *Comparative aspects of reproductive failure.* New York: Springer-Verlag.

118. Hertig, A.T. & Sheldon, W.H. (1983). Minimal criteria required to prove prima facie of traumatic abortion. *Ann Surg, 117,* 596.

119. Hill, E.P., Power, G.G., & Longo, L.D. (1972). A mathematical model of placental O_2 transfer with consideration of hemoglobin reaction rates. *Am J Physiol, 222,* 721.

120. Hill, E.P., Power, G.G. & Longo, L.D. (1973). A mathematical model of carbon dioxide transfer in the placenta and its interaction with oxygen. *Am J Physiol, 224,* 283.

121. Hill, E.P. & Longo, L.D. (1980). Dynamics of maternal-fetal nutrient transfer. *Fed Proc, 39,* 239.

122. Hill, L.M., Kislak, S., & Runco, C. (1987). An ultrasonic view of the umbilical cord. *Obstet Gynecol Surv, 42,* 82.

122a. Hill, R.M. & Stern, L. (1979). Drugs in pregnancy: Effects on the fetus and newborn. *Drugs, 17,* 182.

123. Hillier, S.G. et al. (1980). Intraovarian sex steroid hormone interactions and the regulation of follicular maturation: Aromatization of androgens by human granulosa cells in vitro. *J Clin Endocrinol Metab, 50,* 640.

124. Ho, P.C. et al. (1986). Plasma prolactin, progesterone, estradiol, and human chorionic gonadotropin in complete and partial moles before and after evacuation. *Obstet Gynecol, 67,* 99.

125. Holbrook, R.H. & Ueland, K. (1989). Endocrinology of parturition and preterm labor. In S.A. Brody & K. Ueland (Eds.), *Endocrine disorders in pregnancy* (pp. 81–98). Norwalk, CT: Appleton & Lange.

126. Hollenbach, K.A. & Hickok, D.E. (1990). Epidemiology and diagnosis of twin gestation. *Clin Obstet Gynecol, 33,* 3.

127. Holley, R.W. (1980). Control of animal cell proliferation. *J Supramol Struct, 13,* 191.

128. Houwert-de Jong, M.H. et al. (1989). Habitual abortion: A review. *Eur J Obstet Gynecol Reprod Biol, 30,* 39.

129. Huszar, G. & Bailey, P. (1979). Isolation and characteristics of myosin in the human term placenta. *Am J Obstet Gynecol, 135,* 707.

130. Hutchinson-Williams, K.A. & DeCherney, A.H. (1989). Endocrinology of ectopic pregnancy. In S.A. Brody & K. Ueland (Eds.), *Endocrine disorders in pregnancy* (pp. 437–450). Norwalk, CT: Appleton & Lange.

131. Im, S.S. et al. (1984). Nonimmunologic hydrops fetalis. *Am J Obstet Gynecol, 148,* 566.

132. Jaffe, R.B., Lee, A., & Midgley, A.R. (1969). Serum gonadotropin before, at the inception of, and following human pregnancy. *J Clin Endocrinol Metabol, 29,* 1281.

133. James, W.H. (1981). Dizygotic twinning, marital stage and status, and coital rates. *Ann Hum Biol, 8,* 371.

134. Jones, C.J.P. & Fox, H. (1981). An ultrastructural and ultrahistochemical study of the human placenta in maternal essential hypertension. *Placenta, 2,* 193.

135. Jones, K.L. (1988). *Smith's recognizable patterns of human malformation* (4th ed.). Philadelphia: WB Saunders.

136. Kadar, N. & Romero, R. (1990). Ectopic pregnancy. In R.D. Eden & F.H. Boehm (Eds.), *Assessment and care of the fetus* (pp. 575–599). Norwalk, CT: Appleton & Lange.

137. Kalant, H., Roschlau, W.H.E,. & Sellers, E.M. (1985). *Principles of medical pharmacology* (4th ed.). Toronto: University of Toronto Press.

138. Kaplan, C. (1987). Gross and microscopic abnormalities of the placenta. In J.P. Lavery (Ed.), *The human placenta: Clinical perspectives* (pp. 47–66). Rockville, MD: Aspen.

139. Kaufmann, P. (1982). Development and differentiation of the human placental villous tree. *Bibl Anat, 22,* 29.

140. Kaufmann, P., Sen, D.K., & Schweikhardt, G. (1979). Classification of human placental villi. I. Histology. *Cell Tissue Res, 209,* 409.

141. Key, T.C. & Resnik, R. (1988). Obstetric management of the high risk patient. In G. Burrow & F. Ferris (Eds.), *Medical complications during pregnancy* (pp. 95–135). Philadelphia: WB Saunders.

142. Khong, T.Y. & Pearce, J.M. (1987). In J.P. Lavery (Ed.), *The human placenta: Clinical perspectives* (pp. 25–45). Rockville, MD: Aspen.

143. Knorr, L.J. (1989). Relieving fetal distress with amnioinfusion. *MCN, 14,* 346.

144. Koren, Z. & Spigland, I. (1987). Irrigation technique for detection of mycoplasma intrauterine infection in infertile patients. *Obstet Gynecol Surv, 52,* 588.

145. Krantz, K.E. & Parker, J.C. (1963). Contractile properties of the smooth muscle in the human placenta. *Clin Obstet Gynaecol, 6,* 26.

146. Kubli, F. et al. (1977). Antepartum heart rate monitoring. In R. Bear & S. Campbell (Eds.), *The current status of FHR monitoring and ultrasound in obstetrics* (p. 28). London: Royal College of Obstetrics and Gynaecology.

147. Lage, J.M., Mark, S.D., & Driscoll, S.G. (1987). The twin placenta. In J.P. Lavery (Ed.), *The human*

placenta: Clinical perspectives (pp. 67–77). Rockville, MD: Aspen.

148. Lala, P.K., Kearns, M., & Colavincenzo, V. (1984). Cells of the fetomaternal interface. *Am J Anat, 170,* 501.

149. Larson, B. & Galas, R. (1977). Protection of the fetus against infection. *Semin Perinatol, 1,* 183.

150. Lavery, B.S. (1987). The third stage. In J.P. Lavery (Ed.), *The human placenta: Clinical perspectives* (pp. 155–178). Rockville, MD: Aspen.

151. Lavery, J.P. (1987). Appendages of the placenta. In J.P. Lavery (Ed.), *The human placenta: Clinical perspectives* (pp. 257–279). Rockville, MD: Aspen.

152. Layde, P.M. et al. (1980). Congenital malformations in twins. *Am J Hum Genet, 32,* 69.

153. Leridon, H. (1977). *Human fertility.* Chicago: University of Chicago Press.

154. Leveno, K.J. (1986). Amniotic fluid volume in prolonged pregnancy. *Semin Perinatol, 10,* 154.

155. Lin, C.C. (1989). Perinatal hypoxia in the growth-retarded fetus: Basic pathophysiology and clinical management. In M. Rathi (Ed.), *Current perinatology* (pp. 1–24). New York: Springer-Verlag.

156. Lind, T. (1978). The biochemistry of amniotic fluid. In D.V.I. Fairweather & T.K. Eskes (Eds.), *Amniotic fluid: Research and clinical application* (pp. 59–80). Amsterdam: Excerpta Medica.

157. Longo, L. (1981). Nutrient transfer in the placenta. In *Placental transport* (pp. 15–20). Mead Johnson Symposium on Perinatal and Developmental Medicine No. 18. Evansville, IN: Mead Johnson.

158. Longo, L.D. (1982). Some physiological implications of altered uteroplacental blood flow. In A.H. Moawad & M.D. Lindheimer (Eds.), *Uterine and placental blood flow* (pp. 93–102). New York: Masson Publishing.

159. Longo, L.D. (1985). The role of the placenta in the development in the embryo and fetus. In C.T. Jones & P.W. Nathanielsz (Eds.), *The physiological development of the fetus and newborn* (p. 1–9). Orlando, FL: Academic Press.

160. Longo, L.D. & Power, G.G. (1969). Analysis of P_{O_2} differences between maternal and fetal blood in the placenta. *J Appl Physiol, 26,* 48.

161. Lopata, A. (1983). Concepts in human in vitro fertilizaiton and embryo transfer. *Fertil Steril, 40,* 289.

162. Lotgering, F.K. & Wallenburg, H.C.S. (1986). Mechanisms of production and clearance of amniotic fluid. *Semin Perinatol, 10,* 94.

163. Lubbe, W.F. & Liggins, G.C. (1985). Lupus anticoagulant and pregnancy. *Am J Obstet Gynecol, 153,* 322.

164. MacGillivray, I. (1980). Twins and other multiple deliveries. *Clin Obstet Gynecol, 7,* 581.

165. MacGillvray, I. (1986). Epidemiology of twin pregnancy. *Semin Perinatol, 10,* 4.

166. MacLennon, A.H. et al. (1983). Neonatal water metabolism: An objective postnatal index of intra-uterine fetal growth. *Early Hum Dev, 8,* 21.

167. Maddox, D.E. et al. (1984). Localization of a molecule immunochemically similar to eosinophilic major basic protein in human placenta. *J Exp Med, 160,* 29.

168. Manning, F.A. (1989). Fetal biophysical assessment by ultrasound. In R.K. Creasy & R. Resnik R (Eds.), *Maternal-fetal medicine: Principles and practice* (pp. 357–361). Philadephia: WB Saunders.

169. Manning, F.A. (1989). General principles and application of ultrasound. In R.K. Creasy & R. Resnik (Eds.), *Maternal-fetal medicine: Principles and practice* (pp. 195–253). Philadephia: WB Saunders.

170. Manning, F.A. & Harman, C.R. (1990). Fetal biophysical profile. In R.D. Eden & F.H. Boehm (Eds.), *Assessment and Care of the Fetus* (pp. 385–396). Norwalk, CT: Appleton & Lange.

171. Mannino, F.L., Jones, K.L., & Benirschke, K. (1977). Congenital skin defects and fetus papyraceus. *J Pediatr, 91,* 559.

172. March, C.M. et al. (1979). Roles of estradiol and progesterone in eliciting the midcycle luteinizing hormone and follicle-stimulating hormone surges. *J Clin Endocrinol Metab, 49,* 507.

173. Marrs, R.P. et al. (1984). Effect of variation of in vitro culture techniques upon oocyte fertilization and embryo development in human in vitro fertilization procedures. *Fertil Steril, 41,* 519.

174. Martin, C.B. (1968). The anatomy and circulation of the placenta. In A.C. Barns (Ed.), *Intra-uterine development* (pp. 35–67). Philadelphia: Lea & Febiger.

175. Martin, C.R. & Gingerich, B. (1976). Uteroplacental physiology. *JOGN (Suppl.), 5* (Sept-Oct), 16s.

176. Mascola, L. & Guinan, M.E. (1986). Screening to reduce transmission of sexually transmitted diseases in semen used for artificial insemination. *N Engl J Med, 314,* 1354.

177. McCullough, K. (1988). Neonatal problems in twins. *Clin Perinatol, 15,* 141.

178. McDonough, P.G. (1985). Repeated first trimester loss: Evaluation and management. *Am J Obstet Gynecol, 153,* 1.

179. McNatty, K.P. (1982). Ovarian follicular development from the onset of luteal regression in humans and sheep. In P. Rolland et al. (Eds.), *Follicular maturation and ovulation.* Amsterdam: Excerpta Medica.

180. Masters, W. & Johnson, V. (1966). *Human sexual response.* Boston: Little, Brown.

181. Miller, D.S., Ballon, S.C., & Teng, N.H. (1989). Gestational trophoblastic diseases. In S.A. Brody & K. Ueland (Eds.), *Endocrine disorders in pregnancy* (pp. 451–466). Norwalk, CT: Appleton & Lange.

182. Miller, F.J. et al. (1980). Foetal loss after implantation. *Lancet, 2,* 554.

183. Metcalfe, J., Bartels, H., & Moll, W. (1967). Gas exchange in the pregnant uterus. *Physiol Rev, 47,* 782.

184. Miller, M.E., Higgenbottom, M., & Smith, D.W. (1981). Short umbilical cord: Its origin and relevance. *Pediatrics, 67,* 618.

185. Miller, M.M. & Stiehm, E.R. (1983). Immunity and resistance to infection. In J.S. Remington & J.O. Klein (Eds.), *Infectious diseases of the fetus and newborn infant* (pp. 27–68). Philadelphia: WB Saunders.

186. Miller, P.W., Coen, R.W., & Benirschke, K. (1985). Dating the time interval from meconium passage to birth. *Obstet Gynecol, 66,* 459.

187. Moessinger, A.C. (1983). Fetal akinesia deformation sequence: An animal model. *Pediatrics, 72,* 857.

188. Moessinger, A.C. (1989). Morphological consequences of depressed or impaired fetal activity. In W.P. Smotherman & S.R. Robinson (Eds.), *Behavior of the fetus* (pp. 163–173). Caldwell, NJ: Telford Press.

189. Moessinger, A.C. et al. (1982). Umbilical cord

length as an index of fetal activity: Experimental study and clinical implications. *Pediatr Res, 16,* 109.

190. Moessinger, A.C. et al. (1986). Oligohydramnios-induced lung hypoplasia: The influence of timing and duration of gestation. *Pediatr Res, 20,* 951.

191. Moore, K. (1988). *The developing human: Clinically oriented embryology* (4th ed., pp. 104–130). Philadelphia: WB Saunders.

192. Moriyama, I. et al. (1988). Fetal growth and the placenta-Development of the transport function of the human cell membrane and fetal growth. In G.H. Wiknjosastro, W.H. Prakoso, & K. Maeda K (Eds.), *Perinatology* (pp. 45–54). Amsterdam: Elsevier Science Publishers.

193. Morriss, F.H. & Boyd, R.D.H. (1988). Placental transport. In E. Knobil & J Neill (Eds.), *The physiology of reproduction* (Vol. II, pp. 2043–2083). NY: Raven Press.

194. Muir, B. (1983). *Essentials of genetics for nurses.* New York: John Wiley.

195. Myrianthopolous, N.C. (1976). Congenital malformations in twins. *Acta Genet Med Gemellol, 25,* 331.

196. Myrianthopoulos, N.C. (1970). An epidemiological survey of twins in a large prospectively studied population. *Am J Hum Genet, 22,* 611.

197. Naeye, R.L. (1965). Organ abnormalities in a human parabiotic syndrome. *Am J Pathol, 46,* 829.

198. Naeye, R.L. (1978). Effect of maternal smoking in the fetus and placenta. *Br J Obstet Gynaecol, 85,* 732.

199. Naeye, R.L. (1985). Maternal floor infarction. *Hum Path, 16,* 823.

200. Newton, E.R. (1989). The fetus as patient. *Med Clin North Am, 73,* 517.

201. Nichols, J. & Schrepfer, R. (1966). Polyhydramnois in anencephaly. *JAMA, 197,* 549.

202. Nicolaides, K.H., Thorpe, J.G., & Noble, P. (1990). Cordocentesis. In R.D. Eden & F.H. Boehm (Eds.), *Assessment and care of the fetus* (pp. 291–305). Norwalk, CT: Appleton & Lange.

203. Nielson, T.F., Hagberg, H., & Ljungblad, U (1989). Placenta previa and antepartum hemorrhage after previous caesarean section. *Gynecol Obstet Invest, 27,* 88.

204. Nordenvall M. & Sandstedt, B. (1990). Placental lesions and maternal hemoglobin levels. *Acta Obstet Gynaecol Scan, 69* 127.

205. Nuwayhid, B. (1981). Fetal homeostatis. In L. Iffy & H. Kaminetzkey (Eds.), *Principles and practices of obstetrics and perinatology* (pp. 269–304). New York: John Wiley.

206. Pattillo, R. (1981). Immunology of gestation. In L. Iffy & H. Kaminetzkey (Eds.), *Principles and practices of obstetrics and perinatology* (pp. 101–125). New York: John Wiley.

207. Nylander, P.P.S. (1971). Biosocial aspects of multiple births. *J Biosocial Sci, 3(Suppl.),* 1.

208. Nylander, P.P.S. (1973). Serum levels of gonadotropins in relation to multiple pregnancy in Nigeria. *Br J Obstet Gynaecol, 80,* 651.

209. Nylander, P.P.S. (1979). Perinatal mortality in twins. *Acta Genet Med Gemellol, 28,* 363.

210. Oski, F.A. & Naiman, J.L. (1982). *Hematologic problems in the newborn* (3rd ed.). Philadelphia: WB Saunders.

211. Overstreet, J.W. (1983). Transport of gametes in the reproductive tract of the female mammal. In J.F. Hartmen (Ed.), *Mechanism and control of animal fertilization.* New York:Academic Press.

212. Overstreet, J.W. & Cooper, G.W. (1978). Sperm transport in the reproductive tract of the female rabbit. II. The sustained phase of transport. *Biol Reprod, 19,* 115.

213. Pace-Owens, S. (1985). In vitro fertilization and embryo transfer. *J Obstet Gynecol Neonatal Nurs, 14,* 44s.

214. Page, E.W., Villee, C.A., & Villee, D.B. (1981). *Human reproduction: Essentials of reproductive and perinatal medicine* (pp. 175–207). Philadelphia: WB Saunders.

215. Parer, J.T. (1989). Fetal heart rate. In R.K. Creasy & R. Resnik (Eds.), *Maternal-fetal medicine: Principles and practice* (pp. 314–343). Philadephia: WB Saunders.

216. Parer, J.T. (1976). Normal and impaired placental exchange. *Contemp Obstet Gynecol, 7,* 117.

217. Pauerstein, C.J. (Ed.). (1987). *Clinical obstetrics.* New York: John Wiley.

218. Perrin, E.V.D.K. (1984). Placenta as a reflection of fetal disease. In E.V.D.K. Perrin (Ed.), *Pathology of the placenta.* New York: Churchill Livingstone.

219. Phelan, J.P. (1989). The postdate pregnancy: An overview. *Clin Obstet Gynecol, 32,* 219.

220. Poland, B.J. et al. (1977). Reproductive counseling in patients who have had a spontaneous abortion. *Am J Obstet Gynecol, 127,* 685.

221. Potter, E.L. (1963). Twin zygosity and placental form in relation to the outcome of pregnancy. *Am J Obstet Gynecol, 87,* 566.

222. Pritchard, J.A. (1965). Deglutition by normal and anencephalic fetuses. *Obstet Gynecol, 25,* 289.

223. Pritchard, J.A. (1966). Fetal swallowing and amniotic fluid volume. *Obstet Gynecol, 28,* 606.

224. Pritchard, J., MacDonald, P.C., & Gant, N.F. (1985). *Williams obstetrics* (17th ed.). New York: Appleton-Century-Crofts.

225. Ramsey, E.M. & Donner, M.W. (1980). *Placental vasculature and circulation.* Philadelphia: WB Saunders.

226. Reid, D.E., Ryan, K.J., & Benirschke, K. (1972). *Principles and management of human reproduction.* Philadephia: WB Saunders.

227. Resnik, R. & Wilkes, M. (1982). The effects of nicotine on uterine blood flow. In A.H. Moawad & M.D. Lindheimer (Eds.), *Uterine and placental blood flow* (pp. 171–175). New York: Masson Publishing.

228. Richards, J.S. (1979). Hormonal control of ovarian follicular development. *Recent Prog Horm Res, 35,* 343.

229. Richter, M.A., Haning, R.V., & Shapiro, S.S. (1984). Artificial donor insemination: Fresh versus frozen semen; the patient as her own control. *Fertil Steril, 41,* 227.

230. Robertson, W.B., Brosens, I., & Dixon, G. (1975). Uteroplacental vascular pathology. *Eur J Obstet Gynecol Reprod Biol, 5,* 47.

231. Robertson, W.B., Brosens, I., & Dixon, H.G. (1981). Maternal blood supply in fetal growth retardation. In F.A. Van Assche & W.B. Robertson (Eds.), *Fetal growth retardation* (pp. 126–138). Edinburgh: Churchill Livingstone.

232. Roman, E. (1984). Fetal loss rates and their relation to pregnancy order. *J Epidemiol Community Health, 38,* 29.

233. Ross Laboratories. (1975). *Abnormalities of the placenta.* Clinical Education Aid No. 12. Columbus, OH: Author.

234. Ross, G.T. et al. (1970). Pituitary and gonadal hormones in women during spontaneous and induced ovulatory cycles. *Recent Prog Horm Res, 26,* 1.

235. Roth, S. & Shur, B. (1975). The biochemistry of cell recognition and migration. In *Biological and clinical aspects of malformations* (pp. 24–29). Mead-Johnson Symposium on Perinatal and Developmental Medicine. Evansville, IN: Mead Johnson.

236. Sachs, E.S. et al. (1985). Chromosome studies of 500 couples with two or more abortions. *Obstet Gynecol, 65,* 375.

237. Sadovsky, G. (1990). Fetal movements. In R.D. Eden & F.H. Boehm (Eds.), *Assessment and care of the fetus* (pp. 341–349). Norwalk, CT: Appleton & Lange.

238. Sagar, H.J. & Desa, D.J. (1973). The relationship between hydramnios and some characteristics of the infant in pregnancies complicated by fetal anencephaly. *J Obstet Gynaecol Br Comm, 80,* 429.

239. Sanfilippo, J.S. & Stoelk, E.M. (1987). Endocrinology of the placenta. In J.P. Lavery (Ed.), *The human placenta: Clinical perspectives* (pp. 179–198). Rockville, MD: Aspen.

240. Savona-Ventura, C. (1987). Amniocentesis for fetal maturity. *Obstet Gynecol Surv, 42,* 717.

241. Schinzel, A.A., Smith, D.W., & Miller, J.R. (1979). Monozygotic twinning and structural defects. *J Pediatr, 95,* 921.

242. Schlievert, P., Johnson, W., & Galask, R.P. (1977). Amniotic fluid antibacterial mechanisms: New concepts. *Semin Perinatol, 1,* 59.

243. Schuman, W. (1951). Double sac with secondary rupture of the bag of waters during labor. *Am J Obstet Gynecol, 62,* 633.

244. Seeds, A.E. (1980). Current concepts of amniotic fluid dynamics. *Am J Obstet Gynecol, 138,* 575.

245. Sheppard, B.L. & Bonnar, J. (1976). The ultrastructure of the arterial supply of the human placenta in pregnancy complicated by fetal growth retardation. *Br J Obstet Gynaecol, 83,* 948.

246. Sher, G. et al. (1986). In vitro fertilization and embryo transfer: Two year experience. *Obstet Gynecol, 67,* 309.

247. Short, G.M. (1988). Genetic disorders. In G. Burrow & F. Ferris (Eds.), *Medical complications during pregnancy* (pp. 136–179). Philadelphia: WB Saunders.

248. Sibley, C.P. & Boyd, R.D.H. (1988). Control of transfer across the mature placenta. *Oxford Rev Reprod Biol, 10,* 382.

249. Siler-Khodr, T. (1983). Hypothalmic-like releasing hormones of the placenta. *Clin Perinatol, 10,* 553.

250. Simpson, J.L. & Elias, S. (1989). Prenatal diagnosis of genetic disorders. In R.K. Creasy & R. Resnik (Eds.), *Maternal-fetal medicine: Principles and practice* (pp. 78–107). Philadephia: WB Saunders.

251. Smith, E.B. et al. (1984). Human chorionic gonadotropin levels in complete and partial moles and in nonmolar abortuses. *Am J Obstet Gynecol, 149,* 129.

252. Snyder, A.K., Singh, S.P., & Pullen, G.L. (1986). Ethanol induced intrauterine growth retardation: Correlation with placental glucose transfer. *Alcoholism, 10,* 167.

253. Speirs, A.L. et al. (1983). Analysis of the benefits and risks of multiple embryo transfer. *Fertil Steril, 39,* 468.

254. Speroff, L. & Dorfman, G.S. (1977). Prostaglandins and pregnancy hypertension. *Clin Obstet Gynecol, 4,* 635.

255. Speroff, L., Glass, R.H., & Kase, N.G. (1989). *Clinical gynecologic endocrinology and infertility* (4th ed.). Baltimore: Williams & Wilkins.

256. Spranger, J. et al. (1982). Errors of morphogenesis: Concepts and terms. Recommendations of an international working group. *J Pediatr, 100,* 160.

256a. Stockard, C.R. (1921). Developmental rate and structural expression: An experimental study of twins, "double monsters" and single deformities, and the interaction among embryonic organs during their origin and development. *Am J Anat, 28,* 115.

257. Stray-Pederson, B., Eng, J., & Reikvam, T.M. (1978). Uterine T-mycoplasma colonization in reproductive failure. *Am J Obstet Gynecol, 130,* 307.

258. Strong, S.J. & Corney, G. (1967). *The placenta in twin pregnancy.* Oxford: Pergamon Press.

259. Szulman, A.E. & Surti, U. (1978). The syndrome of hydatidiform mole. I. Cytogenics and morphologic correlation. *Am J Obstet Gynecol, 131,* 665.

260. Teasdale, F. (1980). Gestational changes in the functional structure of the human placenta in relation to fetal growth. *Am J Obstet Gynecol, 137,* 560.

261. Teasdale, F. (1985). Histomorphology of the human placenta in maternal preeclampsia. *Am J Obstet Gynecol, 152,* 25.

262. Terragno, N.A. et al. (1982). Role of naturally occurring vasoactive prostaglandins in pregnancy. In A. H. Moawad & M.D. Lindheimer (Eds.), *Uterine and placental blood flow* (pp. 161–167). New York: Masson Publishing.

263. Tho, P.T., Byrd, J.R., & McDonough, P.G. (1978). Etiologies and subsequent reproductive performance of 100 couples with recurrent abortion. *Fertil Steril, 32,* 389.

264. Thomas, R.L. & Blakemore, K.J. (1990). Evaluation of elevations in maternal serum alpha-fetoprotein: A review. *Obstet Gynecol Surv. 45,* 269.

265. Tropper, P.J. & Petrie, R.H. (1987). Placental exchange. In J.P. Lavery (Ed.), *The human placenta: Clinical perspectives* (pp. 199–206). Rockville, MD: Aspen.

266. Tulchinsky, D. (1982). Endocrine assessments of fetal -placental well being. *Clin Perinatol, 10,* 763.

267. Van Allen, M.J., Smith, D.W., & Shepard, T.H. (1983). Twin reversed artery perfusion (TRAP) sequence: A study of 14 twin pregnancies with acardius. *Semin Perinatol, 7,* 285.

268. Van Der Veen, F. & Fox, H. (1982). The effects of maternal smoking on the human placenta. *Placenta, 3,* 243.

269. Vorherr, H., Thliveris, J.A., & Baskett, T.F. (1978). Fine structure of the human placenta in prolonged pregnancy: Preliminary report. *Gynecol Clin Investigation, 9,* 40.

270. Wallenberg, H. (1977). The amniotic fluid: II. *J Perinat Med, 5,* 233.

271. Wallenberg, H. (1977). The amniotic fluid: I. *J Perinat Med, 5,* 193.

272. Walsh, S.W. (1990). Physiology of low-dose aspirin therapy for the prevention of preeclampsia. *Semin Perinatol, 14,* 152.

273. Warburton, D. (1987). Reproductive loss: How much is preventable? *N Engl J Med, 316,* 158.

274. Warburton, D. & Fraser, F.S. (1964). Spontaneous abortion risks in man: Data from reproductive

histories collected in a medical genetics unit. *Am J Hum Genet*, 16, 1.

275. Wigglesworth, J.S. (1969). Vascular anatomy of the human placenta and its significance for placental pathology. *J Obstet Gynaecol Br Comm, 76*, 979.

276. Wigglesworth, J.S. (1984). The placenta in perinatal pathology. In J.S. Wigglesworth (Ed.), *Perinatal pathology* (pp. 48–83). Philadelphia: WB Saunders.

278. Wilson, J.G. (1973). Mechanisms of teratogenesis. *Am J Anat, 136*, 129.

279. Wilson, J.G. (1977). Current status of teratology: General principles and mechanisms derived from animal studies. In J.G. Wilson & F.C. Fraser (Eds.), *Handbook of teratology: General principles and etiology.* New York: Plenum Press.

280. Wladimiroff, J.W. & Campbell, S. (1974). Fetal urine production rates in normal and abnormal pregnancies. *Lancet, 1*, 151.

281. Wynn, R.M. (1975). Principles of placentation and early human placental development. In P. Gruenwald (Ed.), *The placenta and its maternal supply line* (pp. 18–34). Lancaster, England: Medical and Technical Publishing.

282. Yen, S.S.C. (1989). Endocrinology of pregnancy. In R.K. Creasy & R. Resnik (Eds.), *Maternal-fetal medicine: Principles and practice* (pp. 375–403). Philadelphia: WB Saunders.

283. Yoshida, Y. & Manabe, Y. (1990). Different characteristics of amniotic and cervical collagenous tissue during pregnancy and delivery: A morphologic study. *Am J Obstet Gynecol, 162*, 190.

284. Young, M. & Prenton, M.A. (1969). Maternal and fetal plasma amino acid concentrations during gestation and in retarded fetal growth. *J Obstet Gynaecol Br Comm, 76*, 333.

285. Zielmaker, G.H., Alberta, A.T., & VanGent, I. (1983). Fertilization and cleavage of oocytes from a binovular human ovarian follicle: Possible cause of dizygous twinning and a chimerism. *Fertil Steril, 40*, 841.

CHAPTER 3

Parturition and Uterine Physiology

The Uterus
  Uterine Structure
  Uterine Growth
The Myometrium
  Myometrial Cell Structure
  Changes During Pregnancy
Physiology of Parturition
  Initiation of Labor
  Myometrial Contraction
  The Cervix

Clinical Implications for the Pregnant Woman and Her Fetus
  Maternal Position During Labor
  Maternal Pushing Efforts During the Second Stage
  Preterm Labor
  Pharmacology of Labor
    Control of Cervical Ripening
    Induction of Labor
    Inhibition of Labor
  Dystocia
  Postterm Labor

During parturition the actions of the myometrium, decidua, fetus, placenta and membranes must be integrated in order to achieve expulsion of the fetus without compromising fetal or placental perfusion.[64] Ulmsten compares the process of parturition to an opera:

> . . . where cervical priming [ripening] is the overture to the grand performance by the cervix and uterus. After training and rehearsals, the cervix and uterus are able to act in concert and produce a successful grand finale, delivery. Yet many players and factors in the parturition orchestra are unknown, and remarkably, the director or conductor who starts the event remains unknown. [203, p. 427]

This chapter reviews the structure of the uterus and individual myometrial cells; changes during pregnancy; physiology of parturition, with respect to cervical dilatation, initiation of labor, and myometrial contractions; and clinical implications related to pre- and postterm labor onset, labor induction, and dystocia. Maternal pain during labor is discussed in Chapter 12.

THE UTERUS

The uterus is a major site of physiologic activity during the childbearing years. Alterations in the endometrium occur with the monthly menstrual cycle (see Chapter 1). During pregnancy the uterus supports growth and development of the embryo and fetus. At the end of pregnancy, the uterine myometrium must move from a relatively inactive state to produce the strong, synchronous, coordinated contractile forces needed to expel the fetus and placenta.[50] Knowledge of the physiologic changes that bring about this transition in uterine function is incomplete at present but the focus of much interest and research.

Uterine Structure

The uterine wall consists of three layers: (1) internal endometrium; (2) myometrium; and (3) external serous epithelial layer. The thin serosa protects the uterus and provides a relatively inelastic base upon which the myometrium develops tension to increase intrauterine pressure.[5, 42]

The myometrium consists of two muscle layers separated by a vascular zone. The muscle layers form a web that supports and protects the developing fetus (Fig. 3–1). The inner layer is circular and perpendicular to the long axis of the uterus and runs clockwise and counterclockwise in a spiral. The outer muscle layer runs parallel to the longitudinal axis of the uterus. The muscle layers are composed of smooth muscle cells arranged in interconnected bundles of 10 to 50 partially overlapping cells set in a matrix of collagenous connective tissue or ground substance. [42, 76] The ground substance transmits the contractile forces from individual myometrial cells along the muscle bundle.[42] Around the bundles of smooth muscle cells are fibroblasts, blood and lymphatic vessels, and nerve cells.

The uterus is innervated by adrenergic neurons (postganglionic sympathetic fibers from lumbar and mesenteric ganglia), cholinergic neurons (sparse, primarily innervating the cervix), and peptidergic neurons.[201] Adrenergic fibers are most dense in the area of the fallopian tubes, cervix, and vagina and relatively sparse in the uterine corpus and fundus.[64] In comparison to other smooth muscle cells, which tend to be richly innervated, the uterus has a relatively low density of nerves to smooth muscles cells.[76]

The role of the nervous system in myometrial activity is poorly understood.[40] The adrenergic and peptidergic nerves may play a role in suppressing myometrial contractility during pregnancy.[42, 76, 127, 186] Most of the adrenergic fibers in the uterine wall disappear near term, leaving only those in the cervix and uterine horns.[127] Peptidergic neurons also decrease during pregnancy.[201]

Uterine Growth

The elastic properties of the uterus support its growth during pregnancy. The uterus, which weighs approximately 40 g in the nulliparous woman and 60 to 70 g in the nonpregnant multiparous woman, increases during pregnancy to a weight of approximately 680 g.[153] Uterine growth begins after implantation. Initially it primarily involves hyperplasia and is influenced by estrogen and independent of the effects of stretching from the growing embryo. This early uterine growth occurs regardless of whether the embryo is implanted in the uterus or at an extrauterine site.[153]

Further uterine growth involves hypertrophy from distention of the uterus by the enlarging fetus. As the uterus grows the ratio of RNA to DNA increases owing to increased RNA synthesis and total protein. By 3 to 4 months the uterine wall has thickened from 10 to 25 mm, and with further distention the wall thins to 5 to 10 mm at term. Myometrial smooth muscle cells increase in length from 0.05 mm to 0.2 to 0.6 mm owing to a progressive increase in actin and myosin content.[153] Smooth muscle cell creatinine phosphatase, adenosine triphosphate (ATP), and adenosine diphosphate (ADP) also increase to term.[153]

The height of the uterine fundus reaches the maternal umbilicus by about 20 weeks' gestation and the xiphoid process of the sternum by 8 months (see Fig. 2–1). As the fetal head descends into the pelvis ("lightening") late in gestation, the fundal height becomes slightly lower.

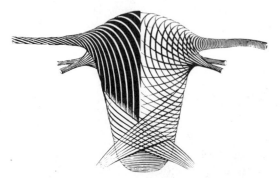

FIGURE 3–1. Interlacing myometrial fibers. (From Bumm, E. (1921). *Grundriss zum Studium der Geburtschilfe* (13th ed.). Wiesbaden: JF Bergmann.)

After 2 to 4 months' gestation when the fundus changes from a spherical to an elliptical (cylindrical) shape, distention occurs primarily in a cephalic direction. The shape of the fundus influences intrauterine pressure. In a sphere, tension is a geometric function of the radius of curvature; whereas in a cylinder, tension is a linear function (and thus is lower).[153] In the absence of contractions, intrauterine pressure peaks at midpregnancy, then decreases to less than 10 mmHg of amniotic fluid pressure when the shape of the fundus changes. The pressure remains low until term in spite of the increasing intrauterine volume. Laceration of the internal cervical os or incompetence of the cervix during the period of higher intrauterine pressure may result in "blowout" of the fetal membranes with late spontaneous abortion or preterm birth.[153]

At mid-gestation contractions of the circular muscles of the uterus are weaker than those of the longitudinal muscles. Contractile strength increases in the circular muscles so that by term these muscles are similar to longitudinal muscles in their contractile ability. The basis for this change is thought to be differences in membranous electrical events, cell-to-cell coupling, and intracellular calcium release.[76]

THE MYOMETRIUM

The myometrium has two basic properties: contractility and elasticity. Contractility is the ability to lengthen and shorten. Elasticity is the ability to grow and stretch to accommodate the enlarging uterine contents, maintain uterine tonus, and permit involution following delivery. Much of what is known about myometrial function is based on knowledge of smooth muscle function in other human organs and knowledge of myometrial function in animals such as the sheep, the rat, and the calf, which may not be analogous to human myometrial function.

Myometrial Cell Structure

The contractile units of the uterus are the smooth muscle cells in a connective tissue matrix. Transmission of contractile forces along the uterus occurs from transmission of tension generated by individual smooth muscle cells to other smooth muscle cells and the connective tissue matrix.[76] Uterine smooth muscles are unique in that active, synchronous contraction of these muscles occurs only during the birth process.

Myometrial cells contain three types of protein myofilaments (actin, myosin, and intermediate) and protein structures called dense bodies. Myosin is a hexamer approximately 160 nm long and is the principal contractile protein. Myosin is laid down in thick (15 to 18 nm) myofilaments that optimize interaction with actin and generation of force.[95] Myosin filaments consist of two heavy and two light chains and a head and tail (Fig. 3–2). The heavy chains form helices that unite at one end of the filament to form two globular heads. These heads contain (1) magnesium adenosine triphosphatase (Mg-ATPase) (an enzyme necessary for the interaction of actin and myosin and subsequent generation of force) sites; (2) the actin binding site; (3) a long light chain (molecular weight 20,000 daltons) that can bind to calcium and magnesium and be phosphorylated; and (4) a smaller light chain (molecular weight 15,000 to 17,000 daltons) whose function is unclear.[41, 42, 95] The helical tail formed by the heavy chains transmits the force (tension) generated by the interaction of myosin and actin. Myosin filaments are unidirectional and longer in smooth muscle than in striated muscle. This allows actin to interact with the myosin heads throughout the length of the myosin increasing the maximum degree of shortening to 5 to 10 times greater than that of skeletal muscle.[42, 95]

Actin is a globular protein monomer that polymerizes into long, thin (6 nm) filaments. These filaments originate in and are distributed between dense bodies.[95, 205] Adenosine triphosphatase (ATPase) activity on the myosin head initiates formation of cross-links or bonds between actin and myosin. The myosin head rotates and as a result pulls on the actin filament. This creates tension (force) and a relative spatial displacement (shortening).[95] Interaction of myosin and actin is illustrated in Figure 3–3.

The dense protein (α-actinin) bodies are scattered throughout the cytoplasm and on the inner surface of the cell membrane and are attached to the poles of the smooth muscle cell by intermediate (10 nm thick) filaments. The dense bodies and their filaments form a supportive structure for the contractile filaments and a network of actin attach-

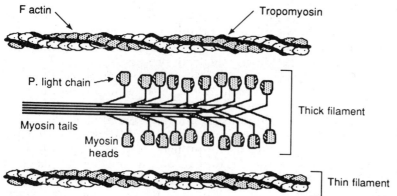

FIGURE 3–2. Schematic structure of myosin (thick) and actin (thin) filaments in smooth muscle. The actin filaments show the helical arrangement of the globular actin molecules and the rod-shaped tropomyosin lying in the long pitched grooves on either side. The myosin molecules aggregate together by means of their tail regions with their heads projecting toward the actin filaments. (From Nuwayhid, B. & Rahabi, M. (1987). Beta-sympathomimetic agents: Use in perinatal obstetrics. *Clin Perinatol, 14,* 757.)

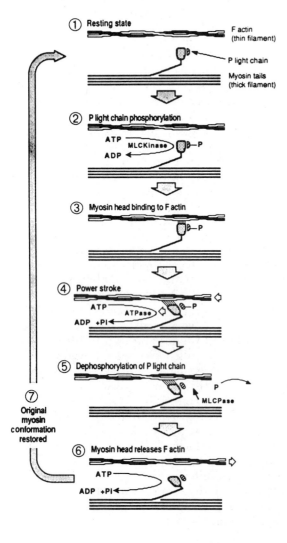

FIGURE 3–3. Mechanisms of smooth muscle contraction and relaxation. Myosin light chain kinase, activated by calcium-calmodulin complex, phosphorylates P-light chain on the myosin head (2). This results in activation and binding of myosin head with F-actin (3) and adenosine triphosphate (ATP) hydrolysis by myosin adenosine triphosphatase (ATPase). The myosin head undergoes a conformational change while it is bound to the actin filament. Movement of actin filament is powered by adenosine diphosphate (ADP) release and myosin conformational change (4). Myosin light chain phosphatase phosphorylates the P-light chain (5) resulting in inhibition of both myosin ATPase and binding of the myosin head with F-actin (6). Binding of an ATP molecule to the myosin head results in restoration of the original conformation of myosin (7) resulting in relaxation. (From Nuwayhid, B. & Rahabi, M. (1987). Beta-sympathomimetic agents: Use in perinatal obstetrics. *Clin Perinatol, 14,* 757.)

ment sites.[40] These structures enable the uterus to enlarge and generate forces sufficient for expulsion of the fetus regardless of the weight or position of the fetus.[95]

In comparison to striated muscle cells, smooth muscle cells are smaller, have a higher ratio of surface area–to–cell volume, and have less myosin. Actin filaments predominate, with approximately 11 to 15 actin filaments per myosin filament versus a 6:1 ratio in skeletal muscle.[40, 42, 105] Filaments in smooth muscle occur in random rather than regular bundles throughout the cell, thus these muscles do not have the striated appearance seen in skeletal muscle. The myofilaments in smooth muscle are oriented obliquely to the long axis of the muscle fibers, which allows the muscle to exert a large force along a short distance at low velocity. This may account for the ability of the myometrium to sustain strong contractions over many hours.[153] The maximal force per area is similar to or greater than that of skeletal muscle.[95, 205] In smooth muscle the pulling force can be exerted in any direction, whereas in skeletal muscle the force generated and the resultant contraction are aligned with the axis of the muscle fibers.[39, 205]

Changes During Pregnancy

Uterine blood flow increases during pregnancy owing to increased vessel diameter and decreased resistance.[195] These changes are described in Chapter 2. The uterus is never completely quiescent; low frequency activity occurs even in the nonpregnant state.[42, 133] The frequency of contractions increases during pregnancy from 0.32/hour at 25 weeks to 2.33/hour at 40 weeks in primiparas.[217] Initially these contractions tend to be mild, irregular, nonsynchronized, and focal in origin and are generally not felt by the pregnant woman. As pregnancy progresses, contractions become more intense and frequent and more are felt by the woman. With the onset of labor, contractions become regular, coordinated, and intense as individual myometrial cells contract in harmony. The contractile force is about five times greater in the pregnant than in the nonpregnant myometrium. Synchronous contraction of the uterus is dependent on formation of gap junctions.[76, 133]

Alterations in the character of uterine contractions are due to structural and functional changes in the myometrium as a result of the extended estrogen-progesterone environment of pregnancy. These changes include:

1. Change in the velocity and timing of action potentials. In the nonpregnant uterus, action potentials occur at the peak of a contraction at a velocity of about 6 cm/second. In pregnancy the action potential occurs much closer to the beginning of the contraction wave and at 1 to 2 cm/second.
2. Hypertrophy and hyperplasia of the myometrial cells, with increased contractile proteins, under the influence of estrogen.
3. Alteration in the arrangement of muscle bundles. In pregnancy these bundles are arranged in closer contact, forming gap junctions.
4. Development of the sarcoplasmic reticulum, enhancing calcium movement.
5. Increased number of mitochondria and cellular ATP, enhancing energy production by the myometrial cell.[76, 100, 133]

The uterus at term seems to have enhanced communication among its cells; at term the action potential covers the entire uterus in 2 to 3 seconds, resulting in nearly simultaneous contraction of the myometrium. This phenomenon may result from the increased velocity of the action potentials, the closer arrangement of muscle bundles with gap junction formation, and the increased number of muscle cells.[76, 133]

PHYSIOLOGY OF PARTURITION

Parturition involves a complex interplay of maternal and fetal factors whose specific interrelationships and significance are still not completely understood. Current knowledge of the etiology of labor consists of a number of hypotheses and theories. Once labor is initiated myometrial contraction and relaxation proceed via the enzymatic phosphorylation and dephosphorylation of myosin and subsequent promotion and inhibition of myosin-actin interaction. Possible pathways for the hormonal control of labor are illustrated in Figure 3–4.

Initiation of Labor

Labor is an all-or-none phenomenon that depends on complicated interaction between the fetus and mother. Factors believed to be influential in the onset of labor include ge-

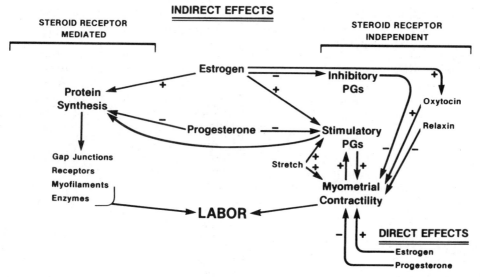

FIGURE 3–4. Model of possible pathways for hormonal control of myometrial contractility and labor (direct and indirect effects of steroid hormones on steroid-dependent and -independent mechanisms). (From Garfield, R.E. (1984). Control of myometrial function in preterm versus term labor. *Clin Obstet Gynecol, 27,* 572.)

netic control, myometrial stretch, increased estrogen levels, progesterone withdrawal (or binding), oxytocin sensitivity, prostaglandins, and fetal and membrane factors.[37] Owing to interspecies differences in the length of gestation and hormonal levels, animal models may not provide accurate data about labor onset in humans.[138, 178]

Estrogen and Progesterone

Progesterone suppresses uterine excitement throughout gestation. As a result, antiprogesterone compounds can induce labor in humans at any stage of gestation.[11, 74–76, 124] Decreases in progesterone may interfere with the stability of lysosomes in the decidua and the fetal membranes by blocking local activity of prostaglandin $F_{2\alpha}$ ($PGF_{2\alpha}$).[133] This increases availability of enzymes that stimulate prostaglandin biosynthesis and activation of cervical collagenase (the enzyme involved in cervical ripening).[95] Although human labor is not preceded by a significant fall in maternal serum progesterone, changes within fetal membranes and decidua may be triggered by localized increases in estrogen synthesis and decreases in progesterone formation.[43] Localized decreases in progesterone may be caused by increased activity of a progesterone-binding protein induced by increased estrogen near term. Decreased availability of progesterone to the myometrial cells allows

estrogen effects to dominate.[136, 173, 180] Possible pathways for hormonal control of myometrial contractility are illustrated in Figure 3–4.

Estrogen levels rise at 34 to 35 weeks. Estrogen promotes formation of gap junctions; increases oxytocin and estrogen receptors in the myometrium; enhances lipase activity and release of arachidonic acid, thus stimulating prostaglandin production; increases binding of intracellular calcium; and increases myosin phosphorylation.[42, 50, 64, 66, 76, 114, 198] Since estrogen production by the placenta comes from fetal adrenal precursors (see Chapter 2), fetal factors may play a critical role in labor onset. Concentrations of estradiol and estrone in amniotic fluid increase 15 to 20 days prior to onset of either term or preterm labor. Estrone produced locally in the chorion and decidua may influence the intrauterine progesterone-to-estrogen ratio, promote production of stimulatory prostaglandins ($PGF_{2\alpha}$), decrease production of inhibitory prostaglandins (PGI_2), and promote formation of oxytocin and prostaglandin receptors as well as gap junction formation.[42]

Prostaglandins

Prostaglandins (Fig. 3–5) are thought to have a central role in the initiation of labor, although their specific functions are still being

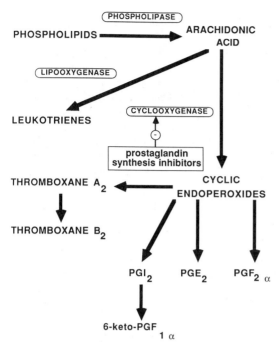

FIGURE 3–5. Metabolism of arachidonic acid and the formation of prostaglandins. (From Holbrook, R.H. & Ueland, K. (1989). Endocrinology of parturition and preterm labor. In S.A. Brody & K. Ueland (Eds.), *Endocrine disorders in pregnancy* (p. 83). Norwalk, CT: Appleton & Lange.)

defined.[4, 18, 36, 37, 39, 42, 90, 92, 203] Levels of PGE_2 and $PGF_{2\alpha}$ increase prior to and during labor, and they mediate labor onset through their role in the formation of gap junctions and by increasing calcium levels in the cytoplasm of myometrial smooth muscle cells. PGE_2 is also involved in ripening of the cervix.[90, 203] Prostaglandin inhibitors (e.g., aspirin, indomethacin) inhibit preterm labor and prolong pregnancy.[85, 158, 211]

The composition and biosynthesis of prostaglandins by the various maternal and fetal tissues, as well as the source of amniotic fluid prostaglandins, are still unclear.[43, 64, 90, 138] In the amnion the major prostaglandin is PGE_2; the decidua produces large amounts of PGI_2 and to a lesser extent $PGF_{2\alpha}$ and PGE_2. The placenta produces PGE_2, PGD_2, PGI_2, and thromboxane A_2 (TXA_2). Placental TXA_2 may be important following delivery in enhancing hemostasis after placental separation.[64]

PGI_2 (prostacyclin) is produced by the pregnant and the nonpregnant myometrium as well as by the placental vasculature and has little uterotonic activity. PGI_2 is a potent vasodilator that inhibits platelet aggregation and protects the vascular epithelium. Pros-

Prostaglandins

Prostaglandins (PGs) are organic compounds that act as chemical mediators or local hormones, exerting their major effect at or near the site of production. They are usually metabolized locally but may enter the blood to be rapidly inactivated by pulmonary and hepatic enzymes. Over 16 PGs have been identified and classified into subgroups based on the configuration of their 5-carbon ring. PGE_2, $PGF_{2\alpha}$, and PGI_2 (prostacyclin) are the most important in reproductive processes. During pregnancy, prostaglandins are important for maternal cardiovascular changes, including preventing hypertension and increasing uteroplacental blood flow, and in cervical ripening and the initiation of labor. PGs are synthesized rapidly, are relatively unstable, and have a short half-life. PGs are formed by enzymatic oxidation of arachidonic acid, a polyunsaturated fatty acid precursor found in an esterified form (glycophospholipid). Formation of PG requires that arachidonic acid be changed to a nonesterified form either directly by cellular phospholipase A_2 or indirectly by phospholipase C. Nonesterified arachidonic acid can be further metabolized by specific microsomal or cytosolic enzymes via several pathways (including cyclooxygenase and lipoxygenase) as illustrated in Fig. 3–5. PGs and thromboxane (TXA_2) are formed via the cyclooxygenase pathway under the influence of prostaglandin synthetase and thromboxane synthetase. TXA_2 is a platelet aggregation factor and vasoconstrictor whose actions are balanced by the opposing actions of prostacyclin. Formation of PGs and TXA_2 is inhibited by nonsteroidal anti-inflammatory agents such as aspirin and indomethacin, which block cyclooxygenase activity. Since PGs mediate the action of the hypothalamus in responding to pyrogens released during an infection, aspirin effectively reduces fever. Arachidonic acid metabolism via the lipoxygenase pathway leads to the production of various acids followed by the formation of leukotrienes (LTs). Leukotrienes are chemotactic and chemokinetic for leukocytes. The fetal membranes, decidua, and placenta produce both prostaglandins and leukotrienes. The role of LTs in gestation and parturition is unclear. In animals exogenous LT has been reported to stimulate contractility and inhibit myometrial prostacyclin (PGI_2) synthesis.[4, 90, 203]

tacyclin is important in maintaining blood flow to the placenta and in ensuring adequate uterine blood flow during labor.[40] Suppression of prostacyclin formation leads to vasoconstriction and is thought to have a role in pregnancy-induced hypertension (PIH) (see Chapter 6).[119, 159] Thromboxanes are platelet aggregation factors and potent vasoconstrictors that oppose the action of prostacyclins. Increased placental TXA_2 is also implicated in the pathogenesis of PIH, and since production is blocked by prostaglandin synthetase inhibitors (Fig. 3–5), that provides a rationale for low-dose aspirin therapy.

Arachidonic acid metabolism via the lipoxygenase pathway (Fig. 3–5) leads to formation of leukotrienes (LTs), which are chemotactic and chemokinetic for leukocytes.[138] The fetal membranes, decidua, and placenta produce both PGs and LTs. The role of LT in gestation and parturition is unclear. In animals exogenous LT has been reported to stimulate contractility and inhibit myometrial prostacyclin synthesis.[42]

Thus the major sources of prostaglandins involved in labor onset are the fetal membranes, decidua, placenta, and uterus (Fig. 3–6). Arachidonic acid is stored in the fetal membranes along with lysosomal enzymes such as phospholipase A_2, which are necessary to convert esterified arachidonic acid to its unesterified form. Release of lysosomal enzymes may be triggered by a local decrease in progesterone, altered estrogen-to-progesterone ratio, or physical and chemical stressors such as hypertonic saline, stripping of the membranes, and stresses of labor.[16, 40, 42, 43] A circular action may occur in which prostaglandins stimulate labor contractions, which stimulate further PG synthesis.

Synthesis of prostaglandins is also stimulated by stretch of the uterus and cervix, estrogens (especially estradiol), and oxytocin. Challis postulates that the critical point in the onset of labor is stimulation of PGE_2 synthesis in the amnion. PGE_2 is then transferred across the chorion and amniotic fluid to the decidua. In the decidua PGE_2 is converted to or acts as a stimulus for production of $PGF_{2\alpha}$. Unlike oxytocin, prostaglandins seem to have similar effects on the myometrium at all stages of pregnancy and thus can be used to initiate labor prior to term.[42] Prostaglandins bind to the cell membrane, increase the frequency of action potentials, and stimulate actual muscle contraction.

Endogenous inhibitors of prostaglandin synthase (EIPS) are found in amniotic fluid and may suppress prostaglandin production by the fetal membranes. EIPS activity decreases gradually during gestation and markedly during labor.[178] The potency of EIPS found in maternal plasma decreases during the third trimester. Since EIPS are still present during labor, they may have a permissive rather than an active role in labor onset.[27, 138]

Oxytocin

Oxytocin is a stimulant that is often used to induce or augment labor. Alterations in myometrial sensitivity are mediated by changes in the concentration of oxytocin receptors, which increase 100 to 200 times by term and parallel the increase in uterine oxytocin sensitivity.[69, 71] Binding of oxytocin to receptors on the cell membrane increases the frequency of pacemaker potentials and lowers the threshold for initiation of action potentials. Failed induction and postdate pregnancies are associated with a decreased concentration of oxytocin receptors. Under the influence of estrogen, the sensitivity of the myometrium to the effects of oxytocin changes markedly during pregnancy, so that oxytocin does not work well as a labor stimulant for induction of labor prior to term. Fetal oxytocin may stimulate prostaglandin production in the decidua.[64]

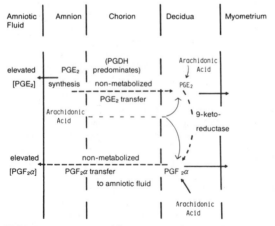

FIGURE 3–6. Possible sources of prostaglandins at term. (From Challis, J.R.G. (1989). Characteristics of parturition. In R.K. Creasy & R. Resnik (Eds.), *Maternal-fetal medicine: Principles and practice* (2nd ed., p. 466). Philadelphia: WB Saunders.)

Relaxin

Relaxin is an insulin-like ovarian hormone produced primarily by the corpus luteum but also by the myometrium, decidua, and placenta. Relaxin levels are greatest during the first trimester but remain detectable in maternal circulation throughout gestation, falling rapidly after delivery.[42] Specific roles of relaxin are still unclear. Relaxin probably acts synergistically with progesterone in blocking uterine activity and maintaining myometrial quiescence during pregnancy and may suppress oxytocin release.[64] Relaxin enhances cervical ripening and may help regulate gap junction permeability.[76]

Myometrial Contraction

Myometrial contraction is mediated via interaction of actin and myosin. In smooth muscle such as myometrium, contraction and relaxation are regulated primarily via enzymatic phosphorylation and dephosphorylation of myosin. The key enzyme is myosin light chain kinase (MLCK). Activity of MLCK is regulated by calcium, calmodulin, and cyclic adenosine monophosphate (cAMP)–mediated phosphorylation, which are in turn influenced by hormones and pharmacologic agents. The exact mechanisms for myometrial contraction are still a subject of speculation and controversy. The following description and Figure 3–7 reflect the current, generally accepted hypothesis.[40, 42, 95, 149]

Contractions are produced by spontaneous electromechanical coupling or are initiated by exogenous hormones or drugs. Initiation of action potentials in uterine smooth muscle is probably primarily dependent on the influx of Ca^{2+} across the cell membrane, although other ions such as Na^+ may also be involved.[38, 105] Intracellular calcium is critical for activation of MLCK. Calcium levels increase significantly with contractions.

MLCK is associated with the long light chain of myosin and activated by changes in intracellular calcium. Excitation of myometrial cell, primarily by hormonal stimuli, increases the concentrations of free calcium in the cytoplasm.[42, 76, 87] The calcium may be released from stores in the sarcoplasmic reticulum or, since the sarcoplasmic reticulum is relatively sparse, from intracellular membrane–bound calcium vesicles, mitochondrial stores, or extracellular calcium.[64, 76, 95, 205]

Mechanisms for transport of extracellular calcium across the cell membrane include (1) membrane potential–dependent Ca^{2+} channels, (2) ATP-dependent pumps (via Ca,Mg-ATPase), (3) Na^+-Ca^{2+} exchange across the membrane, and (4) receptor-controlled calcium gates.[20, 44, 64] Magnesium may trigger further intracellular calcium release.[6] Potential-sensitive channels allow passage of calcium when the potential across the cell membrane falls to a critical level. Influx of calcium across these channels can be blocked by calcium antagonists or slow channel blockers such as nifedipine.[6, 146] Receptor-operated channels are less specific and not effectively blocked by calcium antagonists but can be controlled by drugs acting directly on receptors.[6]

Although the amount of free calcium is critical in determining whether or not the muscle contracts or relaxes, calcium does not act independently.[6] Calcium must first bind with calmodulin, forming a calcium-calmodulin complex, which in turn activates MLCK.[40, 95, 149] Calmodulin is a cytoplasmic protein that is activated by increases in unbound intracellular calcium.[42] Activated MLCK catalyzes phosphorylation (addition of a phosphate group) of the myosin light chain. Phosphorylation activates the ATPase on the myosin head with the release of chemical energy needed for the subsequent binding of myosin and actin (actomyosin). The result is release of ADP and a phosphorus molecule, which changes the configuration of the myosin with flexion of the head on the tail. The flexion pulls on the actin filament and the muscle contracts (see Fig. 3–3).[42, 95, 149, 205]

Myometrial relaxation involves the action of another enzyme, myosin light chain phosphatase. With removal of the phosphate group from the myosin head, the actin no longer recognizes the myosin. Actin-myosin interaction is inhibited and the muscle cell relaxes.[40, 95] Reduction in MLCK activity due to decreased calcium-calmodulin levels also leads to muscle relaxation as does inhibition of phosphorylation by increased levels of cAMP.[40] Cyclic AMP is a second messenger (i.e., it carries the message of a hormone to the site where the hormonal effect is realized) that may lower the affinity of myosin for calcium-calmodulin or reduce intracellular calcium by stimulating calcium return to intracellular stores or extrusion across the cell membrane.[76, 95, 149] Prostaglandins may inhibit cAMP calcium uptake.[3, 6]

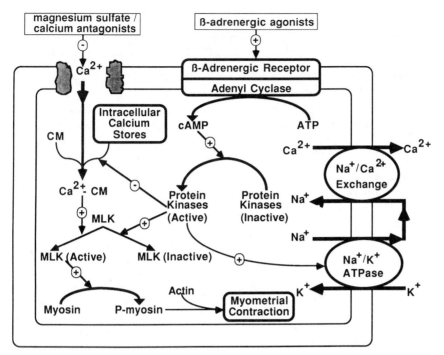

FIGURE 3–7. Cellular mechanisms controlling myometrial contractility. (From Holbrook, R.H. & Ueland, K. (1989). Endocrinology of parturition and preterm labor. In S.A. Brody & K. Ueland (Eds.), *Endocrine disorders in pregnancy* (p. 90). Norwalk, CT: Appleton & Lange, as adapted from Huzar, G., et al. (1984). The myometrium and uterine cervix in normal and preterm labor. *N Engl J Med, 311,* 571, and Fuchs, F. & Stubblefield, P.G. (Eds.). (1984). *Preterm birth: Causes, prevention, and management* (p. 28). New York: Macmillan. Reprinted by permission.)

The relative activity of adenylate cyclase (mediates cAMP synthesis) and phosphodiesterase (mediates cAMP breakdown) influence myometrial contractility by altering cAMP levels within the cell. Adenylate cyclase increases intracellular cAMP, which reduces calcium-calmodulin complexes and intracellular calcium levels and thus MLCK (Fig. 3–7). These enzymes can be altered by pharmacologic agents. For example, adenylate cyclase is activated by β-adrenergic agonists, resulting in increased cAMP and reduced contractility. Substances that inhibit phosphodiesterase, which normally mediates cAMP breakdown, also result in elevated levels of intracellular cAMP. Therefore substances such as theophylline and α-adrenergic agents also decrease myometrial contractility.[39]

Activity of MLCK and cAMP is influenced by hormones and pharmacologic agents. Oxytocin and PGF$_{2\alpha}$ enhance contractility by increasing intracellular calcium levels and the rate of MLCK phosphorylation. Oxytocin also releases calcium from intracellular stores and inhibits calcium uptake by the sarcoplasmic reticulum, extending actin-myosin interaction and thus muscle contraction. Relaxin increases cAMP, which inhibits MLCK phosphorylation and induces muscle relaxation.

Energy (released from ATP by myosin ATPase) is critical for myometrial contraction. ATP is used for both actin-myosin interaction and ion transport. If adequate oxygen and glucose are not available for ATP formation, as may occur with prolonged labor, the contractile process will be inhibited. The myosin head contains Mg-ATPase sites where ATP is hydrolyzed, converting chemical energy to mechanical force.[92] Transport of calcium back across the cell membrane may be mediated by cell membrane Ca,Mg-ATPase. Oxytocin inhibits this enzyme, thus enhancing contractility.[95]

Prostaglandins and oxytocin promote release of calcium from intracellular pools or prevent uptake of calcium into these pools. This promotes contractility. On the other hand, agents that inhibit myometrial activity such as progesterone, relaxin, prostacyclin, and β-agonists promote calcium sequestration or extrusion (via cAMP-dependent enzymes) and thus myometrial relaxation.[39, 40]

In summary, control of myometrial activity is dependent on enzymatic phosphorylation of myosin by MLCK to allow interaction of actin and myosin. Hormonal, biochemical, and physical factors mediate MLCK activity, uterine activity, and myometrial structural and functional alterations. For example, increased estrogens, decreased progesterone, or changes in activity of receptors are involved in activating myometrial cells (see Figs. 3–4 and 3–7). Other factors include prostaglandins, oxytocin, cAMP, energy for contractile processes, and mechanical stretch.

Coordination of Uterine Contractions

Electrical and contractile activity in smooth muscle cells is controlled by myogenic, neurogenic, and hormonal control systems.[40, 73, 74] Myogenic activity, the spontaneous activity of the myometrium that occurs in the absence of any neural or hormonal input, includes the intrinsic excitability of the muscle cell, ability of the muscle to contract spontaneously, and mechanisms that produce rhythmic contractions. Neurogenic and hormonal control systems are superimposed on the muscle's inherent myogenic properties to initiate, augment, and suppress myometrial activity.[74, 76] Myogenic control is dominated by hormonal influences, especially those of estrogen and progesterone, which influence myogenic characteristics through their generally opposing actions.[50] Neurogenic control is not critical, since labor can occur in women with spinal injury, although the length of labor may be altered (see Chapter 12).[13]

PACEMAKER POTENTIAL
Spontaneous cycles of activity in myometrial cells are characterized by (1) slow, rhythmic fluctuations in the magnitude of electrical potential across the cell membrane (pacemaker potential); (2) spikes of electrical activity that occur in bursts at the crests of slow waves (action potentials) and become synchronous at parturition (a single spike can initiate a contraction; multiple spikes are needed to maintain forceful contractions); and (3) prepotential-like pacemaker potentials associated with initiation of action potentials.[76]

Pacemaker potential in the human uterus is not well understood. Specific pacemaker cells have not been identified.[95] The pacemaker potential depolarizes the cell membrane to a critical threshold. This triggers a change in the Na^+, Ca^{2+}, and K^+ conductance (action potential). The action potential increases membrane permeability to calcium

and release of intracellular calcium stores.[76, 95, 205] As long as extracellular K^+ concentrations are high, action potentials increase in frequency. When maximum ion concentrations are reached within the cell, ionic stability is restored by active outward transport of Na^+ and Ca^{2+}, intrallular uptake of calcium, and recapturing of intracellular K^+. The muscle cell returns to a resting state.

Specific cells located near the fallopian tubes were once thought to initiate action potentials and myometrial contractions. Investigations have not supported this hypothesis.[76] While it is likely that a cell initiating depolarization will be located in the fundus near the uterotubal junction, any myometrial cell is now thought to have pacemaker potential.[76, 153]

As action potentials are conducted to neighboring myometrial cells, groups of cells contract, leading to what is perceived by the woman as a uterine contraction. Coordination of uterine contractions occurs when all myometrial cells contract nearly simultaneously. Coordination is mediated by the low resistance gap junctions between myometrial cells that promote propagation of the action potential throughout the uterus.

GAP JUNCTION FORMATION
Smooth muscle bundles normally separated from each other within connective tissue may come into closer approximation to form gap junctions (or low-resistance bridges or intercellular communication channels). Increased gap junction interaction is associated with improved propagation of electrical impulses, increased conduction velocity, and coordinated contractility of the myometrium.[74, 76, 95]

Gap junctions are formed when proteins (called connexons) within the cell membranes of adjacent smooth muscle cells align to create symmetric openings between their cytoplasm. These pores are separated by a narrow gap and provide a pathway for transport of ions, metabolites, and second messengers.[42] Gap junctions can be open or closed, thus controlling intercellular communication.[95] Increased permeability across the junctions increases synchrony of electrical conduction and muscular contraction and subsequently more effective labor.

The number and size of gap junctions increase markedly during gestation to approximately 1000/cell during labor.[76] Gap junctions are absent or infrequent in nonpregnant myometrium and decline markedly within 24 hours of delivery.[40, 42, 72, 76, 79, 80] An increase in gap junctions has been reported in women in preterm labor; delay in the formation of gap junctions is associated with prolonged pregnancy.[40, 72, 76, 79, 80]

Formation of gap junctions in the uterus is under hormonal control.[40, 76, 80, 95] Estrogen stimulates gap junction formation by stimulating synthesis of connexons. One way progesterone functions to inhibit labor and maintain the pregnancy may be by inhibition of estrogen-enhanced connexon synthesis.[76, 84]

The specific role of prostaglandins in gap junction formation is still unclear. Some prostaglandins seem to stimulate whereas others inhibit gap junction formation, either directly or indirectly via estrogen and progesterone activities.[76] Gap junction formation is also inhibited or decreased by indomethacin, relaxin, isoxsuprine, and isoproterenol; oxytocin (Pitocin) has little effect.[95] Lack of adequate concentrations of gap junctions decreases the effectiveness of Pitocin; as a result, Pitocin may not be effective with women experiencing pre- or postterm labor. Increased intracellular calcium reduces coupling, and increased cAMP in the uterus decreases gap junction permeability.[74, 76] One mechanism by which relaxin, prostacyclin and β-agonists are thought to inhibit myometrial contractility is by increasing intracellular cAMP, which uncouples gap junctions, thus preventing synchronous uterine activity.[74]

Physiologic Events During a Uterine Contraction

A normal uterine contraction spreads downward from the cornu within about 15 seconds. Although the actual contractile phase begins slightly later in the lower portion of the uterus, functional coordination of the uterus is such that the contraction peak is attained simultaneously in all portions. The intensity of the contraction decreases from the cornu downward and is essentially absent in the cervix.

Resting baseline tonus in labor is at an intrauterine pressure of approximately 10 to 12 mmHg, which may increase to 30 mmHg with hypertonia.[153] Uterine contractions can be palpated abdominally with intrauterine pressure greater than 10 to 20 mmHg and perceived by the woman at 15 to 20 mmHg (Fig. 3–8).[133] During early first stage, intra-uterine pressure increases 20 to 30 mmHg above resting values, increasing to greater than 50 mmHg in the active phase and to 100 to 150 mmHg during a Valsalva maneuver with maximal expulsive efforts.[133] A laboring woman often perceives pain at pressures greater than 25 mmHg or more, although this varies with individual thresholds. Thus the duration of a contraction assessed from palpation or patient perception will be shorter than the actual contraction, and the duration between contractions will seem longer.[133]

Page and colleagues define hyperactive labor as pressure greater than 50 mmHg at the peak or contractions closer than 2 minutes apart and hypoactive labor as generation of peak pressures less than 30 mmHg or an interval greater than 5 minutes between contractions.[153] Women exhibit marked individual variation in the intensity, frequency, and duration of contractions. Contractions may also be influenced by position and the use of oxytocin, analgesics, and anesthesia.[133]

The Cervix

During pregnancy the cervix increases in mass, water content, and vascularization. The connective tissue of the uterus (particularly the cervix) undergoes changes in its viscoelastic plasticity so that by term "it combines the properties of a rubber band with those of salt water taffy."[153, p.90] Myometrial contractions exert a slow, steady pull on the cervix, resulting in cervical stretching but with little rebound between contractions. This leads to progressive cervical dilatation. In order for the fetus to be expelled, the cervix must first change from a relatively rigid to a soft, distensible structure.

Structure of the Cervix

The cervix is composed primarily of connective tissue covered by a thin layer of smooth muscle that penetrates into the connective tissue matrix.[6] Approximately 85 to 90% of the cervix is connective tissue and 10 to 15% smooth muscle.[40, 153] The amount of smooth muscle varies in the upper (25%), middle (16%), and lower (6%) portions.[174] The connective tissue consists of a dense network of interlacing collagen and elastin fibers embedded in a gel-like ground substance matrix (proteoglycans).

FIGURE 3–8. Correlation between abdominal palpation and intrauterine pressure tracing. (From Page, E.W., Villee, C.A., & Villee, D.B. (1981). *Human reproduction: Essentials of reproductive and perinatal medicine* (3rd ed., p. 322). Philadelphia: WB Saunders.)

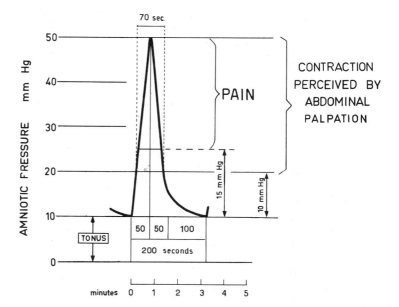

The collagen fibers form a relatively rigid rod-shaped structure (important during pregnancy to retain the fetus) and impart tensile strength to the cervix.[40] Collagen fibers can be of the cross-striated type I (70%) or the reticular type II (30%). Elastin is haphazardly arranged, imparting elasticity to the cervical tissue and contributing to the integrity of the tissue.[53, 76] Elastin may be important in the ability of the cervix to distend in labor and then return to its normal shape post partum.[133]

The connective tissue matrix (ground substance) is composed of glycosaminoglycans attached to a protein core. The major glycosaminoglycans in the cervix are dermatan sulfate (70%), heparan sulfate (15%), and hyaluronic acid (15%).[40, 42] These substances are large charged molecules that bind together, attract water, and coil around and lock the collagen fibrils.[42]

Fibroblasts, leukocytes, macrophages, and eosinophils proliferate in the cervix during pregnancy. These changes may be important in altering vasopermeability to increase cervical water content.[53] The fibroblasts are also involved in the metabolism of collagen and glycosaminoglycans.

Cervical Ripening and Dilatation

The rigid cervix of pregnancy must become distensible in order to expel the fetus.[40] Cervical ripening (softening, effacement, and increased distensibility) involves changes in collagen, proteoglycans, and smooth muscle with enzymatic degradation of collagen by collagenase, elastase, and other enzymes.[153, 202, 203] Collagenase activity increases threefold beginning as early as 10 weeks; elastase activity increases toward the end of pregnancy and post partum.[111, 201] Myometrial contractions have little effect on cervical ripening; considerable ripening usually occurs before the onset of contractions.[42, 53]

Ripening of the cervix involves changes in the solubility of collagen. Collagen is first degraded by collagenase, leukocyte elastase, and other nonspecific proteolytic enzymes, resulting in a loss of collagen fibrils. Hyaluronic acid (which loosely binds collagen fibrils) increases, accompanied by a decrease in dermatan sulfate (which tightly binds collagen fibrils) and an increase in the water content of the cervix.[53, 206] This weakens the structure of the cervix.[40, 64, 83, 93, 143] It has been suggested that similar changes in the amnion enhance membrane rupture, although amnion collagenous tissue was recently reported not to dissociate at term.[187, 214]

Hormonal control of cervical ripening is a complex process that may involve a cascade of changes in estradiol, progesterone, relaxin, prostacyclin, PGE_2, and $PGF_{2\alpha}$ mediated via the fibroblasts.[4, 40, 64, 93, 153, 202] Progesterone inhibits collagen breakdown. Alterations in the estrogen-to-progesterone ratio correlate with increased collagenase activity and collagen degradation.[40, 93] Increased cervical relaxin may activate collagen peptidase and mediate changes in water and mucopolysaccharide content of the cervix.[40]

Uterine activity is enhanced by mechanical stretching of the cervix (Ferguson reflex). This response may be due to stimulation of $PGF_{2\alpha}$ or oxytocin release by the cervical stretching.[63, 64]

PGE_2 and $PGF_{2\alpha}$ have a localized influence on cervical softening. PGE_2 action on the cervix is independent of uterine contractile activity and has been used to improve cervical inductability (i.e., responsiveness of the cervical tissue) prior to induction of labor (e.g., when delivery is indicated because of risk factors).[61, 143, 151, 156, 199] PG levels tend to correlate with the degree of cervical dilatation and to be higher in women with spontaneous initiation of labor than in those delivered by elective cesarean section or who require oxytocin stimulation.[43, 109, 110, 137, 188] Prostacyclin may alter cervical smooth muscle.

CLINICAL IMPLICATIONS FOR THE PREGNANT WOMAN AND HER FETUS

Labor and delivery place additional stressors on the maternal-fetal unit, which may be further increased in high risk situations. Alterations in the physiologic processes of parturition can have a significant impact on the well-being of the mother, fetus, and neonate. Knowledge of these processes is critical in understanding the basis for nursing care and therapies to initiate or inhibit labor and the etiologic factors in dystocia and pre- or post-term labor onset.

Maternal Position During Labor

Position during labor is influenced by cultural factors, obstetric practices, place of delivery, technology, and preference of health care providers.[123, 145, 164] Maternal position during labor influences the characteristics and effectiveness of uterine contractions, fetal well-being, maternal comfort, and course of labor.[1, 29, 32, 81, 132, 164, 167, 169–171]

Historically a variety of positions have been used for labor and delivery. Delivery positions currently used in many U.S. institutions include lithotomy, lateral (Sim's), semi-sitting, dorsal (or modified lithotomy), and occasionally kneeling.[165] Although lithotomy has often been used routinely, primarily for the comfort and convenience of the person delivering the infant, this position has no physiologic advantages and may interfere with expulsive efforts.[162] Currently alternative positions are being used with increasing frequency in many settings.

Several positions have advantages or disadvantages from an anatomic and physiologic standpoint. During the first stage of labor upright positions, such as sitting, standing, squatting, and kneeling, allow the abdominal wall to relax, and the influence of gravity causes the uterine fundus to fall forward. This directs the fetal head into the pelvic inlet in an anterior position and applies direct pressure to the cervix, which helps stimulate and stretch the cervix. Feedback from the cervix to the myometrium may stimulate more intense contractions and shorten labor.[123] The lateral recumbent position reduces pressure on maternal blood vessels and promotes venous return and cardiac output, thus increasing uterine perfusion and fetal oxygenation.[132, 164] Side-lying may be effective during labor with a posterior fetus, by allowing the weight of the uterus and fetus to tip away from the back and permitting application of counterpressure over the lumbosacral area.[169]

Position at delivery should optimize alignment for fetal descent and maximize the capacity of the pelvis and efficiency of maternal expulsive efforts.[165] Squatting during the second stage enhances engagement and descent of the fetal head and increases maternal pelvic diameters. In this position the upper portion of the symphysis pubis is compressed and the bottom part separated slightly. This results in an outward movement and separation of the innominate bones and backward movement of the lower sacrum. The pelvic outlet increases 28% with increased transverse (1 cm) and anteroposterior (0.5 to 2 cm) diameters. Thigh pressure against the abdomen during squatting may also promote fetal descent and correction of unfavorable fetal positions. Sitting or semi-sitting (30-degree angle) may have similar advantages.[123, 165]

Dorsal and supine positions have been associated with adverse effects on maternal hemodynamics and fetal status and with the supine hypotension syndrome.[81, 145, 164, 165] A supine position is a disadvantage during engagement and descent of the fetal head because this position does not optimize fetal alignment, maximize pelvic diameter, or maximize efficiency of maternal expulsive efforts.[123]

Most studies of maternal position during labor have compared the effects of two positions, so findings vary with the positions used. Some general outcomes can be summarized. In the supine position contractions were more frequent but less intense than in the side-lying position. The use of the supine position during the first stage of labor compromised effective uterine activity, prolonged labor, and increased use of drugs to augment labor.[167] Placing a woman in the side-lying position increased the intensity and decreased the frequency of contractions and promoted greater uterine efficiency.[39, 40, 42] Frequency and intensity of contractions and uterine activity increased with sitting or standing.[29] Upright (standing, sitting, squatting, kneeling) positions (versus supine) were associated with more regular and intense contractions and shorter duration of first and second stages and total labor.[123] The lateral recumbent position (versus sitting) led to more intense, less frequent contractions and greater uterine efficiency during the first stage.[170, 171]

Positional effects appear as soon as the maternal position is changed and last as long as the position is maintained. [32, 169, 170] Changes are more marked with spontaneous than with induced labor and do not seem to be affected by parity or fetal position. The effectiveness of contractions can be enhanced by alternating positions after the woman has maintained one position for a period of time. If the woman prefers a supine position, the efficiency of contractions can be increased by alternating this position with standing or side-lying.[170]

Although many studies have not found specific alterations in fetal status associated with maternal position, positions that increase the efficiency of contractions and decrease the duration of labor may reduce fetal stress.[29, 164, 170, 171] For example, semi-sitting positions during delivery may shorten the length of the second stage and reduce fetal acidosis.[29, 122, 165]

Maternal comfort is also an important consideration. Many women prefer lateral or standing positions over supine.[132, 164] Position preferences may change during labor. A woman may prefer sitting or walking during early labor but semi-recumbent or side-lying with pillow support as labor progresses. Roberts and colleagues summarize factors to consider in selecting a position conducive to labor progress and maternal comfort: "potential mechanical advantage of the position; the associated hemodynamic alterations and subsequent uteroplacental perfusion; the position of the fetus; the parturient's perception of her contractions, discomfort, and fatigue; and obstetrical indications for confinement to bed for continuous fetal monitoring, medication, or care."[169, p.115]

Maternal Pushing Efforts During the Second Stage

There have been increasing concerns regarding the effects of bearing down and the Valsalva maneuver on maternal hemodynamics and fetal status (Fig. 3–9).[9, 30, 113, 123, 165, 207, 213] Yeates and Roberts conclude that fetal outcome is probably affected more by maternal position and sustained maternal bearing down than by duration of the second stage per se.[213] Maternal hypotension and fetal hypoxia may develop more rapidly with supine position or epidural anesthesia.[113, 154, 207] Maternal hemodynamic changes with bearing down and the Valsalva maneuver are mediated by sympathetic discharge and catecholamine release, which also increase maternal discomfort and in combination with maternal acidosis may decrease uterine activity.[165]

Several investigations have compared the effects of open-glottis pushing (based on involuntary maternal urges to push) with those of the Valsalva maneuver.[9, 30, 213] With long Valsalva pushing, there were less frequent expulsive contractions and a trend toward a longer second stage.[9] Bearing down (prolonged Valsalva maneuver) lasting greater than 5 to 6 seconds was associated with decreased maternal blood pressure and placental blood flow, alterations in maternal and fetal oxygenation, decreased fetal pH and PO_2, increased fetal PCO_2, an increased incidence of fetal heart rate pattern changes, and delayed recovery of the fetal heart rate with fetal asphyxia.[9, 30, 33, 81, 130] Open glottis pushing was not associated with changes in maternal blood pressure (probably since intrathoracic pressure elevations were not sustained) or increased fetal pH.[9] Involuntary pushing with minimal straining has been associated with fewer episiotomies and forceps deliveries and a shorter second stage.[123, 161, 165] Roberts suggests that a semi-recumbent position with bearing down efforts that are short and in accordance with involuntary

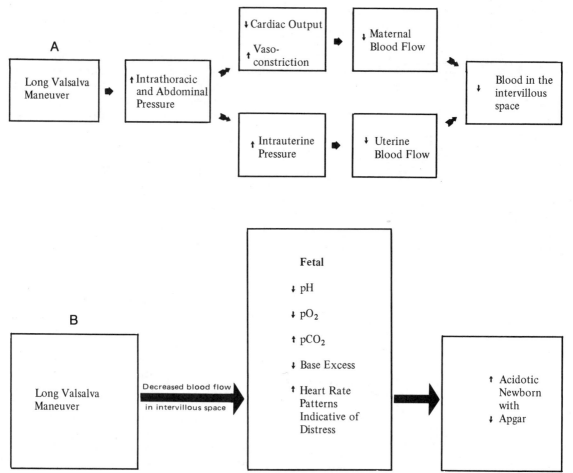

FIGURE 3–9. Possible maternal *(A)* and fetal *(B)* effects of a long Valsalva push. (From Barnett, M. & Humenick, S. (1982). Infant outcome in relation to second stage labor pushing method. *Birth*, *9*(Winter), 221, by permission of Blackwell Scientific Publications, Inc.)

urges to push is most conducive to favorable delivery outcomes.[165]

Sleep and colleagues recently reviewed available research regarding care practices during the second stage and concluded that (1) directed pushing should be abandoned since no data support this practice and some data suggest it is harmful; (2) supine positions tend to lengthen the second stage, reduce the incidence of spontaneous births, increase fetal heart rate abnormalities, and reduce umbilical cord pH; and (3) arbitrary limits on duration of the second stage should be abandoned if mother and fetus are doing well and labor is progressing.[189]

Preterm Labor

Infants born prematurely are at high risk during the neonatal period and for later developmental problems. As a result much effort has been directed toward eliciting the causes for preterm labor and developing intervention strategies to prevent the onset of labor and to terminate uterine contractions that begin prior to term. Preterm labor is defined as the onset of regular contractions with progressive cervical effacement and dilatation prior to 37 weeks.[34] There is still speculation concerning the specific events leading to onset of labor prior to term. Preterm labor is probably not initiated by a single etiologic event, but rather by a group of factors (Table 3–1). These factors probably act by influencing the various pathways involved in control of labor onset (see Figs. 3–4 and 3–7). The role of infection in the initiation of preterm labor is discussed in Chapter 10.

Pharmacology of Labor

Uterine activity can be controlled directly by blocking or stimulating specific hormonal re-

TABLE 3–1
Factors Associated with Preterm Labor and Possible Underlying Mechanisms

FACTOR	HYPOTHESIZED MECHANISMS
Infection	Production of phospholipase A_2 by bacteria that often cause amnionitis and urinary tract infections. This enzyme stimulates formation of nonesterified arachidonic acid, the precursor for formation of prostaglandins (see Fig. 3–5) Premature rupture of membranes
Uterine distention (secondary to multiple pregnancy, polyhydramnios, fibroids, etc.)	Overdistention of the uterus with stretching of myometrial smooth muscle cells
Uterine and cervical anomalies (e.g., incompetent cervix, bicornate or septate uterus, anomalies associated with diethylstilbestrol [DES] exposure)	Uterine overdistention and stretching (smaller space for fetus to grow) Altered endometrium and blood flow Early loss of protective function of cervix
Premature rupture of membranes	Maternal genital infection Other(?)
Maternal substance abuse (especially cocaine)	Maternal hypertension with abrupt elevation of maternal blood pressure and vasoconstriction of placental blood vessels often resulting in abruptio placentae
Maternal illness (e.g., diabetes mellitus, renal and cardiac disorders, hypertension, hyperthyroidism)	Unknown; alteration or interference with placental perfusion may be a factor
Maternal or fetal stress (physical, physiologic, or emotional)	Decreased uteroplacental perfusion secondary to release of catecholamines with redistribution of blood away from uterus
Socioeconomic factors (lack of prenatal care, poor nutrition)	Risk of infection; other predisposing factors or early signs of labor unrecognized owing to lack of early care; altered availability of nutrients for fetoplacental unit; environmental or individual stress
Iatrogenic prematurity	Termination of pregnancy prior to term (by induction or cesarean birth) owing to maternal or fetal illness or electively (miscalculation of dates)

Compiled from references 46, 62, 129, 147, and 173.

ceptors or altering electromechanical coupling, and indirectly via agents that interfere with the synthesis of enzymes and other mediators of myometrial contraction and relaxation.[6] Use of these agents must take into consideration the physiologic properties of as well as the pharmacologic actions on both the cervix and the myometrium. A woman who is post term with altered myometrial contractility and an unripe (resistant) cervix needs an agent that increases and coordinates myometrial activity and decreases cervical resistance. On the other hand, agents used for women in preterm labor lead to myometrial relaxation and increase cervical resistance.[6] This section examines pharmacology of labor related to control of cervical ripening, labor induction, and labor inhibition.

Control of Cervical Ripening

Cervical ripening is not dependent on myometrial contractions and occurs in the absence of regular uterine contractions. Agents that have been clinically evaluated to enhance cervical ripening include estrogen, relaxin, and prostaglandins.[6] Prostaglandins are currently used most frequently. Physiologic ripening is under the control of local mediators, in particular PGE_2, whose action is influenced by other hormones such as estrogens and relaxin. Exogenous PGE_2 has been used to induce significant cervical ripening by relaxing cervical smooth muscle.[61, 143, 151, 156, 199, 204] PGE_2 has little influence on myometrial activation. Conversely, intravenous administration of oxytocin or $PGF_{2\alpha}$ stimulates myometrial contractions but causes no significant changes in cervical resistance.[61] Antiprogesterone agents (RU 486, or mifepristone) are currently being evaluated as alternative cervical ripening agents.[103, 115] Drug-induced inhibition of cervical ripening may be possible with prostaglandin synthetase inhibitors. Use of these drugs for this purpose has not been widely studied to date, and concerns exist regarding their potential fetal hazards.[6]

Induction of Labor

Labor induction is the "initiation of uterine activity by an independent stimulus to achieve vaginal delivery after 28 weeks of gestation before the onset of spontaneous labor."[6, p. 61] Miller and Mattison note that there is little if any rationale for elective induction owing to the risks of unanticipated prematurity.[134] They recommend that induction be used only when continuance of the pregnancy poses a greater risk to the well-being of either the mother or infant than the risks of induction.

Two types of pharmacologic agents used for labor induction or augmentation are oxytocin and prostaglandins. Oxytocin (and synthetic forms such as Pitocin and Syntocinon) is usually the drug of choice to initiate uterine activity if the condition of the cervix is favorable.[3] Since oxytocin has little effect on the cervix, an unripe cervix may resist even forceful oxytocin-induced myometrial contractions. Oxytocin increases myometrial cell membrane spike activity possibly by altering calcium flux through voltage-dependent calcium channels.[6] Effects of oxytocin on uterine activity depend on the concentration of oxytocin receptors on the myometrial cells, number of available receptors, receptor affinity for oxytocin, and metabolic state of the myometrium.[134]

Oxytocin is a potent octapeptide synthesized in the hypothalamus and then transported along the neurons to the posterior pituitary gland via carrier proteins and released episodically. Oxytocin is most effectively administered intravenously via an infusion pump for dosage control (buccal and intranasal oxytocin are not reliably absorbed), and the patient must be carefully, continuously monitored.[175, 176, 183] Oxytocin release can also be stimulated by nipple stimulation (similar to the mechanism with suckling described in Chapter 4).[54, 167, 189]

Side effects include uterine hyperstimulation with fetal hypoxia and asphyxia. Maternal water intoxication (due to the antidiuretic activity of oxytocin) may occur at doses above 45 mIU/min.[6, 111] The risk of water intoxication is increased if oxytocin is given over a prolonged period of time in a dilute, low electrolyte solution. This risk may be reduced by using a balanced electrolyte solution when diluting oxytocin and monitoring maternal fluid and electrolyte status.[134]

Prostaglandins have also been used to induce or augment labor contractions. $PGF_{2\alpha}$ acts similarly to oxytocin, i.e., increasing spike activity of the myometrial cell membrane by altering calcium fluxes. Oxytocin and prostaglandins can be used together in an additive manner to increase intracellular free calcium and myometrial contractions. This is an advantage in coordinating myometrial activity and cervical distensibility, but it increases the risk of hyperstimulation. This risk may be reduced by using intracervical PGE_2 or low infusion rates of $PGF_{2\alpha}$ (<6 μg/min) along with amniotomy during the latent period to promote cervical ripening.[6]

Inhibition of Labor

Inhibition of uterine contractions is used in the management of preterm labor and to reduce uterine activity in the presence of fetal distress.[12] In many women uterine contractions subside with bed rest, hydration, and sedation, although there is a lack of randomized, controlled data to evaluate these therapies.[20] Many other women require tocolytic therapy. Pharmacologic inhibition of labor is used most frequently to prevent preterm birth. Prerequisites for the use of these agents include (1) presence of preterm labor; (2) gestational age at which this therapy will benefit the fetus and at which the fetus is better off in utero than in the extrauterine environment (this point is generally felt to be between 32 and 34 weeks); and (3) absence of maternal or fetal factors that are usually contraindications for labor inhibition (including pregnancy-induced hypertension, abruptio placentae, chorioamnionitis, intrauterine death, and congenital anomalies incompatible with extrauterine life).[34] Labor inhibition has been used successfully in women with chronic abruptions (marginal sinus).[185] Labor inhibition in women with ruptured membranes is controversial.

A variety of uterine activity–inhibiting drugs (tocolytics) have been investigated, including ethanol, β-sympathomimetic agents, magnesium sulfate, and prostaglandin synthetase inhibitors.[6, 12, 20, 34, 46, 64, 90, 166] Characteristics of these groups of drugs are described below; sites of action are illustrated in Figure 3–7. Use of one agent is unsuccessful in 20 to 40% of cases.[34] Since each group of drugs has a different action, combinations of drugs tend to enhance their effectiveness since they act synergistically.[34, 64, 57, 88, 106]

PROGESTERONE

Progesterone has been used with some effectiveness in threatened abortion but has not been demonstrated to be effective in inhibiting labor. Endogenous progesterone promotes uterine relaxation by decreasing smooth muscle contractility and inhibiting prostaglandin release. Progesterone decreases electrical excitement and the number of action potentials and increases resting membrane potential. Progesterone may also stimulate calcium uptake by the mitochondria.[6]

ETHANOL

Ethanol was one of the original therapies used to inhibit preterm labor but is now rarely used.[20] Ethanol inhibits release of oxytocin from the maternal and probably the fetal posterior pituitary gland. This method is more effective nearer to term than at 26 to 27 weeks, possibly owing to the increased sensitivity of the myometrium to oxytocin later in gestation.[6] Maternal side effects (headache, nausea and vomiting, obtundation, and peripheral vasodilation with increased cardiac output) have been a major problem.[6, 48, 65] Ethanol readily crosses the placenta, so fetal and maternal concentrations are similar.[90]

CALCIUM ANTAGONISTS

Calcium antagonists (calcium channel blockers) are organic compounds such as nifedipine, nicardipine, and verapamil that act on the cell membrane to inhibit the influx of extracellular calcium through membrane potential–dependent channels.[26, 59, 60] These agents are less effective in blocking influx through receptor-operated channels that are less specific for calcium.[6, 34, 59, 146] Calcium antagonists may also act by altering calcium-calmodulin binding and inhibiting actin-myosin interaction.[6, 90]

MAGNESIUIM SULFATE

Magnesium affects smooth muscle excitation, excitation-contraction coupling, and the contractile apparatus by modulating calcium uptake, binding and distribution in the cell, competitive blocking of Ca^{2+} influx across the cell membrane, and activation of adenylate cyclase and cAMP.[34] Magnesium sulfate probably acts primarily by regulating and controlling calcium entry into the cell and altering intracellular levels.[6, 90] Magnesium sulfate is effective in inhibiting preterm labor and is being used more often.[20] Maternal and neonatal side effects include impaired renal function, increased urinary calcium excretion, hypocalcemia, peripheral vasodilation (with flushing and a sensation of warmth), decreased deep tendon reflexes, and (at high levels) respiratory depression in the mother and neonatal hypotonia and respiratory depression.[6, 34, 64, 90, 166, 190] However, maternal side effects are reported to be less severe than those associated with use of β-adrenergic agents.[20]

PROSTAGLANDIN SYNTHETASE IHIBITORS

Prostaglandin synthetase inhibitors include nonsteroidal anti-inflammatory agents such as indomethacin, naproxen, flufenamic acid, and aspirin. These agents block prostaglandin synthesis probably by interfering with cyclooxygenase, the enzyme that regulates the production of prostaglandins from arachidonic acid.[6, 34, 64, 147] Since prostaglandins are important in both initiation of myometrial activity and cervical ripening, the potential of this group of agents has generated considerable interest. Although their effectiveness has been documented in both animals and humans, concerns remain over the potential risk for premature closure of the fetal ductus arteriosus and other side effects such as pulmonary hypertension and alterations in renal function.[6, 20, 90, 99, 126, 140, 160, 184, 191] The risk for premature ductal closure is dose dependent and seems greatest in fetuses over 35 weeks' gestation and with long-term therapy.[20, 34, 90, 148]

β-ADRENERGIC AGONISTS

β-Adrenergic agonists (β-sympathomimetics) are the most widely used drugs for inhibition of preterm labor.[20, 34, 46, 64, 90, 204] These agents include ritodrine, terbutaline, fenoterol, isoxsuprine, salbutamol, hexoprenaline, and orciprenaline. β-Adrenergic agonists act to relax myometrial cells by triggering intracellular formation of cAMP. These effects are mediated by β_2-receptors on the outer membrane of the myometrial cell.

Interaction of the β-adrenergic agonist and the β_2-receptor catalyzes the formation of cAMP from ATP by activating adenylate cyclase on the inner surface of the cell membrane (see Fig. 3–7). Cyclic AMP phosphorylates a protein kinase that decreases the affinity of medium light chain kinase for the calcium-calmodulin complex, thus promoting relaxation. It also decreases intracellular calcium possibly by interfering with the Na,K-ATPase exchange pump.[20, 34, 90, 135, 149, 166, 179]

The myometrium contains α- and β-receptors. If the α-receptors are stimulated by prostaglandins or oxytocin, the uterus contracts. Stimulation of the β-receptors inhibits uterine contraction. Two subtypes of β-receptors may be present in the same organ or on the same cell. β_1-Receptors dominate in the heart, small intestine, and adipose tissue; β_2-receptors predominate in the smooth muscle of the uterus, blood vessels, and bronchioles.[149] Since β-adrenergic agonists are not specific for β_2- or β_1-receptors, use of these agents is associated with a variety of side effects. Maternal side effects include hypotension, increased heart rate and cardiac output, cardiac arrhythmias, pulmonary edema, congestive heart failure, hyperglycemia, and hypokalemia; fetal and neonatal side effects include fetal tachycardia and neonatal hypoglycemia, hypocalcemia, and hypotension.*

Prolonged use of β-adrenergic agents results in desensitization (also called down-regulation and refractoriness) and the need to increase dosage to achieve the same therapeutic effect. Desensitization is a multistep process and is thought to result from an agonist-stimulated decrease in the number of β-receptors with a reduction in the effect of the agonist on intracellular processes and myometrial relaxation.[19, 34, 35, 86, 149]

The first step in desensitization is inactivation of the receptor by phosphorylation, which is mediated by a cAMP-independent protein kinase activated by catecholamines. This is followed by uncoupling of the regulator protein and adenylate cyclase. The β-receptors then become sequestered in vesicles within the membrane. Phosphorylation is reversed and the receptor reactivated and recycled back to the outer membrane where it recouples with adenylate cyclase.[149] Discontinuing β-adrenergic agonists with use of an alternative agent allows the myometrial cell to recover responsiveness so these agents can be used later.

Dystocia

Dysfunctional labor can result from problems in the powers (alteration in myometrial function and contraction patterns), passage (obstruction of fetal descent by the maternal bony pelvis or soft tissues), or passenger (fetal malposition or abnormal development).[63] Functional dystocia due to alterations in the physiologic function (powers) results in inadequate contractility and failure of the cervix to dilate. The cellular and molecular basis for weak or ineffective myometrial contractions includes lack of adequate stimulation, depression or the presence of some form of strong inhibitory control, or a combination of these events (Table 3–2).[74]

Stimulation or inhibition of myometrial activity is influenced by myogenic, neurogenic, and hormonal control systems. Dystocia secondary to alterations in myogenic properties arises from factors such as modifications in intracellular ion concentration (due to an inadequate supply of energy or calcium) with depression or absence of myometrial contractility, closure or inadequate function of gap junctions with modifications in the propagation of electrical events, and poor synchronization of contractions across the uterus. Abnormalities in gap junction structure or function may arise from alterations in regulatory hormones or their receptors.

Dystocia can also arise secondary to alterations in neurogenic control (overstimulation by inhibitory neurons or understimulation by excitatory neurons) or in the hormonal control systems. These latter alterations arise directly from inadequate levels of hormones or their receptors or indirectly from alterations in gap junction function or structure.[74]

Supportive interventions with women experiencing dystocia are directed toward preventing or reducing maternal fatigue, providing calories for energy, maintaining hydration, monitoring fluid and electrolyte status, and maintaining fetal homeostasis. Energy (ATP) is essential for labor progression. If adequate calories and ATP are not available, ketoacidosis may develop. With inadequate ATP the effectiveness of uterine contractions is further impeded. Women with dystocia whose labor is not progressing and who are exhausted may be provided with a period of medicated therapeutic rest.[63]

Postterm Labor

Postterm labor (onset of labor aftet 42 weeks) occurs in 3.5 to 15% of all pregnancies.[28]

---

*References 15, 20, 34, 56, 89, 90, 98, 107, 120, 149, and 215.

TABLE 3–2
Possible Reasons for Dystocia

MYOGENIC: INTRINSIC FACTORS
Inadequate depolarization
    Ionic disturbance (local)
    Insufficient stimulation or excessive inhibition by hormonal or neural mechanisms
    Lack of stimulatory receptors or redundant intrinsic inhibitory systems
Deficient propagation of electrical events
    Lack of development of gap junctions
    Suppression of channel opening in gap junctions
Incomplete muscle development
Unsatisfactory energy supply for muscle cells and fatigue

NEUROGENIC: NERVE FACTORS
Depressed neural output by excitatory neurons
Continued dominance by inhibitory nerves
    Failure of inhibitory nerves to degenerate

HORMONAL: HUMORAL FACTORS
Inadequate steroid ratios (estrogen-to-progesterone)
    Progesterone dominance
    Failure of steroid hormones and their receptors to control synthesis of necessary proteins,
        membrane receptors, gap junctions, etc.
Hormonally regulated closure of gap junction channels
Elevated levels of inhibitory prostaglandins, relaxin, etc.
Failure of stimulatory prostaglandins to increase sufficiently

From Garfield, R.E. (1987). Cellular and molecular basis for dystocia. *Clin Obstet Gynecol, 30,* 3.

Fetal and neonatal morbidity increases after 40 weeks to greater than 25% after 42 weeks.[7] Postterm pregnancies are associated with an increased frequency of both intrauterine growth retardation and macrosomia, fetal distress, meconium aspiration, congenital anomalies, and intrauterine death.[28, 45, 142] Several of these disorders are related to the effect of prolonged gestation on placental morphology and functional ability (see Chapter 2).

A specific postmaturity syndrome was de-

TABLE 3–3
Summary of Recommendations for Clinical Practice Related to the Intrapartum Period and Uterine Physiology

Recognize usual changes in the uterine size and shape during pregnancy (pp. 110–111).
Know usual changes in the myometrium during pregnancy and their bases (pp. 111–113).
Recognize factors involved in the initiation of labor and know how these may be altered (pp. 113–117, 130).
Understand the physiologic basis for myometrial contraction and factors that may alter muscular contraction (pp. 117–120, 128–130; Table 3–2).
Assess contractions and document their characteristics (p. 120).
Monitor energy and oxygen needs of the laboring woman (pp. 118, 128).
Understand the basis for cervical ripening and dilatation and factors that may alter this process (pp. 120–122).
Avoid use of the supine position for prolonged periods during the first stage of labor (pp. 122–123).
Alternate supine and side-lying for women who prefer supine positions during the first stage (pp. 122–123).
Promote use of upright positions in first stage (especially early) labor (pp. 122–123).
Assist the woman in selecting a position conducive to labor progress and maternal comfort (p. 123).
Try side-lying position with a posterior fetus (p. 122).
Assist the woman in selecting a position at delivery to optimize alignment for fetal descent and maximize capacity of the pelvis and efficiency of maternal expulsive efforts (pp. 122–123).
Avoid directed pushing and the Valsalva maneuver during the second stage (pp. 123–124; Figure 3–9).
Teach woman to use open-glottis pushing (pp. 123–124).
Avoid supine positions during the second stage (p. 124; Chapter 6).
Recognize factors that increase the risk of preterm labor (Table 3–1).
Understand basis for pharmacologic agents used to control cervical ripening (pp. 121–122, 125–126).
Understand basis for pharmacologic agents used for induction or augmentation of labor (117–118, 126).
Monitor woman for side effects of agents used to induce or augment labor (p. 126).
Understand basis for pharmacologic agents used to inhibit labor (pp. 117–119, 126–128; Fig. 3–7).
Monitor woman for side effects of agents used to inhibit labor (pp. 126–128).
Recognize and monitor for factors that can lead to dystocia (p. 128; Table 3–2).
Monitor woman with postterm labor for fetal distress (pp. 128–130, Chapter 2).

Page numbers in parentheses following each intervention refer to page(s) where rationale for intervention is discussed.

scribed by Clifford.[45] This syndrome is characterized clinically by three progressive stages of alterations in the infant's skin: (1) maceration accompanied by loss of vernix caseosa with dry, wrinkled, parchment-like skin; (2) meconium staining of the skin and amniotic fluid; and (3) yellow staining of the skin (caused by conversion of the meconium to bilirubin).

Brody summarized hormonal causes that may result in failure of initiation of spontaneous labor and postdate gestation: (1) lack of the normal increase in estrogen near term perhaps due to anencephaly and associated adrenal hypoplasia, deficiency in placental sulfatase (necessary for production of estrogen), or fetal adrenal hypoplasia; (2) decreased adrenocortical function leading to reduction in cortisol levels (cortisol promotes hydroxylation of progesterone, reduction in progesterone levels, and increases in estrogen precursors); and (3) decreased fetal adrenocorticotropic factors such as adrenocorticotropic hormone (ACTH) and growth hormone, which stimulate fetal cortisol production.[28]

SUMMARY

An understanding of physiologic processes during the intrapartum period is essential for recognition of the effects of parturition on the pregnant woman and the fetus and in optimizing maternal, fetal, and neonatal outcome. This knowledge provides the basis for assessment of functional and dysfunctional labor patterns and maternal responses to pharmacologic agents used to alter or control uterine activity, for recognition of pre- and postterm labor, and for nursing interventions such as positioning during the first and second stages of labor. Recommendations for clinical practice related to uterine physiology during parturition are summarized in Table 3–3.

REFERENCES

1. Abitbol, M.N. (1985). Supine position in labor and associated fetal heart rate changes. *Obstet Gynecol, 65*, 481.
2. Altura, B.M. & Altura, B.T. (1982). Magnesium ions and contraction of vascular smooth muscles: Relationship to some vascular diseases. *Fed Proc, 40*, 2672.
3. American College of Obstetricians and Gynecologists. (1989). *Guidelines for oxytocin induction.* Washington, DC: Author.
4. Amy, J.J., Calder, A.A., & Kelly, R.W. (1986). Prostaglandins and human reproduction. In E. Phillip, J. Barnes, & M. Newton (Eds.), *Scientific foundations of obstetrics and gynecology* (pp. 255–303). London: Heinemann.
5. Anderson, A.B.M., Turnbull, A.C., & Marray, A.M. (1967). The relationship between amniotic fluid pressure and uterine wall tension in pregnancy. *Am J Obstet Gynecol, 97*, 992.
6. Andersson, K.E., Forman, A., & Ulmsten, U. (1983). Pharmacology of labor. *Clin Obstet Gynecol, 26*, 56.
7. Arias, F. (1987). Predictability of complications associated with prolongation of pregnancy. *Obstet Gynecol, 70*, 101.
8. Avard, D.M. & Nimrod, C.M. (1985). The risks and benefits of obstetric epidural analgesia: A review. *Birth, 12*, 215.
9. Barnett, M. & Humenick, S. (1982). Infant outcomes in relation to second stage labor pushing. *Birth, 9*, 221.
10. Bates, R.G., et al. (1985). Uterine activity in second stage of labour and the effect of epithelial analgesia. *Br J Obstet Gynaecol, 92*, 1246.
11. Baulieu, E.E. (1984). RU486: An antiprogestin steroid with contragestive activity in women. In E.E. Baulieu & S.J. Segal (Eds.), *The antiprogestin steroid RU486 and human fertility control* (p. 1). New York: Plenum Press.
12. Baxi, L.V. & Petrie, R.H. (1987). Pharmacologic effects on labor: Effects of drugs on dystocia, labor and uterine activity. *Clin Obstet Gynecol, 30*, 19.
13. Bell, C. (1972). Autonomic nervous system control of reproduction: Circulatory and other factors. *Pharmacol Rev, 24*, 657.
14. Bell, R. (1983). Antenatal oestradiol and progesterone concentrations in patients subsequently having preterm labour. *Br J Obstet Gynaecol, 90*, 888.
15. Benedetti, T.J. (1983). Maternal complications of parenteral beta-sympathomimetic therapy for premature labor. *Am J Obstet Gynecol, 145*, 1.
16. Bennett, P.R. (1990). Mechanisms of parturition: The transfer of PGE2 and 5-hydroxyeicosatetraenoic acid across fetal membranes. *Am J Obstet Gynecol, 162*, 683.
17. Bennett, P.R., et al. (1987). Preterm labor: Stimulation of arachidonic acid metabolism in human amnion cells by bacterial products. *Am J Obstet Gynecol, 156*, 649.
18. Bennett, P.R., et al. (1988). Mechanisms of parturition: The transfer of prostaglandins across fetal membranes. In C.T. Jones (Ed.), *Fetal and neonatal development* (pp. 407–409). Ithaca, NY: Perinatology Press.
19. Berg, G., Andersson, R.G.G., & Ryden, G. (1983). Beta-adrenergic receptors in human endometrium during pregnancy: Changes in the number of receptors after beta-mimetic treatment. *Am J Obstet Gynecol, 151*, 392.
20. Besinger, R.E. & Niebyl, J.R. (1990). The safety and efficacy of tocolytic agents for the treatment of preterm labor. *Obstet Gynecol Surv, 45*, 415.
21. Bieniarz, J., et al. (1968). Aortocaval compression by the uterus in late pregnancy. II. An aterioradiographic study. *Am J Obstet Gynecol, 100*, 203.
22. Bleasdale, J.E. & Johnston, J.M. (1984). Prostaglandins and human parturition: Regulation of arachidonic acid mobilization. *Rev Perinat Med, 5*, 151.

23. Block, B.S.B., Liggins, G.C., & Creasy, R.K. (1984). Preterm delivery is not predicted by serial plasma estradiol or progesterone concentration measurements. *Am J Obstet Gynecol, 150,* 716.

24. Bolton, T.B. (1979). Mechanisms of action of transmitters and other substances on smooth muscle. *Physiolog Rev, 59,* 606.

25. Bouyer, J., et al. (1986). Maturation signs of the cervix and prediction of preterm birth. *Obstet Gynecol, 68,* 206.

26. Braumwald, E. (1982). Mechanism of calcium-channel-blocking agents. *N Engl J Med, 307,* 1618.

27. Brennecke, S.P., et al. (1982). The prostaglandin synthase inhibiting ability of maternal plasma and the onset of human labor. *Eur J Obstet Gynecol Reprod Biol, 14,* 81.

28. Brody, S.A. (1989). Endocrinology of postdate pregnancy. In S.A. Brody & K. Ueland (Eds.), *Endocrine disorders in pregnancy* (pp. 99–110). Norwalk, CT: Appleton & Lange.

29. Caldeyro-Barcia, R. (1979). The influence of the maternal position on time of spontaneous rupture of membranes, progress of labor, and fetal head compression. *Birth Family J, 6,* 7.

30. Caldeyro-Barcia, R. (1979). The influence of maternal bearing-down efforts during second stage on fetal well being. *Birth Family J, 6*(Spring), 17.

31. Caldeyro-Barcia, R. & Poseiro, J.J. (1960). Physiology of the uterine contraction. *Clin Obstet Gynecol, 3,* 394.

32. Caldeyro-Barcia, R., et al. (1960). Effect of position changes on the intensity and frequency of uterine contractions during labor. *Am J Obstet Gynecol, 80,* 284.

33. Caldeyro-Barcia, R., et al. (1981). The bearing down efforts and their effect on fetal heart rate, oxygenation and acid-base balance. *J Perinat Med, 9*(6), 3.

34. Caritis, S.N., Darby, M.J., & Chan, L. (1988). Pharmacologic treatment of preterm labor. *Clin Obstet Gynecol, 31,* 635.

35. Caritis, S.N., et al. (1987). Myometrial desensitization after ritodrine infusion. *Am J Physiol, 253,* E410.

36. Casey, M.L. & MacDonald, P.C. (1986). The initiation of labor in women: Regulation of phospholipid and arachidonic acid metabolism and of prostaglandin production. *Semin Perinatol, 10,* 270.

37. Casey, M.L. & MacDonald, P.C. (1988). Biomolecular processes in the initiation of parturition: Decidual activation. *Clin Obstet Gynecol, 31,* 533.

38. Casteels, R. (1980). Electro- and pharmacomechanical coupling in vascular smooth muscle. *Chest, 78,* 150.

39. Challis, J.R.G. (1989). Characteristics of parturition. In R.K. Creasy & R. Resnik (Eds.), *Maternal-fetal medicine: principles and practice* (pp. 463–476). Philadelphia: W.B. Saunders.

40. Challis, J.R.G. & Lye, S.J. (1988). Parturition. *Oxf Rev Reprod Biol, 10,* 61.

41. Challis, J.R.G. & Mitchell, B.F. (1981). Hormonal control of preterm and term parturition. *Semin Perinatol, 5,* 192.

42. Challis, J.R.G. & Olson, D.M. (1988). Parturition. In E. Knobil & J. Neill (Eds.), *The physiology of reproduction* (pp. 2177–2216). New York: Raven Press.

43. Challis, J.R.G., et al. (1988). Placental, membrane and uterine interactions in the control of birth. In C.T. Jones (Ed.), *Research in perinatal medicine (VI): Fetal and neonatal development* (pp. 397–406). Ithaca, New York: Perinatology Press.

44. Chan, W.Y. (1983). Uterine and placental prostaglandins and their modulation of oxytocin sensitivity and contractility in the parturient uterus. *Biol Reprod, 29,* 680.

45. Clifford, S.H. (1954). Postmaturity and placental dysfunction: Clinical syndrome and pathologic findings. *J Pediatr, 44,* 1.

46. Cohen, W.R., Acker, D.B., & Friedman, E.A. (1989). *Management of labor* (2nd ed., pp. 333–367). Rockville, MD: Aspen Publishers.

47. Conrad, J.T. & Ueland, K. (1979). The stretch modulus of human cervical tissue in spontaneous, oxytocin-induced, and prostaglandin E2-induced labor. *Am J Obstet Gynecol, 133,* 11.

48. Cook, L.N., Short, R.J., & Andrews, B.J. (1975). Acute transplacental ethanol interaction. *Am J Dis Child, 129,* 1075.

49. Cousins, L.M., et al. (1977). Serum progesterone and estradiol–17 beta levels in premature and term labor. *Am J Obstet Gynecol, 127,* 612.

50. Csaspo, A.I. (1981). Force of labor. In H.A. Kamientzky & L. Iffy (Eds.), *Principles and practice of obstetrics and perinatology* (pp. 761–799). New York: John Wiley & Sons.

51. Dalle, M. (1988). Pituitary-adrenal development and the initiation of birth. In C.T. Jones (Ed.), *Research in perinatal medicine (VII): Fetal and neonatal development* (pp. 389–396). Ithaca, New York: Perinatology Press.

52. Danforth, D.N. (1983). The morphology of the human cervix. *Clin Obstet Gynecol, 26,* 7.

53. Dobson, H. (1988). Softening and dilation of the uterine cervix. *Oxf Rev Reprod Biol, 10,* 491.

54. Elliot, J.P. & Flaherty, J.F. (1983). The use of breast stimulation to ripen the cervix in term pregnancies. *Am J Obstet Gynecol, 145,* 553.

55. Embrey, M.P. (1971). PGE compounds for induction of labor and abortion. *Ann NY Acad Sci, 180,* 518.

56. Epstein, M.F., Nichols, E., & Stubbefield, P.G. (1979). Neonatal hypoglycemia after beta-sympathomimetic tocolytic therapy. *J Pediatr, 94,* 449.

57. Ferguson, J.E., Hensleigh, P.A., & Kredenster, D. (1984). Adjunctive use of magnesium sulate with ritodrine for preterm labor tocolysis. *Am J Obstet Gynecol, 148,* 166.

58. Fitzpatrick, R.J. & Dobson, H. (1981). Softening of the ovine cervix at parturition. In D.A. Ellwood & A.B.M. Anderson (Eds.), *The cervix in pregnancy and labour: Clinical and biochemical investigations* (pp. 40–56). Edinburgh: Churchill Livingstone.

59. Forman, A., Andersson, K.E., & Ulmsted, U. (1981). Inhibition of myometrial activity by calcium antagonists. *Semin Perinatol, 5,* 288.

60. Forman, A., et al. (1979). Relaxant effects of nifedipine on isolated human myometrium. *Acta Pharmacol Toxicol, 45,* 81.

61. Forman, A., et al. (1982). Evidence for a local effect of intracervical PGE2-gel. *Am J Obstet Gynecol, 143,* 756.

62. Friedman, E.A. & Sachtleben, M.R. (1977). Preterm labor. *Am J Obstet Gynecol, 104,* 1152.

63. Friedman, E.A. (1978). *Labor and clinical evaluation* (2nd ed). New York: Appleton-Century-Crofts.

64. Fuchs, A.R. & Fuchs, F. (1984). Endocrinology of

human parturition: A review. *Br J Obstet Gynaecol*, *91*, 948.

65. Fuchs, A.R. & Fuchs, F. (1981). Ethanol for prevention of preterm birth. *Semin Perinatol*, *5*, 236.

66. Fuchs, A.R. (1983). The role of oxytocin in parturition. *Curr Top Exp Endocrinol*, *4*, 231.

67. Fuchs, A.R. (1986). The role of oxytocin in parturition. In G. Huszar (Ed.), *The physiology and biochemistry of the uterus in pregnancy and labor*. Boca Raton, FL: CRC Press.

68. Fuchs, A.R., et al. (1982). Plasma levels of oxytocin and 13,14-dihydro–15 keto prostaglandin F 2- alpha in preterm labor and the effect of ethanol and ritodrine. *Am J Obstet Gynecol*, *144*, 753.

69. Fuchs, A.R., et al. (1982). Oxytocin receptors and human parturition: A dual role for oxytocin in the initiation of labor. *Science*, *215*, 1396.

70. Fuchs, A.R., et al. (1983). Correlation between oxytocin receptor concentration and responsiveness to oxytocin in pregnant rat myometrium: Effect of ovarian studies. *Endocrinology*, *113*, 742.

71. Fuchs, A.R., et al. (1984). Oxytocin receptors in the human uterus during pregnancy and parturition. *Am J Obstet Gynecol*, *150*, 734.

72. Garfield, R.E. (1984). Myometrial ultrastructure and uterine contractility. In S. Bottari, et al. (Eds.), *Uterine contractility* (pp. 81–109). NY: Masson Publishing.

73. Garfield, R.E. (1984). Control of myometrial function in preterm versus term labor. *Clin Obstet Gynecol*, *27*, 572.

74. Garfield, R.E. (1987). Cellular and molecular basis for dystocia. *Clin Obstet Gynecol*, *30*, 3.

75. Garfied, R.E. & Baulieu, E.E. (1987). The antiprogesterone steroid RU486: A short pharmacological and clinical review with emphasis on interruption of pregnancy. *Baillieres Clin Endocrinol Metab*, *1*, 207.

76. Garfield, R.E., Blennerhassett, M.G., & Miller, S.M. (1988). Control of myometrial contractility: Role and regulation of gap junctions. *Oxf Rev Reprod Biol*, *10*, 436.

77. Garfield, R.E. & Hayashi, R.H. (1981). Appearance of gap junctions in the myometrium of women during labor. *Am J Obstet Gynecol*, *140*, 254.

78. Garfield, R.E., Kannan, M.S., & Daniel, E.E. (1980). Gap junction formation in myometrium: Control by estrogens, progesterone and prostaglandins. *Am J Physiol*, *238*, C81.

79. Garfield, R.E., Sims, S.M., & Daniel, E.E. (1977). Gap junctions: Their presence and necessity in myometrium during gestation. *Science*, *198*, 958.

80. Garfield, R.E., et al. (1978). The possible role of gap junctions in activation of the myometrium during parturition. *Am J Physiol*, *235*, C168.

81. Gneiss, F.C. (1965). Effect of labor on uterine blood flow. *Am J Obstet Gynecol*, *93*, 917.

82. Goldkrand, J.W., Schulte, R.L., & Messer, R.H. (1976). Maternal and fetal plasma cortisol levels at parturition. *Obstet Gynecol*, *47*, 41.

83. Golichowski, A.M., King, S.R., & Mascaro, K. (1980). Pregnancy related changes in rat cervical glycosaminoglycans. *Biochem J*, *192*, 1.

84. Gorski, J. & Gannon, F. (1976). Current models of steroid hormone action: A critique. *Ann Rev Physiol*, *38*, 425.

85. Gyory, G., et al. (1974). Inhibition of labor by prostaglandin antagonists in impending abortion and preterm and term labour. *Lancet*, *2*, 293.

86. Harden, T.K. (1983). Agonist-induced desensitization of the beta-adrenergic receptor-linked adenylate cyclase. *Pharmacol Rev*, *35*, 5.

87. Hartshorne, D.J. & Mrwa, U. (1982). Regulation of smooth muscle actomyosin. *Blood Vessels*, *19*, 1.

88. Hatjis, C.G., et al. (1987). Efficacy of combined administration of magnesium sulfate and ritodrine in the treatment of premature labor. *Obstet Gynecol*, *69*, 317.

89. Hendricks, S.K., Keroes, J., & Katz, M. (1986). Electrocardiographic changes associated with ritodrine-induced maternal tachycardia and hypokalemia. *Am J Obstet Gynecol*, *154*, 921.

90. Holbrook, R.H. & Ueland, K. (1989). Endocrinology of parturition and preterm labor. In S.A. Brody & K. Ueland (Eds.), *Endocrine disorders in pregnancy* (pp. 81–98). Norwalk, CT: Appleton & Lange.

91. Humphrey, M., et al. (1973). The influence of maternal position at birth on the fetus. *J Obstet Gynaecol Br Comm*, *80*, 1075.

92. Huszar, G. (1981). Biology and biochemistry of myometrial contractility and cervical maturation. *Semin Perinatol 5* 216.

93. Huszar, G.(1983). Biology of the myometrium and cervix. In J.R. Warshaw (Ed.), *The biological basis of reproductive and developmental medicine*. New York: Elsevier Biochemical.

94. Huszar, G. (1986). *The physiology and biochemistry of the uterus in pregnacy and labor*. Boca Raton, FL: CRC Press.

95. Huszar, G. (1989). Physiology of the myometrium. In R.K. Creasy & R. Resnik (Eds.), *Maternal-fetal medicine: Principles and practice* (pp. 141–148). Philadelphia: WB Saunders.

96. Huszar, G. & Naftolin, F. (1984). The myometrium and uterine cervix in normal and preterm labor. *N Engl J Med*, *311*, 571.

97. Huxley, A.F. (1971). The activation of striated muscle and its mechanical response. *Proc R Soc Lond (Biol)*, *178*, 1.

98. Ingermarsson, I. & Bengtsson, B. (1985). A five year experience with terbutaline for preterm labor: Low rate of severe side effects. *Obstet Gynecol*, *66*, 176.

99. Itskovitz, J., Abramovici, H., & Brandes, J.M. (1980). Oligohydramnios, meconium and perinatal death concurrent with indomethacin treatment in human pregnancy. *J Reprod Med*, *24*, 137.

100. Izumi, H., et al. (1990). Gestational changes in mechanical properties of skinned muscle tissues of human myometrium. *Am J Obstet Gynecol*, *163*, 638.

101. Jacobs, M.M. (1986). Clinical obstetric use of arachidonic acid metabolites and potential adverse effects. *Semin Perinatol*, *10*, 299.

102. Johnson, J.W.C., et al. (1979). High risk prematurity—Progestin treatment and steroid studies. *Obstet Gynecol*, *54*, 412.

103. Johnson, N. & Bryce, F.C. (1990). Could antiprogesterone be used as an alternative cervical ripening agent? *Am J Obstet Gynecol*, *162*, 688.

104. Junqueira, L.C.U., et al. (1980). Morphologic and histochemical evidence for the occurrence of collagenolysis and for the role of neutrophilic polymorphonuclear leukocytes during cervical dilation. *Am J Obstet Gynecol*, *138*, 243.

105. Kao, C.Y. & McCulloch, J.R. (1975). Ionic currents in the uterine smooth muscle. *J Physiol (Lond)*, *246*, 1.

106. Katz, Z., et al. (1983). Treatment of premature labor contractions with combined ritodrine and indomethacin. *Int J Gynaecol Obstet, 21,* 337.

107. Katz, M., Robertson, P., & Creasy, R.K. (1981). Cardiovascular complications associated with terbutaline treatment for preterm labor. *Am J Obstet Gynecol, 139,* 605.

108. Kauppila, A., et al. (1978). Umbilical cord and neonatal cortisol levels. *Obstet Gynecol, 52,* 666.

109. Keirse, M.J.N.C. (1979). Endogenous prostaglandins in human parturition. In M.J.N.C. Keirse, A.B.M. Anderson, & J. Bennebroek-Gravenhorst (Eds.), *Human parturition* (pp. 101–142). The Hague: Martinus Nijhoff.

110. Keirse, M.J.N.C., Mitchell, M.D., & Turnbull, A.C. (1977). Changes in prostaglandin F and 13,14-dihydro–15-keto-prostaglandin F concentrations in amniotic fluid at the onset and during labour. *Br J Obstet Gynaecol, 84,* 743.

111. Kitamura, K., et al. (1979). Changes in the human cervical collagenase with special reference to cervical ripening. *Biochem Med, 22,* 332.

112. Koay, E.S., et al. (1983). Relaxin stimulates collagenase and plasminogen activator secretion by dispersed human amnion and chorion cells in vitro. *J Clin Endocrinol Metab, 56,* 1332.

113. Korner, P.I., Tonkin, A.M., & Uther, J.B. (1976). Reflex and mechanical circulatory effects of graded Valsalva maneuvers in normal man. *J Appl Physiol, 40,* 434.

114. Kuriyama, H. & Suzuki, H. (1976). Changes in electrical properties of rat myometrium during gestation and following hormonal treatments. *J Physiol (Lond), 260,* 315.

115. Lefebvre, Y., et al. (1990). The effects of RU-38483 on cervical ripening. *Am J Obstet Gynecol, 162,* 61.

116. Leppert, P.C., et al. (1982). Conclusive evidence for the presence of elastin in human and monkey cervix. *Am J Obstet Gynecol, 142,* 179.

117. Liggins, G.C. (1969). The foetal role in the initiation of parturition in the ewe. In G.E.W. Wolstenholme & M. O'Connor M (Eds.), *Foetal Autonomy* (p. 218). London: Churchill.

118. Liggins, G.C. (1978). Ripening of the cervix. *Semin Perinatol, 2,* 261.

119. Liggins, G.C. (1981). Cervical ripening as an inflammatory reaction. In D.A. Ellwood & A.B.M. Anderson (Eds.), *The cervix in pregnancy and labor: Clinical and biochemical investigations* (pp. 1–9). London: Churchill Livingstone.

120. Liggins, G.C. (1983). Initiation of spontaneous labor. *Clin Obstet Gynecol, 26,* 47.

121. Liggins, G.C., et al. (1973). The mechanism of initiation of parturition in the ewe. *Recent Prog Horm Res, 29,* 111.

122. Liu, Y.C. (1975). Effects of an upright position during labor. *Am J Nurs, 74,* 2202.

123. Liu, Y.C. (1989). The effects of the upright position during childbirth. *Image J Nurs Sch, 21(Spring),* 14.

124. MacKenzie, L.W. & Garfield, R.E. (1985). Hormonal control of gap junctions in the myometrium. *Am J Physiol, 248,* C296.

125. MacLennan, A.H., et al. (1980). Ripening of the human cervix and induction of labour with purified porcine relaxin. *Lancet, 1,* 220.

126. Manchester, D., Margolis, H.S., & Sheldon, R.E. (1976). Possible association between maternal indomethacin therapy and primary pulmonary hypertension in the neonate. *Am J Obstet Gynecol, 126,* 467.

127. Marshall, J.M. (1981). Effects of ovarian steroids and pregnancy on adrenergic nerves of uterus and oviduct. *Am J Physiol, 240,* C165.

128. Mayberry, L.J. & Inturrisi-Levy, M. (1987). Use of breast stimulation for contraction stress tests. *J Obstet Gynecol Neonatal Nurs, 16,* 121.

129. McGregor, J.A. (1988). Prevention of preterm birth: New initiatives based on microbial-host interactions. *Obstet Gynecol Surv, 43,* 1.

130. McKay, S. & Roberts, J. (1985). Second stage labor: What is normal? *J Obstet Gynecol Neonatal Nurs, 14,* 101.

131. Mendez-Bauer, C. & Newton, M. (1986). Maternal position in labor. In E. Phillip, J. Barnes, & M. Newton (Eds.), *Scientific foundations of obstetrics and gynecology* (p. 209). London: Heinemann.

132. Mendez-Bauer, C., et al. (1975). Effects of standing position on spontaneous uterine contractility, and other aspects of labor. *J Perinat Med, 3,* 89.

133. Miller, F.C. (1983). Uterine motility in spontaneous labor. *Clin Obstet Gynecol, 26,* 78.

134. Miller, F.C. & Mattison, D.R. (1989). Oxytocin for induction of labor. In S.A. Brody & K. Ueland (Eds.), *Endocrine disorders in pregnancy* (pp. 411–425). Norwalk, CT: Appleton & Lange.

135. Miller, J.R., Silver, P.J., & Stull, J.T. (1982). The role of myosin light chain kinase phosphorylation in beta-adrenergic relaxation of tracheal smooth muscle. *Mol Pharmacol, 24,* 235.

136. Mitchell, B.F., et al. (1982). Local modulation of progesterone production in human fetal membranes. *J Clin Endocrinol Metab, 55,* 1237.

137. Mitchell, M.D. (1981). Prostaglandins during pregnancy and the perinatal period. *J Reprod Fertil, 62,* 305.

138. Mitchell, M.D. (1984). The mechanism(s) of human parturition. *J Dev Physiol, 6,* 107.

139. Mitchell, M.D. (1986). Pathways of arachidonic acid metabolism with specific application to the fetus and mother. *Semin Perinatol, 10,* 242.

140. Moise, K.J., et al. (1990). The effect of indomethacin on the pulsatility index of the umbilical artery in human fetuses. *Am J Obstet Gynecol, 162,* 199.

141. Murphy, B.E.P. (1982). Human fetal serum cortisol levels related to gestational age: Evidence of a midgestational fall and a steep late rise, independent of sex or mode of delivery. *Am J Obstet Gynecol, 144,* 276.

142. Naeye, R.L. (1978). Causes of perinatal mortality excess in prolonged gestation. *Am J Epidemiol, 108,* 429.

143. Nager, C.W., Key, T.C., & Moore, T.R. (1987). Cervical ripening and labor outcome with preinduction intracervical prostaglandin E2 (Prepidil) gel. *J Perinatol, 7,* 189.

144. Nakla, S. et al. (1986). Changes in prostaglandin transfer across human fetal membranes obtained after spontaneous labor. *Am J Obstet Gynecol, 155,* 1337.

145. Naroll, F., Naroll, R., & Howard, F.H. (1961). Position of women in childbirth. A study in data quality control. *Am J Obstet Gynecol, 82,* 943.

146. Nayler, W.G. & Poole-Wilson, P.H. (1981). Calcium antagonists: Definition and mode of action. *Basic Res Cardiol, 76,* 1.

147. Niebyl, J.R. (1981). Prostaglandin synthetase inhibitors. *Semin Perinatol, 5,* 274.

148. Niebyl, J.R. & Witter, F.R. (1986). Neonatal outcome after indomethacin treatment for preterm labor. *Am J Obstet Gynecol, 155,* 747.

149. Nuwayhid, B. & Rahabi, M. (1987). Beta-sympathomimetic agents: Use in perinatal obstetrics. *Clin Perinatol, 14,* 757.

150. Nwosu, U.C., et al. (1977). Amniotic fluid cortisol concentrations in normal labor, premature labor, and postmature pregnancy. *Obstet Gynecol, 49,* 715.

151. O'Herlihy, C. & MacDonald, M.B. (1979). Influence of preinduction prostaglandin E2 vaginal gel on cervical ripening and labor. *Obstet Gynecol, 54,* 708.

152. Okasaki, T., et al. (1981). Initiation of human parturition. XII. Biosynthesis and metabolism of prostaglandins in human fetal membranes and uterine decidua. *Am J Obstet Gynecol, 139,* 373.

153. Page, E.W., Villee, C.A., & Villee, D.B. (1981). *Human reproduction: Essentials of reproductive and perinatal medicine* (3rd ed.). Philadelphia: WB Saunders.

154. Page, L. & Young, K. (1986). Uterine activity in the second stage of labour and the effect of epidural analgesia. *Br J Obstet Gynaecol, 93,* 1017.

155. Porter, D.G. (1982). Unsolved problems of relaxin's physiological role. *Ann NY Acad Sci, 380,* 151.

156. Prins, R.P., et al. (1983). Cervical ripening with intravaginal prostaglandin E2 gel. *Obstet Gynecol, 61,* 459.

157. Rajab, M.R., et al. (1990). Changes in active and latent collagenase in human placenta around the time of parturition. *Am J Obstet Gynecol, 163,* 499.

158. Reiss, U., et al. (1976). The effects of indomethicin in labour at term. *Int J Gynaecol Obstet, 14,* 369.

159. Remuzzi, G., et al. (1980). Reduced umbilical and placental vascular prostacyclin in severe preeclampsia. *Prostaglandins, 20,* 105.

160. Repke, J.T. & Niebyl, J.R. (1985). Role of prostaglandin synthetase inhibitors in the treatment of preterm labor. *Semin Reprod Endocrinol, 3,* 259.

161. Reynolds, J. & Yudkin, P. (1987). Changes in the management of labor. I.Length and management of the second stage. *Can Med Assoc J, 136,* 1041.

162. Rhodes, P. (1967). Position in obstetrics. *Physiotherapy, 53,* 158.

163. Riemer, R.K. & Roberts, J.M. (1986). Activation of uterine smooth muscle contraction: Implications for eicosanoid action and interaction. *Semin Perinatol, 10,* 276.

164. Roberts, J. (1980). Alternative positions for childbirth—Part I: First stage of labor. *J Nurse Midwifery, 25*(4), 11.

165. Roberts, J. (1980). Alternative positions for childbirth—Part II. Second stage of labor. *J Nurse Midwifery, 25,* 13.

166. Roberts, J.M. (1984). Current understanding of pharmacologic mechanisms in the prevention of preterm birth. *Clin Obstet Gynecol, 27,* 592.

167. Roberts, J.E. (1989). Maternal positioning during the first stage of labour. In I. Chalmers, M. Enkin, & M.J.N.C. Keirse (Eds.), *Effective care in pregnancy and childbirth* (pp. 883–892). Oxford: Oxford University Press.

168. Roberts, J.M., Insel, P.A., & Goldfien, A. (1981). Regulation of myometrial adrenoreceptors and adrenergic response by sex steroids. *Mol Pharmacol, 20,* 52.

169. Roberts, J., Malasanos, L., & Mendez-Bauer, C. (1981). Maternal positions in labor: Analysis in relation to comfort and efficiency. *Birth Defects, 17*(6), 97.

170. Roberts, J., Mendez-Bauer, C., & Wodell, D. (1983). The effects of maternal position on uterine contractility and efficiency. *Birth, 10*(4), 243.

171. Roberts, J., et al. (1984). Effects of lateral recumbency and sitting on the first stage of labor. *J Reprod Med, 29,* 477.

172. Rodriquez-Escudero, F.J., et al. (1981). Verapamil to inhibit the cardiovascular side effects of ritodrine. *Int J Gynaecol Obstet, 19,* 333.

173. Romero, R. & Mazor, M. (1988). Infection and preterm labor. *Clin Obstet Gynecol, 31,* 553.

174. Rorie, D.K. & Newton, M. (1967). Histologic and chemical studies of the smooth muscle in the human cervix and uterus. *Am J Obstet Gynecol, 99,* 446.

175. Russ, J.S., Rayburn, W.E., & Samuel, M.F. (1983). Uterine stimulants. In W.E. Rayburn & F.P. Zuspan (Eds.), *Drug therapy in obstetrics and gynecology* (pp. 123–133). Norwalk, CT: Appleton-Century-Crofts.

176. Russell, J.G. (1982). The rationale of primative delivery position. *Br J Obstet Gynaecol, 89,* 712.

177. Sachs, B.P. & Ringer, S.A. (1989). Intrapartum and delivery management of the very low birth-weight infant. *Clin Perinatol, 16,* 809.

178. Saeed, S.A., et al. (1982). Inhibition of prostaglandin synthesis by human amniotic fluid: Acute reduction in inhibitory activity of amniotic fluid obtained during early labor. *J Clin Endocrinol Metab, 55,* 801.

179. Scheid, C.R., Honeyman, T.W., & Fay, F.S. (1979). Mechanisms of beta-adrenergic relaxation of smooth muscle. *Nature, 277,* 32.

180. Schwarz, B.E., et al. (1977). Progesterone binding and metabolism in human fetal membranes. *Ann NY Acad Sci, 286,* 304.

181. Seitchik, J., et al. (1984). Oxytocin augmentation of dysfunctional labor. IV. Oxytocin pharmacokinetics. *Am J Obstet Gynecol, 150,* 225.

182. Seitchik, J. (1981). Quantitating uterine contractility in clinical context. *Obstet Gynecol, 57,* 453.

183. Seitchik, J. & Castillo, M. (1983). Oxytocin augmentation in dysfunctional labor. II. Uterine activity data. *Am J Obstet Gynecol, 145,* 526.

184. Seyberth, H.W., et al. (1983). Effect of prolonged indomethacin therapy on renal function and selected vasoactive hormones in very-low-birth-weight infants with symptomatic patent ductus arteriosus. *J Pediatr, 103,* 979.

185. Sholl, J.S. (1987). Abruptio placentae: Clinical management in non-acute cases. *Am J Obstet Gynecol, 156,* 40.

186. Sjoberg, N.O., et al. (1984). Adrenergic, cholinergic and peptidergic innervation of the myometrium: Distribution and effects of sex steroids and pregnancy. In S. Bottari, et al. (Eds.), *Uterine contractility* (pp. 117–126). New York: Masson Publishing.

187. Skinner, S.J.M., Campos, G.A., & Liggins, G.C. (1981). Collagen content of human amniotic membranes: Effect of gestational length and premature rupture. *Obstet Gynecol, 57,* 487.

188. Skinner, K.A. & Challis, J.G.R. (1985). Changes in the synthesis and metabolism of prostaglandins by human fetal membranes and decidua at labor. *Am J Obstet Gynecol, 151,* 519.

189. Sleep, J., Roberts, J., & Chalmers, I. (1989). Care during the second stage of labour. In I. Chalmers, M. Enkin, & M.J.N.C. Keirse (Eds.), *Effective care in pregnancy and childbirth* (pp. 1129–1144). Oxford: Oxford University Press.

190. Spisso, K.R. & Harbert, G.M. (1982). The use of magnesium sulfate as the primary tocolytic agent to prevent premature delivery. *Am J Obstet Gynecol, 142,* 840.

191. Starling, M.B. & Eliot, R.B. (1974). The effects of prostaglandins, prostaglandin inhibitors, and oxygen on closure of the ductus arteriosus, pulmonary arteries and umbilical vessels in utero. *Prostaglandins, 8,* 187.

192. Strickland, D.M., et al. (1983). Stimulation of prostaglandin biosynthesis by urine of the human fetus may serve as a trigger for parturition. *Science, 220,* 521.

193. Tamby Raja, R.L. & Salmon, J.A. (1977). Endocrinology of normal pregnancy and premature labor. *NZ Med J, 86,* 89.

194. Tamby Raja, R.L. & Lun, K.C. (1978). Plasma estriol as a predictor of preterm labor. *Int J Gynaecol Obstet, 15,* 535.

195. Thaler, I., et al. (1990). Changes in uterine blood flow during human pregnancy. *Am J Obstet Gynecol, 162,* 121.

196. Theiry, M. (1979). Induction of labor with prostaglandins. In M.J.N.C. Keirse, A.B.M. Anderson, & J. Bennebroek-Gravenhorst (Eds.), *Human parturition* (pp. 155–164). The Hague: Martinus Nijhoff.

197. Thiery, M. (1985). Stimulation of uterine activity. In T.K.A.B. Eskes & M. Finster (Eds.), *Drug therapy in pregnancy* (pp. 183–194). London: Butterworths.

198. Thornburn, G.D. & Challis, J.R.G. (1979). Endocrine control of parturition. *Physiol Rev, 59,* 863.

199. Toplis, P.J. & Sims, C.D. (1979). Prospective study of different methods and routes of administration of prostaglandin E2 to improve the unripe cervix. *Prostaglandins, 18,* 127.

200. Tulchinsky, D., et al. (1972). Plasma estrone, estradiol, progesterone and 17-hydroxy-progesterone in human pregnancy. I. Normal pregnancy. *Am J Obstet Gynecol, 112,* 1095.

201. Uldbjerg, N., Ulmsted, U., & Ekman, G. (1983). The ripening of the human uterine cervix in terms of connective tissue biochemistry. *Clin Obstet Gynecol, 26,* 14.

202. Uldbjerg, N., et al. (1983). Ripening of the human uterine cervix related to changes in collagen, glycosaminoglycans, and collagenolytic activity. *Am J Obstet Gynecol, 147,* 662.

203. Ulmsten, U. (1989). Prostaglandins in high-risk obstetrics. In S.A. Brody & K. Ueland (Eds.), *Endocrine disorders in pregnancy* (pp. 427–436). Norwalk, CT: Appleton & Lange.

204. Ulmsten, U., Wingerup, L., & Andersson, K.E. (1979). Comparison of prostaglandin E2 and intravenous oxytocin for induction of labor. *Obstet Gynecol, 54,* 581.

205. Vick, R.L. (1984). *Contemporary medical physiology* (pp. 184–191). Menlo Park, CA: Addison-Wesley.

206. Von Maillot, K. & Zimmerman, B.K. (1976). The solubility of collagen of the uterine cervix during pregnancy and labour. *Arch Gynecol, 220,* 275.

207. Weaver, J.B., Pearson, J.F., & Rosen, M. (1977). Response to a Valsalva maneuver before and after an epidural. *Anesthesia, 32,* 148.

208. Weitz, C.M., et al. (1986). Prostaglandin F metabolite concentrations as a prognostic factor in preterm labor. *Obstet Gynecol, 67,* 496.

209. Wesselius-deCasparis, A., et al. (1971). Results of a double-blind, multicentre study with ritodrine in premature labour. *Br Med J, 3,* 144.

210. Wilson, L. (1990). A new tocolytic agent: Development of an oxytocin antagonist for inhibition of uterine contractions. *Am J Obstet Gynecol, 163,* 195.

211. Wiqvist, N., Lundstrom, V., & Green, K. (1975). Premature labor and indomethacin. *Prostaglandins, 10,* 515.

212. Witter, F.R. & Niebyl, J.R. (1986). Inhibition of arachidonic acid metabolism in the perinatal period: Pharmacology, clinical application, and potential adverse effects. *Semin Perinatol, 10,* 316.

213. Yeates, D.A. & Roberts, J.E. (1984). A comparison of two bearing down techniques during the second stage of labor. *J Nurse Midwifery, 29*(1), 3.

214. Yoshida, Y. & Manabe, Y. (1990). Different characteristics of amniotic and cervical collagenous tissue during pregnancy and delivery: A morphologic study. *Am J Obstet Gynecol, 162,* 190.

215. Young, D.C., Toofarian, A., & Leveno, K.J. (1983). Potassium and glucose concentrations without treatment during intravenous ritodrine tocolysis. *Am J Obstet Gynecol, 145,* 105.

216. Young, J.T. & Poppe, C.A. (1987). Breast pump stimulation to promote labor. *MCN, 12,* 126.

217. Zahn, V. (1984). Uterine contractions during pregnancy. *J Perinat Med, 12,* 107.

CHAPTER 4

The Postpartum Period and Lactation Physiology

Involution of the Reproductive Organs
  Uterus
  Cervix and Vagina
  Breasts
  Sexual Function and Activity
Endocrine Changes
  Estrogens and Progesterone
  Pituitary Gonadotropin
  Prolactin
  Oxytocin

Physiology of Lactation
  Structure of the Mammary Glands
  Mammogenesis
  Lactogenesis
  Galactopoiesis
  Milk Production and Composition
  Nutrition During the Postpartum Period and
     Lactation
  Drugs in Breast Milk

The postpartum period is a time of restoration and return to the nonpregnant state. This period is generally defined as the 6-week period beginning with delivery of the placenta. Although some women may experience involution of the reproductive organs as early as 4 weeks post delivery, it may take 10 to 12 weeks for some structures and systems to heal or return to their prepregnancy state. The postpartum period is characterized by significant anatomic, physiologic, and endocrinologic changes as the woman recovers from the stresses of labor and delivery and lactation is initiated. In addition, all of the anatomic and physiologic changes that occurred during the 9 months of pregnancy are reversed for the most part within a 6-week period. Many of these changes occur within the first 10 to 14 days following delivery. This places additional stresses on the woman, who at the same time is undergoing major psychologic, social, and role changes as she attaches to and assumes responsibility for care of her new infant and incorporates him or her into the family system.

The focus of this chapter is on the hormonal and involutional changes associated with return of the reproductive system to its nonpregnant state and on the anatomic, physiologic, and endocrinologic changes involved in the initiation and maintenance of lactation and production of milk. The physiologic and anatomic changes within other body systems as they return to the nonpregnant state are described in Chapters 5 to 17.

INVOLUTION OF THE REPRODUCTIVE ORGANS

The reproductive system (uterus, cervix, vagina, and breasts in the nonlactating woman) gradually returns to its nonpregnant state during the 6-week postpartum period. This process is referred to as involution.

Uterus

Immediately following delivery of the placenta the uterus weighs about 1000 g and lies with its anterior and posterior walls in close approximation in midline about halfway between the umbilicus and symphysis pubis. Over the next 12 hours the fundus of the uterus rises to the level of the umbilicus (or slightly above or below), followed by a gradual decrease in height over the subsequent 2 to 3 days. The height of the fundus usually decreases by about 1 cm/day so that by 3 days the fundus lies 2 to 3 fingerbreadths below the umbilicus or slightly higher in multigravidas. By 5 to 6 days the uterus weighs about 500 g and is 4 to 5 fingerbreadths below the umbilicus. Generally the uterus has descended into the true pelvis by 10 days, and the fundus can no longer be palpated abdominally. The size of the uterus gradually decreases over the next month so that by 6 weeks the uterus has returned to its nonpregnant location and weighs approximately 60 to 80 g (slightly more than a nulliparous uterus). Involution is slower in multiparous women and following multiple gestation, infection, polyhydramnios, delivery of a large infant, or retention of placental or membrane fragments.

Involution of the uterus involves three processes: (1) contraction of the uterus, (2) autolysis of myometrial cells, and (3) regeneration of epithelium.[42, 67] Immediately following delivery, contractions of the uterine myometrium compress the blood vessels supplying the placental site, causing hemostasis. During the first 12 to 24 hours these contractions (afterpains) are relatively strong, gradually diminishing in intensity and frequency over the next 4 to 7 days. Postpartal uterine contractions tend to be stronger and to persist for a longer period in multiparous women. Contractions can also be stimulated by oxytocin release associated with suckling.

Under the influence of estrogen, the myometrium undergoes hypertrophy and hyper-plasia during pregnancy with increases in cell cytoplasm and size. Following delivery excess intracellular proteins (especially actin and myosin) and cytoplasm within the myometrial cells are eliminated by autolysis with degradation by proteolytic enzymes and macrophages. As a result, the size of individual myometrial cells is markedly reduced without a significant reduction in the total number of cells.

Initially the endometrium resembles a large desquamating wound. The upper portion of the spongy endometrial layer is sloughed off with delivery of the placenta. Regeneration of the uterine epithelial lining begins 2 to 3 days post partum with differentiation of the remaining decidua into two layers (a superficial layer and a basal layer). The superficial layer of granulation tissue, which provides a barrier to infection, is formed as leukocytes invade the remaining decidua. This layer gradually degenerates, becoming necrotic, and is sloughed off in lochia. The basal layer, which contains the fundi of the uterine endometrial glands, remains intact and is the source of the new endometrium. Regeneration of the endometrium (except at the placental site) occurs by 2 to 3 weeks. The new endometrium forms from proliferation of the fundi of the endometrial glands and the interglandular connective tissue stroma.[67]

Healing at the placental site occurs more slowly over 6 to 7 weeks. Following delivery the placental site is a raised rough area 4 to 5 cm in diameter and consists of many thrombosed vascular sinusoids.[18] The large blood vessels that supplied the intervillous spaces are invaded by fibroblasts and their lumen obscured. Some of these vessels recanalize later but with smaller lumina. The placental site heals by exfoliation without leaving a scar. This occurs with upward growth of the fundi of the endometrial glands in the decidua basalis under the placental site with simultaneous growth of endometrial tissue from the margins of the site.[67]

Lochia

The process of involution and restoration of the endometrium is reflected in the characteristics of postpartum vaginal discharge, or lochia. Lochia varies in amount and color as healing occurs. Three forms of lochia are observed: rubra, serosa, and alba. Lochia rubra, seen during the first 2 to 4 days post delivery, contains blood from the placental site, pieces of amnion and chorion, and cellular elements from the decidua, vernix, lanugo, and meconium. This form of lochia is dark red or brownish and has a fleshy odor. Lochia serosa is a pinkish-brown discharge seen from day 3 or 4 through about day 10. Lochia serosa contains some blood, wound exudate, erythrocytes, leukocytes, cervical mucus, microorganisms, and shreds of degenerating decidua from the superficial layer. Lochia alba is whitish-yellow in color since it contains primarily leukocytes along with decidual cells, mucus, bacteria, and epithelial cells. This form of lochia initially appears about 10 to 14 days and lasts until 3 to 6 weeks post partum. Most women produce a total of 150 to 400 ml of lochia (average 225 ml).[42, 48] The amount of lochia is greater in multiparous women and increases with activity; decreased flow is seen at night or with lying down and following cesarean delivery. Women who breast-feed tend to have less lochia (probably owing to more rapid healing secondary to hormonal influences), although flow may increase temporarily during feeding. Characteristics of lochia flow and their significance are summarized in Table 4–1.

TABLE 4–1
Characteristics of Lochia

CHARACTERISTIC	SIGNIFICANCE
Amount: 1st hour postpartum, no more than 2 perineal pads; next 8 hours, about 1 pad per 2–4 hours; after first 8 hours, similar to menstrual flow	Excessive flow may indicate hemorrhage or infection
Fleshy odor	Abnormal odor may indicate infection, decomposing clot, retained sponge or packing
Present for at least first 2–3 weeks (usually lasts 3–6 weeks)	Normal flow does not cease until endometrium is healed Early cessation of flow associated with infection
Proceeds from lochia rubra to serosa to alba	Characteristics reflect healing and restoration of endometrium; return to rubra after serosa or alba may indicate hemorrhage or infection

Compiled from Moore, M.L. (1983). *Realities in childbearing* (2nd ed., pp. 876–896). Philadelphia: WB Saunders.

Cervix and Vagina

Immediately following a vaginal delivery the cervix is thin, bruised, and edematous with multiple lacerations, and it hangs into the vagina. Over the next 12 to 18 hours the cervix shortens and becomes firmer ("forming up"). During the first 1 to 2 days the cervix is dilated 3 to 4 cm and two fingers can be inserted into the cervical os. By one week the os barely accommodates one finger, and by 10 to 12 days a finger can barely be inserted into the internal os but no further. By 4 weeks the external os is a small transverse slit characteristic of multiparous women.[67]

After a vaginal delivery the vagina is edematous and relaxed with decreased tone and absence of rugae. The vagina gradually decreases in size and regains tone, although never returning to its prepregnancy state. By 3 to 4 weeks rugae have begun to reappear, and edema and vascularity have decreased. The vaginal epithelium is generally restored by 6 to 10 weeks post partum.[67] Decreased lubrication of the vagina during this period can lead to discomfort with sexual intercourse, as can an episiotomy site.

Episiotomies are commonly used (in 65% of vaginal deliveries and 80% of primiparas) in the United States to prevent tearing of the fascia and muscle during delivery.[69] This technique is controversial and associated with postpartum problems such as pain, infection, alterations in urination, third-degree lacerations, and dyspareunia.[69, 77, 83] Alternative strategies to avoid an episiotomy, such as perineal massage and positioning to enhance perineal stretching, are advocated (and used by many nurse midwives), although their effectiveness has been questioned.[8a, 71, 77] Although initial healing occurs in 2 to 3 weeks, the episiotomy site may take 4 to 6 months to heal completely.[77]

Breasts

The breasts or mammary glands undergo marked changes during pregnancy with development of alveolar tissue and the ductal system in preparation for lactation. Following delivery further anatomic and physiologic changes occur in women who choose to breast-feed (see section on Physiology of Lactation). In women who do not breast-feed, involution occurs. Distention and stasis of the vascular and lymphatic circulations result in primary engorgement by 2 to 4 days following delivery. Secondary engorgement due to distention of the lobules and alveoli with milk may be seen as lactation is established. Without stimulation by suckling and removal of milk, secretion of prolactin decreases and milk production ceases. Glandular tissue gradually returns to a resting state over the next few weeks. Since new alveoli formed during pregnancy never totally disappear, the breasts do not completely return to their prepregnant state.

The treatment of engorgement varies depending on whether or not the woman is lactating. Suckling or manual expression of milk provides relief to the lactating woman but is not indicated in the nonlactating woman since these maneuvers increase milk production. Heat is used with lactating women to promote milk flow, whereas cold is used with nonlactating women to reduce flow.[48]

Sexual Function and Activity

The postpartum period is characterized by alterations in sexual activity and function for many women and their partners. Trauma to the reproductive organs, postpartal anatomic and physiologic problems, lochia flow, the presence and stress of the new baby, leaking or engorged breasts, fatigue, and psychologic factors can modify sexual function. Vaginal lubrication is altered for up to 6 months post delivery owing to reduction of estrogen following removal of the placenta.[59] Prolactin and oxytocin may also alter vaginal lubrication in the lactating woman. Masters and Johnson reported that orgasms in women for the first few months following birth tended to be shorter and less intense with greater latency of response and decreased vasocongestion of the labia majora and minora and vaginal lubrication.[41] These alterations along with decreased tone in the perineal muscles may result in more painful and less fulfilling intercourse. An episiotomy or a laceration, which may take 4 to 6 more months to completely heal depending on the extent of the wound, can also increase discomfort during intercourse.

Many cultures have taboos against resumption of sexual intercourse and other activities during the postpartum period (and sometimes for longer periods). In the United States the timing for resumption of intercourse by individual couples varies from shortly after delivery to several months. Kyndely suggests that the timing for resump-

tion of sexual intercourse be based on maternal physical restoration (cessation of bleeding and absence of perineal discomfort) and the psychological readiness of both partners.[34] Nursing interventions include counseling regarding postpartum sexual function, encouraging alternate forms of sexual intimacy, recommending vaginal lubricants, and teaching Kegel exercises to strengthen the perineal muscles.

ENDOCRINE CHANGES

Endocrine changes post partum primarily occur secondary to removal of the placenta with its hormones and to changes in prolactin secretion. Removal of placental hormones alters the physiologic function of many body systems, thus initiating return of those systems to their nonpregnant state. The rate at which placental hormones disappear from the maternal system depends on the half-life of the particular substance in maternal plasma and involves two components.[59] The "first half-life" involves removal of a substance from blood and is relatively short, resulting in rapid clearance of hormones from maternal plasma. The second component involves removal of substances from extravascular compartments and generally takes longer. The longer this "second half-life," the longer substances remain in maternal plasma post partum.[59] For example, human placental lactogen (hPL) generally disappears by 1 to 2 days, whereas human chorionic gonadotropin (hCG) can be detected for up to 2 weeks.[20] Other proteins such as alpha-fetoprotein are present in maternal plasma for several weeks or longer, suggesting that these substances are derived from maternal as well as placental sources.[59] In general most peptide hormones, enzymes and other circulating proteins of placental origin reach nonpregnant levels by 6 weeks post partum.[59]

Estrogens and Progesterone

Since the placenta is the major source of estrogens and progesterone, these hormones tend to disappear rapidly following delivery. Plasma estradiol (with a first half-life of 20 minutes and second half-life of 6 to 7 hours) reaches levels that are less than 2% of pregnancy values by 24 hours. By 1 to 3 days estradiol levels are similar to those found during the follicular phase of the menstrual cycle, and unconjugated estriol is undetectable.[59, 60] Estrogen levels fall further to day 7 post partum then gradually increase to follicular phase levels over the next few weeks. Although the first and second half-lives of progesterone are quite short, progesterone levels do not fall as rapidly as estradiol levels because the corpus luteum continues progesterone secretion during the first days following delivery.[59, 67] Generally progesterone levels similar to the luteal phase of the menstrual cycle are reached by 24 to 48 hours and follicular phase levels by 3 to 7 days.[59, 60, 67] Ovarian production of estrogens and progesterone is low during the first 2 weeks, maintaining low levels of these hormones. Levels of estradiol and progesterone gradually increase with resumption of gonadotropin secretion by the pituitary and ovarian cycling.

Pituitary Gonadotropin

The pituitary-hypothalamic axis along with production of pituitary gonadotropin, follicle-stimulating hormone (FSH), and luteinizing hormone (LH) is suppressed during pregnancy. Serum levels of FSH and LH remain very low during the first 2 weeks post partum in both lactating and nonlactating women, then gradually increase over the next few weeks with resumption of pituitary function by 4 to 6 weeks. The basis for the initially sluggish pituitary response is unknown. Tulchinsky suggests that this phenomenon may be related to (1) suppression of the pituitary-hypothalamic axis by the high levels of circulating estrogens during pregnancy; (2) need for time in order to reestablish adequate stores of FSH and LH leading to a delay in secretion of gonadotropin-releasing hormone (GnRH) by the hypothalamus; and (3) inhibition of LH release by hCG (which can be found for up to 2 weeks post partum) and prolactin.[59]

Resumption of Menstruation and Ovulation

The postpartum period tends to be a period of relative infertility for many women. Resumption of menstruation and ovulation varies among individual women regardless of whether or not the woman is lactating. Resumption of ovulation is associated with an increase in plasma progesterone. Although for most women the initial menstrual cycle following delivery is anovulatory, up to 25% of these cycles may be preceded by ovulation.[12, 57] The sooner menstruation returns following delivery, the more likely that the cycle will be anovulatory. Anovulatory cycles are more frequent in lactating women.

In nonlactating women, menstruation generally begins by 6 to 10 weeks post partum, with 50% of the first cycles anovulatory.[65] Ovulation rarely occurs prior to 4 weeks and has been reported in only 6% of woman prior to 6 weeks.[12] The average time to the resumption of menstruation and first ovulation in nonlactating women has been reported as 8.1 and 10.8 weeks, respectively.[31] Vorherr noted that in nonlactating women, 40% experienced a resumption of menses by 6 weeks, 65% by 12 weeks, and 90% by 24 weeks post partum; 15% resumed ovulation by 6 weeks, 40% by 12 weeks, and 65% by 24 weeks.[64, 65]

Lactation is associated with a delay in resumption of menstruation and ovulation.[12] Lactating women experience anovulation for varying lengths of time, with 80% of these woman reported to have anovulatory first cycles.[65] Anovulation is related to increased production of prolactin by the anterior pituitary gland. Prolactin reduces the sensitivity of the pituitary to the effects of GnRH from the hypothalamus, reducing FSH and LH secretion. Prolactin also lowers the sensitivity of ovarian follicles to LH and FSH.[59] Hyperprolactinemic states (i.e., during lactation or with infertility-associated abnormalities) tend to inhibit the LH surge and ovulation.

Ovulation usually does not occur in lactating women prior to 10 weeks following delivery but may occur as early as 35 days.[12, 59, 80] Therefore lactation, although associated with decreased fertility, is not a reliable method for preventing pregnancy. Duration of amenorrhea is longer in women who exclusively breast-feed than in those who combine breast-feeding and bottle feeding.[1] Vorherr noted that menses returned in 15% of these women by 6 weeks, 45% by 12 weeks, and 85% by 24 weeks. By 6 weeks 5% of lactating women had resumed ovulation, with 25% ovulating by 12 weeks, and 65% by 24 weeks.[64, 65]

The resumption of menstruation and ovulation in lactating women is influenced by the length of time that they lactate. Howie and colleagues reported that the average time to return of menstruation in lactating women was 30 to 36 weeks, with an average time to first ovulation of 17 weeks in woman who breast-fed for 3 months and 28 weeks in woman breast feeding for 6 months.[31] Women who lactated for less than 1 month tended to follow the pattern of nonlactating women for resumption of menstruation and ovulation. Longer periods of anovulation were noted in women who had more total time breast-feeding per day and more total infant suckling time, who maintained night feedings longer, and who introduced supplements most gradually.[30, 31]

Prolactin

Prolactin is a single-chain peptide hormone secreted by the anterior pituitary gland. Serum levels of prolactin increase during pregnancy, although its effects are suppressed by estrogen. During pregnancy prolactin is one of several hormones acting synergistically to promote development of the mammary alveoli and duct system. Prolactin release from the pituitary is suppressed by prolactin-inhibiting factor (PIF) from the hypothalamus. Prolactin levels are similar in nonlactating females and males and vary diurnally with an increase during sleep. Prolactin levels increase with stress, anesthesia, surgery, exercise, nipple stimulation, and sexual intercourse.[39]

The onset of labor is associated with a decrease in prolactin followed by an increase immediately after delivery that peaks at about 3 hours post partum.[53, 62] Secretion of prolactin post partum is triggered by suckling. In nonlactating women prolactin levels fall into the high end of the nonpregnant range by 7 to 14 days.[59] Patterns of prolactin secretion associated with lactation are described in the section on Physiology of Lactation.

Oxytocin

Oxytocin is an octapeptide hormone produced in the hypothalamus and stored and secreted by the posterior pituitary gland. The uterus becomes increasingly sensitive to oxytocin throughout pregnancy, probably owing to increasing estrogen. The placenta may contain a catabolic enzyme to maintain lower levels during pregnancy.[59] Oxytocin stimulates electrical and contractile activity in the myometrium (see Chapter 3) and is critical in the ejection of milk during lactation.

PHYSIOLOGY OF LACTATION

Lactation is a complex physiologic process involving integration of neuronal and endocrine mechanisms. Lactation can be divided into three phases: mammogenesis (mammary growth), lactogenesis (initiation of milk secretion), and galactopoiesis (maintenance of established milk secretion).[59] Hormonal influences on lactation are summarized in Table 4–2.

Structure of the Mammary Glands

The breasts or mammary glands are modified exocrine glands consisting of epithelial glandular tissue with an extensive system of branching ducts surrounded by adipose tissue and separated from the pectoralis major muscles of the chest and the ribs by connective tissue. The breasts are highly innervated with rich vascular and lymphatic systems. The basic glandular unit is the alveolus, which consists of clusters of epithelial secretory cells, the site of milk production, around a lumen into which the ductules terminate. Myoepithelial cells surrounding the secretory cells form smooth muscle contractile units responsible for ejecting milk from the lumen of the alveoli into the ductules.[39, 68] The structure of milk production and ejection portions of the mammary glands is illustrated in Fig. 4–1.

The branching ductule system from the alveoli gradually merges into larger lactiferous or mammary ducts. At the base of the nipple (mammary papilla) the ducts dilate, forming ampullae, or lactiferous sinuses. The lactiferous sinuses are surrounded by fibromuscular tissue and provide an area for milk storage. The ends of the lactiferous sinuses constrict as the duct system enters the nipple. The breast consists of 15 to 20 lobes arranged in spokes around the nipple and separated from each other by connective tissue. Each lobe terminates in a lactiferous duct that opens onto the nipple and from which milk is ejected. A lobe consists of 20 to 40 lobules each containing 10 to 100 alveoli with their respective ductules.[39] The areolar area

TABLE 4–2
Hormonal Contributions to Breast Development

HORMONE	ORIGIN	FUNCTION Before and During Pregnancy	After Delivery
Prolactin (PRL)	Anterior pituitary	Serum levels rise but estrogen suppresses its effect (see text) during pregnancy	Stimulates alveolar cells to produce milk (is probably of primary importance in initiating lactation but of secondary importance in maintaining lactation); may also cause lactation infertility by suppressing release of FSH and LH from pituitary or by causing ovaries to be unresponsive to gonadotropins; levels rise in response to various psychogenic factors, stress, anesthesia, surgery, high serum osmolality, exercise, nipple stimulation, and sexual intercourse.
Prolactin-inhibiting factor (PIF)	Hypothalamus	Suppresses release of PRL into blood; release stimulated by dopaminergic impulses (i.e., catecholamines)	Suppresses release of PRL from anterior pituitary; agents that increase PRL by decreasing catecholamines and thus PIF include phenothiazides and reserpine
Oxytocin	Posterior pituitary	Generally no effect on mammary function; sensitivity of myoepithelial cells to oxytocin increases during pregnancy	Causes myoepithelial cells to contract, leading to "milk ejection"; release is inhibited by stresses such as fear, anxiety, embarrassment, distraction; also causes uterine contraction and postpartum involution of the uterus

Adapted from Worthington-Roberts, B.W. & Williams, S.R. (Eds.). (1989). *Nutrition during pregnancy and lactation* (4th ed., pp. 256–257). St. Louis, Times Mirror/Mosby College Publishing.

around the nipple contains small sebaceous glands (tubercles of Montgomery) that provide nipple lubrication and antisepsis. Washing the nipple with soap can remove these protective secretions and lead to drying and cracking of the nipples and increase the risk of infection.

Mammogenesis

Mammogenesis involves mammary growth, which begins during fetal life and accelerates at puberty with further development and maturation of the breasts. The breasts undergo additional changes during pregnancy and post partum in order to support lactation. Breast changes begin soon after conception. The weight of the breast increases by about 12 ounces during pregnancy. External changes include increases in size and areolar pigmentation. The tubercles of Montgomery enlarge and become more prominent, and the nipples more erect. The myoepithelial cells hypertrophy. The skin over the breasts appears thinner; the blood vessels are more prominent, and there is a twofold increase in blood flow to the breast.[54]

During the first trimester the ductule system proliferates and branches under the influence of estrogen. The glandular tissues of the alveoli proliferate under the influence of hPL, hCG, and prolactin; lobular formation

TABLE 4–2
Hormonal Contributions to Breast Development *Continued*

HORMONE	ORIGIN	FUNCTION	
		Before and During Pregnancy	**After Delivery**
Estrogen	Ovary and placenta	Stimulates proliferation of glandular tissue and ducts in breast; probably stimulates pituitary to secrete PRL but inhibits PRL effects on breasts	Blood level drops at parturition, which aids in initiating lactation; not important to lactation thereafter
Progesterone	Ovary and placenta	With estrogen, stimulates proliferation of glandular tissue and ducts in breast; inhibits milk secretion	Blood levels drop at parturition, which aids in initiating lactation; probably unimportant to lactation thereafter
Growth hormone	Anterior pituitary		May act with PRL in initiating lactation but appears to be most important in maintaining established lactation
Adrenocorticotropic hormone (ACTH)	Anterior pituitary	Blood levels gradually increase during pregnancy; stimulates adrenal to release corticosteroids	High level is believed necessary for maintenance of lactation
Human placental lactogen (hPL)	Placenta	Like growth hormone in structure; stimulates mammary growth; associated with mobilization of free fatty acids and inhibition of peripheral glucose utilization and lactogenic action	
Thyroxine	Thyroid	Normally no direct effect on lactation	Appears to be important in maintaining lactation either through some direct effect on the mammary glands or by control of metabolism
Thyrotropin-releasing hormone	Hypothalamus	Normally no effect on lactation	Stimulates release of PRL; can be used to maintain established lactation

Adapted from Worthington-Roberts, B.S. & Williams, S.R. (1989). *Nutrition in pregnancy and lactation* (4th ed., pp. 256–257). St. Louis: Times Mirror/Mosby College Publishing.

is enhanced by progesterone (Fig. 4–2). Growth hormone and adrenocorticotropic hormone (ACTH) act synergistically with prolactin and progesterone to promote mammogenesis. Concurrently breast interstitial tissue becomes infiltrated with lymphocytes, plasma cells, and eosinophils. During the second and third trimesters there is further lobular growth with formation of new alveoli and ducts and dilation of the lumina. Ductal arborization begins at mid-gestation. Secretory material similar to colostrum accumulates in the lumina beginning in the second trimester.[18, 37, 59, 68]

During the third trimester the epithelial cells of the alveoli differentiate into secretory cells capable of milk production and release. Fat droplets accumulate in the secretory cells.

Progressive dilation of the breast results from the increase in secretory cells and distention of the alveoli with colostrum.[39] Following birth the alveolar epithelial cells continue to proliferate with synthesis of milk under the influence of increased levels of prolactin and the stimulus of suckling. Initial synthesis of milk components is preceded by an increase in required enzymes within the secretory cells. Upon cessation of lactation, involution of the breasts occurs over several months. The breasts never return to their prelactation size owing to retention of many of the new loboalveolar structures.

Lactogenesis

Lactogenesis, or initiation of milk production, involves a complex neuroendocrine

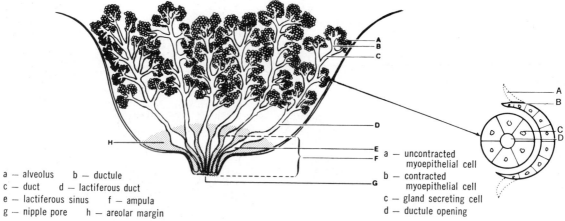

a — alveolus   b — ductule
c — duct   d — lactiferous duct
e — lactiferous sinus   f — ampula
g — nipple pore   h — areolar margin

a — uncontracted
    myoepithelial cell
b — contracted
    myoepithelial cell
c — gland secreting cell
d — ductule opening

FIGURE 4–1. Functional unit of milk production: lobular and alveolar systems. (From Applebaum, R.M. (1975). The obstetrician's approach to the breasts and breastfeeding. *J Reprod Med, 14*(3), 100.)

process with interaction of several hormones. The predominant hormone is prolactin, which acts synergistically with growth hormone, insulin, cortisol, and thyrotropin-releasing hormone (Table 4–2 and Fig. 4–3). Milk production and release are controlled primarily by the effect of suckling on prolactin release via a complex neuroendocrine process. Suckling stimulates prolactin release from the anterior pituitary (Fig. 4–4). Suckling also stimulates sensory nerve endings in the nipple and areola, sending impulses to the hypothalamus via the spinal cord. As a result, hypothalamic secretion of prolactin-inhibiting factor is suppressed, and adenohypophysis secretion of prolactin increases.

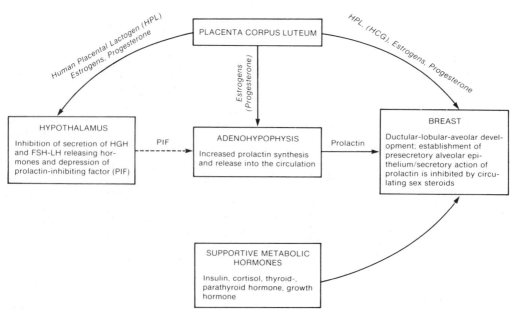

FIGURE 4–2. Hormonal preparation of breast during pregnancy for lactation. (Modified from Vorherr, H. (1974). *The breast* (p. 72). New York: Academic Press, by Lawrence, R. (1985). *Breastfeeding: A guide for the medical profession* (p. 45). St. Louis: CV Mosby.)

POSTPARTUM

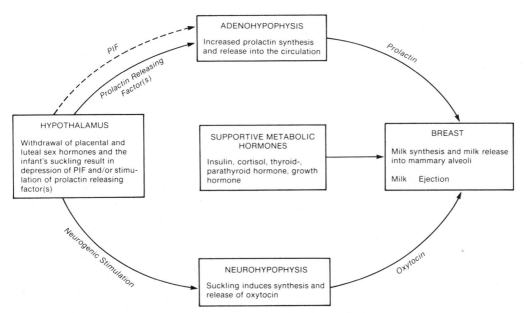

FIGURE 4–3. Hormonal preparation of the breast post partum for lactation.
(Modified from Vorherr, H. (1974). *The breast* (p. 72). New York: Academic Press,
by Lawrence, R. (1985). *Breastfeeding: A guide for the medical profession* (p. 47).
St. Louis: CV Mosby.)

Prolactin levels increase toward the end of a feeding, increasing the volume, fat, and protein content of milk in the next feeding.[59]

Prolactin is important in generating milk for subsequent feedings. Decreased frequency of feedings or bottle supplementation decreases milk production. However, if the frequency of suckling is increased, milk production will again increase. During early lactation increasing the frequency of feedings is especially important in establishing adequate milk production. This can often be accomplished by demand feeding. Increasing maternal fluid intake does not significantly increase milk production.[14] For mothers of preterm or other infants who cannot yet

FIGURE 4–4. The neuroendocrine reflexes that are initiated by suckling. Stimulatory (STIM.) as well as inhibitory (INHIB.) influences leading to milk production (PR.) are shown. PV, paraventricular nucleus; SO, supraoptic nucleus; T, thoracic region. (From Tulchinsky, D. (1980). The postpartum period. In D. Tulchinsky & K. J. Ryan (Eds.), *Maternal-fetal endocrinology* (p. 154). Philadelphia: WB Saunders.)

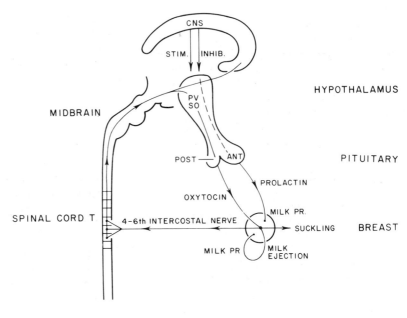

tolerate enteral feedings, increasing the frequency of breast pumping can help to establish and maintain the mother's milk supply. Hopkinson and coworkers found that optimal milk production in mothers of preterm infants was associated with five or more milk expressions per day and pumping durations exceeding 100 min/day.[29]

Prolactin Patterns in Lactating Women

Prolactin acting synergistically with insulin and cortisol, in particular, stimulates the alveolar secretory cells to produce milk proteins and fat. If prolactin is absent, milk secretion will not occur. However, lactation will not begin unless preceded by a fall in plasma estrogens (removing a blocking effect and allowing breast tissue to respond to prolactin) and progesterone (which may have an inhibitory effect on production of α-lactalbumin and consequently lactose).[59] The number of prolactin receptors on breast tissue increases markedly post partum. The decrease in hPL following removal of the placenta may also facilitate prolactin action, since hPL competes with prolactin for the same breast tissue receptors.[59] Bromocriptine mesylate, a substance used to suppress lactation, acts by decreasing the number of specific prolactin receptors.

Three patterns of prolactin secretion are seen in lactating women. During the 1st week following delivery basal prolactin levels are high and increase only slightly with suckling. From approximately 2 weeks to 3 months baseline levels are 2 to 3 times higher. With suckling, prolactin levels increase 10 to 20 times. After 3 months baseline prolactin levels are similar to those of nonlactating women and do not rise significantly with suckling (Fig. 4–5).[39, 59, 61] In lactating women prolactin levels are highest with more frequent suckling and after the last feeding in the day (maintaining the normal diurnal increase in prolactin seen in both males and females).[8, 13]

Galactopoiesis

Galactopoiesis is the maintenance of established milk secretion. This phase of lactation is dependent on establishment of periodic suckling, removal of milk, and an intact hypothalamic-pituitary axis regulating prolactin and oxytocin levels.[39] Other hormones enhancing galactopoiesis include growth hormone, corticosteroids, thyroxine, and insulin (see Fig. 4–3). Prolactin seems most critical during initiation of lactation and less so with long-term maintenance of lactation. Oxytocin stimulates propulsion of milk through the duct system (let-down reflex).

Let-Down Reflex

The let-down or milk ejection reflex is a complex neuroendocrine process important for movement of milk along the duct system to the nipple. Suckling stimulates sensory nerve endings in the nipple and areola. These impulses travel via afferent neural pathways in the spinal cord to the mesencephalon and hypothalamus, stimulating oxytocin release from the posterior pituitary gland (see Fig. 4–4). Oxytocin stimulates contraction of the myoepithelial cells surrounding the alveoli. As a result milk is ejected into the duct system and propelled to the lactiferous ducts and sinuses. Oxytocin also stimulates uterine contractions and involution. The let-down reflex can also be triggered by thinking of the infant, infant crying, and orgasm. Anxiety, pain, and fatigue can reduce the let-down reflex and decrease the amount of milk released to the infant.[39, 68] This reflex is also inhibited by ethanol consumption in amounts greater than 1 g/day.[10]

Milk Production and Composition

The components of milk are synthesized in the secretory cells of the alveoli (protein, fat, lactose) or extracted from maternal plasma (vitamins, minerals) by these same cells. The individual components of milk then pass into the alveolar lumen where the final milk is constituted. The secretory cells proceed through several stages as milk is produced, moving from a resting state to a secretory state and back to a resting state (Fig. 4–6).[39] Milk synthesis occurs at very low levels much of the time, but is most active during infant suckling. The secretory cells change from a cuboidal to club-like appearance immediately prior to milk secretion, reflecting cellular uptake of water.[68]

Proteins, lactose, and fats synthesized within the microsomal fraction of the cell (Fig. 4–7) are packaged into vesicles that migrate through the cytoplasm to the apex of the secretory cells (see Fig. 4–6). These substances are then released into the alveolar lumen via either apocrine or merocrine se-

FIGURE 4–5. Plasma prolactin and human growth hormone (hGH) concentrations (mean ± SE) during nursing in the 8th to 41st and the 63rd to 194th days post partum. (From Noel, G.L., Suh, H.K., & Frantz, A.G. Prolactin release during nursing and breast stimulation in postpartum and nonpostpartum patients. *J Clin Endocrinol Metab, 38,* 413, 1974, © by The Endocrine Society.)

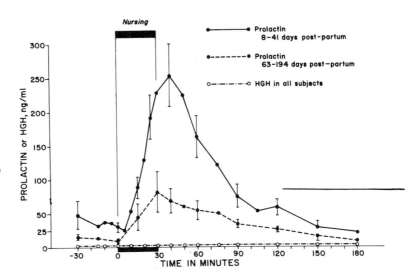

cretion. Merocrine secretion involves release of materials such as newly synthesized proteins through the cell apex without significant loss of cytoplasm. Apocrine secretion also involves expulsion of secretory material such as fat droplets from the cell apex.[39] The fat droplets move through the cytoplasm of the secretory cell to the cell apex, projecting into the alveolar lumen. The droplets are secreted into the lumen accompanied by pieces of cell membrane and surrounding cytoplasm.[39]

Composition of Human Milk

The initial substance produced by the alveolar secretory cells is colostrum. Colostrum appears early in the second trimester and is present during the first few days post partum. Colostrum is a transparent yellow substance (the yellow color comes from its high carotene content). Colostrum is higher in protein than mature milk owing to increased concentrations of globulins, and lower in car-

bohydrate, fat, and calories (mean of 67 versus 75 kcal/dl). Colostrum is gradually replaced by a transitional form of milk after the first few days. This milk contains greater quantities of fat, lactose, and calories than colostrum and is replaced by mature milk over the first 1 to 2 weeks as lactation is established.[34, 68]

The composition of human milk varies with the stage of lactation, gestation, amount of milk secreted, and individual maternal characteristics (age, parity, and health).[39, 54, 68] The vitamin and fat content of human milk is related to maternal nutrition; the content of other substances is generally independent of maternal nutritions. The primary components of human milk are fats (3.8%), proteins (3.2%), carbohydrates (4.8%), water (87.5%), electrolytes, vitamins, and minerals.[51] Each 100 ml of human milk contains 75 kcal (range, 67 to 77).[16] The average volume of milk increases during lactation from about 500 ml/day at 1 week, to

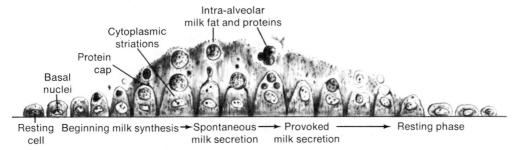

FIGURE 4–6. Diagram of cycle of secretory cells from resting stage to secretion and return to resting stage. (From Grynfeltt, J. 1937. Etude de processus cytologique de la secretion mammaire. *Arch Anat Microsc, 33,* 177; as modified from Vorherr, H. (1974). *The breast.* New York: Academic Press, by Lawrence, R. (1985). *Breastfeeding: A guide for the medical profession* (p. 56). St. Louis: CV Mosby.)

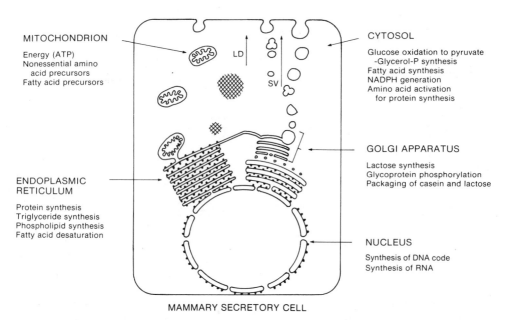

MAMMARY SECRETORY CELL

FIGURE 4–7. Schematic representation of cytologic and biochemical interrelationships of secretory cell of mammary gland. LD, lipid droplet; SV, secretory vesicle. (From Lawrence, R. (1985). *Breastfeeding: A guide for the medical profession* (p. 57). St. Louis: CV Mosby.)

750 to 850 ml/day (up to 1200 ml) by 6 months.[40, 54, 55] Concentrations of substances contained in colostrum, mature human milk, and cow's milk are listed in Table 4–3.

Milk fat, protein, and lactose are synthesized in the secretory cells of the alveoli (see Figs. 4–1, 4–6, and 4–7). Water, electrolytes, and water-soluble compounds cross the alveolar membrane via diffusion through water-filled pores or active transport.[21, 39, 63] Human milk is isosmotic with plasma. Lactose appears in high concentrations in human milk and is the major osmotic component. In order for milk to maintain isosmolarity with plasma, concentrations of other ions, sodium and chloride, in particular, must remain proportionately lower.

Substances such as calcium, amino acids, glucose, magnesium, and sodium are actively transported across the milk-blood barrier.[63] This barrier is analogous in many ways to both the blood-brain barrier and the placental barrier. The milk-blood barrier is a lipid membrane barrier with water-filled pores consisting of tissue layers that separate the lumina of the alveoli from maternal capillary blood. This barrier consists of the capillary epithelium and basement membrane, interstitial space, myoepithelial cells, and alveolar cell basement membrane.[21, 63]

Human milk also contains vitamins, iron, and trace minerals derived from maternal blood. In general, if maternal nutrition is adequate, the vitamin and trace mineral components will meet minimal requirements.[54] Water-soluble vitamins pass readily from maternal blood to breast milk, and levels reflect maternal diet. Minimal amounts of fluoride pass into breast milk so supplementation may be needed if the infant does not receive this mineral from the water supply.[68] Although the iron content of human milk is significantly less than in cow's milk, a much greater proportion of the iron is absorbed, facilitated by lactose and ascorbic acid. Zinc levels are similar in human and cow's milk; however, the bioavailability of zinc in human milk is increased owing to the presence of a zinc-binding ligand that facilitates intestinal absorption.[54]

The total mineral content of human milk is generally stable at any stage of lactation and is not closely related to maternal nutrition. As lactation continues, absorption of iron and zinc decreases regardless of maternal nutritional status or milk content. Calcium is taken up by the alveoli from maternal blood. Much of this calcium comes from maternal bone stores so that the calcium content of milk is not affected by maternal nutritional intake. In healthy women approximately 2.2% of the femoral bone is miner-

TABLE 4–3
**Approximate Concentrations (per dl) of Components of Human Colostrum, Transitional
Human Milk, Mature Human Milk, and Cow's Milk**

COMPONENT	HUMAN COLOSTRUM	TRANSITIONAL HUMAN MILK	MATURE HUMAN MILK	MATURE COW'S MILK
Water (g)	87.0	–	87.5	86.0
Lactose (g)	5.5	6.4	7.0	4.8
Fat (g)	2.9	3.5	3.7	4.3
Protein (g)	4.1	1.6	1.2	3.3
Amino acids (g)	1.2	0.9	1.3	3.3
Nonprotein nitrogen (g)	91.0	48.0	32.0	25.0
Calcium (mg)	39.0	46.0	35.0	130.0
Phosphorus (mg)	14.0	20.0	15.0	120.0
Sodium (mg)	48.0	29.0	15.0	58.0
Potassium (mg)	74.0	64.0	57.0	145.0
Magnesium (mg)	4.0	4.0	4.0	12.0
Iron (μg)	70.0	70.0	100.0	70.0
Copper (μg)	40.0	50.0	40.0	15.0
Vitamin A (μg)	151.0	88.0	75.0	41.0
Thiamine (μg)	1.9	5.9	14.0	43.0
Riboflavin (μg)	30.0	37.0	40.0	145.0
Nicotinic acid (μg)	75.0	175.0	160.0	82.0
Pantothenic acid (μg)	183.0	288.0	246.0	340.0
Biotin (μg)	0.06	0.35	0.60	2.8
Folic acid (μg)	0.05	0.02	0.14	0.13
Vitamin B$_{12}$ (μg)	0.05	0.04	0.10	0.60
Ascorbic acid (mg)	5.9	7.1	5.0	1.1
Vitamin D (IU)	–	–	5.0	2.5
Vitamin E (mg)	1.5	0.09	5.0	0.07
Vitamin K (μg)	–	–	1.5	6.0

Adapted from Vorherr, H. (1978). Human lactation and breast feeding. In B.L. Larson (Ed.), *Lactation* (Vol. IV, pp. 216–217). New York: Academic Press.

alized to provide for milk calcium content during the first 3 months of lactation.[3, 40]

Since levels of protein, calcium, sodium, potassium, phosphorus, and other ions are lower in human than in cow's milk, the potential renal solute load is also lower (about one-third that of cow's milk) and thus puts less stress on the kidneys (see Chapter 8). Human milk is also rich in immunologic substances that protect the infant from infections (especially gastrointestinal and respiratory infections) and provides some protection against the development of allergies both by reducing exposure of the infant to cow's milk allergens and by providing secretory IgA, which reduces intestinal absorption of potentially antigenic proteins prior to gut closure (see Chapter 10) at 6 to 9 months. The antiallergic and anti-infectious properties of human milk are discussed in Chapter 10.

Fat Synthesis and Release

The largest portion of calories in human milk comes from fat. The major constituents of milk fat are triglycerides. Other lipids found in human milk include free fatty acids, cholesterol, phospholipid, and glycolipid. In comparison with cow's milk, human milk has greater concentrations of linoleic acid (an essential fatty acid) and cholesterol, with fewer short-chain saturated fatty acids.[36, 45] The higher cholesterol may benefit the infant by enhancing synthesis of myelin in the central nervous system and stimulating development of the enzyme system essential in later life for cholesterol degradation.[32] Human milk also contains a lipase that initiates fat digestion prior to the time milk enters the infant's intestine, enhancing release of energy and fat digestion and absorption (see Chapter 9).

The concentration of fat in human milk shows marked diurnal variation with lowest levels at 6 A.M. and peaking in midafternoon.[68] In addition, within a given feeding the fat content is highest at the end of a feeding (hindmilk) perhaps facilitating infant satiety.[27] Severe maternal caloric restriction alters the fatty acid composition, as do alterations in the type of fat consumed by the mother.[25, 68] For example, if the maternal diet is altered to include more polyunsaturated fatty acids, her milk will also contain more polyunsaturated fats.

Milk fat is synthesized in the endoplasmic

reticulum (Fig. 4–7) from precursors available within the secretory cell or obtained from maternal blood. Short-chain fatty acids are synthesized from acetate, whereas long-chain fatty acids are obtained from maternal plasma. Triglycerides are either obtained from maternal plasma or synthesized from intracellular carbohydrates (primarily glyceride and glucose). Two enzymes (lipoprotein lipase and palmitoyl-CoA transferase) involved in the production and utilization of triglycerides are stimulated by prolactin. Lipoprotein lipase acts in the capillaries to catalyze the lipolysis and uptake of triglyceride (and its component fatty acids and glycerol) into the secretory cell. Palmitoyl-CoA transferase is involved in intracellular synthesis of triglyceride from glyceride.[39, 68]

Fatty acids are esterified in the endoplasmic reticulum to form triglycerides. The triglycerides accumulate and coalesce to form larger fat droplets. As fat droplets increase in size they migrate to the apex of the secretory cell and are released into the alveolar lumen via apocrine secretion.

Carbohydrate Synthesis and Release

The major carbohydrate found in human milk is lactose. Other carbohydrates found in small quantities include glucose, glucoamines, and nitrogen-containing oligosaccharide. Lactose promotes growth of lactobacilli in the infant's intestine and facilitates synthesis of B complex vitamins. As lactose is metabolized, lactic and acetic acid are produced and increase intestinal acidity to help protect the infant from intestinal infection by reducing growth of enteropathic organisms. The acidic environment enhances absorption of calcium, phosphorus, and magnesium.[37, 68]

Lactose is synthesized in the secretory cell's Golgi apparatus (Fig. 4–7) from glucose and galactose. The glucose is obtained from maternal circulating blood glucose. Production of lactose from glucose and galactose is catalyzed by galactosyl transferase, which in turn is catabolized by α-lactalbumin (a whey protein). The availability of α-lactalbumin is the rate-limiting step in the production of lactose. During pregnancy progesterone inhibits this enzyme. Following delivery reduction in progesterone and estrogens along with the concomitant increase in prolactin result in increased production of α-lactalbumin and therefore lactose.[39, 68]

The concentration of lactose in human milk is constant and independent of maternal nutritional status. Lactose is a critical factor in controlling the volume of milk produced. If less lactose is available, less milk will be produced so that the lactose concentration remains constant. The lactose synthesized in the Golgi apparatus attaches to protein and is released from the surface of the secretory cell into the alveolar lumen via merocrine secretion.

Protein Synthesis and Release

Milk protein consists of casein and whey proteins. The major whey protein is α-lactalbumin. The concentrations of whey protein and casein in human milk are in a 60:40 ratio versus the 20:80 ratio seen in cow's milk. Whey protein is easily digested forming soft, flocculent curds. Casein, the predominant cow's milk protein, is less easily digested and forms tough, rubbery curds. Casein requires a greater energy expenditure to digest, and digestion is more likely to be incomplete.

Protein content decreases slowly during the first 6 months of lactation. Colostrum has three times as much protein as mature milk owing to the addition of several amino acids and antibodies such as secretory IgA and lactoferrin (see Chapter 10). All of the essential amino acids are present in colostrum. Although the total protein content of human milk is less than half that of cow's milk, the infant has adequate nitrogen for growth of new cells owing to increased nonprotein nitrogen in the form of urea, free amino acids, amino sugars, choline, creatinine, nucleic acids, and other substances.[19]

In addition the amino acid content is specific to the unique physiologic characteristics of the human newborn. For example, human milk has lower levels of methionine and increased cystine. As a result the breast-fed infant is less dependent on the enzyme cystathionase, an enzyme which develops late in fetal life. Human milk also has less tyrosine and phenylalanine. Since the enzymes that catabolize these amino acids develop later, low levels prevent excessive concentrations of these substances. Human infants do not synthesize taurine well, and levels of taurine are higher in human as compared with cow's milk. Taurine is involved in bile acid conjugation and as a neurotransmitter and modifier in the brain and retina.[68]

Three major milk proteins, casein, α-lactalbumin (whey), and β-lactalbumin (whey), are formed. These proteins are unique to milk and derived primarily from synthesis in the secretory cells from amino acids. All of the essential and some of the nonessential amino acids come from maternal plasma. Other nonessential amino acids are synthesized in the alveolar secretory cells.[58] A small amount of protein (primarily the proteins found in colostrum) is derived from maternal plasma. The production of milk proteins by the ribosomes of the endoplasmic reticulum of the secretory cell is induced by prolactin acting in conjunction with insulin and cortisol.

Synthesis of milk proteins is similar to synthesis of other proteins by the body. Prolactin induces synthesis of messenger and transfer RNA. Messenger RNA transmits the genetic information to the ribosomes. This information is interpreted by transfer RNA to utilize specific amino acids to assemble appropriate sequences of polypeptide chains to form the specific milk proteins.[39] The milk proteins are then released from the secretory cell into the alveolar lumen via apocrine secretion.

Preterm versus Term Milk

In recent years several differences have been reported in preterm as compared with term breast milk in women delivering prior to 32 to 33 weeks (see Table 9–17).[75] Preterm breast milk has a higher protein content during the 1st month. Nitrogen content of preterm milk is 15 to 20% higher than that of term milk.[4, 28, 33, 66] In addition the energy density of preterm milk has been reported to be 30% higher owing to greater fat concentration, although other investigators have reported either no differences or marked variability in caloric density among individual women.[1, 28, 66] Preterm milk contains slightly less lactose, is higher in sodium and chloride during the 1st month, and has similar levels of calcium, phosphorus, magnesium, and iron as compared with term milk (see Table 9–17).[5, 6, 9, 23] Levels of other minerals such as zinc and copper are similar or slightly higher in preterm milk.[44] Use of human milk for feeding low birth weight infants is discussed in Chapter 9.

Nutrition During the Postpartum Period and Lactation

Maternal nutritional requirements during the postpartum period for nonlactating women are generally similar to those for nonpregnant women. However these women do need adequate protein, vitamins, and minerals to promote healing and restoration. Some women may also need iron supplementation to replenish body stores. Other women may have increased energy requirements to meet the demands and added responsibility of the new infant.

As with pregnancy, there are specific maternal physiologic changes associated with lactation that influence nutritional requirements. These changes include an increased demand for nutrients, redistribution of blood to increase the supply of nutrients and precursors to the mammary glands, increased metabolic rate, and increased cardiac output with increased blood flow to the liver and gastrointestinal system (to meet increased demands for specific nutrients and precursors).[39] Maternal diet must be altered to meet the demands of lactation. The two components that are most affected by lactation are maternal protein intake and energy production.

During lactation the maternal basal metabolic rate increases 60%.[40] Approximately 900 kcal of energy are required to produce a liter of milk.[58] Thus it has been estimated that women need a minimum of 750 kcal/day to support lactation (150 kcal for synthesis and secretion of milk and 600 kcal to provide for the energy content of the milk).[55] These calories come from maternal fat stores and caloric intake. During the initial 3 months of lactation women use the 2 to 4 kg of body fat stored during pregnancy to provide about 200 to 300 kcal/day, or one-third of the additional calories needed each day. The additional 500 kcal is supplied by maternal diet. Increased caloric intake is needed after 3 months (when pregnancy fat stores are depleted), in undernourished women, or if the mother is nursing more than one infant.[40, 55, 68]

Protein intake is generally increased to 65 g/day.[16, 55] Intake of water-soluble vitamins is increased, as are calcium (1200 mg); vitamins A (1300 μg), D (10 μg), and E (12 μg); and folate (280 μg).[16]

Drugs in Breast Milk

Drugs cross into breast milk across the milk-blood barrier via mechanisms similar to those described for movement of substances across the placenta (see Chapter 2). Many pharmacologic agents; environmental pollutants; and alcohol, nicotine, and other abused drugs can be found in human milk. Concentrations of drugs in human milk are affected by factors such as drug dosage and physicochemical characteristics, maternal physiology, and infant physiology and maturity. As a result, drugs should be used with caution and only as absolutely needed in the lactating woman with careful monitoring of both infant and mother. Table 4–4 provides examples of specific drugs contraindicated during lactation.

The use of any pharmacologic agent in the breast-feeding woman should be carefully evaluated. Often little is known about side effects of less commonly used agents. The nurse and the mother should be aware of potential hazards for both mother and infant of any drug, since drugs other than those listed in Table 4–4 may cause potentially harmful side effects in the infant. There are many reviews of drug use during breast feeding and of hazards of specific agents.[7, 15, 22, 49, 56, 63, 70] Voora and Yeh offer several suggestions for reducing the effects of drugs in breast milk on the infant: (1) using a short-acting form of the drug to reduce the risk of accumulation; (2) feeding the infant prior to taking the medication, thus avoiding feeding during high peak plasma levels; (3) using preparations that can be given at longer intervals (once versus 3 to 4 times/day); (4) using single-dose regimens if possible; (5) temporarily discontinuing breast-feeding or using previously expressed milk while the mother is on the medication.[63]

Use of oral contraceptives by lactating women is controversial. Combined estrogen-progestin oral contraceptives suppress lactation probably through inhibition of prolactin by estrogen. These agents are associated with decreases in milk production, shorter overall length of time that the woman lactates, and slower infant weight gain.[39, 72, 82] Combined agents with less than 50 μg ethinyl estradiol and less than 100 μg mestranol when used after the immediate postpartum period appear to have few side effects.[39, 65] Progestin-only agents have less effect on lactation but are slightly less effective contraceptives and are associated with irregular bleeding.[39, 72]

TABLE 4–4
Examples of Drugs Contraindicated During Breast-Feeding*

DRUG	REPORTED SIGN OR SYMPTOM IN INFANT/ EFFECT ON LACTATION
Methotrexate	Possible immune suppression, unknown effect on growth or association with carcinogenesis
Bromocriptine	Suppresses lactation
Cimetidine	May suppress gastric acidity in infant, inhibit drug metabolism, and cause central nervous system stimulation
Clemastine	Drowsiness, irritability, refusal to feed, high-pitched cry, neck stiffness
Cyclophosphamide	Possible immune suppression, unknown effect on growth or association with carcinogenesis
Ergotamine	Vomiting, diarrhea, convulsions (doses used in migraine medications)
Gold salts	Rash, inflammation of kidney and liver
Methimazole	Potential for interfering with thyroid function
Phenindione	Hemorrhage
Thiouracil	Decreased thyroid function (does not apply to propylthiouracil)

*Use of any pharmacologic agent in the breast-feeding woman should be carefully evaluated since, although not contraindicated, other agents may cause potentially harmful side effects in the infant (see text).

From Voora, S. & Yeh, T.F. (1985). Drugs in breast milk. In T.F. Yeh (Ed.), *Drug therapy in the neonate and small infant* (pp. 47–48). Chicago: Year Book Medical Publishers.

SUMMARY

The postpartum period is a time of rapid and complex change as the woman recovers from labor and delivery and undergoes reversal of the anatomic, physiologic, and endocrine changes of pregnancy. For most women these changes occur almost unnoticed, yet they provide the background for the new mother's physical function and sense of well-being and may influence the adaptation of the woman to her infant and new role. Understanding of the physiologic basis of lactation is essential in intervening appropriately to support the lactating woman and in assisting with problems. Clinical recommendations related to postpartum physiologic adaptations are summarized in Table 4–5.

TABLE 4–5
Summary of Recommendations for Clinical Practice Related to Involutional Changes and Lactation

Recognize and monitor the progress of normal involutional changes for each of the reproductive organs (pp. 137–142).

Teach postpartum women the expected physiologic and anatomic changes during the postpartum period (pp. 131–141).

Monitor the fundus and ensure that the uterus remains contracted (pp. 137–138).

Know factors associated with afterpains and institute interventions to promote maternal comfort (p. 137).

Observe for signs of altered or delayed involution (pp. 137–138).

Monitor color and characteristics of lochial flow (pp. 137–138, Table 4–1).

Counsel women and their partners regarding changes in vaginal tone and lubrication post partum (pp. 138–139).

Counsel women regarding actions to increase vaginal lubrication and perineal tone (pp. 138–139).

Counsel women and their partners regarding resumption of sexual activity (p. 139).

Encourage alternative forms of sexual intimacy during the postpartum period (p. 139).

Recognize breast engorgement and implement interventions appropriate for the breast-feeding and non–breast-feeding woman (pp. 138–139).

Teach women interventions to reduce the risk of infection (pp. 137–138, 142).

Counsel women regarding the expected timing for resumption of menstruation and ovulation (pp. 140–141).

Counsel women regarding methods of family planning (pp. 140–141, 152; Chapter 1).

Counsel women who are breast-feeding regarding potential risks of using lactation as a method of fertility control (pp. 140–141).

Teach women the physiology of lactation and milk production (pp. 141–151).

Encourage frequent breast-feeding on demand to assist women to establish their milk supply (pp. 144–145).

Assist women who are pumping to increase their milk volume by increasing frequency of pumping (pp. 145–146).

Teach breast-feeding women nipple and breast care (pp. 141–142).

Counsel women regarding factors that promote or interfere with the let-down reflex (p. 146).

Counsel women to abstain from or limit alcohol intake during lactation (p. 146).

Know the composition of human milk and factors that influence composition and volume (pp. 146–151; Table 4–3).

Know the advantages and limitations of human milk for preterm infants (p. 151; Chapter 9).

Encourage early initiation of breast-feeding after delivery and use of demand feeding (pp. 143–150).

Encourage women to ensure that their infants consume hindmilk or that this milk is included in pumped milk (p. 149).

Counsel lactating women regarding nutritional requirements and effects of their nutritional status on milk production (pp. 147–151).

Assess nutritional status and counsel women regarding nutritional needs post partum (p. 151).

Recognize the risk associated with use of pharmacologic agents in breast-feeding women (pp. 151–152, Table 4–5).

Counsel women regarding use of medications during lactation (pp. 151–159).

Evaluate the need for use of specific drugs and counsel women regarding side effects (pp. 151–152).

Monitor and evaluate maternal and neonatal responses to drugs taken by the breast-feeding woman (pp. 151–152).

Institute interventions as appropriate to reduce the risks associated with specific drugs (p. 152).

Page numbers in parentheses following each intervention refer to the page(s) where the rationale for the intervention is discussed.

REFERENCES

1. Anderson, G.H., Atkinson, S.A., & Bryan, M.H. (1981). Energy and macronutrient content of human milk during early lactation from mothers giving birth prematurely and at term. *Am J Clin Nutr, 34,* 258.

2. Arrata, W.S.M. & Chatterton, R.T. (1974). Human lactation: Appropriate and inappropriate. *Obstet Gynecol Annu, 3,* 443.

3. Atkinson, P.J. & West, R.R. (1970). Loss of skeletal calcium in lactating women. *J Obstet Gynaecol Br Comm, 77,* 555.

4. Atkinson, S.A., Anderson, G., & Bryan, M.H. (1980). Human milk: Comparison of nitrogen composition of milk from mothers of premature infants. *Am J Clin Nutr, 33,* 811.

5. Atkinson, S.A., Radde, I.C., & Anderson, G.H. (1983). Micromineral balances in premature infants fed their own mothers' milk or formula. *J Pediatr, 102,* 99.

6. Avery, G.B. & Fletcher, A.B. (1987). Nutrition. In G.B. Avery (Ed.), *Neonatology: Pathophysiology and management of the newborn* (pp. 1173–1229). Philadelphia: JB Lippincott.

7. Berglund, F., et al. (1984). Drug use during pregnancy and breast-feeding. *Acta Obstet Gynecol Scand, 126,* 1.

8. Bunner, D.L., Vanderlaan, E.F., & Vanderlaan, W.P. (1978). Prolactin levels in nursing mothers. *Am J Obstet Gynecol, 131,* 250.

8a. Chalmers, I., et al. (1989). *Effective care in pregnancy and childbirth.* Oxford: Oxford University Press.

9. Chan, G.M. (1982). Human milk calcium and phosphorus levels of mothers delivering term and preterm infants. *J Pediatr Gastroenterol Nutr, 1,* 201.

10. Cobo, E. (1973). Effect of different doses of ethanol on the milk-ejecting reflex in lactating women. *Am J Obstet Gynecol, 113,* 819.

11. Cowie, A.T. & Tindal, J.S. (1971). *The physiology of lactation.* London: Edward Arnold.

12. Cronin, T.J. (1968). Influence of lactation on ovulation. *Lancet, 2,* 422.

13. Delvoye, P., et al. (1977). The influence of the

frequency of nursing and of previous lactation experience on serum prolactin in lactating mothers. *J Biosoc Sci, 9,* 447.

14. Dusdieker, L.B., et al. (1985). Effect of supplemental fluids on human milk production. *J Pediatr, 106,* 207.

15. Findlay, J.W. (1983). The distribution of some commonly used drugs in human breast milk. *Drug Metab Rev, 14,* 653.

16. Food and Nutrition Board. (1989). *Recommended Dietary Allowances* (10th ed). Washington, DC: National Academy of Sciences, National Research Council.

17. Frantz, A.G. (1978). Prolactin. *N Engl J Med, 298,* 201.

18. Frisoli, G. (1981). Physiology and pathology of the puerperium. In I.L. Iffy & H.A. Kaminetsky (Eds.), *Principles and practice of obstetrics and perinatology* (pp. 1657–1675). New York: John Wiley & Sons.

19. Garza, C., et al. (1987). Special properties of human milk. *Clin Perinatol, 14,* 11.

20. Geiger, W. (1973). Radioimmunological determination of human chorionic gonadotropin, human placental lactogen, growth hormone and thyrotropin in the serum of mother and child during the early puerperium. *Horm Metab Res, 5,* 342.

21. George, G.P. & O'Toole, T.J.A. (1983). A review of drug transfer to the infant by breast feeding: Concerns for the dentist. *J Am Dent Assoc, 106,* 204.

22. Giacoia, G.P. & Catz, C.S. (1988). Drug therapy in the lactating mother: How to decide whether to prescribe or proscribe. *Postgrad Med, 83,* 211.

23. Gross, S.J., et al. (1980). Nutritional composition of milk produced by mothers delivering preterm. *J Pediatr, 96,* 641.

24. Grosvenor, C.E. & Mensa, G. (1974). Neural and hormonal control of milk secretion and milk ejection. In B.L. Larson & V.R. Smith (Eds.), *Lactation* (Vol II, pp. 227–270). New York: Academic Press.

25. Guthrie, H.A., Picciano, M.F., & Sheehe, D. (1977). Fatty acid patterns of human milk. *J Pediatr, 90,* 39.

26. Gyorgy, P. (1971). The uniqueness of human milk: Biochemical aspects. *Am J Clin Nutr, 24,* 970.

27. Hall, B. (1979). Uniformity of human milk. *Am J Clin Nutr, 32,* 304.

28. Hibberd, C.M., et al. (1982). Variation in the composition of breast milk during the first 5 weeks of lactation. *Arch Dis Child, 57,* 658.

29. Hopkinson, J.M., Schanler, R.J., & Garza, C. (1988). Milk production by mothers of premature infants. *Pediatrics, 81,* 815.

30. Howie, P.W., et al. (1982). Fertility after childbirth: Infant feeding patterns, basal prolactin levels and post-partum ovulation. *Clin Endocrinol, 17,* 315.

31. Howie, P.W., et al. (1982). Fertility after childbirth: Post-partum ovulation and menstruation in bottle and breastfeeding mothers. *Clin Endocrinol, 17,* 323.

32. Jelliffe, D.B. (1975). Unique properties of human milk. *J Reproduct Med, 14,* 133.

33. Josimovich, J.B., Reynolds, M., & Cobo, E. (1974). *Problems of human reproduction* (Vol. II). New York: John Wiley & Sons.

34. Kyndely, K. (1978). The sexuality of women in pregnancy and postpartum: A review. *J Obstet Gynecol Neonatal Nurs, 7,* 28.

35. Larson, B.L. & Smith, V.R. (1974). *Lactation; Vol II. Biosynthesis and secretion of milk/diseases.* New York: Academic Press.

36. Larson, B.L. & Smith, V.R. (1974). *Lactation Vol III.*

Nutrition and biochemistry of milk/maintenance. New York: Academic Press.

37. Larson, B.L. (1978). *Lactation; Vol IV. The mammary gland/human lactation/milk synthesis.* New York: Academic Press.

38. Larson, B.L. (1974). *Lactation; Vol I. The mammary gland/development and maintenance.* New York: Academic Press.

39. Lawrence, R. (1989). *Breastfeeding: A guide for the medical profession.* St Louis: CV Mosby.

40. Luke, B. (1979). *Maternal nutrition.* Boston: Little, Brown.

41. Masters, W.H. & Johnson, V.E. (1966). *Human sexual response.* Boston: Little, Brown.

42. McKensie, C.A., Canaday, M.E., & Carroll, E. (1982). Comprehensive care during the postpartum period. *Nurs Clin North Am, 17,* 23.

43. Meites, J. (1974). Neuroendocrinology of lactation. *J Invest Dermatol, 63,* 119.

44. Mendelson, R.A., Anderson, G.H., & Bryan, M.H. (1982). Zinc, copper and iron content of milk from mothers of preterm infants. *Early Hum Dev, 6,* 145.

45. Mepham, T.B. (1987). *Physiology of lactation.* Philadelphia: Open U Press.

46. Miyake, A., et al. (1978). Pituitary LH response to LHRH during the puerperium. *Obstet Gynecol, 51,* 37.

47. Monheit, A., Cousins, L., & Resnick, R. (1980). The puerperium: Anatomical and physiologic readjustments. *Clin Obstet Gynecol, 23,* 973.

48. Moore, M.L. (1983). *Realities in childbearing* (2nd ed.). Philadelphia: WB Saunders.

49. Nice, F.J. (1989). Can a breast-feeding mother take medication without harming her infant? *MCN, 14,* 27.

50. Noel, G.L., Suh, H.K., & Frantz, A.G. (1974). Prolactin release during nursing and breast stimulation in postpartum and nonpostpartum patients. *J Clin Endocrinol Metab, 38,* 13.

51. Patton, S. (1969). Milk. *Sci Am, 221,* 58.

52. Pritchard, J.A., MacDonald, P.C., & Gant, N.F. (1985). *Williams obstetrics* (17th ed.). Norwalk, CT: Appleton-Century-Crofts.

53. Rigg, L.A. & Yen, S.C. (1977). Multiphasic prolactin secretion during parturition in human subjects. *Am J Obstet Gynecol, 128,* 215.

54. Riordan, J. (1983). *A practical guide to breastfeeding.* St. Louis: CV Mosby.

55. Ritchey, S.J. & Taper, L.J. (1983). *Maternal and child nutrition.* New York: Harper & Row.

56. Rivera-Calimlim, L. (1987). The significance of drugs in breast milk: Pharmacokinetic considerations. *Clin Perinatol, 14,* 51.

57. Sharman, A. (1953). Postpartum regeneration of the human endometrium. *J Anat, 87,* 1.

58. Thomson, A.M., Hytten, F.E., & Billewicz, W.Z. (1970). The energy cost of human lactation. *Br J Nutr, 24,* 565.

59. Tulchinsky, D. (1980). The postpartum period. In D. Tulchinsky & K.J. Ryan (Eds.), *Maternal-fetal endocrinology* (pp. 144–166). Philadelphia: WB Saunders.

60. Tulchinsky, D. & Korenman, S.G. (1971). The plasma estradiol as an index of fetoplacental function. *J Clin Invest, 50,* 1490.

61. Tyson, J.E. (1977). Mechanisms of puerperal lactation. *Med Clin North Am, 61,* 153.

62. Tyson, J.E., et al. (1972). Studies of prolactin secre-

tion in human pregnancy. *Am J Obstet Gynecol, 113,* 14.

63. Voora, S. & Yeh, T.F. (1985). Drugs in breast milk. In T.F. Yeh (Ed.), *Drug therapy in the newborn and small infant* (pp. 40–54). Chicago: Year Book Medical Publishers.

64. Vorherr, H. (1973). Contraception after abortion and postpartum. *Am J Obstet Gynecol, 117,* 1002.

65. Vorherr, H. (1974). *The breast.* New York: Academic Press.

66. Wharton, B.A. (1987). *Nutrition and feeding of premature infants.* Oxford: Blackwell Scientific Publications.

67. Williams, J.W. (1931). Regeneration of the uterine mucosa after delivery with especial reference to the placental site. *Am J Obstet Gynecol, 22,* 664.

68. Worthington-Roberts, B.S., Vermeersch, J., & Williams, S.R. (1989). *Nutrition during pregnancy and lactation.* St. Louis: CV Mosby.

69. Banta, H. & Thackers, S. (1982). Risks and benefits of episiotomy: A review. *Birth, 9,* 25.

70 Briggs, G.G., Freeman, R.K., & Yaffe, S.J. (1990). *Drugs in pregnancy and lactation* (3rd ed.). Baltimore: Williams & Wilkins.

71. Bromberg, M. (1986) Presumptive maternal benefits of routine episiotomy. *J Nurse Midwifery, 31,* 121.

72. Committee on Drugs of the American Academy of Pediatrics. (1981). Breast-feeding and contraception. *Pediatrics, 68,* 138.

74. Hamosh, M. & Hamosh, M. (1988). Mother to infant biochemical transfer through breast milk. In G.H. Wiknjosastro, W.H. Prakoso, & K. Maeda (Eds.) *Perinatology.* Amsterdam: Elsevier.

75. Lepage, G., et al. (1984). The composition of preterm milk in relation to the degree of prematurity. *Am J Clin Nutr, 40,* 1042.

76. Liu, J.H. & Yen, S.S.C. (1989). Endocrinology of the postpartum state. In S.A. Brody & K. Ueland (Eds.), *Endocrine disorders in pregnancy.* Norwalk, CT: Appleton & Lange.

77. May, K.A. & Mahlmeister, L.R. (1990). *Comprehensive maternity nursing* (2nd ed.). Philadelphia: JB Lippincott.

78. McNeilly, A.S., et al. (1983). Fertility after childbirth: Pregnancy associated with breastfeeding. *J Endocrinol, 18,* 167.

79. Neville, M.C. & Neifert, M.R. (1983). *Lactation: Physiology, nutrition and breastfeeding.* New York: Plenum Press.

80. Perez, A., et al. (1972). First ovulation after child birth: The effect of breast feeding. *Am J Obstet Gynecol, 11,* 1041.

81. Rassin, D.K. (1990). Quality of human milk versus milk formulas: Protein composition. In N.M. Van Gelder, R.F. Butterworth, & B.D. Drugan (Eds.), *Neurology and neurobiology,* (Vol. 58, pp. 57–64). New York: Wiley-Liss.

82. Tankeyoon, M., et al. (1984). Effects of hormonal contraceptives on milk volume and infant growth. *Contraception, 30,* 505.

83. Wilcox, L.S., et al. (1989). Episiotomy and its role in the incidence of perineal lacerations in a maternity center and a tertiary hospital obstetric service. *Am J Obstet Gynecol, 160,* 1047.

Adaptations in Major Body Systems in the Pregnant Woman, Fetus, and Neonate

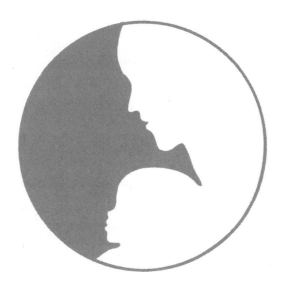

CHAPTER 5

The Hematologic and Hemostatic Systems

Maternal Physiologic Adaptations
  The Antepartum Period
    Changes in Blood and Plasma Volume
    Changes in Blood Cellular Components
    Changes in Plasma Components
    Changes in Coagulation Factors and Hemostasis
  The Intrapartum Period
  The Postpartum Period
Clinical Implications for the Pregnant Woman and Her Fetus
  Hypervolemia of Pregnancy
  Iron Requirements During Pregnancy
  Fetal Oxygenation and Growth
  Severe Anemia and Pregnancy
  Thromboembolism and Pregnancy
  Consumptive Coagulopathies During Pregnancy
Development of the Hematologic System in the Fetus
  Formation of Blood Cells
  Formation of Hemoglobin
  Development of the Hemostatic System

Neonatal Physiology
  Transitional Events
  Changes in Hematologic Parameters
  Alterations in Hemostasis
Clinical Implications for Neonatal Care
  Factors Influencing Hematologic Parameters
  Alterations in Hemoglobin-Oxygen Affinity
  Vitamin K and Hemorrhagic Disease of the Newborn
  Blood Transfusions
  Vitamin E and the Preterm Infant
  Neonatal Polycythemia and Hyperviscosity
  The Infant with a Hemoglobinopathy
  The Infant at Risk for Altered Hemostasis
  Physiologic Anemia of Infancy
    Iron Supplementation
Maturational Changes During Infancy and Childhood

The hematologic system encompasses blood and plasma volume, the constituents of plasma, and the formation and function of blood cellular components. Hemostasis involves mechanisms that result in the formation and removal of fibrin clots. Pregnancy and the neonatal period are associated with significant changes in these processes, increasing the risk for anemia and alterations in hemostasis such as thromboembolism and consumptive coagulopathies. This chapter examines alterations in the hematologic system and hemostasis during the perinatal period and their implications for the mother, fetus, and neonate.

MATERNAL PHYSIOLOGIC ADAPTATIONS

The significant changes in the hematologic system and hemostasis during pregnancy have a protective role for maternal homeostasis and are important for fetal development. These changes are also critical in allowing the mother to tolerate blood loss and placental separation at delivery. The maternal adaptations also increase the risk for complications such as thromboembolism, iron deficiency anemia, and coagulopathies.

The Antepartum Period

Most hematologic parameters, including blood and plasma volume, cellular components, plasma constituents, and coagulation factors, are altered during pregnancy, and this is reflected in progressive changes in many common hematologic laboratory values. As a result it is essential to recognize the normal range of laboratory values and usual patterns of change during pregnancy and to evaluate findings in conjunction with clinical data and previous values in order to distinguish between normal adaptations and pathologic alterations (Table 5–1).

Changes in Blood and Plasma Volume

Among the most significant hematologic changes during pregnancy are increases in blood and plasma volume (Fig. 5–1). These changes result in the hypervolemia of pregnancy, which is in turn responsible for many of the alterations in blood cellular components and plasma constituents. Circulating blood volume increases by 45% (approximately 1½ L), with a usual range of 30 to 50%.[14, 22, 89, 92] Changes in individual women may range from a minimal change to a twofold increase.[2,94] The increased blood volume is due to an increase in plasma volume, followed by an increase in the total red blood cell volume. Blood volume changes begin at 6 to 8 weeks, peak at 30 to 34 weeks to about 1200 to 1500 ml higher than nonpregnant values, then reach a plateau or decrease slightly to term.[8,14,89]

Plasma volume increases by 50% (range, 30 to 60%). This change begins at 6 to 10 weeks and increases rapidly during the second trimester, followed by a slower but progressive increase that levels off at 32 to 34 weeks.[8, 22, 55, 89, 92] Decreases in plasma volume

TABLE 5–1
Normal Laboratory Values in Nonpregnant and Pregnant Women

	NONPREGNANT	PREGNANT
General Screening Assays		
Hemoglobin	12–16 g/dl	11–13 g/dl
Packed cell volume (PCV)	37–45%	33–39%
Red blood cell count (RBC)	4.2–5.4 million/mm³	3.8–4.4 million/mm³
Mean corpuscular volume (MCV)	80–100 fl	70–90 fl
Mean corpuscular hemoglobin (MCH)	27–34 fl	23–31 fl
Mean corpuscular hemoglobin concentration (MCHC)	32–35 fl	32–35 fl
Reticulocyte count	0.5–1.0%	1.0–2.0%
Specific Diagnostic Tests		
Serum iron	50–100 µg/dl	30–100 µg/dl
Unsaturated iron binding capacity	250–300 µg/dl	280–400 µg/dl
Transferrin saturation	25–35%	15–30%
Iron stores (bone marrow)	Adequate ferritin	Unchanged
Serum folate	6–16 µg/ml	4–10 µg/ml
Serum vitamin B$_{12}$	70–85 ng/dl	70–500 ng/dl

Adapted from Morrison, J.C. & Pryor, J.A. (1990). Hematologic disorders. In R.D. Eden & F.H. Boehm (Eds.), *Assessment and care of the fetus* (p. 738). Norwalk, CT: Appleton & Lange.

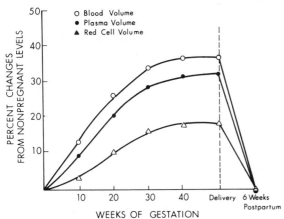

FIGURE 5–1. Changes in blood volume, plasma volume, and red blood cell volume during pregnancy and post partum. (From Peck, T.M. & Arias, F. (1979). Hematologic changes associated with pregnancy. *Clin Obstet Gynecol, 22,* 788.)

after 36 weeks have been reported. However, this decline was related to the supine position of the woman during measurement, with compression of the pelvic veins by the enlarged uterus and sequestering of fluid in the lower extremities. This fluid was not fully accounted for in the volume measurements, and it seemed as if the plasma volume had declined when in fact it had not.[8, 22, 55, 61] The enlarged plasma volume is accommodated by the vasculature of the uterus, breasts, muscles, kidneys, and skin. The increased volume leads to hemodilution with a net decrease in red blood cell (RBC) volume and total circulating plasma proteins.

Plasma volume, placental mass, and birth weight are positively correlated.[42, 55] Fetal growth correlates more closely with maternal plasma volume increases than with changes in RBC volume.[96] Alterations in the usual increase in plasma volume are associated with pregnancy complications. A greater than normal increase in plasma volume has been observed in multiparous women and with maternal obesity, large for gestational age infants, prolonged pregnancy, and multiple gestation.[8, 55]

In twin pregnancies plasma volume increases up to 65% over nonpregnant values, with further elevations seen in women with triplets and other multiple pregnancies.[22, 28, 61] The lower than expected hematocrit seen in these women may be due to hemodilution from excessive plasma volume and may not indicate a problem with erythropoiesis per se.[87] This increased plasma volume may be

the basis for the higher incidence of pulmonary edema reported in women with multiple pregnancy who are treated with β-adrenergic agonists (terbutaline, ritodrine) to inhibit preterm labor.[2] The mechanism for pulmonary edema with use of these agents is unclear, but it may occur secondary to maternal cardiovascular alterations with fluid retention and volume overload. Women already in a relative state of volume overload (multiple pregnancy) would be at greater risk.

Pregnancy-induced hypertension (PIH), intrauterine growth retardation (IUGR), and fetal demise are associated with a reduction in the expected increase in plasma and blood volumes.[8, 14] Physiologic changes in PIH include vasoconstriction and a contracted, but not underfilled, vascular bed. The contracted vascular bed limits the available space for expansion of blood volume and predisposes the woman to edema as fluid is forced out of the vascular space into the interstitial tissues. Since the vascular bed of the woman with PIH is contracted and not underfilled, attempts to expand the blood volume may result in fluid overload.[44]

The reduction in blood volume in PIH is related to the severity of the disorder. Women with severe PIH may experience a 30 to 40% decrease in blood volume.[22] On the other hand, RBC volumes are generally normal or near normal in these women, resulting in hemoconcentration. The combination of vasoconstriction, reduced blood volume, and hemoconcentration leads to increased blood viscosity with resistance to blood flow and a predisposition to sludging. Increased viscosity along with vasoconstriction increases the cardiac force needed to maintain circulation. Diuretics to reduce edema are generally not recommended for use with women with PIH. An initial action of diuretics is to reduce plasma volume. Since plasma volume is already reduced in women with PIH, diuretics will only aggravate the situation.[22] Chapters 6 and 8 further examine relationships between maternal physiologic adaptations and PIH.

The exact etiology of plasma volume changes in pregnancy is poorly understood.[14] These changes are influenced by hormonal effects and are closely linked with the alterations seen in fluid balance and in the renal and cardiovascular systems (Fig. 5–2). Hormonal influences, especially the effects of progesterone, on the vasculature of the venous system lead to decreased venous tone,

TABLE 5–2
Changes in Blood Cellular Components During Pregnancy

COMPONENT	CHANGE	PATTERN OF CHANGE
Red blood cells (RBC)	Increase 33% (450 ml) with iron; increase 18% (250 ml) without iron	Slow, continuous increase beginning in first trimester; may accelerate slightly in third trimester
Hematocrit	Decreases 3–5% to 33.8% at term (range, 33–39%)	Decrease from second trimester as plasma volume peaks
Hemoglobin	Decreases 2–10% to 12.1–12.5 g/dl (range, 11–13) at term	If iron and folate are adequate, little change to 16 weeks; lowest values at 16–22 weeks; slowly increases to term
Reticulocytes	Increase 1–2%	Gradual increase to third trimester
White blood cells	Increase 8% to 5000–12,000 (up to 15,000 seen)/mm³	Begins in second month; increase involves primarily neutrophils
Eosinophils	Increase or decrease	Variable
Basophils	Slight decrease	
Platelets	Increase, decrease, or stay the same; usual range 150,000–400,000/mm³	Variable
Erythrocyte sedimentation rate	Increases	Progressive

increased capacity of the veins and venules, and decreased vascular resistance. These changes allow the vasculature to accommodate the increased blood volume. Estrogen and progesterone influence plasma renin activity and aldosterone levels, resulting in retention of sodium and an increase in total body water (see Chapter 8).[55] Most of this water is extracellular and available to contribute to the increased plasma volume. Changes in plasma volume have also been linked to a mechanical effect with the low resistance uteroplacental circulation acting as an arteriovenous shunt. This shunt provides physical space to accommodate the increased cardiac output and corresponding change in plasma volume.[22, 55]

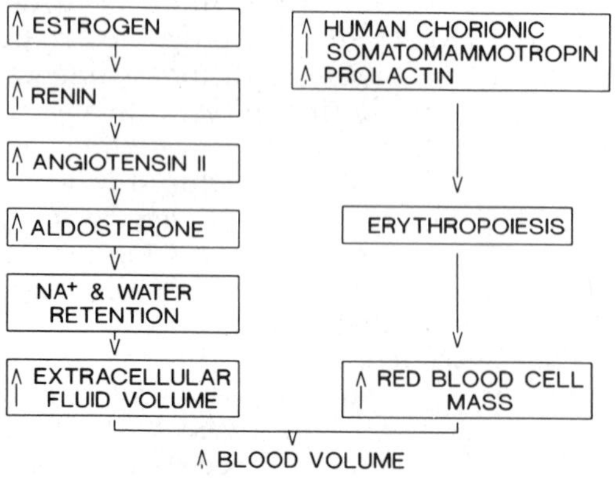

Hypervolemia reduces blood viscosity. The hypervolemia leads to hemodilution and changes in plasma protein and blood cellular components, which further reduce viscosity. Blood viscosity decreases approximately 20% during the first two trimesters. During the third trimester viscosity may increase slightly. The decreased viscosity reduces resistance to flow and the cardiac effort needed, thus conserving maternal energy resources.[22]

Changes in Blood Cellular Components

The principal change in blood cellular components during pregnancy is increased red blood cell volume (Table 5–2). This alteration, in conjunction with changes in plasma volume, is reflected in changes in the hemoglobin and hematocrit.

Changes in Red Blood Cells

The total red blood cell (RBC) volume increases during pregnancy, with an average increase in circulating RBC of 33% (450 ml)

FIGURE 5–2. Possible mechanisms of hypervolemia during pregnancy. (From Gleicher, N. & Elkayam, U. (Eds.), (1990). *Cardiac problems in pregnancy* (2nd ed., p. 7). New York: Alan R. Liss. Reprinted by permission of Wiley-Liss, a division of John Wiley and Sons, Inc.)

TABLE 5–2
Changes in Blood Cellular Components During Pregnancy Continued

BASIS FOR CHANGE	INTRAPARTUM CHANGES	POSTPARTUM CHANGES
Erythropoietin stimulated by human placental lactogen, progesterone, and prolactin	Slight increase due to slight hemoconcentration; 50% of increased RBCs lost at delivery	RBC production ceases temporarily; remainder of increased RBCs lost via normal catabolism
Hemodilution		Returns to nonpregnant levels by 4–6 weeks owing to RBC catabolism
Hemodilution	Slight increase due to stress and dehydration	Initial decrease; stabilizes at 2–4 days; nonpregnant values by 4–6 weeks
Increased RBC production		Increase slightly; nonpregnant values by 4–6 weeks
Estrogen	Increase to 25,000–30,000/mm³	Decrease to 6000–10,000/mm³; normal values by 4–7 days
	Disappear from peripheral blood	By 3 days return to peripheral blood
?Hemodilution	20% decrease with placental separation	Increase by 3–5 days with gradual return to nonpregnant levels
Increased plasma globulin and fibrinogen	Increases	Initially 55–80 mm/hr; peaks 1–2 days post partum

in women on iron supplementation and 18% (250 ml) in women not taking iron.[55, 61] Changes in RBC volume are due to increased circulating erythropoietin and accelerated RBC production.[2] The rise in erythropoietin in the last two trimesters is stimulated by progesterone, prolactin, and human placental lactogen.[54] The magnitude of change varies from a moderate rise to 30 to 35% above values in nonpregnant women.[22, 54]

The increase in total RBC volume begins at the end of the first trimester as erythropoietin begins to rise. The increase occurs at a relatively constant rate, but slower than changes in plasma volume, and may accelerate slightly during the third trimester.[54, 55, 61] The lack of increase in RBC volume early in the first trimester may be related to initial depression of erythropoietin. Levels of placental hormones that stimulate erythropoietin release are low during this period. The increased RBC production results in a moderate erythroid hyperplasia of the bone marrow and an increase in the reticulocyte count.[54]

Red blood cell 2,3-diphosphoglycerate (2,3-DPG) increases beginning early in pregnancy and leads to a gradual shift to the right of the maternal oxygen-hemoglobin dissociation curve (see Chapter 6). This results in an increase in the amount of oxygen unloaded in the peripheral tissues, including the intervillous space, which facilitates oxygen transfer from mother to fetus and fetal growth.[15, 55, 61]

The mean cell volume, diameter, and thickness of the RBC also change, resulting in a cell that is more spherical in shape.[79] Because the increase in plasma volume is three times greater than the RBC volume increase, the net result is a decrease in the total RBC count, hemoglobin, and hematocrit (Table 5–2).

The hemoglobin and hematocrit decrease from the second trimester on as plasma volume peaks. In a group of pregnant women with adequate iron and folate the hemoglobin was relatively stable until 16 weeks, fell to its lowest point at 16 to 22 weeks, then increased slowly to term.[8, 39] Total body hemoglobin increases 85 to 150 g in pregnancy, whereas net hemoglobin decreases. Even with adequate iron supplementation, the hemoglobin decreases about 2 g/dl to a mean of about 11.6 g/dl in the second trimester owing to hemodilution.[56, 114] At term the hemoglobin averages 12.1 to 12.5 g/dl with a range of 11 to 13 g/dl (versus a mean of 14 ± 2 for nonpregnant females).[7,33] The CDC suggests values of 11 (first and second trimesters) and

TABLE 5–3
Changes in Plasma Components During Pregnancy

COMPONENT	CHANGE	TIMING
Total plasma proteins	↓ 10–14%	First trimester
Albumin	Total: 144 g Serum: 3.5 g	First trimester
Fibrinogen	↑ 50–80%	First to third trimesters
Globulin	↑	First to third trimesters
Alpha and beta globulin	↑	Progressive throughout pregnancy
Gamma globulin	↓	Third trimester
Thyroxin binding globulin	↑	First trimester
α_1-Antitrypsin	Doubles	
α_2-Macroglobulin	↑ 20%	
Total serum lipids	↑ 40–60%	Continuous to term
Cholesterol	↑ 40%	Continuous to term
Phospholipids	↑ 37%	Continuous to term
Beta-lipoprotein	↑ Up to 180%	
Serum electrolytes	↓ 5–10 mg/L	First trimester
Serum ferritin	↓ 30%	To 30–32 weeks, then reaches a plateau
Transferrin	↑ 70%	Linear rise
Iron binding capacity	↓ 15%	

ESR = erythrocyte sedimentation rate.

10.5 g/dl (second trimester) as the lowest acceptable values for screening pregnant women.[23] The mean hematocrit is 33.8% (range, 33–39%) at term.[2, 79]

Changes in White Blood Cells

Total white blood cell (WBC) volume increases slightly during early pregnancy beginning in the 2nd month and levels off during the second and third trimesters (Table 5–2). The total WBC count in pregnancy varies with individual women, ranging from 5000 to 12,000/mm³, with values as high as 15,000/mm³ reported.[2, 14, 89] The increased WBC count is due to a neutrophilia with an elevation in mature leukocyte forms. A slight shift to the left may occur with occasional myelocytes and metamyelocytes seen on the peripheral smear.[2] Changes in other WBC forms are minimal (Table 5–2). Alkaline phosphatase activity of the leukocytes rises during pregnancy, falling several days prior to delivery. Changes in leukocytes accompanying pregnancy are similar to changes that occur with physiologic stress, such as vigorous exercise, with return to the circulation of

mature leukocytes that were previously shunted out of the circulatory system.[94]

Changes in Platelets

Reports regarding changes in platelets during pregnancy are conflicting, i.e., platelets are reported to increase, decrease, or stay the same.[2, 49, 74, 89] Recent reports demonstrated a slight decrease in platelet count and increase in platelet aggregation during the last 8 weeks of pregnancy, which suggests a low grade activation and consumption of platelets.[49] Changes in platelet aggregation with release of thromboxane A_2 (vasoconstrictor) have also been implicated in the pathogenesis of PIH and are the basis for low-dose aspirin therapy (see Chapter 6). In healthy pregnant women platelet counts have generally not been reported at values below lower limits for normal nonpregnant women.[2] Mild to moderate thrombocytopenia (<150,000/mm³) has been reported at term in some healthy pregnant women who have no other evidence of idiopathic thrombocytopenic purpura (ITP).[74] The acceptable range for platelet values in pregnancy is

TABLE 5–3
Changes in Plasma Components During Pregnancy Continued

BASIS	SIGNIFICANCE
Estrogen/progesterone	Decrease in colloid osmotic pressure (edema formation)
	Altered protein binding of calcium, drugs, etc.
Estrogen/progesterone	See above
Hemodilution	
Estrogen/progesterone	Alterations in hemostasis
	Decreased ESR
Estrogen/progesterone	Decreased ESR
	See individual globulins
	Facilitate transport of carbohydrates and lipids to placenta and fetus
	Transplacental passage of IgG
	Increased plasma T3 and T4
	Protects lungs from deported trophoblast tissue
	Anti-plasmin effect, which may predispose to DIC
Human placental lactogen and altered metabolism	
	Essential precursor for steroid hormones (estrogen/progesterone)
	Major component of cell membranes needed for maternal and fetal growth
	May increase risk of thrombosis
Hemodilution	Decreased plasma osmolarity
Respiratory system changes	
Hb synthesis (early)	Reflects decreasing iron stores
Fetal uptake (late)	
Altered liver function	Facilitate Fe absorption and transport

150,000 to 400,000/mm³. Values below 100,000/mm³ are considered abnormal.[81]

Changes in Plasma Components

Many components of plasma including plasma proteins, electrolytes, serum iron, lipids, and enzymes change during pregnancy (Table 5–3). Total plasma proteins decrease 10 to 14%, with much of the change occurring in the first trimester. Although there is an absolute increase in albumin concentration during the first trimester, there is a relative decrease due to increased blood volume and hemodilution. Decreased albumin leads to a net decrease in colloid osmotic (oncotic) pressure, reducing the normal forces counteracting edema formation.[5] Although edema formation in pregnancy is primarily due to alterations in venous hydrostatic pressure, decreased oncotic pressure from decreased albumin is an important contributory factor.[5, 76]

Globulin concentration demonstrates both absolute and relative increases, leading to progressive falls in the albumin-to-globulin ratio. Alpha and beta globulins increase progressively during pregnancy, whereas gamma globulin decreases slightly. Fibrinogen also demonstrates both absolute and relative increases of 50 to 80%.[5, 94] The erythrocyte sedimentation rate (ESR) increases progressively during pregnancy, probably owing to the elevation in plasma globulin and fibrinogen levels. Alterations in other plasma proteins are summarized in Table 5–3.

The alterations in plasma proteins alter protein binding of substances such as calcium, drugs, and anesthetic agents. Since many drugs are transported in the blood bound to albumin, drug doses may need to be altered during pregnancy. Increased binding of substances such as calcium reduces the level of free calcium in the maternal plasma. As a result calcium must be actively transported across the placenta to the fetus.

Decreases in serum electrolytes (anions, cations, and buffer base) reduce plasma osmolarity from 290 to 280 mOsm/L during the first trimester.[1, 5] These changes are due to both hypervolemia and the effects of respiratory system alterations, particularly hyperventilation with increased CO_2 loss (see Chapter 7).[1, 22]

Serum iron decreases during pregnancy,

especially after 28 weeks and in women not receiving supplemental iron.[8] Levels of serum ferritin, which is a more precise indicator of reticuloendothelial iron stores, gradually fall until 30 to 32 weeks and then stabilize. With supplemental iron, serum ferritin levels stabilize by 28 weeks or earlier, and may even rise near term.[8, 52, 54] Decreases in serum ferritin in early pregnancy are due to mobilization of iron stores for maternal hemoglobin synthesis; later decreases are due to increased fetal iron uptake. In multiparous women the decrease in serum ferritin occurs earlier and may be greater.[8]

Levels of serum lipids rise with marked elevations in cholesterol and phospholipids. Cholesterol is an essential precursor for steroid hormones by the placenta; phospholipids are major components of cell membranes. The rise in serum lipids begins in the first trimester, increasing to 40 to 60% at term (Table 5–3).

Increases in serum alkaline phosphatase are due to increased placental production. As a result, alkaline phosphatase levels are not useful in evaluating liver disorders during pregnancy. Serum cholinesterase activity decreases by 30%. Increased cholinesterase activity may lead to longer periods of paralysis if substances such as succinylcholine are used during surgical procedures.[5]

Changes in Coagulation Factors and Hemostasis

Pregnancy has been called an acquired hypercoagulable state, reflecting an increased risk for thrombosis and consumptive coagulopathies (e.g., disseminated intravascular coagulation).[96] Hemostatic changes during pregnancy are thought to result in an ongoing low grade activation of the coagulation system within the uteroplacental circulation beginning as early as 11 to 15 weeks. This state of compensated intravascular coagulation is characterized by thrombin formation and local consumption of clotting factors in which component synthesis equals or exceeds consumption.[49, 92, 96, 103]

Intra- and extravascular fibrin deposits are found in the uteroplacental circulation, intervillous spaces, and placental bed. Circulating high-molecular-weight, soluble, fibrin-fibrinogen complexes, which are indicative of uteroplacental fibrin formation, also increase.[30, 104] During pregnancy smooth muscle and elastic tissue within the uterine spiral

arteries are replaced by a fibrin matrix (see Chapter 2). These changes allow for expansion of the vessels to accommodate increased blood flow to the placenta and to facilitate collapse of the terminal portion of the vessel with placental separation.[49, 99] Increased (50 to 80%) fibrinogen, thrombin generation, and inhibition of fibrinolysis during pregnancy may interact to ensure integrity of uteroplacental vessels. Lower levels of fibrinogen have been associated with spontaneous abortion.[104] During late pregnancy, accumulation of mural thrombi in the vessel walls decreases the diameter of the lumen, reducing blood flow, which may result in the placental infarcts and small areas of ischemia often seen at term.[49]

Contact factors (XII, prekallikrein, and high-molecular-weight kininogen) involved in initiation of the clotting cascade are all elevated.[49] (Table 5–4 summarizes properties of major factors.) Factor VIII complex and Factors I (fibrinogen), VII, IX, and X are increased, and Factor II is reported to be either slightly elevated or to remain stable (Fig. 5–3).[2, 103] Factors XI and XIII decrease. The concurrent increase in fibrinogen and decrease in Factor XIII (fibrin stabilizing factor) alters the process of clot stabilization and subsequent lysis during pregnancy.[49] Changes in coagulation factors during pregnancy are reflected in the partial thromboplastin time (PTT) and prothrombin time (PT), which decrease slightly.

Fibrinolytic activity increases during the first two trimesters, then decreases to term.[3] Inhibitors of fibrinolysis produced by the placenta can be found in maternal plasma.[86, 96] The net effect of changes in hemostasis during pregnancy (Fig. 5–3) is increased activity of coagulation factors, except Factors XI and XII (which are not associated with hemorrhagic tendencies), and a lowering of factors that inhibit coagulation. The result is a hypercoagulable state.[49, 96]

The hypercoagulable state of pregnancy is balanced to some extent by changes in plasminogen. Plasminogen is elevated and tissue plasmin inhibitors are decreased, which helps retain the dynamic equilibrium between clotting and clot lysis and thus overall homeostatic balance during pregnancy.[49] The increased tendency toward coagulation during pregnancy may also be partly balanced by pregnancy specific proteins (PSP), which act similarly to heparin to facilitate neutralization

TABLE 5–4
Coagulation Factors

NUMBER	NAME	FUNCTION
I	Fibrinogen	Fibrin precursor
II	Prothrombin	Thrombin precursor (vitamin K)
III	Tissue thromboplastin	Tissue factor formed in plasma or tissues that reacts with VII and calcium to activate X
IV	Calcium	Activator of enzyme activity in all stages of coagulation
V	Proaccelerin	Accelerates conversion of prothrombin to thrombin
VII	Proconvertin	Reacts with III and calcium to activate X (vitamin K)
VIII	Antihemophilic factor (AHF)	Reacts with IX, calcium, and phospholipid to activate X
IX	Plasma thromboplastin component (PTC)	Reacts with VIII, calcium, and phospholipid to activate X (vitamin K)
X	Stuart-Prower factor	Accelerates conversion of prothrombin to thrombin (vitamin K)
XI	Plasma thromboplastin antecedent (PTA)	Contact factor for formation of thromboplastin
XII	Hageman factor	Contact factor for initiation of clotting cascade
XIII	Fibrin stabilizing factor	Maintain firm fibrin clot
	High-molecular-weight kininogen (HMWK)	Contact factor that reacts with prekallikrein and XI
	Prekallikrein	Contact factor that reacts with HMWK and XI
	Protein C, protein S	Coagulation inhibitors of V and VIII (vitamin K)
	Antithrombin III	Coagulation inhibitor of thrombin, II, X, and other factors
	Plasminogen	Fibrinolytic; plasmin precursor

of thrombin by antithrombin III.[96] Many clotting factors are synthesized by the liver and influenced by estrogen.[103] Many of these changes are similar to those with oral contraceptives.[60, 64, 92] Figure 5–3 summarizes hemostatic changes during pregnancy.

The Intrapartum Period

Changes in the hematologic system and hemostasis are crucial in preparing the pregnant woman to tolerate the normal blood loss at delivery and prevent significant bleeding with placental separation. The amount of blood loss with delivery averages up to 500 ml (vaginal delivery) or 1000 ml (cesarean section or a vaginal delivery of twins).[1, 5, 89, 92] This loss at delivery may be underestimated by up to 50%.[50] Blood loss at delivery and in lochia over the first few postpartum days account for about half of the increased RBC volume acquired during pregnancy.[1, 92]

Changes in Hematologic Parameters

Hemoglobin levels tend to increase slightly during labor owing to hemoconcentration. The degree of hemoconcentration is related to increases in erythropoiesis (as a stress response), muscular activity, and dehydration.[92, 94] Leukocyte alkaline phosphatase activity increases with the onset of labor. Increases in this enzyme are often associated with inflammatory responses. The WBC count increases during labor and immediately post partum to values up to 25,000 to 30,000/mm³. This increase is primarily due to an increase in neutrophils and may represent a response to stress.[89, 92] Changes in hematologic parameters are summarized in Table 5–2.

Changes in the hematologic system can complicate diagnosis of infection during this period. The usual increase in WBC count may include release of immature neutrophils, which is similar to findings associated with bacterial infection. Erythrocyte sedimentation rates also rise and are therefore less useful. In addition the laboring woman may experience a relative tachycardia, dehydration, and elevated temperature.

Changes in Hemostasis

The coagulation system undergoes further activation during the intrapartum period both before and after placental separation. The placenta and decidua are rich in thromboplastin, and exposure or release of this tissue factor during placental separation will activate coagulation via the extrinsic system (Fig. 5–3).[96] Concentrations of clotting factors increase during labor. Results of clotting tests, particularly prothrombin time (PT), shorten significantly, especially during the third stage of labor with clotting at the placental site. Levels of fibrinogen and plasminogen may also decrease owing to their

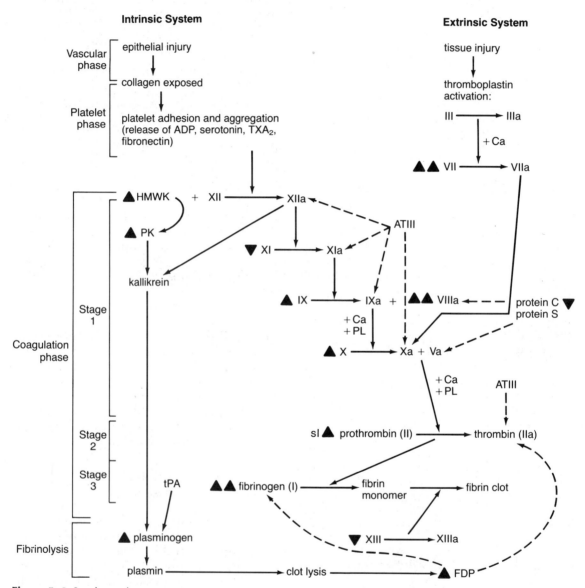

Figure 5–3 *See legend on opposite page*

increased utilization after placental separation.[49] Factor VIII complex increases during labor and delivery. Factor V increases after placental separation, which contributes to activation of clotting via the extrinsic system.

Fibrinolytic activity decreases further during labor and delivery, enhancing formation of clots at the placental site following separation.[5, 49] This promotes development of a hemostatic endometrial fibrin mesh over the wound.[96] About 5 to 10% of the total body fibrin is deposited at this site.[49]

Levels of fibrin-fibrinogen degradation products (FDP) increase after delivery. This change increases the risk of coagulation disorders in the immediate postpartum period by interfering with formation of firm fibrin clots.[5, 49, 100] The number of platelets falls about 20% with placental separation owing to clotting at the placental site. Platelet activation and fibrin formation are maximal at delivery (Fig. 5–4).[43] Thus the hypercoagulable state of pregnancy is further magnified during the intrapartum period. This state protects the woman from hemorrhage and excessive blood loss at delivery by providing

for rapid hemostasis following removal of the placenta.

The Postpartum Period

Changes in Blood Volume

The decrease in blood and plasma volume during the immediate postpartum period corresponds to the amount of blood loss with delivery.[22] This loss usually accounts for over half of the RBC volume accumulated during pregnancy.[1] During the first few days post partum, plasma volume decreases further owing to diuresis. After 3 to 4 days, mobilization of interstitial fluid leads to a slight increase in plasma volume. This hemodilution decreases hemoglobin, hematocrit, and plasma protein by the end of the 1st postpartum week (Fig. 5–5).[1, 22] The volume change may contribute to circulatory embarrassment in women with cardiac problems.[22] Plasma volume continues to decrease after the 1st week, reaching nonpregnant values by 6 to 8 weeks or sooner.

Accurate and consistent assessment of

FIGURE 5–3. Physiology of coagulation and alterations during pregnancy. ADP = adenosine diphosphate; TXA_2 = thromboxane A_2; HMWK = high-molecular-weight kininogen; PK = prekallikrein; PL = phospholipid or platelet factor 3; ATIII = antithrombin III; tPA = tissue plasminogen activator; FDP = fibrin-fibrinogen degradation products; Ca = calcium; sl = slight. Dashed line = inhibitory action. ▲▼ denote changes during pregnancy.

Clotting is divided into three phases: vascular, platelet, and coagulation (followed by fibrinolysis and clot removal). The *vascular phase* follows damage to vascular epithelium, exposure of connective tissue collagen, and vasoconstriction. In the *platelet phase* adherence of platelets to collagen (vessel wall) triggers release of ADP, serotonin, TXA_2 from the platelets, and fibronectin from epithelium, which enhance platelet aggregation. TXA_2 promotes further vasoconstriction. Platelets form a soft pliable temporary plug over the damaged area.

The *coagulation phase* (formation of a fibrin clot) is divided into three stages. In stage 1 thromboplastin or prothrombin activator is formed by intrinsic or extrinsic pathways. These pathways are interdependent and involve a series of enzymatic reactions (coagulation cascade) to convert substrates to active products. The intrinsic (contact) system involves binding of Factor XII to the damaged epithelium, which initiates a series of reactions involving other contact factors that result in activation of Factors XI and X. In the extrinsic system tissue thromboplastin (Factor III) interacts with calcium and Factor VIII complex to form activated Factor X. Stage 2 involves formation of thrombin from prothrombin. Thrombin acts as an enzyme in the formation of fibrin from fibrinogen in stage 3. Fibrin is an insoluble protein consisting of dense interlacing threads that entrap platelets and erythrocytes.

Fibrinolysis is accomplished by activation of plasmin from plasminogen via intrinsic (contact factors) or extrinsic (tissue plasminogen activator) substances. Lysis of the fibrin clot produces fibrin-fibrinogen degradation products (FDP) or fibrin split products (FSP), which can interfere with further clotting by impairing platelet aggregation and thrombin formation. The maintenance of normal hemostasis is also dependent on the presence of naturally occurring coagulation inhibitors (e.g., antithrombin III and protein C).

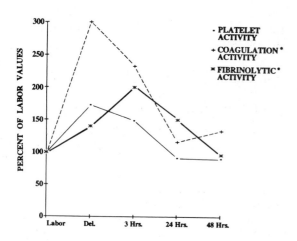

FIGURE 5–4. Platelet, coagulation, and fibrinolytic activity in labor, delivery, and post partum. Hemostasis activity is calculated from β-thromboglobulin, platelet factor 4 (platelet), fibrinopeptide A (clotting), and fibrin-fibrinogen degradation product (fibrinolysis) values. *Scaled to 20% of actual. (From Gerbasi, F.R., et al. (1990). Changes in hemostasis during delivery and the immediate postpartum period. *Am J Obstet Gynecol, 162,* 1158.)

blood loss is essential at delivery and post partum. Blood losses during these periods are reported to be both under- and overestimated. Unit and product-specific standards for estimating losses increase accuracy of these assessments.[51, 68]

Changes in Hematologic Parameters

Increased RBC production ceases early in the postpartum period owing to suppression of erythropoietin.[22] Hemoglobin levels decrease immediately after delivery (owing to blood loss), whereas the hematocrit tends to remain relatively stable (or increase slightly with a vaginal delivery), for the first few days.[89] A 500 ml blood loss such as occurs

with vaginal delivery will usually result in a 1 g reduction in hemoglobin.[52] Hemoglobin levels tend to stabilize by 2 to 3 days.[61] Hematocrit returns to nonpregnant levels by 4 to 6 weeks following usual RBC destruction.

Excess circulating hemoglobin is catabolized, and the iron released is stored in the reticuloendothelial system. Serum ferritin levels increase by 5 to 8 weeks to levels seen early in pregnancy. This increase occurs regardless of whether or not the woman received supplemental iron during pregnancy and is more marked after vaginal delivery.[8, 56, 61]

The WBC count, which increased in labor and immediately post partum, falls to 6000 to 10,000/mm³, then returns to normal values

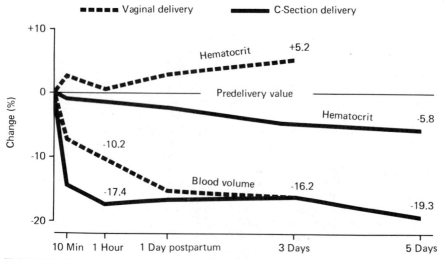

FIGURE 5–5. Estimations of changes in blood volume and hematocrit following vaginal and cesarean births. Values are expressed as percent changes from values immediately prior to delivery. (From Metcalfe, J. & Ueland, K. (1980). Heart disease and pregnancy. In N. O. Fowler (Ed.), *Cardiac diagnosis and treatment* (3rd ed., p. 1159). Hagerstown, MD: Harper & Row.)

by 4 to 7 days. Eosinophils tend to disappear from the peripheral blood during delivery, returning by 3 days post partum.[89] The number of platelets, which fell following placental separation, increases beginning at 3 to 4 days and gradually returns to nonpregnant levels. These changes are summarized in Table 5–2.

Changes in Hemostasis

Fibrinolytic activity is maximal for the first 3 hours after delivery.[43] Return to normal activity reflects removal of the fibrinolytic inhibitors produced by the placenta.[104] Secondary increases in fibrinogen, Factor V, and Factor VIII complex occur during the 1st week, followed by a return to predelivery levels by 3 to 5 days, and a slow decrease to nonpregnant levels.[49] Clotting factors, which increased during labor, slowly decrease, reaching their lowest levels by 7 to 10 days. Factors VII and X return to normal levels by 2 weeks.[30] The hemostatic system has usually returned to nonpregnant status 3 to 4 weeks post partum.[49]

CLINICAL IMPLICATIONS FOR THE PREGNANT WOMAN AND HER FETUS

The changes in the hematologic system and in hemostasis during pregnancy are important for maternal and fetal homeostasis but also increase the woman's need for iron and other nutrients and place her at risk for developing anemia, thromboembolic disorders, and coagulopathies. This section examines maternal-fetal implications related to hypervolemia, hemodilution, and the hypercoagulable state along with implications for women with pathophysiologic states affecting the hematologic system.

Hypervolemia of Pregnancy

The increased blood and plasma volume during pregnancy result in a physiologic hypervolemia that allows the woman to tolerate many of the changes associated with pregnancy and delivery and helps to (1) meet the demands of an enlarged uterus and hypertrophied vascular system while maintaining normal systemic blood pressure, (2) allow the woman to tolerate blood loss at delivery, (3)

protect the woman from impaired venous return and hypotension with position changes late in the third trimester (when a significant proportion of her fluid volume may be sequestered within the venous system of the lower extremities) and thus reduce the risk of supine hypotension, (4) enhance maternal-fetal exchange of gases and nutrients, and (5) increase cutaneous blood flow by four- to sevenfold, thus assisting with heat dissipation via the skin.[5, 8, 22, 61, 89, 92]

The increased RBC volume helps offset hemodilution and maintain blood oxygen carrying capacity and availability of oxygen for the fetus. The increased volume allows for adequate blood flow within the expanding uteroplacental circulation, thus ensuring adequate nutrient availability for the fetus throughout gestation. These changes alter evaluation of hematologic variables in the pregnant woman (see Table 5–1).

Iron Requirements During Pregnancy

Iron requirements increase during pregnancy by about 1 g over the usual body iron stores of 2 to 2.5 g in adult women.[8] This iron is used as follows: 300 to 350 mg go to the fetus and placenta, 200 to 240 mg are lost via usual routes of excretion, and 450 to 600 mg are required for increased maternal RBC volume. An additional 250 mg are lost with the normal blood loss associated with delivery.[46] Most of the increased iron is needed in the second half of pregnancy when maternal needs are 6 to 7 mg/day.[94]

The amount of iron needed by the fetus and placenta and to replace usual maternal losses is an obligatory requirement that is met regardless of the cost to maternal iron stores.[8] Even if the mother is iron-deficient and anemic, the fetus will usually not suffer, since the placenta continues to transport iron to meet fetal needs. If adequate iron is not available for synthesis of additional red blood cells, the maternal RBC volume will not increase to the usual levels and the hematocrit and hemoglobin will decrease further as plasma volume increases.[2, 8, 94]

Although intestinal iron absorption increases in the second half of pregnancy (probably as a compensatory mechanism in response to increased iron demand), dietary sources and maternal stores alone are usually not adequate to meet the increased demands of pregnancy. Iron stores in young, healthy nonpregnant women may be marginal to nonexistent.[30] Even with adequate nutrition, 10 to 20% of pregnant women will develop an iron deficiency.[27, 129] The Institute of Medicine's general recommendations for iron supplementation during pregnancy are 30 mg ferrous iron (which is provided by 150 mg ferrous sulfate, 300 mg ferrous gluconate, or 100 mg ferrous fumarate) daily beginning at 12 weeks along with a well-balanced diet.[56] Iron supplementation does not prevent or correct the normal decline in hemoglobin seen in pregnancy but can prevent depletion of stores, the first stage of iron deficiency anemia.[8, 56]

Fetal Iron Requirements

Fetal and neonatal iron content is 75 mg/kg. The majority (75%) of fetal iron is found in hemoglobin, with about 7 mg/kg in tissues and 10 mg/kg stored in the liver and spleen. The stored iron doubles during the last few weeks of gestation.[84]

The fetus has been called an "efficient parasite" in terms of iron transport across the placenta.[84] Iron passes rapidly against a concentration gradient from mother to fetus via transferrin. Iron bound to maternal serum transferrin will not cross the placenta. The maternal transferrin releases its iron in the intervillous space. The iron is taken up by transferrin receptors located on the surface of trophoblast cells. Iron is transported across the placenta to fetal blood and attaches to fetal serum transferrin. Fetal transferrin is synthesized by the fetal liver after about 29 to 30 days of gestation.[8, 84]

With fetal growth, the rate of iron transfer across the placenta increases. Thus transport of iron from mother to fetus is greatest during the last few months of gestation (up to 4 mg/day at term). Serum iron and ferritin levels in cord blood are higher than in maternal blood. Cord blood serum ferritin levels are lower (but usually still within normal limits) in infants of iron deficient mothers, reflecting lower fetal iron stores.[52]

Fetal Oxygenation and Growth

Increased levels of 2,3-DPG in the pregnant woman shift her oxygen-hemoglobin dissociation curve to the right. This reduces the affinity of maternal hemoglobin for oxygen, favors release of oxygen in the intervillous space, and facilitates transfer to the fetus. Alterations in placental function that occur with maternal disorders such as pregnancy-induced hypertension, chronic renal disease, diabetes, and severe anemia can decrease oxygen transfer across the placenta. The fetus may develop chronic hypoxia, with stimulation of erythropoietin production, increased erythropoiesis, polycythemia, and increased neonatal morbidity.

Severe Anemia and Pregnancy

The most common anemias encountered in pregnancy are iron deficiency anemia, megaloblastic anemia of pregnancy (folic acid deficiency), sickle cell disorders, and β-thalassemia.[61] Anemias caused by iron or folate deficiency are due to underproduction of red blood cells and are associated with decreased reticulocytes. The normal hematologic changes along with altered nutritional needs during pregnancy increase the risk for these nutritional anemias. Sickle cell and β-thalassemia anemia are caused by increased red blood cell destruction and loss and thus are associated with increased reticulocytes in the peripheral blood.[61] Changes in the hematologic system may influence the course of these disorders during pregnancy and alter fetal outcome.

In women with severe anemia (hemoglobin <6 to 8 mg/dl), maternal arterial oxygen content and oxygen delivery to the fetus are decreased. The fetus attempts to adapt through increased uterine and fetal blood flow, redistribution of blood within the fetal organs, increased RBC production (to increase the total oxygen carrying capacity), and a decrease in the diffusing distance for oxygen across the placenta.[6, 8, 21]

Because fetuses have predominantly fetal hemoglobin, they cannot readily increase the availability of oxygen to the tissues by further altering the affinity of hemoglobin for oxygen. Although the fetus adapts, the cost may be high, with decreased growth and an increased mortality due to the lack of an adequate oxygen supply and nutrients.[21] Severe maternal anemia (especially with a maternal Pao_2 <70 torr) has also been associated with placental hyperplasia (perhaps as a compensatory response to fetal anoxia), congenital anomalies, low birth weight, and preterm birth.[6, 8, 79]

Iron Deficiency Anemia

The most common cause of anemia during pregnancy is iron deficiency anemia. Generally this form of anemia is preventable or easily treated with iron supplements. Hematologic changes in pregnancy can make diagnosis of iron deficiency difficult.[61, 87] Total iron binding capacity and serum iron often fall during pregnancy, as well as with iron deficiency anemia. A useful test for iron deficiency in the pregnant woman is serum ferritin levels, which correlate well with iron stores during pregnancy.[8, 61] Serum ferritin levels less than 12 μg/L with a low hemoglobin indicate iron deficiency, which can be treated with 60 to 120 mg of ferrous sulfate until the hemoglobin returns to levels normal for the stage of gestation.[56]

The effects of maternal iron deficiency anemia on the fetus and neonate are unclear. In general, even with significant maternal iron deficiency, the fetus will often be protected and receive adequate stores at cost to the mother. If the mother is severely iron deficient and anemic, the fetus may be affected with decreased RBC volume, hemoglobin, iron stores, and cord ferritin levels and increased risk of iron deficiency in infancy.[22, 61] Maternal hemoglobin levels of less than 10.4 g/dl, especially after 24 weeks, are associated with a risk of low birth weight and preterm infants and increased perinatal mortality.[56, 80]

Megaloblastic Anemia

Megaloblastic anemia in the nonpregnant woman is usually due to folic acid or vitamin B_{12} deficiency. Folic acid deficiency is the most common cause of megaloblastic anemia encountered during pregnancy.[61] Vitamin B_{12} deficiency with pregnancy is rare because (1) stores of vitamin B_{12} are normally large, so deficient states take years to develop; (2) vitamin B_{12} is used for chromosome replication, so a deficiency usually leads to infertility; and (3) vitamin B_{12} deficiency is usually due to pernicious anemia, a disorder seen primarily in older women.[61, 101] Vitamin B_{12} deficiency may be misdiagnosed in a pregnant woman, since serum vitamin B_{12} levels fall with the expanded plasma volume and consequent hemodilution. In addition, the alterations in plasma proteins during pregnancy interfere with vitamin B_{12} assays.[61]

Folate demands increase three-fold during pregnancy. Since folic acid is essential for DNA synthesis and cell duplication, folate is needed for growth of the fetus and placenta as well as for maternal RBC production. Folate requirements increase throughout pregnancy and are higher in multiple pregnancy.[61, 101] Maternal serum folate levels fall during pregnancy, and supplements are needed by women with an inadequate dietary intake. Routine folate supplementation during pregnancy is generally not recommended if dietary intake is adequate.[56]

Severe folic acid deficiency has been associated with fetal malformations, PIH, abruptio placentae, prematurity, and low birth weight, although the causal association between these events is questionable.[61] The fetus has higher levels of folate and elevated folate binding protein, which protects against fetal folate deficiency; even with low maternal folate levels, neonatal cord levels are usually within normal limits.[101]

Sickle Cell Anemia

Sickle cell anemia is a disorder of beta chain structure of the hemoglobin molecule. A woman with sickle cell anemia normally has a lower hemoglobin level (7 to 8 g/dl) and oxygen carrying capacities to which her system has adjusted. Pregnancy places both the woman and her infant at greater risk for complications. As plasma volume increases during pregnancy, the woman may become slightly more anemic. In addition she often experiences an increase in frequency and severity of sickling attacks. Sickle cell crises are triggered by physical or emotional stress, which may be caused by infection, trauma, hypoxia, and pregnancy. Crises in pregnancy may be related to the hypercoagulable state, increased susceptibility to infection, or vascular stress.[90] The rapid hemodynamic changes post partum will often precipitate crises, especially if associated with a long or difficult labor and delivery.[21, 71]

In women with sickle cell anemia, tissue deoxygenation or acidosis triggers structural changes in the sickle hemoglobin (Hb S) so the RBCs take on a half-moon or sickle appearance. The sickled cells can obstruct blood flow in the microvasculature. The areas most susceptible to obstruction are those characterized by slow flow and high oxygen extraction such as the spleen, bone marrow, and placenta. Obstruction leads to venous stasis, further deoxygenation, platelet aggregation, hypoxia, acidosis, further sickling, and eventually infarction.[71]

Fetal and neonatal mortality are increased with a higher incidence of prematurity, stillbirth, IUGR, and neonatal death. The increased fetal wastage is due to placental infarction and fetal hypoxia. Fetal hypoxia results from decreased oxygen transport due to the abnormal biochemistry of the maternal hemoglobin and the loss of functional placental tissue for gas and nutrient exchange caused by infarctions associated with maternal sickling crises.[1, 21]

β-Thalassemia

Thalassemia is a disorder in the synthesis of either the alpha or beta peptide chains of the hemoglobin molecule. This leads to alterations in the RBC membrane and decreased RBC life span. β-Thalassemia minor is the most frequently encountered thalassemia during pregnancy. Females with thalassemia major (Cooley's anemia) usually die in childhood or adolescence; those who survive are often amenorrheic and infertile.[2, 61, 90]

Women with β-thalassemia minor are mildly anemic but generally healthy otherwise. There is controversy as to whether or not this disorder is associated with increased maternal or infant morbidity.[61, 87] Laboratory values normally associated with β-thalassemia minor, which indicate a mild hypochromic microcytic anemia, may lead to the diagnosis of iron deficiency and iron supplementation therapy. This treatment is potentially dangerous in that β-thalassemia is associated with increased iron absorption and storage and a susceptibility to iron overload. Iron therapy can increase morbidity in these women unless a true iron deficiency state (as diagnosed by bone marrow aspiration) is present.[61]

Thromboembolism and Pregnancy

The hypercoagulable state of pregnancy is crucial in protecting the mother against excessive blood loss with delivery and placental separation. However, the hypercoagulable state is also a disadvantage by significantly increasing the risk of thromboembolic disorders (TED) during pregnancy and post partum.

The risk of TED increases sixfold during pregnancy (1 to 3 in 1000 pregnant women).[29, 35] The risk increases with parity and age and is 3 to 16 times higher among women with cesarean than among those with vaginal births, and three to five times higher post partum than ante partum.[96] Pulmonary embolism occurs in 1 in 2000 pregnancies and is a major cause of maternal mortality.[49] Pulmonary emboli usually result from dislodged deep venous thrombi in the lower extremities.

The three factors (Virchow's triad) that predispose to thromboembolic disorders (stasis, altered coagulation, and vascular damage) are all present or potentially present during pregnancy.[120] During pregnancy increased venous capacitance leads to increased distensibility, decreased flow in the lower extremities, and venous stasis. By late pregnancy the velocity of venous blood flow in the lower extremities has been reduced by half, and venous pressure has risen an average of 10 mmHg.[49]

The hypercoagulable state during pregnancy increases the risk of clot formation. If a clot develops, the decreased fibrinolytic activity impedes fibrin removal and clot lysis. An increase in the incidence of TED is seen during the third trimester when fibrinolytic activity decreases.[120] Finally, the potential for localized vascular damage and release of tissue thromboplastin exists with delivery and particularly with cesarean section. Thus the risk of TED is higher in women post partum or following surgical intervention. Once a thrombus develops, it is more likely that it will extend if the predisposing factors persist over time, as occurs with pregnancy.[120]

Women with a history of a TED either prior to or during pregnancy have an increased risk of developing a similar disorder in subsequent pregnancies.[96, 120] Women with a history of TED during a previous pregnancy have a recurrence risk of 5 to 30%.[35, 103] Other women at increased risk are those with anemia, artificial heart valves, or PIH (due to exaggeration of hypercoagulable state) and those who undergo operative deliveries. Ambulation soon after delivery decreases venous stasis and the risk of TED.

Pregnant women with TED present with a clinical dilemma in terms of treatment. Coumarin derivatives (warfarin sulfate) inhibit vitamin K–dependent coagulation factors. These agents cross the placenta, whereas vitamin K–dependent coagulation factors do not, impairing fetal coagulation and increasing the risk of fetal and neonatal hemorrhage.[29] The risk of fetal bleeding and intracranial hemorrhage is especially high during labor. Warfarin has been associated with an increased risk of abortion and with a specific syndrome of fetal anomalies, involving the face, eyes, bones, and central nervous system (CNS), if given in the first 11 to 13 weeks of gestation.[29, 120] These abnormalities may be due to inhibition of vitamin K dependent proteins (osteocalcins) involved in bone development.

Heparin is considered the drug of choice for TED in pregnancy because its molecular weight prevents placental transfer or excretion in breast milk.[29, 103] Heparin is more costly and difficult to regulate than other anticoagulants and is associated with complications such as maternal osteoporosis, thrombocytopenia, and hemorrhage and an increased incidence of prematurity and stillbirth. If used on an outpatient basis, heparin must be self-administered via subcutaneous injections.[29, 81, 94]

Heparin doses often need to be increased as pregnancy progresses, particularly during the third trimester. Changes in heparin requirements have been related to increasing plasma volume and renal clearance and to the presence of a placental heparinase enzyme.[120] Heparin doses may need to be decreased in women who develop significant alterations in renal function or in whom plasma volume changes are reduced, e.g., women with PIH.[29]

Heparin treatment is usually stopped during labor and delivery, then resumed in the early postpartum period. An alternative approach is to use heparin during the first trimester and late third trimester, switching to warfarin in the intervening interval. This approach is often used with women who have artificial heart valves or mitral valve disease, conditions associated with a significant risk of arterial emboli for which heparin is often not an effective anticoagulant.[35, 81, 120] Warfarin is also used during the postpartum period. Warfarin is excreted in breast milk in very small amounts. Although many feel that with careful monitoring the use of warfarin by women who are breast feeding is safe, this is an area of controversy.[29, 120]

Consumptive Coagulopathies During Pregnancy

Pregnancy is characterized by increases in fibrinolytic activity and plasminogen, plasminogen activators in the uterus, and an ongoing low grade activation of the coagulation system within the uteroplacental circulation. As a result, events such as extravasation of blood into the myometrium or rupture of blood vessels in the area can activate the fibrinolytic system and lead to a consumptive coagulopathy.[5] The risk of such coagulopathies such as disseminated intravascular coagulation (DIC) is higher during pregnancy, particularly in association with abruptio placentae, PIH, intrauterine fetal death, amniotic fluid embolism, and septic abortion.[100, 119] These events result in one or more of the processes commonly associated with intravascular coagulation: release of tissue thromboplastin, endothelial injury, or shock and stasis.[63] Many of these complications trigger the formation of tissue thromboplastin, activating the extrinsic coagulation pathway (see Fig. 5–3) with depletion of fibrinogen and increased fibrinolytic activity.[49, 124]

DIC arises from inappropriate activation of normal clotting processes within the circulation with intravascular consumption of procoagulant proteins, clotting factors and platelets, formation of fibrin clots within the vascular bed, and activation of fibrinolysis (Fig. 5–6). Consumption of the clotting factors can lead to hemorrhage and shock. As clots are formed and fibrin is deposited in the microcirculation, further cell (tissue) injury may occur, triggering further coagulation and eventual depletion of plasma clotting factors. These fibrin clots may also cause intravascular obstruction and infarction. Activation of clotting also activates the fibrinolytic system, which leads to formation of fibrin-fibrinogen degradation products (FDP) or fibrin split products (FSP). These fibrin degradation products further inhibit coagulation and decrease platelet function.[63, 75, 119]

SUMMARY

The hematologic and hemostatic systems undergo significant alterations during pregnancy that promote maternal adaptation but also influence interpretation of laboratory values and increase the risk of thromboembolic insults and coagulopathies. Owing to the significant risks associated with these events, appropriate measurement, observation, data gathering, and evaluation are essential. Changes in the hematologic system

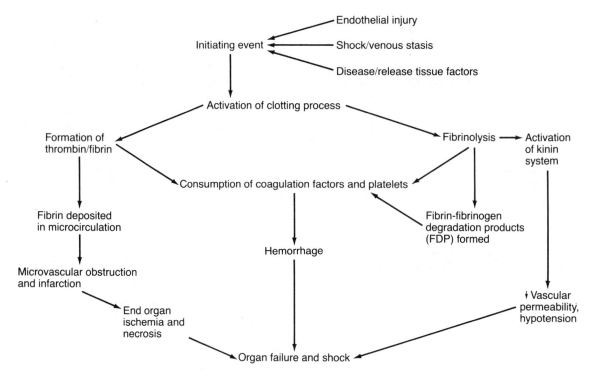

FIGURE 5–6. Pathophysiology of disseminated intravascular coagulation.

during pregnancy are also critical for fetal homeostasis. Maternal hypervolemia promotes delivery of oxygen and nutrients to the fetus, and changes in albumin concentration may influence the availability of both nutrients and potentially harmful substances. The fetus in turn can affect maternal status, as is the case with iron metabolism and needs. Clinical recommendations for nurses working with pregnant women based on changes in the hematologic system are summarized in Table 5–5.

DEVELOPMENT OF THE HEMATOLOGIC SYSTEM IN THE FETUS

The hematologic system arises early in gestation and along with the primitive cardiovascular system is one of the earliest systems to achieve some functional capacity. The hematologic system is critical for the well-being of the fetus through transport of nutrients and oxygen and removal of waste products.

Formation of Blood Cells

Blood cells develop from stem cells derived from mesenchymal tissues. Stem cells first appear in the yolk sac and at about 6 weeks migrate to the developing liver, thymus, lymph nodes, and bone marrow.[88] Hematopoiesis in the fetus can be divided into three periods: mesoblastic, hepatic, and myeloid (Fig. 5–7).

During the mesoblastic period (from 14 to 19 days to a peak at 6 weeks) blood cells are formed in blood islands in the yolk sac. Peripheral cells in these islands form primitive blood vessels; central cells develop into hematoblasts (primitive blood cells).[84] Blood formation in the yolk sac disappears by the 3rd month.

The hepatic period begins during the 5th week. The liver is the major source of blood cells from 3 to 5 months, although some blood formation continues in this site through 1 week post birth. The predominant cells produced by the liver are normoblastic erythrocytes, although some megakaryocytes and granulocytes are also produced. Hematopoiesis can be detected in the spleen and thymus during the 3rd month and shortly

TABLE 5–5
Summary of Recommendations for Clinical Practice Related to Changes in the Hematologic System:
Pregnant Woman

Recognize usual hematologic values and patterns of change during pregnancy and post partum (pp. 160–171; Tables 5–1 to 5–4).

Recognize that isolated lab values must be evaluated in light of clinical findings and previous values (pp. 160, 171; Table 5–1).

Assess maternal nutritional status in relation to iron, folate, and vitamins and provide nutritional counseling (pp. 171–173).

Monitor hematocrit and hemoglobin values throughout pregnancy (pp. 163–164, 170).

Know patterns of change in plasma and blood volume during pregnancy and post partum (pp. 160–162, 169–170).

Monitor and counsel women with cardiac problems with particular attention to periods when blood/plasma volume increases significantly (p. 161; Chapter 6).

Monitor women on tocolytic therapy regarding pulmonary edema with particular attention to women with greater increases in plasma volume (p. 161).

Monitor for and teach pregnant woman to recognize signs of thromboembolism and consumptive coagulopathy (pp. 174–175).

Recognize risk factors for the development of thromboembolism (p. 174).

Ambulate women soon after delivery to reduce the risk of thromboembolism (p. 174).

Recognize risk factors for development of consumptive coagulopathies (pp. 168–169, 175).

Question the use of diuretics in women with PIH (p. 161).

Evaluate maternal responses to prescribed drugs for signs of subtherapeutic levels or side effects (pp. 165–166, 175).

Counsel women regarding the effects of plasma volume increases and decreased plasma proteins on drug levels during pregnancy (pp. 161–162, 165–166).

Recognize factors that may mask signs of infection during the intrapartum and early postpartum period (p. 167).

Know effects of early versus late cord clamping and when early clamping is warranted (pp. 180–181; Table 5–6).

Note timing of cord clamping (p. 180).

Page numbers following each recommendation refer to pages in the text where rationale is discussed.

FIGURE 5–7. Stages of hematopoiesis in the embryo and fetus. (From Wintrobe, M. (1981). *Clinical hematology* (8th ed., p. 49). Philadelphia: Lea & Febiger.)

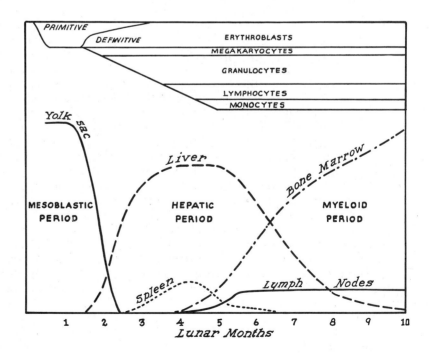

thereafter in the lymph nodes. Blood formation in the spleen, initially producing erythrocytes and later lymphocytes, declines after 4 to 5 months. Some blood formation in the spleen can be seen during the 1st week post birth. The thymus and lymph nodes are primarily involved in lymphopoiesis.[84, 88]

The myeloid period begins at 3 to 4 months. The bone marrow is the major site for blood production after 6 months' gestation. Centers for blood formation arise in mesenchymal tissues and invade cavities produced during bone formation (see Chapter 14). Initially bone marrow produces granulocytes and megakaryocytes. After liver erythropoiesis declines, bone marrow erythropoiesis increases. The major area of blood production is the fatty marrow in the core of the long bones. Large fat cells are not found in fetal marrow as in adults, suggesting that fetal marrow is functioning at full hematopoietic capacity.[129]

The long bones of the fetus and newborn are cartilaginous, and their relative marrow volume is smaller than in older individuals. As a result, the only way the fetus or newborn can significantly increase production of blood cells is by either reactivation or persistence of extramedullary hematopoiesis in the abdominal viscera, such as the liver and spleen.[59] This extramedullary erythropoiesis is responsible for much of the hepatosplenomegaly seen in infants with erythroblastosis fetalis.[10]

Development of Red Blood Cells

The initial RBCs are primitive megaloblasts and appear at 3 to 4 weeks, followed by normative megaloblastic erythropoiesis at 6 weeks. By 10 weeks the latter cells constitute 90% of the RBC volume. The early cells are large nucleated cells with increased deformability. With increasing gestation, hemoglobin, hematocrit, and total red blood cell count increase, whereas the number of nucleated RBCs, mean corpuscular volume, cell diameter, mean corpuscular hemoglobin, reticulocytes, and proportion of immature cell forms decrease.[59, 84] Erythropoietin does not cross the placenta, so fetal erythropoiesis is endogenously controlled.[106] Fetal erythropoietin increases from 19 weeks to term and is produced primarily in the liver rather than in the kidneys.[94, 129] From 32 weeks on, and perhaps earlier, the fetus reacts to hypoxia with increased erythropoietin production.[84]

Development of White Blood Cells and Platelets

Formation of WBCs begins in the liver at 5 to 7 weeks, followed by the spleen (8 weeks), thymus (10 weeks), and lymph nodes (12 weeks). Significant numbers are not produced until the myeloid period. Circulating granulocytes increase rapidly during the third trimester. At birth numbers of WBCs are equal to or greater than those found in adults. T lymphocytes can be detected by 7 weeks and B lymphocytes by 8 weeks. Lymphocytes are formed in the fetal liver and lymphoid plexuses initially, then in the thymus (7 to 10 weeks) and spleen and bone marrow (10 to 12 weeks). The numbers of circulating lymphocytes increase rapidly to peak at 20 weeks (10,000 mm³), then decline to 3000/mm³ by term.[59, 84] Megakaryocytes are first found at 5 to 6 weeks in the yolk sac and liver; platelets appear in the blood by 11 weeks. By 13 weeks megakaryocyte and platelet numbers are similar to those in adults.[84]

Formation of Hemoglobin

Several forms of hemoglobin (Hb) are found in the embryo and fetus (Fig. 5–8). The primitive embryonic forms are Gower 1 and Gower 2 (seen prior to 12 weeks) and Hb Portland. The predominant hemoglobin of the fetus is fetal hemoglobin (Hb F), which consists of a pair of alpha peptide chains and a pair of gamma chains. Adult hemoglobin (Hb A), which consists of pairs of alpha and beta chains, appears after 6 to 8 weeks and increases rapidly after 16 to 20 weeks.[92] By 30 to 32 weeks, 90 to 95% of the hemoglobin is Hb F. After this point the amount of Hb F begins to slowly decline, and levels of Hb A increase along with the total body hemoglobin mass.[84] The switch from fetal to adult hemoglobin synthesis is related to postconceptual, not post birth, age.[106] Synthesis of Hb A and Hb F is not significantly affected by intrauterine transfusions or exchange transfusions after birth.

Fetal hemoglobin is unique in several of its properties. Hb F is more resistant to acid elution and can be oxidized to methemoglobin more readily, increasing the susceptibility of newborns to methemoglobinemia. Hb F has a greater affinity for oxygen because Hb F does not bind 2,3-DPG as effectively as does Hb A. Increased affinity facilitates oxy-

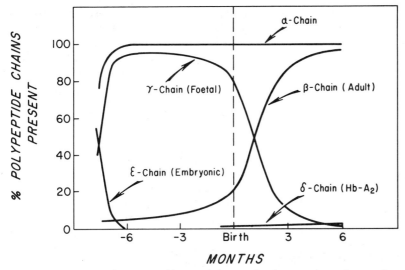

FIGURE 5–8. Development of hemoglobin in the fetus and newborn. The relative proportions of each globin chain produced at each stage of gestation are shown. The α chain, fully expressed throughout life, is expressed as 100%; the percentages of non-α chains produced at each stage are expressed relative to α chain production. (From Nathan, D.G., et al. (1973). The development of hemoglobin in the antenatal diagnosis of the hemoglobinopathies. In *Hematology in the perinatal patient* (p. 11). Mead Johnson Symposium on Perinatal and Developmental Medicine, No. 4. Evansville, IN: Mead Johnson.)

gen transfer across the placenta but reduces oxygen release to the tissues.

The resistance of fetal hemoglobin to acid elution is the basis for tests such as the Kleihauer techniques used to detect fetal cells in maternal blood. These tests may be unreliable as a measure of fetal cells if maternal Hb F is elevated or with ABO incompatibility. In the presence of ABO incompatibility fetal cells may be destroyed by maternal antibody and cleared from the mother's circulation. Altered levels of Hb F are seen in women with sickle cell anemia, thalassemia minor, hydatidiform mole, and leukemia and in a pregnancy-induced elevation of Hb F. Fetal cells may still be identified, since with elevated maternal Hb F there tend to be many cells with varying amounts of Hb F and the fewer fetal cells have consistently high Hb F concentrations.[10]

Development of the Hemostatic System

Hemostatic and fibrinolytic systems develop simultaneously. Fetal blood demonstrates clotting ability by 11 to 12 weeks.[12, 49] Fibrinogen synthesis in the liver begins at 5 weeks. Fibrinogen can be found in the plasma by 12 to 13 weeks, reaching adult values by 30 weeks.[129] The placenta is rich in tissue thromboplastin and thus able to respond rapidly to insults with initiation of the clotting cascade.[49] This helps to protect the fetus from significant blood loss. Vitamin K levels are 30% of adult values by the end of the second trimester and 50% by term.[129]

Fibrinolytic activity can also be demonstrated at 12 to 13 weeks. The whole blood clotting time in the fetus is relatively short, and the fetus is in a hypercoagulable state during the first and second trimesters. Fibrinolytic activity in the fetus is increased even though levels of blood plasminogen are low, owing to increased tissue plasminogen activator (tPA) or decreased inhibitor or both.[49] The elevated fibrinolytic activity may help to protect and maintain the extensive fetal capillary circulation within the placental villi.

NEONATAL PHYSIOLOGY

The neonate experiences significant alterations in the hematologic system and hemostasis. Among the more striking differences are the structural and functional alterations in the neonatal red blood cell and the potential impact of Hb F on oxygen delivery to the tissues. Variations are also seen in blood volume, blood cellular components and in hemostasis parameters. These alterations increase the risk for anemia, thromboembolism, and coagulopathies in the neonate.

Transitional Events

A major transitional event for the neonate is removal of the placental circulation with clamping of the umbilical cord. The timing of umbilical cord clamping influences the amount of placental transfusion and subsequent plasma and RBC volume of the neonate. At term, fetal blood volume is approximately 70 to 80 ml/kg and placental blood volume 45 ml/kg of fetal weight.[65] Blood volume in normal neonates varies from 70 to 125 ml/kg depending on the direction and magnitude of blood transfer between the fetus and placenta at birth.[65, 84, 128]

The umbilical arteries constrict at birth so blood does not flow from the infant to the placenta. The umbilical vein remains dilated, however, so blood flows from the placenta to the infant via gravity.[128] If the newly delivered infant is kept at or below the level of the placenta, transfer of blood from the placenta to the fetus will occur during the first 3 minutes after birth.

The timing of cord clamping and the position of the infant in relation to the placenta influence placental transfusion. Yao and Lind reported that if the infant's position was maintained at the level of the introitus ($\pm$ 10 cm) until the cord was clamped, or held 40 cm below the introitus for no more than 30 seconds, the infant received a placental transfusion of approximately 80 ml.[125, 127] The amount of placental transfusion was negligible if the infant was held 50 to 60 cm above the introitus.

With the infant held at the level of the introitus or slightly below, if the cord is clamped 30 to 60 seconds after delivery, placental transfusion increases the newborn's blood volume by 15 to 20%; clamping at 60 to 90 seconds results in a 25% increase; and clamping at 3 minutes produces a 50 to 60% increase.[65, 126, 127] The timing at which the umbilical cord is clamped and the magnitude of placental transfusion have significant physiologic and clinical effects on many body systems. Table 5–6 summarizes the effects on infants of placental transfusion with late versus early clamping. Although late clamping is associated with increased initial total blood volume, by 3 days post birth differences in blood volume between early versus late clamped infants are actually slight owing to the usual fluid shifts post birth with a decrease in plasma volume.[84]

There is little consensus on when to clamp the umbilical cord. Yao and Lind recommend that following a normal vaginal delivery the cord be clamped by 30 seconds if the infant has not been elevated above the level of the uterus.[127] Linderkamp suggests that in full term infants a medium transfusion of 15 to 20 ml/kg can be achieved when the cord is clamped 30 to 60 seconds after delivery.[65] Oski and Naiman recommend that after a cesarean birth the infant be held 20 cm below the level of the placenta for approximately 30 seconds prior to cord clamping.[84] In examining the advantages and disadvantages of early versus late cord clamping (Table 5–6), there appears to be an optimal median timing for cord clamping with adverse consequences from either too little (early clamping) or too much (late clamping) additional blood volume at birth.

In preterm infants, delayed cord clamping is associated with hyperbilirubinemia, due to the increased volume of RBCs, and respiratory distress. Respiratory distress may result from movement of excess plasma volume that cannot be accommodated in the vascular compartment into extravascular spaces including areas around the lungs, with a decrease in lung compliance and functional residual capacity.[65]

There are other groups of infants for whom even moderate placental transfusion may not be warranted and for whom late cord clamping or milking of the cord should be avoided. Hydropic infants are already fluid overloaded and may not tolerate additional volume. Placental transfusion in the erythroblastotic infant may increase the load of maternal antibodies, which destroy fetal and neonatal RBCs. Even though these infants are often anemic, administration of packed cells after birth is more appropriate than attempting to increase RBCs by placental transfusion.

If the mother has received heavy doses of analgesia or general anesthesia, earlier clamping may be warranted to prevent additional amounts of these agents from reaching the infant. Early clamping is also appropriate for infants at risk for polycythemia, such as infants of diabetic mothers (IDM) or

TABLE 5–6
Effects of Placental Transfusion on Neonatal Adaptation After Birth

ALTERATION	LATE OR EARLY CLAMPING*	BASIS FOR CHANGE
Volume Effects		
↑ Atrial pressure	Late	Volume overload
↑ Systolic blood pressure	Late	Volume overload
↑ Central venous pressure	Late	Volume overload
↑ Pulmonary artery pressure	Late	↑ Pulmonary vascular resistance due to distention of pulmonary capillary-venous bed
↑ Left ventricle afterload	Late	↑ Systemic BP and ↑ vascular resistance
Delayed closure of foramen ovale and ductus arteriosus	Late	↑ Pulmonary artery pressure escape outlet to prevent right ventricle overload
↑ Blood volume in first 4 hours	Late	Compensatory response to overload with transudation of plasma into interstitial space
Left-to-right ductal shunt (?)	Early	↑ Pulmonary artery pressure
↓ Peripheral blood flow	Early	↓ Volume and compensatory mechanisms
↑ Urinary output	Late	↑ Glomerular filtration rate due to systolic BP
Hypovolemia	Early	↓ Blood volume
Heart murmurs	Early	Earlier fall in pulmonary artery pressure
Effects on Hematocrit		
↑ Hematocrit	Late	RBC volume
Polycythemia	Late	↑ RBC volume; hemoconcentration in first 24 + hours due to compensatory fluid shifts
Hyperviscosity	Late	↑ Hematocrit, ↓ deformability
Plethora	Late	Polycythemia, ↑ RBC
Anemia (slight)	Early	↓ RBC volume
↓ Iron stores	Early	↓ RBC, less iron from degraded RBC
Hyperbilirubinemia	Late	↑ RBC volume
Respiratory Effects		
↓ Time to 1st breath	Early	Anoxia with ↓ blood supply and thus ↓ oxygen supply
↓ Lung compliance (1st 6 hours)	Late	Higher cardiac load, pulmonary and capillary filling
↓ Functional residual capacity (FRC) (1st 6 hours)	Late	Higher cardiac load, pulmonary and capillary filling
Mild signs of respiratory distress	Late	Overdistended circulatory system, ?slight pulmonary edema
↑ PaO_2, PCO_2	Early	↓ Transudation of fluid at alveolar-capillary interface
↑ Respiratory distress syndrome (?)	Late	↓ Lung compliance and ↓ FRC
↓ Respiratory distress syndrome (?)	Late	Improved oxygen carrying capacity
Other Effects		
↑ Intraventricular hemorrhage (?)	Early	↓ Blood volume and hypotension
↑ Intraventricular hemorrhage (?)	Late	Rapidly expanded blood volume with ↑ BP after birth; hypertension; ↑ viscosity
↑ Activity, more alert, ↓ crying	Early	Less physiologic stress (?)
↑ Quiet sleep and wakefulness	Late	Greater physiologic stress (?)

*Definitions of late versus early clamping varied among studies reported.
BP = blood pressure; RBC = red blood cell.
Material compiled from Yao, A.C. & Lind, J. (1982). *Placental Transfusion*. Springfield, IL: Charles C Thomas; and Linderkamp, O. (1982). Placental transfusion: Determinants and effects. *Clin Perinatol, 9*, 559.

severely growth retarded infants. With multiple births early cord clamping of the first infant is recommended to protect the unborn fetus(es), since the circulations of these infants may communicate via the placenta. Earlier clamping may also be warranted in the severely asphyxiated infant so that resuscitative efforts can be initiated promptly; however, hypovolemia must also be avoided.

Changes in Hematologic Parameters

Hematologic parameters differ in neonates as compared with adults and change rapidly during the 1st week post birth. Considerable variation may be noted between individual infants and within the same infant over time.[128] Hematologic parameters in preterm and full term neonates are summarized in Table 5–7.

Blood Volume

Blood volume averages about 80 to 100 ml/kg in term infants and 90 to 105 ml/kg in preterm infants. Variations in blood volume at birth are due primarily to placental transfusion and gestational age. The higher blood

TABLE 5–7
Normal Hematologic Values in Newborns

| VALUE | GESTATIONAL AGE (WEEKS) | | FULL-TERM CORD BLOOD | DAY 1 | DAY 3 | DAY 7 | DAY 14 |
	28	34					
Hb (g/dl)	14.5	15.0	16.8	18.4	17.8	17.0	16.8
Hematocrit (%)	45	47	53	58	55	54	52
Red blood cells (mm³)	4.0	4.4	5.25	5.8	5.6	5.2	5.1
MCV (μ^3)	120	118	107	108	99	98	96
MCH (pg)	40	38	34	35	33	32.5	31.5
MCHC (%)	31	32	31.7	32.5	33	33	33
Reticulocytes (%)	5–10	3–10	3–7	3–7	1–3	0–1	0–1
Platelets (1000s/mm³)			290	192	213	248	252

MCV = mean corpuscular volume; MCH = mean corpuscular hemoglobin; MCHC = mean corpuscular hemoglobin concentration.
From Klaus, M.H. & Fanaroff, A.A. (1986). *Care of the High Risk Neonate* (3rd ed., p. 412). Philadelphia: WB Saunders.

volume of the preterm infant is due to increased plasma volume. Plasma volume decreases with gestation.[84]

Red Blood Cells

Red blood cell counts are 4.6 to 5.2 million/mm³ at birth, increasing by about 500,000 in the initial hours post birth, then falling to around 5.2 million/mm³ by the end of the 1st week.[84] Nucleated RBCs are seen in most newborns during the first 24 hours, perhaps as a response to the stresses of delivery, disappearing by 4 days in term infants and by 1 week in most preterm infants. Increased numbers of nucleated RBCs are found in more immature infants (and may persist beyond the 1st week) and in infants with Down syndrome or congenital anomalies.[84] Nucleated RBCs are also seen in the neonate as an acute stress response to asphyxia, with anemia, and following hemorrhage. In older individuals, these cells are rare and associated with abnormal erythropoiesis.[128] The erythrocyte sedimentation rate is decreased in neonates owing to alterations in plasma viscosity, protein content, and hematocrit.[72] The red blood cell of the neonate differs from that of the adult. These differences and their implications are summarized in Table 5–8.

HEMOGLOBIN AND HEMATOCRIT

Hemoglobin levels are higher in newborns, ranging from 13.7 to 20.1 g/dl, with most in the 16.6 to 17.5 g/dl range.[84] Hemoglobin levels increase by up to 6 g/dl within the first 24 to 48 hours post birth. This increase results from a shift in fluid distribution after birth with a decrease in plasma volume and a net increase in RBCs and partially compensates for placental transfusion.[41, 106, 128]

The hemoglobin concentration decreases by the end of the 1st week to values similar to cord blood levels.[106] Higher hemoglobin levels are seen in infants with severe hypoxia and in some IUGR and postterm infants, possibly as a compensatory mechanism to increase oxygen availability to the tissues. Lower hemoglobin levels are found in preterm infants. An elevation of either the reticulocyte count or the number of nucleated RBCs above normal values in any infant, regardless of the hemoglobin level, suggests a compensatory response and may indicate anemia.[84]

Cord blood contains 50 to 85% fetal hemoglobin (Hb F), 15 to 40% adult hemoglobin (Hb A), and less than 1.8% hemoglobin A₂ (a minor normal adult form). A fourth type, Hb Bart's (<0.5%), is seen in small amounts in some infants. Cord blood hemoglobin levels vary with gestational age.[84, 128]

Hb F does not bind 2,3-DPG as readily as does Hb A, shifting the oxygen-hemoglobin dissociation curve of the fetus and newborn to the left. Increased concentrations of Hb F are seen in small for gestational age (SGA) infants and other infants who have experienced chronic hypoxia in utero, probably owing to a delay in the normal switch to synthesis of Hb A at about 32 weeks.[10, 129] Alterations in Hb F are not seen in infants with acute intrapartal hypoxia, since the more recent onset of this condition does not allow the infant sufficient time to compensate.[84] The increased Hb F seen in infants with trisomy 13 during the first 2 years of life is also thought to be due to a delay in Hb A synthesis. Decreased Hb F is seen in infants with Down syndrome. Increased Hb A is found in infants with erythroblastosis fetalis owing to rapid destruction of older RBC

TABLE 5–8
Characteristics of Neonatal Red Blood Cells and Their Implications

RBC CHARACTERISTIC	CLINICAL IMPLICATION
Macrocytosis with increased mean cellular diameter and mean corpuscular volume	More susceptible to damage in small capillaries; increased RBC turnover
Increased permeability to sodium and potassium	Increased risk of cell lysis owing to osmotic changes
Altered enzyme activity with increased glucose utilization	Risk of hypoglycemia, especially in infants with low glucose stores or altered glucose metabolism with a tendency toward polycythemia (i.e., IDM, SGA)
Increased ATP utilization	Higher energy (glucose) needs and oxygen consumption
Decreased survival time (80–100 days for term and 60–80 days for preterm versus 120 days for adult)	Increased RBC turnover rate; proportionately greater amounts of bilirubin produced
Increased receptor sites for substances such as insulin and digoxin	Insulin receptor sites facilitate increased glucose uptake; digoxin sites contribute to greater tolerance for digoxin
Increased fetal hemoglobin, less adult hemoglobin	Increased affinity of hemoglobin for oxygen with less ready release to tissues
Increased RBC count at birth (4.6–5.2 million/mm^3), falling to 3–4 million/mm^3 by 2–3 months	Increased RBC turnover rate and bilirubin production
Increased phospholipid, cholesterol, and total lipid content	Increased risk of lipid peroxidation and hemolysis (cholesterol may provide protection against hemolysis)
Increased fragility, decreased deformability, increased variety and frequency of morphologic abnormalities	Increased susceptibility to damage, especially in microcirculation; increased RBC turnover

ATP = adenosine triphosphate; IDM = infant of a diabetic mother; RBC = red blood cell; SGA = small for gestational age.
Compiled from references 10, 72, 73, 86, and 123.

containing Hb F and replacement by new cells containing higher concentrations of Hb A.[84]

Hematocrit levels at birth normally range from 51.3 to 56%. The hematocrit increases in the first few hours or days owing to the movement of fluid from intravascular to interstitial spaces. The hematocrit falls again to levels near cord blood values by the end of the 1st week.[41, 83, 84]

CHANGES IN 2,3-DPG
Although 2,3-DPG levels at birth in term infants are similar to those in adults, the 2,3-DPG is less stable.[106] Concentrations of 2,3-DPG may fall the 1st week, then increase by the time the infant is 2 to 3 weeks of age.[72, 84] The P$_{50}$ (the PO$_2$ at which 50% of the hemoglobin is saturated with oxygen) is decreased at birth but gradually increases during the 1st week of life.[128] This initial change in the P$_{50}$ is due primarily to an increase in 2,3-DPG rather than in the percentage of Hb F. In comparison with term infants, the preterm infant has a lower P$_{50}$, decreased concentrations of 2,3 DPG, and increased amounts of Hb F. Therefore, in the initial few weeks post birth the functioning DPG fraction in the preterm infant is significantly reduced.[37, 123, 128]

ERYTHROPOIETIN
Erythropoietin levels are higher at birth in term infants than in preterm infants. After the 1st day erythropoietin is not found in the plasma of healthy term infants until 60 to 90 days of age. The return of erythropoietin coincides with the resumption of bone marrow activity and RBC production.[59, 111] Erythropoietin disappears from the plasma for longer periods in the preterm infant. Elevated levels of this hormone are found at birth in infants with Down syndrome, IUGR, or anemia secondary to erythroblastosis fetalis and those born to women with diabetes or PIH. In the first 24 hours erythropoietin is elevated in infants with severe anemia or cyanotic congenital heart defects.[84] The increased levels in the latter group result from low arterial oxygen saturations, which stimulate continued production of erythropoietin.

RETICULOCYTES
The reticulocyte count is elevated at birth, ranging from 3 to 7% in term infants and up to 8 to 10% in preterm infants. The reticulocyte count increases slightly in the initial 2 to 3 days after birth, then falls to less than 1% by 1 week of age.[10]

IRON AND SERUM FERRITIN
Iron status of the neonate is determined by maturity, birth weight, and hemoglobin level. Cord serum ferritin levels at term are five times higher than maternal values and rise further in the 1st 24 hours with RBC catabolism and release of hemoglobin iron.[8] Cord

hemoglobin and serum ferritin levels are inversely related. At birth the serum folate level of the neonate is three times higher than that in maternal blood.[101] Stores in preterm infants are lower and more rapidly depleted in the first months owing to rapid growth.

White Blood Cells

The WBC count ranges from 10,000 to 26,000/mm³ in term infants and from 6000 to 19,000/mm³ in preterm infants. The number of cells increases during the first 12 to 24 hours, then gradually decreases to the level of 6000 to 15,000/mm³ (mean, 12,000/mm³) by 4 to 5 days in both term and preterm infants.[84] The initial increase in WBCs may be due to displacement of cells from the margins of larger vessels and is similar to changes seen in adults following strenuous exercise. The stress of labor and delivery may result in similar changes in the newborn.[49]

Initially up to 60% of the WBCs may be neutrophils with a variety of immature forms. During the first 3 to 4 days the neutrophil count is higher in preterm than in term infants. By the 4th day both groups of infants have neutrophil counts ranging from 2000 to 6000/mm³. These values are stable throughout the 1st month of life.[84] Immature forms of neutrophils (bands, metamyelocytes, myelocytes) may be seen in healthy neonates during the first 2 to 3 days.[70] The number of monocytes increases slightly during the first 12 hours, then gradually decreases.

Eosinophil counts in the neonate show great individual variation, with reported values ranging from 100 to 2500/mm³ at birth and increasing during the first 4 to 5 days of life.[10] Others have reported a progressive increase in eosinophils during the initial 3 to 5 weeks, especially in preterm infants who may have an absence of eosinophils in the first 24 hours post birth.[19] Eosinophilia (>700/mm³) is common in preterm infants during the first 3 to 5 weeks post birth. Disappearance of eosinophils from the peripheral circulation has been noted prior to death.[19]

Alterations in Hemostasis

Platelets

In term and many preterm infants platelet counts are 200,000 to 300,000/mm³, similar to older individuals. About 14 to 15% of preterm infants have counts greater than 150,000/mm³ in the 1st month. Platelet counts may increase to 300,000 to 400,000/mm³ by the end of the 1st month in both term infants and preterm infants. Higher levels may persist for the first 3 months in preterm infants.[84] A marked thrombocytosis has been seen by 2 weeks in offspring of polydrug users, which may persist for several months.[20] Platelet counts less than 100,000/mm³ are abnormal in neonates.[10, 129]

Platelet function is altered along several parameters in some, but not all, infants. Neonatal platelets often have decreased aggregation (i.e., cohesion of platelets to each other to form a temporary plug over a damaged area of a blood vessel). This is due to diminished thromboxane A₂, which normally recruits more platelets. The neonatal platelets also demonstrate decreased adhesion (i.e., adherence of platelets to damaged blood vessel walls, which triggers release of adenosine diphosphate (ADP) to stimulate platelet aggregation), possibly owing to altered membrane reactivity.[17, 18]

Platelet release of substances that enhance the clotting cascade may also be impaired. Oski and Naiman suggest that under normal circumstances platelet dysfunction in the neonate may serve as a protective mechanism against the increased tendency toward thrombosis in these infants.[84] However, if the infant is ill or immature, these limitations increase the risk of bleeding and coagulopathy. Coagulation in the neonate may be impaired by maternal drugs such as aspirin that alter platelet aggregation and Factor XII (contact factor) activity.

Coagulation

Vitamin K–dependent clotting factors II (prothrombin), VII, IX, and X are reduced. This reduction is greater in preterm infants, since concentrations of vitamin K–dependent factors are gestational age dependent.[32] Contact factors involved in the initiation of the clotting cascade (XI, XII, prekallikrein, and high-molecular-weight kininogen) are reduced and may be 30% of adult values in preterm infants.[17, 128] Factors V and VIII are similar to or higher than adult values in term and older preterm infants but reduced in infants less than 31 weeks' gestational age.[12, 49]

Neonatal fibrinogen levels may be at or slightly below those in adults, but there is decreased functional ability of fibrinogen. Activity of all clotting factors involved in activation of the intrinsic clotting system is decreased in the newborn (Fig. 5–9). Activity is further diminished with decreasing gestational age and in severely ill neonates. Levels of antithrombin III (a protease inhibitor that neutralizes activated clotting factors) and protein C (an inhibitor of factors VII and V and the vitamin K–dependent factors) are decreased, which increases the risk for hy-

percoagulable states and thrombi formation.[49, 128, 129]

Prothrombin time (PT), thrombin time (TT), and especially partial thromboplastin time (PTT) are prolonged, more so with decreasing gestational age. Although specific values for these tests vary between laboratories, PT greater than 17 seconds at any gestation or PTT greater than 45 to 50 seconds in a term infant is of concern.[17]

PTT is generally not a useful parameter

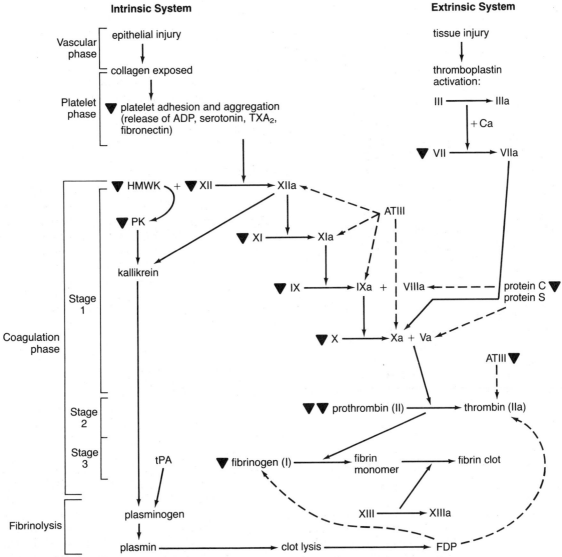

FIGURE 5–9. Alterations in coagulation in the neonate (ADP = adenosine diphosphate; TXA$_2$ = thromboxane A$_2$; HMWK = high-molecular-weight kininogen; PK = prekallikrein; PL = phospholipid or platelet factor 3; ATIII = antithrombin III; tPA = tissue plasminogen activator; FDP = fibrin-fibrinogen degradation products; Ca = calcium. Dashed line = inhibitory action. ▲▼ denote changes in the newborn. See Figure 5–3 for a summary of the physiology of coagulation.

in preterm infants. PTT measures all coagulation factors except VII and XIII and is abnormal if any one factor is 20 to 40% of normal. PTT is influenced unduly by decreases in the contact factors, such as are seen in many healthy preterm infants.[17] Despite the prolonged PTT, PT, and TT, newborn whole blood clotting times are equal to or shorter than adult values. The mechanism for this paradoxical finding is unknown but may represent a slight overbalance of the tendency toward thrombosis (decreased antithrombin III and proteins C and S) in comparison with the physiologic hypocoagulability (low levels of factors II, VII, IX, and X).[7, 32] The degree to which hemostatic and coagulation factors are altered in the preterm and term infant is summarized in Table 5–9.

Fibrinolysis

Activity of the fibrinolytic system is increased at birth, decreasing to adult values by 4 to 6 hours. In addition, clearance of collagen debris, fibrin, and injured cells is delayed secondary to immaturity of the reticuloendothelial activating system and low levels of fibronectin (glycoprotein involved in clearance of debris from tissue injury and inflammation).[83] Alterations in healthy preterm infants are similar to or slightly less than those in term newborns. However, activity of the fibrinolytic mechanism may be significantly depressed in some infants, especially preterm infants with severe respiratory distress syndrome (RDS) and asphyxiated infants, for at least the first 24 hours post birth and possibly longer. Plasminogen levels are half of adult values at birth and are decreased even further in small for gestational age infants and some preterm infants, increasing the risk for hemostatic disorders.[22, 83]

CLINICAL IMPLICATIONS FOR NEONATAL CARE

Alterations in the hematologic system and hemostasis in the neonate have a significant impact on neonatal adaptations to extrauterine life. These alterations along with the changes that occur during the first few months of life can influence interpretation of laboratory test results, lead to alterations such as physiologic anemia or hemorrhagic disease of the newborn, and increase the risk of

thromboembolism and consumptive coagulopathies. This section discusses these implications and two areas of controversy related to the hematologic system, that is, the role of vitamin E and decisions regarding transfusion of preterm infants.

Factors Influencing Hematologic Parameters

Factors that influence blood values and their interpretation in the neonate include the timing, site, and amount of blood sampled; placental transfusion; and infant growth rate.[10,84] The timing of blood sampling in relation to changes in hemoglobin and hematocrit during the 1st week of postnatal life and effects of placental transfusion were discussed earlier in this chapter. The detection of hemolysis can be more difficult owing to the unique characteristics of the neonate's hematologic system.[10, 128]

Site of Sampling

The site of sampling can result in significant variations in values. Capillary hemoglobin values average 2 to 4 g/dl higher than venous values (with differences up to 8 g/dl reported); arterial values average 0.5 g/dl above venous values and are probably of less clinical significance.[10, 84, 116] Capillary hematocrits are 5 to 10% higher than venous hematocrits in newborns.[84] The neonate's hematocrit does not reflect RBC mass as accurately as in an adult, with a correlation of .63 versus .78 in adults.[10] Poorer correlations are reported in ill and preterm infants who are growing rapidly (owing to increased circulating blood volume).

WBC counts can be altered by both sampling site and physical activity. A mean capillary difference of $+1.8 \times 10^9/L$ has been found in neutrophil counts between capillary and arterial samples.[116] Using simultaneously drawn blood samples, venous WBC counts were reported to be 82% and arterial values 77% of capillary values.[25] Intense crying was associated with an increase in WBC counts of up to 146% and a shift to the left in the differential count, with the appearance of more immature forms of WBC in the peripheral circulation.

Differences between capillary and venous blood samples are due to poor circulation and venous stasis in the peripheral circula-

TABLE 5–9
Activity of Hemostatic and Coagulation Factors in Preterm, Term, and Older Infants

FACTOR	PRETERM INFANT	TERM INFANT	AGE AT WHICH ADULT LEVEL IS ATTAINED
Vascular and Platelet Function			
Vasoconstriction	Present	Present	At birth
Capillary fragility	Increased	Normal	At birth
Bleeding time	Normal	Normal	At birth
Platelet count	Normal	Normal	At birth
Platelet function	Markedly decreased aggregative ability	Decreased aggregative ability, clot retraction, and platelet factor 3 availability	Not established
Coagulation			
Whole blood clotting time	Decreased	Decreased or normal	At birth
aPTT (adult normal = 35–45 sec)	70–145 sec	45–70 sec	2–9 months
PT (adult normal = 12–14 sec)	12–21 sec	13–20 sec	3–4 days
TT (adult normal = 8–10 sec)	11–17 sec	10–16 sec	Few days
Thrombotest (II, VII, IX, X)	30–50%	40–68%	2–12 months
XII (Hageman factor)	10–50%	25–60%	9–14 days
IX (PTA)	5–20%	15–70%	1–2 months
IX (PTC)	10–25%	20–60%	3–9 months
VIII (AHF)	20–80%	70–150%	At birth
VII (proconvertin)	20–45%	20–70%	2–12 months
X (Stuart-Power factor)	10–45%	20–55%	2–12 months
V (proaccelerin)	50–85%	80–200%	At birth
II (prothrombin)	20–80%	26–65%	2–12 months
I (fibrinogen (g/dl)	150–300%	150–300%	2–4 days
XII (fibrin-stabilizing factor)	100%	100%	At birth
Fibrin split products (μg/ml)	0–10	0–7	
Antithrombin III	48%	55%	

% = percentage of adult activity; aPTT = activated partial thromboplastin time; PT = prothrombin time; TT = thrombin time; PTA = plasma thromboplastin antecedent; PTC = plasma thromboplastin component; AHF = antihemophilic factor.
Adapted from Bleyer, W.A., Hakami, N., & Shepard, T.H. (1971). The development of hemostasis in the human fetus and newborn infant. *J Pediatr*, 79, 848 with modifications to original table by Shurin, S.B. (1987). Hematologic problems in the fetus and neonate. In A.A. Fanaroff & R.J. Martin (Eds.), *Neonatal-perinatal medicine* (4th ed., p. 853). St. Louis: CV Mosby.

tion. Differences between arterial and venous samples are thought to be due to passage of plasma to the interstitial spaces in the capillary bed with later return to circulation via the lymphatic system.[116] Capillary and venous differences are more marked with decreasing gestational age, after a large placental transfusion, and in infants with acidosis, hypotension, or severe anemia.[10] Prewarming of the heel prior to drawing blood, obtaining a good blood flow, and discarding the initial few drops of blood reduce the magnitude of capillary and venous differences.[84] The site of sampling is critical in interpreting hematologic values in the neonate and should be recorded for all samples. Site-related differences are most marked in those infants for whom accurate determination of hematologic values is most critical.[84]

Iatrogenic Losses

Hematologic parameters are also influenced by iatrogenic losses. Blanchette and Zipursky

note that in the first 6 weeks after birth infants in intensive care nurseries had a mean iatrogenic blood loss equivalent to 22.9 ± 10 ml of packed cells; 46% of these infants had cumulative losses that exceeded their circulating red blood cell mass at birth.[10] Iatrogenic blood losses were greater in ill than in healthy preterm infants (26.9 ± 9 ml versus 14.6 ± 5 ml). In very low birth weight (VLBW) infants these losses were equivalent to a significant proportion of their circulating RBC mass (32.2 to 45.5 ml/kg in the preterm infant). Removal of 1 ml of blood from a 1000 g infant is estimated to be equivalent to removing 70 ml from the average adult.[10] Accurate determination of true anemia versus "anemia" due to blood loss is often dependent on accurate recording of the amount of blood that has been previously drawn for sampling.[10]

Growth Influences

Rapid weight gain results in an obligatory increase in total blood volume that often precedes any change in RBC mass. The ensuing hemodilution can lead to a static or falling hemoglobin even with active erythropoiesis as evidenced by reticulocytosis. [3, 85] The correlation between RBC mass and hemoglobin is low during the first 6 weeks owing to the effects of this hemodilution, so hemoglobin levels do not accurately reflect RBC mass.[128]

Detection of Hemolysis

The detection of hemolytic disease is often problematic in the neonates owing to the characteristics of their hematologic system. The determination of hemolysis usually involves evidence of increased RBC destruction and alterations in morphology.[128] Many of the factors that suggest increased RBC blood cell destruction in the adult (falling hemoglobin, decreased haptoglobin, hemoglobinuria, reticulocytosis, abnormally shaped RBCs, increased production of RBCs, bilirubin, and free plasma hemoglobin) may be present normally in many neonates.[10, 128]

Alterations in Hemoglobin-Oxygen Affinity

The increased affinity of hemoglobin for oxygen is an advantage to the fetus in facilitating oxygen transfer across the placenta but may be a liability for the neonate. Preterm infants who have higher levels of Hb F and lower concentrations of 2,3-DPG are more vulnerable. With increased affinity, oxygen is unloaded less rapidly and efficiently in the peripheral tissues (see Chapter 7). Therefore the newborn may be less able to respond to hypoxia by significantly increasing oxygen delivery to the tissues.[85, 123] The newborn is also lacking in some of the protective responses seen in adults. For example, in adults, but not in neonates, hypoxia tends to stimulate increased production of 2,3-DPG, a response that further facilitates oxygen release to the tissues.[86]

The measurement of arterial hemoglobin saturation (SaO_2) by pulse oximetry is generally as reliable in neonates, who have high levels of Hb F, as it is in adults, whose hemoglobin is predominantly Hb A.[91] This occurs because pulse oximetry is a direct measure of percent saturation, whereas calculating saturation from PaO_2 requires knowledge of the percent concentrations of

Hb A and Hb F in the blood.[36] Pulse oximetry works on a light absorbance principle. The light absorbed by the hemoglobin molecule is absorbed primarily by the heme portion (which is similar in both Hb A and Hb F) and not by the globulin chains (which are different in Hb A and Hb F). Infants with Hb F can have a high SaO_2 (>85%) even with a low PaO_2; therefore, infants on pulse oximeters must also have their PaO_2 levels regularly evaluated. Even if an infant is well saturated, PaO_2 levels must be kept within normal ranges, since this is the driving force for movement of oxygen from the blood to the tissues.

Since the P_{50} of preterm infants is lower than in term infants, the progressive shift to the right of the oxygen-hemoglobin dissociation curve is more gradual in preterm infants and related to postconceptual rather than post birth age.[8, 84] As a result the oxygen unloading capacity in the untransfused preterm infant is reduced for at least the first 3 months.[128] Stockman suggests that there may be some circumstances in which the shift to the left in the oxygen-hemoglobin dissociation curve may be an advantage to the infant by helping to maintain oxygen delivery with severe hypoxemia and low cardiac output.[106]

Vitamin K and Hemorrhagic Disease of the Newborn

The newborn has reduced levels of all the vitamin K–dependent clotting factors (II, VII, IX, X) at birth, leading to a physiologic hypoprothrombinemia. The reduction in these factors is the consequence of poor placental transport of vitamin K to the fetus as well as lack of intestinal colonization by bacteria that normally synthesize vitamin K.[92] The levels of vitamin K–dependent coagulation factors rise at 3 to 5 days post birth, then decrease. This decline is more marked in infants who are breast-fed, have a history of perinatal asphyxia, or are born to mothers on coumarin derivative anticoagulants.[32] Since this decline leads to a bleeding tendency in some newborns, prophylactic vitamin K is given after birth to prevent hemorrhagic disease of the newborn.

Hemorrhagic disease of the newborn (HDN) involves bleeding from the gastrointestinal tract, umbilical cord, or circumcision site; oozing from puncture sites; and generalized ecchymosis. These findings are most commonly manifest 2 to 3 days following birth but may occur earlier, particularly in infants of women on medications such as anticonvulsants, warfarin, and antibiotics. Laboratory findings include reduction in the vitamin K–dependent clotting factors, decreased prothrombin activity, and prolonged clotting and prothrombin times.

A late form of HDN is seen occasionally in infants who do not receive vitamin K at birth and are subsequently breast-fed (breast milk contains very low levels of vitamin K).[128] Prophylactic vitamin K may also be given to preterm and ill infants who are on prolonged antibiotic therapy (particularly with use of the new cephalosporins such as cefotetan). Antibiotics may significantly reduce the normal intestinal bacterial flora essential for vitamin K synthesis and compete for vitamin K in the liver.[48]

Vitamin K is not required for the synthesis of these clotting factors per se but rather for the conversion of precursor proteins synthesized in the liver to activated proteins with coagulant properties.[37, 124] The hypoprothrombinemia commonly present at birth is secondary to decreased levels of these precursor proteins.[32, 84] Term neonates respond to prophylactic vitamin K administration at birth by achieving normal or near normal prothrombin times, although actual values of individual clotting factors may not reach adult values for several weeks or more. The response in preterm infants is less predictable, with minimal response to vitamin K seen in some VLBW infants owing to an inability of the immature liver to synthesize adequate amounts of the precursor proteins.[84, 124]

The need for routine vitamin K prophylaxis in all newborns has been questioned.[32, 77, 78, 129] Recent studies have suggested that although the immunologic and biologic activity of the vitamin K–dependent clotting factors is reduced, the newborn appears to have normal levels of these factors and is not vitamin K deficient.[32, 128] In addition, concentrations of vitamin K–dependent factors do not necessarily increase after vitamin K prophylaxis, especially in healthy infants.[32, 78] Unfortunately, it is difficult to identify which infants need this prophylaxis and which do not, and clinical and research evidence clearly demonstrate the risk of hemorrhage in some infants.[48, 84]

Vitamin K–dependent clotting factors may be further reduced in infants of women taking anticonvulsants such as phenobarbital and diphenylhydantoin (Dilantin) during pregnancy. These agents, especially diphenylhydantoin, tend to concentrate in the fetal liver and inhibit the action of vitamin K in the formation of precursor proteins for Factors II, VII, IX, and X.[33, 113] Women on anticonvulsants are often given vitamin K in the last weeks of pregnancy to reduce the risk of neonatal bleeding. Vitamin K–dependent clotting factors may also be reduced in infants of women on anticoagulants (warfarin) and chronic antibiotic therapy (antituberculosis agents).[48] In addition to receiving the usual dose of vitamin K following birth, these infants must be assessed for signs of bleeding throughout the neonatal period.

Blood Transfusions

Decisions regarding whether or not to transfuse an infant, especially a preterm infant, are often difficult. The advantages of transfusion must be balanced against the consequences and potential risks. Risks of transfusion include infection, metabolic and cardiovascular complications, hypothermia, and graft-versus-host disease.[9, 106]

The major risk from infection arises from blood contaminated with hepatitis B, HIV (human immunodeficiency virus), and cytomegalovirus. Careful screening of donors and blood prior to administration has reduced the risk of infection. Metabolic complications include hypoglycemia (from stimulation of insulin secretion and rebound hypoglycemia due to the high glucose load of transfused citrate-phosphate-dextrose [CPD] or acid-citrate-dextrose [ACD] blood), hyperkalemia (due to transfusion of nonviable cells in blood stored over 5 days), and hypocalcemia (with the use of blood preserved with the anticoagulant citrate, which combines with ionized calcium in the infant's blood). Cardiovascular complications include volume overload, arrhythmias and thromboembolism. Rapid transfusion and volume expansion may increase the risk of intraventricular hemorrhage in VLBW infants. Hypothermia can result from transfusion of unwarmed or inadequately warmed blood. Graft-versus-host disease is an immunologic reaction seen in 0.1 to 1.0% of transfused infants.[16] The risk of graft-versus-host disease can be reduced with irradiation of blood prior to administration.[16, 106] With assessment and monitoring, most complications are preventable.

Following transfusions, particularly exchange transfusions with adult blood, there may be rapid alterations in the oxygen-hemoglobin dissociation curve. These changes are influenced by the characteristics of the blood utilized for the exchange. For example, blood stored over 5 days, especially ACD blood, is characterized by a significant decrease in 2,3-DPG and an increased oxygen-hemoglobin affinity.[128] Transfusion with this type of blood may further impair the infant's oxygen unloading capacity to the tissues.

On the other hand, use of fresh heparinized blood or CPD blood stored for less than 5 days leads to a rapid shift in the P_{50} to adult values.[10] This shift is an advantage to the infant because it improves oxygen release to the tissues but may result in rapid changes in PaO_2, increasing the risk of retinopathy of prematurity (ROP). Following an exchange transfusion or after multiple transfusions, a portion of the infant's Hb F will have been replaced by Hb A, which has a greater ability to unload oxygen. This change can lead to a rapid improvement in the amount of oxygen delivered to the tissues at a given PaO_2 and possible hyperoxia.[106]

Transfusion of Preterm Infants

The major indications for transfusion in preterm infants are (1) to replace significant iatrogenic losses, (2) to treat physiologic anemia, and (3) to improve well-being and weight gain while reducing the incidence of apnea and bradycardia.[62] The most frequent controversies over whether or not to transfuse generally arise with these latter two indicators. Although a low hemoglobin level may be utilized as the criterion for transfusion to treat these forms of anemia, some clinicians suggest transfusions should be used only if the infants are symptomatic.[10, 48, 84, 106, 107, 128] Clinical findings associated with anemia in these infants include tachycardia, tachypnea, lethargy, poor feeding and fatigue with feeding, poor weight gain (<25 g/day), pallor, and possibly apnea or bradycardia.[62, 84, 106, 106] Evidence is conflicting regarding whether or not apnea is a clinical sign of anemia and the effect of transfusion on the incidence of apnea. In many infants transfusion has no effect, while others demon-

strate a decrease in frequency of apnea following transfusion.[11, 38, 57, 62, 106] The basis for a decrease in apnea has been attributed to improvement in the delivery of oxygen to the CNS.[112] Inconsistent findings have also been reported with regard to the effect of transfusion on other parameters such as heart rate, respiratory rate, and growth.[11, 62, 111]

Stockman suggests that a single hemoglobin value is of little clinical use in the decision to transfuse and that one needs to consider the balance between oxygen demand, oxygen supply, and available oxygen.[106] This takes into account the infant's hemoglobin-oxygen affinity, oxygen consumption, blood volume, erythropoietin levels, growth rate, and blood oxygenation. In true anemia, an increase in erythropoietin would be expected.

Clinical findings associated with anemia are seen in preterm infants at widely varying hemoglobin levels, and hematocrit is not a good predictor of RBC mass.[62] Although clinical findings are poorly correlated with hemoglobin levels in the preterm infant, there is a better correlation with available oxygen. Wardrop and colleagues found a linear correlation between available oxygen and gestational age, which they expressed as: available oxygen = $(0.54 + 0.005$ week from conception$) \times$ [Hb] (ml/dl).[118] In general, symptomatic anemia is seen in infants less than 32 weeks, gestational age with an available oxygen value of 7 or less (assuming these infants have not had previous exchange transfusions, or multiple transfusions, which alter their expected Hb F concentration).[106, 118]

Vitamin E and the Preterm Infant

There has been considerable controversy over the existence of vitamin E deficiency anemia in preterm infants. Vitamin E is an antioxidant that prevents lipid peroxidation and hemolysis of RBCs. Highest concentrations of vitamin E occur in membranes with high concentrations of polyunsaturated fatty acids. Vitamin E levels in term and preterm infants are lower than those in adults (0.2 to 0.3 mg/dl versus 0.5 to 2.0 mg/dl). Because of the neonate's lower fat content, the α-tocopherol–to–very-low-density lipoproteins ratio is similar to that in adults. Thus newborns may need less vitamin E than adults and may not be vitamin E deficient per se.[58]

Earlier studies suggested that vitamin E deficiency anemia developed in preterm infants during the 2nd month, and supplemental vitamin E was utilized for many infants.[10, 58, 130] This anemia was most severe in those infants on formulas with high linoleic acid content and concurrent iron supplementation.[130] Recent studies have confirmed that vitamin E deficiency is unlikely to develop in infants who have low intakes of linoleic acid and who are not receiving iron supplements.[58]

Preterm formulas have been modified in recent years to achieve vitamin E–to–linoleic acid ratios of greater than 0.6 mg/g. Mature breast milk has an adequate α-tocopherol–to–total lipid ratio. Preterm breast milk has higher levels of α-tocopherol, which increase over time. Breast-fed infants reach adult vitamin E levels by 2 weeks of age.[58] The American Academy of Pediatrics recommends a minimum vitamin E intake for low birth weight infants of 0.7 IU/100 kcal with at least 1.0 IU α-tocopherol/g of linoleic acid.[28] This is achieved if the infant has a total caloric intake of 100 kcal/kg. If the infant's intake is less, supplementation with an enteral multivitamin complex containing vitamin E may be warranted.[58] Sources of vitamin E in the infant should be evaluated to avoid toxicity, as an infant may be simultaneously receiving supplemental vitamin E in formula, parenteral hyperalimentation, and an enteral multivitamin preparation.

Vitamin E has been suggested for use in the prevention of bronchopulmonary dysplasia (BPD) and ROP.[10, 130] The use of vitamin E with these disorders was based on the rationale that vitamin E is an antioxidant that protects the polyunsaturated lipids of cell membranes from peroxidation by excess free oxygen radicals. (Free oxygen radicals are a toxic by-product of cell metabolism.) Since BPD and ROP are disorders associated with cellular damage from oxygen, the hope was that vitamin E might protect the cells from damage. Results of investigations to date in human infants are conflicting and have not provided adequate evidence to support the efficacy and safety of this therapy.[10, 58, 66, 130] Vitamin E may limit extension of existing intraventricular hemorrhages in very low birth weight (VLBW) infants, but this specific use is still under investigation.[102] The intravenous form of vitamin E (tocopherol acetate or E-Ferol Aqueous Solution) has been linked to a significant increase in neonatal mortality, possibly owing to renal and hepatic damage along with the other toxic effects.[58]

Neonatal Polycythemia and Hyperviscosity

Factors that alter RBC production or neonatal blood volume can lead to polycythemia and hyperviscosity. Neonatal polycythemia is generally defined as a venous hematocrit greater than 65% or hemoglobin greater than 22 g/dl.[4, 45, 83, 128] Oh proposed a model of pathogenesis for polycythemia and hyperviscosity arising from prenatal, intrapartal, and postbirth factors (Fig. 5–10).[83]

Infants who experience chronic hypoxia prior to birth, including infants with IUGR, those born at high altitudes, and possibly infants of diabetic mothers (especially with poor maternal diabetic control during pregnancy) respond to decreased tissue oxygenation by increasing erythropoietin production. Erythropoietin increases erythropoiesis and fetoplacental blood volume.[122] Infants with acute hypoxemia during the intrapartum period may also develop polycythemia owing to fluid shifts from the intravascular to interstitial space and hemoconcentration.

The amount of placental transfusion can rapidly alter the newborn's blood volume, leading to a rise in hematocrit and risk for polycythemia and hyperviscosity. Excessive placental transfusion leads to a total blood volume that exceeds the infant's vascular capacity. Fluid moves from the intravascular to the interstitial space, further increasing RBC volume.[83] Fluid transudation within the lungs can produce respiratory distress, and the increased red blood cell mass leads to hypoglycemia (due to the high glucose utilization of the neonatal red blood cell) and hyperbilirubinemia.

The Infant with a Hemoglobinopathy

Disorders such as thalassemia and sickle cell anemia rarely cause difficulty in the neonatal period because of the neonate's increased levels of Hb F (which consists of two alpha and two gamma chains) in relation to Hb A (two alpha and two beta chains). The neonate with a higher proportion of Hb F has an increased number of gamma chains, fewer beta chains, and similar percentage of alpha chains to those of the adult. Thus disorders of beta chain structure (sickle cell anemia) or synthesis (β-thalassemia) do not manifest themselves until the infant is 1 to 2 months of age or older. On the other hand, alpha

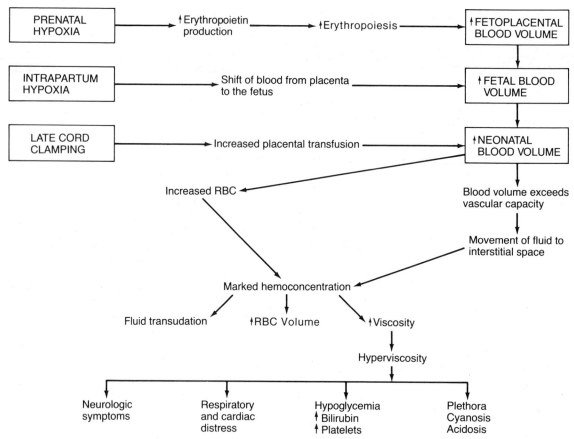

FIGURE 5–10. Neonatal polycythemia and hyperviscosity. (Adapted from Oh, W. (1982). Neonatal polycythemia and hyperviscosity. *Pediatr Clin North Am, 33,* 523.)

chain disorders such as α-thalassemia will be apparent in the neonate.[128]

The Infant at Risk for Altered Hemostasis

Neonates are at increased risk for both thromboembolism and consumptive coagulopathies such as disseminated intravascular coagulation (DIC) owing to alterations in their hemostatic system. The preterm infant, in particular, is at risk for hemostatic problems due to significant decreases in clotting factors, platelet function, and factors protecting against excessive clot formation. Although clotting factors are also decreased in term infants, these infants, unless severely ill, generally do not have impaired hemostasis since only 20 to 30% of most coagulation factors are normally needed for clot formation.[17]

The most common cause of bleeding due to impaired hemostasis in the neonate is DIC

(see Fig. 5–6). The increased risk for this disorder is secondary to decreased levels of antithrombin III and protein C, which normally protect against accelerated coagulation by neutralizing or inhibiting activated clotting factors.[17] Other limitations that make the newborn more susceptible to DIC are a decreased capacity of the reticuloendothelial system to clear intermediary products of coagulation (which stimulate further coagulation and consumption of clotting factors), difficulty in maintaining adequate perfusion of small vessels (resulting in local accumulation of clotting factors and delayed clearance), hepatic immaturity (with delay in compensatory synthesis of essential clotting factors), and vulnerability to pathologic problems known to initiate DIC.[49] Even in preterm infants the major risks for bleeding disorders or thrombosis are not the infant's physiologic limitations per se but rather the presence of other pathologic problems (for DIC) and trauma or indwelling lines (for thrombosis).[18]

Respiratory distress, sepsis, necrotizing enterocolitis, and other severe disease are all associated with one or more of the processes that usually lead to intravascular coagulation: (1) release of tissue thromboplastin (sepsis, severe perinatal asphyxia, and other hypoxic-ischemic events such as severe RDS, necrotizing enterocolitis and CNS hemorrhage), (2) endothelial injury (viral infections), and (3) shock and venous stasis (severe disease that promotes local accumulation of clotting factors and decreased clearance by the liver of activated factors).[63]

Altered hemostasis in the ill VLBW infant, with release of tissue thromboplastin secondary to ischemic events in the germinal matrix microcirculation, may increase the risk of both intraventricular hemorrhage and extension of earlier hemorrhages.[49] Fibrinolytic activity in the periventricular area and germinal matrix is increased, leading to more rapid destruction of fibrin clots that might prevent further hemorrhage.

Thrombosis is more common during the neonatal period than at any other time during childhood.[98] The three factors that predispose to thromboembolism (stasis, altered coagulation, and vascular damage) are present in some neonates.[98, 120] Infants with polycythemia and hyperviscosity have alterations in blood flow with increased platelet adhesion, and thrombi formation in the microcirculation, especially in the bowel, kidneys, and extremities. This may explain the increased risk of renal vein thrombosis in infants of diabetic women, who also have a high incidence of polycythemia.[98] The infant with shock or perinatal asphyxia also has altered flow with hypotension and stasis.[10] Vascular damage can occur prior to birth within placental vessels in association with maternal complications such as PIH or secondary to trauma from indwelling catheters.

The frequency of thrombotic lesions found on autopsy in infants with umbilical artery catheters ranges from 20 to 95%.[10] The umbilical catheter acts as a foreign body along which fibrin is deposited and thrombi form. Infants with these catheters require close observation for vasospasm or emboli formation, especially in the extremities or buttocks. If the extremities or buttocks blanch from vasospasm or emboli the catheter should be removed immediately. If the area becomes blue owing to vasospasm, the contralateral leg can be warmed to induce reflexive vasodilation with removal of the catheter if the vasospasm is not relieved within 10 minutes; others recommend immediate removal. A patent ductus arteriosus may also predispose to thrombi formation.[98]

The newborn is also at risk for thrombi owing to alterations in hemostasis such as the shorter whole blood clotting time, increased levels of factors V and VIII, and altered function along with decreased levels of major naturally occurring anticoagulants (antithrombin III and proteins C and S).[49] Antithrombin III levels are further reduced in small for gestational age (SGA) infants, increasing their risk of thrombosis. The neonatal period is also characterized by decreased fibrinolytic activity, so that once clots develop the infant is less able to remove fibrin and lyse the clots.

Physiologic Anemia of Infancy

Both term infants and preterm infants experience a decline in hemoglobin during the first 2 to 4 months after birth. This process has been termed the physiologic anemia of infancy because the infant is generally able to tolerate the change without any clinical difficulties.[83] Physiologic anemia of infancy results from postnatal suppression of hematopoiesis (Fig. 5–11). Hematopoiesis is controlled by erythropoietin, which increases when oxygen delivery to the tissues is reduced. This hormone stimulates the bone marrow to increase production of RBCs. The low fetal arterial oxygen tension stimulates erythropoietin release, which leads to production of RBCs.

At birth the arterial oxygen saturation rapidly increases, erythropoietin disappears from the plasma, and production of new RBCs is reduced. Owing to the shorter life span of neonatal RBCs, the turnover of these cells is more rapid. Iron released from the destroyed cells is stored in the reticuloendothelial system. With rapid expansion of blood volume due to the infant's rapid growth, hemoglobin levels progressively decrease to 2 to 3 months of age.

Although the decrease in hemoglobin reduces the oxygen carrying capacity of the blood in early infancy, this is balanced by the gradual shift to the right in the oxygen-hemoglobin dissociation curve caused by increasing concentrations of 2,3-DPG and Hb A. As a result the actual amount of oxygen capable of being released to the tissues in-

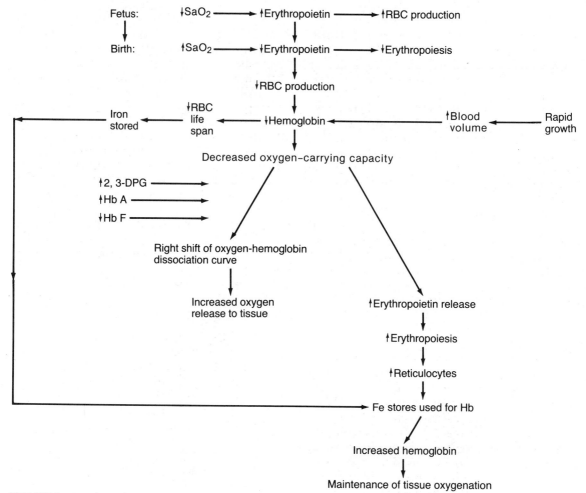

FIGURE 5–11. Physiologic anemia of infancy.

creases.[106] Eventually hemoglobin levels fall to a point where tissue oxygen needs stimulate erythropoietin and resumption of erythropoiesis (Fig. 5–11).

In the term infant the lowest hemoglobin level (11.4 g/dl ± .09) is reached at 8 to 12 weeks; in the preterm infant the lowest levels of 7 to 10 g/dl are reached by 4 to 8 weeks.[84] The decrease in hemoglobin cannot be prevented by nutritional supplements (i.e., iron, vitamin B_{12}, vitamin E) and is not associated with hematologic abnormalities.[84, 112] The lower hemoglobin values in preterm infants are due to decreased iron stores, an altered response of erythropoietin along with a net decrease in RBC mass, RBC survival time and marrow erythroid elements, and rapid

postnatal growth and concomitant increase in circulating blood volume.[84, 128] The drop in hemoglobin may be intensified in sick infants who have had repeated blood sampling.

The resumption of erythropoietin production and erythropoiesis may be delayed in infants who have had exchange transfusion or multiple blood transfusions during the first few weeks post birth. These infants have increased Hb A, which releases oxygen more readily to the tissues, providing less stimulation for erythropoietin production.[128] Strauss points out that the routine use of erythrocyte booster transfusions to maintain hemoglobin levels above 10 g/dl in preterm infants can delay the natural recovery from physiologic anemia by delaying stimulation of erythropoietin and resumption of RBC production (Fig. 5–11), resulting in dependence on further transfusions.[112]

Infants with hemolytic disorders due to isoimmunization may experience a late and often severe anemia that is not physiologic but the result of continued hemolysis. Infants with severe hemolysis who never required an exchange transfusion are at greatest risk for this form of late anemia because of the presence in the infant's blood of maternal antibodies that continue to hemolyze the infant's RBCs. Maternal antibodies are normally removed during an exchange transfusion, reducing the risk of late anemia. The normal hemoglobin decrease after birth is often not seen in infants with cyanotic heart disease, who maintain higher erythropoietin levels and thus higher hemoglobin levels in an attempt to increase oxygen delivery to their tissues.

With resumption of erythropoiesis the reticulocyte count increases to 2 to 8%, followed by a decrease to 1 to 2% after 5 to 6 months. Total body hemoglobin levels also rise. Blood hemoglobin levels may not increase significantly if RBC production only keeps up with growth and the increase in blood volume. In older individuals, the combination of increased production of RBCs (as evidenced by a reticulocytosis) with no change in hemoglobin levels would indicate either hemorrhage or hemolysis. However, during early infancy the infant is growing so rapidly that although total body hemoglobin is increasing, blood hemoglobin values decrease because of hemodilution.[84, 128]

Administration of iron, vitamin E, or folate during this period will not increase the hemoglobin to the level necessary to stimulate erythropoiesis nor diminish the rate of hemoglobin decrease.[128] However, administration of recombinant human erythropoietin (HuEPO) is currently being investigated as a mechanism to maintain the hematocrit level in VLBW infants.[15, 24] Once erythropoiesis is resumed, iron stores are used to produce new red blood cells. The reticuloendothelial system of the term infant has adequate iron stores at this point for another 6 to 12 weeks. After this time hemoglobin levels will again decrease if adequate iron (about 1 mg/kg/day) is not available from dietary sources or as a supplement.[69, 109, 128] In preterm infants or infants who experienced early blood losses, iron stores are reduced and may be depleted by 2 to 3 months of age.

Iron Supplementation

Iron supplementation is generally started prior to the point of depletion to maintain and build up the infant's iron stores. Current recommendations by the American Academy of Pediatrics are for term infants to receive iron supplementation by 4 months and preterm infants by 2 months of age.[28] Supplementation may be in the form of drops or in fortified cereal or milk. Breast milk is low in iron, and although the available iron is more readily absorbed, breast-fed infants still require iron supplementation.

Earlier administration of iron is not recommended in preterm infants owing to the association of early iron administration and anemia in these infants. Iron acts as a catalyst in nonenzymatic oxidation of unsaturated fatty acids, especially in the absence of adequate levels of an antioxidant such as vitamin E, resulting in red blood cell lipid peroxidation and hemolysis. This risk occurs primarily in the first few weeks, when supplemental iron is not needed by the body and vitamin E levels are often low owing to stress and poor fat absorption.[58]

MATURATIONAL CHANGES DURING INFANCY AND CHILDHOOD

Most of the maturational changes in the hematologic system occur during the first 6 to 12 months. The most significant changes are related to the decline in hemoglobin with the resulting physiologic anemia of infancy, accumulation of higher concentrations of 2,3-DPG, and shift of the oxygen-hemoglobin dissociation curve to the left. An awareness of these changes in infancy is necessary for an appropriate evaluation and treatment of anemia and hypoxia.

Changes in Hematologic Parameters

Blood volume values per unit weight are higher than adult values for the 1st month or 2, increasing the risk of hypovolemia.[84] The mean RBC corpuscular volume and mean diameter decrease rapidly during the

1st week, followed by a gradual decrease to diameters similar to those of adult cells by 6 months and to adult volumes by about 1 year.[72] Red blood cell fragility also decreases and is similar to that of adults by 3 months.[84] During the first 2 to 3 months blood and total body hemoglobin levels decrease secondary to decreased RBC production, resulting in the physiologic anemia of infancy discussed previously. Differences between capillary and venous hemoglobin levels persist until 3 months of age.[84] The hematocrit decreases to around 30% by 2 months, then increases to 35% by one year and to adult values in adolescence. Reticulocyte levels reach adult values by 2 years.

Serum ferritin levels rise after birth and remain high for 4 to 6 weeks, with a mean of 356 ng/ml. After this time levels fall to 30 ng/ml (versus 39 in female and 140 in male adults) by 6 months and remain stable until early to mid-adolescence.[8, 84]

With the occurrence of hypoxia, congestive heart failure, or other physiologic stressors, until early childhood the liver and spleen can resume active hematopoiesis and serve as alternate sites for RBC production.[67] Blood tissue in long bones is gradually replaced by adipose tissue beginning at 3 years. By puberty the red marrow in these bones is found only in the upper ends of the humerus and femur and has disappeared by adulthood.[31]

Activity of coagulation factors gradually increases during infancy. Values approach adult levels by 2 weeks to 12 months depending on the individual factor (Table 5–9).

Changes in Oxygen-Hemoglobin Affinity

During the first 3 months after birth the P_{50} gradually increases, and by 4 to 6 months the oxygen-hemoglobin dissociation curve is similar to that of the adult. Hb F concentrations decrease 3 to 4% per week during the first 6 months. By 4 months Hb F accounts for only 5 to 10% of the hemoglobin. The P_{50} gradually increases to adult values by 4 to 6 months of age.[128] From 8 to 11 months the curve may actually be shifted slightly to the right of the adult curve owing to increased blood organic phosphates along with changes in the concentrations of Hb A and 2,3-DPG.[86] Levels of Hb F gradually decrease to adult levels (<2%) by 2 to 3 years. Hb A_2 concen-

TABLE 5–10
Summary of Recommendations for Clinical Practice Related to the Hematologic System: Neonate

Monitor for physiologic effects of early or late cord clamping and to determine whether early clamping is warranted (pp. 180–181; Table 5–6).

Know normal parameters for hematologic values in the preterm and term neonate and patterns of change during the neonatal period (pp. 181–186; Table 5–7).

Recognize changes in hematocrit during the first few days post birth that are due to fluid shifts (versus changes indicating pathologic processes) (pp. 182–183).

Monitor for problems for which the newborn is at increased risk owing to alterations in the neonate's RBC (p. 182; Table 5–8).

Recognize the effects of sampling site and physical activity (especially crying) on hematologic values (pp. 186–187).

Record sampling site and infant activity each time blood is drawn (pp. 186–187).

Prewarm heel prior to drawing blood and discard first few drops (pp. 186–187).

Record amount of blood drawn and other iatrogenic blood loss (p. 187).

Evaluate the amount of iatrogenic blood loss in light of infant's blood volume (p. 187).

Ensure that vitamin K is given following birth (pp. 188–189).

Monitor for signs of hemorrhagic disease of the newborn, especially in infants of mothers on anticonvulsants, anticoagulants, or chronic antibiotic therapy and in infants on long term antibiotic therapy (pp. 188–189).

Recognize laboratory and clinical signs associated with anemia in preterm and term neonates and with anemia of infancy (pp. 182, 190, 193–195).

Recognize laboratory and clinical signs associated with hemolysis in the neonate (p. 188).

Monitor for clinical signs of anemia, anemia of prematurity, and hemolysis (pp. 190, 193–195).

Recognize and monitor for signs of bleeding and disseminated intravascular coagulation, especially in infants at risk (pp. 184–186, 192–193).

Recognize transfusion complications (pp. 189–190).

Monitor PO_2 values regularly in infants on pulse oximetry and maintain within normal limits (p. 188).

Monitor PO_2 and for hyperoxia in infants following transfusions (especially with fresh blood, after multiple or exchange transfusions) (pp. 188, 190).

Monitor intake and ratio of vitamin E and linoleic acid (pp. 190–191).

Evaluate sources of vitamin E and monitor total intake for excess or inadequate amounts (p. 191).

Recognize and monitor for signs of thromboembolism in infants with indwelling lines or who are hypotensive, polycythemic, or in shock (p. 193).

Recognize and monitor infants at risk for polycythemia and hyperviscosity (p. 191, Fig. 5–10).

Ensure that term and preterm infants receive iron supplementation at recommended time points (pp. 193–196).

Page numbers in parentheses following each recommendation refer to pages in the text where rationale is discussed.

trations increase to adult levels of 2 to 3% by 5 months.[84]

The gradual shift of the oxygen-hemoglobin dissociation curve during the first 6 months after birth is determined by the relative proportions of Hb F to Hb A and concentrations of 2,3-DPG. Infants with similar concentrations of Hb F may have different P_{50} values if they have significantly different levels of 2,3-DPG. Similarly, infants with similar levels of 2,3-DPG may have different P_{50} values if concentrations of Hb F are significantly different. Thus an infant with elevated levels of Hb A and low levels of 2,3-DPG may have a P_{50} that is similar to that of another infant with high levels of Hb F and 2,3-DPG.[9, 10, 84, 86] This seeming paradox is explained by what Delivoria-Papadopoulos and colleagues called the functioning DPG fraction: the gradual decrease in affinity of hemoglobin for oxygen during the first 6 months after birth correlates with a fraction derived from multiplying the total RBC 2,3-DPG content by the percentage of Hb A.[37] Thus the two critical factors in determining the position of the oxygen-hemoglobin dissociation curve during infancy are the amounts of Hb A and 2,3-DPG. The rate of postnatal decline in fetal hemoglobin concentrations is generally not affected by persistent cyanosis secondary to cyanotic heart disease.[84]

SUMMARY

The hematologic and hemostatic systems undergo significant alterations during the neonatal period. Because of these changes, the infant is at risk for anemia, thromboembolic insults, and coagulopathies. Many of the changes in the hematologic system encountered in the neonate occur progressively over time. Therefore gestational and post-birth age as well as health status must be considered in evaluating and managing individual infants. Clinical recommendations for nurses working with neonates based on changes in the hematologic system are summarized in Table 5–10.

REFERENCES

1. Aladjem, S., Brown, A.K., & Surreau, C. (1980). *Clinical perinatology.* (pp. 1–31). St. Louis: CV Mosby.
2. Anderson, H.M. (1984). Maternal hematologic disorders. In R.K. Creasy & R. Resnik (Eds.), *Maternal-fetal medicine* (pp. 795–832). Philadelphia: WB Saunders.
3. Arias, F., et al. (1979). Whole blood fibrinolytic activity in normal and abnormal pregnancies and its relation to placental concentrations of urokinase inhibitors. *Am J Obstet Gynecol, 133,* 624.
4. Avery, M.E. & Taeusch, M.D. (1984). *Polycythemia.* Philadelphia: WB Saunders.
5. Bassell, G.M. & Marx, G.F. (1981). Physiologic changes of normal pregnancy and parturition. In E.V. Cosmi (Ed.), *Obstetrical anesthesia and perinatology* (pp. 51–63). New York: Appleton-Century-Crofts.
6. Belscher, N.A. (1971). The effects of maternal anemia on the fetus. *J Reprod Med, 6,* 21.
7. Bennhagen, R. & Holmberg, L. (1989). Protein C activity in preterm and fullterm newborns. *Acta Paediatr Scand, 78,* 31.
8. Bentley, D.P. (1985). Iron metabolism and anaemia in pregnancy. *Clin Haematol, 14,* 613.
9. Blajchman, M.A., Sheridan, D., & Rowls, W.E. (1985). Risks associated with blood transfusion in the newborn infant. *Clin Obstet Gynecol, 28,* 403.
10. Blanchette, V. & Zipursky, A. (1987). Hematologic Problems. In G.B. Avery (Ed.), *Neonatology* (pp. 638–688). Philadelphia: JB Lippincott.
11. Blank, J.P., et al. (1984). The role of red blood cell transfusion in the premature infant. *Am J Dis Child, 138,* 831.
12. Bleyer, W.A., Hakami, N., & Sheppard, T.H. (1971). The development of hemostasis in the human fetus and newborn infant. *J Pediatr, 79,* 853.
13. Bowman, J.M., Pollock, J.M., & Penston, L.E. (1986). Fetomaternal transplacental hemorrhage during pregnancy and post delivery. *Vox Sang, 51,* 117.
14. Brinkman, C.R. (1984). Maternal cardiovascular and renal disorders. In R.K. Creasy & R. Resnik (Eds.), *Maternal-fetal medicine* (pp. 679–690). Philadelphia: WB Saunders.
15. Brown, E.G., et al. (1990). The relationship of maternal erythrocyte oxygen transport parameters to intrauterine growth retardation. *Am J Obstet Gynecol, 162,* 223.
16. Brubaker, D.B. (1986). Transfusion-associated graft-vs-host diseases. *Hum Pathol, 17,* 1085.
17. Buchanan, G.R. (1986). Coagulation disorders in the neonate. *Pediatr Clin North Am, 33,* 203.
18. Buchanan, G.R. (1978). Neonatal coagulation: Normal physiology and pathophysiology. *Clin Haematol, 7,* 85.
19. Burrell, J.M. (1952). A comparative study of the circulating eosinophil levels in babies. *Arch Dis Child, 27,* 337.
20. Burstein, Y., et al. (1977). Thrombocytosis and increased platelet aggregates in newborn infants of polydrug users. *J Pediatr, 94,* 895.
21. Carache, S. & Niebyl, J. (1985). Pregnancy in sickle cell disease. *Clin Haematol, 14,* 729.
22. Chesley, L.C. (1972). Plasma and red cell volumes during pregnancy. *Am J Obstet Gynecol, 112,* 440.
23. CDC. (1989). CDC criteria for anemia in children and childbearing women. *MMWR, 38,* 400.
24. Christensen, R.D. (1989). Recombinant erythropoietic growth factor as an alternative to erythrocyte transfusion for patients with "anemia of prematurity." *Pediatrics, 83,* 793.
25. Christensen, R. & Rothstein, G. (1979). Pitfalls in

the interpretation of leukocyte counts of newborn infants. *Am J Clin Pathol, 72,* 608.

26. Cohen, F., Zuelzer, W., & Gustafsen, D.C. (1964). Mechanisms of isoimmunization. I. The transplacental passage of fetal erythrocytes in homospecific pregnancies. *Blood, 23,* 621.

27. Committee on Iron Deficiency. (1988). Iron deficiency in the United States. *JAMA, 203,* 407.

28. Committee on Nutrition, American Academy of Pediatrics. (1985). Nutritional needs of low birth weight infants. *Pediatrics, 75,* 976.

29. Consumers Association. (1987). Treatment of thromboembolism in pregnancy. *Drug Ther Bull, 25*(1), 1.

30. Corash, L. (1986). Laboratory evaluation of hemostasis. In R.K. Laros (Ed.), *Blood disorders in pregnancy* (pp. 125–149). Philadelphia: Lea & Febiger.

31. Corrigan, J.J. (1989). Neonatal coagulation disorders. In B.P. Alter (Ed.), *Perinatal hematology.* Edinburgh: Churchill Livingstone.

32. Corrigan, J.J. (1981). The vitamin K-dependent proteins. *Adv Pediatr, 28,* 57.

33. Davies, V.A., et al. (1985). Prothrombin status in patients receiving anticonvulsant drugs. *Lancet, 1,* 126.

34. De Boer, K., et al. (1989). Enhanced thrombin generation in normal and hypertensive pregnancy. *Am J Obstet Gynecol, 160,* 95.

35. De Swiet, M. (1985). Thromboembolism. *Clin Haematol, 14,* 643.

36. Deckardt, R. & Steward, D.J. (1984). Noninvasive arterial oxygen saturation versus transcutaneous oxygen tension monitoring in the preterm infant. *Critical Care Medicine, 12,* 935.

37. Delivoria-Papadopoulous, M., Roncevic, N.P., & Oski, F.A. (1971). Postnatal changes in oxygen transport of term, preterm, and sick infants: The role of 2,3-DPG and adult hemoglobin. *Pediatr Res, 5,* 235.

38. DeMaoi, J.G., et al. (1986). The response of apnea of prematurity to transfusion therapy. *Pediatr Res, 20,* 389A.

39. Faxelius, G., et al. (1977). Red cell volume measurements and acute blood loss in high risk newborn infants. *J Pediatr, 90,* 272.

40. Finley, B.E. (1989). Acute coagulopathy in pregnancy. *Med Clin North Am, 73,* 723.

41. Gairdner, D., et al. (1958). The fluid shift from the vascular compartment immediately after birth. *Arch Dis Child, 33,* 489.

42. Garn, S.M., et al. (1981). Maternal hematologic levels and pregnancy outcomes. *Semin Perinatol, 5,* 155.

43. Gerbasi, F.R., et al. (1990). Changes in hemostasis during delivery and the immediate postpartum period. *Am J Obstet Gynecol, 162,* 1158.

44. Gilstrap, L.G. & Gant, N.F. (1990). Pathophysiology of pre-eclampsia. *Semin Perinatol, 14,* 147.

45. Glader, B.E. (1989). Recognition of anemia and red blood cell disorders during infancy. In B.P. Alter (Ed.), *Perinatal hematology.* Edinburgh: Churchill Livingstone.

46. Hallberg, L. (1988). Iron balance in pregnancy. In H. Berger (Ed.), *Vitamins and minerals in pregnancy and lactation.* New York: Raven Press.

47. Halperin, D.S., et al. (1990). Effects of recombinant human erythropoietin in infants with anemia of prematurity: A pilot study. *J Pediatr, 116,* 779.

48. Hathaway, W.E. (1987). New insights on vitamin K. *Hematol Oncol Clin North Am, 1,* 367.

49. Hathaway, W.E. & Bonnar, J. (1987). *Hemostatic disorders of the pregnant woman and newborn infant.* New York: Elsevier.

50. Hayashi, R.H. (1986). Hemorrhagic shock in obstetrics. *Clin Perinatol, 13,* 755.

51. Higgins, P.G. (1982). Measuring nurses' accuracy of estimating blood loss. *J Adv Nurs, 7,* 157.

52. Hiss, R.G. (1986). Evaluation of the anemic patient. In R.K. Laros (Ed.), *Blood disorders in pregnancy* (pp. 1–18). Philadelphia: Lea & Febiger.

53. Holland, B.M., Jones, J.G., and Wardrop, C.A.J. (1987). Lessons from the anemia of prematurity. *Hematol Oncol Clin North Am, 1,* 355.

54. Howells, M.R., et al. (1986). Erythropoiesis in pregnancy. *Br J Haematol, 64,* 595.

55. Hytten, F. (1985). Blood volume changes in normal pregnancy. *Clin Haematol, 14,* 601.

56. Institute of Medicine. (1990). *Nutrition during pregnancy.* Washington, DC: National Academy Press.

57. Joshi, A., et al. (1987). Blood transfusion effect on the respiratory pattern of preterm infants. *Pediatrics, 80,* 79.

58. Karp, W.B. & Robertson, A.F. (1986). Vitamin E in neonatology. *Adv Pediatr Res, 33,* 127.

59. Keleman, E., Calvo, W., & Fliedner, T.M. (1979). *Atlas of human hematopoietic development.* Berlin: Springer-Verlag.

60. Kelleher, C.C. (1990). Clinical aspects of the relationship between oral contraceptives and abnormalities of the hemostatic system. *Am J Obstet Gynecol, 163,* 392.

61. Kelton, J.G. & Cruickshank, M. (1988). Hematologic disorders of pregnancy. In G.N. Burrow & T.F. Ferris (Ed.), *Medical complications during pregnancy* (pp. 65–94). Philadelphia: WB Saunders.

62. Keyes, W.G., et al. (1989) Assessment of the need for transfusion of premature infants and the role of hematocrit, clinical signs and erythropoietin level. *Pediatrics, 84,* 412.

63. Kisker, C.T. (1981). Diagnosis and treatment of coagulopathy in the newborn. *Am J Pediatr Hematol/Oncol, 3,* 192.

64. Kooistra, T. (1990). Studies on the mechanisms of action of oral contraceptives with regard to fibrinolytic variables. *Am J Obstet Gynecol, 163,* 404.

65. Linderkamp, O. (1982). Placental transfusion: Determinants and effects. *Clin Perinatol, 9,* 559.

66. Lloyd, J.K. (1990). The importance of vitamin E in human nutrition. *Acta Paediatr Scand, 79,* 6.

67. Lowrey, G.H. (1986). *Growth and development of children.* Chicago: Year Book.

68. Luegenbiehl, D.L., et al. (1990). Standardized assessment of blood loss. *MCN, 15,* 241.

69. Lundstrom, U., Siimes, M.A., & Dallman, P.R. (1977). At what age does iron supplementation become necessary in the low birth weight infant? *J Pediatr, 91,* 878.

70. Manroe, B.L., et al. (1979) The neonatal blood count in health and disease. I. Reference values for neutrophil cells. *J Pediatr, 95,* 89.

71. Martin, J.N. & Morrison, J.C. (1984). Managing the parturient with sickle cell crisis. *Clin Obstet Gynecol, 27,* 39.

72. Matovcik, L.M. & Mentzer, W.C. (1985). The membrane of the human neonatal red cell. *Clin Haematol, 14,* 203.

73. Matovcik, L.M., et al. (1986). The aging process of

the human neonatal erythrocyte. *Pediatr Res, 20,* 1091.

74. Matthews, J.H., et al. (1990). Pregnancy-associated thrombocytopenia: Definition, incidence and natural history. *Acta Haematol, 84,* 24.

75. McKay, M.L., Martin, J.N., & Morrison, J.C. (1986). Disseminated intravascular coagulation, idiopathic thrombocytopenic purpura, and hemoglobinopathies. In R.A. Knuppell & J.E. Drukker (Eds.), *High risk pregnancy: A team approach* (pp. 440–447). Philadelphia: WB Saunders.

76. Moise, C.P. & Cotton, D.B. (1986). The use of colloid osmotic pressure in pregnancy. *Clin Perinatol, 13,* 827.

77. Molia, R.C., et al. (1990). Evidence against vitamin K deficiency in normal newborns. *Thromb Haemost, 44,* 159.

78. Mori, P.G., et al. (1978). Vitamin K deficiency in the newborn. *Lancet, 2,* 188.

79. Morrison, J.C. & Pryor, J.A. (1990). Hematologic disorders. In R.D. Eden & F.H. Boehm (Eds.), *Assessment and care of the fetus.* Norwalk, CT: Appleton & Lange.

80. Murphy, J.F., et al. (1986). Relationship of haemoglobin levels in the first and second trimesters to outcome of pregnancy. *Lancet, 1,* 992.

81. Nagy, D.A., et al. (1986). Reacting appropriately to thromboembolism in pregnancy. *South Med J, 79,* 1385.

82. Nicholaides, K.H. & Mibashan, R.S. (1989). Fetal red blood cell isoimmunization. In B.P. Alter (Ed.), *Perinatal hematology.* Edinburgh: Churchill Livingstone.

83. Oh, W. (1986). Neonatal polycythemia and hyperviscosity. *Pediatr Clin North America, 33,* 523.

84. Oski, F.A. & Naiman, J.L. (1982). *Hematologic problems in the newborn* (3rd ed.). Philadelphia: WB Saunders.

85. Oski, F.A. (1979). Clinical implications of the oxygen-hemoglobin dissociation curve in the neonatal period. *Crit Care Med, 7,* 412.

86. Oski, F.A. (1973). The unique fetal red cell and its functions. *Pediatrics, 51,* 203.

87. Pauerstein, C.J. (1987). *Clinical Obstetrics* (pp. 593–626). New York: John Wiley & Sons.

88. Pearson, H. (1973). Ontogenesis of blood forming elements. In *Hematology in the perinatal patient* (pp. 3–8). Mead Johnson Symposium on Perinatal and Developmental Medicine, No. 4. Evansville, IN: Mead Johnson.

89. Peck, T.M. & Arais, F. (1979). Hematologic changes associated with pregnancy. *Clin Obstet Gynecol, 22,* 785.

90. Perry, K.J. & Morrison, J.C. (1990). The diagnosis and management of hemoglobinopathies during pregnancy. *Semin Perinatol, 14,* 90.

91. Pologe, J.A. & Raley, D.M. (1987). Effects of fetal hemoglobin on pulse oximetry. *J Perinatol, 7,* 324.

92. Pritchard, J.A. (1965). Changes in blood volume during pregnancy and delivery. *Anesthesiology, 26,* 393.

93. Pritchard, S.L. & Rogers, P.C.J. (1987). Rationale and recommendations for the irradiation of blood products. *CRC Crit Rev Oncol Hematol, 7,* 115.

94. Pritchard, J.A., MacDonald, P.C., & Gant, N. (1985). *Williams' obstetrics* (16th ed., pp. 191–194). New York: Appleton-Century-Crofts.

95. Ramos, J.L.A., et al. (1990). Red cell enzymes and intermediates in AGA term newborns, AGA pre-

term newborns and SGA preterm newborns. *Acta Paediatr Scand, 79,* 32.

96. Rutherford, S.E. & Phelan, J.P. (1986). Thromboembolic disease in pregnancy. *Clin Perinatol, 13,* 719.

98. Schmidt, B. & Zipursky, A. (1984). Thrombotic disease in the newborn infant. *Clin Perinatol, 11,* 461.

99. Sheppard, B.L. & Bonnar, J. (1974). The ultrastructure of the human placenta in early and late pregnancy. *J Obstet Gynaecol Br Comm, 81,* 497.

100. Sher, G. & Statland, B.E. (1985). Abruptio placentae with coagulopathy: A rational basis for management. *Clin Obstet Gynecol, 28,* 15.

101. Shojania, A.M. (1984). Folic acid and vitamin B_{12} deficiency in pregnancy and the neonatal period. *Clin Perinatol, 11,* 433.

102. Sinha, S., et al. (1987). Vitamin E supplementation reduces the frequency of periventricular haemorrhage in very pre-term babies. *Lancet, 1,* 466.

103. Sipes, S.L. & Weiner, C.P. (1990). Venous thromboembolic disease in pregnancy. *Semin in Perinatol, 14,* 103.

104. Stirling, Y., et al. (1984). Haemostasis in normal pregnancy. *Thromb Haemost, 52,* 176.

105. Stockman, J.A. (1981). Red cell transfusion in the newborn: Indications and unique blood banking needs. *Am J Pediatr Hematol Oncol, 3,* 205.

106. Stockman, J.A. (1986). Anemia of prematurity: Current concepts in the issue of when to transfuse. *Pediatr Clin North Am, 33,* 111.

107. Stockman, J.A. & Clark, D.A. (1984). Weight gain: A response to transfusion in selected preterm infants. *Arch Dis Child, 138,* 828.

108. Stockman, J.A. & Oski, F.A. (1978). Erythrocytes of the human neonate. In S. Piomelli & S. Yachnin (Eds.), *Current topics in hematology* (Vol. 1, p. 193). New York: Alan R. Liss.

109. Stockman, J.A. & Oski, F.A. (1978). Physiologic anaemia of infancy and anaemia of prematurity. *Clin Haematol, 7,* 3.

110. Stockman, J.A., et al. (1981). Anemia of prematurity, erythropoietin, and central venous oxygen tension, indicators of adequate tissue oxygenation. *Pediatr Res, 15,* 683.

111. Stockman, J.A., et al. (1984). Anemia of prematurity: Determinants of the erythropoietin response. *J Pediatr, 105,* 786.

112. Strauss, R.G. (1986). Current issues in neonatal transfusion. *Vox Sang, 51,* 1.

113. Svinivasan, G., et al. (1982). Anticonvulsant therapy and hemorrhagic disease of the newborn. *Obstet Gynecol, 59,* 250.

114. Tayler, D.J., et al. (1982). Effect of iron supplementation on serum ferritin levels during and after pregnancy. *Br J Obstet Gynaecol, 89,* 1011.

115. Thomas, R.M., et al. (1983). Erythropoietin and cord blood hemoglobin in the regulation of human fetal erythropoiesis. *Br J Obstet Gynaecol, 90,* 995.

116. Thurlbeck, S.M. & McIntosh, N. (1987). Preterm blood counts vary with sampling site. *Arch Dis Child, 62,* 74.

117. Vander, A.J., Sherman, J.H., & Luciano, D. (1980). *Human physiology: The mechanism of body function* (pp. 319–326). New York: McGraw-Hill.

118. Wardrop, C., et al. (1978). Nonphysiological anemia of prematurity. *Arch Dis Child, 53,* 855.

119. Weiner, C. (1986). The obstetrical patient and

disseminated intravascular coagulation. *Clin Perinatol, 13*, 705.

120. Weiner, C. (1985). Diagnosis and management of thromboembolitic disorders in pregnancy. *Clin Obstet Gynecol, 28*, 107.

121. WHO. (1968). *Nutritional anemias.* Report of a WHO Subcommittee Group, Technical Report Series No. 405. Geneva: WHO.

122. Widness, J.A., Garcia, J.A., & Oh, W. (1982). Cord serum erythropoietin values and disappearance rates after birth in polycythemic newborns. *Pediatr Res, 16*, 218A.

123. Wimberley, P.D. (1982). Fetal hemoglobin, 2,3-diphosphoglycerate and oxygen transport in the newborn premature infant. *Scand J Clin Lab Invest, 160* (suppl.), 1.

124. Yang, Y-M., et al. (1989). Maternal-fetal transport of vitamin K and its effects on coagulation in preterm infants. *J Pediatr, 115*, 1009.

125. Yao, A.C. & Lind, J. (1969). Effect of gravity on placental transfusion. *Lancet, 2*, 505.

126. Yao, A.C., Moinian, M., & Lind, J. (1969). Distribution of blood between the infant and placenta at birth. *Lancet, 2*, 871.

127. Yao, A.C. & Lind J. (1982). *Placental transfusion.* Springfield, IL: Charles C Thomas.

128. Zipursky, A. (1987). Hematology of the newborn infant. In L. Stern & P. Vert (Eds.), *Neonatal medicine* (pp. 681–717). New York: Masson Publishing.

129. Stockman, J.A. (1990). Fetal hematology. In R.D. Eden & F.H. Boehm (Eds.), *Assessment and care of the fetus.* Norwalk, CT: Appleton & Lange.

130. Zipursky, A. (1984). Vitamin E deficiency anemia in newborn infants. *Clin Perinatol, 11*, 393.

CHAPTER 6

Cardiovascular System

Maternal Physiologic Adaptations
    The Antepartum Period
        Hemodynamic Changes
        Oxygen Consumption
        Physical Changes
    The Intrapartum Period
    The Postpartum Period
Clinical Implications for the Pregnant Woman and Her Fetus
    Arrhythmias
    Supine Hypotensive Syndrome of Pregnancy
    Exercise
    Anesthesia and Cesarean Section
    Twins
    Cardiac Disease and Pregnancy
    Pregnancy-Induced Hypertension
    HELLP Syndrome
Development of the Cardiovascular System in the Fetus
    Anatomic Development
        Development of the Primitive Heart
        Septation of the Heart

Functional Development
    Stress-Strain Relationship
    Contractile Properties
    Frank-Starling Relationship
    Afterload
    Inotropy
Neonatal Physiology
    Transitional Events
        Fetal Circulation
        Oxygen Content
        Transition
    Cardiac Physiology
        Metabolic Rate and Oxygen Transport
        Central Mechanisms
        Regulation of Fetal and Neonatal Circulation
Clinical Implications for Neonatal Care
    Fetal Stress Response
    Hydrops Fetalis
    Bronchopulmonary Dysplasia
    Patent Ductus Arteriosus
    Congenital Cardiac Malformations
Maturational Changes During Infancy and Childhood

The circulatory system is the transport system that supplies substrates absorbed from the gastrointestinal tract and oxygen from the lungs to the tissues. It also returns carbon dioxide from the cells to the lungs for disposal; other by-products of metabolism are routed to the kidneys. In addition, the cardiovascular system (CVS) is involved in the regulation of body temperature and the distribution of substances (i.e., hormones) that regulate cellular functioning.

In pregnancy the maternal cardiovascular system must meet the demands of not only the mother but also the dynamically changing fetus. The constant ebb and flow of nutrients and by-products via the uteroplacental system creates a sensitive interdependence between the mother and the fetus. At birth the infant undergoes significant changes in the CVS that if altered may compromise extrauterine existence and postnatal adaptation. This chapter examines alterations in the CVS during the perinatal period and implications for the mother, fetus, and neonate.

MATERNAL PHYSIOLOGIC ADAPTATIONS

Pregnancy is associated with physiologically significant but reversible changes in hemodynamics and cardiac function. These changes are caused by an increased load on the cardiovascular system and increased levels of circulating estrogen, progesterone, and prostaglandin E_1 and E_2. The fetal nutritional requirements, as well as the increased circulating blood mass, placental circulatory system, and gradual increase in body weight over gestation place an increased strain on the cardiovascular system, which is usually met without compromising the mother.

The enlarging uterus limits movement of the diaphragm and causes an increase in intra-abdominal pressure and a change in heart position. All of these influence heart function, but for most women this is not a problem. However, when superimposed upon an existing disease state, in which hemodynamics are already compromised, pregnancy may prove to be a dangerous situation for maternal homeostasis.

On the other hand, if maternal hemodynamics do not change, there can be adverse effects on the uteroplacental circulation and resultant fetal compromise, which may be manifested as fetal malformations (including congenital heart disease), growth retardation, or fetal wastage. Therefore, the maternal cardiovascular system must achieve a balance between fetal needs and maternal tolerance.

During the second stage of labor, expulsive efforts lead to an increase in muscle tension and intrathroacic and intra-abdominal pressure, all of which affect the functioning of the heart and the hemodynamics of the system. Intra-abdominal pressure is abruptly decreased upon delivery and blood pools in the abdominal organs, thereby affecting cardiac return. Blood loss during delivery may also affect hemodynamics.

The Antepartum Period

The major hemodynamic changes that occur during pregnancy are outlined in Table 6–1. The hormonal changes as well as the changes in other organ systems are responsible for these alterations in the cardiovascular system. Anatomic changes such as the upward displacement of the diaphragm by the gravid uterus shift the heart upward and laterally. There is slight cardiac enlargement on x-ray film, and the left heart border is straightened. The size and positioning of the uterus, the strength of the abdominal muscles, and the configuration of the abdomen and thorax determine the extent of these changes.[202]

The hemodynamic changes are partly the result of hormonal influences as well as of the development of the placental circulation and alterations in systemic vascular resistance. These changes include modifications in total body volume, plasma volume, red blood cell volume, and cardiac output.

Hemodynamic Changes

Hemodynamic alterations in pregnancy include changes in blood volume, cardiac output, heart rate, systemic blood pressure, vascular resistance, and distribution of blood flow.

Total Blood Volume. Total blood volume (TBV) is a combination of plasma volume and red blood cell volume, both of which increase during pregnancy. Although there are wide individual variations (20 to 100%), the average TBV increase is between 30 and 50% (1200 to 1500 ml or more) in singleton pregnancies and 50% or above in twin pregnancies.[35, 53, 194] This increase begins early in the first trimester and can be noticed as early as the 6th week of gestation. TBV increases rapidly until mid-pregnancy and then more slowly during the latter half. A plateau or slight decline in circulating volume may occur during the last few weeks of gestation.[8, 79, 118, 168, 179, 194, 204, 227]

The rise in blood volume correlates directly with fetal weight, supporting the concept of the placenta as an arteriovenous shunt on the maternal vascular compartment. Although the degree of hypervolemia varies from woman to woman, subsequent pregnancies in the same woman result in similar increases in circulating volume. Twin pregnancies, however, result in greater increases in blood volume, imposing substantially greater demands on the cardiovascular system.[118, 204]

Red Blood Cell Volume. Red blood cell volume increases throughout pregnancy to a level 33% higher than nonpregnant values (approximately 450 ml).[117, 130] Intravascular expansion is mainly due to an increase in plasma volume, therefore hemodilution oc-

TABLE 6–1
Hemodynamic Changes During Pregnancy

STAGE	HEMODYNAMIC VARIABLE*							
	HR	BP	BV	SV	CO	LVEDP	SVR	PVR
First trimester	Increased	Normal	Increased	Increased	Increased	Normal	Decreased	Decreased
Second trimester	Peaks at 28th week	Slightly decreased	Peaks at 20th week	Peaks at 28th week	Peaks at 20th week	Normal	Decreased	Decreased
Third trimester	Slightly decreased	Normal	Gradually decreased	Gradually decreased	Slightly decreased	Normal	Decreased	Decreased
Labor and delivery	Increased; bradycardia at delivery	Normal	Rises sharply	Decreased	Increased	Normal	Sharply decreased at delivery	Decreased
Postpartum period	Normal within 2–6 weeks	Normal within 2–6 weeks	Normal within 2–6 weeks	Normal within 2–6 weeks	Normal within 2–6 weeks	Normal within 2–6 weeks	Normal within 2–6 weeks	Normal within 2–6 weeks

*HR, heart rate; BP, blood pressure; BV, blood volume; SV, stroke volume; CO, cardiac output; LVEDP, left ventricular end-diastolic pressure; SVR, systemic vascular resistance; PVR, pulmonary vascular resistance.

From Walsh, S. (1988). Cardiovascular disease in pregnancy: A nursing approach. *J Cardiovasc Nurs, 2,* 55.

curs. This physiologic anemia of pregnancy is reflected in a lower hematocrit. Blood hemoglobin levels also fall, reaching levels of 11.6 g/dl.[263] This cannot be prevented with iron supplementation; however, women who are provided exogenous sources of iron do have higher hemoglobin levels in the third trimester than women not receiving supplements.[43, 55, 79, 121a, 203, 263]

Plasma Volume. Seventy-five percent of the TBV increase is in plasma volume. The exact reason for these changes is not completely understood. Alterations in blood and plasma volume are influenced by hormonal effects, mechanical factors (blood flow in uteroplacental vessels), and changes in the renal system and fluid and electrolyte homeostasis (see Chapters 5 and 8 and Fig. 5–2). Fluid balance changes are probably mediated by the hormones of pregnancy.[79]

Plasma renin activity and blood aldosterone levels are increased owing to the action of estrogens and progesterone. An increase in plasma renin activity enhances sodium retention, thereby stimulating aldosterone secretion. Progesterone inhibits aldosterone's renal tubular cell sodium retention activities, thus contributing to sodium retention and an increase in total body water. The degree of fluid retention is influenced by the increased distensibility of the vascular system and the uterine vein capacity present during pregnancy.[63, 79, 140, 141, 150, 163, 239, 262]

Distribution. Fluid distribution changes depending on body position. Supine positioning produces the lowest blood volume, with a decrease being noted after being supine for 1 hour. This is probably due to the trapping of blood in the legs and pelvis as the gravid uterus creates a mechanical impedance to blood flow through the inferior vena cava. This causes an increase in venous pressure in the lower extremities and a sharp rise in hydrostatic pressure in the microcirculation with subsequent leakage of fluid from the vascular bed into the interstitium. The result is edema of the feet and ankles. Venous distensibility contributes to the decreased venous return to the heart.[51, 133, 168, 170, 171, 179, 294]

CARDIAC OUTPUT

Cardiac output is the product of heart rate and stroke volume and is one of the most significant hemodynamic changes encountered during pregnancy. Research conducted in this area over the years is unequivocal owing to the various techniques used in making assessments. For example, impedance measurements underestimate cardiac output by a mean difference of -0.73 L/min.[82] However, some of the more recent research has determined that the majority of pregnancy-induced changes in cardiac output occur during the embryonic period and can be attributed to an increase in stroke volume over heart rate. Capeless and Clapp[45] and Robson and colleagues[220] have demonstrated significant changes in heart rate and stroke volume by 5 weeks' and 8 weeks' gestation, respectively. Cardiac output increases by 1 L/min by 8 weeks, which is a 22% increase over prepregnant values and 57% of the total increase seen at 24 weeks' gestation.[45] By 24 to 28 weeks' gestation, a 30 to 50% increase in cardiac output can be assessed and is associated with an increase in venous return and intensified right ventricular output. An elevated level is then maintained throughout the remainder of the pregnancy.*

The rise in cardiac output early in pregnancy exceeds the heart rate increase and therefore must be due to an increase in stroke volume (30% increase). As pregnancy advances, the heart rate continues to increase (by 10 to 15 beats per minute), becoming a more dominant factor in determining cardiac output. Stroke volume declines during the latter stages of pregnancy, returning to values that are within the normal nonpregnant range. The resting stroke volume is lower at term in the supine position than it is in the postpartum period.[44, 78, 168, 176, 273] Figure 6–1 compares the changes in cardiac output, heart rate, and stroke volume over gestation and into the postpartum period.[167]

During pregnancy (especially the third trimester), the resting cardiac output fluctuates markedly with changes in body position.[181] In the supine position, there is a greater decline in cardiac output than that experienced in the sitting or lateral recumbent position. The compression of the inferior vena cava by the uterus late in gestation (more than 24 weeks) results in a decreased venous return and a markedly decreased cardiac output (20 to 30%). Heart rate changes do not necessarily occur with positional changes, therefore the changes in cardiac output are more likely due to a decrease in stroke volume. There is also no decrease in blood pressure, probably owing to an increase in peripheral vascular resistance.[18, 128, 133, 145, 209, 272, 273]

*References 27, 45, 63, 78, 128, 168, 176, 220, 259, 273, 286, and 298.

The slight decline in cardiac output in the last couple of weeks of pregnancy is more pronounced in the supine position than in the sitting or lateral recumbent position. This lower value is actually less than levels seen 6 to 8 weeks post partum. This decline in cardiac output is another indication of compression of the inferior vena cava by the gravid uterus and is seen even in the sitting position. Tamponade leads to a decreased venous return even in those women with well-established collateral circulation.[18, 78, 79, 109, 168, 272, 273]

Twin and triplet pregnancies have a greater increase in cardiac output than do singletons. The peak is not only greater, but also the decline in cardiac output seen in late pregnancy is smaller. The cardiac output at 20 weeks' gestation is higher than that encountered in a singleton pregnancy and is 15% above normal to the singleton's 10% in late gestation. The maximum cardiac output in multiple pregnancy is also increased by 20%.[78, 168, 229]

The increase in cardiac output is not related to the metabolic requirements of the mother or the fetus, nor to the increase in body mass (which is approximately 13%).[223] At the time the increase occurs, the fetus is relatively small. When fetal growth is accelerated (late in gestation), there is an actual decline in maternal cardiac output. There is, however, a progressive increase in maternal oxygen consumption, which may be due to the metabolic needs of the fetus as well as the demands of the maternal heart and respiratory muscles. However, this increase in oxygen consumption begins at the end of the first trimester and therefore does not help to

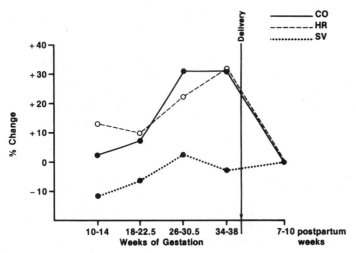

FIGURE 6–1. Percentage of changes in cardiac output (CO), heart rate (HR), and stroke volume (SV) during gestation with the postpartum period used as a control. (From Mashini, I.S., et al. (1987). Serial noninvasive evaluation of cardiovascular hemodynamics during pregnancy. *Am J Obstet Gynecol, 156,* 1208.)

explain the increase in cardiac output seen earlier.

The increased oxygen requirements are most likely the result of the contractility-promoting influences of estrogen and progesterone and the development of the placental circulation. The placenta functions much like an arteriovenous shunt with a concomitant decrease in peripheral vascular resistance. Therefore, despite the increase in cardiac output, there is a decrease in mean blood pressure due to a decrease in diastolic pressure. The concomitant increase in blood volume (either in time or magnitude) probably explains the increase in cardiac output. Both begin to rise as early as 6 to 8 weeks of gestation, peaking toward the end of the second trimester, being 40 to 50% higher than prepregnant levels. Figure 6–2 compares the rise in cardiac output and blood volume over gestation.[78, 95, 99, 119, 168, 223, 267]

Changes in uterine blood flow might also be proposed as an explanation for the increased cardiac output. At the end of the first trimester, uterine blood flow is 100 ml/min, increasing to 500 ml/min by term. The progressive rise in uterine blood flow, however, does not parallel the resting maternal cardiac output changes. Therefore, uterine blood flow can account for only a portion of the increase in cardiac output seen at 20 weeks.[268]

Filling pressures in the heart are not elevated; therefore the increase in circulating blood volume cannot explain the cardiac output changes. Steroid hormones and prolactin may cause changes in hemodynamics by directly affecting the myocardium. Estrogens may alter the actomyosin–adenosine triphosphatase (ATPase) relationship in the myocardium, thereby increasing the contractility of the heart and altering the stroke volume.

This same effect can be seen when oral contraceptives are used.[19, 38, 168, 192, 285] Further research is needed in this area to determine the significance of hormonal influences upon the myocardium and the clinical features of pregnancy.

HEART RATE

Heart rate is the determinant of cardiac output that has the widest range (60 beats per minute to 200 beats per minute in women of childbearing age). The wide range provides stability to the circulatory system under a variety of circumstances (e.g., rest to maximal exercise). Heart rate can be altered in order to maintain blood pressure if changes in vascular resistance or stroke volume are encountered. However, an increased heart rate is insufficient to increase cardiac output; it must be accompanied by an increase in venous return. Both heart rate and venous return are increased in pregnancy, contributing to the increase in cardiac output seen throughout gestation.[181]

The maternal heart rate increases progressively during pregnancy, averaging a 15 to 20 beat per minute increase (20% increase) over the nonpregnant state.[144] Clapp has shown that this increase in heart rate is seen as early as 4 weeks' gestation.[59] This suggests that a hormonal mechanism not normally active is affecting the sinus node and the myometrium.[59, 181] The early augmentation in cardiac output can probably be attributed to this relative maternal tachycardia prior to 20 weeks' gestation.[144]

The increased heart rate results in an elevated myocardial oxygen requirement, which is probably not important in women without cardiac disease, but may become significant in pregnant women with underlying cardiovascular pathology. Beyond this, the

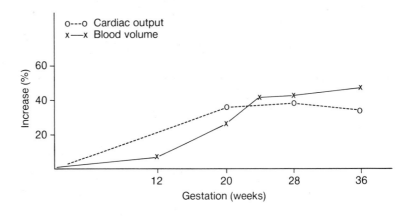

FIGURE 6–2. Changes in cardiac output and blood volume throughout pregnancy. (From Romen, Y., Masaki, D.I., & Mittelmark, R.A. (1991). Physiological and endocrine adjustments to pregnancy. In R.A. Mittlemark, R.A. Wiswell, & B.L. Drinkwater (Eds.), *Exercise in pregnancy* (2nd ed., p. 15). Baltimore: Williams & Wilkins.)

increased resting heart rate decreases the maximal work capacity by diminishing the output increment that can be achieved during maximal exercise.[181]

At term, the heart rate may return to baseline levels in some women. Maternal position may affect heart rate; heart rate is higher in a sitting or supine position and slightly lower in the lateral recumbent position. Twin pregnancies have an earlier acceleration in heart rate, with a maximum increase 40% above the nonpregnant level near term.[44, 79, 202, 258]

STROKE VOLUME

Left ventricular stroke volume is the result of the shortening and thickening of the ventricular muscle against a closed mitral valve. The determinants of muscle shortening are muscle length before shortening (preload), average muscle stress during shortening (afterload), and intrinsic strength of the muscle (contractility). Preload and contractility can be reflexively altered to meet instantaneous demands; however, long-term changes in stroke volume are most affected by altering heart size. Preload is based on Starling's law, which states that lengthening of the filaments of the sarcomere during diastole increases the amount of shortening that occurs during the subsequent systole. This lengthening of filaments, however, could not explain the entire 30% increase in stroke volume that is encountered during pregnancy, in that supine positioning in nonpregnant individuals places them near the top of their Starling curve. The importance of preload changes and their effect on stroke volume are unclear and await futher research.

Afterload is a measure of muscle stress and requires accurate measurements of ventricular dimensions and pressures during systole. These have not been done during pregnancy. However, it is unlikely that reduced afterload is responsible for the increase in stroke volume seen during pregnancy. Intraventricular volume and rate of ejection in pregnancy are increased; however, the effects of these seem to be offset by a diminished aortic impedance (which is determined by systemic vascular resistance and aortic compliance). In pregnancy a large, relatively thin left ventricle delivers a larger stroke volume to a compliant, low-resistance arterial circuit. Therefore, myocardial mechanics and vascular impedance are matched to provide an increased cardiac output at a normal or slightly reduced arterial pressure.[181]

Morton points out that intrinsic contractility measurements during pregnancy have not been done.[181] Therefore, changes in this parameter during pregnancy are not known, although extrapolation of data may indicate a small increase in contractility that would lead to an increase in stroke volume.

Stroke volume increases progressively during the first and second trimesters, to a peak value of approximately 30% above nonpregnant values.[181] After 20 weeks' gestation, stroke volume assumes the primary responsibility for increased cardiac output. This is presumably due to the increased end-diastolic volume changes that are observed on M-mode echocardiography. Left ventricular eccentric hypertrophy has also been observed, being reversible by 6 weeks post partum.[144] Morton and coworkers suggest that this augmented stroke volume is due to a shift to the right of the left ventricular pressure volume curve as a result of the Frank-Starling mechanism and the hypervolemia of pregnancy.[182]

BLOOD PRESSURE

Although there are substantial increases in both blood volume and cardiac output during pregnancy, they are not associated with increases in either venous or arterial pressure.[19, 181] In fact, systolic and diastolic blood pressures begin to fall in the first trimester, decreasing until mid-pregnancy and gradually returning to the nonpregnant baseline by term. Serial observations show that as women advance through their pregnancies there is a slight fall in systolic blood pressure associated with a considerable decrease in the diastolic pressure, leading to an increase in pulse pressure. The magnitude of these changes varies from study to study. The reduction in blood pressure is probably due to hormones that mediate a decrease in peripheral vascular resistance.[56, 90, 121, 128, 176, 291]

Both age and parity have significant effects on blood pressure during pregnancy. Christianson demonstrated that as parity increases (regardless of age) both the systolic and diastolic blood pressures decrease with the greatest difference being between nulliparas and primiparas. As maternal age advances (greater than 35 years), systolic pressure remains unchanged. Diastolic pressure, however, gradually increases with age.[56] A previous study showed that systolic pressures rise steadily from 30 years of age.[164]

There is also a lack of change in venous pressures during pregnancy, which is surprising. The equilibrium pressure in the circulation (mean circulatory filling pressure) is linearly related to blood volume with cessation of cardiac activity. Therefore, given the large increase in blood volume during pregnancy, an increase in venous pressure would be expected. This lack of change can be explained by the increased vascular capacitance and compliance seen during pregnancy. These changes are probably due to the effects of estrogen.[181] Venous pressure below the uterus is increased,[182] which may be caused by the increased capacitance encountered in the large pelvic veins and the veins distal to the uterus. The latter may affect venous return to the heart, especially in the upright position, owing to regional pooling. Late in gestation the gravid uterus may also contribute to reduced venous return and pooling in all positions except the lateral recumbent position. The ability to sustain venous return is crucial in determining maternal exercise capacity (see section on maternal exercise).[181]

SYSTEMIC VASCULAR RESISTANCE

Systemic vascular resistance (mean arterial pressure divided by cardiac output) is decreased during pregnancy. The slight decrease in mean arterial blood pressure and the marked increase in cardiac output indicate a significant decrease in systemic vascular resistance. This is due to the addition of the low-resistance uteroplacental circulation, which receives a large proportion of cardiac output. Although of major impact on vascular resistance, the decline in resistance is not limited to the uteroplacental circulation.[79, 144]

Reductions in systemic vascular resistance can be seen with the administration of estrogen and progesterone in oral contraceptives. Administration of estrogen and prolactin in animals has also lowered vascular resistance. The hormonal activity of pregnancy probably plays a significant role in the reduction of systemic vascular resistance throughout the body and contributes to changes in regional blood flow. Along with this, the increased heat production by the fetus results in vasodilatation of vessels (especially in heat-losing areas such as the hands) and further reductions in resistance.[79]

REGIONAL BLOOD FLOW

The distribution of the increased cardiac output of pregnancy is not well known in humans. Limited research with flow monitoring techniques has led to varied results. However, the increase in cardiac output above the needs of the uteroplacental circulation leads to increased flow to other organ systems. This creates a reservoir that can be tapped as pregnancy progresses.

Mammary blood flow is probably increased; currently no studies have been done documenting this. Clinically increased flow is evident by the engorgement that occurs early in pregnancy and the dilatation of veins on the surface of the breasts. This dilatation is usually accompanied by a sensation of heat and tingling.[176]

The effect of pregnancy on coronary artery blood flow is unknown. With the increased workload of the left ventricle (owing to the increased cardiac output, blood volume, fetal growth, uterus enlargement, and body weight gain), it can be assumed that the coronary blood flow is increased to meet the cardiac myometrial demands. Hepatic and cerebral blood flow are not significantly altered during pregnancy.[78, 121, 169, 186]

Uterine Blood Flow. The decline in uterine vascular resistance allows blood flow to the uterus to increase during gestation. At 10 weeks' gestation the blood flow is approximately 50 ml/min, increasing to 200 ml/min by 28 weeks and 500 to 600 ml/min at term. This indicates that the uterus is receiving between 10 and 20% of the total cardiac output.[17, 99, 144, 173, 225] It is generally believed that the uterine vascular bed is widely dilated and not capable of autoregulation. Therefore, uterine oxygen consumption and fetal oxygenation are maintained by increased oxygen extraction rather than by increases in blood flow. Studies demonstrate that fetal oxygenation can be maintained in this fashion until uterine blood flow decreases by 50%.[144, 160]

The reasons for the increased blood flow are not entirely clear. Early suggestions of endometrial erosion and the development of arteriovenous fistulas as the reason for increased flow were not supported by research. The endometrial arteries undergo marked changes during pregnancy (see Chapter 2) that disrupt their muscular and elastic elements (see Figure 2–15). As a result, the uteroplacental arteries are almost completely dilated and are no longer responsive to circulating pressor agents or influences of the autonomic nervous system. These changes may be mediated by placental production of PGI_2.[284a]

Greiss and Anderson demonstrated a relationship between hormonal activities and hemodynamic changes in the uterus.[99] Oophorectomy led to a reduction in uterine blood flow to barely recordable levels in their research. Injection of estradiol returned flow to the uterus. Intravenous injection of angiotensin II in animals has also resulted in an increase in uterine blood flow. This suggests that both steroid hormones and the renin-angiotensin system may contribute to the changes in uterine blood flow encountered during pregnancy.[47, 79, 85]

Renal Blood Flow. Renal blood flow increases early in gestation, reaching an average peak of about 30% above the nonpregnant state. Once at its peak, the blood flow stays stable or decreases slightly until term (when measured in the lateral decubitus position). However, renal blood flow becomes very sensitive to changes in body position as pregnancy progresses. The decline in flow is probably due to the gravid uterus impeding flow through the vena cava.[50, 52, 144, 152, 175]

The glomerular filtration rate increases to a maximum of 50% over nonpregnant levels. This is the result of increased renin plasma flow. The decrease in renal vascular resistance may be mediated by prostacyclin, allowing for the increase in blood flow.[144]

Skin Perfusion. The research conducted by Katz and Sokal demonstrated a significant increase in skin perfusion during pregnancy. There appears to be a slow but steady rise in perfusion up to 18 to 20 weeks' gestation. This slow rise is followed by a sharp increase between 20 and 30 weeks, with no significant increase after that. This increased flow is measurable for up to 1 week post partum.[40, 50, 61, 129, 144]

Clinically this increased flow can be indicated by an increase in skin temperature and clammy hands, which are the result of dermal capillary dilatation. Vascular spiders and palmar erythema can be seen in approximately 60% of white women during pregnancy. This vasodilatation may facilitate the dissipation of excessive heat created by fetal metabolism. Increased peripheral flow can also be seen in the mucous membranes of the nasal passages, explaining the nasal congestion that is common in pregnancy (see Chapter 7).[22, 121, 144, 148]

Extremity Blood Flow. Studies looking at extremity blood flow (forearm and leg) have provided inconclusive if not conflicting data. More recent studies have indicated that there is a progressive rise in blood flow in both the hands and feet during pregnancy. These changes begin early in gestation and continue into the postpartal period, lasting up to 6 to 8 weeks post partum. The flow in twin pregnancies is somewhat higher after the 30th week as compared to that in single pregnancies.[1, 41, 94, 252]

Pulmonary Vascular Blood Flow. Pulmonary vascular blood flow increases secondary to increased circulating blood volume and increased cardiac output. This can be demonstrated on roentgenogram by increased vascular markings. Pulmonary vascular resistance is decreased, probably in response to hormonal stimulation, and is reflected in a lowered mean pulmonary artery pressure. Pulmonary capillary wedge pressure, however, remains within normal limits throughout pregnancy.[19]

Oxygen Consumption

Oxygen consumption is a reflection of metabolic rate. In pregnancy there is a progressive increase in resting oxygen consumption, with a peak increase of 20 to 30% at term. This increase in oxygen consumption is due to the increased metabolic needs of the mother and the growing fetus.[44, 189, 206]

There is a difference between the changes in cardiac output and oxygen consumption, however. Oxygen consumption increases gradually over gestation, whereas cardiac output increases dramatically in the first and second trimesters. Because the resting cardiac output increases before there is a significant rise in maternal oxygen consumption, the arteriovenous oxygen difference is small in early pregnancy and increases as oxygen consumption increases in the later phases of pregnancy. This provides the embryo with well-oxygenated blood flow during the period of organogenesis, prior to the completed development of the fetoplacental circulation.[19, 101, 175, 192]

Physical Changes

The physiologic hypervolemia of pregnancy results in alterations in the cardiac silhouette, chamber size, pressures, and electrocardiogram. These changes along with the hemodynamic alterations lead to changes in the physical findings encountered during cardiovascular assessment.

The pregnant woman often experiences reduced exercise tolerance, tiredness, and dyspnea. Hyperventilation is common, and basilar rales may give the impression of heart failure. These rales, however, are a normal development during gestation and are caused by the compression and atelectasis of the lower portions of the lungs by the enlarging uterus.

As the uterus grows, the diaphragm is displaced upward and the heart shifts to a more horizontal position. The left ventricular point of maximum impact is easily palpated and may be shifted to the left. A right ventricular impulse can usually be palpated at the mid to lower left sternal border; this is the pulmonary trunk. Difficulty in localizing this point may be caused by the enlarged breast tissue.

The arterial pulse is full, becoming sharp and jerky between 12 and 15 weeks. This finding remains until 1 week after delivery. Jugular vein pulsations are more readily seen, as vein distention appears around 20 weeks' gestation. A venous hum may be associated with the rapid downward flow through the jugular veins. This is indicative of a rapid circulation and high cardiac output state.[71, 73, 104, 195]

Edema of the ankles and legs is a frequent finding during the latter part of pregnancy. As maternal age increases, edema is more common. An increase in capillary permeability and the fall in colloid osmotic pressure in the plasma, along with the increase in femoral venous pressure, are implicated in edema formation.[28, 120, 218, 253]

HEART SOUNDS

Auscultation of the heart reveals an exaggerated split and loudness of both components of the first heart sounds (mitral and tricuspid valve closure). These changes can be heard for the first time between 12 and 20 weeks and continue into the postpartum period (2 to 4 weeks). Nearly 90% of pregnant women will have a split first sound that is best heard at the left sternal border between the third and fifth intercostal spaces. This change is primarily due to the earlier closure of the mitral valve.[71, 79, 144]

There are no significant changes in the aortic and pulmonic elements of the second heart sound during the first 30 weeks of gestation. During the last 10 weeks the interval between aortic and pulmonary closure may increase, varying with respiration. This change may be due to the reduced diaphragmatic movement secondary to uterine size.[71, 79, 120, 144]

Eighty-eight percent of women develop a split first sound during their pregnancy; 92 to 95% demonstrate a systolic murmur. The latter is a common manifestation that is indicative of the increased cardiovascular load. It is especially evident in the last two trimesters.[71, 144]

This is considered an innocent murmur that is usually short, heard in early to midsystole. Such murmurs are best auscultated along the left sternal border in the third intercostal space, although some are more prominent along the lower left sternal border at the apex or aortic area. These murmurs have a musical quality and represent audible vibrations caused by ejection of blood from the right ventricle into the pulmonary trunk or from the left ventricle into the brachiocephalic arteries at the point of branching from the aortic arch. These vibratons usually disappear by postpartum day 8. For approximately 20% of women the systolic murmur persists beyond 4 weeks post partum. The intensity of the murmur does, however, decrease by day 8 even if it does not disappear.[71, 79, 120]

In the normal population, diastolic murmurs are indicative of underlying heart disease. However, in the pregnant population diastolic murmurs can be present without evidence of disease. These murmurs are thought to be due to an increased blood flow through the tricuspid or mitral valve or to the physiologic dilatation of the pulmonary artery in pregnancy. A third heart sound, venous hum, or mammary souffle may be misinterpreted as a diastolic murmur.[79, 120]

Fourteen percent of women have murmurs of mammary vessel origin. Seventy percent are continuous, whereas the other 30% are heard only during diastole. They are more common in lactating women, but can be auscultated during pregnancy as well. Often unilateral, these murmurs are best heard at the right or left second to fourth intercostal space lateral to the left sternal border. They can be changed or obliterated by varying the pressure applied by the stethoscope. The mammary souffle is an indication of the increased blood flow in the mammary vessels. The murmur disappears after the termination of lactation.[79, 120, 195]

ELECTROCARDIOGRAPHIC CHANGES

The electrocardiogram changes as the position of the heart shifts with the enlarging uterus. Electrocardiogram changes include a left axis deviation in some studies and no change in others. A small Q wave and inversion of the P wave are not uncommon. T-wave and ST-segment changes also can be seen.[33, 120, 195, 278]

As the heart size increases, there seems to be an increased incidence of arrhythmias usually of a supraventricular tachycardia nature. Benign arrhythmias that were present prepregnancy may intensify or progress. Labor may lead to an increase in not only the number of arrhythmias but also the variety of arrhythmias. One study conducted during labor showed arrhythmias in every case studied.[278] The arrhythmias identified included premature ventricular contractions, atrial premature beats, premature nodal contractions, sinus bradycardia, sinus tachycardia, and supraventricular tachycardia.[120, 238, 278]

During the second stage of labor, each contraction produces a Valsalva maneuver that leads to a slowing of the heart rate by 35 to 50%. This slowing is followed by a compensatory tachycardia that dissipates to baseline as the uterus and the patient relax.[278]

ECHOCARDIOGRAPHIC CHANGES

Echocardiography demonstrates an increase in left and right end-diastolic dimensions during the second and third trimesters. This is probably due to the expanded blood volume and increased filling during diastole. The increased stroke volume that accompanies this added volume maintains the end-systolic dimensions of the left ventricle at nonpregnant levels. These findings are supported when cardiac catheterization data are reviewed. The right ventricular diastolic pressure is slightly increased over the nonpregnant values. On the other hand, the right ventricular systolic pressure is just below the nonpregnant values (25 to 30 mmHg). This is probably due to the diminished mean pulmonary artery pressure and decreased pulmonary vascular resistance.[35, 79, 230]

These changes in clinical signs and symptoms during pregnancy may lead to inappropriate diagnosis of heart disease. A complete cardiac history, careful physical assessment, and an understanding of the changes, differential diagnosis, and norms related to pregnancy should limit cardiac referrals to those women who warrant specialized evaluation and monitoring.

The Intrapartum Period

During the intrapartum period the repetitive, forceful contractions of the uterus as well as pain, anxiety, and apprehension can have an effect on the cardiovascular system. The pain and anxiety may have more of an impact in primiparous women.[5, 39, 109, 144]

Each contraction contributes approximately 300 to 500 ml of additional volume to the circulation.[259] This results in a significant increase in cardiac output. Hendricks and Quilligan demonstrated a 31% increase in cardiac output over that found in a resting state.[109] They hypothesized that the contractions led to an improved venous return, transient tachycardia, and an increased circulating volume, thereby explaining the increase in cardiac output. The increase in pulmonary arterial-venous oxygen difference also supports this hypothesis, suggesting that there is a sudden influx of blood from the maternal vascular bed into the systemic circulation.[102, 109, 192, 276] The first stage of labor is associated with a progressive rise in cardiac output. Kjeldsen found cardiac output to increase by 1.10 L/min in the latent phase of labor, 2.46 L/min during the accelerating phase, and 2.17 L/min in the decelerating phase.[137]

Other factors that contribute to the increase in cardiac output include pain and anxiety, as well as position and anesthesia. Hendricks and Quilligan noted a 50 to 61% increase in cardiac output in women experiencing pain and anxiety alone.[109] This was accompanied by a rise in both systolic and diastolic blood pressures and heart rate. This suggests that the increase in sympathetic tone due to pain, anxiety, and muscular activity might be the major factor in the increased cardiac output during contractions rather than an increase in circulating volume.

Ueland and Hansen reported that the increase in cardiac output during labor was not as pronounced when the woman was given caudal anesthesia as compared with local anesthesia (paracervical or pudendal blocks).[276] Caudal anesthesia also appeared to prevent progressive increases in cardiac output during labor, as well as limiting the absolute increase in cardiac output when assessed immediately post delivery. This supports the concept that alleviation of pain and anxiety can influence the hemodynamic changes seen during labor.

Supine positioning results in lower cardiac outputs, increased heart rates, and decreased stroke volumes.[272] Movement from the supine to the lateral decubitus position leads to an increase in cardiac output (22%), a fall in pulse rate (6 beats per minute), and an increase in stroke volume by 27%.[3, 272, 275]

Uterine contractions also have an effect on heart rate and blood pressure. There is a variable response in heart rate depending on the research reviewed. Ueland and Hansen demonstrated a 7.6% decrease in heart rate and a 22% increase in stroke volume in supine patients.[276] These changes were less when women were placed in the lateral decubitus position, although cardiac output between contractions in this position was actually higher. These variable responses may be the result of the use of different drugs during labor or the individuals' physiologic variances in response to contractions.[3, 110, 137, 226, 276]

Systolic and diastolic blood pressures increase during uterine contractions. During the first stage of labor there may be a systolic increase of 35 mmHg, which may climb higher during the second stage. The diastolic pressure increases 25 mmHg and 65 mmHg in the first and second stages of labor, respectively. The increase in blood pressure precedes the onset of the contraction by 5 to 8 seconds and returns to baseline once the contraction subsides. Since peripheral vascular resistance increases only slightly during labor, the increase in blood pressure is attributed to the elevated cardiac output. The redistribution of blood flow to the upper body after compression of the distal aorta and common iliac artery probably plays a role in the pressure measured within the arm.[30, 69, 84, 292]

Method of delivery may also influence maternal hemodynamics. The greatest hemodynamic changes are encountered with vaginal deliveries. Ueland and colleagues have demonstrated the greatest changes in cardiac output in vaginal deliveries in which local or caudal anesthesia is used.[270, 271, 275] Balanced general anesthesia allows for reasonable hemodynamic stability, with transient changes occurring during intubation and ex-

tubation. The best results were obtained using epidural anesthesia without epinephrine.[270, 271]

Robson and colleagues in a more recent study concluded that cesarean section under epidural anesthesia resulted in a relatively small change in maternal hemodynamics.[221] Systolic blood pressure showed no significant changes, whereas diastolic pressure was lower at 24 to 48 hours post delivery than preoperatively. Heart rate remained stable during the operation and during the first 48 hours after delivery. After that, the heart rate fell. Stroke volume stayed stable after the epidural was established and then increased after delivery of the placenta. Cardiac output followed the same pattern, with the cardiac output remaining elevated for 15 to 20 minutes after delivery and a return to preoperative values by 1 hour. This reduction in cardiac output occurs earlier than in vaginal deliveries. The rest of the postnatal changes are comparable to those encountered in vaginal deliveries. Therefore, in situations in which changes in maternal hemodynamics during labor may be detrimental (e.g., maternal cardiac disease), cesarean section under epidural anesthesia provides an acceptable alternative.

The Postpartum Period

Delivery of the fetus, placenta, and amniotic fluid results in dramatic maternal hemodynamic alterations that can result in cardiovascular instability during the immediate postpartal period. These changes are due to the loss of blood at delivery and the body's compensatory mechanisms. On the average, 500 ml of blood is lost in vaginal deliveries and 1000 ml in cesarean sections. Despite this "hemorrhage," cardiac output is significantly elevated above prelabor levels for 1 to 2 hours post partum.[201] Immediately post delivery, cardiac output is 60 to 80% higher than prelabor levels. However, within 10 minutes there is a sharp decline to levels that stabilize for the next couple of hours. Cardiac output then remains unchanged for days, even weeks, postpartally. Somewhere between weeks 2 and 4 the cardiac output returns to nonpregnant levels.[3, 29, 109, 276]

Several factors may contribute to this transient increase in maternal cardiac output. These include reduction in gravid uterus pressure and improved venacaval blood flow, autotransfusion of uteroplacental blood back into maternal circulation, and decreased systemic vascular resistance and vascular capacitance due to contraction of the muscular uterus and absence of placental blood flow.[144] Mobilization of extracellular fluid also improves venous return to the heart. The increased return to the heart contributes to the higher central venous pressure seen postpartally.

Maternal hypervolemia acts as a protective mechanism for excessive blood loss at delivery. Normal pregnant women can lose 20 to 30% of their predelivery blood volume with little change in hematocrit. Eclamptic women, who do not expand their vascular space normally, may not tolerate normal delivery blood loss well. In vaginal deliveries there is a steady decline in blood volume over the initial few days post partum. Women who undergo cesarean sections, on the other hand, stabilize their blood volume soon after delivery, and it may remain at the same level for days. Vaginal delivery is associated with a 10% decrease in blood volume as compared to a greater loss by 1 hour post partum in cesarean deliveries (17%). By the 3rd postpartum day, however, both groups had experienced a 16% blood loss.[274]

Despite this comparable blood volume loss, hematocrits in vaginal deliveries rose by 5.2%, whereas women who delivered by cesarean section demonstrated a fall in hematocrit of 5.8%. Therefore, the volume loss in women delivering vaginally was primarily due to diuresis with a rising hematocrit. The falling hematocrit in cesarean sections could be attributed to a compensatory hemodilution from the more extensive blood loss.[144, 274]

Kjeldsen found a 12% decrease in heart rate postpartally that was associated with a 38% increase in stroke volume 2 hours after delivery (as compared to prelabor values).[137] These changes contribute to the 20% increase in cardiac output seen during this time.

During the 1st week following delivery there is a decrease in the sodium space compartment by 2 liters. This results in a 3-kg weight loss. Diuresis in order to dissipate the increased extracellular fluid occurs between day 2 and day 5. Without the diuresis of mobilized extracellular fluid, increased pulmonary wedge pressures and pulmonary edema can result.[54, 144, 202] The latter is encountered in women with preeclampsia or heart disease who do not undergo normal diuretic patterns. Wedge pressures eventually normalize once diuresis occurs.[144]

Most of the cardiovascular system changes resolve by 6 to 8 weeks post partum. Extracellular fluid is mobilized, and the increased load upon the heart has dissipated. As the blood volume returns to normal the cardiac output drops and the signs of a high circulating volume resolve. Hart and colleagues did find that aortic diameters in multiparous women are larger, indicating a failure to return to preconception baselines.[45, 103] Breast-feeding and influence on plasma volume, as well as metabolic demands, can also alter the rate at which a woman's cardiovascular system recovers from pregnancy.[45]

CLINICAL IMPLICATIONS FOR THE PREGNANT WOMAN AND HER FETUS

The stress of pregnancy on the cardiovascular system can result in signifcant alterations in the ability of the woman to carry on the activities of daily living, exercise, or be comfortable in various positions. Because the maternal circulatory system is the life line for the fetus to receive oxygen and nutrients, hemodynamic alterations can impact on the well-being of the fetus. Some of the changes experienced are relatively normal and have little impact on the fetus; however, disease states may result in significant growth alterations or potentiate hypoxic episodes. Fetal heart rate alterations and stress response are discussed on pp. 243–247.

Arrhythmias

Many pregnant women experience rhythm disruptions that become more intense during the second and third trimesters. Most of these are benign and are not indicative of heart disease. The woman may describe skipped beats, momentary pressure in the neck or chest, or extra beats. These are usually representative of premature ventricular contractions and require no further treatment.

Awareness of the increased heart rate can be uncomfortable for some women. True tachycardia, such as paroxysmal atrial tachycardia or paroxysmal atrial fibrillation, may be evident for the first time during pregnancy. This may be frightening for the woman, and she needs to be reassured that she and her infant are at no risk. Taking a deep breath or coughing may result in a slowing or conversion of the heart rate into a more normal pattern.[104]

Supine Hypotensive Syndrome of Pregnancy

Prior to the 1960s the clinical significance of maternal posture and position upon cardiac output was not known. Vorys and associates demonstrated a 17% decrease in maternal cardiac output when the dorsal lithotomy position was assumed; a 14% increase was found in the left lateral decubitus position. The usefulness of this positioning in maintaining uteroplacental perfusion during periods of fetal distress or maternal hypotension was obvious.[280]

Orthostatic stress generated by changes in position (from recumbent to sitting to standing) is associated with acute hemodynamic changes. Blood pools in dependent vessels, which reduces venous return and decreases cardiac output and blood pressure with increasing orthostatic stress. Heart rate and systemic vascular resistance increase; mean arterial pressure changes, however, are not significant. In situations where orthostatic stress is not compensated, the uteroplacental circulation may be compromised and fetal distress experienced.[81]

Further studies have demonstrated that the gravid uterus is also associated with a significant amount of caval blood flow obstruction in the supine position. Approximately 90% of gravid women experience obstruction of the inferior vena cava in the supine position. Late in pregnancy, but before the fetal presenting part becomes engaged, the uterus is mobile enough to fall back against the inferior vena cava in both the supine and lateral recumbent positions. This results in vena caval tamponade. Vascular compression may also be applied to the aorta and its branches. In most women paravertebral collateral circulation develops during pregnancy. This, along with the dilated utero-ovarian circulation, permits blood flow from the legs and pelvis to bypass the vena cava.[132, 133, 144]

In most circumstances the fall in cardiac output due to a posture change is compensated for by an increase in peripheral resistance. This allows systemic blood pressure and heart rate to remain unchanged. The pregnant woman in the supine position, however, may experience a significant decrease in heart rate and blood pressure, leading to symptoms of weakness, lightheadedness, nausea, dizziness, or syncope. This is referred to as supine hypotensive syndrome of pregnancy and is usually corrected when position is changed.[34, 113, 133, 134, 172, 208]

Initially it was felt that the symptoms were due to the occlusion of the vena cava by the uterus. However, the incidence of symptomatology varies from 0.5 to 11.2%. Therefore, it must be more than mechanical impedance of blood flow through the vena cava that causes supine hypotensive syndrome. Currently, it has been suggested that failure to develop adequate collateral circulation may result in a 25 to 30% drop in cardiac output and symptomatology when in the supine position for longer than a few minutes (Figs. 6–3 and 6–4).[24, 132, 133, 137, 208]

Exercise

The current health and fitness awareness in the United States has brought about many concerns and questions regarding exercise during pregnancy. Exercise increases the demand on the cardiorespiratory system. Most of the current research is unclear and controversial regarding the impact of exercise upon the mother and the fetus. The concerns regarding redistribution of weight, effects of hormones, hyperthermia, and increased cardiac workload need to be explored. The differences between women who train and those who do not, along with the difference between exercise and hard labor on pregnancy and fetal outcome, have yet to be evaluated conclusively.

Concerns regarding hyperthermia relate to issues of teratogenicity to the fetus. Can exercise elevate maternal temperatures to a point that might have detrimental effects on the fetus? Animal studies indicate that temperatures greater than 39°C increase risks of neural tube defects. In sheep, researchers have demonstrated that exercise raises fetal temperatures by 1.5°C. This has not been the case in research conducted in women, however. Concerns about hyperthermia in humans have come from the use of hot tubs and the possibility that the increased temperature could lead to decreased fetal umbilical circulation and subsequent decreased fetal cardiac function. These questions have yet to be resolved, although current recommendations encourage women not to let their body temperatures go above 38°C.[7, 15, 106, 125, 159, 185]

The increased energy expenditure that occurs with exercise results in an increased core temperature; the magnitude of this increase is directly related to the intensity of

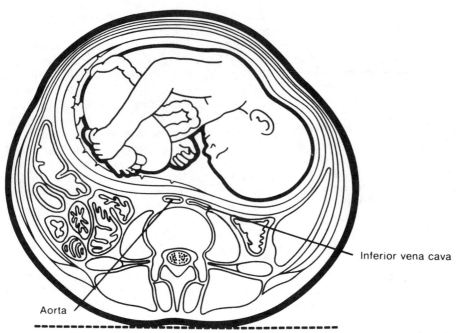

FIGURE 6–3. The pregnant uterus compressing the aorta and the inferior vena cava (aortocaval compression). Patient in supine position. (From Cohen, W.R., Acker, D.B., & Friedman, E.A. (Eds.) (1989). *Management of labor* (2nd ed., p. 80). Rockville, MD: Aspen.)

the exercise.[57, 235] This change in temperature can also be influenced by environmental factors that can alter the ability to dissipate heat (i.e., ambient temperature and humidity). Because of the positive thermal gradient between the mother and fetus, any increase in maternal temperature may result in a rise in embryonic temperature that exceeds the maternal temperature by 0.5 to 1.0°C. Other physiologic changes during pregnancy may decrease the thermal effect of exercise. Both exercise and early pregnancy result in an

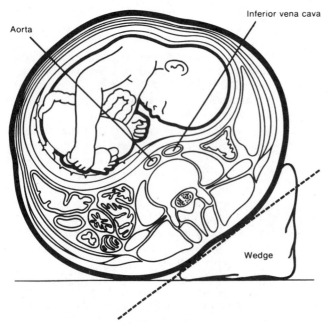

FIGURE 6–4. Uterine displacement with wedge under hip to relieve aortocaval compression. (From Cohen, W.R., Acker, D.B., & Friedman, E.A. (Eds.), *Management of labor* (2nd ed., p. 81). Rockville, MD: Aspen Publication.)

increase in blood flow to the skin. This excessive redistribution of blood flow may actually improve dissipation of heat during exercise in early pregnancy. Early weight gain should contribute to thermal inertia and buffer any rise in core temperature. Along with this, resting core temperature is actually lower in early pregnancy, and this coupled with peripheral venous pooling should decrease the absolute temperature attainable during exercise.[57, 58]

Along with the redistribution of weight that occurs with the anterior displacement of the uterus, the progressive enlargement of the fetus and uterus can lead to alterations in venous blood return and supine hypotensive syndrome. The woman may experience dizziness due to poor venous return and resultant orthostatic hypotension. Altered cardiac return with supine hypotensive syndrome may modify blood flow to the uterus and place the fetus at risk for hypoxia. Therefore certain positions and activities may need to be modified in exercise regimens.[183]

The question of fetal risk with exercise is a complicated one; the potential for preterm labor, acute fetal hypoxia, or intrauterine growth retardation may be increased. Pregnancy increases the workload of the heart, although in most pregnancies the cardiac reserve is adequate to meet these demands. Even with mild exercise, the increase in cardiac output and stroke volume in all stages of pregnancy is greater than that experienced in the nonpregnant state. Also the cardiac output with exercise gets progressively smaller as pregnancy advances. This does suggest a progressive decline in circulatory reserve as pregnancy advances.[19, 226, 273, 277] Bruce and Johnson suggest that the decline is not the result of decreased reserve but instead a function of increased peripheral pooling.[37]

There may be situations, however, in which exercise during pregnancy may exceed the capacity of the cardiovascular system. Blood diverted from the uterus may lead to acute fetal hypoxia or to a chronic hypoxic state and growth retardation. The variables that influence fetal risk include the frequency and length of exposure as well as the degree of alteration in oxygen and nutrient delivery.

Blood flow is redistributed during exercise, moving blood away from the viscera and to the skin and skeletal muscles. This leads to a reduction in utero-ovarian blood flow.

The limitation in substrate delivery to the conceptus could have adverse effects resulting in fetal hypoxia or asphyxia; however, to cause such changes, the reduction in uterine blood flow has to exceed 50%. Given such circumstances, a decrease in oxygen tension and an increase in carbon dioxide tension (respiratory acidosis) could occur. In healthy pregnant women, these occurrences would be rare, being most likely during strenuous and prolonged exercise.[48, 57, 62, 70, 157, 160, 178]

Studies have shown either no reduction or significant alterations in hemodynamics.[48, 61, 70, 180] Lotgering and colleagues demonstrated a 24% decrease in blood flow after 40 minutes of exercise. Whether this reduction affects oxygen availability (transport) or oxygen uptake is unknown.[157]

Wilkening and Meschia demonstrated in ewes that uterine blood flow can fall by approximately 50% without an appreciable effect on either uterine or fetal oxygen uptake.[290] Therefore under normal conditions there is probably enough oxygen available to the uterus to meet and exceed uterine and fetal demands. Lotgering and Longo identify three compensatory mechanisms that help to maintain oxygen availability: blood flow is selectively distributed to the cotyledons, at the expense of the myometrium; maternal hematocrit rises during exercise, therefore there is a smaller reduction in oxygen availability–to–blood flow ratio; and uterine oxygen uptake increases during exercise in order to maintain a stable oxygen consumption level.[158]

Maternal exercise is also associated with a significant increase in circulating catecholamines. The placenta, under normal circumstances, is very efficient in metabolizing the catecholamines, and only 10 to 15% reach the fetus. Elevated catecholamine levels could have an additional restrictive effect on the fetal circulation. The combined effect of redistributed blood flow and restricted blood flow could result in fetal asphyxia and bradycardia. The frequency at which this occurs is unknown.[178]

The usual fetal response to maternal exercise is an increase in heart rate by 10 to 30 beats per minute. These changes are consistent and are independent of either gestational age or intensity of maternal exercise. Immediately after exercise and during the next 5 minutes fetal heart rate remains elevated regardless of the type of exercise.

Within 15 minutes, fetal heart rate drops to pre-exercise values in women engaged in mild to moderate exercise activities. For women engaged in strenuous activities, the fetal heart rate does not return to baseline for 30 minutes.[178]

Fetal distress may be exhibited through alterations in fetal heart rate (FHR); both bradycardia and tachycardia have been observed following exercise. Numerous studies have demonstrated a rise in FHR following exercise, with one study finding 10% of fetuses falling into the lower end of the tachycardiac range.[14, 60, 64, 65, 76, 243] These findings were not confirmed by Sorenson and Borlum, however.[249]

Artal and coworkers found fetal bradycardia (down to 90 beats per minute) in 3 out of 19 fetuses whose mothers were participating in strenuous exercise activities. They suggest that this may be a normal response, possibly to a rapid rise in catecholamine levels.[14] The elevated FHRs seen post exercise may also be a normal physiologic response to compensate for short periods of hypoxia.[161] A study conducted in rhesus monkeys demonstrated that when a rapid rise in catecholamines is delivered, fetal hyoxemia and bradycardia result. In this study the degree of fetal bradycardia was directly related to the initial acid-base status of the fetus, the catecholamine dose delivered, and the maternal response to a given dose. Recovery was rapid once the infusion was discontinued.[4]

Artal and colleagues suggest that fetal response to exercise may be related to gestational age, maternal catecholamine release (and consequently the fetal catecholamine release), maternal stress, and level of fitness. In all three studies the episodes of bradycardia did not compromise fetal outcome.[4, 14] Fetal reserve should be assessed if any abnormalities are suspected, and maternal cardiac as well as fetoplacental reserve should be the basis for determining exercise and work levels and activities during pregnancy.

It is not clear whether brief episodes of fetal bradycardia are common during maternal exercise, and the mechanism by which they can be triggered can only be speculated. Brief episodes of asphyxia seem to be well tolerated by most fetuses. An initial response of tachycardia may lead to bradycardia if hypoxia becomes prolonged and vagal stimulation occurs. There is also the possibility that these brief occurrences are within the normal realm of fetal reflex responses to major maternal hemodynamic and hormonal events.[178] In most situations, fetal bradycardia was mild (100 to 119 beats per minute), and severe bradycardia was reported in one study in which women engaged in one maximal exertion.[46] Concerns are generated because of the inability to predict who may experience an adverse fetal event and what the consequences might be.[178]

It is unclear what the maternal and fetal physiologic and blood chemistry changes are during exercise and what significance should be placed on observed changes. Exercise results in changes in epinephrine, norepinephrine, glucagon, cortisol, prolactin, and endorphin levels. There are concerns that changes in the hormone levels may influence implantation and uterine quiescence in early pregnancy. The catecholamine alterations may contribute to preterm labor in susceptible women. This possibility is supported by observations of uncoordinated uterine contractions during exercise. Women should be trained to recognize signs of preterm labor and cease activities that lead to uterine stimulation so that progression of labor may be stopped.[57]

Both exercise and early pregnancy increase oxygen consumption and the need for energy substrate by different tissues. Until the process of placental vascularization is complete, the conceptus is more subject to diffusional and gradient limitation in substrate availability than it is later in pregnancy. This diffusional limitation, coupled with a sustained reduction in blood flow and the potential for a hypoglycemic response to exercise, could theoretically reduce nutrient availability below a critical level, resulting in an adverse outcome during early pregnancy.[57]

Since current research provides few guidelines regarding activity in pregnancy, clients should be counseled according to the current American Academy of Obstetrics and Gynecology recommendations.[7] Moderate exercise three to four times a week is a good guideline for pregnant women to follow and is preferable to intermittent activity. Competitive activities should be discouraged. Vigorous exercise should not be performed in hot, humid weather or during a period of febrile illness.[7]

Jumping, jerky movements or deep flexion or extension of joints should be avoided because of the joint instability that occurs during pregnancy. Gradual changes in position should be undertaken to avoid orthostatic stress and hypotension. Heart rate should be monitored during peak activity and should not exceed 140 beats per minute, and strenuous activity should be limited to 15 minutes. Caloric intake needs to be high enough to meet not only the demands of exercise but also of pregnancy.[7]

At no time should exercise be continued if pain or contractions are experienced. The physician should be contacted if bleeding, dizziness, shortness of breath, palpitations, faintness, tachycardia, back pain, pubic pain, or difficulty in walking is experienced. Women designated as high risk for preterm labor need to receive special counseling regarding not only appropriate activity levels but also signs and symptoms of labor.[7]

Anesthesia and Cesarean Section

Cesarean section is often performed to reduce or modify the significant hemodynamic alterations that occur with labor. However, the anesthesia and surgical procedure, as well as pain, anxiety, and apprehension, are associated with their own impact on the cardiovascular system (see Fig. 12–1).

Significant hemodynamic changes can be attributed to the pain and anxiety associated with labor and delivery, especially in primiparous women. This is probably due to the release of catecholamines and the increased systemic vascular tone. The greatest hemodynamic changes are seen with vaginal deliveries in which only local anesthesia is used.[39, 109, 275, 299]

These changes include tachycardia during the second stage of labor that is accentuated with uterine contractions. Systolic and diastolic blood pressures rise gradually during the first stage, followed by a marked increase in the second stage. These changes are associated with a progressive increase in stroke volume, which peaks immediately after delivery.

The use of caudal anesthesia does not alter the above hemodynamic changes. However, the progressive rise in cardiac output seen between the contractions of the first and second stages is eliminated, and blood pressure remains more constant throughout labor and delivery. This may indicate that the lack of pain and anxiety reduces the peak increase in cardiac output. Supine positioning, re-gardless of the stage of labor or the anesthetic agent used, increases cardiac output by as much as 20%.[143]

Following delivery of the baby and placenta by cesarean section there is a significant increase in cardiac output probably due to the decompression of the pelvic vessels and the increased circulatory volume. Ueland and co-authors explored the hemodynamic responses to various anesthetic agents used during cesarean section. His group found that following the administration of a subarachnoid block there was a decrease in stroke volume and cardiac output that was associated with a rise in heart rate and a decline in blood pressure. These changes did not correlate with the dose delivered or the level of anesthesia achieved. The significant hypotension and the deleterious effects on the fetus was reversed when the patient was turned to her side.[269]

There are fewer hemodynamic changes when balanced anesthesia without epinephrine is used. Cardiac output does not significantly change, and the heart rate increases only slightly. There is, however, a moderate increase in diastolic pressure. Delivery leads to an increase in stroke volume and cardiac output, whereas heart rate and blood pressure decline slightly.[271]

The greatest degree of hemodynamic stability was achieved with epidural anesthesia without epinephrine. Women undergoing cesarean section with epidural anesthesia demonstrated only minor changes in heart rate, cardiac output, and stroke volume. There was a moderate decline in blood pressure following induction, but then it stabilized. Following delivery, the cardiac output increased by 25%, and there was no change in heart rate.[270]

These researchers felt that the changes encountered when subarachnoid block was used might be deterimental to patients with heart disease and therefore should not be used. Balanced general anesthesia appears to be the technique of choice for many women with cardiac lesions who undergo cesarean section. The combination of epidural opioids and low-concentration local anesthetic seems to work well for pain relief during or after vaginal delivery in cardiac patients; however, careful monitoring is warranted.[124, 269]

Twins

The mother with a twin pregnancy is subject to a higher risk of morbidity and mortality.

There is an increased production of estriol, progesterone, and human placental lactogen (hPL) that results in an increased volume expansion and weight gain. The weight difference can be seen in the first trimester, therefore it must represent more than just the size of the conceptus. Clinically, the increased uterine size is not appreciated until 12 weeks' gestation. Total intrauterine volume is similar for single and twin pregnancies at the beginning of the second trimester. However, by week 18 the total intrauterine volume for twins is double that of a singleton, and at 25 weeks it is equal to the volume encountered at term in single pregnancies.[193, 213]

Whereas plasma volume is increased by about 50% in single pregnancies, in twins there is a further increase of up to 65%. There is also a higher red blood cell (RBC) volume, increased hemodilution of iron and folate, and an exaggerated physiologic anemia. Whether the hemodilution is due to a greater increase in total body volume or a greater demand for iron or folic acid is unclear; however, it is probably some combination of the two.[193, 228, 289]

The increase in maternal cardiac output in twin pregnancies is greater than that found in singletons. The average increase is approximately 0.4 L/min higher at term in twins versus singletons. Beyond this, however, heart rate, stroke volume, and mean circulation time are similar in single and multiple pregnancies.[193, 289]

In twins the characteristic changes in blood pressure include a lowered diastolic pressure at 20 weeks (74% of women with twins have a diastolic pressure less than 80 mmHg), which is followed by a greater rise in diastolic pressure between mid-pregnancy and delivery (95% experience a rise in diastolic pressure of 15 mmHg or more).

Mothers with twins are at greater risk for preterm labor, pregnancy-induced hypertension, placenta previa, placental abruption, anemia, hyperemesis gravidarum, and postpartum hemorrhage. Compression of pelvic vessels during quiet standing has been found to coincide with uterine contractions. This phenomenon occurs earlier in twin pregnancies and may contribute to the onset of preterm labor. Left lateral recumbent positioning decreases the frequency and intensity of contractions.

The length of labor is similar in twin and single pregnancies, although with twins the active phase is longer and the latent phase is shorter. Labor may be more difficult, possibly owing to uterine overdistention and an increased incidence of malpresentation. Blood loss is about double that in a single delivery, and hemorrhage is more frequent owing to uterine atony and sudden decompression of the overdistended uterus. There is also a slightly higher incidence of vasa praevia and placenta previa, increasing the possibility of hemorrhage at delivery.

The risk of proteinuric preeclampsia is five times greater in twin than in single pregnancies. This is probably due to the large placental mass that is to be found with twin pregnancies. The protective nature of previous pregnancies is also negated when twins are carried.[5, 190, 193]

Careful and consistent monitoring of the maternal and fetal status is necessary to identify detrimental changes early. Education regarding the normal changes throughout gestation, nutrition, activity levels, and signs and symptoms of preterm labor is essential in order to facilitate maternal-fetal well-being.

Cardiac Disease and Pregnancy

Pregnancy brings about profound alterations in the cardiovascular system. The hemodynamic changes can result in death or disability to women who have underlying heart disease. Pregnancy is particularly dangerous for women who have specific cardiac lesions, including Eisenmenger's syndrome, primary pulmonary hypertension, Marfan's syndrome, and hemodynamically significant mitral stenosis. In fact, in the presence of a cardiac lesion involving pulmonary hypertension, pregnancy carries a risk of maternal mortality somewhere between 30 and 50%. Pregnancy may also aggravate preexisting cardiac conditions such that damage is extensive and recovery to prepregnancy levels is not possible. In addition, pregnancy may result in maternal heart disease (e.g., peripartal cardiomyopathy).[62, 168, 260]

The fetus must also be monitored closely in order to make decisions regarding treatment during complicated pregnancies. Fetal well-being and growth are dependent upon a continuous flow of well-oxygenated blood to the uterus. When this supply is reduced or interrupted or oxygenation is decreased, the fetus is at risk for altered growth and development and in danger of dying.[168]

Currently, cardiac disease affects 0.5 to 2% of pregnant women. This incidence is steadily increasing as improved management and technical capabilities for both the mother and fetus make it possible to sustain pregnancy in those who previously would have been advised to terminate or avoid pregnancy. Corrective surgery for infants and children with congenital heart disease has increased the number of these women who are now of childbearing age. In addition, the incidence of heart disease increases in women who wait until their thirties or forties to have children.[284]

The fetus is at increased risk of being born with a congenital heart defect if either parent has congenital heart disease. If the mother is the affected parent, she adds an environmental risk as well as a genetic risk for her infant.[168]

All of these factors and the risk to the mother and fetus should be discussed in depth with couples prior to pregnancy. This preconception counseling allows the potential problems and treatment options to be explored and the woman's current health status to be characterized.

Obstructive Lesions

These lesions are basically stenotic in nature, representing a subgroup of the acyanotic heart defect group. The main concern is an obstruction of flow causing an elevation of pressure proximal to the obstructive lesion and a decrease in flow distal to the stenotic area. Pulmonary stenosis without septal defect, coarctation of the aorta, aortic stenosis, mitral stenosis, and tricuspid stenosis are included in this group. Mitral stenosis and mitral regurgitation are presented as examples.

MITRAL STENOSIS
This lesion is caused almost exclusively by rheumatic fever. The stenotic valve restricts cardiac output, resulting in fatigue, which is the most common symptom. The obstruction of left atrial outflow leads to pressure elevations in the left atrium, pulmonary veins, and pulmonary capillaries. These changes usually lead to pulmonary congestion.

The increased cardiac output and heart rate of pregnancy, along with the fluid retention, may lead to an increase in symptoms. Signs of pulmonary congestion usually occur by 20 weeks and stabilize by 30 weeks. An exacerbation may occur at the time of delivery if there is prolonged tachycardia.

Management should include prophylaxis against rheumatic fever during the pregnancy and against endocarditis during labor and delivery. If severe mitral stenosis is diagnosed, mitral commissurotomy should be considered prior to conception. If symptoms develop during the course of pregnancy, activity restrictions to reduce the strain on the heart, sodium intake restrictions, diuretics, and digitalis may be considered. If symptoms of pulmonary congestion persist despite medical therapeutics, surgical intervention to do either a mitral commissurotomy or valve replacement may be necessary. If thromboembolism occurs, anticoagulation therapy with subcutaneous heparin is needed.[168, 248]

MITRAL REGURGITATION
Mitral regurgitation may be due to rheumatic fever; however, there are numerous other conditions that can lead to its development. Prolapse of the mitral valve during systole allows for regurgitation of blood back into the left atrium. Fatigue is the result. If severe, pulmonary congestion can occur. There is a propensity for atrial fibrillation, and left atrial thrombus formation exists.[261]

Individuals with mitral regurgitation may be asymptomatic for extended periods of time. Pregnancy is usually well tolerated, and the development of congestive failure is rare. Prophylactic antibiotics are warranted.

MITRAL VALVE PROLAPSE
Mitral valve prolapse (MVP) is one of the most common congenital heart lesions. It is found in approximately 6% of the general population and may occur in 12 to 17% of women of childbearing age.[334] Most women with MVP are asymptomatic and tolerate pregnancy well; in fact, there is evidence that pregnancy may actually improve hemodynamics and symptoms in some women. Although rare, complications associated with MVP (arrhythmias, infective endocarditis, and cerebral ischemic events) may result in serious complications during pregnancy.

There are two theories used to explain MVP currently. One theory suggests inheritance of an abnormality of the connective tissue that results in a weakness and stretching of the mitral leaflets, chordae tendineae, and annulus, resulting in prolapse. The other theory postulates a minor congenital variance in the valve that allows the leaflets and chordae tendineae to be injured with prolonged systolic stress. Repair and reinjury then lead to progressive weakening.[66, 74]

Although much has been written about MVP in the general population, there is little known about the effect of pregnancy on MVP. Mitral valve prolapse can be both a primary disease function and a secondary pathology associated with connective tissue diseases or cardiac disease that reduces the size of the left ventricle.[66] The latter includes syndromes such as Marfan's syndrome, pseudoxanthoma elasticum, osteogenesis imperfecta, as well as others.

The hemodynamic changes of pregnancy can reduce the clinical signs of MVP by decreasing audible murmurs (usually a late systolic murmur associated with a click), possibly by increasing the left ventricular end-diastolic volume and favorably realigning the mitral valve complex. The decrease in peripheral vascular resistance relieves the mitral insufficiency, thereby reducing the murmur. Once these parameters return to normal in the postpartum period, the auscultatory findings of MVP return.[105] These changes are also reflected on echocardiographic studies.[212]

In most situations, pregnancy is tolerated well in women with MVP, and poor maternal or fetal outcome need not be anticipated. However, there have been anecdotal reports of women experiencing transient thromboembolic ischemia and left hemiparesis and endocarditis.[66] It is more common for women to experience an increase in palpitations, arrhythmias, or chest pains that may require medical intervention with the use of β-blockers. Whether prophylactic antibiotics to prevent bacterial endocarditis are necessary in all pregnant women with MVP is not yet settled. Current recommendations suggest that antibiotics should be used in patients in whom MVP is complicated by mitral insufficiency.[66]

Left-to-Right Shunts

Left-to-right shunts can occur through an atrial septal defect (ASD), ventricular septal defect (VSD), or a patent ductus arteriosus (PDA). Most patients born with these defects either have experienced closing of the defect on its own during childhood or have had corrective surgery to reduce the defect. A residual defect may remain, however.[168]

The magnitude of the left-to-right shunt is dependent upon the ratio of resistance in the systemic and pulmonary vascular circuits. During pregnancy both circuits have a decline in resistance so that there is usually no significant change if shunting occurs. If pulmonary vascular disease exists, the normal fall in pulmonary vascular resistance may not occur. It is rare that cyanosis occurs with these defects unless significant pulmonary hypertension or right ventricular failure develops. Pregnancy does not seem to precipitate these events, however.[142, 168]

ATRIAL SEPTAL DEFECT

This is one of the most common defects seen in adults and therefore is more common during pregnancy. It is usually asymptomatic. The most common complications are arrhythmias and heart failure; however, arrhythmias usually do not appear until the forties.[62]

The hypervolemia of pregnancy increases the left-to-right shunt through the ASD, thereby creating an additional burden on the right ventricle. This additional load is usually tolerated well by most women. If not, right ventricular failure occurs, leading to marked peripheral edema, atrial arrhythmias, pulmonary hypertension, and paradoxic systemic emboli across the septal defect. Death may result if heart failure occurs.[62, 168]

VENTRICULAR SEPTAL DEFECT

Ventricular septal defects can occur either as an isolated lesion or in conjunction with other congenital cardiac anomalies (tetralogy of Fallot, transposition of the great vessels, or coarctation of the aorta). The size of the defect determines the degree of shunting, tolerance to the additional burden of pregnancy, and prognosis. Small defects are usually tolerated well; large VSDs often lead to congestive failure, arrhythmias, or the development of pulmonary hypertension. A large VSD is often associated with some degree of aortic regurgitation, which contributes to the possibility of congestive failure.

PATENT DUCTUS ARTERIOSUS

Patency of the ductus arteriosus is usually identified in the early neonatal period or during infancy. Surgical correction is usually done at that time. Therefore, it is uncommon to find this type of defect in childbearing women. However, if it does exist, it is usually well tolerated during gestation, labor, and delivery. If the PDA is complicated by pulmonary hypertension, the prognosis becomes much worse.

Right-to-Left Shunts

Right-to-left shunting occurs through an ASD, VSD, or PDA when the pulmonary vascular resistance rises so that it exceeds the systemic vascular resistance or when an obstruction to right ventricular outflow exists. These women present with cyanosis, clubbing of the fingers, and right ventricular hypertrophy. Conditions include Eisenmenger's syndrome, tetralogy of Fallot, and primary pulmonary hypertension.

EISENMENGER'S SYNDROME

This syndrome combines the presence of a congenital left-to-right shunt with progressive pulmonary hypertension that leads to shunt reversal or bidirectional flow. It is more commonly associated with VSD or PDA. During pregnancy the decreased systemic vascular resistance increases the degree of right-to-left shunting, which reduces pulmonary perfusion, leading to hypoxemia and maternal and fetal compromise. Systemic hypotension leads to decreased right ventricular filling pressures, which may be insufficient to perfuse the pulmonary bed where high pulmonary vascular resistance exists. The result may be the onset of sudden and profound hypoxemia. Hemorrhage or complications of conduction anesthesia (hypovolemia) may precipitate hypoxemia and lead to death during the intrapartum period.[62, 123, 156]

The mortality rate for pregnant women with Eisenmenger's syndrome can be as high as 65% when pulmonary hypertension is associated with a VSD. Because of this high mortality rate, abortion is usually recommended. If gestation continues, hospitalization, continuous oxygen administration, and the use of pulmonary vasodilators are recommended.

During labor it is essential to maintain an adequate fluid load, and the placement of a pulmonary artery catheter is warranted to monitor fluid status. Maintaining a preload edge to protect against unexpected blood loss may risk tipping the scales toward pulmonary edema.[62]

TETRALOGY OF FALLOT

This is the most common cause of right-to-left shunting and is a congenital defect that includes a combination of VSD, pulmonary valve stenosis, right ventricular hypertrophy,

and rightward displacement of the aortic root. Pulmonary vascular resistance is normal. Surgical correction usually occurs during infancy, although there may be residual shunting following correction. Pregnancy outcome is relatively good for those individuals who have undergone surgical correction.[15, 173, 177]

In pregnant women with uncorrected VSDs, the decrease in systemic vascular resistance leads to worsening right-to-left shunting. This can be complicated by intrapartum blood loss leading to systemic hypotension. Therefore careful monitoring of fluid status is warranted.[62, 122]

PULMONARY ARTERY HYPERTENSION

Severe pulmonary hypertension associated with pregnancy carries a 50% maternal mortality rate and a 40% fetal mortality rate if the mother survives. Significant pulmonary hypertension is a contraindication to pregnancy, and pregnancy should be prevented or terminated if it occurs. If abortion is not possible, physical activity should be curtailed and supine positioning avoided during late gestation. Careful monitoring of oxygenation and fluid status at the time of labor and delivery is essential in order to identify problems early and intervene appropriately.[168]

Marfan's Syndrome

Marfan's syndrome is an autosomal dominant disorder of connective tissue with clinical manifestations in skeletal, ocular, and cardiovascular abnormalities. Aortic dilatation is one of the manifestations and complications that can result in aneurysm formation and rupture, aortic dissection, and aortic regurgitation. Structural changes in the aortic wall due to high estrogen levels predispose pregnant women to aortic dissection. Rupture usually occurs in the third trimester or in the first stages of labor. If there is no preexisting cardiovascular disease, the risk of maternal death is relatively low.[62, 142, 207]

Counseling regarding the risk of inheritance and the potential maternal complications should be given preconceptually if possible. If pregnancy occurs and abortion is not desired, the use of oral propranolol to decrease pulsatile pressure on the aortic wall is indicated. If a surgical delivery is performed the generalized connective tissue weakness must be taken into consideration and the use of retention sutures may be necessary.[62]

Nursing Care

Some cardiac diseases actually benefit from the increase in cardiac output, decrease in systemic vascular resistance, and increased heart rate. On the other hand, cardiac diseases associated with fixed lesions do not tolerate the volume increase because the stenotic area cannot accommodate the increased flow. The increased heart rate shortens the diastolic filling time, thereby preventing adequate filling of the heart. This combined with the decrease in systemic vascular resistance may result in a drop in blood pressure.[284]

When blood volume reaches its peak in the 20th week of pregnancy, the potential for congestive heart failure is increased. At delivery this risk is further increased owing to the 20% increase in blood volume, and acute pulmonary edema may occur. Applying pressure to the abdomen can slow the blood return to the heart and facilitate cardiovascular stabilization. If the heart is unable to compensate for the decrease in systemic vascular resistance, the blood pressure falls. This may increase fatigue and contribute to episodes of dizziness and syncope as well as reduce uterine blood flow. Maintenance of blood pressure can be attempted by administration of chronotropic and alpha pressor agents. Epidural and spinal anesthesia may further decrease systemic vascular resistance and should be avoided in these patients.[284]

Maternal education and counseling about rest, nutrition, exercise, recumbent positioning, medications, signs and symptoms of decompensation, and potential difficulties are necessary to alleviate anxiety. Frequent monitoring with appropriate testing is necessary to assess cardiovascular status and determine psychological well-being. Reassurance regarding feelings of ambivalence about the high-risk nature of the pregnancy and the fetus should be provided, along with opportunities to vocalize fears and concerns. Coping strategies and social support systems need to be continually assessed.

Pregnancy-Induced Hypertension

Pregnancy-induced hypertension (PIH), or preeclampsia, is a hypertensive, multisystem disorder associated with proteinuria, edema, central nervous system irritability, and at times coagulation or liver function abnormalities. The underlying pathology appears to be related to severe peripheral vasospasm with increased alveolar sensitivity to angiotensin II and alterations in the relationships between prostacyclin (PGI_2) and thromboxane. The result is a reduction in visceral blood flow, including renal blood flow, tissue hypoxia, and damage to maternal organs, most significantly the placenta. Decreased placental blood flow leads to hypoxia and inadequate nutritional support of the developing fetus and reduced amounts of amniotic fluid. PIH occurs primarily in primiparous women after 20 weeks' gestation. Approximately 5 to 10% of all pregnancies are complicated by preeclampsia. Rapid onset of seizure activity (eclampsia) occurs in aprroximately 2% of cases.[67, 151]

Although often defined as the onset of hypertension with proteinuria, edema, or both, preeclampsia is further characterized as occurring when there is a systolic rise in blood pressure greater than 30 mmHg or a diastolic rise greater than 15 mmHg or a blood pressure greater than 140/90 measured on two separate occasions that are at least 6 hours apart.[86, 245] The current accepted standard for defining PIH by the American College of Obstetricians and Gynecologists is reflected in Table 6–2.[215] Redman and Jefferies suggest that a first diastolic pressure below 90 mmHg, a subsequent increase of at least 25 mmHg, and a maximum diastolic reading of at least 90 mmHg were more specific for identifying preeclamptic women and separating women with mild chronic hypertension.[214] Consistency in measurement, position, and equipment is necessary in order to correctly identify preeclampsia in a clinical setting.[242]

Severe preeclampsia is diagnosed when one of the following is present: (1) systolic blood pressure greater than 160 mmHg or diastolic pressure greater than 110 mmHg, which must be measured at two different times at least 6 hours apart; (2) proteinuria of levels greater than 5 g in 24 hours, which is roughly equivalent to a 3+ or 4+ on dipstick; (3) oliguria less than 400 ml in 24 hours; (4) cerebral or visual disturbances; or (5) pulmonary edema or cyanosis.[67, 245]

Preeclampsia superimposed upon preexisting hypertension is identified when there is an exacerbation of hypertension with a greater than 30 mmHg rise in systolic pressure or 15 mmHg increase in diastolic pressure with significant proteinuria or general-

TABLE 6-2
Classification of Hypertensive Disorders of Pregnancy

CLASSIFICATION	DEFINITION AND DIAGNOSTIC CRITERIA
Pregnancy-induced hypertension 　Preeclampsia	Hypertension with proteinuria, edema, or both developing after week 20 of gestation
Mild	Blood pressure of 140/90 mmHg or greater or an increase of 30 mmHg systolic or 15 mmHg diastolic over baseline
Severe	One of more of the following symptoms: blood pressure of 160/110 mmHg or greater, proteinuria 5 g/24 hr or 3+ to 4+, oliguria, cerebral or visual disturbances, pulmonary edema or cyanosis, HELLP syndrome
Eclampsia	Extension of preeclampsia with tonic-clonic seizures
Chronic hypertension preceding pregnancy (any cause)	History of hypertension (140/90 mmHg or greater) before conception, discovery of hypertension before week 20 of gestation, or continuation of hypertension indefinitely after delivery
Chronic hypertension with superimposed acute PIH	Preexisting chronic hypertension complicated by elevation of systolic blood pressure 30 mmHg or diastolic blood pressure 15 mmHg above baseline; development of proteinuria, edema, or both
Late or transient hypertension	Transient elevations of blood pressure observed during labor or in the early postpartum period, returning to baseline within 10 days after delivery

From Koniak-Griffin, D. & Dodgson, J. (1987). Severe pregnancy-induced hypertension: Postpartum care of the critically ill patient. *Heart & Lung, 16,* 662. As modified from Gant, N. F. & Worley, R. (1980). Hypertension in pregnancy: Concepts and management (pp. 2–9). East Norwalk, CT: Appleton-Century-Crofts.

ized edema. These changes also usually occur late in the third trimester.[245]

The complications associated with pre-eclampsia are the result of altered hemodynamics that result in underperfusion and damage to maternal organ systems, including the uteroplacental system, which then affects the fetus. All of the complications are the result of the primary labile vasospastic process that, when uncompensated for, leads to tissue hypoxia and ischemia. The vasospasm results in increased vascular resistance, elevated arterial pressures, and vascular damage. Subendothelial fibrin and platelet deposition occurs because of endothelial injury, which with the vasospasm promotes tissue hypoxia, hemorrhage, necrosis, and compromised perfusion to the organ systems.[67, 83]

The heart attempts to compensate for the decrease in blood flow by increasing heart rate or stroke volume (increasing preload or contractility). Increased heart rates can decrease diastolic filling time and therefore preload such that stroke volume is actually decreased. There is also a decrease in coronary perfusion leading to myocardial hypoxia and further decompensation. On the other hand, if preload itself is increased, then cardiac function improves. Of course, there is a limit at which further stretching of the myocardial fibers provides no further benefit (Frank-Starling mechanism). When this is reached, coronary perfusion is compromised. Increasing contractility requires increased ventricular muscle work and greater oxygen consumption. This compensatory mechanism

results in an increased afterload, which only compounds the cycle of events, in that the vascular space is already reduced and a state of higher afterload already exists.[245]

Because the pregnant heart may already be functioning at the limit of preload reserve, an increase in afterload may not be compensated for. This suggests the need to monitor and treat the hypertension of preeclampsia in order to preserve hemodynamic integrity.[245]

Hypertensive disease is one of the major causes of maternal mortality in the United States, usually being associated with an eclamptic event superimposed on chronic hypertension. Death is usually associated with cerebral hemorrhage. Preeclampsia can also result in cardiac failure, pulmonary edema, renal insufficiency with pregnancy-induced glomerular disease, abruptio placentae (10 to 12%), hemorrhage and necrotic lesions in the liver, and retinal ischemia, edema, and potential detachment.[83]

Preeclampsia is also one of the major causes of preterm birth and perinatal death. When preeclampsia is superimposed on chronic hypertension, or when severe preeclampsia or eclampsia occurs, the fetus is at risk for growth abnormalities (intrauterine growth retardation [IUGR]) as well as asphyxia and death (10 to 30% increase). These risks are due to the marked decrease in uterine blood flow and limited placental reserve. The fall in blood flow can occur as much as 3 to 4 weeks before maternal hypertension is detected and is related to alterations in the normal changes seen in endometrial arteries during pregnancy (see Chapter 2).[284a]

Because of these risks to the mother and fetus, the ability to identify and predict women who will develop preeclampsia becomes important for initiating medical therapy. It has been suggested that mean arterial pressure during the second trimester may be useful. However, the specificity and sensitivity varied significantly, therefore reducing the power to predict on a consistent basis.[214]

The supine pressor test (roll-over test) has also been suggested as a relatively simple predictive tool that can be used in the clinical setting. A 20 mmHg or more increase in diastolic blood pressure when the woman turns from a lateral to a supine position is said to be predictive of women who will go on to develop pregnancy-induced hypertension. Variations in study techniques, sample size, and measurement techniques have led to a variety of results. The sensitivity of the test is highly variable, and there is a high incidence of false-positive tests. Therefore the test is not recommended for clinical use.[214]

There is no current testing method that reliably predicts the development of PIH. Therefore, consistent blood pressure evaluation and monitoring of urine for protein as well as physical assessment for edema remain the most useful clinical indicators of PIH.

Current theories regarding pathogenesis of pregnancy-induced hypertension begin with abnormal prostaglandin synthesis (Figs. 6–5 and 6–6). Vasodilatation and enhancement of uteroplacental flow during normal pregnancy may be regulated by prostaglandins (PGs). There is increasing evidence that there are derangements in prostaglandin synthesis, catabolism, or action at the arteriolar level, which may contribute to vasospasticity. Synthesis of prostaglandins PGE_1, PGE_2, and PGI_2 is normally elevated in pregnancy. These vasodilators are potentially responsible for the regulation of uterine blood flow.

Pregnancy is normally characterized by increased synthesis of PGE_2 in the uterus and kidneys as well as increased PGI_2 synthesis in the blood vessels. There is usually an insensitivity to angiotensin, manifested as low to normal blood pressure, high plasma renin activity, and increased urinary PGE_2 excretion. Maternal blood obtained in late pregnancy contains elevated levels of PGE_2 metabolites. In the preeclamptic patient, however, decreased PGE_2 activity has been consistently found.[86, 97, 148, 150, 256]

Preeclampsia is characterized by an increased sensitivity to pressor substances (angiotensin, epinephrine, norepinephrine) possibly owing to a decrease in PG synthesis. This would mean that the balance that usually exists between the aggregatory influence of thromboxane produced in platelets and the antiaggregatory PGI_2 produced in the endothelium would no longer be present. The decreased synthesis of PGI_2 would predispose platelets to aggregation, thereby possibly explaining some of the coagulation complications seen in preeclampsia.[86, 219, 284a, 297]

The lower prostaglandin concentration could also explain the decreased uteroplacental blood flow seen in preeclampsia. PGE_2 synthesis is dependent upon angiotensin II. A reduction in the uterine PGE_2 production may lead to an increase in uterine renin synthesis and a possible increase in uterine renin secretion. A decrease in PGI_2 synthesis in the blood vessels increases vessel sensitivity to angiotensin. Both situations contribute to alterations in uterine and peripheral hemodynamics.[86, 91, 245]

The onset of edema in conjunction with a rise in blood pressure may be indicative of salt retention during diminished vascular capacity and cannot be considered benign during pregnancy. The retention of sodium is a major cause of the developing hypertension because the increased sodium concentration leads to an increase in extracellular volume and increased sensitivity to angiotensin and may increase peripheral vascular resistance by causing arteriolar swelling. The reduced glomerular filtration rate and renal vasoconstriction are probably the reasons for sodium retention in pregnancy-induced hypertension.[83, 86]

Whereas the normal pregnant woman expands her blood volume, women with PIH manifest a decrease in blood volume. The magnitude of this reduction is related to the intensity and the duration of the hypertension. It is currently not known whether this decrease precedes, coincides with, or follows the onset of hypertension. However, it seems logical that vasospasm occurs first, followed by hypertension and then a decrease in blood volume.[93] Therefore reduction in plasma volume reflects the constriction of venous capacitance vessels, causing an increase in capillary hydrostatic pressure.[245] Although the vascular bed is contracted, it is not hypovo-

FIGURE 6–5. Conversion of arachidonic acid to prostaglandins and thromboxanes. (From Ferris, T.F. (1982). Toxemia and hypertension. In G.N. Burrow & T.F. Ferris (Eds.), *Medical complications during pregnancy* (2nd ed., p. 5). Philadelphia: WB Saunders.)

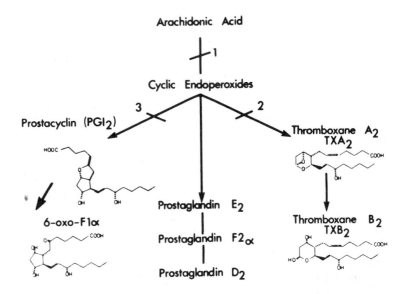

lemic. Treatment with volume expanders is therefore ineffectual and leads to an increase in blood pressure and the possibility of cardiac failure, pulmonary edema, or cerebral hemorrhage.

More recently the use of volume expansion in PIH has been questioned. Studies have continued to be varied in results, but it does appear that some women, under very controlled situations, may benefit from volume expansion. The central hemodynamic status of most women with severe preeclamp-

sia is thought to be made up of a hyperdynamic left ventricle, a variably increased systemic vascular resistance, and a normal pulmonary vascular resistance. Left ventricular function, however, depends on systemic resistance. Therefore it can range widely from a high-output state with a modest increase in systemic resistance to a low-output state, with or without failure, and an extreme rise in systemic resistance. It appears that women with a low cardiac index (output) and very high systemic vascular resistance may

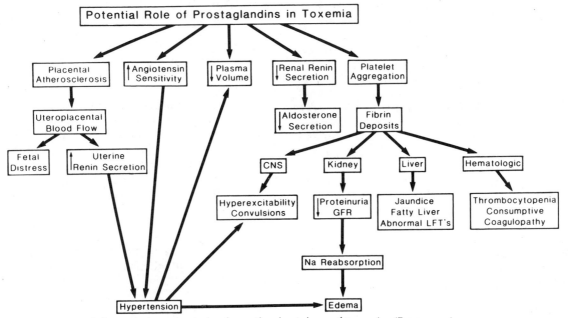

FIGURE 6–6. Schematic hypothesis for the pathophysiology of toxemia. (From Ferris T.F. (1988). Toxemia and hypertension. In G.N. Burrow & T.F. Ferris (Eds.), *Medical complications during pregnancy* (3rd ed., p. 14). Philadelphia: WB Saunders.)

benefit from volume expansion provided there is also vasodilatation. These women may not appear any different and are only recognizable through invasive cardiac monitoring (Swan-Ganz catheter placement).[26, 77] One of the benefits of volume expansion is improved placental perfusion and subsequent fetal growth.

Benedetti and associates have demonstrated an increase in cardiac output in some women with severe PIH and diverse findings in women with less severe PIH. They suggest that an increase in cardiac output is one of the earlier changes in PIH and might lead to an elevation in blood pressure similar to that seen in nonpregnant women with renal hypertension.[27]

The major hematologic change in PIH is thrombocytopenia. Other abnormalities include hemolysis, elevated fibrin-degradation products, decreased plasma fibrinogen, and a protracted thrombin time, which are most often seen in the HELLP syndrome (see later).

Other Organ Systems

Renal function is altered in PIH, with reduction in glomerular filtration and renal blood flow (see Chapter 8). Filtration fraction is also decreased, which is the reverse of the change with primary hypertension. In severe PIH, oliguria, reduced creatinine clearance, and proteinuria are found, probably due to vasospasm and an increased permeability to large molecules such as albumin.[93]

The majority of women do not experience alterations in central nervous system functioning. The most common event is seizure activity, which may be due to vasospasm and the resultant ischemia. Blurred vision and even blindness have been reported on rare occasions; once again this may be due to vasospasm, ischemia, and, rarely, retinal detachment.[93]

The placenta is underperfused in women with PIH. Pharmacologic interventions to improve uteroplacental perfusion have not been successful to date. Antihypertensive therapy also does not appear to improve perfusion. Bed rest does help, and volume expansion may be beneficial in some women.[93] Table 6–3 summarizes changes in organ systems.

Prenatal Therapy

Recognition of the early physiologic changes associated with PIH allows for prompt initiation of treatment. Bed rest in the lateral recumbent position is the first course of action, and evaluation of daily activities, family responsibilites, and support systems can determine whether this regimen will be complied with. Blood pressure, heart rate, and urine output also need to be monitored closely. Evaluation of fetal well-being is essential to determine whether delivery is necessary for fetal survival.

Measures to control further hypertension include sedation, sodium restriction, daily weights, and 24-hour urine collection for volume and total protein excretion. Serum uric acid levels can help determine the severity of the disease process. Antihypertensive therapy may need to be utilized to control intractable hypertension. The definitive treatment for PIH is delivery of the fetus.

Two newer therapies include the use of low-dose aspirin and the administration of prostaglandin A_1. The altered placental production of prostacyclin (vasodilator) and thromboxane A_2 (vasoconstrictor) (thromboxane dominance) increases the risk for platelet aggregation and endothelial damage in the placenta as well as other maternal organs. Women identified early in their second trimester as being at risk for preeclampsia have been able to prevent progression of complications by taking daily low-dose aspirin (see Chapter 2). Low-dose aspirin therapy selectively inhibits thromboxane A_2, resulting in a more normal balance of thromboxane and prostacyclin.[284a] This therapy may alter vascular reactivity, inhibit thrombosis formation, or both. The benefits to the fetus include improved substrate delivery with decreased risk for growth retardation and hypoxic episodes.[216, 266]

Treatment with prostaglandin A_1 is based on replacement therapy for the prostaglandin deficiency that is theorized to exist. The PGE series is unsuitable for this replacement therapy because of its uterine stimulation component. However, PGA_1 is a weak uterine stimulant that has a strong hypotensive (vasodepressant) effect. PGA_1 also improves renal functioning. Continued evaluation of both of these therapies is indicated and may lead to prevention of the disease as well as effective reversible therapy that benefits both mother and fetus.[265, 284a]

Intrapartum Management

During labor, the goal for treatment of women with PIH is to prevent further increases in blood pressure and prevent sei-

TABLE 6–3
Cardiovascular, Renal, and Endocrine Changes During Hypertension and Pregnancy

	UNCOMPLICATED ESSENTIAL HYPERTENSION	NORMAL PREGNANCY	PREGNANCY-INDUCED HYPERTENSION
Cardiovascular			
Arterial pressure	Increased	Reduced	Increased
Cardiac output	Normal or increased	Increased	Increased
Systemic vascular resistance	Increased	Decreased	Increased
Vascular reactivity	Increased	Decreased	Increased
Uterine blood flow		Increased	Reduced
Renal			
Renal blood flow	Increased early Decreases with severity	Increased	Decreased
Glomerular filtration rate	Unchanged	Increased	Decreased
Plasma volume	Contracted	Expanded	Contracted
Total body sodium	Normal	Increased	Increased
Intracellular sodium	Increased	Decreased in 2nd trimester	Normal
Endocrine			
Plasma catecholamines	Normal to increased	Unchanged	Unchanged
Plasma renin activity	High, low, or normal	Increased	Decreased
Plasma aldosterone	Normal	Increased	Decreased
Plasma PGE_2 and PGI_2	Normal	Increased	Decreased
Urinary kallikrein	Decreased	Increased	Decreased

From Sullivan, J. M. (1986). *Hypertension and pregnancy* (p. 70). Chicago: Year Book Medical Publishers.

zures. Therefore intravenous administration of magnesium sulfate to prevent seizures has been recommended along with close monitoring of the mother and fetus. Antihypertensive therapy may be necessary in order to maintain blood pressure control both during labor and post partum. Therapy should be maintained after delivery until spontaneous diuresis occurs and the blood pressure has stabilized below 160/110.[93]

HELLP Syndrome

In 1987 Weinstein described a unique set of findings in some women with severe preeclampsia (or in some situations without clinical symptomatology of severe preeclampsia).[288] These findings include hemolysis (H), elevated liver enzymes (EL), and a low platelet (LP) count (HELLP syndrome). They usually occur during the early part of the third trimester. It is essential that early identification and aggressive treatment be instituted to correct these alterations in order to reduce morbidity and mortality.

Severe preeclampsia is diagnosed when one or more of the following are present: blood pressures of at least 160 mmHg systolic or 110 mmHg diastolic on two readings 6 hours apart; proteinuria of greater than 5 g/24 hours; oliguria (<400 ml in 24 hours); cerebral or visual disturbances; or pulmonary edema or cyanosis. In addition, a platelet count of less than 100,000 mm³ and abnormalities in serum glutamic-oxaloacetic transaminase (SGOT) or serum glutamic-pyruvic transaminase (SGPT) levels with evidence of intravascular hemolysis (schistocytes or burr cells on peripheral smear) are indicative of HELLP syndrome. Hyperbilirubinemia may be present as an indication of hemolysis along with a hematocrit following delivery greater than 10 points out of proportion to observed blood loss. Ascites may be present, and palpation of the liver may reveal a firm well-demarcated border.[288]

Treatment includes delivery if diagnosis occurs in the prenatal period. Intravenous antihypertensive therapy along with a constant infusion of magnesium sulfate should be initiated. Platelet, fresh frozen plasma, or blood transfusion may be necessary to treat the thrombocytopenia and hemolysis (microangiopathic hemolytic anemia) that occur. These findings may lead to a diagnosis of disseminated intravascular coagulation, but when clotting studies are conducted they reveal normal prothrombin times, partial thromboplastin times, and fibrinogen levels.

This indicates that although platelet counts are low, function is normal. Hypoglycemia may be present in these women and can be associated with a high mortality rate if blood glucose levels fall below 40 mg/dl. The worst manifestations of the disease occur during the 48 to 72 hours following delivery.[288] There is increasing evidence that deficient or functionally impaired prostacyclin results in an imbalance of vasodilator-vasoconstrictor factors in the capillary endothelium, which leads to platelet consumption, abnormal platelet forms, microangiopathic hemolytic anemia, and multiple organ dysfunction. On the other hand, antiendothelial cell antibodies, platelet antibodies, or accelerated platelet activation by circulating immune complexes may enhance vasoactivity and lead to increased endothelial damage.[166]

For persistent severe preeclampsia with HELLP syndrome plasma exchange has been proposed. These women fail to show improvement with conventional therapy in the 72 to 96 hours following delivery and have severe thrombocytopenia, persistent hemolytic anemia, elevated concentrations of lactate dehydrogenase (LDH), and continued need for repetitive transfusions. These women have a high mortality rate that is significantly reduced with plasmapheresis with fresh frozen plasma. This therapy not only arrests the disease process but also leads to reversal of symptoms (i.e., pulmonary function, sensorium, and renal function) and progressive improvement in laboratory values.[166]

SUMMARY

The cardiovascular changes associated with pregnancy are highly significant, although well tolerated by most women in their childbearing years. Major maternal and fetal implications can occur when underlying cardiovascular or pulmonary disease processes are compounded with the changes incurred during pregnancy. Cardiovascular pathology–associated pregnancy (PIH and HELLP syndrome) can increase maternal morbidity and mortality and compromise the health and well-being of the fetus. Careful assessment and ongoing monitoring of cardiovascular status throughout the prenatal, intrapartum, and postpartum periods are essential for early identification and prompt intervention, thereby improving maternal and neonatal outcome. Table 6–4 identifies clinical implications related to the cardiovascular system during pregnancy.

DEVELOPMENT OF THE CARDIOVASCULAR SYSTEM IN THE FETUS

The cardiovascular system is the first system in the embryo to begin to function. The need

TABLE 6–4
Summary of Recommendations for Clinical Practice Related to the Cardiovascular System: Pregnant Woman

Recognize usual cardiovascular and hemodynamic patterns of change during pregnancy (pp. 201–210).
Assess maternal cardiovascular changes throughout pregnancy (pp. 208–210).
Counsel women on normal cardiovascular changes and anticipated symptoms associated with those changes (pp. 201–210; 212–215).
Counsel women greater than 24 weeks' gestation to refrain from supine positions and to use lateral recumbent position (p. 213).
Screen women for PIH with each prenatal visit (pp. 222–224).
Assess and closely monitor women with PIH throughout pregnancy for edema, proteinuria, fetal growth, and fetal well-being (pp. 222–223; Table 6–2).
Teach women self–uterine palpation to assess for uterine contractions during exercise (pp. 215–217).
Advise cessation of exercise if contractions or pain occurs (pp. 216–217).
Encourage moderate exercise on a regular basis during pregnancy (pp. 213–217).
Recommend interval-type exercises rather than long continuous exercise (pp. 213–216).
Provide counseling and regularly evaluate pregnant women who start a progressive exercise program during pregnancy (pp. 215–217).
Discourage exercise in pregnant women with threatened miscarriage, PIH, preterm labor, uterine hemorrhage, IUGR (pp. 213–216).
Encourage pregnant women to be careful when first exposed to higher altitudes (above 2500 meters), especially if planning to do exercise (pp. 215–216).
Monitor vascular volume status very carefully during the intrapartum and postpartum periods (pp. 210–212).
Evaluate blood loss and fundal tone postpartally (pp. 210–212).
Monitor for signs of congestive heart failure in women with cardiac disease, especially at about 20 weeks' gestation (pp. 202–204; 217–222; Table 6–1).
Assess maternal activity tolerance in women with cardiac disease and discuss management of daily activities (p. 222).
Teach women with cardiac disease the signs and symptoms of cardiovascular decompensation (pp. 209–222).

Page numbers in parentheses following each recommendation refer to pages in the text where rationale is discussed.

for substrates to support the rapid growth and development of the embryo necessitates the early development of a system that transports nutritional elements and metabolic by-products to and from the cells of the body. Initially, the embryo is small enough so that diffusion of nutrients can meet the demands of the cells; however, this is short lived because of the exponential growth of the embryo. Blood can be seen circulating through the "body" as early as the end of the 3rd week.[24, 179]

At this time, the chorionic sac is approximately 1 cm in diameter, and the distance from the embryo to the nearest maternal blood supply is little more than 3 mm. However, this is too great a distance to allow adequate cellular nutrition by direct diffusion. Each of the developing regions of the embryo requires different amounts of circulatory support at various times throughout gestation, therefore the pattern of vessel development is markedly different from one region to the next depending on the demand.[100]

The cardiovascular system is composed of the heart and the blood vessels. Their development is both independent and contiguous, with the final product being a closed system that continuously circulates a given blood volume. The system is initially formed from endothelial tubes that develop from the mesenchyme in the embryo as well as in the embryonic tissue. Although considered separately here, development of the two elements of the system (heart and vessels) occurs simultaneously.[24]

Anatomic Development

Development of the Primitive Heart

The cardiovascular system arises from mesenchymal cells known as the angioblastic tissue, which is identifiable in the late presomite embryo. These cells appear as scattered small masses at the anterior margin of the embryonic disc in front of the neural plate. The cells coalesce to form a plexus of endothelial vessels that fuse to form two longitudinal cellular strands called cardiogenic cords, which can be seen ventral to the pericardial coelom at the end of the 3rd week. These cords canalize to form two thin-walled tubes, the endocardial heart tubes. As the embryo undergoes lateral folding, the tubes come into proximity and fusion occurs in a cranial to caudal direction. Fusion results in a single tube that will eventually form the internal endothelial lining of the heart (endocardium).[100, 179]

At this stage the mesenchymal tissue around the endocardial tube thickens to form the myoepicardial mantle. Cardiac jelly, a gelatinous connective tissue, separates the simple endothelial tube from the thickened mesenchymal tube, resulting in a tube within a tube appearance. The inner tube becomes the endothelial lining of the heart (endocardium), and the myoepicardial mantle devel-

ops into the myocardium and epicardium (pericardium).[179]

As the head fold occurs, the pericardial cavity and heart rotate on the transverse axis almost 180 degrees to lie ventral to the foregut and caudal to the oropharyngeal membrane. The septum transversum is therefore positioned between the pericardial cavity and the yolk sac, and the heart is now situated in a definitive pericardial cavity.[100, 179]

This primitive heart consists of the endothelial tube and the myoepicardial mantle and is situated such that it passes cranially-caudally through the pericardial cavity and is fixed to the pericardial wall only at the venous entrance (caudal end) and at the arterial outlet (cranial end). It is at this time that differentiation of the heart regions occurs and alternating dilations and constrictions can be identified. The first areas to appear include the bulbus cordis, ventricle, and atrium. The truncus arteriosus and sinus venosus follow.[179]

The truncus arteriosus lies above and is connected to the bulbus cordis. The aortic sac from which the aortic arches arise is included in the truncus arteriosus. The large sinus venosus receives the umbilical, vitelline, and common cardinal veins from the primitive placenta, yolk sac, and embryo, respectively.[100, 179]

During this differentiation stage there is rapid growth of the cardiac tube as well. Because the ends are held fixed and the bulboventricular portion of the tube grows more rapidly than the surrounding cavity (doubles in length from day 21 to day 25), the tube bends upon itself and forms a U-shaped loop that has its convexity directed forward and to the right. Continued growth results in an S-shaped curve that nearly fills the pericardial cavity (Fig. 6–7).

The separation of the atrium and sinus venosus from the septum transversum positions the atrium dorsal and to the left of the bulboventricular loop; the sinus venosus lies dorsal to the atrium. The right and left horns of the sinus venosus now partially fuse to form a single cavity that opens into the atrial cavity via the sinoatrial orifice.

By the end of the somite stage the heart is a single tube except at the caudal end where the remaining unfused portions of the right and left horns of the sinus venosus lie. There are three pairs of symmetric veins that return blood to the horns, including the placental (umbilical), the yolk sac (vitelline),

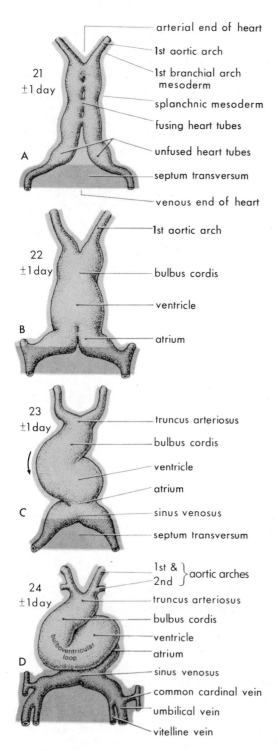

FIGURE 6–7. *A* to *D*, Drawings illustrating the fusion of the heart tubes, which forms a single heart tube, and the bending of the heart tube to form a bulboventricular loop. (From Moore, K.L. (1988). *The developing human* (4th ed., p. 292). Philadelphia: WB Saunders.)

and the embryo body (cardinal) veins. The vitelline vessels soon develop asymmetrically with the left vein undergoing retrogression. At 33 to 34 days the right umbilical vein atrophies and disappears. The left horn of the sinus venosus also becomes much smaller as the veins in the septum transversum re-

arrange. Eventually the left sinus venosus becomes the coronary sinus.[100, 179]

During the rearrangement of vessels the ductus venosus is formed in the liver. This shunt between the left umbilical vein and the right hepatocardiac channel allows most of the blood to bypass the liver sinusoids and flow directly into the heart from the placenta. This results in an enlargement of the right horn of the sinus venosus and a change in the position of the sinoatrial orifice. The latter is positioned to the right side of the dorsal surface and converted to a vertical alignment. The margins are now projected into the atrium and compose the right and left venous valves.[100]

The atrium, ventricle, and bulbus cordis continue to expand rapidly, resulting in a change in position. The atrium expands transversely, extending laterally and ventrally, and appears on either side of the bulbus cordis. This results in the atria being deeply grooved. Further growth results in the right and left auricular appendages being formed. At the same time, the bulboventricular sulcus dissipates with the growth of these structures. Eventually the caudal portion of the bulbus becomes part of the ventricle. The ventricle gradually moves to the left and ends up on the ventral surface of the heart. It is at this time that the atrioventricular canal becomes defined.[100]

Septation of the Heart

Septation of the atrioventricular canal, the atrium, and the ventricle begins in the middle of the 4th week and is complete by the end of the 5th week. The changes in shape and position of the heart tube, as described above, facilitate the partitioning of these structures. The process of septation takes place while the heart continues to pump and blood continues to move unidirectionally through the tube. The subdivision of the heart into right and left compartments occurs simultaneously in the various regions of the heart; however, all of the processes must be integrated so that normal functional development occurs.

The right horn of the sinus venosus becomes incorporated into the right atrium. Most of the wall of the left atrium is derived from the primitive pulmonary vein. The vein develops to the left of the septum primum and is an outgrowth of the dorsal atrial wall. However, as the atrium expands, the vein is progressively incorporated into the wall of the atrium.[100, 179]

ATRIOVENTRICULAR CANAL
The atrium leads into the ventricle via a narrow atrioventricular canal. During the 4th week the endocardium proliferates to produce dorsal and ventral bulges in the wall of the atrioventricular canal. These swellings are the atrioventricular endocardial cushions. The swellings are invaded by mesenchymal cells, which results in the growth of the cushions toward each other. Fusion of the cushions occurs leading to right and left atrioventicular canals.[24, 179]

ATRIUM
A thin crescent-shaped septum (septum primum) begins to grow downward from the roof of the atrium during the 4th week. Initially a large opening exists between the caudal free edge of the septum and the endocardial cushions; this is the foramen primum. This allows oxygenated blood that is returned to the right atrium to pass to the left atrium so that it can be distributed to the systemic circulation. The opening progressively gets smaller and is eventually obliterated when the septum primum fuses with the endocardial cushions.[24]

Before the septum primum reaches the atrioventricular cushions, however, a second interatrial communication forms as the result of multiple perforations that coalesce in the upper part of the septum. This is the foramen secundum.[179]

Late in the 5th week, a second thicker septum begins to develop just to the right of the septum primum. It is also crescent-shaped, but grows only until it overlaps the foramen secundum. The partition is incomplete, and an oval opening, the foramen ovale, is left.[100, 179]

The upper portion of the septum primum regresses, whereas the lower segment (attached to the endocardial cushions) remains, serving as a flap valve for the foramen ovale. Prior to birth this valve allows directed blood to move freely from the right to the left atrium. However, flow from the left to the right is prevented by apposition of the thin flexible septum primum to the rigid septum secundum after birth. This results in fusion of the septa and anatomic closure of the foramen ovale (Fig. 6–8).

VENTRICLES
Division of the bulboventricular cavity is first indicated by a sagittal muscular ridge appearing on the floor of the ventricle near the apex; this is the interventricular septum. At first the septum appears to lengthen owing to the dilation of the lateral halves of the ventricle. Later there is active proliferation of the septal tissue as the muscular portion of the interventricular septum forms.[100, 179]

Communication between the right and left

plane of sections A₁ to H₁

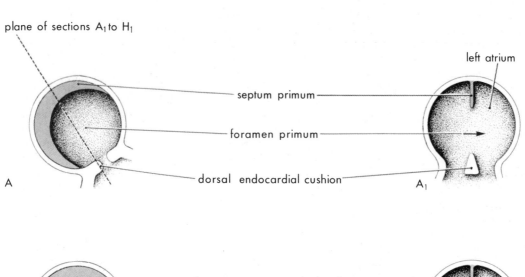

left atrium

septum primum

foramen primum

dorsal endocardial cushion

A   A₁

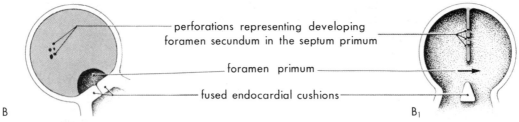

perforations representing developing
foramen secundum in the septum primum

foramen primum

fused endocardial cushions

B   B₁

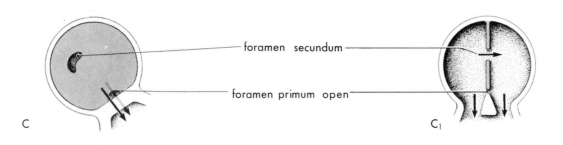

foramen secundum

foramen primum open

C   C₁

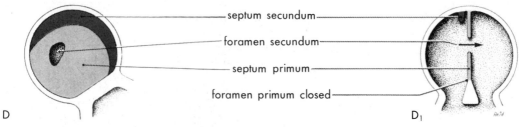

septum secundum

foramen secundum

septum primum

foramen primum closed

D   D₁

FIGURE 6–8 *See legend on opposite page*

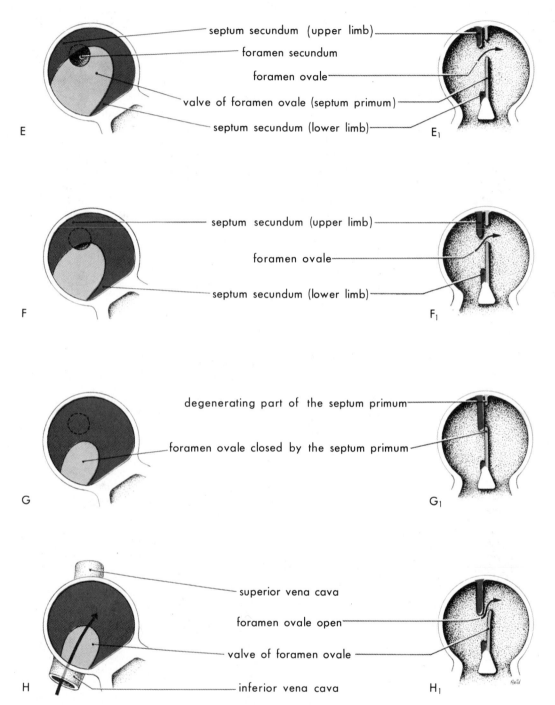

FIGURE 6–8. Diagrammatic sketches illustrating the partitioning of the primitive atrium. *A* to *H* are views of the developing interatrial septum as viewed from the right side. *A₁* to *H₁* are frontal sections of the developing interatrial septum at the plane shown in *A*. (From Moore, K.L. (1988). *The developing human* (4th ed., pp. 298, 299). Philadelphia: WB Saunders.)

sides of the ventricle is maintained until the end of the 7th week. At this time the bulbar ridges fuse. This closure is the result of fusion of subendocardial tissue from the bulbar ridges and the atrioventricular cushions.[179]

The membranous portion of the ventricular septum is derived from tissue that extends from the right side of the endocardial cushions. This eventually fuses with the aorticopulmonary septum of the truncus arteriosus and the muscular interventricular septum. Closure of the interventricular foramen results in the pulmonary trunk being in communication with the right ventricle and the aorta with the left ventricle (Fig. 6–9).[179]

BULBUS CORDIS AND TRUNCUS ARTERIOSUS

Before the interventricular septum has developed completely, spiral subendocardial thickenings appear in the distal part of the bulbus cordis. These are the bulbar ridges and can be seen during the 5th week of gestation. Initially these ridges are composed of cardiac jelly but are later invaded by mesenchymal cells. In the proximal part of the bulbus the ridges are located on the ventral and dorsal walls, whereas in the distal portion they are attached to the lateral walls. The distal portion of the bulbus is continuous with the truncus arteriosus, which develops truncal ridges that match those of the bulbus cordis. The growth and fusion of these ridges

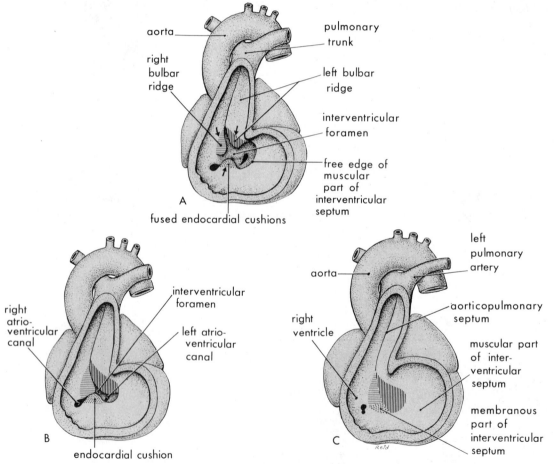

FIGURE 6–9. Schematic diagrams illustrating closure of the interventricular foramen and formation of the membranous part of the interventricular septum. The walls of the truncus arteriosus, the bulbus cordis, and the right ventricle have been removed. *A,* Five weeks, showing the bulbar ridges and the fused endocardial cushions. *B,* Six weeks, showing how proliferation of subendocardial tissue diminishes the interventricular foramen. *C,* Seven weeks, showing the fused bulbar ridges and the membranous part of the interventricular septum formed by extensions of tissue from the right side of the endocardial cushions. (From Moore, K.L. (1988). *The developing human* (4th ed., p. 305). Philadelphia: WB Saunders.)

during the 8th week result in the spiral aorticopulmonary septum. The spiral effect may be due to the streaming of blood from the ventricles through the truncus during septum development. The result is the creation of two channels, the pulmonary trunk and the aorta. The bulbus cordis is gradually incorporated into the ventricles.[100, 179]

CARDIAC VALVES

Part of the septation process involves the development of the cardiac valves. This includes the development of the semilunar valves of the aorta and the pulmonary arteries and the atrioventricular valves (tricuspid and mitral valves). The semilunar valves develop from a swelling of subendothelial tissue that appears on each side of the ventricular end of the bulbar ridges. These swellings consist of loose connective tissue covered by endothelium. Eventually the swellings become hollowed out and reshaped to form the three thin-walled cusps.[100, 179]

The atrioventricular valves similarly develop from local proliferation of subendocardial tissue as well as from connective tissue under the endocardium of the atrioventricular canals. These, too, become hollowed out, but on the ventricular side. The atrioventricular valves remain connected to the ventricular wall via muscular strands that are both papillary muscles and chordae tendineae. The mitral valve develops two cusps; the tricuspid has three.[100, 179]

Conducting System

The initial pacemaker of the cardiac muscle is located in the caudal part of the left cardiac tube. Because the muscle layers of the atrium and ventricle are continuous, this temporary pacemaker is effective in controlling contractions throughout the primitive heart. Once the sinus venosus develops, the excitatory center (sinoatrial node) is found in the right wall. This node will be incorporated into the right atrium along with the sinus venosus, where it will lie near the entrance of the superior vena cava.[100, 179]

Once the sinus venosus is incorporated into the atrium, cells from the left wall of the sinus venosus can be found in the base of the interatrial septum. When combined with cells from the atrioventricular canal, the atrioventricular (AV) node and the bundle of His are formed. These structures can be identified in

embryos early in the 2nd month of gestation.[100, 179]

The Purkinje fibers are one of the most unusual features of the heart muscle. These cells are responsible for the initiation and propagation of the cardiac impulse and the assurance of a regular contraction sequence within the organ. Although they are cardiac muscle cells, they are specialized through differentiation for conduction rather than contraction. These cells have fewer fibrils and are larger in diameter than the rest of the cardiac muscle cells. Purkinje cells are located external to the endocardium and run without interruption from the atrium to the ventricle as the atrioventricular bundle.[100]

The muscles of the atria and ventricles are eventually separated by a fibrous band of connective tissue. This results in the AV node and bundle of His being the only conductive pathways between the upper and lower halves of the heart.

Blood Vessels

Blood vessels consist of an endothelial lining stabilized by an outer coat of connective tissue. The earliest vessels are derived from angioblastic tissue, which differentiates from the mesenchyme that covers the yolk sac and is within the connecting stalk and the wall of the chorionic sac. The impetus for vascular differentiation seems to be the reduction of yolk within the ovum and yolk sac, which leads to an urgent need for a vascular system to supply nutrients to the cells.[100, 179]

Masses of isolated angioblasts come together and form blood islands. Soon spaces can be seen in these islands, around which the angioblasts will arrange themselves. This results in lumen formation and the development of a primitive endothelial layer. The isolated vessels fuse to form a network of channels and extend to adjacent areas either through growth (endothelial budding) or by fusion with other independently formed vessels. Mesenchymal cells surrounding the primitive endothelial vessels differentiate into the muscle and connective layers of the vessels.[179]

Endothelial tissue first appears in the yolk sac wall as isolated cellular cords that develop a lumen. As these vessels join together, a network of endothelial vitelline vessels is formed. By extension and growth the network progressively reaches the embryonic body.[100]

Primitive plasma and blood cells are developed from endothelial cells trapped within the vessels of the yolk sac and allantois. Blood formation in the embryo does not occur until the 5th week.[24, 179]

The endothelial lining of vessels develops before the circulation. However, once circulation begins, the hemodynamics of blood flow influences the growth of the endothelium and the differentiation of the other parts of the vessel wall. The developing organs and the temporal sequence and metabolic demands of those organs also may influence the differentiation of vessels.[100]

The first vessels seen within the embryonic body seem to form from a diffuse network that runs throughout the embryonic mesenchyme. As tissues and organs differentiate, the regional networks elaborate to meet metabolic demands.[100]

The earliest vessels are simple endothelial tubes; differentiation of arteries from veins is not possible. As development continues, the tunica media and tunica adventitia of the definitive arteries and veins arise from mesenchymal tissue.[14, 100]

ARTERIES

The right and left dorsal aortae are the primary embryonic arteries. Initially these vessels are continuations of the endocardial tubes and can be divided into three portions: a short ventral ascending portion that supplies blood to the forebrain, a primitive first aortic arch that lies in the mesenchyme of the mandibular arch (pharynx), and a relatively long descending portion that distributes blood to embyonic body, yolk sac, and chorion via the segmental plexuses, vitelline vessels, and umbilical branches, respectively. The paired dorsal aortae initially run the length of the embryo. As development continues, the two fuse just caudal to the branchial region so that there is only a single midline vessel in the caudal part of the embryo.[24, 100]

There are three major arterial branches that run off the dorsal aorta above the level of right and left aortic fusion. The intersegmental arteries are a group of 30 or more vessels that pass between and carry blood to the somites and their derivatives. In the cervical region, the first seven intersegmental arteries are connected by a longitudinal anastomosis that forms the vertebral artery. The proximal segments of the first six arteries

disappear, and the seventh intersegmental artery becomes the subclavian artery.[24, 179]

The somatic arteries also arise from this group of vessels. Eventually the intercostal arteries, lumbar arteries, common iliac arteries, and lateral sacral arteries can be identified.[24, 179]

The midline branches of the dorsal aorta run to the yolk sac, allantois, and chorion. There are two main groups, the lateral branches and the ventral branches. The ventral or vitelline arteries supply the yolk sac and the gut. These vessels will eventually be reduced to three persisting vessels, the celiac, superior mesenteric, and inferior mesenteric arteries. These vessels service the foregut, midgut, and hindgut, respectively.[24, 179]

The lateral branches supply the nephrogenic ridge and its derivatives. At first there are several branches, but retrogression results in four vessels remaining in the mature organism. These vessels are the phrenic, suprarenal, renal, and gonadal arteries.[24]

By far the largest of the dorsal aortic vessels are the paired umbilical arteries. These vessels pass through the connecting stalk (umbilical cord) and become continuous with the chorionic vessels in the developing placenta. After delivery the proximal portions of these arteries become the internal iliac and superior vesical arteries. The distal portions are obliterated and become the medial umbilical ligaments.

AORTIC ARCHES

The aortic arches are essential in the primitive circulatory system. These vessels arise from the aortic sac and terminate in the dorsal aorta. A total of five pairs develop; however, the third, fourth, and fifth arches are the only ones to contribute to the great vessels. By the end of the 8th week, the adult pattern has been established.[24, 179]

VEINS

There are three sets of paired veins that drain into the heart of the 4-week-old embryo. These are the vitelline veins, which return blood from the yolk sac; the umbilical veins, which bring oxygenated blood from the chorion; and the cardinal veins, which return blood from the body.

Vitelline Veins. The vitelline veins follow the yolk stalk and ascend on either side of the foregut. They then pass through the septum transversum and enter the sinus venosus of the heart. As the primitive liver grows into the septum transversum the hepatic sinusoids become linked with the vitelline veins. As the right vitelline vein begins to disintegrate, parts are incorporated into the developing hepatic vessels. The portal vein develops from the vitelline-derived vessels that surround the duodenum.

Umbilical Vein. The umbilical veins originate as a pair of vessels; however, the right vein and part of the left degenerate so that only a single vessel remains to return blood from the placenta to the fetus. As these vessels degenerate, the ductus venosus develops in the liver and connects the remaining umbilical vein with the inferior vena cava.

At birth the umbilical vein and the ductus venosus are obliterated with the cutting of the umbilical cord and the modifications in the circulation. The remnants of the vessels are identified as the ligamentum teres and ligamentum venosum, respectively.

Cardinal Veins. Very early in the embryonic period the cardinal vessels are the main drainage system. The anterior and posterior cardinal veins bring blood from the cranial and caudal regions and empty into the heart via a common cardinal vein that enters the sinus venosus on each side. By the 8th week, the anterior cardinal veins are connected through an anastomosis that allows for shunting of blood from the left vein to the right. This connection becomes the left brachiocephalic vein. The superior vena cava is formed by the right anterior and right common cardinal veins.

The posterior cardinal veins are transitional vessels. These vessels service the mesonephric kidneys and disappear when the kidneys degenerate. The subcardinal and supracardinal vessels develop gradually and facilitate perfusion of the mesonephric kidneys. These vessels do not degenerate entirely like the posterior cardinal veins.

The inferior vena cava is the result of a series of changes in the embryonic veins of the trunk. The four main segments of the inferior vena cava are derived from the hepatic vein and hepatic sinusoids (hepatic segment), the right subcardinal vein (prerenal segment), the subcardinal and supracardinal anastomosis (renal segment), and the right supracardinal vein (postrenal segment).[179]

Functional Development

The myocardium undergoes structural and functional changes during the fetal and neonatal periods, prior to achieving maturational properties and capabilities. Much of this process is not completely understood. The major physiologic change in the myocardium is the improved ability to generate force and to shorten. Initially the fetal myocyte has a small amount of contractile tissue, which is restricted to the subsarcolemmal region. In the neonate, the amount of contractile tissue increases and extends into the interior of the cell. By the time maturation is achieved, 60% of the myocardial tissue consists of contractile mass, in comparison to the 30% found in the fetus. These changes, along with the number of sarcomeres per gram of ventricular muscle, suggest that the fetus may not be able to generate the same force per unit of area as the adult.[293]

Fetal circulation is characterized by high flow, low vascular resistance, and the relatively passive aspects of the umbilical and placental circulations. The high fetal cardiac output may be necessary in order to meet the high fetal oxygen consumption demands. When compared to the adult, fetal oxygen consumption is 1.5 to 2.0 times higher. This may be an adaptive mechanism for the low oxygen tension found in the fetal state.[13]

Changes in fetal cardiac output seem to be directly related to fetal heart rate changes. A 10% increase in fetal heart rate above the resting level is associated with an increase in both right and left ventricular output; a decrease in heart rate results in a decrease in combined ventricular output.[293]

Stress-Strain Relationship

Cardiac muscle undergoes strain when stress (force) is applied. The usual result is lengthening of the papillary muscles. The relationship between the stress and the lengthening of the tissue is not linear but instead curvilinear. This demonstrates that initially large increases in length can be achieved with small increases in tension. As the muscle continues to be stretched it takes increasingly more tension to achieve smaller increases in length. This is a reflection of myocardial compliance.[10]

Fetal myocardium is stiffer than that of the adult, although the relationship between muscle length and force is qualitatively similar. Compliance increases rapidly during the first few days of extrauterine life. Changes in connective tissue content can be seen during this time and may explain the change in compliance, although additional explanations may lie in collagen, extracellular matrix, or matrix attachment site differences between the fetus and the adult. Further research in this area may provide increased understanding.[31, 32, 72, 89, 191]

As extrauterine growth occurs, the compliance of both ventricles increases. The weeks following birth bring about a change in ventricular mass, with the left increasing more than the right. However, during this process the right ventricle becomes more compliant. As a result, changes in right ventricular volume have a greater impact on left ventricular filling in the fetus than in the adult.[10]

In the fetus an increase in right ventricular volume or afterload interferes with left ventricular filling. The impact of one chamber on another is also more marked with decreasing compliance. So if there are changes in right ventricular diastolic or loading pressures in the fetus, the left ventricle is compromised and stroke volume is reduced. Once the pulmonary vascular resistance drops at delivery and throughout the neonatal period, left ventricular filling is enhanced and stroke volume is improved. Therefore, neonates are more compromised than adults if there is an increase in right ventricular preload or afterload with specific pathologic conditions (papillary muscle dysfunction or pulmonary hypertension).

Contractile Properties

Contractile capabilities are dependent upon the force of contraction, shortening velocity (preload), inotropy, and afterload (load carried at the time of contraction). The maximum shortening of muscle is obtained when there is zero load; however, as the afterload increases, the velocity of muscle shortening decreases. If the load is so great that no external shortening is possible, the contraction is considered isometric. The force of the contraction can be altered by changing the muscle length; force development is related to the number of cross-bridges (the greater the number the greater the force).[10]

An increase in contraction ability and development of force is part of the maturation process of the myocardium. There is no sud-

den change in force-generating ability with birth, but rather a slow progression over time as the entire cardiac system matures into adulthood.

Most of these maturational processes are related to structural changes in the myocardial anatomy. As myofibrillar content increases there is an increase in the number of cross-bridge attachments and therefore greater force. The increased organization of the myofibrils may also contribute to the ability to generate forceful contractions. Whether changes in the responsiveness of the contractile apparatus to calcium facilitate any of these changes is currently unclear. Maturation of membrane systems and calcium control may also affect muscle contractions.

The maturational increase in the force-generating ability of the myocardium begins to be seen in late gestation and continues until adulthood. Ventricular filling, pressure development, and ejection in the fetus are similar to those in the neonate and the adult, except that at birth there is a marked increase in combined ventricular output. Overall, the increase in the left ventricle is larger, although reasons for this are not currently known. It is possible that an increase in pulmonary venous return, improved inotropy (strength of contraction), increased heart rate, and the diastolic and systolic interactions of the right and left ventricles may contribute to the change in combined output.

In the weeks after birth left ventricular output returns to fetal levels or lower, whereas systolic and end-diastolic pressures continue to rise. Other indicators of the increased birth inotropy also return to fetal baselines. A clear explanation for this is currently not known, although it may have to do with the reaccumulation of reserves after the birth process. Therefore diseases that place an additional demand on the heart to produce more cardiac ouput in the first days of extrauterine life can result in cardiovascular compromise for the neonate.[10]

Frank-Starling Relationship

This relationship describes the effect of ventricular end-diastolic volume on ventricular output. This is termed preload and occurs prior to ventricular activation. As the end-diastolic volume increases, the ability of the ventricle to contract and to generate pressure increases initially. A plateau is reached, however, where further increases in ventricular volume do not lead to an increase in pressure. This may be explained by changes in myofilament sensitivity to calcium concentrations or by the length of the sarcomere. When the sarcomere is stretched so thin that the thick and thin filaments no longer overlap, cross-bridge attachments cannot be made and force cannot be generated. The ability to generate force is also decreased when the sarcomere length is so short that double overlap occurs.

In the fetal heart the right and left ventricles have stages of filling that are similar to those in the adult; however, the end-diastolic dimensions of the right ventricle are larger than those of the left. There also seems to be a difference in the rate of filling between the ventricles.

Although the Frank-Starling relationship is present in isolated fetal myocardial tissue, in vivo studies are not definitive. The relationship may be present, but there may be little functional reserve because the fetal heart functions at the apex of the relationship. This has been demonstrated through research that has shown a drop in atrial pressure and a decrease in ventricular output with blood withdrawal, whereas an increase in atrial baseline pressure produces little change in cardiac ouput. This has been contradicted by studies that have shown that a change in end-diastolic volume significantly affects stroke volume.[9, 11, 92, 136, 264]

The differences in these studies may be the result of the variables identified to assess the change in end-diastolic volume. Beyond this, the curvilinear relationship between pressure and end-diastolic volume can mean that a large change in diastolic pressure may produce little change in end-diastolic volume. This may be especially true if the myocardium is relatively stiff (noncompliant). Maturational increases in myocardium compliance have been suggested as a basis for apparent developmental acquisition of the Frank-Starling relationship.[10, 224]

The left ventricular end-diastolic volume increases with birth. This probably contributes to the neonatal increase in output via the Frank-Starling relationship. These changes may be due to the circulatory transition that occurs at delivery and the fall in pulmonary vascular resistance and increased pulmonary venous return. Left ventricular filling may be augmented by a decrease in right ventricular afterload. Therefore, a fall in pulmonary

artery pressure would enhance left ventricular output by decreasing right ventricular afterload, which would improve right ventricular ejection and result in a smaller right ventricular end-diastolic volume. The left ventricle is then able to fill to a larger volume at a comparable filling pressure. This interaction is magnified in the fetus and neonate because of the reduced compliance found in the heart.[10, 232]

Afterload

The ability of the myocardium to shorten leads to ejection of blood and is affected by the load present during the contraction. As afterload is increased, this shortening ability is decreased. The velocity of shortening is correlated to the rate of adenosine triphosphate (ATP) hydrolysis by myosin adenosine triphosphatase (ATPase), which is consistent with ATPase activity controlling the rate of cross-bridge detachment. In the presence of a load, shortening velocity is also dependent upon the number of cross-bridge attachments.

In the fetus the myocardium shortens more slowly when compared with adult tissue. This fetal liability is to be expected given the maturation of the force-generating ability of the myocardium. Arterial pressure is a major component of afterload and has a significant effect on ejection (the higher the pressure, the smaller the stroke volume). This relationship holds throughout development, although the neonate seems to be less tolerant of increases in arterial pressure.[10, 264]

Inotropy

The strength of myocardial contractions is termed inotropy. Changes in inotropy reflect a change in the ability of the myocardium to contract, and maturational development affects inotropy in the fetus and neonate. One of these changes is related to the availability of calcium and the control of cytosolic calcium. The development of the sarcomeres and their intracellular control mechanisms is integrally tied to this process. Therefore the lower calcium concentrations bathing the sarcomere account for the lower sarcomere shortening and reextension velocities seen in the fetus and neonate.

Heart rate also affects the strength of contraction in a positive way in the fetus, neonate, and adult. In fetal lambs, however, as heart rate increases, stroke volume decreases. This is most likely due to a decrease in end-diastolic volume that is a natural consequence of the increased heart rate. Conflicting data have been found in studies of the human fetus, although the majority of the time there seems to be a positive effect on ventricular output. This may be due to additional factors that have inotropic effects.[10, 257]

NEONATAL PHYSIOLOGY

Transitional Events

During birth, the circulation changes from a fetal configuration to that of the adult. The initial phase occurs within 60 seconds of birth; however, completion of this transformation takes up to 6 weeks. At this time, oxygenation is moved from the placenta to the lungs, and air ventilation results in increased oxygen availability with a concomitant rise in fetal PO_2 levels. The major alterations occurring at transition are removal of the placenta, increase in pulmonary blood flow, and closure of the fetal cardiovascular shunts.

Fetal Circulation

Most of the information currently available regarding fetal circulation has been obtained from research on fetal lambs. Although this must be taken into consideration, it appears that the research findings are supported by clinical observations of the human fetus.

In the fetus, who is not dependent upon the lungs to oxygenate the blood, circulation is arranged in a parallel fashion. This arrangement allows for mixing of oxygenated blood with unoxygenated blood at the atrial and great vessel levels. The modifications in the circulation that allow for this mixing divert blood from the immature lungs to the placenta where oxygen–carbon dioxide exchange occurs.[184]

As the blood returns from the placenta via the umbilical vein it passes either into the portal system's microcirculation to later run off into the inferior vena cava (IVC) or into the ductus venosus, which connects directly with the IVC (40 to 60% of the blood flow is shunted across the ductus venosus). This blood joins with the blood that returns from the lower half of the fetal body. The venous duct is a low-resistance channel that allows a significant portion of relatively well oxygenated blood to enter the heart directly.

As the blood enters the right atrium the position of the IVC is aligned with the foramen ovale such that it facilitates blood flow across the latter. The crista dividens (the free edge of the atrial septum) separates the flow into two streams with 50 to 60% being diverted across the foramen ovale into the left atrium.

In the left atrium, the blood from the IVC mixes with the pulmonary venous return and passes through the mitral valve into the left ventricle. Upon contraction, this blood is ejected into the ascending aorta to feed the coronary, carotid, and subclavian arteries. Only 10% of the combined ventricular output passes along the aortic arch into the descending aorta.

The rest of the blood from the IVC joins with blood from the superior vena cava (SVC) and coronary sinus in the right atrium, passing through the tricuspid valve into the right ventricle. Very little of the SVC blood return crosses the foramen ovale to the left atrium. The mixed blood in the right atrium is then ejected into the pulmonary artery, where increased pulmonary vascular resistance (PVR) prevents any more than 5 to 10% of the right ventricular output from entering the pulmonary bed. Consequently 60% of the combined ventricular output is shunted across the ductus arteriosus to enter the descending aorta and the low-resistance systemic circulation.

The communication between the atria, along with the PDA, allows for equalization of pressures between the atria and the great vessels. Because these pressures are equal, the ventricular pressures are also equal, with a systolic pressure of 70 mmHg and an amniotic pressure of zero.[88]

Oxygen Content

The oxygen content of the fetus is lower than that of the neonate, child, or adult. The highest oxygen content is found in the blood returning from the placenta via the umbilical vein, which is 32 to 35 mmHg and 70% saturated. This falls to 26 to 28 mmHg (65% saturation) by the time it reaches the left atrium and mixes with blood from the IVC and pulmonary veins and is ejected into the ascending aorta.

The umbilical return that mixes with the superior vena caval blood (PO$_2$ 12 to 14 mmHg, saturation 40%) is reduced to a PaO$_2$ of 20 to 22 mmHg. This blood is destined for the pulmonary arteries, descending aorta, and placenta. Therefore the blood with the highest oxygen content is delivered to the coronary arteries and brain, whereas the blood with the lowest PaO$_2$ is shunted toward the placenta.

Another fetal adaptation to low oxygen tension is the presence of fetal hemoglobin. This specific type of hemoglobin has a high affinity for oxygen even at low oxygen tensions, thereby improving saturation and facilitating transport of oxygen to the tissues. See Chapters 5 and 7 for a further discussion of the properties of fetal hemoglobin.

Transition

The changeover from fetal to neonatal circulation is linked directly with the development and function of the pulmonary vasculature (see Chapter 7). At delivery the low-resistance placental circulation is removed, leading to an increase in systemic vascular resistance (SVR). The initiation of air breathing leads to lung expansion, an increase in alveolar oxygen concentration, and vasodilatation of the pulmonary vascular bed. As vasodilatation occurs PVR falls by almost 80%, resulting in a dramatic increase in pulmonary blood flow and a fall in ductal shunting. Prior to birth the high PVR and low SVR result in 90% of the right ventricular output going through the ductus. After delivery 90% of flow goes to the pulmonary arteries.

These alterations at birth lead to pressure changes within the cardiac chambers and the movement from parallel circulation to in series circulation. The pressure changes result from the rapid drop in systemic venous return via the IVC and the increase in pulmonary venous return. The left atrial pressure rises, exceeding the right atrial pressure, and the foramen ovale's flap valve shuts, separating the two atria.

The ductus arteriosus begins to close almost immediately; however, it may remain patent for several hours to days following delivery. The PVR may remain higher than the systemic vascular bed for a short time following the first breath. This allows for a small right-to-left shunt to remain and desaturated blood to mix with oxygenated blood

in the descending aorta. If the PVR remains high or is increased during the first hours or days after delivery, the right-to-left shunt may become clinically significant.

As the SVR continues to increase and stabilize and the PVR continues to fall, the movement of blood across the ductus arteriosus reverses (left to right). Within the first 12 hours of extrauterine life, the ductus arteriosus achieves functional closure through constriction. Anatomic closure takes much longer and is achieved within the 1st month of life. During this time, the ductus may be reopened if hypoxia or increased PVR is encountered. This may occur with crying or with pathologic problems.

How the ductus arteriosus closes is not completely understood; however, both oxygen and prostaglandins play a role in the immediate process. Although there is a relative hypoxia present at birth (when compared with adult oxygen levels), within 10 minutes the neonate is hyperoxic with a PaO$_2$ of 50 mmHg. This continues to increase over the first hour to approximately 62 mmHg. Arterial oxygen concentrations stabilize between 75 and 85 mmHg over the first 2 days, with a concomitant fall in PVR and improved ventilation-perfusion ratios. The fall in PVR continues for the next several weeks; however, adult circulation is achieved within the first 2 days.[13]

Prostaglandin E$_2$ seems to be responsible for maintaining the patency of the ductus arteriosus during fetal life. In fact, the ductus arteriosus is extremely sensitive to PGE$_2$, and it is the loss of this reactivity that keeps the ductus closed after birth. Just prior to birth there is a decrease in circulating PGE$_2$ concentrations, which may prepare for or enhance ductal closure at the time the infant converts to air breathing and active ductal constriction occurs.[13] Approximately 80% of ducts are anatomically closed by the end of the 3rd month; however, there may be cases where final closure does not occur until 1 year of age.

The combined ventricular output in the fetal lamb is about 450 ml/kg fetal body weight per minute, with about 300 ml/kg/min being ejected by the right ventricle. Within 24 hours of birth, oxygen consumption triples. To meet this demand, the total cardiac output increases dramatically with each ventricle ejecting approximately 400 ml/kg/min. Although there is little change in the right ventricle, the left must increase output significantly resulting in hypertrophy and remodeling of the muscular walls. This change occurs over the 1st month of life.[13]

The adaptation to neonatal life is characterized by an increase in heart rate, end-diastolic volume, and inotropic state. This implies that even at rest the neonate is functioning at nearly full capacity with little or no reserve in contractility, preload, or afterload. This is to meet the increased vascular loading that occurs with birth. Consequently the newborn heart has less ability to adapt to additional acute pressure (afterload) or volume (preload) stresses.[255]

Myocardial contractility in neonates is high during the 1st week of life, and therefore there is little reserve in contractility. This implies that inotropic drugs will do little to improve the contractile state of the normally functioning neonatal heart. One mechanism for this increased inotropic state and the elevated cardiac output is the high level of adrenergic stimulation that occurs around birth. However, the increased cardiac output that remains for several weeks postnatally cannot be explained by continued catecholamine activity. It has been suggested that the postnatal increase in T_3 concentrations may contribute to the increased left ventricular output.[255]

Because of the high volume load following delivery, the neonate functions at the upper limits of the Starling curve. Moreover, the low compliance of the left ventricle decreases the preload reserve volume. Heart rates in neonates are high, falling during the 6 weeks following delivery. Whether infants can augment cardiac output through further increases in heart rate continues to be debated, as does the effectiveness of inotropic support in the neonate without contractility failure. If increases in afterload or preload are associated with decreased contractility, as with sepsis or asphyxia, inotropic support can improve cardiac output rapidly.[255]

Cardiac Physiology

The cardiovascular system is designed to deliver adequate oxygen and nutrients to the tissues and remove metabolic by-products at all stages of development. The coordinated functioning of respiratory, cardiovascular, and endocrine systems is essential to meet the cellular metabolic needs, especially in times of stress. During fetal, neonatal, and adult life these processes are quite different, and maturational processes continue after birth.

Metabolic Rate and Oxygen Transport

Metabolic rate is measured as oxygen consumption and is much higher in the neonate than in the adult. The neonatal metabolic rate is also higher than that of the fetus, owing to independent extrauterine functioning and growth requirements. The components of oxygen consumption are related to energy expenditure and include basal metabolic rate, growth, heat production, and physical activity. The growth component is approximately 2 to 3% of the total metabolic rate and is higher in premature infants. Oxygen consumption in the neonate increases exponentially with physical activity, placement in a nonthermal environment, therapeutic and diagnostic procedures, and increased work of breathing.[2, 36, 68, 80, 114, 154, 155, 244, 296]

The oxygen availability, which is the product of the cardiac output and the arterial oxygen content, is also elevated in the neonate. The estimated delivery of oxygen in the neonate at rest is 75% higher than in the adult.

Impaired oxygen delivery has been assessed in the lamb; however, its difference from the human neonate must be remembered when reviewing data from research conducted in this area. Three major processes impair oxygen availability: ventilation-perfusion mismatching from either intra- or extrapulmonary sources, reduced oxygen-hemoglobin-binding capacity, and reduced cardiac output. Along with these causes, a cardiovascular system that is unable to respond to an increased metabolic demand can result in decompensation.[281, 282]

Endocrine, respiratory, and cardiovascular responses to altered oxygenation are similar to those found in the adult, the major difference being that the neonate functions close to maximum capacity normally and therefore has little reserve to compensate for further demands. Therefore when impaired oxygen transport results in increased cardiac output (increased heart rate), the maximum is readily reached. Further oxygen demands are associated with an increase in oxygen extraction and a decrease in oxygen saturation.[126, 281, 282]

Hypoxemia results in a decrease in oxygen consumption, oxygen availability, and systemic vascular resistance and an increase in oxygen extraction by the tissues. Heart rate and cardiac output increase, since the ability to deliver and release oxygen to the myocardium is essential for the myocardium to respond to the hypoxemia and compensate for impaired oxygen transport.[87]

Isovolemic anemia results in a significant decrease in arterial and mixed venous oxygen content, mean aortic pressure, and systemic vascular resistance. Cardiac output and stroke volume increase regardless of the hemoglobin content; however, heart rate increases were seen only with a hemoglobin of 6 g/dl. If oxygen affinity is reduced, cardiac output and stroke volume increase to a greater degree. These events, once again, occur only when myocardial function is maintained.[279]

Impaired cardiac output results in redistribution of blood flow, with flow directed to the heart and brain preferentially and shunted away from the peripheral organ systems. This is reflected in an increase in vascular resistance in the lower body, with no change in the upper body.

Over the first 2 to 4 months of life there is a fall in hemoglobin concentration, an increase in Hb A, and a rightward shift in the oxygen-hemoglobin dissociation curve. This enables more oxygen to be released to the tissues at the same capillary oxygen tension. However, the increased metabolic demands of extrauterine life (including physical activity) must be accompanied by an increase in the P_{50} to compensate for the total hemoglobin concentration.

The pattern of changes during these first 2 to 4 months includes a decline in total hemoglobin (reaching its lowest point at 8 to 12 weeks in term infants), a progressive shift in P_{50} to the right, and an early change in 2,3-diphosphoglycerate (2,3-DPG) (see Chapter 5). There may also be an increase in cardiac output and an increase in oxygen extraction. The latter is adjusted depending on the oxygen consumption, total hemoglobin, and P_{50}. Once hemoglobin levels fall below a critical point, however, cardiac output is unable to compensate for the reduced oxygen availability, necessitating a redistribution in cardiac output.[126, 231]

Central Mechanisms

As in the adult, fetal and neonatal cardiovascular functions are presumably influenced by medullary, hypothalamic, and cerebral cortical activity. Studies of fetal heart rate and the variables that influence it provide invaluable information on the functioning of the preterm and full-term neonate and extrauterine functioning. Dawes has stressed the importance of the fetal arousal level and circadian central nervous system (CNS) activity patterns,[72a] noting that bradycardia and respiratory activity frequently accompany fetal sheep EEG patterns that resemble human rapid eye movement states in the neonate. These characteristic behaviors can be seen clinically in the preterm infant.

The medullary centers appear to influence cardiovascular responses in a variable fashion in the fetus; however, higher cortical or hypothalamic activities are associated with an increase in heart rate and hypertension. This stimulation and response are quite different than the baroreflex, which is a peripheral response by the baroreceptors to hypertension that itself is secondary to increased peripheral resistance.

Regulation of Fetal and Neonatal Circulation

Complex neurohumoral and metabolic responses maintain blood pressure, heart rate, and distribution of blood flow in the fetus. These include systemic sensors (stretch receptors and neural and hormonal mediators) as well as local responses that allow an organ to regulate flow. The interaction of the two systems allows the fetus to respond to stress events by redistributing blood flow to spare high-priority organs with specific oxygen requirements.

NEURAL REGULATION

Baroreceptors that are sensitive to changes in blood pressure are located in the aortic arch and the carotid sinuses. These sensors cause changes in heart rate and, in the fetus, may be responsible for stabilizing fetal blood pressure with increasing sensitivity as gestational age advances. Baroreceptor activity has been implicated in the decreasing fetal heart rate baseline seen in later gestation as blood pressure rises. Following delivery, baroreceptor sensitivity increases. Chemoreceptors can be found in both the peripheral and central nervous systems and may alter fetal heart rate in response to hypoxemia and acidosis. Their role in the normal fetus is unclear. Present in the latter half of gestation they appear to be responsive to changes in pH and carbon dioxide tension and give rise to bradycardia while cardiac output and umbilical blood flow are perserved. Following birth, hypoxia leads to tachycardia and an increase in cardiac output associated with increased respiratory effort.[13, 293]

Sympathetic intervention is present and functional in the fetus, increasing responsiveness with increasing gestational age. Stimulation results in tachycardia, augmented myocardial contractility, and increased systemic arterial blood pressure.

Parasympathetic input also increases with advancing gestational age. The major effector is the vagus nerve, which provides an inhibitory effect on fetal heart rate. Short-term variability of the fetal heart rate is modulated by impulses from the vagus nerve. Studies looking at the relative contributions of the parasympathetic and sympathetic nervous systems seem to indicate that the parasympathetic nervous system matures more quickly than the sympathetic system. Functional balance is achieved in the neonate.[293]

HUMORAL REGULATION

Humoral regulation of the cardiovascular system is related to the impact of catecholamines, vasopressin, renin-angiotensin, and prostaglandins on the heart and vascular bed. Catecholamines are secreted by the adrenal medulla and may be involved in fetal cardiovascular system regulation prior to the development of the sympathetic nervous system. Fetal myocardium appears to have equal responsiveness to catecholamines when compared with that of the adult.[13, 293]

Arginine vasopressin is produced by the fetal pituitary gland early in gestation. Although usually undetectable, during hypoxia, hypotension, or hypernatremia the concentration of vasopressin increases. This results in vasoconstriction of the vessels in the musculoskeletal system, skin, and gut while increasing flow to the brain and heart. Prostaglandins may also play a role in augmenting blood flow to the brain during hypoxic episodes. These humoral mechanisms may play a major role in the redistribution of blood flow seen in the fetus during significant hypoxia.[13]

Stimulation of the renin-angiotensin system leads to an increase in fetal heart rate, blood pressure, and combined ventricular output. Blood flow to the lungs and myocardium increases; flow to the renal system falls

off. Angiotensin II seems to exert a vasotonic effect on the peripheral circulation. These effects may support the fetus during episodes of significant blood loss.[13]

BASELINE HEART RATE

The average baseline heart rate in the normal fetus at 20 weeks is 155 beats per minute; at 30 weeks, 144 beats per minute; and at term, 140 beats per minute.[13] Variations of 20 beats per minute above or below these levels are considered normal.[13, 127] This baseline rate is determined by the intrinsic depolarization rate of the sinoatrial node, which is actively inhibited by tonic parasympathetic input. As the parasympathetic system matures with advancing gestational age, the resting heart rate decreases.[13]

Fetal tachycardia (>160 beats per minute) is usually seen with nonasphyxial events that lead to cataecholamine release, sympathetic stimulation, or parasympathetic withdrawal. Tachycardia is considered physiologic in the extremely premature fetus in whom the sympathetic nervous system dominates control of cardiac function. This change in baseline can be mediated by a host of fetal and maternal conditions, of which maternal infection is the most common. The extrauterine infection may result in an increased fetal body temperature in response to maternal fever.[13, 127]

Other sources of fetal tachycardia may be the use of β-sympathomimetic agents (to inhibit uterine contractions), fetal anemia (Rh isoimmunization), acute fetal blood loss (placental abruption), or abnormal fetal conduction system (Wolff-Parkinson-White disease). Tachycardia may also be a fetal compensatory or recovery response to an acute asphyxial episode or mild hypoxemia and is probably due to a rise in catecholamine levels.[127]

A sustained fetal heart rate of less than 120 beats per minute is defined as bradycardia. Bradycardia is the initial fetal response to asphyxia. Nonasphyxial causes of bradycardia include heart block, changes in cardiac afterload (seen with cord compression), and head compression. In the last case, vagal nerve stimulation caused by mild cerebral ischemia or increased intracranial pressure seems to explain the bradycardia.[13, 127]

Severe bradycardia (below 100 beats per minute) is the result of acute fetal distress. The fetal hypertension following a hypoxic insult leads to a baroreceptor reflex, which leads to a vagal response and a fall in fetal heart rate. The duration and severity of the bradycardia are correlated to the length and severity of the asphyxial event. These events are related to an interruption in blood flow either through cord compression, decreased placental exchange area (abruptio placentae), or impaired uterine blood flow (hypertonic contractions).[127]

End-stage bradycardia associated with the second stage of labor is thought to be due to cord entanglement or impaired placental perfusion. If associated with metabolic acidosis, fetal well-being is jeopardized.[127]

BEAT-TO-BEAT VARIABILITY

The time interval between two heart beats in a healthy fetus is seldom the same and may be caused by the interaction of the sympathetic and parasympathetic reflexes or by rapidly oscillating vagal impulses. Normal, short- and long-term variability is accepted as an indicator of anatomic and functional integrity of the pathways regulating cardiac function. Short-term variability is considered normal when fetal heart rate (FHR) oscillations are between 6 and 20 beats per minute. Reduced or absent variability exists when oscillations are less than 6 beats per minute or less than 2 beats per minute, respectively. Long-term variability occurs in cycles of 3 to 6 cycles per minute and consists of irregular waves that resemble a sine wave. The FHR pathway starts in the cerebral cortex and travels through the midbrain to the vagus nerve and the cardiac conductive system. Fetuses with anomalies, such as anencephaly, demonstrate alterations in variability without the presence of hypoxia.[127]

Other factors affecting parasympathetic activity include fetal breathing, fetal movement, and fetal sleep state. The use of local or general anesthetics as well as other maternal drugs (i.e., magnesium sulfate or meperidine) also can affect beat-to-beat variability.[13]

Periodic changes in FHR are associated with uterine contractions or fetal activity. They are usually described as decelerations that may be early, variable, or late and accelerations. Early decelerations are the result of a physiologic chain of events that begins with head compression during a uterine contraction; this leads to a reduction in cerebral blood flow, hypoxia, and hypercapnia. Hypercapnia results in hypertension with triggering of the baroreceptors. This results in bradycardia mediated by the parasympathetic nervous system. The fall and rise of

the FHR are matched to the rise and fall of the uterine contraction. These changes usually do not exceed 40 beats per minute and are not indicative of fetal distress.[13, 127]

Variable decelerations imply an inconsistent time of onset when compared with uterine contractions. The clinical implications are related to the depth and duration of the decelerations. Partial compression or stretching of the umbilical cord with blood flow interruption decreases the blood return to the right heart and causes hypotension. This results in sympathetic nervous system stimulation, catecholamine release, and compensatory fetal tachycardia following the deceleration.[127]

Late decelerations begin characteristically within a few seconds of the peak of a contraction, reach their nadir 20 to 90 seconds later, and have a slow recovery phase. These decelerations mirror the image of the uterine contractions, are repetitive and persistent, and occur with each contraction. Their depth is related to the intensity and frequency of the uterine contraction. These decelerations represent fetal hypoxia and are related to an interruption in oxygen supply at the uteroplacental level.[127]

During contractions the blood in the intervillous space (IVS) is sluggish and stagnant. The transfer of nutrients and waste products is reduced. In situations in which the respiratory reserve (oxygen content) in the IVS is reduced, which can occur with suboptimal replacement between contractions or with contractions that come too frequently, the fetal oxygen supply is diminished. The removal of waste products is also reduced, which can result in lactic acid and carbon dioxide buildup within the fetus. This contributes to the development of fetal acidosis.

The reduced oxygen supply in the fetus leads to stimulation of the carotid and aortic chemoreceptors, resulting in activation of the cardiac centers in the brain stem. The sinoatrial node is affected, and FHR is slowed. If hypoxia is prolonged, fetal myocardium is affected, leading to a further decrease in FHR and hypotension. Recovery will be slower as well.

As noted earlier, in the fetus the beat-to-beat variability is an indicator of total central nervous system activity; and the loss of this variability can be a sign of anything from normal sleep to impending death. Certain drugs as well as catecholamine bursts can also affect the CNS and be reflected in heart rate variability. Therefore this one parameter cannot be used as an independent measure of fetal well-being, but instead can provide valuable information when combined with other indicators. Many of these same measures hold true in the neonatal state as well.

CLINICAL IMPLICATIONS FOR NEONATAL CARE

Cardiovascular disturbances in the fetus can be seen with fetal hypoxia and hydrops fetalis. Both of these have implications for delivery and transition and are therefore included in this discussion. In the neonate, cardiovascular disorders are manifest in only a limited number of ways. These include congestive heart failure, cyanosis, murmurs, and dysrhythmias. Cardiac malformations occur in about 8 of every 1000 live births and represent about 10% of all congenital malformations. Murmurs that are due to the normal turbulence of transitional circulation (i.e., ductal closure) or physiologic turbulence in the pulmonary artery are considered benign. Gestational age and disease also affect the cardiovascular system and are factors in patent ductus arteriosus and bronchopulmonary dysplasia.

The fetus lives and grows in a relatively hypoxic environment and yet has enough oxygen to meet basal metabolic and growth needs. It is the integrity of the maternal, fetal, and placental circulations that maintains the continual flow of nutrients to meet the demands of the products of conception. If any interruption in flow occurs, the fetus experiences a reduction or loss of available oxygen and nutrient substrates.

Fetal Stress Response

Factors affecting oxygen transfer to the fetus can be of environmental, maternal, placental, umbilical, or fetal origin. Substrate consumption by the fetus provides fuel for oxidative metabolism and building materials for tissue growth. When substrate availability or transfer is limited, both processes are in jeopardy. This can occur by reducing arterial oxygen content, restricting uterine blood flow, or reducing umbilical blood flow through cord compression. Maternal hypoxemia reduces only the oxygen supply available to the fetus;

however, interruption of uterine or umbilical blood flow interferes not only with oxygen transfer but also with carbon dioxide elimination.[233]

Cardiac output may be affected by hypoxemia, depending on the severity of the event. Maternal hypoxemia of a mild nature usually does not have an effect on fetal combined ventricular output. However, as the severity increases, a drop of 20% can be anticipated. Acute uterine blood flow interruption of a significant degree is associated with a fall in fetal ventricular output. When umbilical blood flow is interrupted and venous return is affected, there is always decreased ventricular output. If there is a 50% interruption in umbilical flow, there is a 20% drop in output.[233]

Oxygen delivery from the placental circulation to the fetal body can be reduced by either maternal hypoxemia or flow disruption. When oxygen delivery is reduced by 40%, the fetal arterial PO_2 is decreased to 12 to 13 mmHg; however, blood flow is maintained. On the other hand, when blood flow is reduced by 50%, there is little change in umbilical venous oxygen content owing to the mismatching of uterine and umbilical flow rates.[233]

The distribution of blood flow and oxygen to fetal organs is quite different in the two types of stress. During maternal hypoxemia, blood flow is directed to the myocardium, adrenal gland, and cerebral circuits. Blood flow to the skin, lungs, gastrointestinal system, muscles, liver, and kidneys is markedly reduced. Cord compression, on the other hand, leads to only a moderate increase in blood flow to the myocardium and brain. There is a marked increase in blood flow to the adrenals, however. The pulmonary system does experience a decrease in blood flow, but blood flow to the kidneys, gastrointestinal tract, and peripheral circulation is maintained or increased.[96, 233, 234]

The percentage of blood flow and therefore oxygen delivery is also altered with the two types of hypoxia. With maternal hypoxia, a 40% reduction in total fetal oxygen uptake coincides with a 40% increase in oxygen delivery to the brain; 100% increase to the myocardium; 60% reduction to gastrointestinal, pulmonary, and peripheral circuits; and 40% reduction to the renal system. Umbilical cord compression, on the other hand, is associated with a minimal reduction of cerebral and myocardial oxygen delivery and only a 25% fall in gastrointestinal, peripheral, and renal oxygen delivery. The pulmonary system, however, experiences a 70% cut in oxygen.[233, 234]

Heart rate, blood pressure, and combined ventricular output are affected by hypoxia. Unlike the adult, the fetus responds to hypoxia not with tachycardia but with bradycardia. Along with this, there is a rise in systemic arterial pressure. Which of these responses comes first is unknown, because both develop slowly over 2 to 3 minutes.

The onset of bradycardia is earlier and the duration prolonged if the baseline arterial blood oxygen saturation is lower. The heart rate does return to baseline values when the hypoxemia is prolonged, although when the initial oxygen saturation is lower, recovery from the bradycardia is more protracted.[233]

During umbilical vein occlusion there are insignificant changes in arterial pressure. The onset of bradycardia is delayed and occurs only after the PaO_2 has fallen. In the sudden, complete occlusion of the umbilical cord, however, there is an immediate rise in arterial pressure because of arterial occlusion, and bradycardia is instantaneous.[96, 217, 233, 234]

The fall in combined ventricular output due to hypoxia is the result of a decrease in left and right ventricular output. This reduced output is mainly due to the fall in heart rate. Output returns to normal once the fetal heart rate is restored to baseline level.[233]

In addition to interruptions in oxidative metabolism due to hypoxia or asphyxia on a short-term basis, long-term reductions in oxygenation lead the fetus to shut down oxygen-consuming processes (i.e., growth or behavioral changes). With acute reductions in oxygenation, fetal glucose consumption may fall and glycogen mobilization increase. These alterations ensure a continuous glucose supply to the placenta. If lactate concentrations rise, this may be another substrate source for maintaining the placenta over time.

In order to maintain the placenta, oxygen-consuming activities such as protein synthesis must be curtailed so as to direct limited resources to more vital functions. Metabolic normality may be maintained by the fetus, which suggests that the fetus is capable of rapid adaptation to limited substrate delivery by decreasing the growth rate. This results in intrauterine growth retardation (IUGR) for the fetus, which can be continued over a protracted period of time. The length of time normal growth patterns are interrupted can change from being protective to being pathologic for some organ systems. These alterations can influence future extrauterine growth and development.[217]

Along with physiologic changes, behavioral state changes can be seen during acute short-term hypoxemia as well as in sustained acute hypoxemia and graded prolonged hypoxemia. Rapid eye movement sleep states are decreased with hypoxemia and may be indicative of changes in oxygen consumption. The development of well-defined behavioral states may be delayed in IUGR infants as compared with normal infants.[217]

There is also a reduction in fetal movements with hypoxia. Acute asphyxia may result in a brief increase in extremity movement that falls off quickly if oxygenation is not restored. This cessation in fetal breathing movements and gross body movements can contribute to reducing fetal oxygen consumption. The number and duration of general body movements are decreased in IUGR infants. This is an indication of decreased energy expenditure.[217, 250]

Although the fetus is capable of reducing its oxygen needs and compensating for limited substrate availability over a protracted period of time, this may end up being detrimental to organ development and functioning on a long-term basis. Acute responses can decrease mortality but may lead to morbidity that becomes evident after delivery.

Hydrops Fetalis

Accumulation of excess interstitial tissue water is termed edema. In the fetus, excessive edema formation is termed hydrops fetalis and may be due to immune or nonimmune causes. The major cause of Rh isoimmunization (immune hydrops fetalis) is anti-D antibodies, although other antibodies are becoming increasingly important as causes of isoimmunization and hydrops. Further discussion of Rh isoimmunization can be found in Chapter 10. Multiple causes are associated with nonimmune hydrops fetalis. These include congenital anomalies, in utero cardiac arrhythmias, anemia, polycythemia, and hypoproteinemia associated with liver damage, among other causes.

The movement of water within the body occurs via random molecular movement (diffusional flow), hydrostatic and osmotic gradients (bulk flow), and electrochemical forces. Intracellular water is under the control of osmotic pressure and the sodium pump. The availability of ATP and glucose as well as the presence of acidosis and hypoxia can affect the functioning capacity of the sodium pump. The integrity of the capillary endothelium, Starling forces, the affinity of interstitial gel for water, and lymphatic drainage determine the distribution of extracellular water.[20, 192, 283]

It is very unlikely that there is a single pathologic process to explain hydrops fetalis. There are several factors that can contribute to fetal development of edema. These factors are delineated in Table 6–5.

The most common maternal conditions correlated with fetal edema are premature delivery (90%) and polyhydramnios (75%). Maternal anemia (hemoglobin less than 11 g/dl) is associated with 39% of the cases of hydrops, and preeclampsia is noted in 34% of hydropic deliveries. All of these conditions may result in maternal hypoproteinemia, which leads to alterations in maternal hydrostatic pressure and colloid osmotic pressure. This would favor water transfer to the fetus.[115]

The severity of immune hydrops fetalis is reflected in the degree of reticulocytosis and anemia that is present. In isoimmunization this is assessed through amniocentesis evaluation of amniotic fluid bilirubin concentration. Although not common, bilirubin may also be found in some cases of nonimmune hydrops fetalis.[16, 236, 295]

The usual findings associated with immune hydrops fetalis include generalized edema, ascites, pleural effusions (possibly with hyaline membranes), hepatosplenomegaly, cardiomegaly, pancreatic islet cell hyperplasia, swelling of the adrenal glands (fetal zone), and villous edema with subsequent enlargement of the placenta. There may be evidence of persistence of the cytotrophoblastic layer. Reticulocytosis and thrombocytopenia are common, with disseminated intravascular coagulation being associated with the latter.[116]

In nonimmune hydrops fetalis, the incidence of chromosomal and genetic abnormalities is high. In one study of 61 cases, a congenital basis was found in 65% of those fetuses older than 28 weeks' gestation. Of those 65%, 40% were considered lethal. The remainder of the cases were classified as idiopathic. The incidence increased by 100-fold if there was a fetal cardiac malformation present.[25, 115, 135]

Of the idiopathic cases, fetal cardiac arrhythmias leading to congestive heart failure may account for a large percentage. Fetal supraventricular tachycardia has been identified as a cause of hydrops fetalis, usually associated with Wolff-Parkinson-White syndrome. This arrhythmia is not present all the time and may explain the transient nature of hydrops in some fetuses. Fetal supraventricular tachycardia has also been associated with the use of tocolytics. Underlying structural cardiac anomalies are not usually encountered.*

Supraventricular tachycardia results in high-output cardiac failure and may lead to hypoproteinemia, although studies demonstrate that hypoproteinemia is not essential to the development of hydrops fetalis in these cases. Left atrial pacing may be more detrimental to the fetus owing to closure of the foramen ovale.[116, 187, 197, 210, 254]

High-output cardiac failure may also result from anemia, polycythemia, or large arteriovenous shunts. However, obstructed venous return (both above and below the diaphragm) leading to low cardiac output has

---

TABLE 6–5
Factors Contributing to the Development of Fetal Edema

Heart failure or venous obstruction can result in alterations in hydrostatic pressure.

Liver damage (due to portal hypertension, which can lead to venous obstruction) results in hypoproteinemia, which alters colloid osmotic pressure.

Membrane permeability may be altered because of inflammation or metabolic, genetic, or neoplastic reasons.

Alterations can occur in water balance between the fluid compartments of the fetal, placental, and amniotic units.

Alterations in the interstitial gel may result in changes in its affinity for water.

Congenital abnormalities or obstructive lesions in the lymph system can alter drainage.

Compiled from Barnes, S.E., et al. (1977). Oedema in the newborn. *Mol Aspects Med, 1,* 187; and Hutchinson, A.A. (1990). Pathophysiology of hydrops fetalis. In W.A. Long (Ed.), *Fetal and neonatal cardiology* (pp. 197–210). Philadelphia: WB Saunders.

---

*References 6, 75, 108, 131, 138, 161, 210, 211, 237, 240, and 287.

also been implicated in the development of fetal edema. Beyond this, decreased colloid oncotic pressure secondary to liver damage or dysfunction (e.g., syphilis) or plasma protein loss (into serous fluid) and its concomitant reduction in colloid osmotic pressure can result in hydrops.[198, 199]

Nonimmune hydrops fetalis has been associated with a poor fetal and neonatal prognosis. Exhaustive fetal evaluation may identify a specific etiology in only 55% of cases. In some cases an exact diagnosis is never found, even after the birth of the infant. Perinatal mortality rates range from 50 to 98%.[49, 251]

An accurate diagnosis helps to determine the course of action that needs to be taken during the perinatal period. There are some causes of hydrops fetalis that can be treated in utero (e.g., arrhythmias). If the primary cause is not treatable or compatible with life and the diagnosis is made prior to 24 weeks' gestation, the mother should be given the option to terminate the pregnancy. If the diagnosis is made after 24 weeks, the primary concern should be the welfare of the mother throughout the pregnancy. Early delivery may also be necessary in certain circumstances (twin-to-twin transfusion, fetomaternal hemorrhage) in order to enhance fetal survival.

Specific interventions should include weekly or biweekly nonstress tests from 30 weeks to determine fetal heart rate responses with fetal movement. This can be done in conjunction with daily kick counts by the mother, with instructions to come in for evaluation in the event of any decrease in movement. Bed rest can facilitate uteroplacental blood flow.

Delivery decisions depend on maternal and fetal well-being. The goal is to maximize fetal development without compromising maternal homeostasis. At delivery the infant may be profoundly depressed and have difficulty expanding the lungs. Shoulder dystocia and soft-tissue trauma due to generalized edema may compound these difficulties. The mother, on the other hand, is at risk for postpartum hemorrhage due to an enlarged placenta, as well as the increased risks associated with a vaginal delivery.

Continued close management is required during the neonatal period. Ventilatory efforts may be hampered because of prematurity, pleural effusions, pulmonary edema with congestive heart failure, or compression of the lungs from ascites. Management of fluid status can be extremely dangerous, and specific interventions need to be undertaken cautiously. Rapid fluid shifts from one vascular compartment to another can occur, and exchange transfusions, vasopressor support, and diuretics may be necessary to stabilize the vascular bed. Adequate nutrition and prevention of skin breakdown can facilitate homeostasis while preventing infection.[16, 49, 188, 200]

Bronchopulmonary Dysplasia

No single factor can be identified as the cause of bronchopulmonary dysplasia (BPD); instead it is most likely due to the interaction of immaturity, disease process (hyaline membrane disease), oxygen toxicity, prolonged positive-pressure ventilation, patency of the ductus arteriosus, and pulmonary air leaks (see Chapter 7). The pulmonary circulation as well as the cardiac system is affected by BPD.

The neonatal pulmonary vascular bed contains more smooth muscle than that of adults. Owing to this, these immature vessels are more reactive and more sensitive to stimuli. Hypoxia, acidemia, hypercapnia, and low mixed venous oxygen tension can lead to significant pulmonary vasoconstriction. Some of these factors are interactive and most occur in BPD.

Pulmonary vascular resistance is variable depending on lung volume. At low lung volumes, the small arterioles and venules constrict, reducing their lumen size and increasing their resistance. At high lung volumes, stretching of the alveolar capillary sheet increases its resistance. In BPD the lung contains areas of alveolar collapse and overinflation combined with scarring and fibrosis. Because of this, extra-alveolar vessels are collapsed, stretched, or compressed in fibrotic areas. All of these reduce the cross section available for gas exchange.

Pulmonary edema can further increase pulmonary vascular resistance by reducing gas exchange and predisposing the lung to fibrotic changes. The increased number of neuroendocrine cells within the lung tissue of infants with BPD can lead to higher concentrations of vasoactive mediators (serotonin, bombesin, calcitonin) and could contribute to pulmonary vasoconstriction. The presence of microemboli (as seen on autopsy after prolonged mechanical ventilation) may also lead to further pulmonary hypertension.

In addition, the smaller cross section found in the neonate may reduce the infant's compensatory ability when flow and pressure changes are encountered. The ductus arteriosus may remain open, and the increased pulmonary vascular resistance can lead to right-to-left shunting through it and the foramen ovale. This shunting will result in worsening hypoxemia and respiratory acidosis, which can further increase pulmonary vascular resistance, creating a vicious circle.

Elevations in pulmonary vasuclar resistance necessitate increased right ventricular work. However, the rather muscular right ventricle of the neonate may cope better with this increased pressure than would the adult heart (the thinner wall copes better with a volume load). Unfortunately, the hypoxemia experienced with BPD may compromise the oxygen available to the myocardium, resulting in right ventricular hypertrophy to which the increased work may contribute. Left ventricular hypertrophy may be the result of PDA and left-to-right shunting or systemic hypertension that is sometimes associated with BPD.

BPD survivors are at increased risk for systemic hypertension, sudden infant death syndrome, and cor pulmonale. Possible etiologic factors in systemic hypertension include thrombosis of renal arteries or arterioles related to umbilical artery catheterization, intermittent hypoxemia elevating systemic vascular resistance, and increased pulmonary angiotensin-converting enzyme activity as a consequence of hypoxia. Serial evaluation of systemic blood pressure should be done so that early treatment with diruetics can be instituted.

The development of cor pulmonale is a major contributing factor to the death of these infants, along with the development of thickened walls in the small pulmonary arteries and arterioles. Infants with BPD may develop severe pulmonary vascular disease that becomes irreversible and results in the infant's succumbing to the disease. Periods of repeated infections and hypoxemic episodes may be the hallmark of progressive disease and contribute to increasing pulmonary vascular resistance and a poor prognosis.

Patent Ductus Arteriosus

There are three general physiologic characteristics of a patent ductus arteriosus: (1) increased flow through the lungs with diastolic volume overload; (2) increased flow through the left atrium, left ventricle, and aorta; and (3) left-to-right shunting to the pulmonary circulation. Blood is shunted from the upper and lower aortic circulations with a large ductus and multiorgan effects.

The preterm infant has less pulmonary arterial muscle and an immature pulmonary parenchyma. The presence of a PDA is associated with interstitial edema and decreased compliance of the lung owing to pulmonary edema. Ductal closure results in an increased compliance and a decreased need for ventilatory support (especially end-expiratory pressure). Prolonged ventilatory support due to a PDA increases the risk of BPD, and therefore early intervention is recommended.

Perfusion of peripheral organ systems is dependent upon adequate systolic and diastolic flow. If a large PDA exists, systemic diastolic arterial flow is compromised and may even be reversed in the descending aorta. This can lead to decreased renal perfusion and contribute to the development of volume overload and congestive heart failure. Treatment with furosemide may actually potentiate ductal opening by altering prostaglandin metabolism.

Gastrointestinal effects are also related to a decrease in flow and intestinal ischemia. Preterm infants with intestinal ischemia due to a PDA can develop necrotizing enterocolitis. Cerebral ischemia may also occur as blood is diverted from the upper body. Cerebral blood flow changes can also increase the incidence of intraventricular hemorrhage.

A large left-to-right shunt through the PDA increases the left atrial and ventricular volume, leading to enlargement of these two chambers. The increased left ventricular size also increases the myocardial wall stress, which could lead to myocardial ischemia in the preterm infant. If left ventricular compromise exists, inotropic support may be needed until PDA closure is achieved.

Treatment includes fluid restriction, ventilatory support, diuretics, prostaglandin inhibitors, and surgical ligation. Early ductal closure may improve outcome and alter the clinical course. In some cases, this may require exposing the infant to the risks of surgery.

Congenital Cardiac Malformations

Currently there is no clear understanding of the etiology of most congenital heart diseases. In about 8% of children with heart disease there is a clear genetic cause; most are associated with obvious chromosomal anomalies (e.g., Down syndrome and trisomy 18). Many of the single mutant gene syndromes are associated with heart disease, but these syndromes account for only 3% of all congenital heart disease.

Environmental factors may also play a role in the etiology of congenital cardiac malformations. Fetal exposure to teratogens through maternal ingestion of drugs or alcohol, as well as viral infections (such as rubella), can result in alterations in cardiac development. These variables account for no more than 2% of congenital heart disease.

In the remaining 85% there is no clear cause. There is probably some type of multifactorial inheritance in which there may be a heritable predisposition for cardiac anomalies. This combined with some type of environmental trigger during a vulnerable period results in abnormal development. Congenital anomalies can be the result of one or more of the causes listed in Table 6–6. A brief review with examples of cyanotic and acyanotic congenital heart disease is included here.

Cyanotic Congenital Heart Disease

Cyanosis is a physical sign characterized by blue-gray mucous membranes, nail beds, and skin. It is the result of deoxygenated hemoglobin in the blood at a concentration of at least 5 g/dl. Hypoxemia is a state of abnormally low arterial blood oxygen concentration. The degree of hypoxemia may or may not correlate with cyanosis, depending on the blood hemoglobin concentration and the abil-

TABLE 6–6
Alterations that May Result in Cardiac Anomalies

Aplasia or agenesis (failure of development)
Hypoplasia (incomplete or defective development)
Dysplasia (abnormal development)
Malposition
Failure of fusion of adjoining parts
Abnormal fusion
Incomplete resorption
Abnormal persistence of a vessel
Early obliteration of a vessel

ity of the observer to detect cyanosis. The most common causes of cyanosis in the neonate are cardiac disease and pulmonary disease. The ability to be able to distinguish between these two is essential. Therefore, when congenital heart disease is suspected, the degree of hypoxemia must be related to the volume of pulmonary blood flow.

Hypoxemia in these infants is due to right-to-left shunting (diversion of blood from the lungs), therefore ventilation and oxygen delivery do not improve oxygenation. This is the basis for the hyperoxia challenge test. With adequate ventilation and 100% oxygen the PaO_2 should rise above 150 mmHg. If the PaO_2 does not increase above 100 mmHg, cyanotic congenital heart disease is most likely the cause of the cyanosis. Between 100 and 150 mmHg, cardiac disease is possible but further diagnostic testing needs to be conducted (e.g., echocardiography). Selected congenital anomalies are discussed in this section to demonstrate these principles.

TOTAL ANOMALOUS PULMONARY VENOUS RETURN

In this condition none of the pulmonary veins connect with the left atrium. Rather, some or all of the pulmonary veins form a confluence or collecting vessel that usually lies posterior to the left atrium. There may be one or more sites of connection between the pulmonary venous collecting vessel or individual pulmonary veins and the systemic venous circuit. Usually the pulmonary veins drain directly or, more commonly, indirectly into the right atrium via one of the normal embryonic channels.

The embryonic defect seems to be a failure of development of the common pulmonary vein normally connecting the developing pulmonary venous plexus with the posterior aspect of the left atrium.

The postnatal presentation depends on the degree of obstruction of pulmonary venous drainage. If obstruction is severe, presentation occurs within the 1st week of life. If mild, presentation may not occur until the latter half of the 1st year. The presence of an interarterial communication, either a patent foramen ovale or a true atrial septal defect (ASD), is necessary to sustain life postnatally.

The hemodynamic impact of total anomalous pulmonmary venous return does not occur until pulmonary blood flow increases at the time of delivery. Pulmonary edema is the usual result. Oxygenation is interrupted because of edema, right-to-left shunting, and increased pulmonary resistance.

TRUNCUS ARTERIOSUS

Truncus arteriosus is a single great artery that arises from the base of the heart and supplies the coronary, pulmonary, and systemic arteries. It is thought to result from septation failure. The truncal valve usually resembles a normal aortic valve.

In utero, the main consequence of truncus arteriosus is complete mixing of the systemic and pulmonary venous return above the truncal valve. The truncus is usually quite large, and the ductus arteriosus arising from the pulmonary arteries may be smaller than normal. Since blood flow through the heart is normal, the rest of the heart develops normally.

Postnatally the flow of the pulmonary arteries and systemic arteries is a function of the relative resistances in the two circuits. Initially, the pulmonary resistance is high and pulmonary flow will equal or slightly exceed systemic flow. Over the first hours or days of life, however, the pulmonary arteriolar resistance decreases and pulmonary blood flow increases. As the pulmonary venous return increases, the left ventricle must eject an increasing volume load, which eventually leads to congestive failure. Since there is common mixing of systemic and pulmonary venous blood above the truncal valve, the degree of hypoxemia decreases as the pulmonary flow increases so that these infants are only mildly cyanotic until left heart failure and pulmonary edema interfere with oxygen exchange and pulmonary venous desaturation ensues.

TRICUSPID ATRESIA

In tricuspid atresia there is a failure in the development of the right atrioventricular valve; therefore an intra-atrial communication is necessary for survival. This communication is usually in the form of a patent foramen ovale. Along with this, there is usually a ventricular septal defect (VSD) connecting a large left ventricular cavity with a hypoplastic chamber that is the outflow portion of the right ventricle. The great arteries may be either normally related or transposed. There may also be an atresia.

Fetal growth and development are uncompromised, so the alterations in cardiovascular status must be compatible with normal de-

velopment. All systemic venous return is diverted across the foramen ovale into the left atrium and left ventricle. If there are no further abnormalities the entire ventricular volume is ejected into the aorta. If the VSD is large, some of the left ventricular output passes through the VSD into the hypoplastic right ventricle, exiting the pulmonary artery if the vessels are normally related or the aorta if transposition is present.

Following delivery there is little change in the circulation, but the normal postnatal alterations impose significant liabilities. Neonates with pulmonary atresia or severe pulmonary stenosis continue to depend on the ductus arteriosus for pulmonary blood flow. When the ductus arteriosus begins to close, severe hypoxemia, acidosis, and eventually death follow. In infants with a large VSD and no pulmonary stenosis, the pulmonary blood flow increases as the pulmonary arteriolar resistance drops and congestive heart failure ensues, usually in the 1st month of life.

Acyanotic Congenital Heart Disease

COARCTATION OF THE AORTA

A constriction in the aorta distal to the left subclavian artery, usually at the site of the ductus arteriosus, is defined as coarctation of the aorta. There may be tubular hypoplasia of the aortic arch and intracardiac anomalies, and these must be ruled out during evaluation. The exact etiology of the constriction is currently unknown.

Since there is normally very little flow across the aortic isthmus in utero, the tubular hypoplasia of the arch does not affect fetal growth and development and blood is shunted across the ductus arteriosus. After birth the constriction in the aorta increases the left ventricular afterload. If a VSD exists, this increased systemic resistance leads to a large left-to-right shunt. As the PVR falls, the left-to-right shunt increases, resulting in a volume as well as a pressure overload of the left ventricle. In addition to congestive heart failure, there is failure of the blood to pass from ascending to descending aorta if the coarctation is severe. The results are tissue hypoxia, lactic acidosis, and eventual death after the ductus arteriosus closes.

Those neonates with a juxtaductal coarctation but no other associated anomalies have a slightly different hemodynamic makeup. Closure of the ductus arteriosus leads to an acute increase in afterload to the left ventricle, as blood must be pumped through the narrowed segment. Since no obstruction was present in utero, no collateral vessels have developed. The neonatal myocardium is unable to respond to the increased workload, consequently congestive heart failure with elevation of left ventricular end-diastolic, left atrial, and pulmonary venous pressures follows.

VENTRICULAR SEPTAL DEFECTS

Ventricular septal defects (VSDs) may be isolated defects or associated with other congenital cardiac defects. The most common site for a VSD is the membranous portion of the septum that lies betwen the crista supraventricularis and the papillary muscle of the conus when the heart is viewed from the right ventricular side. Less common sites are the area above the crista, the muscular portion of the septum below the tricuspid valve, and the anterior trabecular portion of the ventricular spetum near the apex of the right ventricle (RV).

Since the right and left sides of the heart are arranged in a parallel fashion before birth, the presence of a large communication at the ventricular level in addition to the normal ductus connection at the great vessels does not significantly alter the fetal circulation. After birth, however, the hemodynamics depend on the size of the defect and the pulmonary and systemic vascular resistances. If the defect is large it offers no resistance to flow. The systolic pressure in the ventricles and great vessels is approximately equal and the degree of intracardiac shunting is determined by the systemic and pulmonary vascular resistances. As the PVR gradually falls, the volume of blood in the left ventricle (LV) increases. Therefore more blood is ejected through the VSD into the pulmonary artery. When the pulmonary blood flow is about three times greater than the systemic flow, the LV can no longer accommodate the volume load, and congestive heart failure develops. This usually occurs during the 1st or 2nd week of life. The right atrium and RV are not volume overloaded, but in the presence of a large defect the RV must generate pressures equal to those of the LV so there is usually right ventricular hypertrophy without significant dilation.

If the VSD is small, it does offer resistance to flow, and the pressures in the two ventricles may differ. Infants with this type of defect are a heterogeneous group, with the hemodynamics depending on the size of the hole rather than the PVR. If the defect is very small, the right ventricular and pulmonary artery pressures may be normal and the the pulmonary blood flow less than twice the systemic flow. These infants are rarely symptomatic but usually exhibit a murmur.

MATURATIONAL CHANGES DURING INFANCY AND CHILDHOOD

The changes in the heart at birth include a redistribution of workload between the right and left ventricles. The change to in series circulation results in an increase in cardiac output, with the right ventricle ejecting blood against a lower afterload and the left ventricle ejecting against a higher afterload. The ventricular mass changes in response to these new demands with the left ventricle wall thickness increasing significantly while the right remains unchanged.

This change in wall thickness is secondary to an increase in cell number and size. Hyperplasia can occur soon after birth, followed by an increase in cell size. Owing to the increased workload of the left ventricle, cell replication occurs more rapidly in the left myocardium.[12, 139] Ventricular size and compliance change gradually during infancy and childhood, so cardiac function parallels that of adults by adolescence.

The myocardial cells change in size, shape, and architecture following birth. The left ventricle matures more rapidly after birth, which can be seen in myocyte shape changes. The immature cells are rounder and have a smoother surface. As cells mature, their shape becomes increasingly irregular with identifiable step changes along their lateral borders.[112, 146, 147, 165, 221]

The myocytes become longer and acquire a larger cross-sectional area. Stimulation for these changes may be related to the sympathetic nervous system. During the neonatal period α-adrenoceptors and circulating norepinephrine levels are higher than at any other stage of development. In tissue cultures stimulation of α_1 receptors (e.g., with norepinephrine) results in cell growth. Therefore, it can be inferred that the presence of increased receptors and stimulant results in induction of myocardial cell growth.[246, 247]

Myofilament and sarcomere changes also occur with delivery. The sarcomere A-I bands are more irregular; the Z band disc is thicker, although more variable; and the M band is acquired with maturation. The myofibrils are more disorganized and often are not oriented in the same direction as the long axis. Instead they are arranged around a large central mass of nuclei and mitochondria, which may persist for weeks following birth. Eventually the myofibrils assume the adult position and are distributed across the cell.

The increase in the proportion of cell volume that contains myofilaments, organizational changes, and modification of the sarcomeres lead to improved contraction abil-

TABLE 6–7
Summary of Recommendations for Clinical Practice Related to the Cardiovascular System: Neonate

Monitor cardiovascular adaptation to extrauterine life (pp. 240–242).

Assess and evaluate the neonate for changes in cardiovascular volume and symptomatology related to those changes (pp. 240–242).

Conduct a thorough cardiovascular assessment of any infant presenting with a murmur during the transitional period, especially if associated with cyanosis (pp. 250–253).

Provide continuous physiologic monitoring for infants suspected of cardiac disease (pp. 250–253).

Perform oxygen challenge test to determine if oxygenation problems are potentially of cardiac origin (p. 251).

Develop an understanding of the embryonic mechanisms that may result in cardiac congenital anomalies (pp. 228–237).

Understand fetal and neonatal responses to stress, their impact on the functioning of the cardiovascular system, and appropriate therapy to support cardiac output and perfusion (pp. 246–247).

Monitor infants with PDA for signs of increasing respiratory distress and congestive heart failure (p. 250).

Recognize that fetal arrhythmias may result in hydrops fetalis without underlying congenital anomalies; anticipate delivery of a neonate who is edematous, in congestive heart failure, and anemic (pp. 247–249).

Monitor fluid status of hydropic infants carefully (pp. 247–249).

Evaluate blood pressure routinely in infants with bronchopulmonary dysplasia to identify hypertension and need for diuretics (pp. 249–250).

Recognize the complications associated with repeated infections and hypoxemia in the infant with BPD and promote interventions to reduce potential causes (pp. 249–250).

Monitor for signs of PDA or pulmonary edema in the infant with BPD (pp. 249–250).

Evaluate all preterm infants for signs of a PDA on a serial basis (p. 250).

Determine cardiovascular deterioration associated with a PDA (p. 250).

Page numbers in parentheses following each recommendation refer to pages in the text where rationale is discussed.

ity. Other changes that are indicative of maturation include a postnatal mitochondrial increase, which is most likely in response to metabolic changes in the muscle tissue. Initially there is a dramatic increase in the number of mitochondria; with further maturation the mitochondria become highly ordered in their arrangement. This occurs weeks after delivery. The arrangement facilitates energy transfer to the sarcomere during contraction.

Heart growth as reflected in weight gain is very slow for the first 4 months of gestation. After that it is much more steady until birth. After the 1st month to 6 weeks, there is steady weight gain until the growth spurt associated with puberty. There is a final growth spurt at the end of adolescence, at which time the heart reaches its adult weight.

Many of the other maturational changes have been discussed in the functional development section. There is a similarity between the functioning of the fetus, neonate, and adult although it appears that the fetus functions in a much narrower homeostatic range. Stressful events may result in fluctuations outside this range and may compromise the infant's survival.

SUMMARY

Fetal heart rate patterns are useful indicators of fetal well-being during pregnancy and are helpful in identifying infants that are intolerant of the stresses of labor and delivery. In order to achieve extrauterine stability, the newborn undergoes significant alterations in cardiovascular status that convert it from a parallel system to an in series system that must integrate with the respiratory system in order to maintain oxygenation. The complex development of the heart and cardiovascular system makes the neonate at greater risk for alterations in normal development that can lead to postnatal compromise affecting multiple systems. Close assessments during the transitional period result in early identification and treatment of cardiovascular disease, while promoting normal growth and development. Table 6–7 summarizes recommendations for clinical practice.

REFERENCES

1. Abramson, D.I., Flacks, K., & Fierst, S.M. (1943). Peripheral blood flow during gestation. *Am J Obstet Gynecol, 45,* 666.

2. Adams, F.H. & Lind, J. (1957). Physiologic studies on the cardiovascular status of normal newborn infants (with special reference to the ductus arteriosus). *Pediatrics, 19,* 431.

3. Adams, J.Q. & Alexander, A.M. (1958). Alterations in cardiovascular physiology during labor. *Am Obstet Gynecol, 12,* 542.

4. Adamsons, K., Mueller-Heubach, A., & Meyers, R. (1971). Production of fetal asphyxia in the rhesus monkey (administration of catecholamines to the mother). *Am J Obstet Gynecol, 109,* 248.

5. Ahn, M.O. & Phelan, J.P. (1988). Multiple pregnancy: Antepartum management. *Clin Perinatol, 15,* 55.

6. Allan, L.D., et al. (1986). Aetiology of non-immune hydrops: The value of echocardiography. *Br J Obstet Gynaecol, 93,* 223.

7. ACOG guidelines: Exercise during pregnancy and the postnatal period. (1991). In R.A. Mittelmark, R.A. Wiswell, & B.L. Drinkwater (Eds.), *Exercise in pregnancy* (2nd ed.). Baltimore: Williams & Wilkins.

8. Anderson, H.M. (1984). Maternal hematologic disorders. In R.K. Creasy & R. Resnik (Eds.), *Maternal-fetal medicine* (pp. 795–832). Philadelphia: WB Saunders.

9. Anderson, P.A.W., et al. (1987). In utero right ventricular output in the fetal lamb: The effect of heart rate. *J Physiol* (Lond), *387,* 297.

10. Anderson, P.A.W. (1990). Myocardial development. In W.A. Long (Ed.), *Fetal and neonatal cardiology.* Philadelphia: WB Saunders.

11. Anderson, P.A.W., et al. (1986). The effect of heart rate on in utero left ventricular output in the fetal sheep. *J Physiol* (Lond), *372,* 557.

12. Anversa, P., Olivetti, G., & Loud, A.V. (1980). Morphometric study of early postnatal development in the left and right ventricular myocardium of the rat. I. Hypertrophy, hyperplasia, and binucleation of myocytes. *Circ Res, 46,* 495.

13. Arnold-Aldea, S.A. & Parer, J.T. (1990). Fetal cardiovascular physiology. In R.D. Eden & F.H. Boehm (Eds.), *Assessment and care of the fetus: Physiological, clinical, and medicolegal principles.* Norwalk, CT: Appleton & Lange.

14. Artal, R., et al. (1984). Fetal bradycardia induced by maternal exercise. *Lancet, 2,* 258.

15. Artal, R. & Wiswell, R. (1986). *Exercise in pregnancy.* Baltimore: Williams & Wilkins.

16. Ascari, W.Q. (1977). Serology of erythroblastosis fetalis. In J.T. Queenan (Ed.), *Modern management of the Rh problem* (2nd ed.). New York: Harper & Row.

17. Assali, N.S., Rauramo, L., & Peltonen, T. (1960). Measurement of uterine blood flow and uterine metabolism. VIII. Uterine and fetal blood flow and oxygen consumption in early human pregnancy. *Am J Obstet Gynecol, 79,* 86.

18. Bader, M.E. & Bader, R.A. (1968). Cardiovascular hemodynamics in pregnancy and labor. *Clin Obstet Gynecol, 11,* 924.

19. Bader, R.A., et al. (1953). Hemodynamics at rest and during exercise in normal pregnancy as studied by cardiac catheterization. *J Clin Invest, 34,* 1524.

20. Barnes, S.E., et al. (1977). Oedema in the newborn. *Mol Aspects Med, 1,* 187.

21. Baum, J.D. & Harris, D. (1972). Colloid osmotic pressure in erythroblastosis fetalis. *Br Med J, 1,* 601.

22. Bean, W.B., Dexter, M.W., & Cogswell, R.C. (1949). Vascular changes of skin in pregnancy. *Surg Gynecol Obstet, 88,* 739.

23. Beary, J.F., Summer, W.R., & Bulkley, B.H. (1979). Postpartum acute myocardial infarction: A rare occurrence of uncertain etiology. *Am J Cardiol, 43,* 158.

24. Beck, F., Moffat, D.B., & Davies, D.P. (1985). *Human embryology* (2nd ed.). Oxford : Blackwell/ Year Book Medical Publishers.

25. Beischer, N.A., Fortune, D.W., & Macafee, J. (1971). Nonimmunologic hydrops fetalis and congenital abnormalities. *Obset Gynecol, 38,* 86.

26. Belfort, M., et al. (1989). Haemodynamic changes in gestational proteinuric hypertension: The effects of rapid volume expansion and vasodilator therapy. *Br J Obstet Gynaecol, 96,* 634.

27. Benedetti, T. J. (1990). Pregnancy-induced hypertension. In U. Elkayam & N. Gleicher (Eds.), *Cardiac problems in pregnancy* (pp. 323–340). New York: Alan R. Liss.

28. Bickers, W. (1942). The placenta: A modified arteriovenous fistula. *South Med J, 35,* 393.

29. Bieniarz, J., Mapueda, E., & Caldeyro-Barcia, R. (1966). Compression of aorta by the uterus in late human pregnancy. I. Variations between femoral and brachial artery pressure with changes from hypertension to hypotension. *Am J Obstet Gynecol, 95,* 795.

30. Bieniarz, J., et al. (1968). Aortocaval compression by the uterus in late human pregnancy. II. An angiographic study. *Am J Obstet Gynecol, 100,* 203.

31. Borg, T.K., et al. (1985). Connective tissue of the myocardium. In V.J. Ferrans, G. Rosenquist, & C. Weinstein (Eds.), *Cardiac morphogenesis.* New York: Elsevier Science Publishing.

32. Borg, T.K., et al. (1984). Recognition of extracellular matrix components by neonatal and adult cardiac myocytes. *Dev Biol, 104,* 86.

33. Boyle, D.M. & Lloyd-Jones, R. (1966). The electrocardiographic S-T segment in pregnancy. *J Obstet Gynaecol Br Comm, 73,* 986.

34. Brigden, W., Howarth, S., & Sharpey-Schafer, E.P. (1950). Posture and peripheral blood flow. *Clin Sci, 9,* 79.

35. Brinkman, C.R. (1984). Maternal cardiovascular and renal disorders. In R.K. Creasy & R. Resnik (Eds.), *Maternal-fetal medicine.* Philadelphia: WB Saunders.

36. Brooke, O.G., Alvear, J., & Arnold, M. (1979). Energy retention, energy expenditure and growth in healthy immature infants. *Pediatr Res, 13,* 215.

37. Bruce, R.A. & Johnson, W.P. (1961). Exercise tolerance in pregnant cardiac patients. *Clin Obstet Gynecol, 4,* 665.

38. Bryant, E.E., Douglas, B.H., & Ashburn, A.D. (1973). Circulatory changes following prolactin administration. *Am J Obstet Gynecol, 115,* 53.

39. Burch, G.E. (1977). Heart disease and pregnancy. *Am Heart J, 93,* 104.

40. Burt, C.C. (1949). Peripheral skin temperature in normal pregnancy. *Lancet, 2,* 787.

41. Burt, C.C. (1950). The peripheral circulation in pregnancy. *Trans Edinb Obstet Soc (Edinb Med J), 57,* 18.

42. Burwell, C.A., et al. (1938). Circulation during pregnancy. *Arch Intern Med, 62,* 979.

43. Butler, E.F. (1968). The effect of iron and folic

acid on red cell and plasma volume in pregnancy. *J Obstet Gynaecol Br Comm, 75,* 497.

44. Campbell, W.A., et al. (1987). Maternal-fetal reproductive physiology and clinical management. In D.H. Riddick (Ed.), *Reproductive physiology in clinical practice.* New York: Thieme Medical Publishers.

45. Capeless, E.L. & Clapp, J.F. (1989). Cardiovascular changes in early phase of pregnancy. *Am J Obstet Gynecol, 161,* 1449.

46. Carpenter, M.W., et al. (1988). Fetal heart rate response to maternal exertion. *JAMA, 259,* 3006.

47. Caton, D., et al. (1974). The effect of exogenous progesterone on the rate of blood flow of the uterus of ovariectomized sheep. *Q J Exp Physiol, 59,* 225.

48. Chandler, K. & Bell, A. (1981). Effects of maternal exercise on fetal and maternal respiration and nutrient metabolism in the pregnant ewe. *J Dev Physiol, 3,* 161.

49. Chescheir, N.C. & Seeds, J.W. (1990). Management of hydrops fetalis. In W.A. Long (Ed.), *Fetal and neonatal cardiology.* Philadelphia: WB Saunders.

50. Chesley, L.C. & Duffus, G.M. (1971). Preeclampsia, posture, and renal function. *Obstet Gynecol, 38,* 1.

51. Chesley, L.C. & Duffus, G.M. (1971). Posture and apparent plasma volume in late pregnancy. *J Obstet Gynaecol Br Comm, 78,* 406.

52. Chesley, L.C. (1960). Renal functional changes in normal pregnancy. *Clin Obstet Gynecol, 3,* 349.

53. Chesley, L.C. (1972). Plasma and red cell volumes during pregnancy. *Am J Obstet Gynecol, 122,* 440.

54. Chesley, L.C., Valenti, C., & Uichano, L. (1959). Alterations in body fluid compartments and exchangeable sodium in early peurperium. *Am J Obstet Gynecol, 77,* 1054.

55. Chisholm, A. (1966). A controlled clinical trial of prophylactic folic acid and iron in pregnancy. *J Obstet Gynaecol Br Comm, 73,* 191.

56. Christianson, R.E. (1976). Studies on blood pressure during pregnancy. I. Influence of parity and age. *Am J Obstet Gynecol, 125,* 509.

57. Clapp, J.F. (1991). Maternal exercise performance and early pregnancy outcome. In R.A. Mittelmark, R.A. Wiswell, & B.L. Drinkwater (Eds.), *Exercise in pregnancy* (2nd ed.). Baltimore: Williams & Wilkins.

58. Clapp, J.F., et al. (1988). Maternal physiological adaptations to early human pregnancy. *Am J Obstet Gynecol, 159,* 1456.

59. Clapp, J.F. (1985). Maternal heart rate in pregnancy. *Am J Obstet Gynecol, 152,* 659.

60. Clapp, J.F. (1985). Fetal heart rate response to running in midpregnancy and late pregnancy. *Am J Obstet Gynecol, 153,* 251.

61. Clapp, J.F. (1980). Acute exercise stress in the pregnant ewe. *Am J Obstet Gynecol, 136,* 489.

62. Clark, S.L. (1987). Structural cardiac disease in pregnancy. In S.L. Clark, J.P. Phelan, & D.B. Cotton (Eds.), *Critical care obstetrics.* Oradell, NJ: Medical Economics Books.

63. Clark, S.L., et al. (1989). Central hemodynamic assessment of normal term pregnancy. *Am J Obstet Gynecol, 161,* 1439.

64. Collings, C., Curret, L., & Mullings, J. (1983). Maternal and fetal responses to a maternal aerobic exercise program. *Am J Obstet Gynecol, 145,* 701.

65. Collings, C. & Curret, L. (1985). Fetal heart rate response to maternal exercise. *Am J Obstet Gynecol, 157,* 498.

66. Cowles, T. & Gonik, B. (1990). Mitral valve prolapse in pregnancy. *Semin Perinatol, 14,* 34.

67. Creasy, R.K. & Resnik, R. (1984). *Maternal-fetal medicine.* Philadelphia: WB Saunders.

68. Crone, R.K. (1983). The respiratory system. In G.A. Gregory (Ed.), *Pediatric anesthesia.* New York: Churchill Livingstone.

69. Cunningham, I. (1966). Cardiovascular physiology of labor and delivery. *J Obstet Gynaecol Br Comm, 73,* 498.

70. Curret, L., et al. (1976). Effect of exercise on cardiac output and distribution of blood flow in pregnant ewes. *J Appl Physiol, 40,* 725.

71. Cutforth, R. & MacDonald, M.B. (1966). Heart sounds and murmurs in pregnancy. *Am Heart J, 71,* 741.

72. Davies, P., et al. (1975). Postnatal developmental changes in the length-tension relationship of cat papillary muscles. *J Physiol (Lond), 253,* 95.

72a. Dawes, G.S. (1968). *Foetal and neonatal physiology.* Chicago: Year Book Medical Publishers.

73. Demakis, J.G. & Rahimtoola, S.H. (1971). Peripartum cardiomyopathy. *Circulation, 44,* 964.

74. Devereux, R.B., et al. (1987). Diagnosis and classification of severity of mitral valve prolapse: Methodologic, biologic and diagnostic considerations. *Am Heart J, 113,* 1265.

75. Donnerstein, R.L. & Allen, H.D. (1986). Cardiac therapeutic implications from fetal echocardiography. *Am J Dis Child, 140,* 198.

76. Dressendorfen, R. & Goodlin, R. (1980). FHR response to maternal exercising testing. *Physiol Sports Med, 8,* 90.

77. Duncan, S.L. (1989). Does volume expansion in pre-eclampsia help or hinder? *Br J Obstet Gynaecol, 96,* 631.

78. Eliseev, O.M. (1988). *Cardiovascular diseases and pregnancy.* New York: Springer-Verlag.

79. Elkayam, U. & Gleicher, N. (1982). Cardiovascular physiology in pregnancy. In U. Elkayam & N. Gleicher (Eds.), *Cardiac problems in pregnancy: Diagnosis and management of maternal and fetal disease.* New York: Alan R. Liss.

80. Emmanouilides, G.C., et al. (1970). Cardiac output in newborn infants. *Biol Neonate, 15,* 186.

81. Easterling, T.R., Schmucker, B.C., & Benedetti, T.J. (1988). The hemodynamic effects of orthostatic stress during pregnancy. *Obstet Gynecol, 72,* 550.

82. Easterling, T. R. & Benedetti, T. J. (1990). Measurement of cardiac output by impedance technique. *Am J Obstet Gynecol, 163,* 1104.

83. Feinberg, L.E. (1983). Hypertension and preeclampsia. In R.S. Abrams & P. Wexler (Eds.), *Medical care of the pregnant patient.* Boston: Little, Brown.

84. Ferris, E.B. & Wilkins, R. W. (1937). The clinical value of comparative measurements of the pressure in the femoral and cubital veins. *Am Heart J, 13,* 431.

85. Ferris, T.F., Stein, J.H., & Kauffman, J. (1972). Uterine blood flow and uterine renin secretion. *J Clin Invest, 51,* 2827.

86. Ferris, T.F. (1982). Toxemia and hypertension. In G.N. Burrow & T.F. Ferris (Eds.), *Medical complications during pregnancy* (2nd ed.). Philadelphia: WB Saunders.

87. Fisher, D.J. (1984). Oxygenation and metabolism in the developing heart. *Semin Perinatol, 8,* 217.

88. Freed, M.D. (1984). Disorders of the cardiovascular system. General considerations. In M.E. Avery &

H.W. Taeusch (Eds.), *Schaffer's diseases of the newborn* (5th ed.). Philadelphia: WB Saunders.

89. Friedman, W.F. (1972). The intrinsic physiologic properties of the developing heart. *Prog Cardiovasc Dis, 15,* 87.

90. Gallery, E.D.M., et al. (1977). Predicting the development of pregnancy associated hypertension: The place of standardized blood pressure measurement. *Lancet, 1,* 1273.

91. Gant, N.F., et al. (1971). Study of the metabolic clearance rate of dehydroisoandrosterone sulfate in pregnancy. *Am J Obstet Gynecol, 11,* 555.

92. Gilbert, R.D. (1978). Venous return and control of fetal cardiac output. In L.D. Longo & D.D. Reneau (Eds.), *Circulation in the fetus and newborn.* New York: Garland Publishing.

93. Gilstrap, L.C. & Gant, N.F. (1990). Pathophysiology of preeclampsia. *Semin Perinatol, 14,* 147.

94. Ginsburg, J. & Duncan, S.L.B. (1967). Peripheral blood flow in normal pregnancy. *Cardiovasc Res, 1,* 132.

95. Glaviano, V.V. (1963). Evidence for an arteriovenous fistula in the gravid uterus. *Surg Gynecol Obstet, 117,* 301.

96. Goodlin, R.C. (1979). *Care of the fetus.* New York: Masson Publishing.

97. Goodman R.P., et al. (1982). Prostacyclin production during pregnancy: Comparison of production during normal pregnancy and pregnancy complicated by hypertension. *Am J Obstet Gynecol, 142,* 817.

98. Gray, M.J., et al. (1964). Regulation of sodium and total body water metabolism in pregnancy. *Am J Obstet Gynecol, 89,* 760.

99. Greiss, F.C. & Anderson, S.G. (1970). Effect of ovarian hormones on the uterine vascular bed. *Am J Obstet Gynecol, 107,* 829.

100. Hamilton, W.J., Boyd, J.D., & Mossman, H.W. (1972). *Human embryology: Prenatal development of form and function.* Baltimore: Williams & Wilkins.

101. Hamilton, H.F.H. (1949). The cardiac output in normal pregnancy as determined by the Cournand right heart catheterization technique. *J Obstet Gynaecol Br Emp, 56,* 548.

102. Hamilton, H.F.H. (1950). Blood viscosity in pregnancy. *J Obstet Gynaecol Br Emp, 57,* 530.

103. Hart, M.V., et al. (1986). Aortic function during normal human pregnancy. *Am J Obstet Gynecol, 154,* 887.

104. Harvey, W.P. (1975). Alterations of the cardiac physical examination in normal pregnancy. *Clin Obstet Gynecol, 18,* 51.

105. Haas, J.M. (1976). The effect of pregnancy on the midsystolic click and murmur of the prolapsing posterior leaflet of the mitral valve. *Am Heart J, 92,* 407.

106. Hauth, J., Gilstrap, L., & Widmer, K. (1982). Fetal heart rate reactivity before and after maternal jogging during the third trimester. *Am J Obstet Gynecol, 142,* 545.

107. Heckel, G.P. & Tobin, C.E. (1956). Arteriovenous shunts in the myometrium. *Am J Obstet Gynecol, 71,* 199.

108. Hedvall, G. (1973). Congenital paroxysmal tachycardia—a report of three cases. *Acta Paediatr Scand, 62,* 550.

109. Hendricks, C.H. & Quilligan, E.F. (1956). Cardiac output during labor. *Am J Obstet Gynecol, 71,* 953.

110. Hendricks, C.H. (1958). The hemodynamics of uterine contraction. *Am J Obstet Gynecol, 76,* 969.

111. Herbert, C.M., Banner, E.A., & Wakim, K.G. (1958). Variations in the peripheral circulation during pregnancy. *Am J Obstet Gynecol, 76,* 742.

112. Hoerter, J., Mazet, F., & Vassor, G. (1981). Perinatal growth of the rabbit cardiac cell: Possible implications for the mechanism of relaxation. *J Mol Cell Cardiol, 13,* 725.

113. Holmes, F.A. (1960). Incidence of the supine hypotensive syndrome in late pregnancy. A clinical study in 500 subjects. *J Obstet Gynaecol Br Emp, 67,* 254.

114. Hommes, F.A., et al. (1975). The energy requirement for growth: An application of Atkinson's metabolic price system. *Pediatr Res, 9,* 51.

115. Hutchinson, A.A., et al. (1982). Nonimmunologic hydrops fetalis: A review of 61 cases. *Obstet Gynecol, 59,* 347.

116. Hutchison, A.A. (1990). Pathophysiology of hydrops fetalis. In W.A. Long (Ed.), *Fetal and neonatal cardiology.* Philadelphia: WB Saunders.

117. Hytten, F.F. (1985). Blood volume changes in normal pregnancy. *Clin Haematol, 14,* 601.

118. Hytten, F.F. & Paintin, D.B. (1963). Increase in plasma volume during normal pregnancy. *J Obstet Gynaecol Br Comm, 70,* 402.

119. Hytten, F.F. & Leitch, I. (1964). *The physiology of human pregnancy.* Philadelphia: FA Davis.

120. Hytten, F.E., Thomson, A.M., & Taggart, N. (1966). Total body water in normal pregnancy. *J Obstet Gynaecol Br Comm, 73,* 553.

121. Hytten, F.E. & Leitch, I. (1971). *The physiology of human pregnancy* (2nd ed.). Oxford: Blackwell Scientific Publications.

121a. Institute of Medicine. (1990). *Nutrition during pregnancy.* Washington, DC: National Academy Press.

122. Jacoby, W.J. (1964). Pregnancy with tetralogy and pentalogy of Fallot. *Am J Cardiol, 14,* 866.

123. Jones, A.M. & Howitt, G. (1965). Eisenmenger syndrome in pregnancy. *Br Med J, 1,* 1627.

124. Jones, M.M. & Joyce, T.H. (1987). Anesthesia for the patient with pregnancy-induced hypertension and the pregnant cardiac patient. In S.L. Clark, J.P. Phelan, & D.B. Cotton (Eds.), *Critical care obstetrics.* Oradell, NJ: Medical Economics Books.

125. Jones, R., et al. (1985). Thermoregulation during aerobic exercise in pregnancy. *Obstet Gynecol, 65,* 340.

126. Kafer, E.R. (1990). Neonatal gas exchange and oxygen transport. In W.A. Long (Ed.), *Fetal and neonatal cardiology.* Philadelphia: WB Saunders.

127. Katz, M., Meizner, I., & Vaclav, I. (1990). *Fetal well-being: Physiological basis and methods of clinical assessment.* Boston: CRC Press.

128. Katz, R., Karliner, J.S., & Resnik, R. (1978). Effects of a natural volume overload state (pregnancy) on left ventricular performance in normal human subjects. *Circulation, 58,* 434.

129. Katz, M. & Sokal, M.M. (1980). Skin perfusion in pregnancy. *Am J Obstet Gynecol, 137,* 30.

130. Kelton, J.G. & Cruickshank, M. (1988). Hematologic disorders of pregnancy. In G.N. Burrow & T.F. Ferris (Eds.), *Medical complications during pregnancy* (pp. 65–94). Philadelphia: WB Saunders.

131. Kerenyi, T.D., et al. (1980). Transplacental cardioversion of intrauterine supraventricular tachycardia with digitalis. *Lancet, 2,* 393.

132. Kerr, M.G., Scott, D.B., & Samuel, E. (1964).

Studies of the inferior vena cava in late pregnancy. *Br Med J, 1*, 532.

133. Kerr, M.G. (1965). The mechanical effects of the gravid uterus in late pregnancy. *J Obstet Gynaecol Br Comm, 72*, 513.

134. Kim, Y.I., Chandra, P., & Marx, G.F. (1975). Successful management of severe aortocaval compression in twin pregnancy. *Obstet Gynecol, 46*, 362.

135. King, C.R. (1982). Hydrops fetalis and genetic disease. *Birth Defects, 18*, 101.

136. Kirkpatrick, S.E. & Friedman, W.F. (1978). Myocardial determinants of fetal cardiac output. In L.D. Longo & D.D. Reneau (Eds.), *Fetal and newborn cardiovascular physiology*, New York: Garland Press.

137. Kjeldsen, J. (1979). Hemodynamic investigations during labor and delivery. *Acta Obstet Gynecol Scand* (Suppl.), *89*, 1.

138. Kleinman, C.S., et al. (1982). Fetal echocardiography for evaluation of in utero congestive heart failure. *N Engl J Med, 306*, 568.

139. Korecky, B. & Rakusan, K. (1978). Normal and hypertrophic growth of the rat heart. Changes in cell dimensions and number. *Am J Physiol, 234*, H123.

140. Landau, R.L. & Lugibihl, K. (1958). Inhibition of the sodium-retaining influence of aldosterone by progesterone. *J Clin Endocrinol Metab, 18*, 1237.

141. Landau, R.L., et al. (1955). The metabolic effects of progesterone in man. *J Clin Endocrinol Metab, 15*, 1194.

142. Lang, R.M. & Borow, K.M. (1985). Pregnancy and heart disease. *Clin Perinatol, 12*, 551.

143. Lee, W. & Cotton, D.B. (1987). Cardiorespiratory changes during pregnancy. In S.L. Clark, J.P. Phelan, D.B. Cotton (Eds.), *Critical care obstetrics*. Oradell, NJ: Medical Economics Books.

144. Lee, W. & Cotton, D.B. (1990). Maternal cardiovascular physiology. In R.D. Eden and F.H. Boehm (Eds.), *Assessment and care of the fetus: Physiological, clinical, and medicolegal principles*. Norwalk, CT: Appleton & Lange.

145. Lees, H.M., et al. (1967). The circulatory effect of recumbent postural change in late pregnancy. *Clin Sci, 32*, 453.

146. Legato, M.J. (1970). Sarcomerogenesis in human myocardium. *J Mol Cell Cardiol, 1*, 425.

147. Legato, M.J. (1979). Cellular mechanisms of normal growth in the mammalian heart. II. A quantitative and qualitative comparison between the right and left ventricular myocytes in the dog from birth to five months of age. *Circ Res, 44*, 263.

148. Lewis, P.J., et al. (1980). Prostacyclin in pregnancy. *Br Med J, 280*, 1581.

149. Lewis, B.V. & Parsons, M. (1966). Chorea gravidarum. *Lancet, 1*, 284.

150. Lewis P.J., et al. (1981). Prostacyclin and preeclampsia. *Lancet, 1*, 559.

151. Lindheimer, M.D. & Katz, A.I. (1985). Hypertension in pregnancy. *N Engl J Med, 313*, 675.

152. Lindheimer, M.D. & Katz, A.I. (1972). Renal function in pregnancy. *Obstet Gynecol Annu, 1*, 139.

153. Lipsett, M.B., Combs, J.W., & Seigel, D.G. (1971). Problems in contraception. *Ann Intern Med, 74*, 251.

154. Lister, G., et al. (1984). Effects of alterations of oxygen transport on the neonate. *Semin Perinatol, 8*, 192.

155. Lister, G., et al. (1979). Oxygen delivery in lambs: Cardiovascular and hematologic development. *Am J Physiol, 237*, H668.

156. Loffer, F.D. (1967). Eisenmenger's complex and pregnancy. *Obstet Gynecol, 29*, 235.

157. Lotgering, F., Gilbert, R., & Longo, L. (1985). Maternal and fetal responses to exercise during pregnancy. *Physiol Rev, 65*, 1.

158. Lotgering, F. & Longo, L. (1984). Exercise and pregnancy—How much is too much? *Cont Obstet Gynecol, 123*, 63.

159. Lotgering, F., Gilbert, R., & Longo, L. (1984). The interactions of excercise and pregnancy: A review. *Am J Obstet Gynecol, 149*, 560.

160. Lotgering, F.K. & Wallenburg, H.C.S. (1986). Hemodynamic effects of caval and uterine venous occlusion in pregnant sheep. *Am J Obstet Gynecol, 155*, 1164.

161. Lubinsky, M. & Rapoport, P. (1983). Transient fetal hydrops and "prune belly" in one identical female twin. *N Engl J Med, 308*, 256.

162. Lund, C.J. & Donovan, J.C. (1967). Blood volume during pregnancy. *Am J Obstet Gynecol, 98*, 393.

163. MacGillivray, I. & Buchanan, T.J. (1958). Total exchangeable sodium and potassium in non-pregnant women and in normal and pre-eclamptic pregnancy. *Lancet, 2*, 1090.

164. MacGillivray, I. (1961). Hypertension in pregnancy and its consequences. *J Obstet Gynaecol Br Comm, 68*, 557.

165. Markwald, R.R. (1973). Distribution and relationship of precursor Z material to organizing myofibrillar bundles in embryonic rat and hamster ventricular myocytes. *J Mol Cell Cardiol, 5*, 341.

166. Martin, J.N., et al. (1990). Plasma exchange for preeclampsia. I. Postpartum use for persistently severe preeclampsia-eclampsia with HELLP syndrome. *Am J Obstet Gynecol, 162*, 126.

167. Mashini, I.S., et al. (1987). Serial noninvasive evaluation of cardiovascular hemodynamics. *Am J Obstet Gynecol, 156*, 1208.

168. McAnulty, J.H., Metcalfe, J., & Ueland, J. (1982). Cardiovascular disease. In G.N. Burrow & T.F. Ferris (Eds.), *Medical complications during pregnancy*. Philadelphia: WB Saunders.

169. McCall, M. (1949). Cerebral blood flow and metabolism in toxemias of pregnancy. *Surg Gynecol Obstet, 89*, 715.

170. McCausland, A.M., et al. (1961). Venous distensibility during pregnancy. *Am J Obstet Gynecol, 81*, 472.

171. McLennan, C.E. (1943). Antecubital and femoral venous pressure in normal and toxemic pregnancy. *Am J Obstet Gynecol, 45*, 568.

172. McRoberts, W.A., Jr. (1951). Postural shock in pregnancy. *Am J Obstet Gynecol, 62*, 627.

173. Metcalfe, J., et al. (1955). Estimation of uterine blood flow in normal human pregnancy at term. *J Clin Invest, 34*, 1632.

174. Metcalfe, J. & Parer, J.T. (1966). Cardiovascular changes during pregnancy in ewes. *Am J Physiol, 71*, 821.

175. Metcalfe, J. & Ueland, K. (1978). The heart and pregnancy. In J.W. Hurst, et al. (Eds.), *The heart arteries and veins*. New York: McGraw-Hill.

176. Metcalfe, J. & Ueland, K. (1974). Maternal cardiovascular adjustments to pregnancy. *Prog Cardiovasc Dis, 16*, 363.

177. Meyer, E.C., et al. (1964). Pregnancy in the pres-

ence of tetralogy of Fallot. Observation on two patients. *Am J Cardiol, 14*, 874.

178. Mittelmark, R.A. & Posner, M.D. (1991). Fetal responses to maternal exercise. In R.A. Mittelmark, R.A. Wiswell, & B.L. Drinkwater (Eds.), *Exercise in pregnancy*, (2nd ed.). Baltimore: Williams & Wilkins.

179. Moore, K.L. (1988). *The developing human: Clinically oriented embryology* (4th ed.). Philadelphia: WB Saunders.

180. Morris, N., et al. (1956). Effective uterine blood flow during exercise in normal and pre-eclamptic pregnancies. *Lancet, II*, 418.

181. Morton, M.J. (1991). Maternal hemodynamics in pregnancy. In R.A. Mittelmark, R.A. Wiswell, & B.L. Drinkwater (Eds.), *Exercise in pregnancy* (2nd ed.). Williams & Wilkins.

182. Morton, M., et al. (1984). Left ventricular size, output, and structure during guinea pig pregnancy. *Am J Physiol, 246*, R40.

183. Morton, M., Paul, M., & Metcalfe, J. (1985). Exercise during pregnancy. *Med Clin North Am, 69*, 97.

184. Morton, M.J., Pinson, C.W., & Thornburg, K.L. (1987). In utero ventilation with oxygen augments left ventricular stroke volume in lambs. *J Physiol (Lond), 383*, 413.

185. Mullinax, K. & Dale, E. (1986). Some considerations of exercise during pregnancy. *Clin Sports Med, 5*, 559.

186. Munnell, E.W., & Taylor, H.C., Jr. (1947). Liver blood flow in pregnancy—Hepatic vein catheterization. *J Clin Invest, 26*, 952.

187. Naeye, R.L. & Blanc, W.A. (1964). Prenatal narrowing or closure of the foramen ovale. *Circulation, 30*, 736.

188. Nathan, E. (1968). Severe hydrops foetalis treated with peritoneal dialysis and positive-pressure ventilation. *Lancet, 1*, 1393.

189. Novy, M.J. & Edwards, M.J. (1967). Respiratory problems in pregnancy. *Am J Obstet Gynecol, 98*, 1024.

190. O'Grady, J.P. (1987). Clinical management of twins. *Cont Obstet Gynecol, 129*, 126.

191. Olivetti, G., Anversa, P., & Loud, A,V. (1980). Morphometric study of early postnatal development in the left and right ventricular myocardium of the rat. II. Tissue composition, capillary growth, and sarcoplasmic alterations. *Circ Res, 46*, 503.

192. Palmer, A.J. & Walker, A.H.C. (1949). The maternal circulation in normal pregnancy. *J Obstet Gynaecol Br Comm, 56*, 537.

193. Parsons, M. (1988). Effects of twins: Maternal, fetal, and labor. *Clin Perinatol, 15*, 41.

194. Peck, T.M. & Arias, F. (1979). Hematologic changes associated with pregnancy. *Clin Obstet Gynecol, 22*, 785.

195. Perloff, J.K. (1980). Pregnancy and cardiovascular disease. In E. Braunwald (Ed.), *Heart disease*. Philadelphia: WB Saunders.

196. Persianinov, L.S. & Demidov, V.N. (1977). *Circulatory function during pregnancy, labour, and puerperium*. Moscow: Meditsina.

197. Pesonen, E., et al. (1983). Intrauterine hydrops caused by premature closure of the foramen ovale. *Arch Dis Child, 58*, 1015.

198. Phibbs, R.H., et al. (1976). Cardiorespiratory status of erythroblastotic newborn infants. III. Intravas-

cular pressures during the first hours of life. *Pediatrics, 58*, 484.

199. Phibbs, R.H., Johnson, P., & Tooley, W.H. (1974). Cardiorespiratory status of erythroblastotic newborn infants. II. Blood volume, hematocrit, and serum albumin concentration in relation to hydrops fetalis, *Pediatrics, 53*, 13.

200. Phibbs, R.H., et al. (1972). Cardiorespiratory status of erythroblastotic infants. I. Relationship of gestational age, severity of hemolytic disease, and birth asphyxia to idiopathic respiratory distress syndrome and survival. *Pediatrics, 49*, 5.

201. Pritchard, J.A., et al. (1972). Blood volume changes in pregnancy and the puerperium. II. Red blood cell loss and changes in apparent blood volume during and following vaginal delivery, cesarean section, and cesarean section plus total hysterectomy. *Am J Obstet Gynecol, 84*, 1271.

202. Pritchard, J.A., MacDonald, P.C., & Gant, N. (1988). *Williams obstetrics* (17th ed.). New York: Appleton-Century-Crofts.

203. Pritchard, J.A. (1960). Hematologic aspects of pregnancy. *Clin Obstet Gynecol, 3*, 378.

204. Pritchard, J.A. & Rowland, R.C. (1964). Blood volume changes in pregnancy and the puerperium. III. Whole body and large vessel hematocrits in pregnant and non-pregnant women. *Am J Obstet Gynecol, 88*, 391.

205. Pritchard, J. (1965). Changes in blood volume during pregnancy and delivery. *Anesthesiology, 26*, 393.

206. Prowse, C.M. & Galnslar, E.A. (1965). Respiratory and acid-base changes during pregnancy. *Anesthesiology, 33*, 414.

207. Pyeritz, R.E. & McKusick, V.A. (1979). The Marfan's syndrome: Diagnosis and management. *N Engl J Med, 300*, 772.

208. Quilligan, E.J. & Tyler, C. (1978). Postural effects on the cardiovascular status in pregnancy. *Am J Obstet Gynecol, 130*, 194.

209. Quilligan, E.J. (1982). Maternal physiology. In D.N. Danforth (Ed.), *Obstetrics & Gynecology*. Philadelphia: Harper & Row.

210. Radford, D.J., Izukawa, T., & Rowe, R.D. (1976). Congenital paroxysmal atrial tachycardia. *Arch Dis Child, 51*, 613.

211. Ramzin, M.S. & Napflin, S. (1982). Transient intrauterine supraventricular tachycardia associated with transient hydrops fetalis. Case report. *Br J Obstet Gynaecol, 89*, 965.

212. Rayburn, W.F., et al. (1987). Mitral valve prolapse: Echocardiographic changes during pregnancy. *J Reprod Med, 32*, 185.

213. Redford, D.H.A. (1982). Uterine growth in twin pregnancy by measurements of total intrauterine volume. *Acta Genet Med Gemellol, 31*, 145.

214. Redman, C.W.G. & Jefferies, M. (1988). Revised definition of pre-eclampsia. *Lancet, 386*, 809.

215. Remich, M.C. & Youngkin, E.Q. (1989). Factors associated with pregnancy-induced hypertension. *MCN, 14*, 20.

216. Remuzzi, G., et al. (1980). Reduction of fetal vascular prostacyclin activity in pre-eclampsia. *Lancet, 2*, 310.

217. Richardson, B.S. (1989). Fetal adaptive responses to asphyxia. *Clin Perinatol, 16*, 595.

218. Robertson, E.G. (1968). Increased erythrocyte fragility in association with osmotic changes in pregnancy serum. *J Reprod Fertil, 16*, 323.

219. Robertson W.B., Brosens I., & Dixon G. (1976). Maternal uterine vascular lesions in the hypertensive complications of pregnancy. In M.D. Lindheimer, A.I. Katz, & F.P. Zuspan (Eds.), *Hypertension in pregnancy*. New York: John Wiley & Sons.

220. Robson, S.C., et al. (1989). Serial study of factors influencing changes in cardiac output during human pregnancy. *Am J Phsyiol, 256*, H1060.

221. Robson, S.C., et al. (1989). Haemodynamic changes associated with caesarean section under epidural anaesthesia. *Br J of Obstet Gynaecol, 96*, 642.

222. Casella, E.S., Rogers, M.C., & Zahka, K.G. (1987). Developmental physiology of the cardiovascular system. In R.C. Rogers (Ed.), *Textbook of pediatric intensive care*. Baltimore: Williams & Wilkins.

223. Romen, Y., Masaki, D.I., & Mittelmark, R.A. (1991). Physiological and endocrine adjustments to pregnancy. In R.A. Mittelmark, R.A. Wiswell, & B.L. Drinkwater (Eds.), *Exercise in Pregnancy* (2nd ed.). Baltimore: Williams & Wilkins.

224. Romero, T.E. & Friedman, W.F. (1979). Limited left ventricular response to volume overload in the neonatal period: A comparative study with the adult animal. *Pediatr Res, 13*, 910.

225. Romney, S.L., et al. (1955). Oxygen utilization by the human fetus in utero. *Am J Obstet Gynecol, 70*, 791.

226. Rose, D.J., et al. (1956). Catheterization studies of cardiac hemodynamics in normal and pregnant women with reference to left ventricular work. *Am J Obstet Gynecol, 72*, 233.

227. Rovinsky, J.J. & Jaffin, H. (1965). Cardiovascular hemodynamics in pregnancy. I. Blood and plasma volumes in multiple pregnancy. *Am J Obstet Gynecol, 93*, 1.

228. Rovinsky, J.J. & Raffin, H. (1966). Cardiovascular hemodynamics in pregnancy. II. Cardiac output and ventricular work in multiple pregnancy. *Am J Obstet Gynecol, 95*, 781.

229. Rovinsky, J.J. & Jaffin, H. (1966). Cardiovascular hemodynamics in pregnancy. III. Cardiac rate, stroke volume, total peripheral resistance, and central blood volume in multiple pregnancy. Synthesis of results. *Am J Obstet Gynecol, 95*, 787.

230. Rubler, S., Prabodhkumar, M.D., & Pinto, E.R. (1977). Cardiac size and performance during pregnancy estimated with echocardiography. *Clin Obstet Gynecol, 40*, 534.

231. Rudolph, A.M. (1984). Oxygenation in the fetus and neonate—a perspective. *Semin Perinatol, 8*, 158.

232. Rudloph, A.M., et al. (1989). Ventilation is more important than oxygenation in reducing pulmonary vascular resistance at birth. *Pediatr Res, 20*, 493A.

233. Rudolph, A.M. (1984). The fetal circulation and its response to stress. *J Dev Physiol, 6*, 11.

234. Rudolph, A.M., et al. (1988). Fetal cardiovascular responses to stress. In G.H. Wiknjosastro, W.H. Prakoso, & K. Maeda (Eds.), *Perinatology*. New York: Elsevier Science Publishers.

235. Saltin, B. & Hermansen, L. (1966). Esophageal, rectal and muscle temperature during exercise. *J Appl Physiol, 21*, 1757.

236. Schanfield, M.S. (1981). Antibody-mediated perinatal diseases. *Clin Lab Med, 1*, 239.

237. Schreiner, R.L., et al. (1978). Atrial tachy-arrhythmias associated with massive edema in the newborn. *J Perinat Med, 6*, 274.

238. Schwartz, D.B. & Schamroth, L. (1979). The effect

239. Seitchik, J. (1967). Total body water and total body density of pregnant women. *Obstet Gynecol, 29*, 155.

240. Shenker, L. (1979). Fetal cardiac arrhythmias. *Obstet Gynecol Surg, 34*, 561.

241. Sheridan, D.J., Cullen, M.J., & Tynan, M.J. (1979). Qualitative and quantitative observations on ultrastructural changes during postnatal development in the cat myocardium. *J Mol Cell Cardiol, 11*, 1173.

242. Sibai, B.M. (1988). Pitfalls in diagnosis and management of preeclampsia. *Am J Obstet Gynecol, 159*, 1.

243. Sibley, L., et al. (1981). Swimming and physical fitness during pregnancy. *J Nurse Midwifery, 26*, 3.

244. Sidi, D., et al. (1983). Effects of ambient temperature on oxygen consumption and the circulation in newborn lambs at rest and during hypoxemia. *Pediatr Res, 12*, 254.

245. Silver, H.M. (1989). Acute hypertensive crisis in pregnancy. *Med Clin North Am, 73*, 623.

246. Simpson, P. (1985). Stimulation of hypertrophy of cultured neonatal rat heart cells through an alpha 1–adrenergic receptor and induction of beating through an alpha 1– and beta 1–adrenergic receptor interaction: Evidence for independent regulation of growth and beating. *Circ Res, 56*, 884.

247. Simpson, P. (1983). Norepinephrine-stimulated hypertrophy of cultured rat myocardial cells in an alpha1–adrenergic response. *J Clin Invest, 72*, 732.

248. Slaughter, C.L. (1985). Rheumatic heart disease and pregnancy. *NAACOG Update Series, 3*, 21.

249. Sorenson, K. & Borlum, K. (1986). Fetal heart function in response to short-term maternal exercise. *Br J Obstet Gynaecol, 93*, 310.

250. Sorokin U. & Dierker, L.J. (1982). Fetal movement. *Clin Obstet Gynecol, 25*, 719.

251. Spahr, R., et al. (1980). Non-immunologic hydrops fetalis: A review of 19 cases. *Int J Gynaecol Obstet, 18*, 303.

252. Spetz, S. (1964). Peripheral circulation during normal pregnancy. *Acta Obstet Gynecol Scand, 43*, 309.

253. Spetz, S. (1965). Capillary filtration during normal pregnancy. *Acta Obstet Gynecol Scand, 44*, 227.

254. Stevens, D.C., et al. (1982). Supraventricular tachycardia with edema, ascites and hydrops in fetal sheep. *Am J Obstet Gynecol, 142*, 316.

255. Stopfkuchen, H. (1987). Changes of the cardiovascular system during the perinatal period. *Eur J Pediatr, 146*, 545.

256. Stuart, M.J., et al. (1981). Decreased prostacyclin production: A characteristic of chronic placental insufficiency syndromes. *Lancet, 1*, 1126.

257. Sugimoto, T., Sagawa, K., & Guyton, A.C. (1966). Effect of tachycardia on cardiac output during normal and increased venous return. *Am J Physiol, 22*, 288.

258. Sullivan, J.M. (1986). *Hypertension and pregnancy*. Chicago: Year Book Medical Publishers.

259. Sullivan, J.M. & Ramanathan, K.B. (1985). Management of medical problems in pregnancy—severe cardiac disease. *N Engl J Med, 313*, 304.

260. Szekely, P. & Snaith, L. (1974). *Heart disease and pregnancy*. Edinburgh: Churchill Livingstone.

261. Szekely, P., Turner, R., & Snaith, L. (1973). Pregnancy and the changing pattern of rheumatic heart disease. *Br Heart J, 35*, 1293.

262. Tapia, H.R., Johnson, C.E., & Strong, C.G. (1973). Effect of oral contraceptive therapy on the renin-

of pregnancy on the frontal plane QRS axis. *J Electrocardiol, 12*, 279.

angiotensin system in normotensive and hypertensive women. *Obstet Gynecol, 41,* 643.

263. Tayler, D.J., et al. (1982). Effect of iron supplementation on serum ferritin levels during and after pregnancy. *Br J Obstet Gynaecol, 89,* 1011.

264. Thornburg, K.L. & Morton, M.J. (1983). Filling and arterial pressures as determinants of RV stroke volume in the sheep fetus. *Am J Physiol, 244,* H656.

265. Toppozada M.K., et al. (1988). Treatment of preeclampsia with prostaglandin A$_1$. *Am J Obstet Gynecol, 159,* 160.

266. Trudinger B.J. (1988). Low-dose aspirin therapy improves fetal weight in umbilical placental insufficiency. *Am J Obstet Gynecol, 159,* 681.

267. Ueland, K. & Parer, J.T. (1966). Effects of estrogens on the cardiovascular system of the ewe. *Am J Obstet Gynecol, 96,* 400.

268. Ueland, K. & Metcalfe, J. (1966). Acute rheumatic fever in pregnancy. *Am J Obstet Gynecol, 95,* 586.

269. Ueland, K., Gills, R.E., & Hansen, J.M. (1968). Maternal cardiovascular dynamics. I. Cesarean section under subarachnoid block anesthesia. *Am J Obstet Gynecol, 100,* 42.

270. Ueland, K., et al. (1972). Maternal cardiovascular dynamics. VI. Cesarean section under epidural anesthesia without epinephrine. *Am J Obstet Gynecol, 114,* 775.

271. Ueland, K., et al. (1970) Maternal cardiovascular dynamics. V. Cesarean section under thiopental, nitrous oxide, and succinylcholine anesthesia. *Am J Obstet Gynecol, 108,* 615.

272. Ueland, K. & Hansen, J.M. (1969). Maternal cardiovascular dynamics. II. Posture and uterine contractions. *Am J Obstet Gynecol, 103,* 1.

273. Ueland, K., et al. (1969). Maternal cardiovascular dynamics. IV. The influence of gestational age on maternal cardiovascular response to posture and exercise. *Am J Obstet Gynecol, 104,* 856.

274. Ueland, K. (1976). Maternal cardiovascular dynamics. VII. Intrapartum blood volume changes. *Am J Obstet Gynecol, 126,* 671.

275. Ueland, K. & Metcalfe, J. (1975). Circulatory changes in pregnancy. *Clin Obstet Gynecol, 18,* 41.

276. Ueland, K. & Hansen, J.M. (1969). Maternal cardiovascular dynamics. III. Labor and delivery under local and caudal analgesia. *Am J Obstet Gynecol, 103,* 8.

277. Ueland, K., Novy, J.M., & Metcalfe, J. (1973). Cardiorespiratory responses to pregnancy and exercise in normal women and patients with heart disease. *Am J Obstet Gynecol, 115,* 4.

278. Upshaw, C.B., Jr. (1970). A study of maternal electrocardiograms recorded during labor and delivery. *Am J Obstet Gynecol, 107,* 17.

279. Van Amerigan, M.R., et al. (1981). Oxygenation in anemic newborn lambs with high or low oxygen affinity red cells. *Pediatr Res, 15,* 1500.

280. Vorys, N., Ullery, J.C., & Hanusek, G.E. (1961). The cardiac output changes in various positions in pregnancy. *Am J Obstet Gynecol, 82,* 1312.

281. Wagner, P.D. (1977). Recent advances in pulmonary gas exchange. *Int Anesthesiol Clin, 15,* 81.

282. Wagner, P.D. (1974). The oxyhemoglobin dissociation curve and pulmonary gas exchange. *Semin Hematol, 11,* 405.

283. Wallenburg, H.C.S. (1978). Water and electrolyte homeostasis of the amniotic fluid. In *Developmental aspects of fluid and electrolyte homeostasis* (pp. 9–17). Mead Johnson Symposium on Perinatal and Developmental Medicine, No. 10. Evansville, IN: Mead Johnson.

284. Walsh, S. (1988). Cardiovascular disease in pregnancy: A nursing approach. *J Cardiovasc Nurs, 2,* 53.

284a. Walsh, S.W. (1990). Physiology of low-dose aspirin therapy for the prevention of preeclampsia. *Semin Perinatol, 14,* 152.

285. Walters, W.A.W. & Lim, Y.L. (1969). Cardiovascular dynamics in women receiving oral contraceptive therapy. *Lancet, 2,* 879.

286. Walters, W.A.W., MacGregor, W.G., & Hills, M. (1966). Cardiac output at rest during pregnancy and the puerperium. *Clin Sci, 30,* 1.

287. Wedermeyer, A.L. & Breitfeld, V.. (1975). Cardiac neoplasm, tachyarrhythmia, and anasarca in an infant. *Am J Dis Child, 129,* 738.

288. Weinstein, L. (1987). The HELLP syndrome: A severe consequence of hypertension in pregnancy. *J Perinatol, 6,* 316.

289. Wenstrom, K.D. & Gall, S.A. (1988). Incidence, morbidity and mortality, and diagnosis of twin gestations. *Clin Perinatol, 15,* 1.

290. Wilkening, R. & Meschia, G. (1983). Fetal oxygen uptake, oxygenation, and acid-base balance as a function of uterine blood flow. *Am J Physiol, 244,* 749.

291. Wilson, M., et al. (1980). Blood pressure, the renin-aldosterone system, and sex steroids throughout normal pregnancy. *Am J Med, 68,* 97.

292. Winner, W. & Romney, S.L. (1966). Cardiovascular responses to labor and delivery. *Am J Obstet Gynecol, 95,* 1104.

293. Wolfson, R.N., Sorokin, Y., & Mortimer, G.R. (1982). Autonomic Control of Fetal Cardiac Activity. In U. Elkayam & N. Gleicher (Eds.), *Cardiac problems in pregnancy: Diagnosis and management of maternal and fetal disease.* New York: Alan R. Liss.

294. Wood, J.E. (1972). The cardiovascular effects of oral contraceptives. *Mod Concepts Cardiovasc Dis, 41,* 37.

295. Wynn, R.J. & Schreiner, R.L. (1979). Spurious elevation of amniotic fluid bilirubin in acute hydramnios with fetal obstruction. *Am J Obstet Gynecol, 134,* 105.

296. Yeh, T.F., et al. (1984). Increased O$_2$ consumption and energy loss in premature infants following medical care procedures. *Biol Neonate, 46,* 157.

297. Ylikorkala, O. & Viinikka, L. (1980). Thromboxane A2 in pregnancy and puerperium. *Br Med J, 281,* 1601.

298. Zatikyan, E.P. (1983). Changes in venous return in pregnancy. (in Russian). *Krovoobrasheniie, 3,* 44.

299. Zimmerman, H.A. (1950). A preliminary report on intracardiac catheterization studies during pregnancy. *J Lab Clin Med, 36,* 1007.

CHAPTER 7

The Respiratory System

Maternal Physiologic Adaptations
    The Antepartum Period
        Mechanical Changes
        Biochemical Changes
        Lung Volumes
        Changes in Lung Function
    The Intrapartum Period
    The Postpartum Period
Clinical Implications for the Pregnant Woman and Her Fetus
    Dyspnea
    Upper Respiratory Capillary Engorgement
    Respiratory Infection
    Exercise
    Asthma
    Smoking
    Inhalation Anesthesia
Development of the Respiratory System in the Fetus
    Anatomic Development
    Functional Development

Neonatal Physiology
    Transitional Events
    Control of Respiration
    The Respiratory Pump
    Mechanical Properties of the Respiratory System
    Ventilation
    Lung Volumes
    Perfusion
    Ventilation-Perfusion Matching
    Alveolar-Capillary Membrane
Clinical Implications for Neonatal Care
    Respiratory Risk Factors
    Physiologic Basis for Clinical Findings
    Nursing Interventions to Promote Respiratory Stability
    Asphyxia
    Resuscitation
    Transient Tachypnea
    Respiratory Distress Syndrome
    Bronchopulmonary Dysplasia
    Meconium Aspiration Syndrome
    Persistent Pulmonary Hypertension
Maturational Changes During Infancy and Childhood

Respiration is the totality of those processes that ultimately result in energy being supplied to the cells. In pregnancy, the respiratory system undergoes significant changes. The increased metabolic needs of the pregnant woman, fetus, and placenta require increased maternal respiratory efficiency in order to ensure adequate oxygenation during the antepartum, intrapartum, and postpartum periods.

The placenta functions as the respiratory system for the fetus, providing nutrients and oxygen and removing waste products. This makes the relationship between the mother and fetus not only intimate but interdependent.

At birth, tremendous energy is expended by the neonate to generate sufficient negative pressure to convert to an air-liquid interface in the alveoli. Transitional events continue over the 1st week of life as the neonate adjusts to the new environment, more alveoli are recruited, and the surfactant system stabilizes.

MATERNAL PHYSIOLOGIC ADAPTATIONS

Changes in the respiratory system during pregnancy are mediated by hormonal and biochemical changes as well as the enlarging uterus. As the muscles and cartilage relax in the thoracic region, the chest broadens and tidal volume is improved. The normal changes that occur during pregnancy are in conjunction with a conversion from abdominal to thoracic breathing. This leads to a 50% increase in air volume per minute. These changes result in a mild respiratory alkalosis. For the fetus, this respiratory alkalosis is essential for the exchange of gases across the placenta.[362]

The Antepartum Period

Pregnancy is associated with major changes in the respiratory system in both lung volumes and ventilation. Both biochemical and mechanical factors interact to increase the delivery of oxygen and the removal of carbon dioxide.

Mechanical Changes

The gradual enlargement of the uterus leads to changes in abdominal size and shape, shifting the resting position of the diaphragm up to 4 cm above its usual position. The transverse diameter increases about 2 cm in response to the increased intra-abdominal pressure, and a flaring of the lower ribs occurs. The subcostal angle progressively increases from 68.5 to 103.5 degrees in late gestation. Not all of these changes can be attributed to intra-abdominal pressure, since the increase in the subcostal angle occurs prior to the increasing mechanical pressure.[28, 88, 352]

Although the above changes suggest that diaphragmatic motion decreases, the reverse is actually true. Results of studies indicate that diaphragmatic movement actually increases during pregnancy, with the major work of breathing being accomplished by the diaphragm rather than by the costal muscles.[28, 352]

The modification in abdominal space through changes in thoracic structures may be in preparation for the increase in uterine size. These changes in thoracic configuration have a major impact on lung volumes, however, to which the increasing intra-abdominal pressure contributes.

Biochemical Changes

Hormones and other biochemical factors are important in stimulating changes in the respiratory system in pregnancy. These substances can act centrally via stimulation of the respiratory center or directly on smooth muscle and other tissues of the lung. The most important influences are mediated by progesterone and prostaglandins.

Serum progesterone levels increase progressively throughout pregnancy and have been implicated as a major factor in the changes seen in ventilation. The administration of progesterone to normal subjects in a study cited by Weinberger and Weiss led to an increase in minute ventilation as well as an enhanced response to hypercapnia.[352] This suggests that there is an increased sensitivity to carbon dioxide (CO_2) by the respiratory center and that progesterone lowers the CO_2 threshold of the respiratory center. This increased sensitivity most likely contributes to the sensation of dyspnea that is experienced by a large percentage of pregnant women and may also lead to some of the hyperventilation that occurs during the second stage of labor after pushing efforts (as CO_2 levels increase during breath holding).[103, 352]

Other hypotheses suggest that progesterone alters ventilation through direct stimulation of the respiratory center rather than by altering sensitivity to existing stimuli. These theories have received very little support. Currently, it has been postulated that progesterone exerts a local effect on the lung, causing water retention in the lung that results in decreased diffusion capacity. Therefore hyperventilation is an attempt to maintain normal PO_2 levels.[108, 191, 219, 234]

Progesterone may also play a role in decreasing airway resistance (up to 50%), thereby reducing the work of breathing and facilitating a greater airflow in pregnancy. Hormonal relaxation of bronchiole smooth muscle has been attributed to progesterone. This counteracts the expected increase in airway resistance that would be the result of lungs that are less distended.[139, 216]

Prostaglandins may also play a role in ventilatory changes by affecting the smooth muscle tissue of the bronchial airways. Prostaglandin $F_{2\alpha}$ ($PGF_{2\alpha}$) has been identified as a bronchial smooth muscle constrictor, whereas PGE_1 and PGE_2 have been found to exert a bronchodilator effect. Several studies have demonstrated an increase in prostaglandin F levels throughout pregnancy; increases in prostaglandin E concentrations are found only in the third trimester.[138, 193]

The lack of clarity surrounding the specific functions of prostaglandins carries over to the influence these substances have on airway tone, especially in women with airway diseases such as asthma. Studies have demonstrated increased bronchial constriction with precipitation of asthmatic attacks when PGF_2 was used to induce abortion in women with underlying reactive airway disease. In healthy women and those without underlying pathology, there is little evidence to indicate that these alterations in prostaglandin levels result in clinically significant symptomatology.[123, 138, 213]

The effects of these chemicals on ventilation seem to both counteract some of the results of the necessary structural changes (decreased lung distention due to elevated diaphragm) and modify respiration in order to meet fetal requirements (maternal respiratory alkalosis promotes CO_2 transfer from the fetus). More research needs to be conducted in this area in order to understand the balance that is created between biochemical and structural changes in pregnancy.

Lung Volumes

During the middle of the second trimester changes in lung volumes can be seen. The most significant change is a 25 to 40% increase in tidal volume (V_T) with a progressive decrease in expiratory reserve volume (ERV), residual volume (RV), and functional residual capacity (FRC). Along with the change in V_T, there is a concomitant increase in inspiratory capacity (IC), thereby allowing the total lung capacity (TLC) to remain unchanged. Vital capacity (VC) and inspiratory reserve volume (IRV) are essentially unaltered, although some literature notes a change in IRV (Fig. 7–1 and Table 7–1).[88, 344]

All of the above changes result from the elevation of the diaphragm and the changes in the configuration of the chest. The alter-

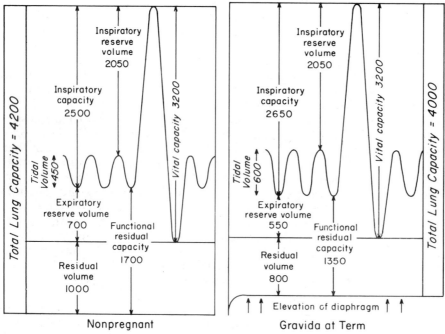

FIGURE 7–1.   Changes in lung volumes with pregnancy. (From Bonica, J. J. (1967). *Principles and practice of obstetric analgesia and anesthesia* (p. 24). Philadelphia: FA Davis.)

TABLE 7–1
Lung Volume and Capacity Changes During Pregnancy

	ALTERATION
Volume	
Inspiratory reserve volume (IRV)	None or sl ↑
Tidal volume (V_T)	↑ 150–200 ml
Residual volume (RV)	↓ 200–300 ml
Expiratory reserve volume (ERV)	↓ 150–200 ml
Capacity	
Total lung capacity (TLC)	None or sl ↓
Vital capacity (VC)	Unchanged
Inspiratory reserve capacity (IRC)	↑ up to 500 ml
Functional residual capacity (FRC)	↑ up to 500 ml

ation in RV is also the result of decreased chest wall compliance, which is partially caused by hormonal influences. This reduction in stiffness allows for more inward movement of the chest wall and reduces the amount of trapped air (residual trapped volume) that contributes to the RV. Therefore the RV decreases 200 to 300 ml. This along with the 200 ml decrease in ERV brings the total deficit in the FRC to 500 ml. There is a progressive drop in FRC from 20 weeks' gestation for a total change of 18% by term.[352]

Changes in Lung Function

Changes in lung function are related to three major factors: ventilation, air flow, and diffusing capacity. Oxygen consumption increases during pregnancy; however, the arterial oxygen pressure (PaO_2) does not significantly change even though the arteriovenous oxygen difference decreases. This indicates that there must be a change in ventilation.[103]

VENTILATION

A major change in ventilation during pregnancy is the result of a 30 to 50% increase in minute ventilation ($V_T \times RR$ [respiratory rate]), culminating in an increased minute volume from 6.5 L/min to 10 L/min at term. The elevated resting ventilation exceeds the demands in oxygen consumption (which increases by approximately 20%), indicating that women hyperventilate during pregnancy.[27, 103, 216]

The increase in minute ventilation is usually attributed to a 40% increase in V_T and a 15% increase in respiratory rate. Others, however, have found no change in respiratory rate. Therefore, the change in minute ventilation may be a function of V_T alterations alone. DeSwiet notes that it is much more efficient to increase alveolar ventilation through an increase in V_T than with a proportionately equal increase in respiratory rate. This may explain some of the differences found in studies in the current body of literature.[42, 103, 352]

Alveolar ventilation is further enhanced by the reduced RV. This change in RV decreases the amount of dilution (mixing) that occurs with each tidal exchange in the alveolus, thereby improving gas exchange at the alveolar level. Alveolar ventilation increases by 70% during pregnancy.[103, 191]

AIR FLOW

Despite the changes in minute ventilation and the concomitant increase in alveolar ventilation, the work of breathing (airway resistance and lung compliance) remains unchanged. A reduction in airway resistance may explain this. Air flow is dependent upon resistance encountered in the bronchial tree. Two of the important determining factors for resistance are smooth muscle tone in the bronchi and the degree of congestion encountered in the bronchial wall capillaries.

In the larger airways, congestion has very little to do with resistance. Studies measuring airway resistance during pregnancy provide conflicting results, with either a decrease in resistance and concomitant increase in airway conductance or no change in resistance. Several factors influencing airway resistance act in opposition and may result in no net change. For example, PGF_2 is a potent bronchoconstrictor, whereas PGE_1 and PGE_2 as well as progesterone function as bronchodilators. It is most likely the balance of forces within individuals that determines what is seen upon testing.[103, 193, 352]

Assessment of small airway function is most often determined by the evaluation of closing volume (CV) and closing capacity (CC). Closing volume is the point at which the small airways close (collapse and cease to ventilate) in the lowest part of the lung. Small airway (<1 mm) patency is believed to be the result of transpulmonary pressure, compliance of the airway walls, and the presence of sufficient surfactant. Closure in the lung bases normally occurs somewhere between the RV and FRC. Closing volume is usually expressed as a percentage of vital capacity (CV/VC%). Closing capacity is the term applied to the sum of the closing volume and residual volume (CC = CV + RV) and is expressed as a percentage of total lung capacity (CC/TLC%).[138, 267, 357]

Under normal circumstances closure does not occur during tidal breathing. When closure occurs at a higher than normal volume, however, gas exchange may be affected because ventilation to the lung bases is decreased. In pregnancy, airway closure above the FRC has been reported and is attributed to the 20% decrease in ERV. This alteration changes gas distribution and results in a fall in PaO_2.[103, 263]

Whether closing volumes are normally altered in pregnancy is unclear; however, small airway dysfunction is not a feature of normal pregnancy pulmonary dynamics. If airway closure is at or above FRC, there is the possibility of altering PaO_2 owing to ventilation-perfusion $(\dot{V}/\dot{Q})$ differences in the bases. If these differences are significant, compensatory maternal physiologic responses such as an increase in respiratory rate may result.

DIFFUSING CAPACITY

Diffusing capacity refers to the ease with which gas is transferred across the pulmonary membrane. In the early stages of pregnancy, diffusion capacity is decreased. Pecora and coworkers suggest that the mucopolysaccharides in the capillary walls may be affected by estrogen and increase the thickness of the capillary walls, although a direct relationship between these two is not definitive.[280] This reduced diffusion capacity may last up to 12 months post partum.[259, 280]

Interestingly, this is the one factor that counteracts the efforts of the mother to improve gas exchange at a time when oxygen consumption by numerous maternal systems is high. As noted earlier, the hyperventilation of pregnancy exceeds these demands. In fact, maximum hyperventilation can be seen as early as the 2nd or 3rd month of gestation. This suggests that there is some other source (e.g., progesterone) of stimulus for the increased minute ventilation or that a percent-

age of the hyperventilation serves to compensate for this reduction in diffusion.

ACID-BASE CHANGES

The normal pregnant woman is in a compensated respiratory alkalosis, thought to be the result of progesterone's effects on the respiratory system and lung volume changes. The result is a reduction in arterial and alveolar CO_2 and an increase in PaO_2. The purpose of the respiratory alkalosis seems to be facilitation of CO_2 transfer from the fetus to the mother by increasing the arterial carbon dioxide pressure ($PaCO_2$) gradient. Hyperventilation leads to average $PaCO_2$ values of 30 to 32 mmHg and a concomitant decrease in serum bicarbonate levels between 18 and 21 mEq/L with a base deficit of -1 to -3 mEq/L. The latter is a consequence of increased renal excretion of bicarbonate, reflecting a metabolic compensation for the low $PaCO_2$. The pH, therefore, increases to the high end of normal (7.40 to 7.45). The reduction in blood buffer reduces the mother's ability to compensate for the metabolic acidosis that could develop during prolonged labor or other states in which tissue perfusion may be reduced. These changes are stable throughout pregnancy until the onset of labor. Table 7–2 provides a comparison of arterial acid-base values in pregnant and nonpregnant women.[64, 263, 352]

In contrast, PaO_2 levels increase from those of prepregnancy (95 to 100 mmHg) owing to the increase in alveolar ventilation. During the first trimester PaO_2 levels range from 106 to 108 mmHg, dropping to 101 to 104 mmHg by the third trimester. Even though the PaO_2 level remains elevated, the alveolar-arterial PO_2 gradient ($AaDO_2$) may not increase until term, which may result from an attempt to offset hyperventilation. Whether there is clinical significance to these changes is unknown at the present. However, supine positioning versus sitting in late pregnancy does decrease PaO_2 levels and increase the $AaDO_2$ gradient.[352]

TABLE 7–2
Comparison of Acid-Base Values in Arterial Blood of Pregnant and Nonpregnant Women

WOMEN'S CLINICAL STATE	$PaCO_2$ (mmHg)	SERUM BICARBONATE (mEq/L)	BASE EXCESS (mEq/L)	BLOOD pH
Pregnant	32.8 ± 1.5	17.97 ± 2.99	−1.2 ± 1.02	7.43 ± 0.005
Nonpregnant	40.0 ± 0.6	25.00 ± 1.00	+1.0 ± 0.059	7.38 ± 0.007

From Burgess, A. (1979). *The nurse's guide to fluid and electrolyte balance* (p. 96). New York: McGraw-Hill.

Oxygen-Hemoglobin Dissociation Curve

The oxygen-hemoglobin dissociation curve demonstrates the equilibrium between oxygen and hemoglobin. The curve relates the partial pressure of oxygen to the percentage of hemoglobin that is saturated. There are two aspects of the curve that must be considered: its shape and its position.

The shape of the curve is sigmoid, indicating that at higher levels (>50 mmHg) the curve flattens and an increase in Po_2 produces little increase in saturation. This upper region is the Po_2 range in which oxygen binds to hemoglobin in the lungs. At low Po_2's the curve is steep and small changes in Po_2 result in large changes in hemoglobin saturation. In this range oxygen is released from hemoglobin and cellular activities occur. A small drop in Po_2 here allows a large amount of oxygen to be unloaded to the tissues.

The position of the curve, whether it is shifted to the right or the left, depends on the oxygen affinity for the hemoglobin molecule. The affinity of hemoglobin for oxygen must be sufficient to oxygenate the blood during its movement through the pulmonary circulation. However, it must be weak enough to allow release of oxygen to the tissues.

This affinity is expressed as the P_{50}, the oxygen tension at which hemoglobin is half saturated. The higher the affinity the lower the P_{50} and vice versa, indicating an inverse relationship. The P_{50} for adult blood at a pH

of 7.40 and a temperature of 37°C is normally 26 mmHg. Numerous factors, both genetic and environmental, can influence the affinity of hemoglobin and shift the oxygen-hemoglobin dissociation curve (see Fig. 7–13).

A shift to the right implies a lowered affinity; a shift to the left indicates that oxygen is more tightly bound to hemoglobin. The structure of the hemoglobin molecule regulates the affinity and can be affected by pH, Pco_2, and temperature.

Increasing amounts of carbon dioxide reduce hemoglobin affinity for oxygen. This is termed the Bohr effect. Because of the Bohr effect the reciprocal exchange of oxygen for carbon dioxide is facilitated. Elevations in temperature also shift the curve to the right such that saturation is decreased at any given Po_2. The pH increases with release of CO_2, and the curve shifts to the left. The shift indicates an increased affinity for oxygen and favors the uptake of oxygen by hemoglobin.

Because of the sigmoid shape of the curve, a shift in position has little effect on the saturation when the Po_2 is within the normal arterial range (95 to 100 mmHg). However, in the venous system, in which the Po_2 range is around 40 mmHg, there is a right shift in the curve, leading to an increased unloading of oxygen to the tissues and improving tissue oxygenation.

The oxygen-hemoglobin dissociation curve demonstrates that once the plateau of the curve is achieved it takes large changes in oxygen concentration in order to make small changes in PaO_2.[57] The question here is whether the small changes seen in PaO_2 levels during pregnancy are significant to the maternal-fetal oxygen gradient and therefore to the fetus. Considering that fetal PaO_2 levels are between 25 and 35 mmHg, this seems unlikely. However, this increase may reflect an increased pulmonary circulation, with a greater volume of blood contained within the pulmonary vasculature at any given point in time. This may be very significant at higher altitudes.

With increasing altitude, increases in PaO_2 can be seen as compensatory in nature. The change in altitude has a significant effect on oxygen saturation, and a change in the oxygen-hemoglobin dissociation curve can be seen. The hyperventilation of pregnancy is also accentuated, therefore patients need to

be given assurance that it is normal. All these factors are an attempt by the maternal system to maintain higher PaO_2 levels under relatively hypoxic conditions. Women who travel by airplane may also experience an increase in dyspnea and respiratory rate as their bodies attempt to compensate for the increased altitude.[145]

The Intrapartum Period

The major impact of labor upon the respiratory system is related to the increased work of the muscles, metabolic rate, and oxygen consumption. Consequently, alterations in ventilation and acid-base status can be anticipated.

With the onset of labor there is an increased demand for oxygen, and oxygen consumption increases with uterine muscle activity. If there is insufficient time for uterine relaxation and restabilization after a contraction, oxygen content is low and myometrial hypoxia as well as metabolic acidosis may occur with the next contraction. Over time this can lead to inadequate oxygenation, which increases the severity of the pain experienced. Most studies have evaluated respiratory system changes during active and painful labor. There are few studies evaluating the labor process with the use of sporadic analgesia and psychoprophylaxis. This limits some of the conclusions that can be drawn from the data in the literature.

The pain experienced during labor is the result of the interaction of a number of factors (see Chapter 12). The subjective component includes the discomfort that is perceived by the mother. Objective factors are related to changes in the functioning of the cardiorespiratory system, alterations in the autonomic nervous system, and physical changes that occur during labor and delivery.

Ventilatory alterations related to pain vary significantly from patient to patient, therefore each laboring woman must be evaluated independently. Changes seen during the intrapartum period include an increase in RR and a change in V_T, with a tendency toward hyperventilation. Hyperventilation is a natural response to pain and becomes evident as the pain and apprehension of labor increase. It has been demonstrated that when pain is alleviated by lumbar epidural anesthesia, the hyperventilation is greatly diminished, if not completely eliminated.[187]

Although pain seems to be the major cause of this hyperventilatory response, anxiety, drugs, and oxygen mask application as well as voluntary use of psychoprophylactic breathing exercises can contribute to the elevated RR. Tidal volumes may be further increased during the second stage of labor as hyperventilation following breath holding with expulsive efforts is encountered.

This increase in ventilation can lead to a progressive and substantial decline in $PaCO_2$. Once again there are wide variations in values between patients; however, a $PaCO_2$ level of 25 mmHg is representative of what might be encountered during the first stage of labor. It has been suggested that there is a transient decline in $PaCO_2$ with each contraction until cervical dilatation is complete, at which time the decline in $PaCO_2$ can be seen even between contractions. Arterial carbon dioxide levels as low as 17 mmHg have been recorded in some women experiencing painful contractions. Most of the changes in $PaCO_2$ are

eliminated when continuous lumbar epidural anesthesia is used during labor. Variables affecting $PaCO_2$ levels that need to be considered include breath holding (which elevates $PaCO_2$ levels), compensatory hyperventilation following breath holding, length of contractions, and frequency of contractions. The timing of analgesia administration as well as the frequency and efficacy of the analgesia may also alter $PaCO_2$ values.[78, 263]

The respiratory alkalosis that ensues from hyperventilation is normally associated with a drop in base excess and possibly a decrease in arterial pH according to some researchers. Other investigators have documented a rise in pH to above 7.6. In either case, the degree of change indicates that labor and hyperventilation are highly significant events that may lead to dramatic alterations in physiologic parameters.[42, 78, 248, 263, 275]

Labor studies demonstrate that maternal acidosis is not uncommon and can be attributed to isometric muscular contractions which reduce the blood flow to working muscles, leading to tissue hypoxia and anaerobic metabolism in the face of a normal PaO_2. The degree of maternal acidosis is dependent upon the extent of maternal anxiety and tension, intensity of muscular workload, degree of isometric contractions, and duration of labor. Studies have shown that changes in pH may also be minimized through the use of epidural anesthesia throughout labor.[78, 246, 300]

In the first stage of labor, the maternal and fetal $PaCO_2$ levels parallel each other. This may reflect the respiratory nature of these changes. As labor progresses this paralleling of values is lost, which may be an indication of the difficulty charged ions have in crossing the placental membrane.[300]

Fetal $PaCO_2$ levels rise when maternal acidosis occurs, reflecting not only fetal base deficit alterations but also the hypoxia within the uterine muscle. Contractions not only decrease the blood flow within the intervillous space but also reduce the oxygen supply to the uterus as well. The longer and stronger the contractions, the more pronounced the effects. The local buildup of $PaCO_2$ decreases the fetal elimination of CO_2, which may lead to significant fetal acidosis.[300]

During the second stage of labor, maternal $PaCO_2$ levels may rise during pushing efforts. It is during this stage that a further increase in blood lactate levels owing to voluntary muscle activity during bearing down is seen. This is reflected in a substantial decline in blood pH and a fall in blood buffering capability (base excess).[246]

Bonica has suggested that the changes in acid-base status due to hyperventilation and oxygen consumption are unphysiologic and potentially hazardous to mother and fetus.[42] Extremely low $PaCO_2$ levels result in cerebral vasoconstriction and possibly reduce intervillous perfusion and blood flow. The alkalemia that results shifts the oxygen-hemoglobin dissociation curve to the left. This shift impairs the release of oxygen from maternal blood to fetal blood, thereby decreasing the availability of oxygen to the fetus during a time when oxygenation may already be impaired owing to uterine contractions.[28, 42, 57]

In order to modify the consequences of labor on the mother and fetus, the nurse should conduct an ongoing assessment of the mother's cardiorespiratory status. Hyperventilation may lead to dizziness and tingling due to low $PaCO_2$ levels. Interventions can include counting respirations out loud to help the mother slow her respiratory rate, letting her know when the contraction is ending so that she can begin to relax, encouraging her to breathe when breath holding is inappropriate, and promoting deep breathing between contractions to cleanse the system and promote oxygenation and restabilization.

The acid-base changes encountered in the first and second stages of labor quickly reverse in the third stage and postpartum period with compensatory respiratory efforts. These efforts are largely due to a decrease in respiratory rate. Within 24 hours post delivery acid-base levels return to pregnancy values and to nonpregnant levels in several weeks. Table 7–3 summarizes the changes in arterial blood gases during the intrapartum period.[60]

Although it may appear that the use of epidural anesthesia is being advocated here, it is not. Research on the effects of labor on acid-base status has been conducted in conjunction with the delivery of epidural analgesia. Psychoprophylaxis (psychoanalgesia) has been shown to reduce the need for medication, to reduce tension and pain by self-report, and to engender a positive attitude toward the labor and delivery experience. Lamaze psychoprophylaxis is based on the hypothesis that childbirth is a natural physiologic process and that pain can be minimized through education and specified exercises. Education and antenatal preparation are designed to reduce anxiety through knowledge of the processes of labor. Relaxation techniques are designed to reduce skeletal muscle spasm and tension that may contribute to pain. Reduction of pain sensations and perception is achieved through distraction by utilizing conditional responses such as breathing patterns.[71, 99, 107, 311]

Psychoprophylactic research, however, has failed to substantiate its therapeutic benefits from an empirical perspective. The lack of control groups and statistical analysis as well as knowledge regarding therapeutic benefits of component parts make research in this area more difficult to interpret.

The Postpartum Period

The respiratory tract rapidly returns to its prepregnant state after delivery. This is a direct result of the separation of the placenta and consequential loss of progesterone production as well as the immediate reduction in intra-abdominal pressure with delivery of the neonate and concomitant increased ex-

TABLE 7–3
Maternal Blood Gas Alterations During Intrapartum Period

STAGE OF LABOR	PARAMETER	RANGE VALUE	ACID-BASE STATUS
Early	$PaCO_2$ Plasma base deficit Blood pH	21–26 mmHg −0.9 to −6.9 mEq/L 7.43–7.49	Respiratory alkalosis
End of first stage	$PaCO_2$ Plasma base deficit Blood pH	21–35 mmHg −1.2 to −9.2 mEq/L 7.41–7.54	Mild metabolic acidosis compensated by respiratory alkalosis Mild respiratory acidosis during bearing down
End of second stage (delivery)	$PaCO_2$ Plasma base deficit Blood pH	16–24 mmHg −2.3 to −12.3 mEq/L 7.37–7.45	Metabolic acidosis uncompensated by respiratory alkalosis

From Burgess, A. (1979). *The nurse's guide to fluid and electrolyte balance* (p. 99). New York: McGraw-Hill.

cursion of the diaphragm. Chest wall compliance returns to normal immediately post delivery owing to relief of diaphragmatic pressure. A 25% increase in static compliance was noted by Marx and associates following vaginal delivery and was attributed to the descent of the diaphragm.[247] This increase in compliance was confirmed in studies conducted on women undergoing cesarean section, in which a 20% increase in total respiratory compliance post delivery was documented. These researchers attributed this change not only to a decrease in pressure on the diaphragm but also to a reduction in pulmonary blood volume. Further research may clarify these findings. This modification in compliance post delivery can be seen in the need to decrease inflation pressures when providing intermittent positive-pressure ventilation (IPPV) following the delivery of the infant.[77, 119, 247]

Tidal volume and RV return to normal soon after delivery whereas ERV may remain in an abnormal state for several months. As progesterone levels fall, a in rise $PaCO_2$ levels can be seen during the first 2 days post delivery. Diffusing capacity, which at term is slightly below postpartum levels, increases during the postpartum period. Overall, anatomic changes and ventilation return to normal 1 to 3 weeks post delivery.[77, 114, 181, 254, 260]

CLINICAL IMPLICATIONS FOR THE PREGNANT WOMAN AND HER FETUS

The respiratory changes that occur with pregnancy can be annoying as well as limiting in some circumstances. Common complaints and experiences include, among others, dyspnea and capillary engorgement of the upper respiratory tract. As a result, modifications in activity levels as well as in the activities themselves may need to be considered. Discussions with women regarding their usual activities are necessary in order to provide them with sufficient information for determining when change is needed.

In addition, changes in the maternal respiratory system can impact on other disease processes (e.g., asthma), affecting not only the mother but also the fetus. Specific areas addressed in this section include dyspnea of pregnancy, upper respiratory capillary engorgement, respiratory infections, asthma,

smoking, and anesthesia. Exercise is discussed briefly; further information can be found in Chapter 6. Implications for both mother and fetus are explored.

Dyspnea

The sensation of dyspnea is a common complaint of women during pregnancy (60 to 70%), especially in the first or second trimester. Since abdominal girth has not increased significantly at this time, intra-abdominal pressure cannot be ascribed as the cause. The actual cause remains unclear. One of the earliest studies suggested that a decreased diffusion capacity was the cause of dyspnea; this theory has not received much support, however.[88, 147, 218, 287]

Other more accepted theories explain the dyspnea of pregnancy in relation to the hyperventilation of pregnancy. Decreased $PaCO_2$ levels and an increased awareness of the V_T changes that occur in normal pregnancy have been implicated in these theories. As early as 1953, it was suggested that the heightened awareness of the normal hyperventilation of pregnancy might result in the sensation of dyspnea. The frequent improvement in symptoms with increasing gestation suggests an adjustment to the normal process.[92]

A later study correlated dyspnea with altered $PaCO_2$ levels, suggesting a physiologic basis for this sensation. The women most likely to experience dyspnea had relatively high $PaCO_2$ levels prior to pregnancy, and the researchers felt that the marked change in $PaCO_2$ (from nonpregnant to pregnant levels) might account for the dyspnea. Follow-up work by these researchers demonstrated that women who experienced dyspnea had an increased ventilatory response to CO_2 and that this altered response led to a heightened awareness of the hyperventilation associated with pregnancy.[146, 147]

For whatever reasons this process occurs, it can be quite uncomfortable and anxiety provoking for some women. Early descriptions of dyspnea to the patient are appropriate and encouraged.

Upper Respiratory Capillary Engorgement

Hormonal changes (especially the increase in estrogens) result in capillary engorgement throughout the respiratory tract. Progesterone may contribute to engorgement by inducing vascular smooth muscle relaxation and nasal vascular pooling. Of course, increased circulating blood volume may also play a role in the latter. Some of the results of this change can be uncomfortable to some women and in certain situations can be hazardous.[194]

The gums become edematous and soft during pregnancy and may bleed after brushing (see Chapter 9). Consistent attention to dental and mouth care can reduce if not eliminate this frequent complaint, making dental intervention unnecessary.

Along with this, the nasopharynx, larynx, trachea, and bronchi may become swollen and reddened. For some individuals this may be uncomfortable but usually does not pose any unusual difficulties. These symptoms can be markedly aggravated with minor upper respiratory infections and in pregnancy-induced hypertension. The swelling can lead to inflammation (noninfective in nature) causing changes in the voice, making nose breathing difficult, and increasing the incidence of nosebleeds. The swelling can increase the hazard of intubation, if necessary. Abrasions and lacerations of the mucosa may occur, and bleeding may ensue.[42]

Patients need to be warned of these changes and advised not to use over-the-counter drugs to relieve symptoms or reduce the swelling to make breathing easier. Moisture can be delivered to the nares with the use of a normal saline spray, however, and may reduce some of the discomfort experienced.

Respiratory Infection

The altered cell-mediated immunity in the pregnant woman may place her at risk for upper respiratory infections (see Chapter 10). These changes along with hypererythema and edema can not only make having an upper respiratory infection more uncomfortable but also potentiate its movement into the lungs. Hyperventilation is accentuated, and the woman may become more aware of dyspnea. The combination of these factors can lead to a decreased ability to maintain usual activity levels.

Nurses should discourage the client with an upper respiratory infection from self-medication or using over-the-counter drugs. Initial treatments include rest, adequate hydration, and good nutrition. If symptoms persist or dyspnea increases, evaluation and pharmacologic treatment may be needed.

Infections associated with lung involvement could potentially increase airway resistance, thereby increasing the work of breathing, and lead to decreased V_T and RV. This may lead to decreased PaO_2 levels possibly leading to fetal hypoxemia.

Although difficult to accomplish for some women, avoidance of those situations in which infections might be contracted and avoidance of individuals carrying infections is a good practice. Most upper respiratory infections are an annoyance but do not lead to significant consequences for mother or fetus.

Exercise

The impact of exercise on the respiratory system is related to alveolar ventilation and is dependent upon the age, body weight, body composition and physical condition of the individual. Cardiovascular function, uterine blood flow, respiratory function, blood gases, aerobic capacity, metabolism, temperature, and psychological state are all affected by exercise (see Chapter 6). Maternal respiratory function, aerobic capacity, oxygen consumption, and blood gases are considered here along with fetal blood gases, activity, and breathing movements.[348]

Maternal Respiration and Blood Gases

Studies of respiratory rates with exercise in pregnant and nonpregnant women demonstrate that respiratory rates in pregnant women are higher than those in nonpregnant women during mild exercise, but this difference disappears during moderate exercise. Tidal volume and minute volume remain higher in pregnant subjects during all levels of exercise, however.[11, 165, 209]

The efficiency of gas exchange does not seem to be impaired in the pregnant woman during exercise. In sheep (in which temperature correction has occurred) blood gas values remain stable during short-term exercise. During prolonged exercise, however, PaO_2 increases and $PaCO_2$ decreases. This decrease in $PaCO_2$ is most likely due to the effects of progesterone on the respiratory center, which persist during moderate exercise.[76, 230, 231]

Oxygen Consumption

Oxygen consumption (VO_2) increases during exercise. In pregnancy, oxygen consumption also increases with advancing gestational age. Part of this increase is due to the increased work of carrying the extra weight associated with pregnancy.[8, 345]

Non–weight bearing exercise seems to result in little or no increased energy cost (difference between resting and exercising VO_2) during pregnancy, with a slight increase occurring during late gestation. These same findings hold true in weight bearing exercise, with some investigators finding no change in oxygen consumption during treadmill exercise, whereas others reported an increase. Artal and associates noted no change during mild to moderate activity patterns, but during strenuous exercise they documented an actual decrease in oxygen consumption.[11] These investigators speculated this change was either the result of decreased fuel availability or a protective mechanism on the mother's part to prevent hypoxia. Obviously, further research is needed to clarify these issues.[11, 165, 209, 345]

Aerobic Capacity

Aerobic capacity (the measure of an individual's ability to perform exercise) is dependent upon the intake, circulation, and utilization of oxygen. Aerobic capacity is also known as maximum oxygen consumption (VO_2max) and is the maximum oxygen volume that can be extracted from the air during exercise. Alexander noted that aerobic capacity is influenced by age, sex, heredity, hemoglobin content, inactivity (or conversely exercise), and disease.[8] He also reported that aerobic capacity can be increased by as much as 33% with exercise conditioning.[8, 348]

Studies have demonstrated that VO_2max did not increase significantly in sedentary pregnant animals. Collings and coworkers noted an actual decline in VO_2max in nonexercising pregnant women.[79] The same study documented an increase in VO_2max in women starting an exercise program during their second trimester. Other studies have demonstrated an increase in work rate with a concomitant decrease in VO_2max when exercise was instituted during pregnancy; for nonexercising women work rate and VO_2max decreased. This suggests that overall fitness was maintained during pregnancy with ex-

ercise, whereas not exercising led to a decline in fitness levels.[79, 314, 364]

Changes in VO_2max over the trimesters have been discussed in one study that discovered a decrease in VO_2max regardless of exercise patterns (including nonexercise). The decline in aereobic capacity was progressive over the trimesters even though the fit group maintained a higher VO_2max in the first and second trimesters, as well as postpartally. Whether these changes reflect a decrease in activity during the course of the pregnancy or the effect of pregnancy itself is unclear and requires further exploration. It does appear that maintaining a moderate level of exercise throughout pregnancy can be recommended, beginning slowly for nonexercising women.[314, 348]

Fetal Blood Gases

In the fetus, PaO_2 and $PaCO_2$ tensions decrease with the intensity and duration of exercise. These are not significantly different from control groups, unless exercise was prolonged and exhaustive. In sheep, one study reported a progressive decline in PaO_2 with exercise. Statistical significance was not achieved until after 30 minutes of exercise, and these levels remained stable over the next 15 minutes. A return to baseline was achieved by 30 minutes after completion of the exercise activity.[230, 244]

Although fetal PaO_2 does provide information about fetal status, it is not a good indicator of fetal oxygen consumption or whether tissue requirements are being met. In this light, changes in PaO_2 without further indications of hypoxia may be indicative of adjustments in the oxygen-hemoglobin dissociation curve.[231]

Fetal Activity and Breathing Movements

The effect of maternal exercise patterns on the fetus has not been explored extensively, and results of current research are variable. Under various conditions, fetal breathing movements have been found to be unchanged, to have increased irregularity, or to have decreased apnea and periodic breathing episodes. Fetal activity response to exercise has also been reported as variable.[75, 199, 244, 282]

Asthma

Asthma is an obstructive disease characterized by increased airway resistance, decreased expiratory flow rates, and hyperinflation with premature airway closure. There is some loss of lung compliance. These factors lead to an increase in the work of breathing. Along with this, hyperinflation and exaggerated negative pleural pressures can lead to increased demands on the right ventricle. This can be seen as a rise in pulmonary arterial pressure. These factors decrease left stroke volume, arterial systolic pressure, and pulse pressure.[51]

The restrictive processes in asthma are usually reversible and are due to an increased responsivity of the airways to a variety of stimuli. When stimulated, the characteristic responses include contraction of the bronchial smooth muscle, mucous hypersecretion, and mucosal edema. The mechanism for this responsiveness is unclear and may be different from patient to patient.[352]

Several mechanisms have been implicated in the etiology of the disease. These include an immunologic response, blocked β-adrenergic function, β-adrenergic amine deficiency, cholinergic dominance, intrinsic smooth muscle defect, and some combination of two or more of these. Other possibilities include an imbalance in cyclic nucleotides. Cyclic adenosine monophosphate (cAMP) and cyclic guanosine monophosphate (cGMP) are involved in the modulation of airway tone, the former contributing to bronchodilation and the latter to bronchoconstriction.[354]

Asthma may improve, worsen, or remain unchanged during pregnancy (Table 7–4). Trying to predict an individual's course during pregnancy is extremely difficult. Women with more severe asthma before pregnancy are more likely to have severe asthma during pregnancy, although this is not always the case and therefore is not a reliable indicator.

TABLE 7–4
Effect of Pregnancy on Asthma

May improve, worsen, or remain unchanged during pregnancy

Often similar to prepregnancy course, especially in severe asthmatics

Tends to worsen between the 28th and 36th weeks

Highest risk for exacerbation is after 16 weeks' gestation

Tends to improve during the last 4 weeks

During labor and delivery, severe asthma is rare

Delivery tends to improve maternal status

Often reverts back to prepregnancy course within 3 months post partum

Generally similar from pregnancy to pregnancy

Taken from references 93 (p. 120), 188, and 150.

In certain women, changes in IgE levels may be helpful in predicting improvement as well as deterioration during pregnancy; however, current research is not conclusive. Close monitoring, good education, and consistent therapy remain essential to maternal-fetal well-being.[150, 309, 365]

Statistically, asthma complicates approximately 1% of all pregnancies, which is equivalent to the percentage of women experiencing cardiovascular disease but greater than the incidence of most other medical diseases encountered in pregnant women. Of those women afflicted, 10 to 15% require hospitalization for status asthmaticus or recurrent episodes of asthma. Uncontrolled asthma during pregnancy can result in maternal and fetal morbidity and mortality.[102, 156, 188, 307, 324]

Retrospective studies have suggested asthmatics risk serious adverse effects during pregnancy, including hyperemesis, hemorrhage, toxemia, premature delivery, and even death. Fetal risks include prematurity or low birth weight. A more recent study, however, demonstrated no change in perinatal mortality when asthma was methodically managed, although preeclampsia and neonatal hypoglycemia occurred more frequently.[29, 156, 324, 325]

Asthma may lead to maternal hypoxia or hyperventilation with resultant hypocapnia and alkalosis, potentially affecting fetal well-being. Wulf and colleagues demonstrated that maternal hypoxia (PaO_2, 65 mmHg) just prior to delivery led to decreased fetal PaO_2 (26 mmHg) but did not compromise infants (as reflected in normal pH values and Apgar scores).[368] Transient hypoxia, therefore, is not as great a concern as chronic hypoxia, in which prematurity, small for gestational age, and mortality rates are all increased.[93, 308, 368]

The hypocapnia and alkalosis, however, can contribute to fetal depression by reducing umbilical and uterine blood flow secondary to vasoconstriction. Alkalosis also increases maternal hemoglobin affinity for oxygen, thereby reducing availability to the fetus.[93, 223]

The normal alterations of the respiratory system during pregnancy may influence asthma in both positive and negative ways. The increase in circulating cortisol levels may augment cAMP functioning as well as reduce inflammation through steroid action. Progesterone levels decrease bronchomotor tone, relaxing smooth muscle tissue, and thereby decrease airway resistance. Elevated serum cAMP levels may also promote bronchodilation (Table 7–5).

Pharmacologic treatment and the selection of an appropriate agent are based on the risk-to-benefit ratio of bronchodilator effect and hypoxia avoidance versus possible teratogenic consequences. General management includes careful history taking and medical evaluation, patient education, avoidance of known precipitants, and medical therapy. The nurse's role includes assessment and evaluation of the patient status. Education about the medical regimen and recognition of early symptoms so that treatment may be initiated early and hypoxia prevented are essential. Patients need to be told to use only those medications prescribed and to avoid over-the-counter medications. Prescribed medications should be taken only as directed; maternal and fetal side effects need to be explained clearly and concisely.[51, 188]

Smoking

Although there continues to be much controversy regarding the consequences for the fetus of cigarette smoking and studies are inconclusive about its impact, there is general consensus regarding some areas. Smoking

---

TABLE 7–5
Factors Affecting Asthma in Pregnancy

IMPROVE
Increased progesterone-mediated bronchodilation
β-Adrenergic–stimulated bronchodilation
Decreased plasma histamine levels
Increased free cortisol levels
Increased glucocorticoid-mediated β-adrenergic responsiveness
Increased PGE-mediated bronchodilation
PGI$_2$-mediated bronchial stabilization
Increased half-life of bronchodilators
Decreased protein-binding of bronchodilators

WORSEN
Pulmonary refractoriness to cortisol effects
Increased PGF$_{2\alpha}$-mediated bronchoconstriction
Decreased FRC, causing airway closure and altered $\dot{V}/\dot{Q}$ ratios
Increased incidence of viral or bacterial respiratory infection
Increased gastroesophageal reflux
Increased stress

Data from Schatz, M. & Hoffman, C. (1987). Interrelationships between asthma and pregnancy: Clinical and mechanistic considerations. *Clin Rev Allergy, 5*, 301.

---

may interfere with a woman's ability to conceive, which may need to be addressed if fertility problems are present. Additional risks for the mother include a spontaneous abortion rate two times greater than in the nonsmoking population, an increased risk of abruption, placenta previa, early or late bleeding, premature rupture of membranes and prolonged rupture of membranes, and preterm labor. These are relatively significant consequences, and mothers who smoke need to be informed of the possibilities and that the effects of cigarette smoking are also dose related. The risk of preeclampsia to the mother is decreased with cigarette smoking; however, if it does occur, the risk of perinatal mortality is greatly increased.[1, 313, 315]

Abel provided an excellent review of the studies conducted on fetal consequences of maternal smoking, and the reader is referred to this source for further information.[1] His conclusions include an increased risk of intrauterine growth retardation, low birth weight, and slower growth rates (although the difference is very small) for infants of smokers. There is a twofold increase in deaths related to sudden infant death syndrome, and the incidence of respiratory disorders is higher owing to an impairment of the immunologic system. An increased risk of malformations has been reported, although there is some controversy as to what kind of malformations are seen most frequently. Lastly, children of smokers may have some behavioral difficulties and learning problems.[1]

Placentas of smokers are proportionately greater in weight (as related to fetal weight) than are placentas of nonsmokers. This is thought to be evidence that smoking results in hypoxia and that compensatory hypertrophy occurs. In order to maintain the efficiency of oxygen transfer that is needed for the well-being of the fetus, the diffusing distance in the placenta is decreased, whereas the surface area and vascularity increase. In this way the fetus is assured of an adequate oxygen supply. Women who experience chronic anemia or live at high altitudes have similar compensatory mechanisms because of the chronic intrauterine hypoxia.[74, 365]

The placentas of smokers have more areas of calcification, an increased incidence of fibrin deposits, and an increased frequency of necrosis and inflammation in the margin. In addition, an increased risk of placental lesions has also been identified. These findings suggest that smoking causes some direct damage to the blood vessels of the placenta that may lead to placental underperfusion.[1, 74, 268]

If the alterations seen in the placenta are due to a decrease in uterine blood flow, the fetal consequences may be acidosis and hypoxemia. Since diffusion of oxygen to the fetus is blood flow dependent, a decrease in flow could lead to hypoxia; therefore, heavy smoking may subject the fetus to frequent periods of hypoxia that may have a cumulative effect on development.[1] This decrease in uterine blood flow may be mediated through the release of catecholamines from the adrenals when exposed to nicotine.

An increased maternal heart rate and an elevation of blood pressure are clinical indications of catecholamine release. The catecholamines trigger peripheral vasoconstriction, which leads to a decrease in perfusion of the uteroplacental vasculature (underperfusion). Chronic underperfusion leads to fibrin deposition in arteries, inflammation and necrosis of tissue, and the development of lesions and calcifications. The perimeter of the placenta would be affected first since perfusion is lower in these regions. The reduction of blood flow brought about by these defects could impact on the placenta such that it would not be able to sustain itself, leading to an increased incidence of abruption. The overall impact of these changes would be a reduction in placental blood flow, leading to a decrease in available oxygen to the fetus and hypoxia.[1, 323, 339]

The risk of hypoxia is further increased by carbon monoxide, a by-product of smoking. Since carbon monoxide has a higher affinity for hemoglobin than does oxygen, the oxygen-carrying capacity of the blood in smokers is reduced. These effects have been demonstrated by highly elevated levels of carboxyhemoglobin in the fetus at birth.[167] Along with this, carbon monoxide greatly increases the affinity of oxygen for hemoglobin. With increased affinity oxygen is less readily unloaded to the fetal tissues.[1] This, in turn, reduces fetal oxygenation further.

One of the indicators of fetal hypoxia is decreased fetal breathing movements (FBM). Observations have demonstrated that there is a significant increase in fetal apnea after smoking. These effects are sustained, lasting up to as long as 90 minutes post inhalation.[1]

Controversy regarding these observations currently exists, because improved equipment and techniques have found that FBM are not consistently affected by maternal smoking. It has been suggested that the fetal apnea is due to smoking-induced hypoxia. This is supported by data that indicate that FBM are decreased with hypoxia unrelated to smoking.[167]

Other fetal behavior changes that have been associated with cigarette smoking are changes in fetal heart rate (FHR) and fetal movements.[1, 167] Fetal tachycardia has long been believed to occur with maternal smoking. More recent studies have indicated that FHR does not change during or after smoke inhalation; however, beat-to-beat variability is reduced, as is the number of accelerations.[155] A reduction in fetal movements[333] and an increase in the number of epochs without fetal movement have also been reported.[116] Continued research into these effects is important in determining potential outcomes.

Following delivery the neonate may continue to be exposed to the effects of nicotine through breast milk. Once again, concentrations are related to cigarette consumption but can be detected in breast milk up to 8 hours after smoking. Depending on the concentration infants may experience a toxic reaction to the nicotine (vomiting, diarrhea, insomnia, elevated heart rate), or once breast feeding is discontinued, withdrawal behavior may be noted.[1]

Inhalation Anesthesia

The use of inhalation anesthesia in obstetrics usually occurs during an emergency situation. The effect on the maternal respiratory system is related to maternal cardiorespiratory status prior to induction and the type and adequacy of ventilation following induction. Owing to the reduced functional residual capacity and increased closing volumes[330] as well as the higher metabolic requirements,[10] the pregnant woman is less tolerant of apnea or a difficult or failed intubation. Oxygen partial pressure levels drop rapidly in these situations leading to hypoxia, hypoxemia, and acidosis. These events not only place the mother at risk, but also jeopardize the status of the fetus. Light to moderate anesthesia with adequate oxygen mixing should provide no difficulties to the well-hydrated, stable pregnant woman.[41]

Use of anesthesia can place the fetus at risk for depression and asphyxia. Fetal metabolic acidosis may be encountered following the administration of certain intravenous agents used for induction. If depression does occur, it is an indication of impaired placental blood flow, possibly owing to decreased maternal cardiac output.[41, 187, 263] Most of the time no serious depression occurs.

Light anesthesia has been found to lead to progressive fetal metabolic acidosis in animals.[187, 277] This is felt to be due to an increased catecholamine output by the maternal adrenals, leading to uterine vascular constriction. This results in a decreased nutrient flow to the fetus.

Inhalation agents are dose- and time-dependent compounds[85] affecting the fetus directly through transplacental crossing of drugs or indirectly by altering maternal homeostasis or changing uteroplacental blood flow. Uteroplacental blood flow may be altered through several mechanisms: (1) change in perfusion pressure, (2) modification of vascular resistance, (3) alterations in uterine contractions and basal tone, and (4) interference in fetal cardiovascular function (umbilical circulation). Uterine blood flow varies directly with perfusion pressure across the uterine vascular bed (uterine arterial pressure minus uterine venous pressure) and inversely with uterine vascular resistance. The balance between perfusion pressure and vascular resistance is the primary basis for acute changes in uterine blood flow.[87]

Adverse responses or heavy anesthesia can precipitate a hazardous sequence of events. Maternal cardiac output may fall, precipitating a fall in blood pressure and an increased likelihood of maternal acidosis and decreased uterine blood flow. The result is a decreased uteroplacental blood flow with decreased nutrient supply to the fetus. Fetal heart rate and blood pressure may fall owing to direct fetal cardiovascular depression (drug response) or the indirect effect of decreased uteroplacental perfusion. The decreased cardiac output and low blood pressure culminate in fetal hypoxia and acidosis, as reflected in low oxygen saturations, elevated PCO_2 levels, and falling base excess. Fetal status prior to induction affects the severity of the response.[87, 187]

This same sequence of events may occur with severe maternal hyperventilation, which may be the result of psychoprophylaxis, maternal response to the pain of labor, or high inflation pressures with IPPV. Maternal PCO_2 values of 17 mmHg or less (average PCO_2 in pregnancy is 30 to 31 mmHg) can directly reduce uteroplacental blood flow through vasoconstriction. This vasoconstriction along with the decreased maternal cardiac output can result in fetal hypoxemia and acidosis.[263]

Induction time in conjunction with time to placental separation may influence fetal outcome and neonatal response. Prolonged induction to delivery time allows accumulation of the anesthetic agent within the fetus. This may result in progressive depression, culminating in asphyxia. Caval occlusion may also contribute to these events (see Chapter 6).[263] A left lateral tilt surgical table can reduce the possibility of caval occlusion.

Awareness of the potential effects of anesthesia, especially when combined with a compromised mother or fetus (the usual case in an emergency), allows for anticipatory preparation as well as appropriate assessment and intervention. Stability of maternal cardiac and respiratory systems is essential to the health and well-being of the fetus and will improve neonatal outcome.

SUMMARY

The maternal respiratory alterations that occur during pregnancy ensure an adequate supply of oxygen to the developing fetus and its supporting structures. These demands are increased with activity and labor and are usually compensated for without difficulty. However, subjective interpretation of labor and the pain experienced can trigger maternal hyperventilation and place the fetus in jeopardy. Adequate education of the mother about the normal physiologic changes and the labor experience is essential to maternal-fetal well-being. Psychoprophylaxis, analgesia, and anesthesia can moderate the experience and can be used safely during the intrapartum period. Careful monitoring with all these methods is important to safeguard the fetus from deleterious effects. Clinical implications for the pregnant woman and her fetus are summarized in Table 7–6.

DEVELOPMENT OF THE RESPIRATORY SYSTEM IN THE FETUS

An overview of the embryonic development of the lung and the role of lung fluid and

TABLE 7–6
Summary of Clinical Implications for the Respiratory System: Pregnant Woman and Fetus

Understand the normal respiratory changes that occur during pregnancy (pp. 263–270).

Explain to the pregnant woman the changes that can occur in the respiratory system early in pregnancy and how they can impact on daily activities and exercise tolerance (pp. 263–267).

Encourage prelabor preparation in order to reduce discomfort, hyperventilation, and anxiety and promote a positive attitude about labor (pp. 267–269).

Reduce hyperventilation during labor by counting respirations slowly, discouraging breath holding, and encouraging deep breathing between contractions (pp. 267–269).

Discuss upper airway changes that may lead to nasal congestion (pp. 270–271).

Discourage the use of any over-the-counter medications (pp. 270–271).

Discuss usual exercise routines and changes that may be necessary owing to reduced tolerance and increased dyspnea (pp. 271–272).

Counsel asthmatic women who are pregnant to follow their medical regimen as directed, to avoid known precipitating factors, and seek medical intervention when symptoms persist (pp. 272–274).

Encourage and support pregnant women in reducing or eliminating cigarette consumption both during and after pregnancy (pp. 274–275).

Page numbers in parentheses following each intervention refer to pages where rationale for intervention is discussed.

fetal breathing movements in that development, as well as surfactant synthesis and secretion, sets the stage for understanding the changes that occur within the fetal respiratory system. First breath events and the concomitant changes in pulmonary perfusion are also presented, along with a discussion of lung physiology. The application of these principles is discussed in the section on Clinical Implications for Neonatal Care, which explores frequently encountered disease processes and the needs of the neonate during resuscitation.

Anatomic Development

Prenatal lung growth occurs in four stages: embryonic stage, pseudoglandular stage, canalicular stage, and terminal air sac stage. The embryonic stage begins with conception and ends with the 5th week of gestation. At around day 24 a ventral diverticulum (outpouching) can be seen developing from the foregut. This groove extends downward and is gradually separated from the future esophagus by a septum. Between 2 and 4 days later the first dichotomous branches can be seen. At the end of this stage, three divisions are evident on the right and two on the left (lobar and segmental bronchi).[46, 237]

Between 5 and 17 weeks' gestation a tree of narrow tubules forms. New airway branches arise through a combination of cell multiplication and necrosis.[1] These tubules have thick epithelial walls made of columnar or cuboidal cells. This morphologic structure along with the loose mesenchymal tissue surrounding the tree give the lungs a glandular appearance, hence the term pseudoglandular stage.[46, 237]

By 16 weeks, branching of the conducting portion of the tracheobronchial tree is established. These preacinar airways can from this point forward increase only in length and diameter, not in number.[56, 115, 237]

The mesenchymal tissue surrounding the airways holds an inductive capacity for the branching that occurs. Removal of this tissue interrupts epithelial branching until regeneration occurs.[15, 34] This mesenchyme is of two types. The cellular type surrounds the endodermal tree and contributes to the nonepithelial elements of the tree. Less cellular tissue fills the remainder of the space and develop into the pleura, subpleural connective tissue, intralobular septa, and cartilage of the bronchi.[15] It is toward the end of the pseudoglandular period that the rudimentary forms of cartilage, connective tissue, muscle, blood vessels, and lymphatics can be identified.[63, 195, 237]

The epithelial cells of the distal air spaces (future alveolar lining) flatten some time between weeks 13 and 25, signaling the beginning of the canalicular stage.[356] A rich vascular supply begins to proliferate, and with the changes in mesenchymal tissue the capillaries are brought closer to the airway epithelium. Primitive respiratory bronchioles begin to form during this stage, delineating the acinus (gas exchanging section of the lung) from the conducting portion of the lung.

This development continues until 24 weeks' gestation. At that time, terminal air sacs appear as outpouchings of the terminal bronchioles. As the weeks progress, the number of terminal sacs increases, forming multiple pouches off a common chamber (the alveolar duct). The surface epithelium thins considerably as vascular proliferation increases. As the vessels develop, they stretch and thin the epithelium that covers them even more, bringing the capillaries into proximity with the developing airways.[14, 94, 181]

Eventually this leads to fusion of the basement membrane between the endothelium and the epithelium, thus creating the future blood-gas barrier.[292] At term shallow indentations in the saccule walls can be detected. These are primitive alveoli and will deepen and multiply postnatally.[94]

Lung structures and cells are differentiated to the point that life can be supported at between 26 and 28 weeks. Although the normal number of air spaces has not developed, the epithelium has thinned enough and the vascular bed has proliferated to the point that oxygen exchange can occur. The 28-week lung, however, is markedly different than that of the term neonate, just as the term infant's lung is different from that of the child or adult.

The respiratory portion of the lung has a continuous epithelial lining mainly composed of two cell types, type I and type II pneumocytes. The type I pneumocyte (squamous pneumocyte) covers approximately 95% of the alveolar surface with its long cytoplasmic extensions.[53, 62, 169, 255] The thinnest area of the alveolus is composed of these extensions, and it is here that gas exchange occurs most rapidly.

The type II pneumocytes (granular pneumocyte), although more numerous than type I, occupy less than 5% of the alveolar surface.[53, 169] These cells are more cuboidal in shape and contain more organelles than does type I. Mitochondria are larger, and the Golgi apparatus, rough endoplasmic reticulum, ribosomes, and multivesicular bodies are more extensive.[255] Osmiophilic, lamellated bodies are characteristic of these cells. It is here that surfactant is thought to be produced and secreted.

The first type II cells are seen during the terminal sac stage, between 20 and 24 weeks' gestation. Once they appear, the number of cells increase with a concomitant increase in the number of lamellar bodies within the cells. The organelles migrate toward the luminal plasma membrane (alveolar duct surface), which form prominent microvilli extending into the alveolar duct toward the end of gestation.[169] It is along this border that surfactant secretion occurs.

Surfactant secretion is detectable between 25 and 30 weeks' gestation, although the potential for alveolar stability does not occur until later, between 33 and 36 weeks.[24, 196, 204, 336] Along with surfactant production and

secretion type II pneumocytes appear to be the chief cells involved in the repair of the alveolar epithelium. This suggests that type I cells are more susceptible to injury and differentiate from type II pneumocytes (possibly after mitosis). Meyrick and Reid have suggested that either cell type may transform into the other, depending on the needs of the lung.[255] This is an area that needs further exploration.

Pulmonary Vasculature

Pulmonary vessel development occurs in conjunction with the branching of the bronchial tree.[171, 182, 292] The arteries have more branches than the airways; the veins develop more tributaries. The preacinar region has an arterial branch that runs along each conducting airway (termed conventional artery); supernumerary arteries feed the adjacent alveoli. All the preacinar arteries are present by 16 weeks' gestation. If for any reason there is a decrease in the number of airways, there is a concomitant decrease in conventional and supernumerary arteries.[171, 292] From 16 weeks on, the preacinar vessels increase in length and diameter only.[195]

With movement into the canalicular and terminal air sac stages, intra-acinar arteries appear and continue their development through the postnatal period.[171, 182, 195] The conventional arteries continue their development for the first 18 months of life,[113, 115, 292] and the supernumerary arteries continue to be laid down for the first 8 years.[115, 182, 292] These latter vessels are smaller and more numerous, servicing the alveoli directly.[195] If blood flow is reduced or blocked through the conventional arteries, the supernumerary arteries may serve as collateral circulation, thereby maintaining lung function during periods of ischemia or increased pulmonary vascular resistance.[336] Postnatally, the intra-acinar vessels multiply rapidly as alveoli appear.[111, 195]

The pulmonary veins develop more slowly. By 20 weeks pre-acinar veins are present, however.[182] The development of the veins parallels that of the arteries and conducting airways, although supernumerary veins outnumber supernumerary arteries. Both types of veins (supernumerary and conventional) appear simultaneously.[195] Formation of additional veins as well as lengthening of existing veins continues postnatally.

Further development of the pulmonary

circulation is related to the changes in muscle wall thickness and extension of muscle into arterial walls. Because of the low intrauterine oxygen tension, the pulmonary artery wall is very thick. The wall thins as oxygen tension rises at birth. This is caused by the medial layer elastic fibrils becoming less organized. The pulmonary vein, in contrast, is found to be deficient in elastic fibers at birth and progressively incorporates muscle and elastic tissue over the first 2 years of life.[11, 115, 182]

The intrapulmonary arteries have thick walls as well. The smaller arteries have increased muscularity[171] and dilate actively with the postnatal increase in oxygen tension. There is a concomitant fall in pulmonary vascular resistance.[195] Between 3 and 28 days postnatally these vessels achieve their adult wall thickness–to–external diameter ratio; the larger arteries take longer achieving adult levels (4 to 18 months).[111, 182]

The arteries of the fetus are more muscular than those of the adult or child. Muscle thickness–to–external diameter ratio decreases postnatally based on postnatal age and the size of the vessel.[195] After delivery muscle distribution changes, and this process continues over the first 19 years of life. Prenatally, muscle development can be seen in the arteries of the terminal bronchioles; by 4 months postnatal age the arteries of the respiratory bronchioles have incorporated muscle tissue. From 10 months to 11 years the arteries grow and enlarge; the small arteries are mostly nonmuscular or minimally muscular during this time. At the end of this growth period, the muscular arteries have reached the level of the alveolar duct, Here the vessels are 130 μ in diameter. Between 11 years and maturation, which occurs around 19 years of age, muscle extension continues, reaching the alveolus and the vessels 75 μ in diameter.[111, 115, 182] Intrapulmonary veins, on the other hand, are thinner than their counterparts, and muscle extension does not spread as far peripherally.[306] Once this is achieved, the system is considered mature.

Controversy regarding the development and differentiation of lung tissue as well as lung function is evident when reading various sources. Although knowledge regarding lung function has increased tremendously over the past several decades, there continues to be much to learn. Some of these discrepancies are highlighted as the functional development of the lung is discussed.

Functional Development

The functional development of the lung revolves around the biochemistry of surfactant. However, the lung does secrete other substances and has its own particular macrophage function.

Macrophages are found in groups of three or four cells lying free within the alveolar space. Ingested foreign bodies are seen as osmiophilic inclusions within the cell. These cells are spherical in shape and are derived from hematopoietic tissue.[255]

Larger particles not swept away by ciliary action (e.g., bacteria) are thought to be removed and destroyed by pulmonary macrophages. Foreign material, once identified, is engulfed and destroyed by the macrophage. These cells are critical for maintaining the sterility of the lung environment and removing surfactant from the alveolar surface.

Surfactant is of major importance to the adequate functioning of the lung. Pulmonary surfactant is a lipoprotein with 90% of its dry weight composed of lipid (Fig. 7–2).[169] The majority of the lipid is saturated phosphatidylcholine (PC), of which dipalmitoyl phosphatidylcholine (DPPC) is the most abundant (Fig. 7–3). The latter is the component responsible for decreasing the surface tension to almost zero when compressed at the surface during inspiration. Phosphatidylglycerol (PG) accounts for another 8% of the phospholipids present in surfactant. This is a substantial quantity and is unique to lung cells, bronchoalveolar fluid, and amniotic fluid. This makes PG a good marker for surfactant. The rest of the compound is involved in intracellular transport, storage, exocytosis, adsorption, and clearance at the alveolar lining.[37, 52, 169, 198]

The biosynthesis of surfactant entails a series of events including glycerophospholipid production, apoprotein synthesis, glycosylation and surfactant apoprotein processing, integration of surfactant component parts, and transport of components from synthesis sites to integration sites. The components of surfactant are generally thought to be synthesized in the membranes of the rough and smooth endoplasmic reticulum, although the mitochondria have been suggested as an alternative production site. Assembly of the components is not well understood but may occur in the multivesicular bodies intracellularly. Once assembled, surfactant is transported intracellularly to the

Golgi apparatus and then on to the lamellar bodies. It is in the latter structure that transformation occurs, although controversy regarding this exists. Others suggest that transformation occurs outside the pneumocyte during the process of adsorption. This structural change enhances spreadability and adsorption. Once it is synthesized and transformed, surfactant storage is a function of the lamellar body. Secretion occurs by exocytosis; the outer membrane of the lamellar bodies fuses to the cell membrane, and the extrusion of the contents into the aqueous film overlying the alveolar epithelium occurs. The surfactant must migrate to the surface of the liquid layer in order to be physiologically functional. This migration is considered part of the adsorption process.[37, 169, 198, 319]

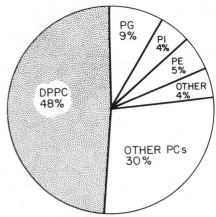

FIGURE 7–3. The glycerophospholipid composition of a typical mammalian lung surfactant. PC, phosphatidylcholine; DPPC, dipalmitoyl phosphatidylcholine; PG, phosphatidylglycerol; PI, phosphatidylinositol; PE, phosphatidylethanolamine. (From Bleasdale, J. E. & Johnston, J. M. (1985). Developmental biochemistry of lung surfactant. In G. H. Nelson (Ed.), *Pulmonary development* (p. 48). New York: Marcel Dekker.)

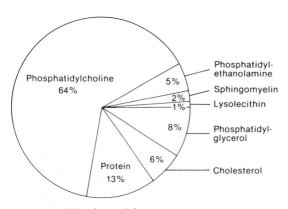

% Composition by Weight

Phospholipids	85
Saturated phosphatidylcholine	60
Unsaturated phosphatidylcholine	20
Phosphatidylglycerol	8
Phosphatidylinositol	2
Phosphatidylethanolamine	5
Sphingomyelin	2
Others	3
Neutral lipids and cholesterol	5
Proteins	10
Contaminating serum proteins	8
Surfactant Protein 35 (32–36,000 daltons)	~1
Lipophilic proteins (6–12,000 daltons)	~1

FIGURE 7–2. Composition of pulmonary surfactant. (From Farrell, P. M. & Ulane, R. E. (1981). The regulation of lung phospholipid metabolism. In A. Minkowski & M. Monset-Couchard (Eds.), *Physiological and biochemical basis for perinatal medicine* (p. 31). New York: S Karger; and Jobe, A. (1987). Questions about surfactant for respiratory distress syndrome (RDS). In *Respiratory distress syndrome and surfactant.* Mead Johnson Symposium on Perinatal and Developmental Medicine, No. 30 (p. 43). Evansville, IN: Mead Johnson.)

Two unique proteins have been identified in the surfactant structure. One of the proteins has an affinity for phospholipids, especially PG, and is thought to improve its functioning. PG improves the adsorption of DPPC, as does phosphatidylinositol (PI). The combination of PG and protein has an additive effect on DPPC. Therefore, the presence of component parts is not enough; it is the way in which they are transformed by each other that maximizes lung functioning.

PC and PG are composed of a three-carbon glycerol backbone with fatty acids esterified to the hydroxyl groups. The asymmetric arrangement of these molecules results in a hydrocarbon-rich fatty acid tail, which is nonpolar, and a phosphodiester region, which is polar. This allows for a monolayer film to be established at the air-liquid interface within the alveoli.[169, 319]

There are two pathways for phosphatidylcholine synthesis (Fig. 7–4). Key precursors for PC synthesis include glycerol, fatty acids, choline, glucose, and ethanolamine. The major pathway is the cytidine diphosphate (CDP) choline system, which provides the maturity necessary for alveolar structural integrity and stability. The other pathway leads to phosphatidylethanolamine (PE) formation and is termed the methyltransferase system. This has minor significance in the adult lung and seems to play a relatively insignificant

FIGURE 7–4. Major pathways for phosphatidylcholine synthesis. (From Farrell, P. M. & Ulane, R. E. (1981). The regulation of lung phospholipid metabolism. In A. Minkowski & M. Monset-Couchard (Eds.), *Physiological and biochemical basis for perinatal medicine* (p. 32). New York: S Karger.)

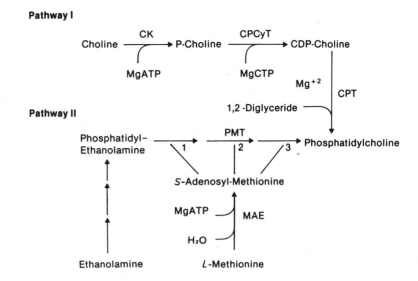

role in fetal lung development. This may be because choline is incorporated more effectively into PC than is methionine. It has been suggested that the ability of the human fetus to synthesize PC by N-methylation of PE early in gestation may contribute to survival with premature delivery. This suggests that further investigation is needed to evaluate the physiologic contribution of this pathway.[346]

Figure 7–5 depicts the biosynthesis of phosphatidylcholine, phosphatidylinositol, and phosphatidylglycerol and demonstrates the dependency of the system upon the biosynthesis of phosphatidic acid. The increased production of phospholipids seen in late gestation is dependent upon the increased synthesis of this acid. The majority of phospholipid produced is PC, and Figure 7–6 illustrates the biosynthesis and remodeling of this critical phospholipid.[37]

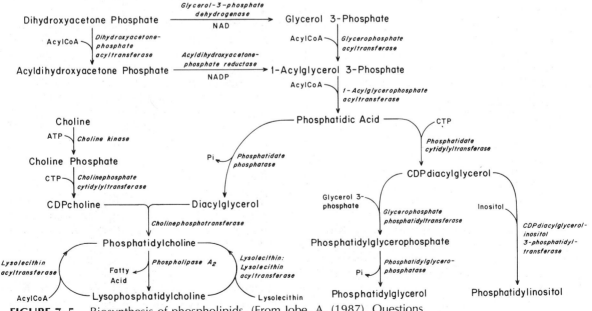

FIGURE 7–5. Biosynthesis of phospholipids. (From Jobe, A. (1987). Questions about surfactant for respiratory distress syndrome (RDS). In *Respiratory distress syndrome and surfactant.* Mead Johnson Symposium on Perinatal and Developmental Medicine, No. 30 (p. 13). Evansville, IN: Mead Johnson.)

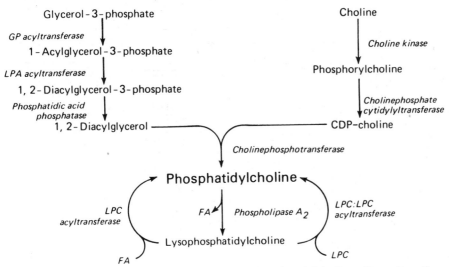

FIGURE 7–6. Biosynthesis and remodeling of phosphatidylcholine. (From Farrell, P. M. & Ulane, R. E. (1981). The regulation of lung phospholipid metabolism. In A. Minkowski & M. Monset-Couchard (Eds.), *Physiological and biochemical basis for perinatal medicine* (p. 33). New York: S Karger.)

Figure 7–6 also demonstrates the interaction of the choline pathway and the diglyceride synthesis mechanisms that yield increased PC synthesis in late gestation. Although this interaction yields increased quantities of PC, it is not the highly saturated version identified in the final surfactant compound. The remodeling of PC that occurs in the phosphatidylcholine-lysophosphatidylcholine cycle provides the DPPC required for surfactant.[51, 120]

As gestation advances, phospholipid content and saturation increase. This is accompanied by an increase in osmiophilic inclusion bodies within the type II pneumocytes. Choline incorporation, which is low in early gestation, has been noted to increase abruptly in rhesus monkeys when 90% of gestation is completed.[346] This suggests that pathway regulatory mechanisms are enhanced in order to meet postnatal needs. Figure 7–7 demonstrates the changes in glycerophospholipids in response to system maturation.

Enzymatic changes in the phospholipid synthesis pathway are discussed in several review articles.[37, 346] The correlation of these changes to the surge in saturated PC and increase in PG with concomitant decrease in PI (Fig. 7–7) is not yet understood. Whether this surge is due to a change in enzyme or substrate concentration, an adjustment in catalytic efficiency, a change in substrate affinity, or the activation of latent enzymes is not known and is currently being investigated.

In addition to enzymes, hormonal regulation of surfactant biosynthesis and secretion has been (and continues to be) investigated. Those hormones that have been implicated include glucocorticoids, adrenocorticotropic hormone, thyroid hormone, estrogens, prolactin, thyrotropin-releasing hormone, catecholamines, insulin, fibroblast pneumocyte factor, prostaglandins, and epidermal growth factor. Factors such as pregnancy-induced hypertension, intrauterine growth retardation, premature rupture of membranes, and other maternal-fetal events that lead to stress and increased fetal catecholamine and corticosteroid levels have been associated with accelerated lung maturity.

Glucocorticoids

Glucocorticoids are probably the best known of the hormones affecting surfactant. Liggins' observations in 1969 set off a flurry of research in the area of hormonal control of fetal lung development that has continued to the present.[226] Glucocorticoids such as betamethasone accelerate the normal pattern of fetal lung development by increasing the rate of glycogen depletion and glycerophospholipid biosynthesis. The depletion in glycogen leads to direct anatomic changes in alveolar

FIGURE 7–7. Changes in phospholipids across gestation. Lung profile defining the maturity of the fetal lung based on amniotic fluid analysis of phosphatidylcholine (lecithin)-to-sphingomyelin ratio *(upper panel),* the percentage of disaturated phosphatidylcholine using cold acetone precipitation, and the percentages of phosphatidylinositol and phosphatidylglycerol, respectively. Gestational age is the ordinate. Phosphatidylglycerol appears at 35 to 36 weeks and heralds lung maturity. (From Merritt, T. A. (1984). Respiratory distress. In M. Zidi, T. A. Clark, & T. A. Merritt (Eds.), *Assessment of the newborn: A guide for the practitioner* (p. 177). Boston: Little, Brown.)

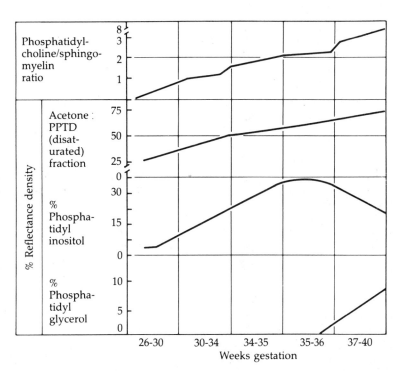

structures by thinning the interalveolar septa and increasing the size of the alveoli. Morphologic changes include an increase in the number of type II pneumocytes and an increase in the number of lamellar bodies within those cells. These changes occur in conjunction with functional maturation, leading to an accelerated synthesis of surfactant phospholipid.[21, 37, 122, 186, 205, 214, 226]

It is unclear how glucocorticoids influence surfactant synthesis. It is evident that glucocorticoid action is centered on synthesis rather than secretion and that it effects more than surfactant synthesis. Acting directly on lung tissue, the number of β-adrenergic receptors increases, and elastin and collagen production is enhanced, the latter improving lung compliance.[122, 171] What is not evident is whether glucocorticoids act independently or in conjunction with other compounds, or whether there is a direct effect on type II pneumocytes. Smith suggests that glucocorticoids may act upon fibroblasts by increasing the production of fibroblast pneumocyte factor, which then affects surfactant production.[317] Of course, there is the possibility that it is not strictly one or the other but some combination of these actions that occurs.[20, 50, 284, 299, 317, 358]

Thyroid Hormones

Thyroxine (T_4) and triiodothyronine (T_3) have also been shown to increase the rate of phospholipid synthesis.[20, 37, 153, 162] Thyroid hormones, like glucocorticoids, enhance production of phosphatidylcholine through choline incorporation. They do not, however, increase phosphatidylglycerol synthesis or stimulate the production of surfactant-specific proteins.[19, 214] Whereas glucocorticoids increase fatty acid synthetase activity, thyroid hormone seems to decrease its activity.[285] These differences suggest different sites of action for these hormones as well as the need for action in conjunction with other hormones.[214]

Low levels of T_3 and T_4 have been associated with respiratory distress syndrome, although the exact mechanisms are unclear.[21, 91, 346] Ballard and associates have shown that the effects of thyroid hormones are mediated by a specific thyroid receptor to which T_3 has a higher affinity and which is a more potent phospholipid synthesis stimulator.[18, 20]

Clinical application of this information is aimed at maximizing beneficial effects through the delivery of hormones or hormone-inducing or -activating substances without direct contact with the fetus. Naturally occurring thyroid hormones do not normally cross the placenta. However, thyrotropin-releasing hormone (TRH) does cross the placenta. It stimulates the fetal pituitary gland to produce thyroid-stimulating hormone (TSH), which leads to an increase in

PC production.[21, 298] The use of 3,5-dimethyl–3-isopropyl-L-thyronine (DIMIT), a synthetic thyroid analogue, produces similar results.[20, 21] Intra-amniotic injections of T_4 to accelerate lung maturation are also being investigated.

Continued investigation of the precise mechanisms of thyroid hormone action and the synergistic interaction between glucocorticoids and thyroid hormones is essential. This interaction occurs at the level of messenger RNA,[214] with significant increases in stimulation occurring when these agents are used together rather than individually and in a shorter period of time.[18, 153, 162] These findings may have significant clinical implications for future therapeutic interventions.

Insulin

One factor that appears to inhibit the development of surfactant can be seen in neonates born to diabetic mothers whose disease is not well controlled. Whether it is the hyperglycemia or the hyperinsulinemia, or both, is unclear, and research continues to provide conflicting results. Maturation of surfactant synthesis occurs at the same time that glycogen is depleted from the lungs and liver. Insulin inhibits glycogen breakdown, thereby decreasing the substrate available for PC synthesis as well as altering the natural anatomic changes that occur with glycogen depletion.[37, 214] Smith and colleagues found that the effect of cortisol on choline incorporation is reduced by insulin, even though its effects on cell growth were not.[318] Gross and coworkers documented no insulin influence and no antagonistic action on the usual dexamethasone response.[161] Mendelson and associates, in comparison, actually reported a synergistic effect when cortisol and insulin were combined.[250]

Recent in vivo studies have shown that hyperglycemia seems to be the cause, whereas tissue cultures implicate hyperinsulinemia.[144, 161, 318] The mechanism remains unclear, although it has been suggested that insulin may antagonize glucocorticoids at the level of the fibroblast, affecting the production of fibroblast pneumocyte factor.[320] Clinically, the incidence of respiratory distress syndrome (RDS) has decreased as the need for stricter control of glucose levels has been recognized and monitoring has been made easier.

Catecholamines

Glucocorticoids and thyroid hormones play a role in enhancing the synthesis of phospholipids; catecholamines stimulate the secretion of surfactant into the alveolar space. This appears to be a direct action of adrenergic compounds on type II cells.[106] The response is prompt, occurring in less than an hour. Further research has shown that there is an increase in surfactant and saturated phosphatidylcholine in lung fluid and improved lung stability. This is demonstrated in an increased lecithin-to-sphingomyelin (L/S) ratio. An added benefit is the inhibition of fetal lung fluid secretion and possible reabsorption of the fluid within the alveoli at the time of delivery. These two effects (increase in surfactant and decrease in lung fluid) work together in preparing for respiratory conversion.[21, 83, 106, 179, 349]

At present, it seems that there is a complex interaction of several hormones and factors controlling surfactant synthesis. There continues to be much to learn about surfactant, its synthesis, and its removal. However, it is apparent that normal lung function is dependent upon the presence of surfactant, which permits a decrease in surface tension at end-expiration and an increase in surface tension during lung expansion. This activity prevents atelectasis at end-expiration and facilitates elastic recoil on inspiration. Surfactant provides the lung with the stability required for maintenance of homeostatic blood gas pressures while decreasing the work of breathing.[172, 312]

Assessment of Fetal Lung Maturity

In order to manage preterm labor it is important to accurately assess fetal lung maturity. This is especially true when the date of the last menstrual period is not known or if PIH, placenta previa, multiple pregnancy, Rh isoimmunization, diabetic pregnancy, or intrauterine growth retardation is present.[105]

The presence of surfactant phospholipids in the amniotic fluid allows determination of lung maturity, because their concentrations change toward the end of delivery. Gluck and associates demonstrated that the L/S ratio is a reliable index and a good predictor of whether RDS will develop within the 48 hours following amniocentesis. This is still the most widely used assessment tool in obstetrics.[105, 151, 274]

Sphingomyelin levels remain constant throughout gestation. Phosphatidylcholine (PC) levels rise sharply at around 34 to 35 weeks' gestation, thereby providing the basis for achieving a ratio between the two. If the L/S ratio is greater than or equal to 2, it indicates lung maturity and a negligble risk for RDS. A ratio less than 1.5 indicates lung immaturity. A higher incidence of inaccurate readings is found in complicated pregnancies.

Factors that influence phospholipid concentrations in the amniotic fluid include volume of amniotic fluid (varies inversely) and contamination with blood, meconium, or antiseptics. PC levels are falsely high with blood contamination (fetal or maternal). PG is only slightly affected, however, because blood does not contain PG in significant amounts. The presence of PG is an indication that the major synthesis pathway for surfactant is present and functioning. Therefore, when PG is present in the amniotic fluid, there is little risk for RDS regardless of what the L/S ratio is.[70, 81, 86, 121, 170, 288, 342] Other techniques for assessing fetal lung maturity include the complete lung profile (see Fig. 7–7), a modified profile (L/S ratio and PG only), and techniques such as the fluorescent polarization (FP) assay.

A low L/S ratio is not an absolute indication that RDS will develop and may in fact predict RDS in only 50% of cases.[170] The presence of PG, however, makes it unlikely that the infant will develop RDS even when diabetes or perinatal asphyxia is present.[104, 276, 359] This has been disputed by other researchers.[25] Regardless, the use of fetal lung maturity tests has decreased the incidence of RDS by 10 to 30%.[166]

Oxygen Antioxidants

The other biochemical system that develops prenatally and is needed for successful adaptation to extrauterine life is the antioxidant system (AOS). The AOS is designed to scavenge or detoxify the highly reactive oxygen metabolites produced during aerobic respiration.[130, 190] The potentially cytotoxic oxygen metabolites (superoxide radical, hydrogen peroxide, hydroxyl radical, singlet oxygen, and peroxide radical) are produced intracellularly in excess amounts under hyperoxic conditions.[134, 135] The detoxifying antioxidant enzymes include superoxide dismutase, catalase, and glutathione peroxidase.

The transition to the extrauterine environment is a move from a relatively hypoxic state to a hyperoxic one. In utero the fetal lung is exposed to low PaO_2 levels, with even lower oxygen tensions existing in the fetal lung fluid that fills the alveolar spaces and bronchiole tubes. At delivery, the alveolar and airway cells are abruptly exposed to hyperoxic tensions. Therefore it is important to have an AOS in place that can reduce damage by oxygen radicals.[128]

The development of the antioxidant enzymes occurs late in gestation.[129, 131] Antioxidant levels appear to be strongly correlated to the degree of protection that can be expected from oxygen radical–induced lung injury. When enzyme levels are increased (as with exogenous treatment), there is increased tolerance to hyperoxia.[100, 130, 132, 190]

Although there are other protective mechanisms (Table 7–7) in place, it does not appear that increased amounts of these will result in an increased level of protection. However, deficiencies within these other pathways will result in an increased susceptibility to cellular damage. This suggests that the other antioxidants play a secondary role in providing protection.[100, 132, 190]

Antioxidant enzymes provide primary protection by direct detoxification of reactive oxygen radicals. This prevents damage to cell proteins and DNA structure.[125, 130, 133, 190] The other systems terminate reactions already initiated by oxygen radical attack.

Lung Fluid

Lung fluid is secreted beginning in the canalicular stage. The site and specific mechanism for formation are unclear, although it is thought to be derived from alveolar epithelium secretions. It is not an ultrafiltrate or mixture of plasma or amniotic fluid. Active transport is required to attain the final ion concentrations found in the fluid; this is probably achieved by the active transport of chloride with sodium following passively. The water flux can be attributed to the osmotic force of sodium chloride (NaCl).[236, 328]

Osmolarity and sodium and chloride levels are lower in amniotic fluid than in tracheal fluid, whereas pH and glucose and protein levels are higher (Table 7–8).[261] The rate of secretion is approximately 2 to 4 ml/kg/min in lambs,[252] which at term is equivalent to

TABLE 7–7
Antioxidant Protective Mechanisms

REACTIVE O_2 SPECIES	ANTIOXIDANT ENZYMES	CELL COMPONENTS ATTACKED BY REACTIVE O_2 SPECIES
O_2^- superoxide radical	$O_2^- + O_2^- + 2 H^+ \xrightarrow{(SOD)} O_2 + H_2O_2$	Lipids: peroxidation of unsaturated fatty acids in cell membranes
H_2O_2 hydrogen peroxide	$2 H_2O_2 \xrightarrow[(GP)]{(CAT)} O_2 + 2 H_2O$	Proteins: oxidation of sulfhydryl-containing enzymes (enzyme inactivation)
ROO • peroxide radical	$2 ROO • + 2H^+ \xrightarrow{(GP)} 2 ROH + O_2$	Carbohydrates: depolymerization of polysaccharides
$^1O_2$ singlet oxygen	$'O_2$ (scavenged by β-carotene)	Nucleic acids: base hydroxylation, cross-linkage, scission of DNA strands
OH • hydroxyl radical	OH • (scavenged by ?vitamin E ?GSH)	(Also, inhibition of protein, nucleotide, fatty acid biosynthesis)

CAT, catalase; GP, glutathione peroxidase; GSH, glutathione; R, lipid; ROH, nontoxic lipid alcohol; SOD, superoxide dismutase.
From Frank, L. & Sosenko, I. R. S. (1987). Development of lung antioxidant enzyme system in late gestation: Possible implications for the prematurely born infant. *J. Pediatr, 110,* 11.

approximately 250 ml/day in infants.[327] Of the fluid produced, some is swallowed and some moves into the amniotic fluid. The amount of lung fluid contributed to the amniotic pool is relatively insignificant when compared to that contributed by micturition. The volume of fluid in the lungs is equal to the FRC; this means at term there is 10 to 25 ml/kg body weight of liquid that must be either expelled or absorbed.[195, 236, 252]

Although the functional importance of lung fluid is not entirely known, it does play an important part in cell maturation and development as well as in determining the formation, size, and shape of the developing air space. Alterations in fluid dynamics affect pulmonary cell proliferation and differentiation. Alcorn and coworkers demonstrated that in fetuses whose tracheas were ligated, the lungs were relatively large but were immature when type II cells were assessed.[7] For those fetuses whose lungs were drained the alveolar walls were thick, lung size was decreased, and type II cells were more abundant.[7] This was substantiated by Perlman and colleagues, who found a reduced number of alveoli in human infants who experienced amniotic fluid leakage.[281] Therefore, if pro-

TABLE 7–8
Composition of Lung Fluid as Compared with Plasma and Amniotic Fluid*

	LUNG FLUID	PLASMA	AMNIOTIC FLUID
Sodium	150 ±1.3	150 ±0.7	113 ±6.5
Potassium	6.3 ±0.7	4.8 ±0.2	7.6 ±6.5
Chloride	157 ±4.1	107 ±0.9	87 ±5.0
Bicarbonate	2.8 ±0.3	24 ±1.2	19 ±3.0
Phosphates	0.02	2.3 ±0.17	3.2
pH	6.27 ±0.05	7.34 ±0.04	7.02 ±0.09
Urea	7.9 ±2.7	8.21 ±1.4	10.5 ±2.4
Protein osmotic pressure (mmHg)	1.0	28.2 ±1.2	1.0
Protein (g/dl)	0.027 ±0.002	3.09 ±0.26	0.10 ±0.01

*Results are means.
From Maloney, J. E. (1987). Lung liquid dynamics in the perinatal period. In J. Lipshitz, et al. (Eds.), *Perinatal development of the heart & lung.* Ithaca, NY: Perinatology Press.

duction of lung fluid is decreased or leakage of amniotic fluid is experienced, there is risk of lung hypoplasia.[73, 204] In comparison, tracheal obstruction of a chronic nature leads to hyperplasia, with an increase in the number of alveoli, although functionally immature.[73, 336]

At birth the lungs must move from secretion to absorption of lung fluid or the infant would rapidly succumb, drowning in his or her own secretions. Secretion ends with birth, and ventilation of the lungs leads to liquid dispersion across the pulmonary epithelium during the absorptive period. At this time, the pulmonary epithelium undergoes a reversible increase in solute permeability, leading to a rapid transfer of lung liquid solutes.[327] This is confirmed clinically, as the interstitial spaces and lymphatics become distended during the first 5 to 6 hours of life and an increase in pulmonary lymph flow can be seen.[351]

Beyond this increase in absorption though, there seems to be a decrease in the rate of secretion. In lambs, it was noted that the administration of epinephrine led to a decrease in fluid secretion. This effect is mediated by β-adrenergic receptors in the alveolar epithelium [361] and may either suppress the chloride pump or activate a second pump that triggers the absorption process.[327] Avery and co-authors suggested that resorption is a sodium pump–dependent mechanism, as the infusion of amiloride can modify the process.[15] This supports the second pump theory.

It is known that the rate of absorption increases as gestation progresses and this can be correlated with an increase in catecholamine levels.[227] Fetal adrenal glands are probably not able to produce sufficient amounts of catecholamines to trigger this mechanism. Labor, however, is sufficient stimulus to release enough epinephrine to switch from secretion to absorption.[327] The catecholamine surge that occurs with delivery is probably the final mechanism that assures that the change is completed.[261]

The drop in pulmonary vascular resistance with aeration and the rise in oxygen tension increase the number of alveolar capillaries perfused, resulting in an increase in blood flow and fluid removal capacity. With the increased lymphatic flow and the dramatic change in the pulmonary blood flow, lung fluid is dispersed within the first few hours following delivery.

Fetal Blood Gases

The factors that affect maternal-to-fetal diffusion of oxygen include maternal and fetal PO_2 relationships, maternal and fetal oxygen-hemoglobin dissociation curves (see box on p. 267), maternal and fetal hemoglobin concentrations, and the Bohr effect. Carbon dioxide transfer is affected by hydrogen ion concentration and the Haldane effect.

OXYGEN TRANSFER

The placenta is separated into cotyledons, which are subdivided into lobules. The lobules are fed by uteroplacental arteries that spurt blood toward the apex of the intervillous space. Depending on where blood is located in the cavity, the maternal-fetal oxygen gradient varies. The PaO_2 of the blood within these arteries is at the most 100 mmHg. By the time blood reaches the apex of the lobule the PaO_2 is 17 mmHg and the maternal-fetal gradients are the greatest. At the rim of the cavity, the maternal PaO_2 is approximately 33 mmHg and fetal PaO_2 is around 28 mmHg. This gradient facilitates the transfer of oxygen from the mother to the fetus.[253, 256]

As noted earlier, the fetal oxygen-hemoglobin dissociation curve is placed to the left of the adult curve, indicating that fetal hemoglobin has a higher affinity for oxygen. This can be seen in the larger quantity of oxygen each gram of fetal hemoglobin carries. Besides the higher affinity, the fetus has an increased number of red blood cells and therefore an increased hemoglobin content. This leads to a higher oxygen carrying capacity when compared with the mother.

When the maternal blood releases oxygen to the fetus, it accepts fetal metabolites in return, leading to a fall in maternal pH. This shifts the maternal oxygen-hemoglobin dissociation curve to the right (the Bohr effect), which increases the movement of oxygen from the mother to the fetus. As the fetus gives up CO_2, the pH rises, shifting the fetal dissociation curve to the left. This allows the fetus to accept more oxygen as the affinity increases.

This movement of hydrogen ions results in a displacement of both dissociation curves, moving them further apart (double Bohr effect). As the distance between the two curves increases, oxygen transfers at a faster rate from maternal blood to fetal blood. This process is unique to the placenta.

CARBON DIOXIDE TRANSFER

The carbon dioxide combining power of blood is dependent upon the amount of hemoglobin that is not combined with oxygen. This uncombined hemoglobin is free to buffer the hydrogen ions formed by the dissociation of carbonic acid. This means that as maternal blood gives up oxygen it is able to accept increased amounts of carbon dioxide (the Haldane effect). The fetus gives up carbon dioxide as oxygen is accepted, without altering the local $PaCO_2$ levels. This double Haldane effect is unique to the placenta and is probably responsible for half the transplacental carbon dioxide transfer.

NORMAL FETAL BLOOD GASES

Table 7–9 lists the expected changes in fetal blood gases during the intrapartum period and the normal (acceptable) range for fetal blood gases. The wide range can be attributed to inaccuracies of measurement and variations in the composition of scalp blood during labor. Of course, the skill of the individual performing the procedure also makes a difference. In order to arrive at the currently accepted upper and lower limits, Lumley and associates looked at blood gases obtained from 600 abnormal patients and calculated that the lower limit for pH is 7.25, the upper limit for $PaCO_2$ is 60 mmHg, and the lower limit for base excess is −8.[233] These limits do not presuppose fetal asphyxia, however.

Saling proposed the concept of preacidosis when the pH was between 7.20 and 7.25. Acidosis was defined as a pH less than 7.20.[305] These values are currently accepted and used for clinically managing patients. However, Saling cautioned that a pH greater than 7.20 does not guarantee that the fetus is not experiencing asphyxia. Further discussion of asphyxia and its impact upon the fetus and neonate can be found in the Clinical Implications for Neonatal Care section of this chapter.

Fetal Breathing Movements

Fetal breathing movements (FBM) can be seen on ultrasound as early as 11 weeks' gestation.[39, 97, 242] They are rapid and irregular, occurring intermittently early in gestation. As gestation progresses, the strength and frequency of FBMs increase, and they occur between 40 and 80% of the time, with a rate of 30 to 70 breaths per minute.[72, 96, 242, 261] Large movements (gasping) occur 5% of the total breathing time, one to four times per minute.[242]

The rapid and irregular respiratory activity may contribute to lung fluid regulation, thereby influencing lung growth. The diaphragm seems to be the major structure involved, with minimal chest wall excursion encountered (4 to 8 mm change in transverse diameter).[39, 241] Movement of the diaphragm is necessary for chest wall muscle and dia-

TABLE 7–9
Fetal Blood Gases

TIME	pH	PO_2	PCO_2	BASE EXCESS
Early labor	7.30	19.7	45.5	6.4
	±.05	±2.9	±6.8	±2.1
Mild labor	7.30	21	45.1	5.4
	±.04	±3	±5.5	±2.6
Full dilation	7.28	19.1	47.8	6.1
	±.05	±3.8	±7.8	±2.5
Before birth	7.26	17.3	50.4	7.3
	±.07	±4.2	±7.8	±2.6
Umbilical artery	7.24	17.6	48.7	8.8
	±.05	±4.6	±7.3	±2.5
Umbilical vein	7.32	27.8	38.9	6.6
	±.05	±5.5	±5.8	±2.9

LOWER AND UPPER LIMITS OF NORMAL RANGE		
	Lower Limit	**Upper Limit**
pH	7.15 to 7.30	7.33 to 7.47
PCO_2 mmHg	22 to 34	50 to 67
PO_2 mmHg	7 to 17	23 to 36
Base excess	−14 to −5.3	−4.3 to +3.0

Compiled from San Francisco General Hospital House Officers Manual (1989); and Pearson, J.F. (1976). Maternal and fetal acid-base balance. In R.W. Beard & P.W. Nathanielsz (Eds.), *Fetal physiology and medicine: The basis of perinatology* (p. 502). Philadelphia: WB Saunders.

phragm training and development, building adequate strength for the initial breath.[96, 97]

The movement of the diaphragm also influences the course of lung cell differentiation and proliferation. Bilateral phrenectomy results in altered lung morphology with an increase in type II over type I cells. Presumably the innervated diaphragm increases the size of the thorax and thereby increases tissue stress, affecting morphology. In addition, however, hypoplastic lungs are found when fetal breathing movements do not occur.[16]

Initially FBMs are infrequent, increasing with gestational age and becoming more organized and vigorous.[261] Even with these gestational changes, tracheal fluid shifts are negligible; the pressure generated being no more than 25 mmHg.[16] Fetal maturation leads to the appearance of FBM cycles, with an increase during daytime hours.[242] Patrick and coworkers noted the peak in FBMs to be in late evening with the nadir being in the early morning hours.[278]

Although the patterns of FBMs vary according to rate, amplitude, and character, they seem to be correlated mostly with fetal behavioral states and occur the most often during active sleep.[72, 96, 242] In sheep, these are periods of electroencephalographic desynchronization and rapid eye movement (REM) that correspond to the active sleep periods seen in newborns and adults.[242] This gives credence to the theory of sleep–wake cycles in the fetus; fetal wakefulness and arousal states are associated with sustained respiratory efforts, whereas quiet sleep often leads to cessation of FBMs.[96]

The mechanism for the initiation of FBMs is unknown, although they seem to be stimulated by maternal inhalation of carbon dioxide, adrenergic and cholinergic compounds, and prostaglandin synthesis inhibitors. Other factors affecting FBMs include maternal glycemia, nicotine and alcohol ingestion, and labor.[40, 240, 279] These are summarized in Table 7–10.

Abnormal breathing patterns can be seen during periods of fetal hypoxia. Mild hypoxemia decreases the incidence of FBMs, while severe hypoxemia may lead to cessation of FBMs for several hours. The onset of asphyxia leads to gasping, which persists until death.[4, 279] Interestingly, the onset of mild hypoxemia (as with umbilical artery occlusion of short duration) may lead to quiet sleep, which for the fetus decreases activity expenditure and oxygen consumption.[242] Although paradoxical in nature, this conservation mechanism may save the fetus while cardiac output is redistributed toward the placenta.

The reduction and cessation of FBMs seen during labor correspond to the increase in prostaglandin E concentrations seen during the last days before delivery. These findings suggest that prostaglandin metabolism may play a role in respiratory conversion at birth.[206] It remains unknown why or if irregular FBMs lead to the sustained respirations of postnatal life.

TABLE 7–10
Factors Affecting Fetal Breathing Movements

FACTOR	EFFECT
Hypoglycemia	↓
Hyperglycemia	↑
Cigarette smoking	↓ for up to 1 hour or cessation
Alcohol consumption (1 oz)	↓
Accelerated labor	↓
Drugs	
Stimulants	↑
Depressants	↓

NEONATAL PHYSIOLOGY

Transitional Events

Transitional events are all those activities that must occur within organ systems to achieve appropriate functioning in the extrauterine environment. The most critical of these is the establishment of an air-liquid interface at the alveolar level and the acquisition of sustained rhythmic respirations by the neonate. This must occur within seconds of placental separation, or pulmonary and cardiovascular changes will not occur and resuscitation will be necessary.

Respiratory Conversion

Before discussing first breath events, a brief review of intrauterine status is warranted. At term, the acinar portion of the lung is well established, although "true" alveoli are only now beginning to develop. The pulmonary blood vessels are narrow; only 5 to 10% of the cardiac output perfuses the lungs to meet cellular nutrition needs. This low volume circulation is in part due to the high pulmonary vascular resistance created by constricted arterioles.

At term the lung holds approximately 20 ml/kg of fluid. Lung aeration is complete when this liquid is replaced with an equal volume of air and an FRC is established. A substantial amount of air is retained from the early breaths, and within an hour of birth 80 to 90% of the FRC is created. The retention of air is due to surfactant and a decrease in surface tension. Surfactant decreases the tendency toward atelectasis; promotes capillary circulation by increasing alveolar size, which indirectly dilates precapillary vessels; improves alveolar fluid clearance; and protects the airway.[169] Therefore, the concentration and adsorption properties of surfactant must be sufficient to react during the short first breaths (1 to 10 seconds). Exactly how all this happens is not known.[327]

The gas tension levels that are encountered in the fetal state would result in intensive hyperventilation if encountered postnatally. This indicates a diminished responsiveness of the respiratory centers to chemical stimuli in the blood in the prenatal period. Postnatal breathing is responsive to stimuli from arterial and central chemoreceptors (O_2 and CO_2 tension in the blood); stimuli from the chest wall and lungs, musculoskeletal system, and skin; and emotions and behavioral stimuli. The change that takes place at birth and the increase in aerobic metabolism are not only rapid but irreversible. Within a few hours of birth, the full-term neonate is responsive to hypoxia and hypercapnia in much the same manner as an adult.[327]

The actual mechanics of respiratory conversion begins with the passage of the fetus through the birth canal. The thorax is markedly depressed during this passage, and external pressures of 160 to 200 cm H_2O[261, 262] and intrathoracic pressures of 60 to 100 cm H_2O pressure are generated.[201, 269] With face or nares exposed to atmospheric pressure, variable amounts of lung fluid are expressed.[269] As much as 28 ml of fluid has been expelled during the second stage of labor,[261] leading to the creation of a potential air space. Recoil of the chest to predelivery proportions allows for passive inspiration of air. This initial step helps to reduce viscous forces that must be overcome in order to establish an air-liquid interface in the alveoli.[269]

The forces that must be overcome in the first breaths include the viscosity of the lung fluid column, the tissue resistive forces (compliance), and surface tension forces at the air-liquid interfaces. The viscosity of lung fluid provides resistance to movement of fluid in the airways.[212] The maximal resistance takes place at the beginning of the first breath, and the greatest displacement occurs in the trachea.[66, 269] The dissipation of tracheal fluid during the vaginal squeeze reduces the amount of pressure that must be generated to move the liquid column down the conducting airways.

As the column progresses down the conducting branches, the total surface area of the air-liquid interface increases as the bronchiole diameter is progressively reduced. The surface tension, however, increases.[212, 261] It is the surface tension forces that are the most difficult to overcome during the first breath events. The maximal forces are encountered where the radial curvature of the airways is smallest (terminal bronchioles); here the viscous forces are at their nadir.[261, 269, 316] In this locality the intraluminal pressure must be at its peak in order to prevent closure by tension in the intraluminal walls (Laplace relationship).[316] If these smaller airways were fluid-filled only (no air-liquid interface), the pressures needed would be considerably less; however, this would make alveolar expansion more difficult. Surface tension forces drop again once air enters the terminal air sacs.[261, 316]

Tissue resistive forces are unknown at birth. However, the fluid within the terminal air sacs enhances air introduction, possibly by modifying the configuration of the smaller units of the lung. The fluid enlarges the radius of the alveolar ducts and terminal air sac, thereby facilitating expansion (Laplace relationship). The lung fluid also reduces the possibility of obstruction of the small ducts by cellular debris.

During the interval between recoil and the generation of first breath pressures, the infant may generate a positive pressure within the mouth by glossopharyngeal breathing. This "frog breathing" may build enough pressure to facilitate lung expansion and reduce the pressure needed during the first inspiration. This is probably not a significant source of pressure in most infants, however.[261, 269]

Another possible contributor to lung expansion is the small increase in pulmonary blood flow that may occur during this time.

This flow may lead to capillary erection as pulmonary capillaries uncoil and may increase transpulmonary pressure and lung stability.[197, 269] This, once again, is not significant enough pressure to produce lung expansion but may contribute modestly to air entry.

The first diaphragmatic inspiration has been noted to begin within 9 seconds of delivery and generates very large positive intrathoracic pressures (mean of 70 cm H_2O). Air enters as soon as the intrathoracic pressure begins to drop, with mean inspiratory pressures of 30 to 35 cm H_2O pressure.[261] These findings confirm similar research conducted on postmortem examination, by calculation, and on other full-term infants.[14, 163, 202]

The large transpulmonary pressure generated by the diaphragm lasts only 0.5 to 1.0 second, pulling in 10 to 70 ml of air.[202] The alveolar lining layer becomes established after the first breath, allowing the molecules of surfactant to reduce the surface tension during expiration.[269] The first expiration is also active, leaving a residual volume of up to 30 ml. The magnitude of the expiratory pressure contributes to FRC formation, even distribution of air, and elimination of lung fluid.[261] The second and third breaths are similar to the first, but require less pressure in that the small airways are open and surface active forces are diminished.[269] Lung expansion augments surfactant secretion, providing alveolar stability and FRC formation.[12]

By 10 minutes of age the FRC is equal to 17 ml/kg, and at 30 minutes it is equal to 25 to 35 ml/kg.[12, 175] The return of muscle tone after the first breath helps to maintain FRC by providing chest wall stability.[261, 262]

Lung compliance is four times greater by day 1 and continues to increase gradually over the 1st week. Flow resistance decreases by one half to one fourth during this time, and the distribution of ventilation is as even after day 1 as it is on day 3.[261] The total work of the first breath is equivalent to the cry of an infant who is several days old.

Structural changes in the pulmonary circulation occur in three overlapping phases according to Haworth and Hislop.[175] The first phase is one of digitation and recruitment and occurs in the first 24 hours of life in nonmuscular and partially muscular arteries. The external diameter of these vessels increases, and the swollen endothelial lining cells flatten. These endothelial cells may play a role in the relaxation of smooth muscle cells by metabolizing substances such as acetylcholine. These enzymatic processes are responsive to changes in oxygen concentrations, with hypoxia leading to inhibition of converting enzymes and causing vasoconstriction. There may also be filaments within the endothelial cells that contract in low oxygen tensions and relax in normoxic environments. The latter constrictive properties may also contribute to increased pulmonary vascular resistance or failed transition when hypoxia occurs.[303]

The second phase is a time of reduced muscularity, occurring in the first 2 weeks. During this time partially muscular and wholly muscular vessels become nonmuscular and partially muscular respectively. Larger vessel muscle coats also become thinner, contributing further to the decrease in pulmonary vascular resistance. These changes are probably associated with a decreased pulmonary artery vasoconstriction ability.[303]

The filaments in the pericytes (nonmuscular vessels) and the intermediate cells of the partially muscular vessels may play a significant role in the increased pulmonary vascular resistance needed during fetal life. These cells atrophy or at least become smaller and less specialized during these initial postnatal weeks.[175]

After the first 2 weeks a growth phase begins. Muscle tissue begins to reappear in the acinus and continues to develop slowly during childhood. The initial two phases allow for the functional adaptation necessary for extrauterine life; the third phase brings about structural remodeling. The growth creates the relationships seen in the mature system between the external vessel diameter and muscle wall thickness.[175]

In conjunction with the local vascular changes in the pulmonary bed, there are major reorganizational changes within the cardiovascular system. The first breath events and cardiovascular events (see Chapter 6) are interdependent and must occur in order for transition to be successful. Therefore, a brief review of fetal circulation and transitional changes is included here.

Cardiovascular Conversion

In the fetus, oxygenated blood returns from the placenta via the umbilical vein with a PaO_2 of 35 mmHg. It enters the liver with a small percentage feeding the liver microcirculation and ending up in the inferior vena cava. The majority of the returning blood is shunted directly into the inferior vena cava via the ductus venosus.

The inferior vena cava enters the right atrium; the majority of its blood flow (approximately 60%) is deflected across the right atrium and through the foramen ovale into the left atrium. Here it mixes with the blood returning from the fetal lungs (unoxygenated), enters the left ventricle, and is ejected into the ascending aorta to feed the cerebral arteries and upper extremities.

The remainder of the right atrium blood mixes with the returning superior vena caval blood (unoxygenated blood returning from the upper body) and enters the right ventricle. This mixed blood is ejected through the pulmonary arteries toward the lungs. The high pulmonary vascular resistance allows only 5 to 10% of the blood to enter the lungs; the majority is shunted across the ductus arteriosus into the thoracic aorta and directed to the lower segments of the body.

The placental circulation acts like a reservoir that contributes to the low systemic vascular resistance found in the fetal state. When the umbilical cord is clamped the systemic vascular resistance increases and there is systemic blood return. This change along with the pulmonary vasodilatation modifies the pressures within the atria. Left atrial pressure increases above pressure in the right atrium and leads to functional closure of the foramen ovale. The increase in PaO_2 and decrease in prostaglandin levels facilitate functional closure of the ductus arteriosus. These modifications in blood flow and pressures indicate the change from in series to parallel circulation and herald cardiovascular conversion.

Once the first breath is taken and cardiovascular conversion is initiated, the infant must be able to sustain rhythmic respirations. This requires that the central nervous system be "turned on" and take over the regulation of respiratory activity.

Control of Respiration

The goal of respiration is to meet the O_2 and CO_2 metabolic demands of the organism through extraction of O_2 from the atmosphere and removal of CO_2 produced by the organism. The brain's respiratory center is responsible for matching the level of ventilation to the metabolic demand. The assessment of metabolic needs and alteration of ventilation is accomplished by the chemoreceptors.

Chemoreceptors

The peripheral chemoreceptors (carotid and aortic bodies) sense PaO_2 and $PaCO_2$, and the central chemoreceptors (medullary) are sensitive to PCO_2-[H^+] in the extracellular fluid of the brain. When the PaO_2 falls below the acceptable range, the chemoreceptors increase the efferent neural activity to the respiratory center (brain) resulting in an increase in ventilation. At birth, the fetal PaO_2 of 25 mmHg (sufficient for intrauterine growth) increases to 50 mmHg with the first few breaths and then to 70 mmHg in the first hours.[326] This increase in oxygen tension exceeds the fetal demands for oxygen yielding a relative neonatal hyperoxia at birth. This change in oxygen tension causes the chemoreceptors to become less responsive to stimuli during the first few days of life.[35, 67] This implies that fluctuations in oxygen tension levels may not lead to a chemoreceptor response during these early days of neonatal life.[96] After this lag time, however, the chemoreceptors reset and become oxygen-sensitive and a major controller of respiration.[59, 148]

Sustained hyperventilation efforts during hypoxia cannot be maintained by the neonate. Studies in infants and animals have demonstrated that an initial hyperventilatory response is achieved but is followed by a subsequent fall in ventilation and oxygen tensions.[6, 58] The reason for this lack of sustained response is unknown. Davis and Bureau[96] speculated that it may be due to feeble chemoreceptor output, a central inhibitory effect of hypoxia on ventilation, or changes in pulmonary mechanics.

The neonate's response to carbon dioxide is also limited in the early neonatal period. Although this is more mature than the response to hypoxia, the neonate can only increase ventilation by 3 to 4 times baseline ventilation in comparison to the 10- to 20-fold increase that can be achieved by adults.[95, 164] Along with this, the threshold of tolerance is initially higher, progressively declining over the 1st month of life.[95, 257] This too may be due to the increased $PaCO_2$ levels found in the fetal state (45 to 50 mmHg) and the need to reset chemoreceptors.

Modification of ventilatory patterns is dependent upon inspiratory muscle strength, rib cage rigidity and compliance, airway resistance, and lung compliance. The status of these parameters at any given time as well as their integrative functioning affects the performance of the respiratory pump and is mediated by specific reflex arcs.[96]

Chest Wall Reflexes

Most of the reflexes for the respiratory pump arise from the chest wall via the muscle spindles through local spinal reflex arcs and centrally mediated reflexes. The diaphragm is scantily innervated; however, the intercostal muscles have abundant fibers from which this information is obtained.[54, 257, 270] These stretch-sensitive mechanoreceptors detect chest wall and workload forces.

Excessive stretch is modulated by alpha motoneuron activity altering respiratory muscle activity or recruiting more muscles.[84, 158] Further sensory information is obtained by proprioreceptors that sense changes in rib position and tension applied across the joint space,[96] and cutaneous stimulation of the thoracic wall causes a generalized increase in sensory and motoneuron stimulation of the respiratory muscles augmenting muscle contractions and ventilation.[243]

Chest wall distortion during inspiration stimulates muscle spindles that trigger central reflex arcs leading to reflex inhibition of intercostal, phrenic, and laryngeal neurons. This is possibly a protective mechanism in the neonate. Termination of distorted inefficient breathing may lead to energy conservation and reduce the possibility of muscle fatigue.[168, 293]

Lung Reflexes

The mechanoreceptors of the large lung airways include stretch receptors, irritant receptors, and C receptors. The sensory feedback mechanisms for these receptors are along the vagus nerve to the central respiratory center.

The stretch receptors sense lung inflation and deflation, with neural output proportional to lung volume or tension.[96] Lung inflation initiates inhibitory impulses that terminate inspiration and prolong expiratory time. This is termed the Hering-Breuer reflex. Once triggered, respiratory frequency slows. Although not found in adults, this reflex is active in the neonate for reasons

that are currently unknown.[44] It may be a protective mechanism for the neonate, since inspiratory occlusion results in an increase in inspiratory effort and inspiratory time in the full-term neonate. Responses in premature infants vary.[141, 208]

The irritant receptors of the mucosal lining in the airways are extremely sensitive to mechanical stimulation and are responsible for the cough reflex seen clinically. In infants over 35 weeks' gestation there is the typical adult response to stimulation, increased breathing, coughing, arousal, and gross body movement. For infants under 35 weeks, however, these responses are not usually elicited.[54] Flemming and coworkers found either no response or a brief cough followed by apnea, slowing of respiration, or immediate respiration.[124] The reason for this difference is unknown but may be due to a functional immaturity or the possibility that unmyelinated irritant receptors may be inhibitory in nature.[54]

C receptor endings lie in close relationship to the capillaries. They seem to be activated by tissue damage, accumulation of interstitial fluid and release of various mediators.[270] The dyspnea of pulmonary vascular congestion and ventilatory response to exercise and pulmonary embolization may be attributed to C receptors. Although characterized in physiologic studies, C receptors have not been identified histologically in humans and little is known about their presence or function in the neonate.[273]

The chemoreceptors provide information about the metabolic needs of the infant, and the mechanoreceptors provide information about the status of the respiratory pump. It is the central respiratory center that integrates this information and establishes the ventilatory pattern that efficiently meets the infant's needs. Each respiratory cycle during a stable state (e.g., quiet sleep) is uniform for amplitude, duration, and wave form. Behavioral influences as well as active sleep states (REM sleep) alter the regularity of breathing. The information received from the various receptors helps to determine the inspiratory time, the expiratory time, the lung volume at which the breath should occur (FRC), the rate of inspiration, and the braking of the expiration.[257, 360] The recruitment and adjustment of the various respiratory muscle groups result in the predetermined lung volume being achieved.[96]

The information described above is received by the respiratory controller in the brain stem, which is responsible for initiating automatic respiration and adjustments.[33] This respiratory control center is divided into three areas: the apneustic center, the pneumotaxic center, and the medullary center. The pneumotaxic center may be responsible for switching inspiration to expiration. The apneustic center seems to be responsible for cutting off inspiration. Both centers are located in the pons and neither seems to be necessary for rhythmic expiration. However, destruction of the medullary center results in apnea and is therefore thought to be responsible for respiratory rhythm.[271]

These centers are connected to the cerebral cortex via the spinal cord, thereby allowing voluntary control of respiration. The spinal cord is responsible for the integration and relay of commands to the muscles of the respiratory pump via the phrenic and intercostal muscles.

The Respiratory Pump

The movement of gas in and out of the lungs is based on the functioning of the respiratory pump, which is composed of the rib cage and respiratory muscles. The pump must move sufficient oxygen and carbon dioxide into and out of the lungs to replace the oxygen consumed and wash out the carbon dioxide that accumulates in the alveoli. Ventilatory efforts in the neonate are dependent upon the strength and endurance of the diaphragm. When the diaphragm is unable to generate the necessary energy to sustain ventilatory efforts, ventilatory assistance is required.[96]

Diaphragm

The diaphragm inserts on the lower six ribs, the sternum, and first three lumbar vertebrae. It is innervated bilaterally by the phrenic nerves and expends its work on the lung, the rib cage, and the abdomen. In order to maximize diaphragmatic work, the intercostal muscles must stabilize the rib cage and the abdominal muscles should stabilize the abdomen.[96, 117] In the full-term infant the coordination of these efforts is almost nonexistent; the preterm infant is even less effective at coordinating these events. During REM sleep (the most predominant sleep state

in the neonate) the intercostal and abdominal muscles are less efficient, contributing to respiratory instability.[117]

The diaphragm works most efficiently when the dome is high in the thorax (relaxed position, optimal fiber length), increasing the thoracic volume while compressing the abdominal contents and moving the abdominal wall.[101] The neonatal diaphragm is situated differently than that of the adult. In its relaxed state it is located higher in the thorax, favoring more efficient generation of inspiratory pressures. In the adult, the diaphragm is flatter and generally lower, making it more inefficient mechanically. This "handicap" is made up for by the stability of the chest wall in the adult.

The composition of the muscle fibers in the neonate is also different. In adults, 60% of the fibers are fast oxidative, fatigue-resistant type I fibers; 30% are type IIa fast oxidative fatigue-sensitive fibers; and the rest are type IIb slow oxidative, fatigue-resistant.[203] In contrast, the neonatal diaphragm and intercostal muscles have a lower proportion of fatigue-resistant muscle fibers (20% type I fibers) and more type IIa fibers.[96, 117, 203] Type I fibers increase in number from 24 weeks' gestation on. At 24 weeks, they comprise 10% of the total fiber content, reaching the adult proportion at 8 months postnatal age.[117] Because of this developmental pattern, the infant is particularly vulnerable to diaphragmatic muscle fatigue, especially when the work of breathing is increased.[96, 117] This worsens with lower gestational age.

The above theory has been disputed by Maxwell and associates who did not find a paucity of oxidative muscle fibers in premature baboons.[249] They suggested that the contraction and relaxation times as well as the latent period were longer in premature babies when compared with adults. Upon further evaluation, it was found that there was a lack of sarcoplasmic reticulum in the diaphragmatic muscle, and this may result in a slower initiation as well as termination of contractions. Therefore when high respiratory rates occur, there may be ischemia of the muscle with fatigue related to inadequate substrate availability. Further research is indicated in this area to determine the actual cause of fatigue that results in respiratory failure in premature infants.

The diaphragm is attached to a chest wall

that is more pliable than that of the adults. This can lead to distortion of the lower portion of the chest wall during contraction, especially if it is forceful. The decreased efficiency of the contraction and reduced tidal volume can make ventilation less effective requiring adjustments in the respiratory pattern.[96]

Rib Cage and Chest Wall Muscles

The muscles of the rib cage include the external intercostal muscles (inspiration), the internal intercostal muscles (expiration), and the accessory muscles including the sternocleidomastoid, pectoral, and scalene muscles. The major role of these muscles is to fixate the chest wall by tonic contraction during diaphragmatic excursion. If they are unable to accomplish this goal, collapse and distortion of the chest wall is likely to occur during inspiratory efforts.

If the needed stability is provided, the contraction of the inspiratory muscles of the rib cage can contribute to the thoracic volume by elevating the anterior end of each rib. During sighing, the increase in tidal volume is largely due to this increased chest wall excursion.[332]

Rib Cage Compliance

The chest wall in the infant is cartilaginous, soft, and pliable. This design allows for compression during passage through the birth canal without rib fractures and for further growth and development.[5, 13, 22] Nelson described it as a loose fitting glove surrounding the neonatal lung.[269] The high compliance dictates that for any given change in volume there is almost no change in pressure.[271] This increased compliance is highest in the preterm infant but is significant in the full-term infant as well.

Elastic recoil is that property of a body that causes it to return to its resting position after having been stretched or deformed.[271] In the older child and adult, once the chest wall has reached the FRC it tends to recoil outward; however, the tendency of the lung to collapse toward the RV provides a counterbalance.[271, 273] In other words, at resting lung volumes (FRC) the elastic recoil of the chest wall is equal and opposite to that of the lungs.

At V_T the chest wall of the neonate is

nearly infinitely compliant. The lack of opposition by the thorax to the recoil of the lung causes the newborn's respiratory system to come to equilibrium at a resting volume very close to the collapse volume (Fig. 7–8).[269] The activity of the intercostal muscles during normal breathing is a major determinant of the elastic characteristics of the chest wall and therefore the functional residual capacity. Therefore, during tidal breathing some of the dependent airways fall into their closing volume range and the bronchioles collapse and are not in communication with the main stem bronchus.[5, 13] Bronchiole compliance contributes to these dynamics.

Elastic recoil of the chest wall increases during the 2 weeks after birth although it remains considerably less than that of the adult for a long period of time. The continued change in recoil pressures is presumed to be the result of progressive ossification, improvement in intercostal muscle tone, and development of a negative pressure on the abdominal side of the diaphragm.[271]

For the infant (with a small abdomen) lying in the supine position, the outward recoil of the chest is presumably inhibited. Once the infant learns to stand and the abdomen has grown, the contents of the abdominal cavity shift away from the upper abdomen thereby creating an increase in negative subdiaphragmatic pressure. This change in pressure favors outward recoil of the chest wall.[271]

The clinical implications of this highly compliant chest are related to the ease at which lung collapse is possible in the neonate. The low elastic recoil pressure of the neonatal lung and the high compliance of the thorax result in the majority of tidal breathing in the infant occurring near the closing capacity of the lung. This contributes to the possibility of collapse and affects gas distribution.

The mechanical liabilities of a highly compliant chest wall post delivery include a compromised ability to produce large tidal volumes, requiring the generation of greater pressures. This requires the infant to perform more work to move the same amount of tidal volume.[271] This is especially true in preterm infants with lung diseases associated with decreased lung compliance. Lung disease causes the respiratory drive (response to stimulus) to increase in an attempt to gener-

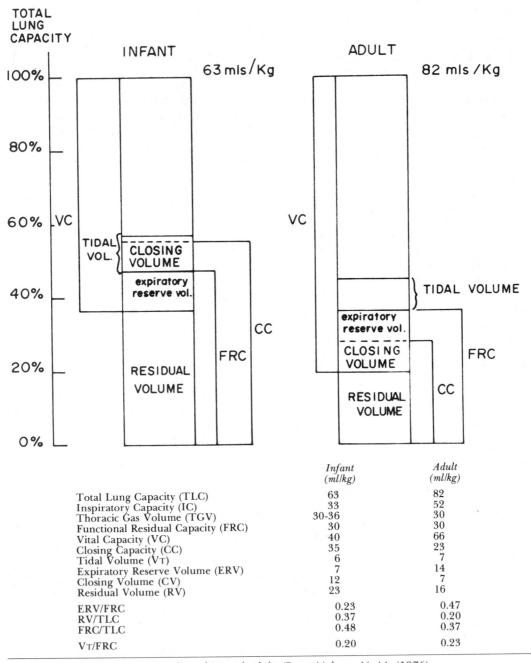

	Infant (ml/kg)	Adult (ml/kg)
Total Lung Capacity (TLC)	63	82
Inspiratory Capacity (IC)	33	52
Thoracic Gas Volume (TGV)	30-36	30
Functional Residual Capacity (FRC)	30	30
Vital Capacity (VC)	40	66
Closing Capacity (CC)	35	23
Tidal Volume (V_T)	6	7
Expiratory Reserve Volume (ERV)	7	14
Closing Volume (CV)	12	7
Residual Volume (RV)	23	16
ERV/FRC	0.23	0.47
RV/TLC	0.37	0.20
FRC/TLC	0.48	0.37
V_T/FRC	0.20	0.23

FIGURE 7–8. Lung volumes in the infant and adult. (From Nelson, N. M. (1976). Respiration and circulation after birth. In C. A. Smith & N. M. Nelson (Eds.), *The physiology of the newborn infant* (p. 207). Springfield, IL: Charles C Thomas.)

ate stronger contractions with high inspiratory pressures in order to expand stiff, noncompliant lungs.

Increased diaphragmatic force and the pliable chest wall lead to chest distortion.[96, 265] Therefore, a portion of the energy and force of the contraction is wasted. Retractions are the clinical signs of these distortions and are indications of the degree of inward rib cage collapse during forceful diaphragmatic contractions.[271] This increase in work of breathing can lead to fatigue and eventually apnea.

The compliance of the chest wall combined with the compliance of the lungs affects the closing volume, closing capacity, expiratory reserve volume, and functional residual capacity. For the neonate, this means that a high closing volume and high closing capacity combine with a low expiratory reserve volume and FRC, culminating in a propensity toward lung collapse.[269]

Mechanical Properties of the Respiratory System

The work of breathing is the cumulative product of the pressure and volume of air moved at each instant. The work is done by the muscles as energy is expended to overcome the elastic and resistive forces (compliance and resistance) of the lung and thorax as well as the frictional resistance to air movement. The respiratory muscles expend about half their energy on inspiration. The rest is stored within the tissues (which have been stretched) as potential energy. As the potential energy is released, expiration occurs passively.

There are two major sources of resistance that the respiratory muscles must overcome during each breath. These are tissue elastic resistance that is created by displacement of the lung and chest wall from their resting positions (compliance) and resistance presented by gas molecules flowing through the airways.

The system is most efficient when the respiratory rate and tidal volume are set to require the minimum expenditure of work. This can be assessed by evaluating the amount of oxygen used in performing the work. Under normal circumstances the oxygen consumed is only a small fraction of the total metabolic requirement. The newborn infant expends the least amount of energy when breathing 30 to 40 breaths per minute.[82]

Lung Compliance

The pressure gradient necessary to overcome the elastic recoil force encountered in the lung depends on tidal volume and lung compliance. Compliance is the measurement of the elastic properties opposing a change in volume (ml) per unit of change in pressure (cm H_2O) (Hooke's law). This can be demonstrated in a pressure-volume curve that relates a change in lung volume to the change in the alveolar-to-intrapleural pressure gradient (i.e., transpulmonary pressure). The slope of the curve indicates the compliance. The flatter the curve, the stiffer the lung is.[269]

Lung compliance depends on the tissue elastic characteristics of the parenchyma, connective tissue, and blood vessels, as well as the surface tension in the alveoli and the initial lung volume before inflation. When the lung must be inflated from a very low lung volume the required pressure gradient is greater.

For the healthy preterm infant lung compliance is similar to that of the full-term infant. The change in lung compliance is sensed by the stretch receptors of the lung. These receptors along with the muscle spindle fibers from the respiratory muscles transmit information to the respiratory center in order to modify the drive necessary to maintain ventilation. Lung disease usually leads to a decrease in lung compliance, which translates to a smaller volume change for pressure change.

The most significant determinant of elastic properties is the air-liquid interface. When molecules are aligned at an air-liquid interface they lack opposing molecules on one side; this means that the intermolecular attractive forces are unbalanced and there is a tendency for the molecules to move away from the interface. This reduces the internal surface area of the lung and therefore augments elastic recoil.

Surfactant varies surface tension, allowing for high surface tensions at large lung volumes and low tensions at low volumes. Surfactant forms an insoluble folded surface film upon compression and thereby lowers surface tension. This tends to stabilize air spaces of unequal size and prevents their collapse. Without surfactant, smaller alveoli tend to empty into larger ones, resulting in microatelectasis alternating with hyperaeration.

Alveolar collapse occurs in a number of diseases, probably the most notable is respiratory distress syndrome (RDS). In RDS, surfactant deficiency is directly related to gestational age and developmental immaturity of the lungs. Surfactant synthesis, however, is also dependent on normal pH and pulmonary perfusion. Therefore any disease or event that interferes with these processes may lead to surfactant deficiencies (e.g., asphyxia, hemorrhagic shock, and pulmonary edema).[14, 80, 232, 251]

Lung Resistance

Lung resistance is dependent upon the size and geometric arrangements of the airways, viscous resistance of the lung tissue, and the proportion of laminar to turbulent airflow. Resistance varies inversely with lung volume, meaning the greater the lung volume the less resistance is encountered, and vice versa. This is because the diameter of the airways increases with the expansion of the parenchyma.

Gas flows through a tube from a point of higher pressure to a point of lower pressure. Two patterns of flow have been identified based on the magnitude of the pressure drop and its relationship to the rate of gas flow. These patterns are termed laminar and turbulent. In laminar flow, resistance is determined by the radius and length of the tube during the flow. Laminar flow can become turbulent if the flow rate rises excessively or when the angle or diameter of the tube changes abruptly (e.g., at branch points).

In the adult, the upper airways (especially the nose) account for the major portion of total airway resistance.[271] In neonates and children under 5 years of age, it is the peripheral airways that contribute the most to airway resistance.[260] The decreased diameter of airways, especially in the periphery, is the reason for this increased resistance. The distal airway growth in diameter and length lags behind proximal growth during the first 5 years of life. Therefore, a small decrement in the caliber of airways can lead to a very large increase in peripheral airway resistance.[271]

Cartilage provides the support for stability of the conducting airways. With ongoing development, there is an increase in number of cartilage rings during the first 2 months of life and an increase in total area of support over the remainder of childhood. The lack of support in the neonate can lead to dynamic compression of the trachea during situations associated with high expiratory flow rates and increased airway resistance (e.g., crying).[336, 261]

In disease states, resistance is increased either by a decrease in the intraluminal size of the airway or through compression or contraction of the walls of the airway.[271] Peripheral airways are tethered open by the elastic mesh of the pulmonary parenchyma and the transmural pressure gradient (intraluminal airway pressure greater than the intrapleural pressure). During forced expiration intrapleural pressure rises significantly; this is transmitted to the alveoli and increased

even further by the pulmonary parenchyma elastic recoil pressure. Initially this maintains a favorable pressure gradient. However, a pressure drop must occur from alveolus to mouth during active expiration, and there will be a point in the airway at which intraluminal pressure will equal intrapleural pressure (equal pressure point). As the gas continues to move toward the mouth, the forces maintaining airway patency are overwhelmed and the airway will collapse.[271] If the elastic parenchyma meshwork is destroyed, as with bronchopulmonary dysplasia (BPD), airway collapse is even more likely.

Resistance increases with decreasing gestational age and with specific lung diseases that are more prominent in low birth weight infants (RDS, BPD). The increased resistance is sensed by respiratory muscles, leading to an increase in ventilatory drive. In the infant with BPD, this may lead to a change in pleural pressure to as much as 20 to 30 cm H_2O pressure.[367] Changes in the radius of the larynx or trachea because of edema (e.g., with repeated intubation for meconium aspiration) or as a result of intubation also increase resistance. This effect may be quite pronounced because the resistance is generated in the large airways where resistance should be at its lowest.[239]

Time Constants

Time constants reflect the combined effect of resistance and compliance on the lung. The time needed for a given lung unit to fill to 63% of its final capacity is the product of resistance and compliance. Nichols and Rogers noted that if the resistance and compliance are equal in two adjacent lung units (alveoli), the time constant will be the same and there will be no redistribution of gases between the alveoli.[271] If the time constant of one unit is longer, but the compliances remain equal, the two alveoli will eventually reach the same volume. However, the longer the time constant the slower the filling will be owing to the increased resistance. In this instance, the intraluminal pressure in the alveolus with the least resistance will be higher and lead to redistribution of its gases into the adjacent slower filling alveolus.

The time constant can also be lengthened when compliance is increased, but resistance remains the same. In this circumstance, the less compliant alveolus will fill faster than its adjacent more compliant neighbor. This is due to the decreased volume the less compliant alveoli can hold. Redistribution of gases will occur if inflation is interrupted prematurely owing to the increased pressure in the less compliant alveolus as compared to the adjacent lung unit.[271]

This redistribution of gases in the lung is not a major factor in the normal lung, in that the alveoli are relatively stable and do not change much in size.[271] This is a result of the effect of surfactant upon the lung.

Ventilation

Once air enters the lungs, it must come in contact with the blood in order to effect gas exchange. The drop in negative pressure causes air to move by bulk flow down the air passages to the level of the bronchioles. From this point forward, the movement of air into the acinar portion of the lungs is due to the random movement of the molecules from a higher area of concentration to a lower area of concentration (diffusion). Any factor that impedes the flow of gas to the acinus reduces gas exchange and influences the partial pressure of gas within the blood.

It is therefore the effective interface of ventilation with blood flow that is responsible for the adequacy of oxygen uptake and carbon dioxide removal. In this section, the factors that affect ventilation at the alveolar level are discussed.

Dead Space Ventilation

A variable portion of each breath is not involved in gas exchange and is therefore wasted; this is considered dead space ventilation. There are two types of dead space; anatomic dead space and alveolar dead space. Anatomic dead space is that volume of gas within the conducting airways that cannot engage in gas exchange. Alveolar dead space is the volume of inspired gas that reaches the alveolus but does not participate in gas exchange because of inadequate perfusion of that alveolus. The total dead space (anatomic and alveolar) is termed physiologic dead space. Physiologic dead space is usually expressed as a fraction of the tidal volume, and is approximately 0.3 in infants and adults.[271] Patients experiencing respiratory failure have elevated dead space–to–tidal volume ratios, which result in hypoxia and hypercarbia unless counteracted by an increase in the amount of air expired per minute.[271]

Pleural Pressure

The differences in pleural pressure within the lung play a significant role in determining the distribution of gases. During spontaneous breathing, a greater proportion of gas is distributed to the dependent regions of the lung.[109] It is assumed that the difference in subatmospheric (negative) intrapleural pressure at the base and at the apex is the reason for this distribution pattern. Interestingly, alveolar pressure remains constant in all regions of the lung. Subsequently, the transpulmonary distending pressure in the dependent regions is decreased, leading to a reduced lung volume in these areas. As Nichols and Rogers point out, the smaller alveoli in the dependent lung regions lie on the steeper slope of the transpulmonary pressure–to–lung volume curve (Fig. 7–9), resulting in a greater portion of the tidal volume being directed to the dependent alveoli during normal breathing.[271] A greater portion of the pulmonary perfusion goes to the dependent regions as well, thereby matching ventilation and perfusion more closely.

Lung Volumes

Functional Residual Capacity

The FRC is established during the first breaths, forming the alveolar reservoir at end expiration and allowing for continuous gas exchange between respiratory efforts and stabilization of PaO_2. Normally the FRC composes 30 to 40% of the total capacity of the lung and may change volume from breath to breath. Immediately following birth the FRC is low, increasing rapidly with successive breaths. In preterm infants with lung disease, the FRC stays low until lung disease resolves. The goal is to keep the FRC above the passive resting volume of the lung, which may be difficult for neonates owing to their pliable chest wall.

The role of the FRC is crucial in the energy expenditure of the respiratory musculature. It minimizes the work of breathing while optimizing the compliance of the system and maintaining a gas reservoir during expiration.[96]

Closing Capacity

As noted earlier, in the neonate (especially the preterm infant) it is possible for lung

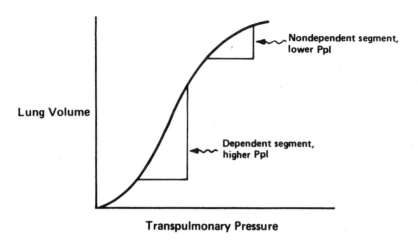

FIGURE 7–9. Transpulmonary pressure–to–volume curve. Effect of the changes in pleural pressure from the apex to the base of the lung. Pleural pressure increases from the apex to the base of the lung. With the increase in pleural pressure, alveoli become smaller at the base. Smaller alveoli are on the steep portion of the pressure-volume (compliance) curve, and thus a given change in transpulmonary pressure produces a greater increase in volume in the smaller alveoli. (From Nichols, D. G. & Rogers, M. C. (1987). Developmental physiology of the respiratory system. In M. C. Rogers (Ed.), *Textbook of pediatric intensive care* (Vol. 1, p. 88). Baltimore: Williams & Wilkins.)

volumes to be reduced below the FRC during quiet breathing, with dependent regions of the lung being closed to the main bronchi (closing capacity). When the closing capacity exceeds the FRC, the ventilation-perfusion ratio drops and hypoxia and hypercarbia occur. If total atelectasis exists, then the closing capacity exceeds not only the FRC but also the tidal volume, and these portions of the lung are closed during expiration and inspiration. The use of end-expiratory pressure is designed to raise the FRC above closing capacity.[271] Continuous distending pressure is used in the neonatal population when chest wall compliance leads to marked distortion and altered lung volumes, as well as during disease states associated with alveolar collapse (e.g., RDS).

The greater closing capacity seen in children under 6 years and in adults over 40 years is probably due to decreased elastic recoil in the lung.[264, 265] Elastic recoil is that property of the lung that allows it to retract away from the chest wall, creating a subatmospheric pressure in the intrapleural space. The decrease in elastic recoil results in the subatmospheric pressure in the intrapleural space being raised, leading to increased airway closure in dependent regions.[271]

Perfusion

Alveolar ventilation is not only dependent upon the functioning of the airways, but also on the functioning of the pulmonary vasculature. Pulmonary vascular muscle thickness is a function of gestational age, with the preterm infant having less well developed smooth muscle. This incomplete development results in a drop in pulmonary vascular resistance much sooner after delivery, predisposing the infant to a faster onset of congestive heart failure and left-to-right shunting.[271]

Normal Pulmonary Blood Flow

The majority of pulmonary blood flow is distributed to the dependent regions of the lungs owing to gravitational forces (Fig. 7–10). In zone 1 (apex of the lung) the alveolar pressure is greater than the pulmonary artery and venous pressures. As a result, the pulmonary vessels collapse with concomitant loss of gas exchange and wasted ventilation.[271]

In zone 2, pulmonary artery pressure exceeds alveolar pressure, and blood flow resumes. The perfusion pressure increases as blood flows downward; this results in a linear increase in blood flow. Slowing of blood occurs when the pulmonary venous pressure and alveolar pressure are equal.[271]

Pulmonary venous pressure and pulmonary artery pressure increase, exceeding alveolar pressure in zone 3. In the more dependent regions of this zone, the transmural pressure increases, with resultant dilation of the vessels, and blood flow increases.[271]

Posture differences between the upright adult and supine lying infant probably affect pulmonary blood distribution; however, these have not been explicated. The general principles in all likelihood still apply, but maybe to a lesser extent. Wasted ventilation in the apices due to lack of perfusion is

FIGURE 7–10. Lung zones. Normal distribution of pulmonary blood flow. Gravitational force makes flow greatest in the base. At the apex (zone 1), there is no flow because alveolar pressure (P_A) exceeds pulmonary arterial (P_a) and venous (P_v) pressures. Flow begins in zone 2 and is determined by the P_a-P_A driving pressure gradient. In zone 3, vessels dilate because of an increased transmural pressure (P_a-P_{PL} and P_v-P_{PL} [P_{PL}, pleural pressure]). Therefore flow increases even though driving pressure (P_a-P_v) is constant throughout zone 3. (From West, J. B., Dollery, C. T., & Naimark, A. (1964). Distribution of blood flow in isolated lung: Relation to vascular and alveolar pressure. *J Appl Physiol, 19,* 713.)

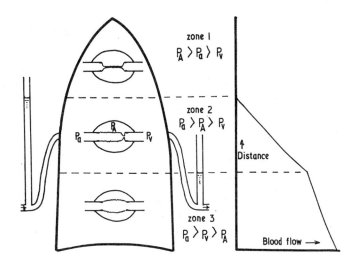

probably much less likely in the supine position, helping to balance some of the limitations encountered in the neonatal lung.

Abnormal Distribution of Pulmonary Blood Flow

There are numerous factors that may influence the distribution of pulmonary blood flow in the lung. One of the most significant to the neonate is hypoxia. Vasoconstriction occurs when alveolar hypoxia is encountered. If diffuse, hypoxia may result in an increase in intravascular pulmonary artery pressure, which is more intense in infants than in adults.[273]

Ventilation-Perfusion Matching

Mismatching of ventilation and perfusion is the most common reason for hypoxia and a frequent result of the neonatal respiratory system's liabilities. Efficient gas exchange in the lungs requires matching of pulmonary ventilation and perfusion. The relationship between ventilation and perfusion is expressed as a ratio and reflects the correlation between alveolar ventilation and capillary perfusion for the lung as a whole.

The ventilation of the air space should be adequate to remove the carbon dioxide delivered to it from the blood, and the perfusion of the air space should be no greater than that which allows oxygenation and complete saturation of the blood on its brief passage through the alveolar capillaries. Ideal efficiency would occur if ventilation were perfectly matched to perfusion, yielding a ratio of 1 (Fig. 7–11).

In the healthy adult, capillary blood spends 0.75 second in the alveolus, and O_2/CO_2 exchange occurs across the 0.5 μ alveolar-capillary membrane. As the blood leaves the alveolus, the blood gas tensions are identical with those of the alveolar gas. The gas tensions achieved at equilibrium are dependent upon rate of ventilation, membrane thickness, membrane area, capillary blood flow, venous gas tensions, and inspired gas tensions.[273, 290, 291] In order for equilibrium to be achieved rapidly the area for exchange must be large enough to allow the blood to be spread thinly over the vessel wall and blood and gas must actively mix together.[273]

Matching of ventilation to perfusion is dependent upon gravity to a large extent. Both ventilation and perfusion increase as air and blood move down the lung, with perfusion increasing more than ventilation. Right ventricular pressure is inadequate to fully perfuse the apices of the lung. On the other hand, lung weight leads to a relatively greater negative intrapleural pressure at the apex than at the base, resulting in the apical alveoli being better expanded but receiving a smaller portion of each tidal volume than the bases. Along with this, there is reduced perfusion in the apices creating a high ventilation-perfusion ($\dot{V}/\dot{Q}$) ratio.[271, 273]

Ventilation-perfusion ratios of zero are characteristic of shunts. In this situation, no ventilation takes place during the passage of blood through the lungs. The pulmonary capillary blood arrives in the left atrium with the same gas tensions it had when it was mixed venous blood. Examples of shunts include the normal bronchial and thebesian circulations, perfusion of an atelectatic area,

Ventilation-Perfusion Ratios

Ventilation-perfusion ($\dot{V}/\dot{Q}$) ratios are based on the distribution of gases, the distribution of the pulmonary circulation, and the interrelationship between these two factors. This interrelationship is affected by the rate of air flow into the lungs (which is a function of depth of inspiration, rate of inspiration, airway resistance, and lung compliance) and pulmonary circulation (which is influenced by cardiac output and pulmonary vascular resistance). The ideal ratio occurs when ventilation and perfusion are matched such that the sites available on the hemoglobin molecules are equal to the concentration of oxygen molecules in the alveoli and there is sufficient time for the diffusion of oxygen across the membranes and attachment of hemoglobin. The "ideal" lung is depicted in Figure 7–11. In this instance neither ventilation (oxygen) nor blood flow is wasted. Interestingly, the usual distribution of gases and blood is neither equal nor ideal.

Maldistribution of pulmonary blood flow is the most frequent cause of reduced oxygenation of arterial blood. The degree of nonuniformity of distribution is probably greater for pulmonary circulation than it is for gas distribution. The uneven distribution not only occurs between the two lungs but also between lobes and alveolar segments. This is usually manifested by a reduction in the Pao_2.

Distribution can range from the unventilated to the unperfused alveoli, with all degrees of variation in between. Ventilated alveoli that are not perfused compose the alveolar dead space and have Pao_2 and $Paco_2$ values that are essentially equivalent to those of inspired air. This is because there is no alveolar gas exchange with the blood to modify the gas concentrations in the alveoli (see Fig. 7–12). On the other hand, alveoli that are perfused but not ventilated result in intrapulmonary shunts in which Pao_2 and $Paco_2$ values are the same as those in mixed venous blood. In this situation, the air trapped within the alveoli equilibrates with the venous blood traversing the capillaries of the alveoli (see Fig. 7–12). Some degree of gas exchange occurs in all other situations.

When there is a low ventilation-perfusion ratio (<1) the alveoli are underventilated with respect to perfusion or overperfused with respect to ventilation. In circumstances in which the alveoli are overventilated for the perfusion available, there is a high ventilation-perfusion ratio (>1). In these abnormal or disease states the ventilation-perfusion inequalities may increase in magnitude, involving greater and greater numbers of alveoli. The net result is a significant impact on gas exchange and blood gases.

venoarterial shunts, and cyanotic congenital heart disease with blood flow directly from the right to the left side of the heart.

High $\dot{V}/\dot{Q}$ ratios are the result of increased dead space and may occur if the blood is spread in an extremely thin film over a very large surface area or if blood is vigorously mixed with large volumes of air. Rapid equilibration occurs, but a large amount of ventilation is required.[273] Here there is wasted ventilation, either in anatomic conducting airways or in poorly perfused alveoli (alveolar dead space). Thus a large amount of ventilation is wasted on a relatively small amount of blood without significantly changing the oxygen content. This inefficient gas exchange will eventually result in CO_2 retention.[271]

On the other hand, alveolar underventilation results in low $\dot{V}/\dot{Q}$ ratios. In this situation, ventilation is low in relation to perfusion but not entirely absent. This is the normal state for the lung bases in an erect position. It is also found in disease in which airway obstruction reduces ventilation to alveolar units (e.g., asthma, cystic fibrosis).

The blood perfusing the underventilated alveoli is incompletely oxygenated and a lower amount of carbon dioxide is removed. Partial venoarterial shunts contribute incomplete arterialized blood to the arterial stream; this is termed venous admixture. This is reflected in an elevated partial pressure of CO_2 upon blood gas evaluation.

Abnormalities of $\dot{V}/\dot{Q}$ ratios may be secondary to either too much or too little ventilation to an area with normal blood flow, too much or too little blood flow with normal ventilation, or some combination of the two. Whichever occurs, the lung's regulatory mechanisms work to achieve and maintain the ideal. In areas where $\dot{V}/\dot{Q}$ ratio is high and CO_2 levels are low, local airway constriction occurs in order to reduce the amount of ventilation going to the area. When the opposite occurs, the airways dilate in an attempt to increase ventilation to the area and improve CO_2 exchange. When oxygenation is also affected and low alveolar oxygen concentrations are found, the lung reduces blood flow to the region. These mechanisms are finite, however.

In the newborn, most of the ventilated

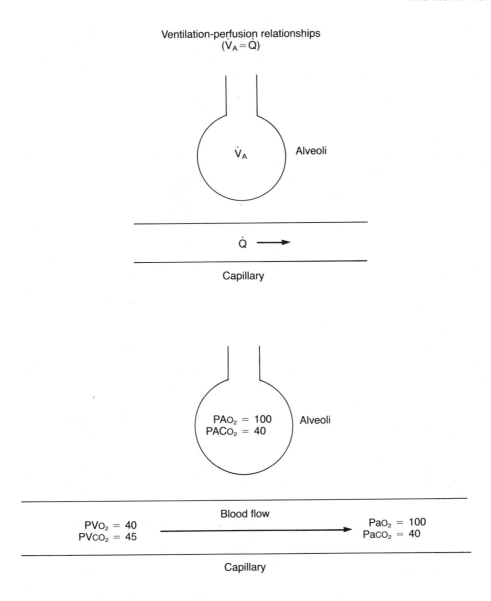

Ventilation-perfusion relationships
$(\dot{V}_A = \dot{Q})$

$\dot{V}_A$ Alveoli

$\dot{Q} \longrightarrow$

Capillary

$PAO_2 = 100$ Alveoli
$PACO_2 = 40$

Blood flow

$PVO_2 = 40$ $PaO_2 = 100$
$PVCO_2 = 45$ $PaCO_2 = 40$

Capillary

Gas exchange in an ideal alveolar capillary unit

FIGURE 7–11.   Ideal lung ventilation-perfusion.

areas are well perfused and there is little dead space. However, in newborn infants significant amounts of perfusion are wasted on unexpanded air spaces (intrapulmonary shunts) as transitional events progress. The lower PaO_2 in the newborn demonstrates the widened alveolar to arterial PO_2 gradient, reflecting the increased venous admixture. Although perfusion of unexpanded air spaces may play a significant role in this, the continued right-to-left shunting through transitional circulatory circuits is another contributory factor. The premature infant is at even greater risk for shunting and venous

admixture owing to developmental immaturity.[211]

Shunting and wasted ventilation are normal features of the newborn lung. The latter results from transition from fluid-filled to air-filled lungs, in which alveoli are underventilated but normally perfused. These effects begin to dissipate after 1 to 2 hours of air breathing. During the first few days of life the neonatal lung has a greater shunt component and a larger proportion of low $\dot{V}/\dot{Q}$ areas as compared with the adult. Tidal volume, alveolar volume, and dead space volume/breath are similar (when expressed in ml/kg), however. These arterial-alveolar differences in both O_2 and CO_2 persist in the full-term infant for about a week owing to the venoarterial shunting. These gradually dissipate and adult values are achieved.[210, 269]

Effect of $\dot{V}/\dot{Q}$ Mismatching on O_2

As inspired gas moves to the level of the arterial circulation there is a stepwise decrease in oxygen tension. This results in a reduced oxygen content in the alveoli; however, alveolar oxygen levels remain higher than those in the arterial blood. This maintains a concentration gradient that supports oxygen diffusion. If the ideal were maintained, at the end of equilibration the alveolar and arterial oxygen concentrations would be the same. This, however, is not the case. There remains a difference between the two ($AaDO_2$), which is reflective of the imperfect matching of ventilation to perfusion (Fig. 7–12).

Under normal circumstances this difference is relatively small and is secondary to the anatomic shunts through the thebesian and bronchial circulations. The hypoxemic patient, however, may have additional shunts (congenital heart disease) or increased $\dot{V}/\dot{Q}$ mismatching. Both situations result in an increased venous admixture.

$\dot{V}/\dot{Q}$ mismatching affects oxygenation by lowering the arterial PO_2 and widening the $AaDO_2$. This occurs for two reasons, the first being an increased blood flow through low $\dot{V}/\dot{Q}$ segments rather than high $\dot{V}/\dot{Q}$ segments. This results in an increased volume of desaturated blood. The second reason is the sigmoid shape of the oxygen-hemoglobin dissociation curve. This implies that the alveolar PO_2 is not proportional to oxygen content or saturation.

On the oxygen-hemoglobin dissociation curve, low $\dot{V}/\dot{Q}$ segments, with lower alveolar PO_2 values, will have a proportionately greater drop in O_2 content. This is because of their position on the steep portion of the curve. The high $\dot{V}/\dot{Q}$ segments will have higher alveolar PO_2 values but will not exhibit the expected increase in oxygen content because they lie on the flat portion of the curve. In this area of the curve, changes in PO_2 have very little effect on oxygen content or saturation.

The net effect is one of low $\dot{V}/\dot{Q}$ segments negating high ones. Although the O_2 content is higher in the latter, it is not high enough to compensate for the markedly lower O_2 content found in the low $\dot{V}/\dot{Q}$ segments. Therefore, arterial desaturation occurs.

Currently, measurement of $\dot{V}/\dot{Q}$ mismatching as it relates to desaturation is difficult. Venous admixture is a convenient way to describe the amount of mixed venous blood it would take to obtain the observed arterial oxygen content. Venous admixture can be expressed as the ratio of shunted blood to total pulmonary blood flow, reflecting the efficiency of the lung in oxygenating the blood.

The magnitude of this ratio determines in part what effect an increase in fractional inspired oxygen (FIO_2) will have on PaO_2. If the ratio is equal to zero, there will be a linear increase in PaO_2 with increasing inspired oxygen. Once the ratio is 0.5 or greater, increasing the FIO_2 will have no effect on PaO_2.[271]

Effect of $\dot{V}/\dot{Q}$ Mismatching on CO_2

$PaCO_2$ is determined mainly by the degree of alveolar ventilation in relation to the CO_2 produced by the cells. When alveolar ventilation is reduced secondary to an increase in alveolar dead space (alveoli are ventilated but not perfused or underperfused), CO_2 levels in the blood begin to rise. This is reflected in the widened gradient between end-expiratory PCO_2 and alveolar PCO_2, with end-expiratory PCO_2 being lower owing to the addition of alveolar dead space gas, which does not contain CO_2.[271]

The difference between alveolar and capillary PCO_2 is usually low owing to the diffusibility of CO_2. This means that even with a large venous admixture load there would be only a slight increase in arterial PCO_2. The small change occurs because the CO_2 dissociation curve is linear and relatively steep (within the normal range), meaning that large changes in CO_2 content produce small changes in CO_2 tension.

Developmental Differences in $\dot{V}/\dot{Q}$ Matching

In the full-term infant, markedly lower PaO_2 levels are found. This is indicative of a widened alveolar to arterial PO_2 gradient and an increase in venous admixture being added to the arterial blood. The persistent right-to-left shunting through fetal vascular channels along with atelectatic areas of the lung

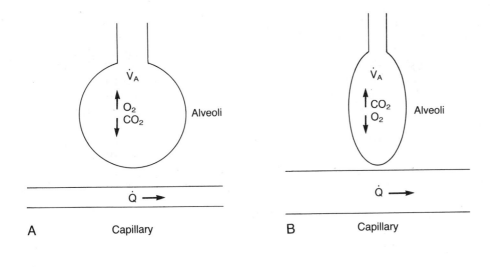

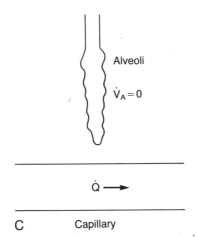

FIGURE 7–12. Ventilation-perfusion mismatching. *A*, High $\dot{V}/\dot{Q}$; *B*, low $\dot{V}/\dot{Q}$; *C*, shunt.

being perfused is the source of the admixture.[210, 211] In the adult, the major component of venous admixture is due to the maldistribution of ventilation.[271]

This alteration stabilizes as transition progresses, lasting a week or so in the full-term infant. The preterm infant, however, is at greater risk for desaturation because of increased chest wall deformation and increased ductal shunting. For the preterm infant it may be several weeks before complete transition and stabilization occur.[269]

Hypoxemia and thermal stress may result in ductal opening and shunting during the early transitional period for both full-term and preterm infants. It is not until late infancy and early childhood that venous ad-

mixture falls to adult levels. Beyond 7 years of age the PaO_2 does not vary much, stabilizing between 95 and 100 mmHg.[271]

Alveolar-Capillary Membrane

The alveolar-capillary membrane is the physical barrier separating the alveolar gases from the pulmonary capillary blood. The barrier also helps prevent liquid movement from the circulation to the alveolus, thereby avoiding alveolar flooding and collapse. Transudation of fluid resulting in pulmonary edema is a major cause of respiratory failure in all age groups.

Diffusion is the movement of gases from an area of high concentration to an area of lower concentration until equilibrium is achieved. This is the mechanism by which gas exchange occurs at the alveolar-capillary membrane. The rate of diffusion is directly proportional to the surface area available and the solubility of the gases and is inversely proportional to the diffusion distance. The diffusion capacity for oxygen is greatly affected by the time it takes for the oxygen to combine with hemoglobin. The surface area in the normal lung is determined by the amount of ventilated and perfused tissue available, increasing with age, height, and body surface area.[55]

Oxygen-Hemoglobin Dissociation Curve

Because of the low oxygen environment in which the fetus lives, the need for an increased affinity for oxygen is essential to survival. Fetal hemoglobin alters this affinity, and 2,3-diphosphoglycerate (2,3-DPG) regulates it.[31, 69] When 2,3-DPG binds with fetal gamma chains it does not lower oxygen affinity as it does with adult hemoglobin beta chains. The fetal oxygen-hemoglobin dissociation curve therefore lies to the left of the adult curve (Fig. 7–13). This means that in the fetus and neonate the affinity of oxygen for hemoglobin is greater and the release of oxygen to the tissues is somewhat less than in the adult at any given Po_2.

Oxygen Consumption

Oxygen consumption in the newly born infant is twice that of the adult in relation to weight. One of the major factors affecting oxygen consumption in the neonate is temperature. The neutral thermal environment is that environmental temperature at which oxygen consumption is minimal. Small changes in environmental temperature can result in dramatic increases in oxygen consumption. A decrease of 2° C in environmental temperature can double oxygen requirements. If the infant is unable to increase delivery to meet these needs, tissue oxygenation falls and may become insufficient. When oxygen consumption is no longer possible, the cell switches to anaerobic metabolism to meet energy and work needs.

Tissue Respiration

The ultimate purpose of oxygenation of arterial blood is for consumption by the cells during aerobic metabolism. Aerobic metabolism is desirable because 20 times more energy is made available when substrates are metabolized aerobically versus anaerobically.[271] Molecular oxygen is used in oxidation-reduction reactions in cells, in which oxidation is the loss of electrons from an atom or molecule and reduction is the gain of electrons.[264]

When one substance is oxidized, another is reduced. Reducing agents give up electrons; electron acceptors are oxidizing agents. Oxygen is an oxidizing agent. Food molecules (substrate), such as glucose, are reducing agents. Within the cells of the body, oxygen serves as final acceptor in the process of cell respiration. Energy is derived from this process and is used to form adenosine triphosphate (ATP) from adenosine diphosphate (ADP) and inorganic phosphate. When energy is later released, ATP is hydrolyzed to ADP. It is the hydrolysis reaction and cellular work activities that allow ATP to provide the energy to accomplish cellular functions.

CONSEQUENCES OF HYPOXIA IN THE CELL

When tissue hypoxia occurs, aerobic metabolism is impaired and there is a subsequent depletion in the supply of ATP available. Therefore those processes that require energy will not occur. If the hypoxic event is not too severe or too long, cellular activities may be disrupted only for a period of time, and any damage is reversible.

Cell death occurs when the loss of ATP leads to failure of the sodium pump. Once pump failure develops, sodium is free to flow into the cell, bringing water with it. The cell and intracellular structures swell with this increased fluid volume. Along with this, anaerobic metabolism is activated, leading to a fall in cellular pH. The lowered pH interferes with enzyme activities and alters the permeability of the cell membrane. Increased permeability allows calcium to diffuse into the cell, resulting in oxidative phosphorylation uncoupling and a further reduction in ATP formation. As the fluid influx increases, the ribosomes located on the endoplasmic reticulum are shed, and protein synthesis is disrupted.[264, 271]

Cell rupture and death may occur if enzymes leak from the intracellular lysosomes. Once released into the intracellular fluid, the enzymes are activated by the low pH, and cell disintegration is inevitable. Enzyme levels

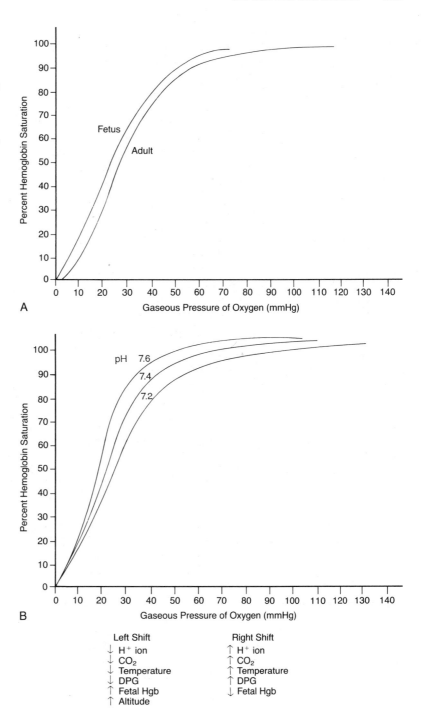

FIGURE 7–13. Oxygen-hemoglobin dissociation curve. *A,* Comparison between fetal and adult curves. *B,* Shift of the curve to the right by increases in hydrogen ions, CO_2, temperature, or DPG. (*B* redrawn from Guyton, A.C. (1991). *Textbook of medical physiology* (8th ed., p. 438). Philadelphia: WB Saunders.)

(e.g., creatine phosphokinase) can be measured once cellular disintegration occurs and the enzymes are released into the extracellular fluid.

SYSTEMIC MANIFESTATIONS OF CELLULAR HYPOXIA

Abnormal functioning of the organ systems is due to the energy-dependent cellular activities. In the brain, aerobic metabolism is necessary for maintaining the sodium-potassium pump, which allows for nerve impulse transmission and synthesis of the synaptic chemicals. Decreased mental activity, impaired judgment, and neuromuscular incoordination may occur when cellular hypoxia is present.

Muscle weakness and fatigue are signs of

muscle cell hypoxia. Skeletal muscles have increased compensatory mechanisms and are therefore less susceptible to hypoxic damage than other organ systems.

Respiratory responses include an increase in frequency and depth of respiration. This is an attempt to provide an increased oxygen supply to the blood. Acidosis may occur, contributing to the respiratory compensation. Heart rate and cardiac output also increase, as the cardiovascular system attempts to deliver more oxygenated blood to the tissues.

Hematologic responses include stimulation of erythropoietin by low circulating oxygen levels through the kidneys. This results in stimulation of the bone marrow with formation and maturation of red blood cells, which are then released into vascular circulation. In acute hypoxia, immature red blood cells are released. If a chronic hypoxic state exists, the marrow produces more cells and the volume of mature cells increases. This response is an attempt to increase the oxygen-carrying capacity of the blood, thereby improving the oxygen availability to the tissues.

CAUSES OF HYPOXIA

There are several factors that affect the availability of oxygen to the cells. Hypoxia can be categorized depending on which of these factors is responsible for the alterations in tissue oxygenation. Hypoxic hypoxia occurs when tissue oxygenation is inadequate because the PaO_2 is reduced and hemoglobin is only partially saturated. This situation may be the result of decreased inspired oxygen (altitude), impaired pulmonary diffusion (pulmonary edema), altered perfusion of the lung (persistent pulmonary hypertension), or some combination of these.[264]

Anemic hypoxia indicates that the hemoglobin available to transport oxygen is reduced although completely saturated. PaO_2 levels are usually normal in this situation. Anemia may be the result of excessive loss or destruction of red blood cells or impaired production of hemoglobin or red blood cells. Physiologic compensation for anemia includes an increased heart rate and cardiac output. Hypoxia results in vasodilatation and decreased blood viscosity, thereby increasing blood flow in an attempt to maintain normal tissue oxygenation.[264, 271]

When tissue oxygenation is decreased owing to inadequate blood flow, as with hyperviscosity syndrome, the infant is at risk for circulatory hypoxia. The oxygen content of the blood may be normal, but the blood flow to the tissues is reduced, consequently oxygen availability is also reduced.

Histotoxic hypoxia is the term for the reduced oxygen uptake capacity of cells or the reduced oxygen utilization of the cells. Blood flow and oxygen tensions are usually not disturbed. Some toxins (e.g., cyanide, arsenic, and some barbiturates) may interfere with oxidative phosphorylation. Deficiencies in thyroid hormone or niacin also can impair cellular energy production and oxygen use, thereby potentiating cellular hypoxia and altered cellular activity levels.[264]

CONSEQUENCES OF CELLULAR HYPEROXIA

Oxygen can be a toxic agent when too much is available. Prolonged exposure in high concentrations (as in ventilatory support) or increased oxygen pressure (e.g., deep sea diving) can lead to oxygen toxicity. In either situation, time is a critical factor. Toxic responses require prolonged exposure to hyperoxia.

For the premature infant hyperoxia is a relative term and must be evaluated in light of the PaO_2 levels that are normally encountered in utero. Therefore, small increases in PO_2 may represent a hyperoxic state and place the infant at risk for oxygen injury. Currently, the pulmonary system, central nervous system, and retina have been identified as being susceptible to oxygen injury. In the neonate the organ systems that are affected are the pulmonary system and the retina.

Hyperoxia results in excessive production of highly reactive metabolites of oxygen called free radicals. These metabolites are normally produced during oxidation-reduction reactions within the cells and are detoxified by the antioxidant system. In hyperoxic states this system is overwhelmed and unable to keep up with the generation of free radicals. This can result in cellular damage through irritation (lungs, see section on BPD) or vasoconstriction (retina).

In the eye, high concentrations of PaO_2 cause reversible vasoconstriction. In premature infants this constriction of blood vessels leads to obliteration of the immature vessels and retinal hypoxia (retinopathy of prematurity). Capillary development is stimulated but is abnormal. There is a lack of organization and the blood vessels may actually extend beyond the retinal surface into the vitreous body. Once the hyperoxia is resolved there can be resolution with normal retinal development. However, in severe cases retinal hemorrhages can occur and fibrous scar tissue forms, causing buckling of the retina, leading to detachment and blindness. Similar changes have been reported in severely hypoxic term infants. Transfusion of preterm infants with adult blood rapidly increases the amount of adult hemoglobin, altering the oxygen-carrying capacity and increasing the risk of retinopathy of prematurity.

CLINICAL IMPLICATIONS FOR NEONATAL CARE

Respiratory Risk Factors

Although there are many liabilities within the neonatal respiratory system, the healthy term infant achieves transition to the extrauterine environment without any difficulties. However, the developmental stage of the system does increase the possibility of respiratory distress and failure above that seen in older individuals. Both anatomic and functional development are required to achieve adult functioning, therefore both contribute to the risk of distress.

Anatomic risk factors include the incomplete development of the bone and cartilage that make up the thoracic cavity and are a part of the respiratory pump. The increased compliance of the thorax makes it extremely important that the intercostal muscles be able to contract and fixate the chest so that adequate pressure can be generated and inspiration occurs. Although full-term infants appear to compensate well, the intercostal muscles and accessory muscles are still not completely developed. This contributes to diaphragmatic breathing and chest wall instability, which can lead to higher closing volumes and a decreased FRC. In disease states in which decreased resistance occurs, the inspiratory pressures necessary to fill the lungs may result in deformation of the chest wall.

The ability to stabilize the chest wall is directly related to increasing gestational age. Therefore, premature infants are highly susceptible to chest wall deformation and atelectasis during tidal breathing. This may result in hypoxemia, hypercarbia, and apnea, necessitating supplemental oxygen or ventilatory support.

The full-term infant has a short neck and a tongue that is not well supported. Such factors can result in partial obstruction when the infant is in the supine position. These are characteristics that require the infant to be placed in the prone or lateral lying position when asleep or lying down or be seated in an infant seat when awake.

Airway resistance is increased owing to the smaller nares, shorter airways with multiple bifurcations, and peripheral airway diameter. Therefore upper airway congestion and minor small airway infections may create tremendous resistance and place the infant at risk for respiratory distress, muscle fatigue, and respiratory failure. Edema secondary to trauma or infection of upper airway passages can easily result in obstruction with a marked increase in resistance to airflow. This distress can be seen in nasal flaring, retractions, and tachypnea.

Until the age of 5 years, the small peripheral airways contribute 50% of the airway resistance that must be overcome. This is compared with 20% in the adult, who has a much larger cross-sectional area for flow. Bronchi constrict in response to numerous factors including inhaled irritants, hypoxemia, hypercarbia, and cold. This constriction significantly increases airway resistance and the work of breathing.

The surface area of the lung is also decreased because of the characteristic structure of the chest. The ribs are rounder, giving the typical barrel chest configuration seen in the full-term infant. However, this results in thoracic crowding due to the relative size of the abdominal organs. The surface area of the lung is consequently decreased and lung expansion is reduced.

The lung is smaller and because of this the compliance is decreased. If compounded by disease states that reduce elasticity (e.g., pulmonary congestion and pulmonary fibrosis), the compliance drops even further and the work of breathing must increase in order to compensate.

Cartilaginous support is essential for the stability of the conducting airways. This too is a function of gestational age and development. Cartilage rings continue to increase in number for up to 2 months in age. Weakness secondary to lack of support can result in dynamic compression of the trachea in situations associated with high expiratory flow rates and increased airway resistance. Although bronchiolitis and asthma are common disease entities that cause this, it can occur during episodes of crying resulting in reduced saturations.

The gas exchanging portion of the lung in the full-term infant is made up of terminal air sacs and alveoli. Terminal air sacs lack the cupped shape of alveoli and are longer and narrower. They require higher pressures in order to maintain expansion, and once collapsed, increased pressures must be generated in order to open them. The alveoli that are present are smaller and predisposed to collapse.

The surface area available for diffusion is reduced in the neonate. During disease states this may be reduced even further, requiring an increase in minute ventilation. Much of neonatal disease may be related to an alteration in functional residual capacity, closing capacity, or both. When the closing capacity is high, the pleural pressure exceeds the intraluminal pressure resulting in early closure of bronchi, making them unavailable for gas exchange. A reduction in FRC can lead to unstable blood gases between respiratory efforts.

Without collateral ventilation the neonate cannot divert ventilation to distal airways when obstruction occurs. Currently no anatomic pathways have been found on histologic sectioning of neonatal lungs. However, radiologic evidence suggests that these alternative pathways may exist.[297] Without channels for collateral ventilation there is an increased risk for atelectasis or emphysematous change and ventilation-perfusion mismatching.[271]

Biochemical immaturity of the surfactant system can result in progressive atelectasis. Primary surfactant deficiency is found in premature infants, resulting in respiratory distress syndrome. However, surfactant production may be interrupted by numerous causes, including cytogenic oxygen toxicity, ischemia of the pulmonary bed, pulmonary edema, and hemorrhagic shock. Synthesis of surface active material is dependent upon a normal pH and adequate pulmonary perfusion.

Prematurity may also result in increased susceptibility to oxygen-induced cytotoxicity. This AOS parallels the maturation of the surfactant system, both occurring late in gestation. Without the ability to detoxify reactive oxygen metabolites, the metabolites are released into the immediate environment where they can injure normal cells.[331, 353] This

may lead to cell death and cause pulmonary edema, surfactant synthesis disruption, and scarring of lung tissues.

Physiologic Basis for Clinical Findings

The presence of increased work of breathing indicates a primary pulmonary disorder. The signs of increased work of breathing are chest wall retractions (subcostal, intercostal, suprasternal) and the use of accessory muscles (alar flare). Patients with respiratory failure have elevated dead space volume to tidal volume ratios, which result in hypoxia and hypercarbia unless counteracted by an increase in expired minute ventilation.[283] Respiratory patterns change with increased respiratory work.

In mild to moderate disease there is tachypnea, slight substernal and intercostal retractions, slight increase in anterior-to-posterior diameter, and intermittent expiratory grunting without cyanosis. Retractions occur because of the increased compliance of the chest wall, the immaturity of the intercostal muscles, and the increased inspiratory pressure generated. As the severity of the disease increases, the retractions become more marked. Deformation of the chest leads to paradoxical breathing (asynchrony of chest and abdominal movements), which is the result of diaphragm fatigue, inability of the intercostal muscles to fixate the chest wall, and increased inspiratory pressures.

Expiratory grunting elevates the end-expiratory pressure and slows the expiratory flow rate. This is accomplished by laryngeal braking through partial closure of the glottis. These maneuvers help maintain expansion and preserve oxygenation between respirations. The severity of lung disease can be determined by the frequency and loudness of the grunting. Nasal flaring results from increased inspiratory pressure.

Tachypnea may be the only sign of abnormalities in lung functioning. It is the most efficient way for neonates to increase ventilation and compensate for hypoxia and hypercarbia. Respiratory rates drop as fatigue sets in.

Nursing Interventions to Promote Respiratory Stability

It is evident that the preterm infant is extremely vulnerable to respiratory problems associated with disease states and immaturity of the respiratory system and its control centers. Nursing interventions can help to stabilize the chest wall and promote oxygenation. Use of transcutaneous oxygen monitors and oxygen saturation monitors provides immediate feedback about infant oxygen status and interventions. Nursing staff are encouraged to use these tools in all situations in which the infant is at risk for hypoxemia.

Positioning of infants can facilitate oxygenation, whether the infant is intubated or not. Abdominal positioning supports the chest wall, allows for greater posterior lung inflation and improved air entry, and improves oxygenation by splinting the chest, thereby decreasing chest deformation during inspiration.

If the infant is lying in the supine position, a small roll under the shoulders can keep the head aligned correctly and keep the airway open. In preterm infants, airway occlusion can result from hyperextension or underextension of the neck. Premature infants often remain as positioned; therefore careful attention to head and neck positioning is important.

Head position can also affect endotracheal tube (ETT) placement, resulting in airway obstruction and soft tissue damage if ETT abutment against the tracheal wall occurs.[49] Hypoxia can also occur with movement of the ETT within the trachea owing to vagal stimulation. Flexion of the head may result in the ETT sliding down the trachea into the right main stem bronchus. Extension, on the other hand, leads to movement upward, with the possibility of displacement of the ETT entirely. The ETT may have to be replaced if the tube comes out during extension.[109, 215] Careful attention to the original confirmed placement and taping can reduce the possibility of ETT shifts.

Suctioning of the ETT can result in hypoxemia either through direct interference or obstruction of the airway and gas flow or by vagal stimulation through vigorous, deep suctioning at the carina. This can be reduced by measuring the length of the ETT and adaptor and suctioning only 0.5 cm below the tip of the ETT. Along with this, gas flow interruption can be reduced by using a ventilator-ETT manifold adaptor that allows the ventilator tubing to remain connected during suctioning.[157, 343]

Suctioning can also result in hypoxia. Routine suctioning of the ETT is probably more traumatic to the infant than beneficial. Tube plugging is less of a concern now than in the past because of improved humidification techniques. Suctioning should be based on assessment of clinical status, including breath sounds, oxygenation status, and infant cuing behaviors.

Preoxygenation, sighing following suctioning, and two-person suctioning are all techniques utilized during the suctioning procedure to reduce the possibility of hypoxemia. Preoxygenation increases the PaO_2, thereby providing a wider tolerance range before hypoxemia sets in. Sighing restores the FRC, opens up atelectatic alveoli, and restores the alveolar gas gradient. This reduces the length of the hypoxic episode, promotes oxygenation, and improves ventilation-perfusion ratios.

Two-person suctioning allows for quick efficient suctioning that reduces airway and gas flow disruption to a short period of time. It also lets one person concentrate on the sterile suctioning technique itself while the other can manipulate the infant and equipment while maintaining oxygenation. Any of these techniques may be used alone or in conjunction with others, depending on the frequency and infant's tolerance of the procedure.

Handling and caregiving procedures can also result in hypoxemia in the preterm infant. The infant may not be able to maintain physiologic homeostasis during stimulation owing to developmental immaturity and lack of organization. Grouping activities and limiting the time of interventions can decrease the degree of hypoxemia and maximize coping abilities. Decisions regarding grouping and length of time must be based on the individual infant's tolerance and response. Responses to interventions can occur several minutes after the precipitating event; therefore careful evaluation of infant patterns and responses is essential to care planning. Structuring rest periods and assessing recovery can help to reduce the episodes of hypoxemia to a minimum.[108, 219]

Asphyxia

There are two categories of asphyxia most frequently encountered in the fetus and neonate; these are perinatal asphyxia and intrauterine asphyxia. Intrauterine asphyxia is the reduction or cessation of placental gas exchange that occurs either prior to or during delivery. This type of event places the infant at greater risk for perinatal asphyxia secondary to central nervous system depression, respiratory depression, and cardiac compromise. Perinatal asphyxia is failure of the newly born infant to establish adequate alveolar ventilation at birth with subsequent hypoxemia and respiratory and metabolic acidosis.

Intrauterine asphyxia is the most frequent cause of acidosis encountered in the neonate. The obstetric risk factors that can result in asphyxia are subdivided into three general categories: altered placental gas exchange, altered maternal perfusion of the placenta, and maternal hypoxemia. Specific risk factors are listed in Table 7–11.

Intrauterinely, the maintenance of a normal fetal acid-base balance requires the maternal and fetal systems to balance the production and elimination of CO_2. Certain

TABLE 7–11
Risk Factors for Fetal Asphyxia

PRENATAL/MATERNAL RISK FACTORS
Toxemia of pregnancy
Hypertension
Diabetes mellitus
Elderly (>35 years) or young (<15 years) primigravida
Chronic renal disease
Maternal malnutrition or severe obesity
Sickle cell disease
Anemia (<9 g Hgb)
Rh or ABO incompatibility
Heart disease
Pulmonary disease
Third trimester bleeding
Drug or ethanol abuse
Maternal infection
Uterine or pelvic anatomic abnormalities
Prolonged rupture of membranes
Previous fetal or neonatal deaths

FETAL RISK FACTORS
Premature delivery
Postmaturity (≥43 weeks' gestation)
Intrauterine growth retardation
Multiple births
Polyhydramnios
Meconium stained amniotic fluid

INTRAPARTUM RISK FACTORS
Breech or other abnormal presentations
Forceps delivery (other than low)
Cesarean section
Prolapsed umbilical cord
Nuchal cord
Prolonged general anesthesia
Excessive sedation or analgesia
Anesthetic complications (hypotension or hypoxia)
Prolonged or precipitous labor
Uterine hypertonus
Abnormal heart rate or rhythm

factors favor the release of CO_2 from the fetus to the mother; these include the increased affinity of fetal hemoglobin for oxygen. This means that as hemoglobin becomes oxygenated at the placental barrier the affinity for CO_2 is driven lower, increasing the release of CO_2 to the mother. At the same time, as maternal blood releases O_2 to the fetus, affinity for CO_2 is enhanced. Figure 7–14 provides a schematic representation of the movement of CO_2 across the placenta.[139, 286, 300]

The driving force behind CO_2 diffusion from fetal to maternal blood is the difference between maternal and fetal $PaCO_2$ levels. Fetal $PaCO_2$ values are higher than those in the maternal system. The hyperventilation of pregnancy creates a mild maternal alkalosis, which helps maintain a gradient that facilitates CO_2 transfer to the maternal system by driving maternal $PaCO_2$ levels lower. This gradient is estimated to be between 14 and 17 mmHg.[171, 300]

When fetal hypoxemia occurs owing to disturbances in base excess production (anaerobic metabolism) or circumstances in which CO_2 concentrations are altered (uterine contractions, placental infarcts, placental abruption), alterations in fetal heart rate minute volume and redistribution of fetal circulation occur. Increased fetal cardiac minute volume, seen clinically as fetal tachycardia, increases the delivery of CO_2 to the placenta in much the same way as hyperventilation increases the delivery of CO_2 to the alveoli. Fetal tachycardia is frequently encountered after the hypoxic episodes of labor. Uterine contractions are repetitive stress events that impede intervillous blood flow by shutting off venous outflow and compromising the exchange of CO_2 between maternal and fetal systems. $PaCO_2$ levels subsequently rise, and hypoxemia and metabolic acidosis may result.

Conversely, a decrease in cardiac minute volume (fetal bradycardia) secondary to hypoxia or anoxia also results in impaired gas exchange and an increase in fetal CO_2 levels. The fetus can tolerate these episodes only for brief periods if protracted hypoxic metabolic acidosis ensues.[300]

During asphyxial episodes fetal blood flow is redistributed in order to spare the brain, heart, and adrenals as much as possible. The sequelae of intrauterine asphyxia are cardiovascular deterioration with hypotension, bradycardia, and central nervous system depression. The latter may affect the infant's

Fetus

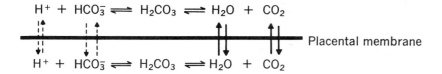

Mother

FIGURE 7–14. Movement of CO_2 across the placenta. (From Roux, J. F., Nakamura, J., Brown, E. G. (1973). Further observations on the determination of gestational age by amniotic fluid analysis. *Am J Obstet Gynecol, 116*, 633.)

ability to establish spontaneous respirations following delivery. A characteristic pattern of fetal response to asphyxia has been extrapolated by Dawes from his work with monkeys and has been translated to neonates.[98]

Once an asphyxial event occurs (in utero, during delivery, or immediately post delivery) there is an initial period of rapid gasping with a concomitant rise in heart rate and flailing movements of arms and legs. Blood pressure begins to slowly rise. These events last approximately a minute and are followed by a cessation of respirations (primary apnea), a falling heart rate, and a gradual decrease in blood pressure. During this period spontaneous respirations can usually be induced by tactile stimulation.

If the asphyxial episode continues for another 2 to 4 minutes, gasping begins again. Initially the gasping is deep and sporadic. Gasping efforts increase briefly and then begin to slow. The heart rate falls to below 100 beats per minutes (bpm), and blood pressure rapidly declines. Respiratory efforts completely cease in another 7 to 8 minutes. This is secondary apnea. The heart rate continues to fall, and bradycardia becomes pronounced.

At this time sensory stimulation will not lead to recovery. Brain damage begins after 8 minutes of total asphyxia and is maximal after 12 to 13 minutes. Death usually follows.[288]

Resuscitative efforts need to be initiated quickly when the infant is in secondary apnea. The longer the delay the less effective the interventions will be. Every minute delay in initiating resuscitation adds 4 minutes before the onset of spontaneous respirations.

The oxygen content of the blood falls to almost zero during the first 2 minutes of asphyxia. Anaerobic metabolism leads to lactic acid buildup and metabolic acidosis. At the same time, CO_2 accumulates and respiratory acidosis sets in. If ventilation is not established at this time, glucose administration in conjunction with buffers is necessary to increase cardiac output and heart rate, while improving serum glucose levels and improving pH.[2, 3, 160]

The maintenance of cardiac output is essential to survival. If substrate can be delivered to the brain and efforts to increase the pH are successful, gasping activity will be extended and secondary apnea will be postponed.[160]

The respiratory system experiences ischemia during asphyxial events because blood flow is shunted away from the lungs. This ischemia results in cellular damage to the alveoli with cell membrane disruption and concomitant leakage of fluid into the alveolar space. Death of the type II cells destroys the surfactant-producing ability of the lung, leading to RDS. Supplemental oxygen and possible ventilatory support may be necessary in order to prevent hypoxia.

Pulmonary hypoxia can also lead to pulmonary vasoconstriction and the persistence of high pulmonary vascular resistance. This reduces blood flow to the pulmonary vascular bed and compounds the local hypoxia. The hypoperfusion, hypoexpansion, and hypoxia can delay the normal closure of fetal shunts, and right-to-left shunting persists.

Not only does intrauterine asphyxia place neonates at risk for RDS and persistent pulmonary hypertension, but intrauterine stress events can result in the passage of meconium into the amniotic fluid (fetuses greater than 35 weeks) with subsequent aspiration during gasping efforts or with spontaneous respirations. This increases the risk of pneumonitis and pneumonia during the early neonatal period and may necessitate respiratory support.

Resuscitation

Neonates are more susceptible to asphyxia and need resuscitation more frequently than any other age group. Therefore appropriate intervention is necessary to preserve quality of life and prevent infant mortality and morbidity. The basic goals of resuscitation are

1. to promote and maintain adequate ventilation and oxygenation.
2. to initiate and maintain adequate cardiac output and tissue perfusion.
3. to maintain a normal core temperature and adequate serum glucose.

High-risk factors during the mother's pregnancy as well as problems or abnormalities during labor may be used to identify a fetus or neonate prone to asphyxia. However, any normal pregnancy may become high risk when unexpected or undetected complications occur during the intrapartum period (Table 7–11). Therefore, there should always be at least one individual skilled in neonatal resuscitation at the delivery of every infant, regardless of the size or type of facility providing services.

Protocols about who is to perform resuscitation, how it is to be performed, and when it is to be carried out need to be developed and mutually agreed upon by obstetric and pediatric personnel. Mechanisms for skill acquisition and maintenance should be designed and evaluated on an ongoing basis.

Anticipation and preparation are key to the success of resuscitative efforts. Most infants tolerate labor and delivery without difficulty. For those that do not, the majority can be identified prior to delivery. However, the unexpected must always be prepared for and emergency equipment must be available for all deliveries. Table 7–12 outlines the minimum equipment that needs to be available for all deliveries.

Every delivery room staff member should be able to prepare for the delivery of a low-risk full-term newborn. These steps include preheating the radiant warmer, ensuring appropriate equipment is available and functioning, identifying the availability of at least two individuals who can work as a team to provide all aspects of resuscitation. Nursing personnel should be skilled in the initial steps of resuscitation, including drying; establishing an airway; suctioning; providing tactile stimulation; evaluating the heart rate, respirations, and color; initiating bag and mask

TABLE 7–12
Equipment Necessary for Resuscitation

External overhead heat source
Suction setup
Suction catheters (6, 8, 10 F.)
Stethoscope
Oxygen source (warm and humidified)
Resuscitation bag with pressure manometer
Flowmeter
Mask
Clock
Orogastric tube (5, 8 F.)
Syringe (20 ml)
Endotracheal tubes (2.5, 3.0, 3.5, 4.0)
Laryngoscope with size 0 and 1 Miller blade
Laryngoscope bulb (extra)
Tape
Stylet
Epinephrine 1:10,000
Volume expanders
   whole blood
   5% albuminated saline
   normal saline
   Ringer's lactate
Sodium bicarbonate 0.5 mEq/ml
Narcan
Umbilical vessel catheterization tray

ventilation; and performing cardiac massage. In addition, there should be someone immediately available who can intubate and intitiate biochemical resuscitation.

When an infant at risk for asphyxia is about to be delivered, two individuals skilled in resuscitation should be present, whose sole responsibility is the neonate. They should be familiar wtih the prenatal and intrapartum history of the mother and fetus, since this could affect the preparations that need to be made. Equipment necessary for complete resuscitation should be set up, operational, removed from its packaging, and so forth. In the event of a multiple pregnancy, a setup for each infant should be available and a separate team(s) should be arranged.

Steps in Resuscitation

There are several steps that should be taken routinely following the delivery of any infant. The external warmer should be turned on either continuously or at the time the mother is pushing. As the infant is delivered, special attention to drying the infant with warm blankets to decrease heat loss is essential.

An airway should be established by positioning the infant in the supine position. The neck should be slightly extended. A small blanket or towel roll can be placed under the shoulders in order to maintain the appropriate position. The roll is especially helpful with an infant who has substantial molding or large occipital caput. The nose and mouth should be suctioned gently either with a bulb syringe or suction catheter (do not exceed 100 mmHg pressure). The mouth should be suctioned first to prevent aspiration of secretions if gasping occurs during nasal suctioning. Vigorous suctioning needs to be avoided, excessive stimulation of the posterior pharynx in the first few minutes after birth can result in a vagal response leading to severe bradycardia, apnea, or both.[38]

Drying and suctioning of the infant often provide sufficient stimulation for most infants to initiate respirations. For those infants who do not breathe immediately, additional stimulation should be provided by either slapping or flicking the soles of the feet and rubbing the infant's back. One or two rubs or flicks are usually enough to initiate respirations in the infant experiencing primary apnea. If the infant does not respond immediately with respiratory efforts sufficient to maintain the heart rate above 100, then IPPV needs to be instituted. Continued tactile stimulation of an infant who is not responding is not warranted and is potentially harmful.

The entire process to this point should take not more than 30 seconds. If at 30 seconds the infant is not breathing or the heart rate is not 100, then bag and mask ventilation should be started and maintained for at least 15 to 30 seconds at a rate of 40 breaths per minute with pressures ranging between 15 and 40 cm H_2O (depending on whether it is the initial breath and the lungs are normal or diseased).[38]

If the heart rate is above 100 and the infant is able to establish sustained respirations but remains cyanotic, free flow oxygen should be provided until the infant is centrally pink.

After the initial period of ventilation, the infant's heart rate should be reassessed. If the heart rate is 60 to 100 and increasing, ventilation should be continued. If the heart rate is not increasing, check for adequacy of ventilation (chest moving, 100% oxygen being delivered) and start chest compressions if the heart rate is less than 80. Continue support until acceptable levels are reached. If this does not occur, consider additional interventions, including intubation and biochemical resuscitation.[38]

External cardiac massage should be instituted whenever the heart rate is below 60, or between 60 and 80 and not improving after 30 seconds of effective ventilation with 100% oxygen. Once the heart rate is 80 or better, chest compressions can be discontinued.[38]

Endotracheal intubation is indicated when bag and mask ventilation is ineffective, airway obstruction is suspected, meconium aspiration is suspected, abdominal wall defects or diaphragmatic hernia is present, and prolonged resuscitation is necessary.[38]

Biochemical resuscitation begins when the infant's heart rate remains below 80 despite adequate ventilation with 100% oxygen and chest compressions for 30 seconds or more or when the heart rate is zero. Medications include epinephrine (cardiac stimulant), volume expanders (for acute bleeding with signs of hypovolemia), sodium bicarbonate (for documented metabolic acidosis), and dopamine (improves cardiac contractility). Narcan (naloxone hydrochloride) is utilized with respiratory depression only if narcotic analgesics have been administered to the mother and may cause seizures in infants of substance-abusing mothers. Atropine and calcium are no longer recommended for use in the acute phase of resuscitation for the asphyxiated infant.[38]

Transient Tachypnea

The population that is most likely to experience transient tachypnea is full-term infants born by cesarean section or having suffered some sort of perinatal hypoxic stress event. The exact cause is unknown. Possible explanations include alteration in permeability of the pulmonary capillary vessels, aspiration of amniotic fluid during gasping efforts in utero, and lack of or decreased vaginal thoracic squeeze. The first two explanations would result in an increased protein concentration in the lung fluid, preventing transfer of fluid into the pulmonary circulation. A vaginal thoracic squeeze during a vertex delivery facilitates removal of upper airway fluid and reduces viscous forces that must be overcome with the first inspiration. The net result is a delay in physiologic adjustment and respiratory transition, with an increase in diffusion distance, a decrease in tidal volume, and an increased risk of $\dot{V}/\dot{Q}$ mismatching.

The most common clinical sign is tachypnea with respiratory rates in the range of

80 to 100 breaths per minute. Mild to moderate retractions and grunting may be exhibited. Cyanosis is not a prominent finding; if oxygen supplementation is necessary, it rarely needs to be greater than 40%. Air exchange is good; breath sounds may initially be moist but clear quickly.

Radiographic findings demonstrate vascular engorgement with increased pulmonary vascular markings. Central markings are ill defined, but there is branching outward toward the periphery. Moderate cardiomegaly may be evident, and occasional air bronchograms can be identified. The overall lung volume is increased indicating hyperaeration. The diaphragm is depressed, and the anterior-to-posterior diameter is increased.

Symptoms and findings clear within 1 to 5 days. Treatment modalities are supportive in nature and based on symptomatology exhibited. Sepsis must be ruled out.

Respiratory Distress Syndrome

Respiratory distress syndrome (RDS) is a developmental deficiency in surfactant synthesis whose incidence is inversely related to gestational age. It is the most common cause of respiratory failure in the preterm infant and is exacerbated by asphyxia.

RDS is a disorder in surface tension, in which increased pressure is required to keep the alveoli open. Pressures in adjacent alveoli are unequal, therefore time constants are changed, with some alveoli taking longer to fill and others filling normally. This leads to overdistention of the normal alveoli. As the alveoli reach their elastic limit, the infant must generate greater transpulmonary pressure in order to inspire the same amount of volume. The loss of elasticity and the progressive collapse of smaller alveoli reduce lung compliance. This results in uneven $\dot{V}/\dot{Q}$ ratios with concomitant hypoventilation, decreased functional residual capacity, and increased closing capacity.

When the closing capacity exceeds the functional residual capacity, some segments of the lung are closed during a portion of tidal breathing. As a result, the $\dot{V}/\dot{Q}$ ratio falls and hypoxemia and hypercarbia ensue. The hypoxemia and CO_2 retention are usually progressive, culminating in metabolic and respiratory acidosis, which further affect the ability of the type II cells to produce surfactant.[307, 308, 309, 310]

If the closing capacity exceeds both the functional residual capacity and tidal volume, lung segments are closed during inspiration and expiration. This represents complete atelectasis and is characterized as a "white out" on chest x-ray film. The use of continuous positive airway pressure (CPAP) and positive end-expiratory pressure (PEEP) prevents alveolar collapse during expiration and increases FRC above closing capacity.

Atelectatic areas of the lung contribute to the dead space within the entire lung. This changes the dead space–to–tidal volume ratio and leads to hypoxia and hypercarbia unless there is a concomitant increase in expired minute ventilation. An increase in respiratory rate reflects the infant's attempt to compensate. If dead space has increased to the point that alveolar ventilation is compromised, respiratory failure may be the result. Dead space may increase up to 70% in severe RDS.[283, 271]

As hypoxemia and hypercarbia become more severe, pulmonary artery vasoconstriction occurs. Pulmonary perfusion is compromised, and right-to-left shunting occurs through the foramen ovale and ductus arteriosus. Hypoperfusion and hypoxemia compound local ischemia leading to continued alveolar and capillary epithelial damage.[47]

The increased subatmospheric intrapleural pressure created by the infant in an attempt to maintain adequate air flow, along with the low serum protein that is common in preterm infants, causes the shift of alveolar and interstitial fluid toward the alveolar space. Combined with the increased alveolar surface tension, pulmonary edema and alveolar flooding ensue. Fibrinogen in the exudate is converted to fibrin. Fibrin lines the alveoli, and binds blood products and cellular debris found in the alveoli resulting in formation of hyaline membranes.[36, 340]

The excess alveolar fluid and membrane formation result in an increased diffusion distance and reduced lung surface area. Gas exchange is hampered, and ventilation-perfusion mismatching is compounded. Further hypoxemia and hypercarbia are the end result.[36, 329, 340] This becomes a vicious circle that may increase in severity over the first 3 days of life. Recovery is characterized by regeneration of alveolar tissue and concomitant increase in surfactant activity.[200]

Pathogenesis

Pathogenesis may be due to an ischemic injury that occurs either in utero or at the time of delivery, resulting in hypoperfusion of the lung. The more immature the lung and smaller the capillary bed the greater the ease with which the nutritional blood supply to the developing lung can be compromised. At 35 weeks, the type II cells are presumably differentiated to the point that the pathway for PC synthesis is more resistant to fetal stress and the nutritional blood supply is more abundant and therefore more difficult to compromise.

A second theory assumes deficient production of surface active material (surfactant). This deficiency is due to a decrease in the number of type II pneumocytes secondary to gestational age. Surfactant must not only be present at the time of delivery, but also must be regenerated at a rate consonant with its use. This implies that type II cells must be present, viable, and intact in order to maintain normal surface tension.

Inadequate amounts of surfactant at birth may be due to a variety of problems. These include extreme immaturity of the alveolar lining cells, diminished or impaired production rates resulting from transient fetal or neonatal stress, impaired release mechanisms from within the cell, and death of type II cells. The extreme immaturity and impaired release mechanisms probably explain the inability of the very early fetus to survive.

Clinical Symptoms

Clinically the infant attempts to compensate for the progressive respiratory and metabolic acidosis by increasing both inspiratory pressures and respiratory rate. Grunting occurs in an attempt to slow expiratory flow rates and maintain a higher FRC. All of the clinical signs appear early and usually increase in severity over the first 72 hours. The infant may also present with pitting edema, cyanosis, and diminished breath sounds.

Cyanosis is due to an excessive concentration of deoxygenated hemoglobin in the capillaries, although hypoxia can occur without cyanosis. Factors contributing to cyanosis include the alveolar hypoventilation, impaired diffusion across the alveolar-capillary membrane, and right-to-left shunting through fetal channels or through completely atelectatic lungs. Usually cyanosis (hypoxia) is progressive, requiring increasing concentrations of oxygen.

Grunting is forced expiration against a partially closed glottis so that end-expiratory pressure is increased and expiratory flow is retarded. This maintains the lung at a slightly higher volume for a longer period of time, thereby increasing gas exchange time. There is usually a very short expiratory phase, this reduces the time in which the lung can become airless before the next inspiratory effort. The tachypnea and grunting help to maintain a more normal FRC.

Retractions are indicative of the increased inspiratory pressure, decreased lung compliance, and increased chest wall compliance. They can be quite marked in RDS, with substernal retractions pulling to the backbone. This dysfunctional respiratory effort results in cephalocaudal expansion only (paradoxical breathing) with increased negative pressures being generated in the bases. Therefore, hyperinflation occurs in the bases and atelectasis in the apices. Marked abnormalities in $\dot{V}/\dot{Q}$ ratios are the result.

Those factors that increase the risk of RDS include prematurity, maternal diabetes (especially if poorly controlled), antepartum hemorrhage, second of twins, asphyxia, and male gender (RDS is two times more frequent in males than in females).[26, 47, 296] Sparing factors include chronic hypertension and chronic placental insufficiency resulting in intrauterine growth retardation, prolonged rupture of membranes (greater than 24 hours), maternal toxemia, maternal heroin addiction, and the administration of glucocorticoids.[30, 47, 149, 225, 369]

Prolonged rupture of membranes is only beneficial if asphyxia and signs and symptoms of sepsis are not present. Glucocorticoid treatment is recommended between 24 and 34 weeks' gestation. Tocolytics need to be instituted to stop labor for a minimum of 24 hours in order to obtain any benefit from glucocorticoid administration; 72 hours is ideal.[17, 225]

Treatment

Neonatal interventions are supportive as well as active in nature. Adequate, effective resuscitation with maintenance of body temperature is essential for reducing the incidence and severity of the disease. Therapy is aimed at maintaining oxygenation, adequate ventilation, normal pH, and adequate perfusion and tissue oxygenation. Hydration is important, but overhydration increases the risk of congestive heart failure. A systolic murmur, bounding pulses, active precordium, tachycardia, tachypnea, apnea, and CO_2 retention as well as worsening ventilatory requirements are indications of patent ductus arteriosus and congestive heart failure.[47, 89, 137, 341]

Active interventions include the use of continuous distending pressure or continuous negative pressure in an attempt to keep FRC above closing capacity. Cycled ventilation may be needed if the infant is unable to compensate for hypoxemia, hypercarbia, and acidosis by generating sufficient negative pressure and increasing minute ventilation.[61, 189] Currently, exogenous surfactant replacement therapy to stabilize the lung until postnatal surfactant synthesis occurs is being utilized. Prophylactic administration from birth has been associated with a reduction in mortality and a reduction in complications in most, but not all, infants.

Bronchopulmonary Dysplasia

Northway and colleagues originally described a sequence of radiographic changes in infants with RDS that came to be known as bronchopulmonary dysplasia (BPD).[272] This discrete sequence was divided into four stages: Stage I (between 2 and 3 days of life) was indistinguishable from RDS; Stage II (seen between day 4 and day 10) consisted of opacification (white out) of the lung fields; Stage III (until day 20) began with the development of small bubbles that alternated with areas of irregular density; and in Stage IV the bubbles coalesced into hyperaerated cysts. This sequence of events is rarely seen in current clinical practice. Instead, there is a slower subtler onset, with the gradual development of lung abnormalities that persist after 20 to 30 days of life.[48, 272]

Currently, the most consistent findings include a "generalized hyperinflation and a peristent haze followed by multiple lacy infiltrates that obscure the pulmonary vessels."[404, p.20] Therapies used to treat other disease processes (e.g., viral pneumonia) may result in characteristic radiographic changes that can make interpretation difficult. Therefore, other clinical criteria have been identified to delineate BPD from other disease processes. These criteria include IPPV during the 1st week of life; tachypnea, auscultatory rales, and retractions lasting longer than 28 days; supplemental oxygen for more than 28 days in order to maintain PaO_2 above 50; and radiographic evidence of persistent

strands of density bilaterally, alternating with areas of hyperlucency.[23] Although better, these additional criteria are still problematic, in that all infants who acquire BPD may not have been ventilated during the 1st week of life.[48]

The risk of BPD is greatest in the very low birth weight infant. Other infants at risk, however, include those with apnea of prematurity requiring ventilation, pneumonia, meconium aspiration, cyanotic heart disease, and persistent pulmonary hypertension. The incidence varies depending on the diagnostic criteria, patient population, and ventilatory management.[48]

Pathogenesis

Although not completely understood, the pathogenesis of BPD seems to be intimately tied to exposure to high concentrations of oxygen and barotrauma from positive pressure ventilation. The risk factors for BPD are identified in Table 7–13; Figure 7–15 provides a schematic representation of the interaction of factors.

Infants who do not receive oxygen do not acquire BPD, and those infants who are treated for longer periods of time with higher concentrations of oxygen are at greater risk. However, oxygen exposure itself is not sufficient to induce BPD. Oxygen therapy must be combined with IPPV for BPD to develop. The barotrauma associated with high peak inspiratory pressures and exposure time seems to be required before BPD is seen.

Recently, Goetzman has developed a model of BPD pathogenesis that brings all the risk factors together.[152] The model proposes that there must be a susceptible host

---

TABLE 7–13
Risk Factors for Bronchopulmonary Dysplasia

Immaturity of the pulmonary parenchyma
Surfactant deficiency
Exposure to elevated concentrations of inspired oxygen
Barotrauma from positive pressure ventilation
Systemic-to-pulmonary shunt through a patent ductus
  arteriosus
Pulmonary edema
Pulmonary air leak
Protease-antiprotease imbalance
Family history of reactive airway disease
Tissue type HLA-A2
Vitamin A deficiency

From Boynton, B. R. (1988). The epidemiology of bronchopulmonary dysplasia. In T. A. Merritt, W. H. Northway, Jr., & B. R. Boynton (Eds.), *Bronchopulmonary dysplasia* (p. 26). Boston: Blackwell Scientific Publications.

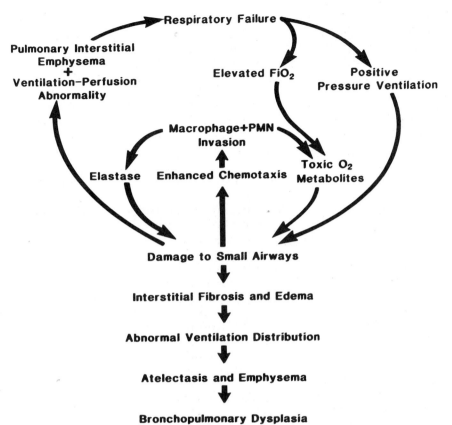

FIGURE 7–15. Factors affecting the development of bronchopulmonary dysplasia. (From Boynton, B. R. (1988). The epidemiology of bronchopulmonary dysplasia. In T. A. Merritt, W. H. Northway, & B. R. Boynton (Eds.), *Contemporary issues in fetal and neonatal medicine: Bronchopulmonary dysplasia* (p. 27). Boston: Blackwell Scientific Publications.)

with an immature respiratory system and a genetic predisposition who has experienced an asphyxial insult. The lungs undergo an acute injury from the lack of surfactant and barotrauma. This injury allows the release of toxic oxidants (antioxidant system enzymes) and proteolytic enzymes that act upon local tissue to cause further damage. As the lungs heal they do so abnormally, which may be compounded by continued oxygenation, inadequate nutrition, and possibly vitamin E or A deficiency.[152]

Examination of the lungs in BPD reveals alterations in bronchi, bronchioli, alveoli, and vessels depending on the severity of the disease. In mild cases, membranous exudates line dilated alveolar transitional ducts and respiratory bronchioles. These hyaline membranes are absorbed quickly. If high oxygen concentration exposure occurs, there is a loss of cilia with mucosal denudation of the airway lining. With the reparative process, edema of the interstitial space of bronchi,

vessels, and lobular and alveolar septa occurs. This results in a decreased exchange surface with an increased diffusion distance, leading to hypoxemia and hypercarbia.[9]

In moderately severe cases, there is extensive loss of cilia with sloughing of bronchial and bronchiolar lining cells. There is also necrosis of alveolar cells and marked edema of the peribronchial spaces, perivascular spaces, and alveolar septa. Focal atelectasis can be seen, contributing to the increased dead space and altered $\dot{V}/\dot{Q}$ patterns.

Extensive necrosis of the airway lining in severe BPD leads to an accumulation of eosinophilic debris in the bronchiole lumina. The alveolar space contains increased numbers of alveolar macrophages. The focal atelectasis now alternates with areas of hyperinflated air sacs. Hyperplasia of the vascular medial layer and metaplasia of bronciolar epithelium increase resistance to both air and blood flow.

These patterns can become quite widespread, resulting in peribronchiolar fibrosis, obliterative fibroproliferative bronchiolitis, and severe derangement of the alveolar architecture (severe hyperinflation alternating with irregular scars and atelectasis). Hypertrophy of the medial layer of the vascular bed along with endothelial cell hyperplasia and adventitial fibrosis leads to a reduced capillary and precapillary vascular volume. Ventilation-perfusion mismatching is pronounced in this case and "normal" blood gases may not be achievable.[43]

Treatment

Treatment for BPD has been multifaceted. Some modalities are centered on primary prevention, and others are employed after the disease process is diagnosed. Primary prevention includes reducing the incidence of premature births through patient education and recognition of early labor, the use of drugs to inhibit premature labor, using glucocorticoids to mature surfactant synthesis pathways, provision of effective resuscitation, and providing exogenous surfactant. Secondary treatment modalities include ventilatory support (either negative or positive pressure); adequate nutrition for growth and healing, facilitating closure of the ductus arteriosus through pharmacologic or surgical treatment; diuretic therapy to mobilize fluids and reduce pulmonary edema; bronchodilators and anti-inflammatory agents to decrease resistance to airflow and improve distribution of ventilation; and various ventilatory techniques (e.g., high-frequency ventilation-jet and oscillation).

Research has focused on enhancing or modifying lung maturation through the antioxidant and surfactant pathways and thereby improving adaptation to extrauterine life. There is little known about the regulatory mechanisms for the development of the AOS. Continued research in this area is essential if there is to be any hope of manipulating the AOS activity in the neonate and reduce the possibility of lung damage secondary to hyperoxia. There are several nonenzymatic antioxidant defenses in cells; the most thoroughly investigated and best understood is vitamin E (α-tocopherol).[366]

Vitamin E is a lipid-soluble antioxidant that is integrated into membrane lipids and provides antioxidant activity. There is very little support for the efficacy of vitamin E supplementation in the prevention of hyper-

oxic lung damage. Clinical trials have not shown any protective mechanism against the development of BPD or modification of the course of RDS.[112, 304] Ward did show early epithelial protection in rabbits exposed to hyperoxia, however, and other studies do show that vitamin E may support the surfactant pathway by preventing a decrease in phospholipid content within the airways when exposed to oxygen.[350, 355] Continued research into these areas is needed to determine whether normal levels of vitamin E can help to maintain surfactant synthesis pathways during the course of RDS and BPD.

The newest therapy in treating RDS and thereby reducing the incidence of BPD is exogenous surfactant replacement. Direct tracheal instillation at the time of delivery has shown that lung mechanics can be altered and improved oxygenation can be achieved. The course of RDS can be modified and the need for ventilatory support can be reduced and the infant weaned at a faster rate. In this way, barotrauma and length of exposure time to oxygen can be reduced. This may limit the injury that occurs and disrupt the vicious circle of factors associated with the development of BPD.[229]

Nursing Care

Nursing care of BPD infants begins with the acutely ill patient requiring ventilatory support. Many supportive measures are necessary for these infants, and careful monitoring of ventilatory and blood gas parameters is essential. The very low birth weight infant can tolerate lower oxygen levels and higher carbon dioxide levels than previously thought; therefore evaluation of the infant's tolerance to these parameters should be undertaken.

Modification of the environment to reduce stimuli and the hypoxia that they can produce needs to be instituted. Infant tolerance to procedures and individualization of care should be determined based on infant cues and physiologic responses.

Special attention to nutritional status and growth requirements is essential for survival and for normal development of lung tissue. Hospitalization is usually prolonged; therefore growth and development of the infant are important in the overall care plan. Helping these infants to achieve normal developmental milestones should be a multidisciplinary team focus. Assessment of the infant's readiness for interaction and activity is necessary if the infant is going to gain any benefit from the stimulus.

These infants are a challenge to both medical and nursing caregivers. They require careful consideration of all aspects of their development and physiologic status. Family needs and promotion of the family unit must also be maintained throughout a lengthy hospitalization. Careful monitoring and creative approaches to each infant result in the best outcome.

Meconium Aspiration Syndrome

Meconium aspiration is a frequent cause of respiratory failure in term and postmature infants. Elimination of meconium into amniotic fluid is commonly associated with some degree of fetal distress, but may occur in normal or breech delivery without evidence of asphyxia.[22, 136, 217, 258]

Meconium is passed in utero owing to hypoxic stress. The hypoxia and acidosis are probably responsible for the gasping activity that leads to aspiration of meconium prior to delivery. Approximately 10% of all babies delivered release meconium into the amniotic fluid; however, less than half these infants have meconium that can be retrieved from below the vocal cords.[22, 159]

If gasping does not occur, there is very little chance that meconium will be aspirated into the lower airways prior to delivery. Aspiration deep into the pulmonary tree can be prevented most of the time with tracheal suction performed before the first breath.[338] If the first breath does occur, the large negative pressure generated will move any fluid present in the nasopharynx or trachea down into the smaller airways.

When the aspirate is thick, the lower airways become partially obstructed resulting in air trapping and over inflation distal to the obstruction. Small airway obstruction produces an alteration in $\dot{V}/\dot{Q}$ ratios and reduced lung compliance. The alveolar hypoventilation leads to CO_2 retention, hypoxemia, and acidosis.

When the obstruction is complete, the distal alveoli collapse, increasing the intrapulmonary shunt and compounding arterial hypoxemia. Obstruction may also be potentiated by epithelial inflammation in the bronchi and alveoli. This results in a chemical pneumonitis with increased airway resistance and decreased diffusing capacity. Both of these events contribute to the hypoxemia seen clinically. The pneumonitis may also explain the decreased lung compliance, because elasticity is lost with inflammation.

Minute ventilation is increased in order to compensate for the $\dot{V}/\dot{Q}$ alterations. The increase is usually due to an increase in respiratory rate; however, CO_2 retention continues because the tidal volume is reduced, thereby increasing dead space and reducing alveolar ventilation.

Clinically these infants present with a history of fetal distress and meconium-stained fluid. They are usually full-term or postterm infants whose initial Apgar scores are low. Early in the neonatal period there is tachypnea, retractions, and even cyanosis. The chest may be overdistended and barrel-shaped. Breath sounds are decreased with coarse bronchial sounds. Expiration may be prolonged.

The chest radiograph demonstrates patchy areas that have reduced aeration. There are sometimes confluent areas alternating with hyperlucent ones. The diaphragm may be depressed.[154] Blood gas levels show a metabolic acidosis and hypoxemia that are dependent upon the degree of pulmonary bed involved. These findings are more pronounced if persistent pulmonary hypertension is present. The infant may be able to compensate initially; therefore $PaCO_2$ levels may be normal. However, this usually does not last.

If the process continues, respiratory failure is likely. Pneumothorax or pneumomediastinum may also occur because of the alveolar distention that occurs with air trapping. Right-to-left shunting is common, especially if persistent pulmonary hypertension is present. Secondary bacterial infections frequently occur but may be difficult to diagnose by chest x-ray film especially during the acute phase of the syndrome.

In order to reduce the amount of meconium fluid in the nasopharynx, suctioning on the perineum of the nares, mouth, and pharynx via catheter and wall suction should be performed. Once delivery has occurred, the vocal cords should be visualized, and any meconium should be suctioned from the oropharynx and trachea with a suction catheter and endotracheal tube. This may necessitate repeated endotracheal tube placement. In order to reduce the risk of trauma and edema and facilitate further meconium removal, the endotracheal tube should be left in place with the third pass.

Assisted ventilation may be necessary in these infants in order to ensure adequate oxygenation, drive the $PaCO_2$ level toward normal, and facilitate transitional events. Cord gases and arterial gas should be assessed in order to evaluate the asphyxial insult and determine adequate recovery. Chest percussion, postural drainage, and suctioning should be done in order to continue the removal of meconium from lung passages. ECMO (extracorporeal membrane oxygenation) may be used to treat critically ill infants who do not respond to conventional therapy.

Persistent Pulmonary Hypertension

Persistent pulmonary hypertension (PPHN), or persistent fetal circulation (PFC), is a syndrome of acute respiratory distress with hypoxemia and acidemia caused by decreased pulmonary blood flow due to elevated pulmonary vascular resistance (PVR). There is central cyanosis associated with right-to-left shunting across the fetal shunts (foramen ovale and ductus arteriosus). This syndrome may represent failure to achieve transition to air breathing or may be secondary to cardiomyopathies, meconium aspiration, alveolar hypoventilation, pulmonary hypoplasia, polycythemia, and hypoglycemia.[126, 127, 142, 173, 289, 295, 302]

Rudolph has identified three anatomic variations that account for PPHN. These are maladaptation, excessive muscularization, and underdevelopment of the pulmonary artery bed.[301, 302] Each of these variations presents with a different pattern of airway and vessel development (Table 7–14) and may occur simultaneously.

Maladaptation of the Pulmonary Vascular Bed

The neonatal pulmonary bed is highly reactive to hypoxic episodes, as compared with the adult. This may be due to the increased medial wall thickness or the lower density of arteries encountered in the newborn versus the adult. This may also explain the PPHN syndrome seen after surgical procedures.[140]

During maladaptation PPHN, either the normal increase in pulmonary artery compli-

ance does not occur or vasoconstriction occurs during the transition process. Hypoxia for any reason (hypoventilation, upper airway obstruction, or interstitial disease) may contribute to these mechanisms. If acidosis or hypercarbia exists, they may react synergistically to contribute to the increase in PVR. A vicious circle may be set up in which hypoxia leads to reactive vasoconstriction, which in turn leads to increased right-to-left shunting, thereby increasing the degree of hypoxemia and decreasing the normal postnatal transition events that result in pulmonary artery vasodilatation.[140, 143, 224, 245, 294]

Elevated PVR can be present with an increased blood viscosity caused by polycythemia or elevated plasma fibrinogen levels.[126, 142, 302] Partial exchange transfusion resolves this situation. Increased PVR can also be found in some infants with large ventricular septal defects (VSD). These infants have normal or reduced pulmonary flow and intermittent right-to-left shunting, and do not develop congestive heart failure (common in infants with VSD without PPHN). This seems to be related to remodeling of the pulmonary arteries to increase medial wall thickness and extend muscularization to the alveolar wall vessels. The reason for some infants not being able to reduce PVR upon delivery is unknown but may be related to increased sensitivity to vasoconstrictor stimuli, increased availability of pulmonary vasoconstrictors, or decreased availability of pulmonary vasodilators.[140, 178, 184, 222]

Excessive Muscularization of the Pulmonary Vascular Bed

There are three categories of PPHN that fit under this heading; these include idiopathic PPHN, meconium aspiration, and congenital heart disease. Idiopathic PPHN is characterized by precocious muscularization of the intra-acinar arteries during intrauterine life. Apart from the increased muscularization there are no other abnormalities in lung growth. Medial smooth muscle is found in the arteries at the alveolar wall level at the time of birth (there is normally no muscle at this level). The arterial external diameter is normal, but the cross section of the internal lumen is reduced owing to medial coat encroachment on the lumen, leading to an increased resistance to flow. If the pulmonary artery pressure is higher than the systemic pressure, right-to-left shunting of blood from

TABLE 7–14
Patterns of Airway and Vessel Development in Persistent Pulmonary Hypertension

CAUSE	AIRWAY		INTRA-ACINAR ARTERY			
	Number of Bronchial Generations	Number of Alveoli Per Acinus	Muscle Extension by Position	External Diameter	Medial Wall Thickness	Number
Excessive Muscularization						
PPHN—idiopathic	N	N	↑	N	↑	N
Meconium aspiration—fatal	N	N	↑	N	↑	N
TAPVC—SD	N	N	↑	↑	↑	N
TAPVC—ID	N	N	↑	N	↑	N
AA/AS	N	N	↑	N	↑	↑
Coarctation, VSD, PDA	N	N	↑	↑	↑¹ (↓²)	N
Underdevelopment						
CDH	↓	N	N, ↑	↓³	↑	↓
Renal agenesis	↓	↓	↑, ↓	↓⁴	↓, N	↓
Renal dysplasia	↓	↓	↑, N	↓⁴	N, ↑	↓
Rhesus isoimmunization	↓	N, ↓	N	↓³	N⁵	↓
Idiopathic (primary)	↓	↓	NA	NA	NA	NA
Diaphragmatic amyoplasia and phrenic nerve agenesis	↓	N	↑	↓	↑	↓
Maladaptation						
VSD	N	N	↑	↓	↑	↓, N

AA, aortic atresia; AS, aortic stenosis; CDH, congenital diaphragmatic hernia; ID, infradiaphragmatic; PDA, patent ductus arteriosus; PPHN, persistent pulmonary hypertension of the newborn; SD, supradiaphragmatic; TAPVC, total anomalous pulmonary venous connection; VSD, ventricular septal defect; N, normal; NA, not available; ↑, increase; ↓, decrease.

1, dependent on severity of coarctation; 2, preacinar arteries; 3, small for age but appropriate for lung volume; 4, small for age but large for lung volume; 5, preacinar medial hypertrophy.

From Geggel, R.L. & Reid, L.M. (1984). The structural basis of PPHN. *Clin Perinatol, 3*, 526.

the pulmonary to systemic circulations occurs.[140, 174, 266]

Increased muscular coats have been seen in animals when pulmonary artery pressure is elevated secondary to partial occlusion of the ductus arteriosus, systemic hypertension with a patent ductus arteriosus, or pharmacologic constriction of the ductus arteriosus with prostaglandin inhibitors (e.g., indomethacin, acetylsalicylic acid). This last instance has been documented in human infants as well.[90, 180, 220, 221, 238]

Meconium aspiration has been attributed to hypoxic pulmonary artery vasoconstriction. However, in studies that examined the dissected lungs of infants who died of PPHN secondary to meconium aspiration, the infants had increased muscularization of arteries. This would indicate that idiopathic PPHN was the primary cause of death in these infants rather than meconium aspiration. Whether there is a connection between the two events has yet to be determined.[140]

Those congenital heart diseases that are clinically similar to PPHN include interrupted aortic arch (IAA), obstructed total anomalous pulmonary venous connection (TAPVC), and left heart obstructive lesions

(aortic atresia, aortic stenosis, coarctation of the aorta with ventricular septal defect and patent ductus arteriosus). Bronchial and alveolar development is normal in these situations, but the pulmonary vasculature, both arterial and venous, has undergone remodeling. The remodeling results in peripheral extension of muscle in the arteries and the appearance of muscle in usually nonmuscular veins with medial hypertrophy of arteries and veins. Prenatal alterations occur in all these anomalies; however, further remodeling can continue after delivery.[117, 118, 140, 176, 337]

Underdevelopment of the Pulmonary Vascular Bed

Congenital diaphragmatic hernia; oligohydramnios associated with renal agenesis, renal dysplasia, or chronic leakage of amniotic fluid; pleural effusion; Rh isoimmunization; vascular anomalies; and diaphragmatic amyoplasia and phrenic nerve agenesis are all associated with pulmonary hypoplasia in the neonatal period. The severity of the abnormality is dependent upon the gestational age at which the interruption in lung development occurs. By 16 weeks' gestation preacinar branching is complete; after that, acinar development continues into the postnatal period. Interruptions in early gestation result in a reduced number of bronchial generations. If the number or size of the alveoli is reduced, the disruption occurred later in gestation.[32, 65, 68, 173, 183, 185, 281, 289, 334]

Pathogenesis

Persistent pulmonary hypertension is a transitional event that is due to either the failure of pulmonary vessels to dilate or an inadequate number of vessels to handle the entire cardiac output at normal pressures. This results in inadequate oxygenation secondary to $\dot{V}/\dot{Q}$ abnormalities. The continued elevated PVR and increased right heart pressure, combined with the resulting hypoxemia and acidosis, lead to maintenance of fetal circulatory channels. Blood flow tends to bypass the lungs and follow the fetal pathways; therefore the pulmonary hypoperfusion, hypoxia, and acidosis continue. This sets up a cyclic, downward spiral, with a negative feedback loop that escalates the problems. Unless aggressive intervention occurs, death due to inadequate oxygenation is the result.[321, 322]

The fetal pulmonary vessels have a greater proportion of smooth muscle tissue than do adult vessels. This results in an increase in tone in these vessels, thereby contributing to the increased PVR present in the fetus. During the 1st week of life the amount of muscle tissue decreases rapidly, reaching the adult level by 4 to 8 weeks of age.

The reactivity of these vessels is also increased during fetal life. Hypoxemia is the greatest stimulus for this vasoconstrictive response. The low fetal PO_2 within these vessels results in constriction and augments the increased PVR created by the increased muscle tissue. As gestational age advances the constrictor response becomes stronger.

At birth constriction of the vessels continues if oxygen levels do not rise so that systemic and pulmonary vascular pressures change. This constriction results in the persistence of fetal circulatory patterns without the benefit of the placenta, the result being hypoxia secondary to transition failure and altered ventilation and perfusion.

Treatment

The goals of PPHN medical and nursing treatment are the relief of the hypoxemia,

correction of the acidosis, promotion of pulmonary vascular dilation, and support of the extrapulmonary systems. The methods most commonly used are hyperventilation, vasodilating drugs, and vasopressors.[110] ECMO may be used with critically ill infants who do not respond to other therapies.

The goal in using hyperventilation with PPHN is to keep the infant hyperoxic and alkalotic. The increased oxygenation is enhanced by the alkalosis and together they facilitate pulmonary vasodilatation. Hyperoxia may be necessary for days to weeks in order to maintain vasodilatation. These infants have extremely sensitive vasoconstrictive responses; therefore withdrawal of oxygen and ventilatory support should be done cautiously to prevent relative hypoxia and vasoconstriction.

The use of volume expanders and vasopressors is designed to maintain systemic blood pressure and prevent complications from hypotension. Infusion of tolazoline hydrochloride (Priscoline) may also be used in an attempt to dilate the pulmonary vasculature. Although the drug may result in pulmonary vasodilation, it is not pulmonary specific, and vasodilation of peripheral vessels can compound the hypotension that already exists. Vasopressors and volume expanders should be readily available when vasodilators are considered.

Anticipation of respiratory problems and monitoring of transitional events are critical to the neonate's successfully achieving adequate ventilatory status. Nurses provide the essential skills to facilitate this critical stage in the neonate's transition to extrauterine existence.

MATURATIONAL CHANGES DURING INFANCY AND CHILDHOOD

The functional and anatomic maturation of the respiratory system continues through childhood until the bony thorax stops growing. Functional development is essentially secondary to anatomic development and is tied to the continued growth of the airways and multiplication of the alveoli.

At the time of birth there are 20 million air spaces, a combination of terminal air sacs and alveoli.[45] From then on alveoli beget alveoli, gradually replacing all of the terminal air sacs. By 8 years of age the alveolar number has increased to 300 million.[111] It is unclear if after this time alveolar multiplication continues or whether further lung growth is related only to alveoli enlarging in size.[335, 336]

Alveolar diameter doubles in size during maturation. At 2 months of age, alveoli measure 150 to 180 μ and by adulthood are 250 to 300 μ.[111] This indicates that there is a steady increase in surface area during childhood. Measurements show that the surface area increases from 2.8 m² at birth, to 32 m² at 8 years, reaching 75 m² by adulthood.[111] This improves the oxygen diffusing capacity of the organ system.

Collateral ventilation also develops during childhood, thereby providing protection against obstruction of small airways and atelectasis. The pores of Kohn appear sometime between the 1st and 2nd years of life. Lambert's channels begin to be evident by 6 years of age. Interbronchiolar channels are not found in normal lungs but may develop in disease situations.[235]

Oxygen affinity continues to increase over the first 6 months of life owing to conversion from fetal hemoglobin. At that time over 90% of the hemoglobin is adult in nature. This improves the diffusion of oxygen to the tissues, meeting the increased metabolic needs of the cells. Maturation of the pulmonary vasculature was discussed on p. 279.

By 8 months the muscle fiber content of the diaphragm reaches adult proportions.[117] Rib cage compliance remains altered during infancy. The peripheral airways contribute the most to airway resistance until 5 years, when the upper airways predominate (as in adults).[260] Cartilage support for the conducting airways increases rapidly in the first 2 months, then more slowly throughout childhood. Closing capacity decreases after 6 years.[264] Venous admixture does not reach adult values until early childhood.[271]

SUMMARY

Although the respiratory system of the newly born infant is not fully developed at birth, the infant does demonstrate capabilities and strategies necessary to achieve sustained respirations, blood gas tension, and acid-base homeostasis and compensatory mechanisms to maintain that balance even in disease states. Transition must be seen as a process that takes several days, with initial responses

relating to the fetal state. Knowledge of these differences and the progression toward extrauterine stability can guide therapeutic interventions and determine clinical assessment.

Recognizing that the infant has prepared throughout gestation for this transition can provide us with an appreciation of the accom-

TABLE 7–15
Summary of Clinical Implications for Respiratory System: Neonate

Understand the normal anatomic and functional development of the respiratory system (pp. 277–289).
Know what factors accelerate fetal lung development, what factors inhibit functional development, and what therapies are utilized with potential preterm delivery (pp. 277–285).
Discuss the various tests utilized to assess fetal lung maturity (pp. 284–285).
Describe the expected changes in fetal blood gases over the intrapartum period (pp. 287–288; Table 7–9).
Identify various steps in respiratory conversion (pp. 289–291).
Understand the consequences of asphyxia (pp. 311–313).
Maintain the appropriate equipment needed for resuscitation at all deliveries (pp. 314–315; Table 7–12).
Acquire and maintain resuscitation skills (pp. 314–315).
Identify high risk deliveries that nursery personnel will attend (pp. 314–315).
Position preterm infants on abdomen with head of the bed elevated in order to promote oxygenation (pp. 294–296, 309–311).
Monitor head and neck positioning in preterm infants in order to either keep airway open or keep ETT positioned correctly (pp. 309–311).
Utilize a ventilator-ETT manifold adapter that allows suctioning without removal from the ventilator (pp. 309–311).
Assess breath sounds on a regular basis in order to determine the need for ETT suctioning (pp. 309–311).
Restore FRC following suctioning by sighing the infant (pp. 309–311).
Evaluate the critically ill infant's tolerance of handling and therapeutic procedures and structure care activities based on this information (pp. 310–311).
Identify the infant population at risk for transient tachypnea (pp. 315–316).
Describe the risk factors and clinical symptomatology associated with RDS (pp. 316–318).
Identify those infants at risk for developing BPD and the radiographic signs of BPD (pp. 318–321).
Monitor blood gases and ventilatory parameters in infants with BPD (pp. 318–321).
Assess, evaluate, and monitor caloric intake for infants with respiratory illnesses on a daily basis (pp. 320–321).
Monitor somatic growth and head circumference changes regularly in infants with BPD (pp. 320–321).
Identify and monitor infants who either are at risk for or who have meconium aspiration or PPHN (pp. 321–324).

Page numbers in parentheses following each intervention refer to pages where rationale for intervention is discussed.

plishment. The respiratory muscles have exercised and trained to take over the function of the respiratory pump itself, although fatigue may be encountered quite quickly. Intercostal muscles can stabilize the chest wall, so that effective ventilation can be achieved. The difficulties come when disease or immaturity is encountered. There is little reserve to increase ventilatory efforts or sustain increased respiratory activity. The ability to recruit accessory muscles, the use of laryngeal braking (grunting), and the recruitment of new alveoli help to improve gas exchange and increase the pulmonary surface area.[30]

For those infants more than 28 weeks' gestational age, these mechanisms may be employable. To what degree and efficiency we do not know. Each infant responds uniquely to the process of transition and to pathology. The development of refined clinical skills and further research may give us more clues as to when and how the respiratory system prepares and achieves its sustained activity. Clinical implications for the neonate are identified in Table 7–15.

REFERENCES

1. Abel, E.L. (1983). *Marihuana, tobacco, alcohol, and reproduction.* Boca Raton, FL: CRC Press.
2. Adamson, K., et al. (1963). The treatment of acidosis with alkali and glucose during asphyxia in foetal rhesus monkeys. *J Physiol, 169,* 679.
3. Adamsons, K., et al. (1964). Resuscitation by positive pressure ventilation and trishydroxymethylaminomethane of rhesus monkeys asphyxiated at birth. *J Pediatr, 65,* 807.
4. Adamsons, K., Mueller-Heubach, A., & Meyers, R. (1971). Production of fetal asphyxia in the rhesus monkey (administration of catecholamines to the mother). *Am J Obstet Gynecol, 109,* 248.
5. Agostini, E. (1959). Volume pressure relationships of the thorax and lung in the newborn. *J Appl Physiol, 14,* 909.
6. Albersheim, S., et al. (1976) Effect of CO_2 on the immediate response to O_2 in preterm infants. *J Appl Physiol, 41,* 609.
7. Alcorn, D., et al. (1977). Morphological effects of chronic tracheal ligation and drainage in fetal lamb lung. *J Anat, 123,* 649.
8. Alexander, S. (1984). Physiologic and biochemical effects of exercise. *Clin Biochem, 17,* 126.
9. Anderson, W.R. & Engel, R.R. (1983). Cardiopulmonary sequelae of reparative stages of bronchopulmonary dysplasia. *Arch Pathol Lab Med, 107,* 603.
10. Archer, G.W. & Marx, G.F. (1974). Arterial oxygen tension during apnoea in parturient women. *Br J Anaesth, 46,* 358.
11. Artal, R., et al. (1986). Pulmonary responses to exercise in pregnancy. *Am J Obstet Gynecol, 154,* 378.
12. Auld, P.A., et al. (1963). Measurement of thoracic gas volume in the newborn infant. *J Clin Invest, 42,* 476.
13. Avery, M.E. & Cook, C.D. (1961). Volume pressure relationship of lungs and thorax in fetal, neonatal, and adult goats. *J Appl Physiol, 16,* 1034.
14. Avery, M.E. & Mead, J. (1959). Surface properties in relation to atelectasis and hyaline membrane disease. *Am J Dis Child, 97,* 517.
15. Avery, M.E., Fletcher, B.D., & Williams, R.G. (1981). *The lung and its disorders in the newborn infant.* Philadelphia: WB Saunders.
16. Avery, M.E. & Taeusch, H.W. (1984). *Schaffer's diseases of the newborn* (5th ed.). Philadelphia: WB Saunders.
17. Bada, H.S., Alojipan, L.C. & Andrews, B.F. (1977). Premature rupture of membranes and its effect on the newborn. *Ped Clin North Am, 24,* 491.
18. Ballard, P.L., Hovey, M.L., & Gonzales, L.K. (1984). Thyroid hormone stimulation of phosphatidylcholine synthesis in cultured fetal rabbit lung. *J Clin Invest, 74,* 898.
19. Ballard, P.L., et al. (1986). Human pulmonary surfactant apoprotein: Effects of development, culture and hormones on the protein and its mRNA. *Pediatr Res, 20,* 422A.
20. Ballard, P.L., et al. (1980). Transplacental stimulation of lung development in the fetal rabbit by 3,5 dimethyl–3-isopropyl-L-thyronine. *J Clin Invest, 65,* 1407.
21. Ballard, P.L. (1979). Hormonal regulation of the surfactant system. In A. Minkowski & M. Monset-Couchard (Eds.), *Physiological and biochemical basis for perinatal medicine.* New York: Karger.
22. Bancalari, E. & Berlin, J.A. (1978). Meconium aspiration and other asphyxial disorders. *Clin Perinatol, 5,* 317.
23. Bancalari, E., et al. (1979). Bronchopulmonary dysplasia: Clinical presentation. *J Pediatr, 95,* 819.
24. Bangham A.D., Morley J.C., & Phillips M.C. (1979). The physical properties of an effective lung surfactant. *Biochim Biophys Acta, 573,* 552.
25. Barnes, D.A., et al. (1984). Respiratory distress syndrome and presence of phosphatidylglycerol: Report of three cases. *Am J Obstet Gynecol, 148,* 347.
26. Barrett, C.T. & Oliver, T.K. (1968). Hypoglycemia and hyperinsulinism in erythroblastosis fetalis. *New Engl J Med, 278,* 1260.
27. Bartels, H., et al. (1972). *Perinatale Atmung.* Berlin: Springer-Verlag.
28. Bassell, G.M. & Marx, G.F. (1984). Physiologic changes of normal pregnancy and parturition. In E.V. Cosmi (Ed.). *Obstetric anesthesia and perinatology.* New York: Appleton-Century-Crofts.
29. Batina, S.L. & Bherkedal, T. (1972). The course and outcome of pregnancy in women with bronchial asthma. *Acta Allergol, 27,* 397.
30. Bauer, C.R., Stern, L., & Colle, E. (1974). Prolonged rupture of membranes associated with a decreased incidence of respiratory distress syndrome. *Pediatrics, 53,* 7.
31. Benesch, R. & Benesch, R.E. (1967). Effect of organic phosphates from human erythrocytes on the allosteric properties of hemoglobin. *Biochem Biophys Res Commun, 26,* 162.
32. Berdon, W.E., Baker, D.H. & Amoury, R. (1968). The role of pulmonary hypoplasia in the prognosis

of newborn infants with diaphragmatic hernia and eventration. *AJR, 103*, 413.

33. Berger, A.J., Mitchell, R.A., & Severinghaus, J.W. (1977). Regulation of respiration. *N Engl J Med, 297*, 92.

34. Bertalanffy F.D. & LeBlond C.P. (1955). Structure of respiratory tissue. *Lancet, 2*, 1365.

35. Blanco, C.E., Hanson, M.A., & McCooke, H.B. (1985). Studies in utero of the mechanisms of chemoreceptor resetting. In C.T. Jones & P.W. Nathaniel (Eds.), *The physiologic development of the fetus and the newborn*. London: Academic Press.

36. Bland, R.D. (1972). Cord blood total protein level as a screening aid for the idiopathic respiratory distress syndrome. *New Engl J of Med, 287*, 9.

37. Bleasdale, J.E. & Johnston, J.M. (1985). Developmental biochemistry of lung surfactant. In G.H. Nelson (Ed.), *Pulmonary development: Transition from intrauterine to extrauterine life*. New York: Marcel Dekker.

38. Bloom, R.S. & Cropley, C. (1989). *Textbook of neonatal resuscitation*. Dallas, TX: American Heart Association.

39. Boddy, K. & Robinson, J. (1971). External method for detection of fetal breathing in utero. *Lancet, 2*, 1231.

40. Boddy, K., Dawes, G.S., & Robinson, J. (1975). Intrauterine fetal breathing movements. In L. Gluck (Ed.), *Modern perinatal medicine*. Chicago: Year Book Medical Publishers.

41. Bonica, J.J. (1974). Maternal physiologic changes during pregnancy and anesthesia. In S.M. Shnider & F. Moya (Eds.), *The anesthesiologist, mother, and newborn*. Baltimore: Williams & Wilkins.

42. Bonica, J. (1984). Maternal physiologic and psychologic alterations during pregnancy and labor. In E.V. Cosmi (Ed.), *Obstetric anesthesia and perinatology*. New York: Appleton-Century-Crofts.

43. Bonikos, D.S. & Bensch, K.G. (1988). Pathogenesis of bronchopulmonary dysplasia. In T.A. Merritt, W.H. Northway, & B.R. Boyton (Eds.), *Contemporary issues in fetal and neonatal medicine: Bronchopulmonary dysplasia*. Boston: Blackwell Scientific Publications.

44. Boychuk, R.B., Rigatto, H., Sheisha, M.M.K. (1977). The effect of lung inflation on the control of respiratory frequency in the neonate. *J Physiol* (Lond), *243*, 599.

45. Boyden, E.A. & Tompsett, D.H. (1965). The changing patterns in the developing lungs of infants. *Acta Anat, 61*, 164.

46. Boyden, E.. (1977). Development and growth of the airways. In W.A. Hodson (Ed.), *Lung biology in health and disease* (Vol. 6). New York: Marcel Dekker.

47. Boyle, R.J. & Oh, W. (1978). Respiratory distress syndrome. *Clin Perinatol, 5*, 283.

48. Boyton, B.R. (1988). The epidemiology of bronchopulmonary dysplasia. In T.A. Merritt, W.H. Northway, & B.R. Boyton (Eds.), *Contemporary issues in fetal and neonatal medicine: Bronchopulmonary dysplasia*. Boston: Blackwell Scientific Publications.

49. Brasch, R., Heldt, G., & Hecht, S. (1981). Endotracheal tube orifice abutting the tracheal wall: A cause of infant airway obstruction. *Pediatr Radiol, 141*, 387.

50. Brehier, A., et al. (1977). Corticosteroid induction of phosphatidic acid phosphatase in fetal rabbit lung. *Biochem Biophys Res Commun, 77*, 883.

51. Brown, W. (1982). Respiratory problems. In F.M. James & A.S. Wheeler (Eds.), *Obstetric anesthesia: The complicated patient*. Philadelphia: FA Davis.

52. Brumley, G.W. (1971). Lung development and lecithin metabolism. *Arch Intern Med, 127*, 413.

53. Brumley G.W., et al. (1967). Correlations of mechanical stability, morphology, pulmonary surfactant, and phospholipid content in the developing lamb lung. *J Clin Invest, 46*, 863.

54. Bryan, A.C. & Bryan, M.H. (1978). Control of respiration in the newborn. *Clin Perinatol, 5*, 269.

55. Bucci, G., Cook, C., & Barrie, H. (1961). Studies of respiratory physiology in children. *J Pediatr, 58*, 820.

56. Bucher U. & Reid L. (1961). Development of the intrasegmental bronchial tree: The pattern of branching and development of cartilage at various stages of intra-uterine life. *Thorax, 16*, 207.

57. Bunn, H.F. & Forget, B.G. (1986). *Hemoglobin: Molecular, genetic and clinical aspects*. Philadelphia: WB Saunders.

58. Bureau, M.A., et al. (1985). The ventilatory response to hypoxia in the newborn lamb after carotid body denervation. *Respir Physiol, 60*, 109.

59. Bureau, M.A. (1985). Postnatal maturation of the respiratory response to O_2 in awake newborn lambs. *J Appl Physiol, 52*, 428.

60. Burgess, A. (1979). *The nurse's guide to fluid and electrolyte balance*. New York: McGraw-Hill.

61. Burgess W.R. & Chernick V. (1982). *Respiratory therapy in newborn infants and children*. New York: Thieme-Stratton.

62. Burri, P.H. & Weibel, E.R. (1977). Ultrastructure and mophometry of the developing lung. In W.A. Hodson (Ed.), *Development of the lung*. New York: Marcel Dekker.

63. Burri P.H. & Weibel E.R. (1977). Ultrastructure and morphometry of the developing lung. In W.A. Hodson (Ed.), *Development of the lung*. New York: Marcel Dekker.

64. Burrows, G.N. & Ferris, T.F. (1982). *Medical complications during pregnancy*. Philadelphia: WB Saunders.

65. Carroll, B. (1977). Pulmonary hypoplasia and pleural effusions associated with fetal death in utero: Ultrasonic findings. *AJR, 129*, 749.

66. Cassin S., et al. (1964). The vascular resistance of the foetal and newly ventilated lung of the lamb. *J Physiol* (Lond), *171*, 61.

67. Ceruti, E. (1966). Chemoreceptor reflexes in the newborn infant: Effect of cooling on the response to hypoxia. *Pediatrics, 37*, 556.

68. Chamberlain, D., et al. (1977). Pulmonary hypoplasia in babies with severe rhesus isoimmunization: A quantitative study. *J Pathol, 122*, 43.

69. Chanutin, A. & Curnish, R. (1967). Effect of organic and inorganic phosphates on the oxygen equilibrium of human erythrocytes. *Arch Biochem Biophys, 121*, 96.

70. Charles, D., Jacoby, H.E., & Burgess, F. (1965). Amniotic fluid volume in the second half of pregnancy. *Am J Obstet Gynecol, 93*, 1042.

71. Charles, A.G., Norr, K.L., & Block, C.R. (1978). Obstetric and psychological effects of psychoprophylactic preparation for childbirth. *Am J Obstet Gynecol, 131*, 44.

72. Chernick, V. (1978). Fetal breathing movements and the onset of breathing. *Clin Perinatol, 5*, 257.

73. Chernick, V., Halson, W.A., & Greenfield, L.J. (1966). Effect of chronic pulmonary artery ligation on pulmonary mechanics and surfactant. *J Appl Physiol, 21,* 1315.

74. Christenson, R. (1979). Gross differences observed in the placentas of smokers and nonsmokers. *Am J Epidemiol, 110,* 178.

75. Clapp, J.F. (1985). Fetal heart rate response to running in midpregnancy and late pregnancy. *Am J Obstet Gynecol, 153,* 251.

76. Clapp, J.F. (1985). Maternal heart rate in pregnancy. *Am J Obstet Gynecol, 152,* 659.

77. Cohen, S. & Mazze, R. (1985). Physiology of pregnancy. In J. M. Baden & J.B. Brodsky (Eds.), *The pregnant surgical patient.* New York: Futura Publishing.

78. Cole, P.V. & Nainby-Luxmoore, R.C. (1962). Respiratory volumes in labour. *Br Med J, 1,* 1118.

79. Collings, C., Curret, L., & Mullins, J. (1983). Maternal and fetal responses to a maternal aerobic exercise program. *Am J Obstet Gynecol, 145,* 702.

80. Comroe, J.H., et al. (1968). Die Lunge. *Klinische Physiologie und Lungenfunktionsprufungen.* Stuttgart: Schattauer-Verlag.

81. Condorelli, S., Cosmi, E.V., & Scarpelli, E.M. (1974). Extrapulmonary source of amniotic fluid phospholipids. *Am J Obstet Gynecol, 118,* 842.

82. Cook, C.D., et al. (1957). Studies of respiratory physiology in the newborn infant. III. Measurement of mechanisms of respiration. *J Clin Invest, 36,* 440.

83. Corbet, A.J., et al. (1978). Effect of aminophylline and dexamethasone on secretion of pulmonary surfactant in fetal rabbits. *Pediatr Res, 12,* 797.

84. Cosgrove, J.F., Neuberger, N., Levison, H. (1976). The ventilatory response to CO_2 in asthmatic children measured by mouth occlusion pressure. *Pediatrics, 57,* 952.

85. Cosmi, EV. (1984). Effect of anesthesia on labor and delivery. In C.V. Cosmi (Ed.), *Obstetric anesthesia and perinatology.* New York: Appleton-Century-Crofts.

86. Cosmi, E.V. & Di Renzo, G.C. (1983). Diagnosis of fetal lung maturity. In E.V. Cosmi & E.M. Scarpelli (Eds.), *Pulmonary surfactant system.* Amsterdam: Elsevier Biomedical.

87. Cosmi, E.V. (1984). Effects of anesthesia on the uteroplacental blood flow and fetus. In C.V. Cosmi (Ed.), *Obstetric anesthesia and perinatology.* New York: Appleton-Century-Crofts.

88. Cruikshank, D. & Hays, P. (1986). Maternal physiology in pregnancy. In S. Gabbe, J. Niebyl, & J. Simpson (Eds.), *Obstetrics: Normal and problem pregnancies.* New York: Churchill Livingstone.

89. Cruz, A.C., et al. (1976). Respiratory distress syndrome with mature L/S ratio: Diabetes mellitus and low Apgar scores. *Am J Obstet Gynecol, 126,* 78.

90. Csaba, I.F., Sulyok, E., & Ertl, T. (1978). Relationship of maternal treatment with indomethacin to persistence of fetal circulation syndrome. *J Pediatr, 92,* 484.

91. Cuestas, R.A., Lindall, A. & Engel, R.R. (1976). Low thyroid hormones and respiratory distress syndrome of the newborn: Studies on cord blood. *N Eng J Med, 295,* 297.

92. Cugell, D.W., et al. (1953). Pulmonary function in pregnancy: Serial observations in normal women. *Am Rev Tuberc, 67,* 568.

93. D'Alonzo, G.E. (1990). The pregnant asthmatic patient. *Semin in Perinat, 14,* 119.

94. Davies, G. & Reid, L. (1970). Growth of the alveoli and pulmonary arteries in childhood. *Thorax, 25,* 669.

95. Davis, G.M., Hobbs, S., & Bureau, M.A. (1986). Limitation of the ventilatory response to CO_2 in newborn lambs. *Am Rev Respir Dis, 133* (Suppl), A136.

96. Davis, G.M. & Bureau, M.A. (1987). Pulmonary and chest wall mechanics in the control of respiration in the newborn. *Clin Perinatol, 14,* 551.

97. Dawes, G.S. (1974). Breathing before birth in animals and man. *New Engl J Med, 290,* 557.

98. Dawes, G.S. (1968). *Foetal and neonatal physiology.* Chicago: Year Book Medical Publishers.

99. Delke, I., Minkoff, H., & Grunebaum, A. (1985). Effect of Lamaze childbirth preparation on maternal plasma beta-endorphin immuno-reactivity in active labor. *Am J Perinatol, 2,* 317.

100. Deneke, S.M., Bernstein, S.P. & Fanburg, B.L. (1979). Enhancement by disulfiram (Antabuse) of toxic effect of 95 to 97% O_2 on the rat lung. *J Pharmacol Exp Ther, 208,* 377.

101. Derenne, J.P., Macklem, P.T., & Roussos, C.H. (1978). State of the art: The respiratory muscles: mechanics, control and pathophysiology. Part I. *Am Rev Respir Dis, 118,* 119.

102. DeSwiet, M. (1977). Diseases of the respiratory system. *Clin Obstet Gynecol, 4,* 287.

103. DeSwiet M. (1984). Maternal pulmonary disorders. In R. Creasy and R. Resnik (Eds.), *Maternal-fetal medicine.* Philadelphia: WB Saunders.

104. Di Renzo, G.C., et al. (1986). The measurement of amniotic fluid phosphatidylglycerol for the assessment of fetal lung maturity. In M. Vignali, E.V. Cosmi, & M. Luerti (Eds.), *Diagnosis and treatment of fetal lung immaturity.* Milan-Paris: Masson Publishing.

105. Di Renzo, G.C., Anceschi, M.M., & Cosmi, E.V. (1988). Diagnosis of fetal lung maturity. In G.H. Wiknijosastro, W.H. Prakoso, & K. Maeda (Eds.), *Perinatology.* New York: Excerpta Medica.

106. Dobbs, L.G. & Mason, R.J. (1979). Pulmonary alveolar type II cells isolated from rats. Release of phosphatidylcholine in response to beta-adrenergic stimulation. *J Clin Invest, 63,* 378.

107. Doering, S.G. & Entwisle, D.R. (1975). Preparation during pregnancy and ability to cope with labor and delivery. *Am J Orthopsychiatry, 45,* 825.

108. Doering, G.K., Loeschke, H.H., & Ochwadt, B. (1950). Weitere Untersuchungen uber die Wirking der Sexualhormone auf die Atmung. Pfleug. *Archiv ges Physiol, 252,* 216.

109. Donn, S. & Kuhns, L. (1980). Mechanism of endotracheal tube movement with change of head position in the neonate. *Pediatric Radiology, 9,* 37.

110. Drummond, W.H., et al. (1981). The independent effects of hyperventilation, tolazoline and dopamine on infants with persistent pulmonary hypertension. *J Pediatr, 98,* 603.

111. Dunnill, M.S. (1962). Postnatal growth of the lung. *Thorax, 17,* 329.

112. Ehrenkranz, R.A., Ablow, R.C., & Warshaw, J.B. (1979). Prevention of bronchopulmonary dysplasia with vitamin E administration during the acute stages of respiratory distress syndrome. *J Pediatr, 95,* 873.

113. Elliott, F.M. & Reid, L. (1965) Some new facts about the pulmonary artery and its branching pattern. *Clin Radiol, 16*, 193.

114. Elrad, H. & Gleicher, N. (1985). Physiologic changes in normal pregnancy. In N. Gleicher (Ed.), *Principles of medical therapy in pregnancy*. New York: Plenum Press.

115. Emery J.L. (1970). The postnatal development of the human lung and its implications for lung pathology. *Respiration, 27* (Suppl), 41.

116. Erickson, P.S., et al. (1983). Acute effects of maternal smoking on fetal breathing and movements. *Obstet Gynecol, 61*, 367.

117. Escobedo, M.B. (1982). Fetal and neonatal cardiopulmonary physiology. In R.L. Schreiner & J.A. Kisling (Eds.), *Practical neonatal respiratory care*. New York: Raven Press.

118. Fakhrae, S.H., et al. (1980). Obstructed total anomalous pulmonary venous return confused with persistent pulmonary hypertension of the newborn. *Clin Pediatr, 19*, 644.

119. Farman, J.V. & Thorpe, M.H. (1969). Compliance changes during caesarean section. *Br J Anaesth, 41*, 999.

120. Farrell, P.M. & Morgan T.E. (1977). Lecithin biosynthesis in the developing lung.

121. Feijen, H.W.H., et al. (1982). Evaluation of the fetal lung profile including the two dimensional L/S ratio for the establishment of fetal lung maturation. *Gynecol Obstet Invest, 14*, 142.

122. Fiascone, J., et al. (1986). Differential effect of beta methasone on alveolar surfactant and lung tissue of fetal rabbits. *Pediatr Res, 20*, 428A

123. Fishburne, J., et al. (1972). Bronchospasm complicating intravenous prostaglandin $F_2\alpha$ for therapeutic abortion. *Obstet Gynecol, 39*, 892.

124. Flemming, P., Bryan, A.C., & Bryan, M.H. (1978). Functional immaturity of pulmonary irritant receptors and apnea in newborn preterm infants. *Pediatrics, 61*, 515.

125. Forman, H.J. & Fisher, A.B. (1981). Antioxidant defenses. In D.L. Gilbert (Ed.), *Oxygen and living processes: An interdisciplinary approach*. New York: Springer-Verlag.

126. Fouron, J.C. & Herbert, F. (1973). The circulatory effects of hematocrit variations in normovolemic newborn lambs. *J Pediatr, 82*, 995.

127. Fox, W.W., et al. (1977). Pulmonary hypertension in the perinatal aspiration syndromes. *Pediatrics, 59*, 205.

128. Frank, L. & Sosenko, I.R.S. (1987). Development of lung antioxidant enzyme system in late gestation: Possible implications for the prematurely born infant. *J Pediatr, 110*, 9.

129. Frank, L. & Sosenko, I.R.S. (1987). Prenatal development of lung antioxidant enzymes in four species. *J Pediatr, 110*, 106.

130. Frank, L. & Massaro, D. (1980). Oxygen toxicity. *Am J Med, 69*, 117.

131. Frank, L., Lewis, P., & Sosenko, I.R.S. (1987). Dexamethasone stimulation of fetal rat lung antioxidant enzyme activity in parallel with surfactant stimulation. *Pediatrics, 74*, 569.

132. Frank, L. & Neriishi, K. (1984). Endotoxin treatment is able to protect vitamin E deficiency rats from pulmonary O_2 toxicity. *Am J Physiol, 247*, R520.

133. Freeman, B.A. & Crapo, J.D. (1982). Biology of disease: Free radicals and tissue injury. *Lab Invest, 47*, 412.

134. Freeman, B.A., Topolosky, M.K., & Crapo, J.D. (1982). Hyperoxia increases oxygen radical production in rat lung homogenates. *Arch Biochem Biophys, 216*, 477.

135. Fridovich, I. (1976). Oxygen radicals, hydrogen peroxide, and oxygen toxicity. In W.A. Prior (Ed.), *Free radicals in biology* (Vol. 1). New York: Academic Press.

136. Fujikura, T. & Klionsky, B. (1975). The significance of meconium staining. *Am J Obstet Gynecol, 121*, 45.

137. Gandy, G.M., et al. (1964). Thermal environment and acid base homeostasis in human infants during the first hours of life. *J Clin Invest, 43*, 751.

138. Ganong, W.F. (1981) *Review of medical physiology* (10th ed.). Los Altos, CA: Lange Medical.

139. Gee, J.B.L., et al. (1967). Pulmonary mechanics during pregnancy. *J Clin Invest, 46*, 945.

140. Geggel, R.L. & Reid, L.M. (1984). The structural basis of PPHN. *Clin Perinatol, 3*, 525.

141. Gerhardt, T. & Bancalari, E. (1981). Maturational changes of reflexes influencing inspiratory timing of newborns. *J Appl Physiol, 50*, 1282.

142. Gersony, W.M. (1973). Persistence of the fetal circulation: A commentary [editorial]. *J Pediatr, 82*, 1103.

143. Gersony, W.M., et al. (1976). The hemodynamic effects of intrauterine hypoxia: An experimental model in newborn lambs. *J Pediatr, 89*, 631.

144. Gewolb, I.H., et al. (1982). Delay in pulmonary glycogen degradation in fetuses of streptozotocin diabetic rats. *Pediatr Res, 16*, 869.

145. Gibson, R.M. (1979). Hyperventilation in aircrews: A review. *Aviat Space Environ Med, 50*, 725.

146. Gilbert, R., Epifano, L., & Auchincloss, J.H. (1962). Dyspnea of pregnancy; A syndrome of altered respiratory control. *JAMA, 182*, 1073.

147. Gilbert, R. & Auchincloss, J.H. (1966). Dyspnea of pregnancy: Clinical and physiological observations. *Am J Med Sci, 252*, 270.

148. Girard, F., Lacaisse, A., & Dejours, P. (1960). Le stimulus O_2 ventilatoire a la periode neonatale chez l'homme. *J Physiol* (Paris), *52*, 108.

149. Gluck, L. & Kulovic, M. (1973). Lecithin/sphingomyelin ratios in amniotic fluid in normal and abnormal pregnancy. *Am J Obstet Gynecol, 115*, 539.

150. Gluck, J.C. & Gluck, P.A. (1976). The effects of pregnancy on asthma: A prospective study. *Ann Allergy, 37*, 164.

151. Gluck, L., et al. (1971). Diagnosis of the respiratory distress syndrome by amniocentesis. *Am J Obstet Gynecol, 109*, 440.

152. Goetzman, B.W. (1986). Understanding bronchopulmonary dysplasia. *Am J Dis Child, 140*, 332.

153. Gonzales, L.W., et al. (1986). Glucocorticoids and thyroid hormone stimulate biochemical and morphological differentiation of human fetal lung in organ culture. *J Clin Endocrinol Metab, 62*, 678.

154. Gooding, C.A. & Gregory, G.A. (1971). Roentgenographic analysis of meconium aspiration of the newborn. *Pediatr Radiol, 100*, 131.

155. Goodman, J.D.S., Visser, F.G.A., & Dawes, G.S. (1984). Effects of maternal cigarette smoking on fetal trunk movements, fetal breathing movements,

and the fetal heart rate. *Br J Obstet Gynecol, 91,* 657.

156. Gordon, M., et al. (1970). Fetal morbidity following potentially anoxigenic obstetric conditions. VII Bronchial asthma. *Am J Obstet Gynecol, 106,* 421.

157. Graff, M. (1987). Prevention of hypoxia and hyperoxia during endotracheal suctioning. *Crit Care Med, 15,* 1133.

158. Greenough, A., Morley, C.J., & Davis, J.A. (1983). Respiratory reflexes in ventilated premature infants. *Early Hum Dev, 8,* 65.

159. Gregory, G.A., et al. (1974). Meconium aspiration in infants—a prospective study. *J Pediatr, 85,* 848.

160. Gregory, G.A. (1975). Resuscitation of the newborn. *Anesthesiology, 43,* 225.

161. Gross, I., et al. (1980). The influence of hormones on the biochemical maturation of fetal rat lung in organ culture. II. Insulin. *Pediatr Res, 14,* 834.

162. Gross, I. & Wilsson, C.M. (1982). Fetal lung in organ culture. IV. Supra-addictive hormone interactions. *J Appl Physiol, 52,* 1420.

163. Gruenwald, P. (1963). Normal and abnormal expansion of the lungs of newborn infants obtained at autopsy. *Lab Invest, 12,* 563.

164. Guthrie, R.D., et al. (1981). Development of CO_2 sensitivity: Effects of gestational age, postnatal age, and sleep state. *J Appl Physiol, 50,* 956.

165. Guzman, C.A. & Caplan, R. (1970). Cardiorespiratory response to exercise during pregnancy. *Am J Obstet Gynecol, 108,* 600.

166. Hack, M., et al (1976). Neonatal respiratory distress following elective delivery: A preventable disease. *Am J Obstet Gynecol, 126,* 3447.

167. Haddon, W., Nesbit, R.E., & Garcia, R. (1961). Smoking and pregnancy and its effect on the fetus. *Obstet Gynecol, 18,* 262.

168. Hagan, R., et al. (1977). Neonatal chest wall afferents and the regulation of respiration. *J Appl Physiol, 42,* 362.

169. Hallman, M. (1984). Development of pulmonary surfactant. In K. Ravio, et al. (Eds.), *Respiratory distress syndrome.* London: Academic Press.

170. Hallman, M. (1984). Antenatal diagnosis of lung maturity. In B. Robertson, L.M.G. Van Golde, & J.J. Batenburg (Eds.), *Pulmonary surfactant.* Amsterdam: Elsevier Science Publishers.

171. Harned, H.S. (1978). Respiration and the respiratory system. In U. Stave (Ed.), *Perinatal physiology.* New York: Plenum Press.

172. Harris, T.R. (1981). Physiological principles. In J.P. Goldsmith & E.H. Karotkin (Eds.), *Assisted ventilation of the neonate.* Philadelphia: WB Saunders.

173. Harrison, M.R. & de Lorimier, A.A. (1981). Congenital diaphragmatic hernia. *Surg Clin North Am, 61,* 1023.

174. Haworth, S.G. & Reid, L. (1976). Persistent fetal circulation: Newly recognized structural features. *J Pediatr, 88,* 614.

175. Haworth, S.G. & Hislop, A.A. (1981). Normal structural and functional adaptation to extrauterine life. *J Pediatr, 98,* 915.

176. Haworth, S.G. & Reid, L. (1977). Quantitative structural study of pulmonary circulation in the newborn with aortic atresia, stenosis or coarctation. *Thorax, 32,* 121.

177. Haworth, S.G. & Reid, L. (1977). Structural study of pulmonary circulation and of heart in total anomalous pulmonary venous return in early infancy. *Br Heart J, 39,* 80.

178. Haworth, S.G., et al. (1977). Development of the pulmonary circulation in ventricular septal defect: A quantitative structural study. *Am J Cardiol, 40,* 781.

179. Hayden, W., Olson, E.B., & Zachman, R.D. (1977). Effect of maternal isoxsuprine on fetal rabbit lung biochemical maturation. *Am J Obstet Gynecol, 129,* 691.

180. Heymann, M.A. & Rudolph, A.M. (1976). Effects of acetylsalicylic acid on the ductus arteriosus and circulation in fetal lambs in utero. *Circ Res, 38,* 418.

181. Hislop, A. & Reid, L. (1981). Growth and development of the respiratory system: Anatomical development. In J.A. Davis & J. Dobbings (Eds.), *Scientific foundations of paediatrics* (2nd ed.). London: Heinemann Medical.

182. Hislop, A. & Reid, L.M. (1977). Formation of the pulmonary vasculature. In W.A. Hodson (Ed.), *Development of the lung.* New York: Marcel Dekker.

183. Hislop, A., Sanderson, M., & Reid, L. (1973). Unilateral congenital dysplasia of lung associated with vascular anomalies. *Thorax, 28,* 435.

184. Hislop, A., et al. (1975). Quantitative structural analysis of pulmonary vessels in isolated ventricular septal defect in infancy. *Br Heart J, 37,* 1014.

185. Hislop, A., Hey, E., & Reid, L. (1976). The lungs in congenital bilateral renal agenesis and dysplasia. *Arch Dis Child, 54,* 32.

186. Hitchcock, K.R. (1979). Hormones and the lung. I. Thyroid hormones and glucocorticoids in lung development. *Anat Rec, 194,* 15.

187. Hodgkinson, R. & Marx, G.F. (1984). Effects of analgesia-anesthesia on the fetus and neonate. In C.V. Cosmi (Ed.), *Obstetric anesthesia and perinatology.* New York: Appleton-Century-Crofts.

188. Holbriech, M. (1982). Asthma and other allergic disorders in pregnancy. *Am Fam Physician, 25,* 187.

189. Hubbell, K.M. & Webster, H.F. (1986). Respiratory management of the neonate. In N.S. Streeter (Ed.), *High risk neonatal care.* Rockville, MD: Aspen Publications.

190. Huber, G.L. & Drath, D.B. (1981). Pulmonary oxygen toxicity. In D.L. Gilbert (Ed.), *Oxygen and living processes: An interdisciplinary approach.* New York: Springer-Verlag.

191. Huch, R. (1986). Maternal hyperventilation and the fetus. *J Perinat Med, 14,* 3.

192. Hung, K.S., Hertweck, M.S., Hardy, J.D. & Loosli, C.G. (1972). Innervation of pulmonary alveoli of the mouse lung: An electron microscopic study. *Am J Anat, 135,* 477.

193. Hyman, A., Spannhake, E., & Kadowita, P. (1978). Prostaglandins and the lung: State of the art. *Am Rev Respir Dis, 117,* 111.

194. Incaudo, G.A. (1987). Diagnosis and treatment of rhinitis during pregnancy and lactation. *Clin Rev Allergy, 5,* 325.

195. Inselman L.S. & Mellins R.B. (1981). Growth and development of the lung. *J Pediatr, 98,* 1.

196. Jacob, J., Hallman, M., & Gluck, L. (1980). Phosphatidylinositol and phosphotidylglycerol enhance surface active properties of lecithin. *Pediatr Res, 14,* 644A.

197. Jaykka, S. (1954). A new theory concerning the

mechanism of the initiation of respiration in the newborn. *Acta Paediatr Scand, 43,* 399.

198. Johnston, J.M., et al. (1975). Phospholipid biosynthesis: The activity of phosphatidic acid phosphohydrolase in the developing lung and amniotic fluid. *Chest, 67*(Suppl.), 195.

199. Jones, R., et al. (1985). Thermoregulation during aerobic exercise in pregnancy. *Obstet Gynecol, 65,* 340.

200. Kanto, W.L., et al. (1976). Tracheal aspirate lecithin/sphingomyelin ratios as predictors of recovery from respiratory distress syndrome. *J Pediatr, 89,* 612.

201. Karlberg, P. (1975). The first breaths of life. In L. Gluck (Ed.), *Modern perinatal medicine year book.* New York: Year Book Medical Publishers.

202. Karlberg, P., et al. (1962). Respiratory studies in newborn infants. II. Pulmonary ventilation and mechanics of breathing in the first minutes of life, including the onset of respiration. *Acta Paediatr Scand, 51,* 121.

203. Keens, D.H. & Ianuzzo, C.D. (1979). Development of fatigue-resisitant muscle fibers in human ventilatory musculature. *Am Rev Respir Dis, 119*(Suppl.), 139.

204. Kikkwa, Y. (1975) Morphology and morphologic development of the lung. In E.M. Scarpelli (Ed.), *Pulmonary physiology of the fetus, newborn, and child.* Philadelphia: Lea & Febiger.

205. Kitterman, J.A., et al. (1981). Preparum maturation of the lung in fetal sheep: Relation to cortisol. *J Appl Physiol, 51,* 384.

206. Kitterman, J. & Liggins, G.C. (1980). Fetal breathing movements and inhibitors of prostaglandin synthesis. *Semin Perinatol, 4,* 97.

207. Klaus, M., et al. (1962). Alveolar epithelial cell mitochondria as a source of the surface-active lung lining. *Science, 137,* 750.

208. Knill, R. & Bryan, A.C. (1976). An intercostal-phrenic inhibitory reflex in the human newborn infant. *J Appl Physiol, 40,* 352.

209. Knuttgen, H.G. & Emerson, K. (1974). Physiological response to pregnancy at rest and during exercise. *J Appl Physiol, 36,* 549.

210. Koch, G. & Wendel, H. (1968). Adjustment of arterial blood gases and acid base balance in the normal newborn infant during the first week of life. *Biol Neonate, 12,* 136.

211. Koch, G. (1968). Alveolar ventilation, diffusing capacity, and $AaPO_2$ difference in the newborn infant. *Respir Physiol, 4,* 168.

212. Kotas, R.W. (1979). Surface tension forces and liquid valance in the lung. In G.A. Gregory & D.W. Thibeault (Eds.), *Neonatal pulmonary care.* Reading, MA: Addison-Wesley.

213. Kreisman, H., Van de Wiel, W., & Mitchell, C. (1975). Respiratory function during prostaglandin-induced labor. *Am Rev Respir Dis, 111,* 564.

214. Kresch, M.J. & Gross, I. (1987). The biochemistry of fetal lung development. *Clin Perinatol, 14,* 481.

215. Kuhns, L. & Poznaski, A. (1971). Endotracheal tube position in infants. *J Pediatr, 78,* 991.

216. Lavery, J.P. & Kochenour, K. (1982). Asthma. In I.T. Queenan (Ed.), *Management of high-risk pregnancy.* Oradell, NJ: Medical Economics.

217. Leake, R.D., Gunther, R., & Sunshine, P. (1974). Perinatal aspiration syndrome: Its association with intrapartum events and anesthesia. *Am J Obstet Gynecol, 118,* 271.

218. Lehmann, V. (1975). Dyspnea in pregnancy. *J Perinat Med, 3,* 154.

219. Lehmann, V. (1974). Veranderungen der Lungendiffusionskapizitat als mogliche Ursache der Hyperventilation in der Schwangerschaft. In J.W. Dudenhausen & E. Saling (Eds.), *Perinatale Medizin 5.* Stuttgart: Georg Thieme-Verlag.

220. Levin, D.L., Mills, L.J., & Weinberg, A.G. (1979). Hemodynamic pulmonary vascular and myocardial abnormalities secondary to pharmacologic constriction of the fetal ductus arteriosus. *Circulation, 60,* 360.

221. Levin, D.L., et al. (1978). Fetal hypertension and the development of increased pulmonary vascular smooth muscle. A possible mechanism for persistent pulmonary hypertension of the newborn infant. *J Pediatr, 92,* 265.

222. Levin, D.L. (1979). Primary pulmonary hypoplasia (editorial). *J Pediatr, 95,* 550.

223. Levinson, G., et al. (1974). Effect of maternal hyperventilation on uterine blood flow and fetal oxygenation and acid-base status. *Anesthesiology, 40,* 340.

224. Lewis, A., Heymann, M., & Rudolph, A. (1976). Gestational changes in pulmonary vascular responses in fetal lambs in utero. *Circul Res, 39,* 536.

225. Liggins, G.C. & Howie, R.N. (1972). A controlled trial of antepartum glucocorticoid treatment for prevention of the respiratory distress syndrome in premature infants. *Pediatrics, 50,* 515.

226. Liggins, G.C. (1969). Premature delivery of foetal lambs infused with glucocorticoids. *Endocrinology, 44,* 515.

227. Liggins G.C. & Kitterman J.A. (1981). Development of the fetal lung. In *The fetus and independent life.* Ciba Foundation Symposium. London: Pitman.

228. Loosli, C.G. & Hung, K.S. (1977). Development of pulmonary innervation. In W.A. Hodson (Ed.), *Development of the lung.* New York: Marcel Dekker.

229. Loper, D.L. (1986). Surfactant replacement therapy. *Neonatal Network, 4,* 14.

230. Lotgering, F.K., Gilbert, R.D., & Longo, L.D. (1983). Exercise responses in pregnant sheep: Blood gases, temperatures, and fetal cardiovascular system. *J Appl Physiol, 25,* 295.

231. Lotgering, F., Gilbert, R., & Longo, L. (1985). Maternal and fetal responses to exercise during pregnancy. *Physiol Rev, 65,* 1.

232. Lough, M., Williams, T., & Rawson, J. (1979). *Newborn respiratory care.* Chicago: Year Book Medical Publishers.

233. Lumley, J., McKinnon, L., & Wood, C. (1971). Lack of agreement and normal values for fetal scalp blood. *J Obstet Gynaecol Br Comm, 78,* 13.

234. Machida, H. (1981). Influence of progesterone on arterial blood and CSF acid-base balance in women. *J Appl Physiol, 51,* 1433.

235. Macklem, P.T. (1971). Airway obstruction and collateral ventilation. *Physiol Rev, 51,* 368.

236. Maloney, J.E. (1987). Lung liquid dynamics in the perinatal period. In J. Lipshitz, et al. (Eds.), *Perinatal development of the heart & lung,* New York: Perinatology Press.

237. Maloney J.E., et al. (1980). Development of the

future respiratory system before birth. *Semin Perinatol, 4*, 251.

238. Manchester, D., Margolis, H.S., & Sheldon, R.E. (1976). Possible association between maternal indomethacin therapy and primary pulmonary hypertension of the newborn. *Am J Obstet Gynecol, 126*, 467.

239. Mann, D.G. & Kirchner, J.A. (1982). Bronchopulmonary dysplasia (or subglottic stenosis?). *Laryngoscope, 92*, 976.

240. Manning, F., Wyn Pugh, E., & Boddy, K. (1975). Effect of cigarette smoking on fetal breathing movements in normal pregnancies. *Br Med J, 1*, 552.

241. Mantell, C.D. (1976). Breathing movements in the human fetus. *Am J Obstet Gynecol, 125*, 530.

242. Marchal, F. (1987). Neonatal apnea. In L. Stern & P. Vert (Eds.), *Neonatal medicine*. New York: Masson Publishing.

243. Marlot, D. & Duron, B. (1976). Cutaneous stimulation and spontaneous respiratory activity in the newborn kitten. In B. Duron (Ed.), *Respiratory centres and afferent systems*. Paris: INSERM.

244. Marsal, K., Lofgren, O., & Gennser, G. (1979). Fetal breathing movements and maternal exercise. *Acta Obstet Gynecol Scand, 58*, 197.

245. Martin, T.C., Bower, R.J., & Bell, M.J. (1982). Postoperative fetal circulation: POFC. *J Pediatr Surg, 17*, 558.

246. Marx, G.F. & Greene, N.M. (1964). Maternal lactate, pyruvate, and excess lactate production during labor and delivery. *Am J Obstet Gynecol, 90*, 786.

247. Marx, G.F., Murthy, P.K., & Orkin, L.R. (1970). Static compliance before and after vaginal delivery. *Br J Anaesthiol, 42*, 1100.

248. Marx, G.F. & Orkin, L.R. (1969). *Physiology of obstetric anesthesia*. Springfield, IL: Charles C Thomas.

249. Maxwell, L.C., et al. (1983). Development of the histochemical and functional properties of baboon respiratory muscles. *J Appl Physiol, 54*, 551.

250. Mendelson, C.R., et al. (1981). Multihormonal regulation of surfactant synthesis by human fetal lung in vitro. *J Clin Endocrinol Metab, 53*, 307.

251. Merritt, T.A. & Farrell, P.M. (1976). Diminished pulmonary lecithin synthesis in acidosis: Experimental findings as related to the respiratory distress syndrome. *Pediatrics, 57*, 32.

252. Mescher, E.J., et al. (1975). Ontogeny of tracheal fluid, pulmonary surfactant, and plasma corticoids in the fetal lamb. *J Appl Physiol, 39*, 1020.

253. Metcalf, J., Bartels, H., & Moll, W. (1967). Gas exchange in the pregnant uterus. *Physiol Rev, 47*, 782.

254. Metcalfe, J., Stock, M., & Banon, P. (1988). Maternal physiology during gestation. In E. Knobil, et al. (Eds), *The physiology of reproduction*. New York: Raven Press.

255. Meyrick, B. & Reid, L.M. (1977). Ultrastructure of alveolar lining and its development. In W.A. Hodson (Ed.), *Development of the lung*. New York: Marcel Dekker.

256. Michel, C.C. (1974). The transport of oxygen and carbon dioxide by the blood. In J.G. Widdicombe (Ed.), *Physiology series one: Volume 2 respiratory physiology*. Baltimore: University Park Press.

257. Milic-Emili, J. (1982). Recent advances in clinical assessment of control of breathing. *Lung, 160*, 1.

258. Miller, F.C., et al. (1975). Significance of meconium during labor. *Am J Obstet Gynecol, 122*, 573.

259. Milne, J., Pack, A., & Coutts, J. (1977). Maternal gas exchange and acid-base status during normal pregnancy. *Scott Med J, 22*, 108.

260. Milne, J.A., et al. (1977). The effect of human pregnancy on the pulmonary transfer factor for carbon monoxide as measured by the single-breath method. *Clin Sci Mol Med, 53*, 271.

261. Milner, A.D. & Vyas, H. (1982). Lung expansion at birth. *J Pediatr, 101*, 879.

262. Milner, A.D., Saunders, R.A., & Hopkin, I.E. (1978). Effects of delivery by caesarean section on lung mechanics and lung volume in the human neonate. *Arch Dis Child, 53*, 545.

263. Moir, D.D. (1980). *Obstetric anesthesia and analgesia* (2nd ed.). London: Bailliere Tindall.

264. Muir, B.L. (1988). *Pathophysiology* (2nd ed.). New York: John Wiley.

265. Muller, N.L. & Bryan, A.C. (1979). Chest wall mechanics and respiratory muscles in infants. *Pediatr Clin North Am, 26*, 502.

266. Murphy, J.D., et al. (1981). The structural basis of persistent hypertension of the newborn infant. *J Pediatr, 98*, 962.

267. Murray, J.F. (1976). *The normal lung: The basis for diagnosis and treatment of pulmonary disease*. Philadelphia: WB Saunders.

268. Naeye, R.L. (1980). Abruptio placentae and placenta previa: Frequency, perinatal mortality and cigarette smoking. *Obstet Gynecol, 55*, 701.

269. Nelson, N.M. (1976). Respiration and circulation after birth. In C.A. Smith & N.M. Nelson (Eds.), *The physiology of the newborn infant*. Springfield, IL: Charles C Thomas.

270. Newsom-Davis, J. (1974). Control of muscles of breathing. In J. Widdicombe (Ed.), *Respiratory Physiology*. MTP International Review of Science. London: Butterworth.

271. Nichols, D.G. & Rogers, M.C. (1987). Developmental physiology of the respiratory system. In M.C. Rogers, (Ed.), *Textbook of pediatric intensive care* (Vol 1). Baltimore: Williams & Wilkins.

272. Northway, W.H., Rosan, R.C., & Porter, D.Y. (1967). Pulmonary disease following respiratory therapy of hyaline membrane disease: Bronchopulmonary dysplasia. *N Engl J Med, 276*, 357.

273. Nunn, J.F. (1987). *Applied respiratory physiology*. London: Butterworth.

274. Oultan, M., et al. (1982). Assessment of fetal pulmonary maturity by phospholipid analysis of amniotic fluid lamellar bodies. *Am J Obstet Gynecol, 142*, 684.

275. Oxron, D.C. (1986). Obstetric analgesia and anesthesia. In H. Oxron (Ed.), *Human labor and birth*. Norwalk: Appleton-Century-Crofts.

276. Painter, P.C. (1980). Simultaneous measurement of lecithin, sphingomyelin, phosphatidylglycerol, phosphatidylinositol, phosphatidylethanolamine and phosphatidylserine in amniotic fluid. *Clin Chem, 26*, 1147.

277. Palahniuk, R.J. & Cumming, M. (1977). Foetal deterioration following thiopentone-nitrous oxide anaesthesia in the pregnant ewe. *Can Anaesth Soc J, 24*, 361.

278. Patrick, J.E., et al. (1978). Human fetal breathing movements and gross body movements at weeks 34–35 gestation. *Am J Obstet Gynecol, 130*, 693.

279. Patrick, J. (1977). Measurement of human fetal

breathing movements. In Mead Johnson Symposium on Perinatal and Developmental Medicine, No. 12. Evansville, IN: Mead Johnson.

280. Pecora, L., Putnam, L., & Baum, G. (1963). Effects of intravenous estrogen on pulmonary diffusing capcity. *Am J Med Sci, 246*, 48.

281. Perlman, M., Williams, J., & Hirsch, M. (1976). Neonatal pulmonary hypoplasia after prolonged leakage of amniotic fluid. *Arch Dis Child, 51*, 349.

282. Platt, L.D., et al. (1983). Exercise in pregnancy II. Fetal responses. *Am J Obstet Gynecol, 147*, 487.

283. Polgar, G. & Weng, T.R. (1979). The functional development of the respiratory system. *Am Rev Respir Dis, 120*, 625.

284. Pope, T.S. & Rooney, S.A. (1987). Effects of glucocorticoid and thyroid hormones on regulatory enzymes of fatty acid synthesis and glycogen metabolism in developing fetal rat lung. *Biochim Biophys Acta, 918*, 141.

285. Pope, T.S. & Rooney, S.A. (1986). Opposing effects of glucocorticoid and thyroid hormones on fatty-acid synthatase activity in culture fetal rat lung. *Fed Proc, 46*, 64.

286. Power, G.G., et al. (1967). Uneven distribution of maternal and fetal placental blood flow, as demonstrated using macroaggregates, and its response to hypoxia. *J Clin Invest, 46*, 2053.

287. Prowse, C.M. & Gaensler, E.A. (1965). Respiratory and acid-base changes during pregnancy. *Anesthesiology, 26*, 381.

288. Quirk, J.G. & Bleasdale, J.E. (1986). Fetal lung maturation in the pregnancy complicated by diabetes mellitus. In G.C. Di Renzo & D.F. Hawkins (Eds.), *Perinatal medicine: Problems and controversies*. New York: Raven Press.

289. Reale, F.R. & Esterly, J.R. (1973). Pulmonary hypoplasia: A morphometric study of the lungs of infants with diaphragmatic hernia, anencephaly, and renal malformations. *Pediatrics, 51*, 91.

290. Rehder, K., et al. (1979). Ventilation-perfusion relationship in young healthy awake and anesthetized-paralyzed man. *J Appl Physiol, 296*, 25.

291. Rehder, K., et al. (1972). The function of each lung of anesthetized and paralyzed man during mechanical ventilation. *Anesthesiol, 37*, 16.

292. Reid L.M. (1984). Structural development of the lung and pulmonary circulation. In K. Raivio, et al. (Eds.), *Respiratory distress syndrome*. London: Academic Press.

293. Remmers, J. & Bartlett, D. (1977). Reflex control of expiratory airflow and duration. *J Appl Physiol, 42*, 80.

294. Rendas, A., et al. (1982). Response of the pulmonary circulation to acute hypoxia in the growing pig. *J Appl Physiol, 52*, 811.

295. Riemenschneider, T.A., et al. (1976). Disturbances of the transitional circulation: Spectrum of pulmonary hypertension and myocardial dysfunction. *J Pediatr, 89*, 622.

296. Robert, M.F., et al. (1976). The association between maternal diabetes and the respiratory distress syndrome in the newborn. *N Engl J Med, 294*, 357.

297. Robotham, J.L., et al. (1980). A physiologic assessment of segmental bronchial atresia. *Am Rev Respir Dis, 121*, 533.

298. Rooney, S.A., et al. (1979). Thyrotropin-releasing hormone increases the amount of surfactant in lung lavage from fetal rabbits. *Pediatr Res, 13*, 623.

299. Rooney, S.A., et al. (1986). Glucocorticoid stimulation of choline-phosphate cytidyltransferase activity in fetal rat lung: Receptor-response relationships. *Biochim Biophys Acta, 888*, 208.

300. Rooth, G. (1980). Fetal homeostasis. In S. Aladjem, A.K. Brown, & C. Surreau (Eds.), *Clinical perinatology*. St. Louis: CV Mosby.

301. Rudolph, A. (1984). Regulation of pulmonary circulation in the fetus and newborn. In K. Raivio, et al. (Eds.), *Respiratory distress syndrome*. London: Academic Press.

302. Rudolph, A.M. (1980). High pulmonary vascular resistance after birth. *Clin Pediatr, 19*, 585.

303. Rudolph, A.M. & Yuan, Ss (1966). Response of the pulmonary vasculature to hypoxia and hydrogen ion concentration changes. *J Clin Invest, 45*, 399.

304. Saldenha, R.L., Cepeda, E.E. & Poland, R.L. (1980). Effect of prophylactic vitamin E on the development of bronchopulmonary dysplasia in high-risk neonates. *Ped Res, 14*, 650.

305. Saling, E. (1966). Amnioscopy and fetal blood sampling: Observations on foetal acidosis. *Arch Dis Child, 41*, 472.

306. Samuelson, A., Becker, A.E., & Wagenvoort, C.A. (1970). A morphometric study of pulmonary veins in normal infants and infants with congenital heart disease. *Arch Pathol, 90*, 112.

307. Schaefer, G., & Silverman, F. (1961). Pregnancy complicated by asthma. *Am J Obstet Gynecol, 82*, 182.

308. Schatz, M. & Hoffman, C. (1987). Interrelationships between asthma and pregnancy: Clinical and mechanistic considerations. *Clin Rev Allergy, 5*, 301.

309. Schatz, M., et al. (1985). Distinguishing clinical and biochemical characteristics associated with improvement or deterioration of asthma during pregnancy [abstract]. *J Allergy Clin Immunol, 75*, 133.

310. Schurch, S., Goerke, J., & Clements, J.A. (1976). Direct determination of surface tension in the lung. *Proc Nat Acad Sci, 73*, 4698.

311. Scott, J.R. & Rose, N.B. (1976). Effects of psychoprophylaxis (Lamaze preparation) on labor and delivery in primiparas. *N Engl J Med, 294*, 1205.

312. Selkurt, E.E. (1982). Respiration. In E.E. Selkurt (Ed.), *Basic physiology for the health sciences* (2nd ed.). Boston: Little, Brown.

313. Shiono, P.H., Klebanoff, M.A., & Berendes, H.W. (1986). Congenital malformations and maternal smoking during pregnancy. *Teratology, 34*, 65.

314. Sibley, L., et al. (1981). Swimming and physical fitness during pregnancy. *J Nurse Midwifery, 26*, 3.

315. Simpson, R.J. & Smith, N.G. (1986). Maternal smoking and low birthweight: Implications for antenatal care. *J Epidemiol Community Health, 40*, 223.

316. Slonin, N.B. & Hamilton, L.H. (1976). *Respiratory physiology*. St. Louis: CV Mosby.

317. Smith, B.T. (1979). Lung maturation in the fetal rat: Acceleration by injection of fibroblast-pneumocyte factor. *Science, 204*, 1094.

318. Smith, B.T., et al. (1975). Insulin antagonism of cortisol action on lecithin synthesis by cultured fetal lung cells. *J Pediatr, 87*, 953.

319. Smith, B.T. (1979). Biochemistry and metabolism of pulmonary surface-active material. In *The surfactant system and the neonate*. Mead Johnson Sym-

posium on Perinatal and Developmental Medicine, No. 14. Evansville, IN: Mead Johnson.

320. Sosenko, I.R.S, Hartig-Beecken, I., & Frantz, I.D. (1980). Cortisol reversal of functional delay of lung maturation in fetuses of diabetic rabbits. *J Appl Physiol, 49*, 971.

321. Southwell, S. (1982). Persistent fetal circulation: Part I. *Neonatal Network, 1*, 41.

322. Southwell, S. (1982). Persistent fetal circulation: Part II. *Neonatal Network, 1*(2), 30.

323. Spira, A., et al. (1977). Smoking during pregnancy and placental pathology. *Biomedicine, 27*, 266.

324. Stablein, J.J. & Lockey, R.F. (1984). Managing asthma during pregnancy. *Compr Ther, 10*, 45.

325. Stenius-Aarniala, B., Pirila, P., & Teramo, K. (1988). Asthma and pregnancy. A prospective study of 198 pregnancies. *Thorax, 43*, 12.

326. Strang, L.B. (1978). *Neonatal respiration: Physiological and clinical studies*. Philadelphia: Lippincott.

327. Strang, L.B. (1978). Pulmonary circulation at birth. In L.B. Strang (Ed.), *Neonatal respiration: Physiological and clinical studies*. Philadelphia: Lippincott.

328. Strang, L.B. (1967). Uptake of liquid from the lungs at the start of breathing. In A.V.S. DeReuck & R. Porter (Eds.), *Development of the lung*. Ciba Foundation Symposium. London: JA Churchill.

329. Straub, N.C. (1966). Effects of alveolar surface tension of the pulmonary vascular bed. *Heart J, 7*, 386.

330. Sykes, M.K. (1975). Arterial oxygen tension in parturient women. *Br J Anaesth, 47*, 530.

331. Tate, I.M. & Repine, J.E. (1983). Neutrophils and the adult respiratory distress syndrome. *Am Rev Respir Dis, 128*, 552.

332. Thach, B.T. & Taeusch, H.W. (1976). Sighing in newborn human infants: Role of the augmenting reflex. *J Appl Physiol, 41*, 502.

333. Thaler, I., Goodman, J.D.S., & Dawes, G.S. (1980). Effects of maternal cigarette smoking on fetal breathing and fetal movements. *Am J Obstet Gynecol, 138*, 282.

334. Thomas, I.T. & Smith, D.W. (1974). Oligohydramnios, cause of the nonrenal features of Potter's sundrome, including pulmonary hypoplasia. *J Pediatr, 84*, 811.

335. Thurlbeck, W.M. & Angus, G.E. (1975). Growth and aging of the normal human lung. *Chest, 67* (Suppl.), 3S.

336. Thurlbeck, W.M. (1975). Postnatal growth and development of the lung. *Am Rev Respir Dis, 111*, 803.

337. Tibbits, P.A., et al. (1981). Interruption of aortic arch masquerading as persistent fetal circulation with definitive diagnosis by two-dimensional echocardiography. *Am Heart J, 102*, 936.

338. Ting, P. & Brady, J.P. (1975). Tracheal suction in meconium aspiration. *Am J Obstet Gynecol, 122*, 767.

339. Tominaga, T. & Page, E.W. (1966). Accommodation of the human placenta to hypoxia. *Am J Obstet Gynecol, 94*, 679.

340. Tooley, W.H. (1977). Hyaline membrane disease. *Am J Dis Child, 126*, 611.

341. Tooley, W.H. (1977). Hyaline membrane disease. *Am Rev Resp Dis, 115*, 9.

342. Tsao, F.H. & Zachman, R.D. (1982). Prenatal assessment of fetal lung maturation: A critical review of amniotic fluid phospholipid tests. In P.M. Farrell (Ed.), *Lung development: Biological and clinical perspectives*. New York: Academic Press.

343. Turner, B. (1983). Current concepts in endotracheal suctioning. *J Calif Perinatal Assoc, 3*, 28.

344. Turner, E.S., Greenberger, P.A., & Patterson, R. (1980). Management of the pregnant asthmatic patient. *Ann Intern Med, 6*, 905.

345. Ueland, K., Novy, M.J., & Metcalfe, J. (1973). Cardiorespiratory responses to pregnancy and exercise in normal women and patients with heart disease. *Am J Obstet Gynecol, 115*, 4.

346. Van Golde, L.M.G. (1976). Metabolism of phospholipids in the lung. *Am Rev Respir Dis, 114*, 977.

347. Vander, A.J., Sherman, J.H., & Luciano, D.S. (1980). *Human physiology: The mechanisms of body function*. New York: McGraw-Hill.

348. Wallace, A.M. & Engstrom, J.L. (1987). The effects of aerobic exercise on the pregnant woman, fetus, and pregnancy outcome: A review. *J Nurse Midwifery, 32*, 277.

349. Walters, D.V. & Over, R.E. (1978). The role of catecholamines in lung liquid absorption at birth. *Pediatr Res, 12*, 239.

350. Ward, J.A., Bucher, J.R., & Roberts, R.J. (1981). The role of nutrition in hyperoxia toxicity in the newborn rat. *Pharmacologist, 23*, 217.

351. Weibel, E.R. & Gil, J. (1977). Structure-function relationships at the alveolar level. In J.B. West (Ed.), *Bioengineering aspects of the lung*. New York: Marcel Dekker.

352. Weinberger, S. & Weiss, S. (1982). Pulmonary diseases. In G.N. Burrow & T.F. Ferris (Eds.), *Medical complications during pregnancy* (2nd ed.). Philadelphia: WB Saunders.

353. Weiss, S.J. & LoBuglio, A.F. (1982). Phagocyte-generated oxygen metabolites and cellular injury. *Lab Invest, 47*, 5.

354. Weiss, E.B. (1975). Bronchial asthma. *Clinical Symposia, 27*, 3.

355. Wender, D.F., et al. (1981). Vitamin E affects lung biochemical and morphological response to hyperoxia in the newborn rabbit. *Pediatr Res, 15*, 262.

356. Wessels, N.K. (1977). *Tissue interactions and development*. Menlo Park, CA: Benjamin & Cummings.

357. West, J.B. (1978). *Pulmonary pathophysiology—the essentials*. Baltimore: Williams & Wilkins.

358. Whisett, J.A., et al. (1987). Induction of surfactant protein in fetal lung: Effects of cAMP and dexamethasone on SAP–35 RNA and synthesis. *J Biol Chem, 262*, 5256.

359. Whittle, M.J., Wilson, A.I. & Whitfield, C.R. (1983). Amniotic fluid phosphatidylglycerol: An early indicator of fetal lung maturity. *Br J Obstet Gynaecol, 90*, 134.

360. Widdicombe, J.G. (1981). Nervous receptors in the respiratory tract. In T.F. Hornbein (Ed.), *Regulation of breathing* (Part I). New York: Marcel Dekker.

361. Wigglesworth, J.S. & Desai, R. (1979). Effect on lung growth of cervical cord section in the rabbit fetus. *Early Hum Dev, 3*, 51.

362. Wilkening, R. & Meschia, G. (1983). Fetal oxygen uptake, oxygenation, and acid-base balance as a function of uterine blood flow. *Am J Physiol, 244*, 749.

363. Williams, D.A. (1967). Asthma and pregnancy. *Allergy, 22*, 311.

364. Wilson, N.C. & Gisolfi, C.V. (1980). Effects of exercising rats during pregnancy. *J Appl Physiol, 48*, 34.

365. Wingerd, J., et al. (1976). Placental ratio in white

and black women: Relation to smoking and anemia. *Am J Obstet Gynecol, 124*, 671.

366. Wispe, J.R. & Roberts, R.J. (1988). Development of antioxidant systems. In T.A. Merritt, W.H. Northway, & B.R. Boyton (Eds.), *Contemporary issues in fetal and neonatal medicine: Bronchopulmonary dysplasia*. Boston: Blackwell Scientific Publications.

367. Wolfson, M.R., et al. (1984). Mechanics and energetics of breathing helium in infants with bronchopulmonary dysplasia. *J Pediatr, 104*, 752.

368. Wulf, K.H., Kunze, L.W., & Lehmann, V. (1972). Clinical aspects of placental gas exchange. In L.D. Long & H. Barkels, (Eds.), *Respiratory gas exchange and blood flow in the placenta*. Bethesda, MD: National Institutes of Health, Public Health Service.

369. Yoon, J.J. & Harper, R.G. (1973). Observations on the relationship between duration of rupture of the membranes and the development of the idiopathic respiratory distress syndrome. *Pediatrics, 52*, 161.

CHAPTER 8

The Renal System and Fluid and Electrolyte Homeostasis

Maternal Physiologic Adaptations
  The Antepartum Period
    Structural Changes
    Changes in Renal Hemodynamics
    Changes in Glomerular Filtration
    Alterations in Tubular Function
    Fluid and Electrolyte Homeostasis
  The Intrapartum Period
  The Postpartum Period
Clinical Implications for the Pregnant Woman and Her Fetus
  Urinary Frequency and Nocturia
  Dependent Edema
  Inability to Void Post Partum
  Risk of Urinary Tract Infection
  Fluid Needs in Labor
  Measurement of Renal Function During Pregnancy
  Hypertension and the Renal System
  Renal Disease and Pregnancy
  Maternal-Fetal Fluid and Electrolyte Homeostasis
Development of the Renal System in the Fetus
  Anatomic Development
  Developmental Basis for Common Anomalies
  Functional Development

Neonatal Physiology
  Transitional Events
  Body Composition
  Urine Output
  Renal Blood Flow and Glomerular Filtration
  Tubular Function
  Water Balance
  Hormonal Regulation
  The Bladder
Clinical Implications for Neonatal Care
  Management of Fluid and Electrolyte Balance
    Insensible Water Loss
    Urine Water Loss
    Estimating Fluid and Electrolyte Needs
    Sodium Requirements of Preterm Infants
    Risk of Overhydration and Dehydration
    Electrolyte Imbalances
  Measurement of Renal Function and Hydration Status
  Renal Handling of Pharmacologic Agents
  Renal Function During Neonatal Illness
Maturational Changes During Infancy and Childhood

The kidneys are critical organs in maintaining body homeostasis by regulation of water and electrolyte balance, excretion of metabolic waste products and foreign substances, regulation of vitamin D activity and erythrocyte production (via erythropoietin), and gluconeogenesis.[144] The kidneys also have an important role in control of arterial blood pressure through the renin-angiotensin system and regulation of sodium balance. This chapter examines the alterations in basic renal processes and regulation of fluids and electrolytes observed in the pregnant woman, fetus, and neonate along with discussion of the implications of these changes in clinical practice.

MATERNAL PHYSIOLOGIC ADAPTATIONS

The renal system undergoes a variety of structural and functional changes during pregnancy with many of the structural changes persisting well into the postpartum period. Pregnancy is characterized by sodium retention and increased extracellular volume, both of which are mediated by alterations in renal function. Many parameters normally used to evaluate renal function and fluid and electrolyte homeostasis are altered in pregnancy, and subclinical renal problems may not be recognized. Understanding of the significance and underlying mechanisms of many renal system changes is still limited.[147]

The Antepartum Period

The renal system must handle the effects of increased maternal intravascular and extracellular volume and metabolic waste products as well as serve as the primary excretory organ for fetal wastes. Changes in the renal system are related to hormonal effects (particularly the influence of progesterone on smooth muscle), pressure from the enlarging uterus, effects of position and activity, and alterations in the cardiovascular system. Cardiovascular system changes that interact with alterations in renal hemodynamics include increased cardiac output, increased blood and plasma volume, and alterations in the venous system and plasma proteins (see Chapters 5 and 6). The predominant structural change in the renal system during pregnancy is dilation of the renal pelvis and ureters; functional changes include alterations in hemodynamics, glomerular filtration, and tubular handling of certain substances. Changes in fluid and electrolyte homeostasis result from changes in renal handling of water and sodium and alterations in the renin-angiotensin system. Table 8–1 summarizes changes in the renal system during pregnancy and their clinical implications.

Structural Changes

Pregnancy is characterized by physiologic hydroureter and hydronephrosis with significant dilation of the renal calyces, pelvis, and ureters, which begins in the first trimester but becomes more prominent after 20 weeks.[11] Hydronephrosis occurs in 80 to 90% of pregnant women.[13, 18, 58, 122] The diameter of the ureteral lumen increases with hypertonicity and hypomotility of the ureteral musculature.[122] Decreased ureteral peristaltic movements have also been reported, perhaps mediated by prostaglandin E (PGE).[18, 25, 58, 113]

The ureters elongate and become more tortuous during the last half of pregnancy as they are laterally displaced by the growing uterus.[18] These changes are seen in the renal pelvis and the upper portion of the ureters to the pelvic brim. The portion of the ureters below the pelvic brim (linea terminalis) is usually not enlarged. The volume of the ureters may increase 25 times and contain as much as 300 ml of urine.[58] This reservoir of urine can interfere with accuracy of 24-hour urine collections. These changes increase the risk of urinary tract infection.

The etiology of physiologic hydroureter is unclear. The major contributing factor is probably external compression of the ureters at the pelvic brim by the uterus, iliac arteries, and enlarging ovarian vein complexes.[58] Hormonal influences early in pregnancy may induce hypertrophy of the longitudinal smooth muscles surrounding distal portions of the ureters and hyperplasia of periurethral connective tissue.[18, 58] This may lead to a temporary stenosis and mild dilation of the upper portion of the ureters similar to that seen in women on oral contraceptives and in postmenopausal women given estrogen and progesterone.[58] As pregnancy progresses, the ureters are compressed at the pelvic brim by blood vessels in the area and by the growing uterus, leading to further, marked dilation and urinary stasis. Dilation is more promi-

TABLE 8–1
Summary of Changes in the Renal System During Pregnancy

PARAMETER	ALTERATION	SIGNIFICANCE
Renal calyces, pelvis, and ureters	Dilation (more prominent on right)	Increased risk of urinary tract infection in pregnancy and post partum
	Elongation, decreased motility, and hypertonicity of ureters	Alter accuracy of 24-hour urine collections
	May last up to 3 months post partum	
Bladder	Decreased tone, increased capacity	Risk of infection
		Urinary frequency
		Alteration in accuracy of 24-hour urine collections
	Displaced in late pregnancy	Urinary frequency
	Mucosa edematous and hyperemic	Risk of trauma and infection
	Incompetence of vesicoureteral valve	Risk of reflux and infection
		Alteration in accuracy of 24-hour urine collections
Renal blood flow	Increases 35–60%	Increased GFR
		Increased solutes delivered to kidney
Glomerular filtration rate (GRF)	Increases 40–50%	Increased filtration and excretion of water and solutes
		Increased urine flow and volume
		Decreased serum BUN, creatinine, uric acid
		Altered renal excretion of drugs with risk of subtherapeutic blood and tissue levels
Renal tubular function	Increased reabsorption of solutes (may not always match increase in filtered load)	Maintenance of homeostasis
		Avoid pathologic solute or fluid loss
	Increased renal excretion of glucose, protein, amino acids, urea, uric acid, water soluble vitamins, calcium, H⁺ ions, phosphorus	Tendency for glycosuria, proteinuria
		Compensation for respiratory alkalosis
		Increased nutritional needs (i.e., calcium, water-soluble vitamins)
	Net retention of sodium and water	Accumulation of Na and water to meet maternal and fetal needs
Renin-angiotensin-aldosterone system	Increase in all components	Maintain homeostasis with expanded extracellular volume
	Resistance to pressor effects of angiotensin II	Retention of water and sodium
		Balance forces favoring sodium excretion
		Maintain normal blood pressure
AVP and regulation of osmolarity	Retention of water	Expansion of plasma volume and other extracellular volume
	Osmostat reset	Maintenance of volume homeostasis in spite of reduction in plasma osmolarity

nent in the primipara whose firmer abdominal wall may increase resistance and pressure on the ureters.[18, 124] Increased urine flow in pregnancy results in some ureteral dilation even without any obstruction to flow.[47]

In up to 86% of women the right ureter is dilated to a greater extent than the left.[128] The right ureter makes a right angle turn as it crosses the iliac and ovarian veins at the pelvic brim; the turn of the left ureter is less acute, and it parallels rather than crosses the left ovarian vein. The iliac vessels are more rigid on the right than on the left, thus further compressing the ureters.

The sigmoid colon, which lies between the left ureter and the pelvis, probably does not have a cushioning effect, as has been proposed.[58] The sigmoid colon does contribute

to dextroversion of the uterus and may increase ureteral compression on the contralateral side during the last trimester.[18, 52, 58, 128] The position of the fetus does not seem to influence ureteral dilation. The site of placental attachment may increase venous flow on that side with subsequent compression of the ureters by the dilated vessels.[40, 58] The decreased incidence of ureteral dilation reported in women with pregnancy-induced hypertension (PIH) may reflect reduction in uteroplacental blood flow and therefore in venous dilation.[83]

The mean kidney length increases by 1 to 2 cm, probably because of increased renal blood flow and vascular volume. Bladder tone decreases owing to the effects of progesterone on smooth muscle. Bladder capacity doubles to about 1 L by term. The bladder becomes displaced anteriorly and superiorly by the end of the second trimester. Under the influence of estrogen the trigone becomes hyperplastic with muscle hypertrophy. The bladder mucosa becomes hyperemic with increased size and tortuosity of the blood vessels. The mucosa becomes more edematous and vulnerable to trauma or infection after engagement of the presenting part.[18]

The decreased bladder tone and flaccidity lead to incompetence of the vesicoureteral valve and reflux of urine. Alterations in bladder placement by the growing uterus stretch the trigone and displace the intravesical portion of the ureters laterally. This shortens the terminal ureter and decreases intravesical pressure. If intravesical pressure subsequently increases with micturition, urine regurgitates into the ureters.[18]

Changes in Renal Hemodynamics

Significant hemodynamic changes occur within the kidneys of the pregnant woman. Renal blood flow (RBF) increases 35 to 60% by the end of the first trimester then decreases from the second trimester to term.[25, 38, 90, 122] The increased flow is due to increased cardiac output and blood volume and decreased renal vascular resistance. Increased flow is enhanced by vasodilation of pre- and postglomerular capillaries. The decrease in renal vascular resistance may be mediated by PGI_2.[59]

Another measure of renal hemodynamics

is the effective renal plasma flow (ERPF), which increases 60% or more by mid-pregnancy.[37, 134, 137] This may then gradually decrease to values 40% greater than controls by term; others have reported that the ERPF falls significantly between 26 and 36 weeks, returning to nonpregnant values by term.[37, 49, 134, 147] The decrease in ERPF in late pregnancy is not a function of positional factors but may be due to the increase in systolic and diastolic blood pressure seen in later pregnancy (versus the relative hypotension seen at mid-gestation).[49] An increase in blood pressure would increase systemic vascular resistance and reduce renal blood flow.

Changes in Glomerular Filtration

The glomerular filtration rate (GFR) increases 40 to 50% during pregnancy (Fig. 8–1).[28, 37, 38, 40, 50] The rise begins soon after conception, peaks at 9 to 16 weeks, then remains relatively stable to term.[38, 49, 147] Values for GFR in pregnancy average 120 to 150 ml/min or higher.[47] Differences in reported values for RBF and GFR during pregnancy relate to the method of measurement. The increased GFR is related to increased glomerular blood flow (and glomerular capillary hydrostatic pressure) and decreased colloid osmotic (plasma oncotic) pressure due to a reduction in the concentration of plasma proteins. Failure of the GFR to increase early in pregnancy has been associated with pregnancy loss.[147]

The increased renal plasma flow (RPF)

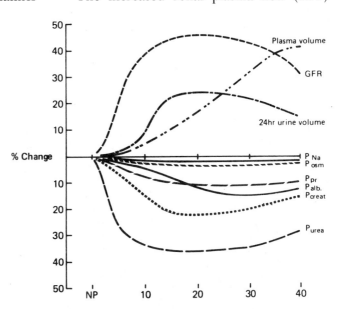

FIGURE 8–1. Physiologic changes in renal function and plasma values during pregnancy. Changes in various parameters are illustrated by percentage of increase or decrease from nonpregnant baseline. GFR, glomerular filtration rate; P_{Na}, plasma sodium; P_{osm}, plasma osmolality; P_{pr}, plasma proteins; P_{alb}, plasma albumin; P_{creat}, plasma creatinine; P_{urea}, plasma urea; NP, nonpregnant; 10–40, weeks of pregnancy. (From Davison, J.M. (1983). The kidney in pregnancy: A review. *J R Soc Med, 76,* 485.)

TABLE 8–2
Changes in Laboratory Values Associated with Renal Function During Pregnancy

VARIABLE	NONPREGNANT VALUES	VALUES DURING PREGNANCY	CRITICAL VALUES
Creatinine clearance	85–120 ml/min	120–180 ml/min	
Plasma creatinine	0.65 ± 0.14 mg/dl	0.46 ± 0.13 mg/dl	>0.80 mg/dl
BUN	13.0 ± 3.0 mg/dl	8.7 ± 1.5 mg/dl	>14 mg/dl
Urinary protein	<150 mg/24 hr	<250–300 mg/24 hr	>300 mg/24 hr
Urinary glucose	20–100 mg/24 hr	>100 mg/24 hr (up to 10 g/24 hr)	
Plasma urate	4–6 mg/dl	2.5–4 mg/dl	>5.8 mg/dl
Urinary amino acids		up to 2 g/24 hr	>2 g/24 hrs

and GFR increase the filtration fraction (GFR/RPF) or the portion of the renal blood flow that is filtered.[108, 122] As a result renal excretion of amino acids, glucose, protein, electrolytes, and vitamins increases, whereas urea, creatinine, blood urea nitrogen (BUN),

and uric acid levels decrease (Table 8–2). Twenty-four-hour urine volumes are 25% higher during pregnancy (Fig. 8–1).[146] The degree to which renal handling of substances is altered during pregnancy depends on the renal process involved (Fig. 8–2).[14] For ex-

FIGURE 8–2. Basic renal processes: (1) glomerular filtration, (2) tubular reabsorption, and (3) tubular secretion. Substances are processed by a combination of filtration, secretion, and reabsorption.
Glomerular filtration. Plasma is filtered from blood moving through the glomerulus into Bowman's capsule. The glomerulus is freely permeable to water and small molecules but impermeable to colloids and larger molecules, including most protein-bound substances. Filtration is influenced by hydrostatic and colloid osmotic pressure.
Tubular reabsorption. Water and other substances appear in the urine in smaller quantities than were originally filtered owing to reabsorption in the tubules. Tubular reabsorption of substances from the tubular lumen back into the blood in the peritubular capillaries occurs through simple diffusion, facilitated diffusion, and active transport. These mechanisms can only transport limited amounts (transport maximum, or Tm) of certain substances, such as glucose, owing to saturation of the carriers. Any amount filtered in excess of this quantity cannot be reabsorbed and appears in the urine. The proximal tubule is the major site for reabsorption of glucose, amino acids, sodium, protein, and other organic nutrients. The movement of water, sodium, and chloride through the kidneys is interrelated and affected by concentration gradients within various segments of the nephron and the surrounding interstitial spaces. These substances are freely filtered and 99% of the amount filtered is reabsorbed, 65 to 80% in the proximal tubule, 20 to 25% in the ascending limb of the loop of Henle, and the remainder in the distal and collecting tubes. The processes through which sodium is reabsorbed vary in different portions of the tubule. Reabsorption of sodium in the proximal tubule is an active, carrier-mediated process. In the ascending limb of the loop of Henle, chloride is actively reabsorbed and sodium follows passively. Sodium reabsorption is mediated by aldosterone in the distal tubule and collecting duct, where sodium is exchanged for potassium and hydrogen ions. Water reabsorption by passive diffusion or osmosis is sodium dependent but also depends on permeability of the tubular membrane (which is altered by arginine vasopressin).
Tubular secretion involves the movement of substances from the peritubular capillaries into the lumen of the tubules. (From Vander, A.J., et al. (1985). *Human physiology: Mechanisms of body function* (3rd ed., p. 426). New York: McGraw-Hill.)

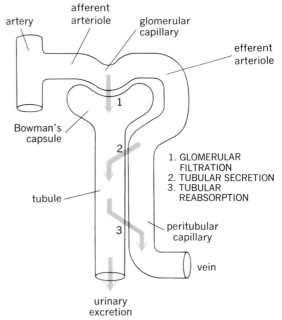

1. GLOMERULAR FILTRATION
2. TUBULAR SECRETION
3. TUBULAR REABSORPTION

ample, since urea and creatinine are processed only by glomerular filtration, the increased GFR leads to a significant decrease in serum urea and creatinine levels.[108]

The increased GFR also alters renal excretion of drugs. Drugs may be eliminated more rapidly, leading to lower and at times subtherapeutic blood and tissue levels. For example, pregnant women with paroxysmal atrial tachycardia may experience an increased frequency of attacks even though maintained on their usual doses of digoxin. These women may require up to a 50% increase in doses during pregnancy.[122] Serum levels and half-life of many antibiotics are reduced during pregnancy (see Chapter 10) primarily because of a more rapid excretion associated with the increased GFR. Drug doses and frequency of administration may need to be altered in pregnancy and the women must be regularly evaluated for signs of drug toxicity and subtherapeutic drug levels.

Alterations in Tubular Function

The elevated GFR increases the concentration of solutes and volume of fluid within the tubular lumen by 50 to 100%. Tubular reabsorption increases in order to prevent rapid depletion from the body of sodium, chloride, glucose, potassium, and water. There is actually a net retention of many of these substances during pregnancy. Conversely, tubular reabsorption rates cannot always accommodate the increased filtered load and lead to excretion of substances such as glucose or amino acids. Changes in tubular clearance are summarized in Fig. 8–3.

Renal glucose excretion increases soon after conception and remains high to term. Urinary glucose values may be up to 10 times greater than nonpregnant values of 20 to 100 mg/24 hours.[38] Glycosuria is more common during pregnancy and can vary from day to day and within any 24 to hour period. Glycosuria is discussed in the clinical implications section.

Excretion of amino acids, urea, and protein increases in pregnancy. Protein excretion rises from less than 150 mg/24 hours to up to 300 mg/24 hours with marked day-to-day variation.[38, 49] Increased urea clearance leads to decreased plasma urea nitrogen levels by 8 to 10 weeks.[35, 38]

Proteinuria occurs more frequently during pregnancy. The filtered load of amino acids during pregnancy may exceed tubular reabsorptive capacity with small amounts of protein lost in the urine. Values of 1+ protein on dipsticks are common and do not necessarily indicate the presence of glomerular pathology or pregnancy-induced hypertension.[122] Urinary protein excretion during pregnancy is not considered abnormal until values exceed 300 mg/24 hours. Protein excretion does not correlate with the severity of renal disease, and increased protein excretion in a pregnant woman with known renal disease does not necessarily indicate progression of the disease.[37, 38] However, proteinuria associated with hypertension in the pregnant woman is associated with a greater risk of an adverse pregnancy outcome.[76a]

Uric acid is normally handled by filtration, secretion, and reabsorption (see Fig. 8–2) so less than 10% of the filtered load appears in urine. During pregnancy, filtration of uric acid increases up to 30% in the first 16 weeks, and net reabsorption is decreased and secre-

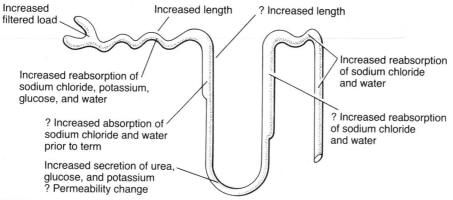

FIGURE 8–3. Tubular changes during pregnancy. (From Green, R. & Hatton, T. M. (1987). Renal tubular function in gestation. *Am J Kid Dis, IX,* 265.)

tion enhanced.[51, 147] As a result uric acid excretion is increased and serum levels are reduced. Serum uric acid levels decrease up to 25% as early as 8 weeks. Levels gradually increase toward nonpregnant levels by the third trimester as tubular reabsorption of uric acid increases, possibly because of increases in RPF with an increased filtration fraction at this stage of gestation.[38, 51, 59, 122]

Potassium excretion is decreased with retention of an additional 350 mEq. Serum potassium levels do not rise, since the additional potassium is used for maternal tissues and by the fetus. The mechanisms for increased potassium reabsorption in pregnancy are not well documented.[66] The altered potassium excretion may be due to antagonistic action of progesterone on renal tubular actions of aldosterone (Fig. 8–4).[12]

Renal acid-base balance is altered to compensate for the respiratory alkalosis that develops secondary to an increased loss of carbon dioxide from hyperventilation (see Chapter 7). The respiratory alkalosis is compensated for by increased renal loss of bicarbonate. This is accomplished by renal retention of H^+ ions and a decrease in serum bicarbonate. As a result serum bicarbonate levels fall 4 to 5 mEq/L to 18 to 22 mEq/L.[12, 108, 127]

Urinary calcium excretion is increased, possibly owing to the increased GFR, and serum calcium and phosphorus levels decrease. In order to maintain homeostasis, meet fetal demands, and avoid depletion of maternal reserves, women need 1200 mg of calcium per day in their diet.[44, 108, 110] Excretion of water-soluble vitamins also increases, so maternal diet must be evaluated to ensure adequate supplies of vitamins B_1, B_2, B_6, and C, folate, and niacin.

Fluid and Electrolyte Homeostasis

The pregnant woman must retain additional fluid and electrolytes to meet her needs and those of her growing fetus. In order to do this, renal excretory responses are modified and a new balance achieved. Since fluid and electrolyte balance is mediated predominantly by sodium and water homeostasis, pregnancy changes involve primarily alterations in these substances. The hormonal systems involved in regulation of sodium and water homeostasis, arginine vasopressin or antidiuretic hormone (ADH) and the renin-angiotensin-aldosterone system, must also be altered in order to react appropriately to the new equilibrium.

SODIUM HOMEOSTASIS

The filtered load of sodium increases up to 50% as a result of the increased GFR. The nonpregnant woman filters approximately 20,000 mEq of sodium/day; the pregnant woman filters 30,000.[59] In order to prevent excessive urinary sodium loss, tubular reabsorption of sodium also increases (see Fig. 8–3). Not only does tubular sodium reabsorption increase so that 99% of the filtered sodium is reabsorbed, but there is a net retention of up to 900 to 950 mOsm (3 to 6 mEq/day) of sodium during pregnancy.[37, 147] Most of the sodium retention occurs during the last 8 weeks, when levels of exchangeable sodium increase by 40 mEq/week.[21] About 60% of the sodium is used by the fetus and placenta; the rest is distributed in maternal blood and extracellular fluid.[122, 147]

Despite these alterations, the pregnant woman remains in sodium balance and responds normally to changes in both sodium and water balance.[60] The specific mechanisms for sodium retention during pregnancy are unclear. The maintenance of sodium balance during pregnancy is multifactorial and related to a balance between natriuretic factors favoring sodium excretion (increased GFR, decreased renal vascular resistance, decreased plasma oncotic pressure, decreased serum albumin, vasodilating prostaglandins, and the diuretic-like and aldosterone-antagonistic actions of progesterone) and antinatriuretic factors favoring sodium conservation (increased renin, aldosterone, deoxycorticosterone, and possibly human placental lactogen [hPL] and estrogen).[8, 25, 56, 66, 90, 116, 144, 147] As a result sodium retention in pregnancy is proportional to water accumulation and the woman remains in homeostatic balance.

RENIN-ANGIOTENSIN-ALDOSTERONE SYSTEM

Pregnancy is characterized by increases in components of the renin-angiotensin-aldosterone system (Fig. 8–4) and decreased sensitivity to the pressor effects of angiotensin II. These changes are mediated by estrogens, progesterone, prostaglandins, and alterations in renal processing of sodium.[122]

Renin peaks at levels two to three times higher than normal during the first trimester and remains elevated with a tendency to reach a plateau by about 32 weeks. The increase in renin is due primarily to increases

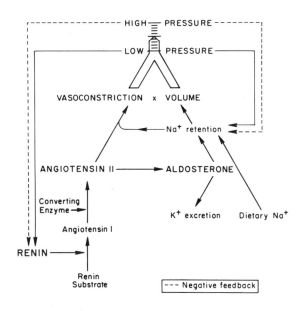

FIGURE 8–4. The renin-angiotensin-aldosterone system. Angiotensinogen (plasma renin substrate) is produced in the liver and is always present in the blood. Renin is a proteolytic enzyme found in blood in active and inactive forms. Renin is secreted and stored primarily in the juxtaglomerular cells surrounding afferent arterioles of cortical nephron glomeruli. Renin is also synthesized in extrarenal sites such as the brain, vascular smooth muscle, the genital tract, and the fetoplacental unit. Stretch receptors in the juxtaglomerular cells sense changes in renal perfusion and afferent arteriole pressures and increase renin release.

Renin release is also influenced by the sympathetic nervous system and concentrations of circulating potassium, angiotensin II, and possibly sodium. Renin acts on angiotensinogen to form angiotensin I, whose actions include stimulating catecholamine release, facilitating norepinephrine release from peripheral sympathetic veins, and reducing renal blood flow in the cortex and the medulla. Angiotensin I is broken down by angiotensin converting enzyme (ACE) to angiotensin II in the pulmonary circulation. Angiotensin II is a potent vasoconstrictor that stimulates adrenal production and release of aldosterone and constriction of the renal vasculature to reduce glomerular filtration rate (GFR) and the effective renal plasma flow (ERPF).

Aldosterone is a mineralocorticoid secreted by the outer zona glomerulosa cells of the adrenal cortex. The two major activities of aldosterone are regulation of extracellular fluid balance by altering sodium retention and excretion and regulation of potassium balance. Aldosterone regulates fluid volume via a direct effect on renal distal tubular transport of sodium to increase sodium reabsorption and decrease potassium reabsorption. As sodium is reabsorbed, potassium and hydrogen ions are secreted into the tubular lumen. Increased reabsorption of sodium results in increased water retention, since water is passively reabsorbed along with the sodium, thus increasing body extracellular fluid volume. Aldosterone is regulated via feedback mechanisms involving potassium and extracellular fluid volume.

A "third factor" influencing sodium balance has been proposed, because there are times when even though GFR is low and aldosterone secretion elevated (conditions that would be expected to increase sodium reabsorption and decrease excretion) sodium excretion is normal.[73,141,144] (From Resnick, L.M. & Laragh, J.W. (1983). The renin-angiotensin-aldosterone system in pregnancy. In F. Fuchs & A. Klopper (Eds.), *Endocrinology of pregnancy* (3rd ed., p. 196). Philadelphia: Harper.)

in inactive renin; however, both active renin and plasma renin activity (a measure of the capacity of plasma to generate angiotensin I) also increase.[3,141] Plasma renin activity increases four to ten times during the first trimester and may remain elevated to term or decrease in the third trimester.[27,141,146]

Renin release is stimulated by estrogens (which increase the concentrations of angiotensinogen), decreased blood pressure, increased levels of plasma and urinary PGE, and aldosterone-antagonizing effects of progesterone. Progesterone stimulates renal sodium loss, which stimulates release of renin and aldosterone.[27,122,146] Increases in plasma renin are also seen during the later part of the secretory phase of the menstrual cycle, peaking at twice normal levels with the luteinizing hormone surge and persisting until midway into the luteal phase. These changes coincide with progesterone release.[141]

Angiotensinogen (plasma renin substrate) levels double by 8 to 10 weeks and increase three to five times by 20 weeks.[116,146] Increases in angiotensinogen are due to the effects of estrogen on the liver, which synthesizes this alpha globulin.[3] Low angiotensinogen levels are associated with spontaneous abortion and may reflect reduced placental estrogen production.[65]

Angiotensin I converting enzyme (ACE) levels may be similar or slightly lower than nonpregnant values, although significant increases after 30 weeks have been reported.[3,141] Angiotensin II increases early in pregnancy and peaks at three to four times nonpregnant levels by mid-pregnancy.[141] Angiotensin II levels fall in the third trimester but are still above nonpregnant values.[122]

Plasma aldosterone levels increase with advancing gestation and reach a plateau at 24 weeks at levels two to five times (or more) those in nonpregnant women. Aldosterone increases again later in gestation, peaking at about 36 weeks at levels eight to ten times higher than nonpregnant values.[60, 116] The increased aldosterone opposes the sodium-losing effects of progesterone and allows a progressive accumulation of sodium in maternal and fetal tissues.

Despite these changes the pregnant woman remains responsive to both sodium depletion and loading, suggesting that a new equilibrium has been established.[108, 141] The expanded intravascular and extracellular fluid compartments are sensed as "normal" by the woman's vascular and renal volume-regulating mechanisms. The elevated levels of aldosterone may be necessary to maintain the expanded extracellular volume. This new equilibrium is protected against further increases or depletion in a manner similar to that in nonpregnant individuals.[122]

Angiotensin II is also a potent vasopressor. Yet despite markedly elevated levels during pregnancy, the blood pressure does not rise and in fact actually decreases along with the peripheral vascular resistance (see Chapter 6). The basis for resistance of the pregnant woman to the pressor effects of angiotensin II and other vasoactive substances is unclear. This refractoriness may be due to decreased vascular smooth muscle responsiveness to angiotensin II, perhaps mediated by local action of vasodilating prostaglandins or to activation of the renal kallikrein-kinin system.[3, 62, 149] The result is an estimated 60% decrease in sensitivity of the systemic vasculature to the pressor effects of angiotensin II during pregnancy.[27]

VOLUME HOMEOSTASIS AND REGULATION OF OSMOLARITY

The amount of water filtered by the kidneys increases 50% or more during pregnancy owing to the increased GFR. Pregnant women accumulate 6.2 to 8.5 L of water to meet their needs and those of the fetoplacental unit.[8, 25, 66] About 70 to 75% of maternal weight gain is due to increased body water in the extracellular spaces. Interstitial fluid volume increases 1.5 to 5 L beginning at 6 weeks and peaking at 24 to 30 weeks, with the greatest accumulation during the second half of pregnancy.[92, 147] Accumulation of greater than 1.5 L of interstitial fluid is associated with edema.[25, 92, 103] Alterations in blood volume are discussed in Chapters 5 and 6.

The exact mechanisms for water retention in pregnancy are not known. The increase in plasma volume occurs despite decreases in plasma osmolarity and colloid osmotic pressure, changes which would normally stimulate decreases in intravascular volume. Estrogen and progesterone may play a role through dilation of the venous capacitance vessels so that they can accommodate additional volume without stimulation of atrial baroreceptors to alter arginine vasopressin (AVP) and aldosterone release.[37]

Plasma osmolarity decreases from conception, reaching 8 to 10 mOsm/kg below nonpregnant values by 10 weeks' gestation and remaining low (273 ± 3 mOsm/kg) to term (see Fig. 8–1).[93] This change is due to decreased urea, sodium, and other solutes and probably arises from the decrease in PCO_2 and subsequent compensatory adjustments in renal ion excretion.[93, 123] A decrease in plasma osmolarity of this magnitude in a nonpregnant person would significantly reduce the osmotic threshold for thirst, suppress AVP release, and lead to a massive water diuresis (as occurs in diabetes insipidus). However, the pregnant woman senses this change in osmolarity as normal. At this new baseline, she responds to water loading and deprivation and concentrates and dilutes urine in a similar manner as nonpregnant individuals.[12, 93]

ARGININE VASOPRESSIN

Arginine vasopressin (antidiuretic hormone) secretion and its effect on renal reabsorption of water are similar in pregnant and nonpregnant women, as is AVP secretion in response to changes in baseline plasma osmolarity.[147] During pregnancy the osmostat for AVP is reset so the threshold at which the osmoreceptors signal the need for increased release is reduced from 280 to 270 mOsm/kg.[122]

Nonosmotic factors regulating AVP secretion in pregnancy are poorly understood. In nonpregnant individuals, a decrease in arterial blood pressure stimulates AVP secretion. In pregnancy the fall in plasma osmolarity occurs weeks before the fall in blood pressure, and the lowered osmolarity is still sensed as normal at term when the blood pressure has returned to nonpregnant values. AVP release is also influenced by plasma volume (decreased plasma volume increases AVP release and increased plasma volume decreases AVP release). During pregnancy the threshold for the release of ADH is reset to accommodate the increase in extracellular volume at a lower baseline plasma osmolarity.[37, 93]

The Intrapartum Period

The renin-angiotensin systems of both the fetus and the mother are altered during labor and delivery. At delivery maternal renin, plasma renin activity, and angiotensinogen as well as fetal renin and angiotensinogen levels are elevated.[3] These changes may be important in control of uteroplacental blood flow during the intrapartum and early postpartum periods.

Since the changes in renal function may also affect handling and excretion of drugs, drug doses and responses must be carefully monitored. General anesthesia decreases GFR, RPF, and sodium excretion and is associated with renal vasoconstriction, which may be magnified by the effects of stress with catecholamine release.[112] Thus monitoring of fluid and electrolyte status is especially important following use of general anesthesia for cesarean birth or with nonobstetric surgery during pregnancy.

The pregnant woman is also at risk for iatrogenic water intoxication during late pregnancy and the intrapartum period. This risk may result from the loss of electrolytes by use of saluretics, forcing fluids in a woman with pregnancy-induced hypertension and compromised renal function, or oxytocin infusion during labor, since the antidiuretic action of oxytocin reduces water excretion.[25]

The Postpartum Period

Renal plasma flow, GFR, plasma creatinine, and BUN return to nonpregnant levels by 6 weeks post partum. Urinary excretion of calcium, phosphate, vitamins, and other solutes returns to normal by the end of the 1st week.[141] Immediately after delivery the creatinine clearance increases and by 6 days is similar to nonpregnant levels.[37, 38, 40, 41] Plasma renin activity and angiotensin II concentrations fall to nonpregnant values immediately after delivery then rise again and remain elevated for up to 14 days.[26, 141] These changes may reflect the loss of renin from the fetoplacental unit with subsequent "overshooting" by the maternal system.[141] Urinary

glucose excretion returns to nonpregnant patterns by 1 week post partum, and pregnancy-associated proteinuria is resolved by 6 weeks.[18, 38, 44, 122]

The postpartum period is characterized by a rapid and sustained natriuresis and diuresis, especially prominent on days 2 to 5, as the sodium and water retention of pregnancy is reversed.[37] Fluid and electrolyte balance is generally restored to nonpregnant homeostasis by 21 days post partum and often earlier.[80] Persistence of more than a trace of edema after this time is indicative of sodium retention or a protein-losing state.

The decrease in oxytocin contributes to diuresis since oxytocin acts similarly to AVP in promoting reabsorption of free water. As oxytocin levels decrease, the diuresis becomes more pronounced, with up to 3000 ml of urine excreted per 24 hours on the 2nd through 5th days post delivery.[34, 35, 56, 99] A normal voiding for the postpartum woman may be 500 to 1000 ml, several times greater than a nonpostpartum individual.[77] Water may also be lost via night sweats.

Women with PIH may become hypervolemic during the postpartum period as excessive water accumulated in the interstitial spaces returns to the vascular compartment. If the woman's renal function remains impaired, the normal diuresis may be delayed. She may be unable to rapidly excrete this increased fluid volume and may develop congestive heart failure or pulmonary edema.

The alterations in tone of the ureters and bladder during pregnancy do not permanently impair function of these structures unless infection has incurred.[18] Morphologic changes in the urinary tract may last up to 3 months. In many women the dilation of the bladder, ureters, and renal pelvis has decreased significantly by the end of the 1st week, although the potential for distensibility of these structures may persist for several months.[11] In most women these structures return to their nonpregnant state by 6 to 8 weeks; in some women these changes may persist for 12 to 16 weeks or longer.[33, 37, 44, 84, 103] Bailey and Rolleston noted that return of the kidney to normal size took place over a 6-month period.[11] In some women mild residual dilation, especially on the right side, may persist for years with no pathologic significance.

The decreased tone, edema, and mucosal

hyperemia of the bladder can be aggravated immediately post partum by prolonged labor, forceps delivery, analgesia, or anesthesia.[18] These events may also lead to submucosal hemorrhages. Pressure of the fetal head on the bladder during labor can result in trauma and transient loss of bladder sensation in the first few days or weeks post partum. This can lead to overdistention of the bladder with incomplete emptying and an inability to void. Sphincter tone may remain altered following birth, with an increased frequency of stress incontinence with events such as coughing.

CLINICAL IMPLICATIONS FOR THE PREGNANT WOMAN AND HER FETUS

Changes in the renal system and fluid and electrolyte homeostasis during pregnancy are associated with common events such as urinary frequency, nocturia, dependent edema, and an inability to void post partum that are experienced by many pregnant women. These events are usually not pathologic but can be annoying and are often amenable to nursing interventions. Renal changes are, however, also associated with an increased risk of pathologic events such as urinary tract infection (UTI) and pyelonephritis and can interfere with the recognition and evaluation of renal disease during pregnancy. In addition renal system changes interact or are aggravated by pregnancy-induced hypertension and other renal and hypertensive disorders.

Urinary Frequency and Nocturia

Urinary frequency is most common during the first and third trimesters owing to compression of the bladder by the uterus. During the second trimester the bladder is displaced upward and over the pelvis so the incidence of frequency diminishes. Alterations in bladder sensation post partum can lead to overdistention with incomplete emptying and overflow incontinence.[18] Nocturia results from increased sodium excretion with an obligatory, concomitant loss of water. During the day water and sodium are trapped in the lower extremities because of venous stasis and pressure of the uterus on the iliac vein and inferior vena cava. At night when the

pregnant woman lies down, pressure on the iliac and inferior vena cava is reduced, promoting increased venous return, cardiac output, renal blood flow, and glomerular filtration with subsequent increase in urine output. Nursing interventions for women experiencing urinary frequency and nocturia are summarized in Table 8–3.

Dependent Edema

Dependent edema is seen in 35 to 80% of pregnant women and is more common as pregnancy progresses.[92, 122] Edema is more common in obese women and is associated with larger babies and a slight decrease in perinatal mortality.[143] The forces resulting in the movement of fluid out of the vascular space include capillary hydrostatic pressure and colloid osmotic (plasma oncotic) pressure, which is generated primarily by albumin.[102] Compression of the iliac vein and inferior vena cava by the growing uterus increases capillary hydrostatic pressure below the uterus, with filtration of fluid into the interstitial spaces of the lower extremities. The net reduction in plasma albumin during pregnancy reduces plasma colloid osmotic pressure, interfering with return of fluid to the vascular compartment.

Dependent edema is more likely to develop in women who are in supine or upright positions for prolonged periods. The development of edema in pregnancy is associated with the amount of water accumulation. Women with no visible edema have an accumulation of approximately 1.5 L. Pedal edema is associated with an accumulation of 2 or more liters; women with generalized edema have accumulated 4 to 5 or more liters of water.[92, 102, 117] Edema in the lower legs increases the risk of varicosities and thromboembolitic complications (see Chapter 5). Nursing interventions are summarized in Table 8–3.

Effects of Position on Renal Function

Position can markedly alter renal function during pregnancy, especially during the third trimester (Table 8–4). These postural effects are magnified in women with pregnancy-induced hypertension.[93] As pregnancy progresses there is pooling of blood in the pelvis and lower extremities while sitting, lying su-

TABLE 8–3
Nursing Interventions for Common Problems During Pregnancy Related to the Renal System

PROBLEM	NURSING INTERVENTIONS
Urinary frequency	Restrict fluids in evening
	Ensure adequate intake over 24-hour period
	Encourage to void when there is sensation in order to reduce accumulation of urine
	Limit intake of natural diuretics (i.e., coffee, tea, cola with caffeine)
	Teach mother signs of UTI
Nocturia	Left lateral recumbent position in evening to promote diuresis
	Reduce fluid intake in evening
	Ensure adequate fluid intake over 24-hour period
	Avoid coffee, tea, cola with caffeine in evening
Dependent edema	Avoid supine position
	Avoid upright position for extended periods
	Rest periods in left lateral recumbent position with legs slightly elevated
	Elevate legs and feet at regular intervals and when sitting
	Use of support hose or elastic stockings
	Avoid tight clothing on lower extremities (pants, socks, girdles, garter belts, knee-high stockings)
	Regular exercise
	Restrict intake of high-salt foods and beverages
	Assess for signs of PIH (increased blood pressure, proteinuria, generalized edema)
Inability to void post partum	Assess for bladder distention and urine retention
	Promote adequate hydration
	Early ambulation
	Provide privacy
	Administer analgesic prior to voiding attempt
	Place ice on perineum to reduce swelling and pain
	Pour warm water over perineum
	Turn on water in bathroom
	Provide fluid during voiding attempt
Risk of UTI	Screen urine culture on initial prenatal visit
	Encourage use of left lateral position to maximize renal output and urine flow
	Teach perineal hygiene
	Encourage adequate fluid intake

pine, or standing. The pooling of blood leads to a relative hypovolemia and decreased cardiac output. In order to compensate and maintain adequate perfusion of vital organs such as the heart and brain, blood vessels supplying less vital organs such as the kidneys are constricted.[25]

During the second half of pregnancy, the supine and upright positions are associated with a reduction in GFR and in urine output.[25, 108] As a result, pregnant women excrete water poorly and have a reduced urine volume when lying supine and, to a lesser extent, when upright.[89] For example, renal ex-

cretion of a water load while in the supine position may be decreased by 40% in late pregnancy.[25] Water excretion is enhanced by the lateral recumbent position. However, this position interferes with the ability of the woman to concentrate urine, possibly because of mobilization of fluid from the lower extremities with increased intravascular volume and subsequent suppression of AVP.[89]

Renal handling of sodium is also affected by postural changes. Moving from a lateral recumbent to a supine or sitting position is associated with sodium retention and, in some cases, with an increase in plasma renin

TABLE 8–4
Physiologic and Pathophysiologic Changes in GFR, RPF, and Sodium Excretion

Function	Normal Pregnancy(*)	Postural Effect	PIH	Essential Hypertension
GFR	50%	17%	33%	30%
RPF	35%	20%	20%	26%
Sodium excretion	50%	60%	50%	30%

(*)The standard for the percent changes in normal pregnancy is normal nonpregnant values; other percentages represent changes from the normal pregnant values.

GFR, glomerular filtration rate; RPF, renal plasma flow; PIH, pregnancy-induced hypertension.

From Brinkman, C.R. & Meldrum, D. (1979). Physiology and pathophysiology of maternal adjustments to pregnancy. In S. Aladjem, A.K. Brown, & C. Surreau (Eds.), *Clinical perinatology* (2nd ed., p. 16). St. Louis: CV Mosby.

and aldosterone levels.[147] Sodium excretion may be decreased in the supine and upright positions.[89] This sodium retention is associated with weight gain and occasional ankle swelling that comes and goes rapidly depending on the woman's activity patterns and position and does not necessarily indicate pathology. Therefore in evaluating sudden weight gain and edema in the extremities during pregnancy, data regarding recent activity patterns are essential.

Inability to Void Post Partum

Immediately post partum the woman has a hypertonic bladder with an increased capacity and decreased sensation leading to incomplete emptying. Women should void within 6 to 8 hours of delivery. Inability to void post partum is related to the following factors: (1) trauma to the bladder from pressure of the presenting part during labor with transient loss of bladder sensation; (2) edema of the urethra, vulva, and meatus and spasm of the sphincter from the forces of delivery; (3) decreased intra-abdominal pressure immediately post partum due to continuing distention of the abdominal wall; (4) decreased sensation of the bladder due to regional anesthesia and catheter use; and (5) hematomas of the genital tract.[99] Nursing interventions are summarized in Table 8–3.

Risk of Urinary Tract Infection

Urinary tract infection (UTI) occurs with increased frequency during pregnancy and is related to anatomic changes in the renal system. The incidence of asymptomatic bacteriuria (ASB) in pregnancy is 2 to 6%; acute pyelonephritis occurs in 1 to 4% of pregnant women.[25, 33a, 113] If left untreated, 16 to 30% of women with asymptomatic bacteriuria at their initial prenatal visit develop pyelonephritis.[33a]

Dilation of the urinary tract along with partial obstruction of the ureters from ureteral compression at the pelvic brim results in urinary stasis. Large volumes of urine may be sequestered in the ureters and hypotonic bladder during pregnancy. These static pools increase the risk of asymptomatic bacteriuria, especially since the urine may contain glucose, protein, and amino acids, which provide additional substrates for bacterial growth. Edema and hyperemia of the bladder mucosa also increase susceptibility to infection. The static column of urine in the hypoactive ureters also facilitates ascending bacterial migration, increasing the risk of pyelonephritis.[58, 108]

UTIs are also more common during the postpartum period. Factors that increase the risk of UTIs post partum include pregnancy-induced changes in the bladder (hypotonia, edema, mucosal hyperemia), which may be aggravated by the trauma of labor and delivery. Decreased bladder sensation from pressure of the fetal head during labor leads to incomplete emptying and urinary stasis, further predisposing to UTI for the first few weeks post partum.[18] Recommendations to reduce the risk of infection during pregnancy and the postpartum period are summarized in Table 8–3.

Urinary Tract Infection and Prematurity

The relationship between asymptomatic bacteriuria (ASB) and prematurity is controversial. In general, ASB per se has not been directly associated with an increased frequency of prematurity; however, 20 to 40% of women with ASB will develop acute pyelonephritis if untreated.[86] The incidence of prematurity when pyelonephritis is present in late pregnancy is as high as 25%.[25] Therefore prevention of pyelonephritis is an important step in reducing the incidence of prematurity. Routine screening of women during their initial prenatal visit will detect 99% of women with ASB and reduce the incidence of acute pyelonephritis by 70 to 80%. These women at risk can then be treated and closely monitored for recurrence.[86] The incidence of women whose cultures are initially negative who later become infected is 1 to 2%.[33a, 86]

In addition, ASB may be a marker of colonization in the rectovaginal area. Bacteria may ascend from this area through the cervix and cause an infection at the choriodecidual junction. Bacterial proteases or substances produced by the maternal host defense system in response to this infection may cause the membranes to rupture or stimulate prostaglandin synthesis and initiation of labor. Either of these events can result in prematurity.[33a]

Fluid Needs in Labor

Fluid needs of women in labor are controversial, and the routine use of intravenous infusions is questioned.[85, 105] Although intravenous administration of fluids and glucose is often used routinely to provide fluid and calories to prevent dehydration and ketosis, there is little documentation supporting the benefits of this therapy for most women. Complications such as infection, phlebitis, and fluid overload can occur with intravenous therapy.[105] For example, Cotton and associates found that the amount of intravenous fluid given during the intrapartum period was often double that ordered.[33] In addition, it may be harder for the woman to change her position during IV therapy, leading to increased use of the supine position and of medications since there is an accessible line.[85]

The use of hypertonic glucose infusions can lead to elevations in maternal blood glucose, which can in turn result in fetal hyperglycemia and hyperinsulinemia and eventually neonatal hypoglycemia.[85, 105] Lower cord blood sodium values and increased neonatal weight loss in the first 48 hours have been reported following the administration of 5% dextrose solutions to laboring women.[34] Conditions associated with intravenous fluid administration during labor are summarized in Table 8–5.

Oxytocin infusions have been associated with water intoxication and maternal and fetal hyponatremia.[25] The risk of water intoxication is increased when oxytocin is administered with large volumes of hypertonic dextrose solution. The hypertonic solution pulls fluid into the vascular compartment from the interstitial space, resulting in hemodilution. However, the additional fluid cannot be readily excreted owing to the antidiuretic effects of oxytocin. Water intoxication results in electrolyte imbalances such as hyponatremia, which can affect both mother and fetus and in severe cases can lead to seizures and hypoxia.[25] Therefore not only must oxytocin infusions be carefully monitored, but maternal electrolyte and fluid status and urine output must also be carefully evaluated for any woman receiving this type of infusion.

Maternal-Fetal Interactions

The fluid and electrolyte status of the infant reflects maternal balance during labor. A reduction in fetal plasma volume with increased fetal osmolarity occurs in most infants during labor. These changes are more pronounced following prolonged labor, with administration of hyperosmolar glucose solutions to the mother, or during fetal hypoxia because fluid is redistributed from the extracellular to intracellular fluid compartments.[25] Maternal electrolyte imbalances result in similar alterations in the fetus. For example, infants of mothers who receive large volumes of fluid during the 6 hours preceding birth have increased extracellular fluid and a higher incidence of hyponatremia.[24] In addition, mothers receiving intravenous fluids are more likely to have hyponatremic newborns than women who received only oral fluids.[53, 142]

Rapid administration of intravenous fluids has been used by some as a method to inhibit preterm labor. Administration of hypotonic fluid to the mother can, by increasing the maternal extracellular fluid volume, lead to decreases in fetal osmotic pressure and serum sodium and has resulted in maternal and neonatal hyponatremia and an increased risk of neonatal complications.[53] If this therapy is

TABLE 8–5
Conditions Associated with Intravenous Fluid Administration During Labor

USE OF INTRAVENOUS DEXTROSE (GLUCOSE OR SORBITOL)	USE OF INTRAVENOUS LACTATED RINGER'S SOLUTION
Maternal and fetal hyperglycemia	Fewer problems than with dextrose, glucose, or sorbitol
Maternal hyponatremia	When combined with dextrose, problems with maternal and fetal hyperglycemia, fetal hyperinsulinism, neonatal hypoglycemia, and jaundice
Fetal hyperinsulinism	
Neonatal hypoglycemia	
Neonatal hyponatremia associated with transient tachypnea	Possible fluid shifts from mother when large amounts of intravenous fluids are given
Neonatal jaundice associated with maternal hyperglycemia	
Fluid shift from mother to baby with greater weight loss in the neonate in the first 48 hours	

From Keppler, A.B. (1988). The use of intravenous fluids during labor. *Birth*, 15(2), 75, by permission of Blackwell Scientific Publications, Inc.

used, the fluid and electrolyte status of both mother and infant must be carefully monitored.

Measurement of Renal Function During Pregnancy

The marked increase in GFR during pregnancy significantly reduces serum BUN and creatinine by the end of the first trimester. As a result values that are normal for nonpregnant individuals may actually be elevations for the pregnant woman and reflect pathologic alterations in renal function. Thus it is critical for health care providers to know the normal values for these parameters during pregnancy (see Table 8–2) so that early signs of renal impairment are not missed. In a pregnant woman plasma creatinine levels greater than 0.80 mg/100 ml, plasma urea nitrogen levels greater than 14 mg/100 ml, or plasma BUN and creatinine levels that do not decrease to expected values by mid-gestation may indicate a significant reduction in renal function and require further investigation.[21, 38, 147]

GFR is usually measured by either inulin or endogenous creatinine clearance. The 24-hour creatinine clearance is generally a good index of GFR in both pregnant and nonpregnant women but is less valid in women with severe renal impairment or diminished urine production. In the latter case the amount of creatinine secreted by the proximal tubule can markedly alter urinary creatinine values.[38, 49] The creatinine clearance rises approximately 45% by 6 to 8 weeks and remains elevated to or near term, when it may begin to fall.[38, 40] Creatinine clearance (Ccr) can be approximated by several formulas[47]:

$$C_{cr} = 70 \, \frac{\text{24-hour urinary creatinine (mg)}}{\text{plasma creatinine (mg)}}$$

or (if only the serum creatinine is known):

$$C_{cr} = \frac{140 - \text{age}}{\text{serum creatinine}} \times 0.88 \text{ (for females)}$$

Dilation of the urinary tract with stasis and retention of large volumes of urine can lead to collection errors. Accuracy of clearance measures in pregnancy can be improved by using 24-hour collections to avoid "washout" from diurnal changes in urine flow, ensuring that the woman is well hydrated to ensure a high urine flow rate, discarding the first morning specimen, and having the woman assume a lateral recumbent position for 1 hour before the start and 1 hour prior to the end of the collection. Dietary intake has to be evaluated in the timing of blood samples during a clearance period since recent ingestion of cooked meat can increase plasma creatinine levels up to 0.18 mg/100 ml. Plasma creatinine levels, used to estimate GFR, are influenced by age, height, weight, and gender. In the pregnant woman body size and weight may not accurately reflect kidney size.[37, 38]

Since structural changes in the urinary system may persist for 12 to 16 weeks post delivery, these alterations also need to be considered when evaluating renal function postpartum. Evaluation of renal function is considered if the GFR during the postpartum period decreases more than 25 to 30% from predelivery values or if the serum creatinine rises above nonpregnant levels.[15]

Glycosuria

Chemically detectable glycosuria is found in the majority of pregnant women.[122, 147] Glucose excretion may be up to 10 times greater than the nonpregnant levels of 20 to 100 mg/24 hours.[94] About 70% of pregnant women excrete more than 100 mg of glucose/24 hours; in up to 50% glucose excretion is greater than 150 mg/24 hours.[37, 132, 147] Large day-to-day variation in glucose excretion is reported with little correlation between excretion rate, plasma glucose levels, and the stage of pregnancy.[37, 147] Few women with glycosuria have abnormal glucose tolerance test results. Thus glycosuria in pregnancy does not reflect alterations in carbohydrate metabolism but rather alterations in renal function.[147]

The basis for glycosuria in pregnancy is not well understood. For many years it was thought that glycosuria developed from a decrease in the transport maximum for glucose in the proximal tubules. Recent evidence demonstrates that this is not the case. The transport maximum (T_m) for glucose is not a constant value but varies with changes in extracellular volume and GFR and with hyperglycemia.[10, 37] As the GFR increases during pregnancy, renal reabsorptive capacity for glucose also increases but not to the same extent. As the filtered load of glucose increases more glucose is excreted, leading to glycosuria at normal plasma glucose levels.[122, 147] When increased glucose excretion occurs, alterations in reabsorption seem to occur primarily in the portion of the glucose load (usually 5% of the filtered glucose) that escapes reabsorption in the proximal tubules and is normally reabsorbed in the loops of Henle and collecting duct.[10, 37, 66]

Glycosuria during pregnancy has not been associated with alterations in perinatal mortality or morbidity or with subsequent development of diabetes or renal disorders.[122] However, Davison suggests that women with greater than the usual degree of glycosuria during pregnancy may have sustained renal tubular damage from earlier untreated urinary tract infections.[37, 38] How this alters renal handling of glucose is unclear. Infection is known to cause a temporary impairment of distal tubular function. In some women sites for glucose reabsorption may not be completely healed and thus are unable to deal with the stresses imposed by the increased filtered load of glucose during pregnancy.

IMPLICATIONS FOR THE DIABETIC WOMAN

Because of the high incidence of glycosuria in normal pregnant women, random testing of urine samples is not useful in the diagnosis and control of diabetes during pregnancy. In addition, urinary glucose may not be a reliable indicator of plasma glucose control in pregnant diabetics, thus decreasing the usefulness of urinary glucose concentrations for monitoring these women.[37, 66, 122] In the pregnant diabetic any elevation of blood glucose results in a greater urinary loss of glucose than in the nonpregnant state. Since water and electrolytes are normally lost along with glucose, volume depletion and polydypsia occur sooner in the pregnant than in the nonpregnant diabetic woman (see Chapter 13).[122]

Hypertension and the Renal System

The kidneys play a critical role in the regulation of blood pressure (Fig. 8–5), therefore alterations in renal function often lead to hypertension. During the perinatal period renal disorders associated with hypertension often have a poorer outcome for both mother and infant. Further discussion of vascular changes associated with pregnancy and the impact of hypertension can be found in Chapter 6.

Women with Pregnancy-Induced Hypertension

Pregnancy-induced hypertension (PIH) involves specific lesions and functional alterations in the renal system. The renal lesion usually seen in PIH is glomerular capillary endotheliosis, which decreases the diameter of the glomerular capillary lumina, resulting in decreased GFR and RPF.[25] This lesion is seen more frequently in primiparas. The contraction of plasma volume and vasospasm including constriction of the preglomerular arterioles seen with PIH further reduce RPF and GFR. In women with PIH the GFR and RPF are decreased significantly from values seen in healthy pregnant women (see Table 8–4).[25]

Women with PIH have an increased reactivity to vasoactive substances with a decreased rate of relaxation following stimulation.[141] Worley and coworkers noted that these women begin to lose this refractoriness up to 18 weeks prior to the onset of hypertension.[149] As a result the woman may develop vasospasm with contraction of the vascular space and movement of fluid to extravascular spaces. Regional perfusion, including perfusion of the intervillous spaces, decreases with progressive vasospasm. Eventually blood pressure increases to maintain perfusion of vital organs.[149] Perfusion of the intervillous spaces may be reduced to 35 to 50% and may remain low in spite of interventions such as bed rest and return to a normotensive state.[149, 150]

An impaired response to infusion of angiotensin II, which antedates the onset of clinically detectable hypertension, has been noted in women with PIH.[26, 61, 141] This altered response has been used to identify women at risk for developing PIH later in pregnancy. Although the false-positive rate (identifying women as at risk for PIH who do not develop the disorder) for this test is around 50%, the false-negative rate (failing to identify women who will subsequently develop PIH) is low.[141] However, the angiotensin infusion test is invasive and cumbersome and thus impractical for routine screening.[76a] As a clinical corollary to the angiotensin infusion response, Gant and colleagues developed the "roll over" test.[61] This test proposed to identify women at high risk for developing PIH based on the degree of rise in blood pressure as the woman moved from a lateral to a supine position. Others have not been

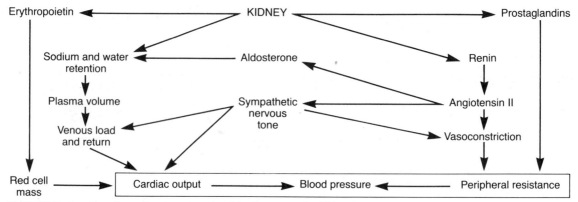

FIGURE 8–5.   Renal mechanisms involved in the control of blood pressure. (From Gabert, H.A. & Miller, J.M. (1985). Renal disease in pregnancy. *Obstet Gynecol Surv, 40,* 449.)

able to replicate the findings of the original investigators (see Chapter 6).[12, 116]

Information on alterations in the renin-angiotensin system in women with PIH is conflicting. Since PIH is associated with sodium retention, overproduction of angiotensin II or aldosterone might be expected.[3] However, the response of women with PIH is paradoxical, and the converse is found. In women with mild PIH, renin, angiotensin II, and aldosterone levels are decreased but still above nonpregnant levels, whereas in women with severe PIH these substances fall to nonpregnant values or lower.[60, 149]

Sodium excretion is reduced in women with PIH (see Table 8–4) owing to the decreased GFR, increased vascular resistance, decreased RPF (with decreased perfusion of the peritubular capillaries), decreased plasma and blood volume, and possibly inadequate tubular reabsorptive mechanisms.[25, 60] Serum uric acid is increased in women with PIH and in those whose fetuses exhibit intrauterine growth retardation (IUGR), perhaps because of decreased plasma volume, decreased RPF, and hemoconcentration.[59] Since levels can be elevated in some healthy women, serial monitoring of values is essential. Serum uric acid values above 5.8 mg/dl are associated with increased perinatal mortality in women with pregnancy-induced or chronic hypertension.[37]

Women with Essential Hypertension

Nonpregnant women with essential hypertension generally have decreased RPF and GFR with an exaggerated excretion of sodium in response to a salt load. During early pregnancy RPF and GFR increase, but the total increase by late pregnancy is less than in normotensive pregnant women (see Table 8–4).[25] With increased blood pressure, fluid moves from the vascular to the extravascular spaces, and the blood becomes hemoconcentrated with further reductions in RPF and GFR. The pregnant woman with essential hypertension also has a 20 to 30% decrease in sodium excretion.[25] Vasoconstriction may reduce uteroplacental perfusion with alterations in fetal growth.

DIURETICS AND PREGNANCY

The use of diuretics in pregnant women, especially to prevent or treat PIH, is controversial.[76a] Diuretics are generally contraindicated in women with PIH whose plasma volume is already contracted (see Chapter 5) unless they develop pulmonary edema.[59] Some clinicians support the use of diuretics in women with chronic hypertension if the woman has been on the drug prior to pregnancy, since her fluid status has had a chance to equilibrate on these drugs, or if needed to stabilize her blood pressure.[59, 115] The use of diuretics may prevent the woman from experiencing the normal volume expansion necessary for normal fetal growth and development.[115] Diuretic use is also associated with fetal volume depletion and thrombocytopenia, maternal hyperglycemia, and elevated uric acid levels.[59]

Renal Disease and Pregnancy

As the severity of renal disease and reduction in renal function increase, the ability to conceive and sustain a pregnancy also decreases.[38] A normal pregnancy is rare if prior to conception the woman has a plasma creatinine greater than 3 mg/dl or a urea nitrogen above 30 mg/dl, values representing 50 to 75% decreases in renal function.[37] Women with severe renal disease rarely have a successful pregnancy outcome. Table 8–6 summarizes the effects of pregnancy on chronic renal problems.

Women with chronic renal problems often have increased RPF and GFR early in pregnancy, with a percentage increase similar to that in healthy pregnant women. However, since these women start from lower baseline levels, the absolute levels are lower. These early changes are followed by a fall to levels at or below those seen in nonpregnant individuals later in gestation.[8, 25] Alterations in RPF and GFR are also associated with decreased uteroplacental perfusion with an incidence of preterm birth and IUGR of 20 to 25% or more.[59] In general, women with mild alterations in renal function prior to pregnancy tend to have a successful pregnancy outcome, and pregnancy does not adversely affect their disease.[8, 59] Women with moderate to severe renal disorders are more likely to develop hypertension during pregnancy and subsequent deterioration of renal function.[112] Women with chronic renal problems are at increased risk to develop PIH; however, early signs may be missed owing to their chronic disease state.[8, 109]

Perinatal outcome in women with chronic renal disease is related to the degree of hypertension.[25] For example, Gabert and Miller report that fetal loss is 4% in women with only proteinuria (reflecting altered renal function), but 45% in women with proteinuria and hypertension (reflecting altered renal function plus decreased RPF and uteroplacental perfusion).[59] Management of women with chronic renal problems includes careful monitoring of maternal functional status and signs of increasing severity of the disease and fetal assessment.

Pregnancy Following Renal Transplant

Over 1000 women have conceived following renal transplants.[39] Approximately 40% miscarried or chose to terminate the pregnancy. Of those women who carried the pregnancy beyond the first trimester, 90% have had a successful pregnancy outcome, although there is an increased frequency of PIH, preterm birth, and IUGR. Renal hemodynamics often improve with pregnancy, but about 15% of these women have permanent impairment of renal function.[8, 39] Pregnancy is

TABLE 8–6
Effects of Pregnancy on Chronic Renal Disease

RENAL DISEASE	EFFECTS
Chronic pyelonephritis	Bacteriuria in pregnancy may lead to exacerbation.
Urolithiasis	Ureteral dilation and stasis do not seem to affect natural history, but infections can be more frequent.
Permanent urinary diversion	Depending on original reason for surgery, there may be other malformations of urogenital tract. UTI is common, and renal function may undergo reversible decrease. No significant obstructive problem but cesarean section may be necessary for abnormal presentation.
Chronic glomerulonephritis and noninfectious tubulointerstitial disease	Some feel disorder is adversely affected by coagulation changes of pregnancy. UTI may occur more frequently. Usually no adverse effect in the absence of hypertension.
Systemic lupus erythematosus (SLE)	Controversial; prognosis most favorable if disease is in remission prior to pregnancy. Steroid dose should be increased post partum.
Periarteritis nodosa	Fetal prognosis is poor. Maternal death often occurs. Therapeutic abortions should be considered.
Scleroderma	If onset during pregnancy, there can be rapid, overall deterioration. Reactivation of quiescent scleroderma can occur post partum.
Diabetic nephropathy	No adverse effects on the renal lesion. Increased incidence of infection, edema, or preeclampsia.
Polycystic disease	Functional impairment and hypertension are usually minimal in childbearing years.
After nephrectomy, solitary and pelvic kidneys	Pregnancy well tolerated. May be associated with other malformations of the urogenital tract. Dystocia rarely occurs with a pelvic kidney.

From Davison, J.M., et al. (1985). Kidney disease and pregnancy: Obstetric outcome and long term prognosis. *Clin Perinatol, 12,* 497.

generally not recommended for 1 to 3 years following transplant to ensure that the transplant is successful and able to function under the increased demands of pregnancy. The frequency of rejection is not altered by pregnancy.[8, 59] Concerns regarding teratogenicity of immunosuppressive drugs, which must be continued during pregnancy, have generally not been realized to date, although long-term follow-up data are still sparse.[39, 60]

Maternal-Fetal Fluid and Electrolyte Homeostasis

Fetal fluid and electrolyte balance is dependent on maternal homeostasis and placental function. Since serum osmolarity is similar in the fetus and the mother, changes in maternal or fetal osmolarity will lead to transfer of water from the opposite compartment to achieve homeostasis. Water is continuously exchanged between mother and fetus with a net flux in favor of the fetus, placenta, and amniotic fluid.[123] Factors that influence the rate and direction of water exchange between the mother and the fetus include maternal and fetal blood flow to and from the placenta, osmotic and hydrostatic pressure gradients across the placenta, and availability of cellular transport mechanisms.[91]

Fetal balance is affected by any maternal or fetal conditions that alter the supply, demand, and transfer of water. Maternal events such as altered nutrition, electrolyte imbalance, diabetes, hypertension, or the excessive use of diuretics are associated with alterations in fetal fluid and electrolyte status, amniotic fluid volume, and fetal growth.[23] For example, fetal urine flow can be increased by volume loading of maternal blood or administration of diuretics, since acute changes in maternal plasma osmolarity induce parallel changes in the fetus owing to transplacental movement of fluid with decreased urine flow and increased AVP.[23] In addition, since fetal free water is derived from the mother, net movement of water to the fetus is decreased when maternal osmolarity increases; this leads to decreased fetal urine flow and increased tubular reabsorption of water.[97]

SUMMARY

The renal system is critical to maintenance of fluid and electrolyte homeostasis within the body. Relatively small changes in renal function can significantly alter this homeostasis, leading to a variety of volume and electrolyte disorders. Renal function and many related laboratory parameters are altered significantly during pregnancy to levels that would be considered pathologic in a nonpregnant individual. In most cases the pregnant woman readily adapts to these changes and establishes a new equilibrium for volume and electrolyte homeostasis. At this new equilibrium she responds to alterations in fluid and electrolyte intake in a manner similar to that of a nonpregnant individual. Pathophysiologic conditions that alter renal function or volume homeostasis affect the health of both the pregnant woman and her infant. Monitoring and health counseling related to fluid and electrolyte status are essential during pregnancy. Clinical recommendations for nurses working with pregnant women based on alterations in the renal system and fluid and electrolyte balance are summarized in Table 8–7.

DEVELOPMENT OF THE RENAL SYSTEM IN THE FETUS

Although functionally different, the renal system and genital systems (see Chapter 1) are closely linked embryonically and anatomically. Both develop from a common ridge of mesodermal tissue and end in the cloaca. Anatomic development of the kidneys begins early in gestation, with formation of the adult number of nephrons by 32 to 36 weeks. Urine formation begins by 9 to 10 weeks; during the second half of gestation urine production by the fetus is a major component of amniotic fluid. Renal function does not reach levels comparable to adults until about 2 years of age.

Anatomic Development

Development of the Kidneys

The kidneys arise from a ridge of mesodermal tissue called the nephrogenic cord that runs along the posterior wall of the abdominal cavity on either side of the primitive aorta. The kidney develops through three successive, overlapping stages. The initial steps involve formation of transient nonfunctional structures called the pronephros and mesonephros on either side of midline from

TABLE 8–7
Summary of Recommendations for Clinical Practice Related to Changes in the Renal System and
Fluid and Electrolyte Homeostasis: Pregnant Woman

Recognize usual values for renal function tests and patterns of change during pregnancy and post partum (pp. 337–346, 350–351, Tables 8–1 and 8–2).

Recognize that individual laboratory values must be evaluated in light of clinical findings and previous values (pp. 339–342, 350–351, Table 8–2).

Teach women to recognize and reduce the risk of urinary tract infection during pregnancy and post partum (pp. 337–339, 348).

Monitor and teach women with pyelonephritis to recognize signs of initiation of preterm labor (p. 348).

Recognize the effects of altered renal function on pharmacokinetics of drug eliminated by glomerular filtration (pp. 339–341, 452–454).

Monitor and evaluate maternal responses to drugs taken prior to pregnancy for evidence of subtherapeutic doses (pp. 339–341).

Monitor and evaluate maternal responses to antibiotics (pp. 341, 452–454).

Know or verify usual doses for antibiotics and other medications given during pregnancy (pp. 341, 452–454).

Assess maternal nutritional status in relation to calcium and water-soluble vitamins and provide nutritional counseling (p. 342, Chapters 9 and 14).

Know the influences of position on renal function (pp. 346–348, Table 8–4).

Counsel women regarding appropriate positions and activity patterns (pp. 346–348, Table 8–4).

Assess activity patterns and position in evaluating changes in weight gain and edema (pp. 346–348).

Monitor fluid and electrolyte status and renal function following use of general anesthetics (pp. 345, 349–350).

Monitor oxytocin and intravenous infusions during labor and delivery to avoid overload (pp. 345, 349–350, Table 8–5).

Use clear fluids, ice chips, and other alternatives to use of intravenous infusions with women with uncomplicated labors (pp. 349–350).

Know the benefits and risks for the mother, fetus, and neonate of different types of intravenous fluids (pp. 349–350, Table 8–5).

Avoid use of hypertonic solutions during labor (pp. 349–350).

Know indications for intrapartum intravenous therapy (pp. 349–350).

Monitor maternal fluid and electrolyte status and urine output (especially in women receiving an oxytocin infusion or with PIH or compromised renal function) during labor and delivery for development of water intoxication (pp. 349–350).

Teach women the common experiences associated with changes in renal system (urinary frequency, dependent edema, nocturia) and implement appropriate interventions (pp. 346–348, Table 8–3).

Monitor women with dependent edema for varicosities and thromboembolism (p. 346).

Teach women involved in 24-hour urine collections strategies to enhance the accuracy of the collection (p. 350).

Know usual values and monitor for glycosuria and proteinuria in the pregnant woman (pp. 341, 350–351).

Monitor fluid and electrolyte status of women with PIH and diabetes, recognizing that alterations may occur more rapidly than in other pregnant women (pp. 350–354).

Question use of diuretics during pregnancy (p. 352).

Monitor fluid and electrolyte status, renal function, amniotic fluid volume, and fetal growth in women on diuretics (p. 352).

Counsel women with renal disorders regarding the impact of their disorder on pregnancy and of pregnancy on their disorder (pp. 352–354, Table 8–6).

Monitor women with chronic renal problems for signs of initiation of preterm labor, intrauterine fetal growth retardation, hypertension, and alterations in maternal renal function (pp. 352–354, Table 8–6).

Monitor amniotic fluid volumes and fetal growth in women with altered renal function, diabetes, or hypertension (pp. 350–354).

Evaluate bladder function and voiding post partum (pp. 345–346, 348).

Implement interventions to encourage postpartum voiding (pp. 345–346, 348, Table 8–5).

Observe for signs of pulmonary edema and congestive heart falure post birth in women with PIH and impaired renal function (p. 345).

Recognize that structural changes in the urinary system may persist for 6 months or more following birth (pp. 345–346, 350).

Page numbers following each intervention refer to pages where rationale for intervention is discussed.

which the metanephros, or permanent kidney, develops (Fig. 8–6A). The pronephros arises in the cervical region in the 3rd week, extends in a cranial to caudal direction, then degenerates beginning in the 4th week. Each pronephros consists of 7 to 10 solid cell groups. The pronephric ducts are incorporated into the mesonephric kidneys.

The mesonephros appears late in the 4th week, forming a large ovoid organ on either side of midline next to the developing gonads in the thoracic and lumbar regions (Fig. 8–6A). The mesonephros and gonad form the urogenital ridge. The mesonephros consists of S-shaped tubules with glomeruli and collecting ducts that enter a common large duct. This mesonephric duct persists in the male as the wolffian duct and gives rise to the male

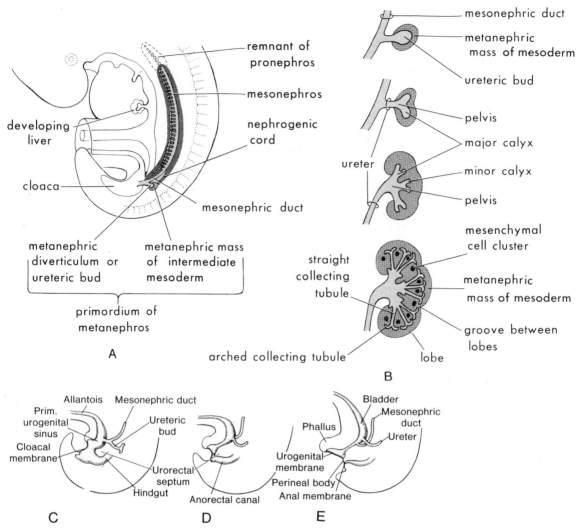

FIGURE 8–6. Embryology of the kidney. *A*, formation of the ureteric bud (5th week); *B*, formation of nephrons (5th to 8th weeks); partitioning of the cloaca into the urogenital sinus and anorectal canal with formation of the bladder at end of the 5th week (*C*), 7 weeks (*D*), and 8 weeks (*E*). (*A* and *B*, From Moore, K.L. (1988). *The developing human* (p. 250). Philadelphia: WB Saunders. *C* to *E*, From Sadler, T.W. (1985). *Langman's medical embryology* (5th ed., p. 255). Baltimore: Williams & Wilkins.)

genital ducts (see Chapter 1). The rest of the mesonephros regresses by 8 to 10 weeks as the metanephros begins to function.[100, 152]

The permanent kidneys (metanephroi) arise during the 5th week from the ureteric bud at the caudal end of the mesonephric duct (Fig. 8–6A). Formation of the permanent kidney involves two separate interrelated processes. The ureteric bud grows out into the surrounding mesoderm (metanephric blastema), dilates, and subdivides to form the ureters, renal pelvis, and collecting ducts (Fig. 8–6B). The growth of the ureteric bud into the surrounding mesoderm induces for-

mation of small vesicles that elongate to form primitive renal tubules. The proximal ends of these tubules form the Bowman's capsule. The distal end comes into contact with the blind ends of the collecting ducts and fuses (Fig. 8–6B).[53, 100, 152] Nephron formation begins at about 8 weeks in the juxtamedullary area and progresses toward the cortex. Nephrons continue developing until 35 to 36 weeks (in both the fetus and the preterm infant), when adult numbers of nephrons are reached. Maturation and hypertrophy of the nephrons continue into infancy with growth of glomeruli and tubules.[53, 100]

Initially the kidneys are in the pelvic area. With straightening of the embryo and growth of the sacral and lumbar areas, the kidneys undergo a series of positional changes and migrate upward. During this process the kidneys rotate 90 degrees so that the renal pelvises face midline.[53] Failure of the kidneys to ascend leads to pelvic kidneys. Abnormal ascent and rotation can result in configurations such as horseshoe-shaped kidneys (the kidneys are pushed together and fuse).

The Urinary System

The urinary system develops following division of the cloaca. The cloaca is the dilated end of the hindgut and is involved in the development of the terminal portions of the genital (see Chapter 1), urinary, and gastrointestinal (see Chapter 9) systems. Downward growth of the urorectal septum at 5 to 6 weeks divides the cloaca into the posterior anorectal canal and anterior primitive urogenital sinus (Fig. 8–6C, D). The upper and largest part of the urogenital sinus becomes the bladder and is initially continuous with the allantois (Fig. 8–6E). The allantois eventually becomes a thick fibrous cord (the urachus or median umbilical ligament). The ureters are incorporated into the bladder wall. The urethra develops from the lower urogenital sinus along with portions of the external genitalia.[100, 152]

Developmental Basis for Common Anomalies

Major malformations of the renal system and urinary tract can be divided into three broad categories: agenesis-dysplasia of the renal system, polycystic kidneys, and malformations of the lower urinary tract.[63] Several events are critical for the normal development of the kidneys. If the ureteric bud does not arise from the end of the mesonephric duct or if the ureteric bud does not induce formation of the renal cortex and nephrons, unilateral or bilateral renal agenesis, aplasia, or hypoplasia results. If the ureteric bud splits early or if two buds arise on one side, there may be duplication of the kidneys or ureters. Renal agenesis and hypoplasia are often associated with oligohydramnios. The marked decrease in amniotic fluid with bilateral renal agenesis is thought to result in adverse effects on extrarenal fetal development (see Chapter 2).[53]

Polycystic kidneys are a heterogeneous group of disorders that arise from environmental and genetic causes. The specific embryologic basis for these defects is unknown. Theories that have been proposed include (1) failure of the collecting ducts to develop, with subsequent cystic degeneration; (2) failure of the developing nephrons to unite with the collecting tubules; and (3) persistence of remnants of early rudimentary nephrons, which normally degenerate but instead remain and form cysts.[63, 100] The last theory has been proposed as a possible cause of adult onset polycystic kidneys.

Malformations of the lower urinary tract include obstructive uropathy and exstrophy. Obstructive uropathy arises from obstructions at the uteropelvic junction due to adhesions, aberrant blood vessels, or strictures or in the urethra from posterior urethral valves. Severe forms result in fetal renal damage from hydronephrosis. Anomalies of other systems may occur secondary to oligohydramnios (see Chapter 2). Fetal surgery has been utilized to promote drainage of the urinary tract and prevent irreversible renal damage prior to birth. Exstrophy of the bladder arises from incomplete midline closure of the inferior part of the anterior abdominal wall, with concurrent abnormalities in the mesoderm of the bladder wall.[100] Timing for development of renal and urinary system anomalies is summarized in Table 8–8.

Functional Development

Urine production and glomerular filtration in the fetus begin at 9 to 10 weeks. Renal blood flow (RBF) and the glomerular filtration rate (GFR) are low throughout gestation, owing to the high renal vascular resistance (RVR) and low systemic blood pressure, but increase rapidly between 20 and 35 weeks then level off to birth.[70] This increase is concurrent with increases in numbers and growth of nephrons. In adults 20 to 25% of the cardiac output goes to the kidneys. In the fetus 40 to 60% of the cardiac output goes to the placenta and only 3 to 7% to the kidneys.[152]

Although RBF and GFR are low, this does not lead to low fetal urine output.[53] Fetal urine is a major component of amniotic fluid. Fetal urine output and amniotic fluid production both increase with gestation. Mean hourly flow rates of urine are about 2 ml at 20 weeks, 10 ml at 30 weeks, 17 ml at 35

TABLE 8–8
Stages of Developmental Abnormalities of the Kidney and Urinary Tract

STRUCTURE FORMED	TIME (WK)	MORPHOLOGIC ABNORMALITIES
Pronephros and mesonephros	3–4	Renal agenesis, unilateral and bilateral (Potter's syndrome)
Ureteric bud and initiation of metanephros	5	Renal agenesis or hypoplasia
Urogenital sinus	6	Urorectal abnormalities
Cephalad migration of kidney	7–9	Renal ectopia, horseshoe kidney
Major calyces, pelvis, ureter, urinary bladder, fetal urine formed	8–11	Ureteral abnormalities, posterior urethral valves, abnormal pelvis and calyces, multicystic dysplasia
Minor calyces, collecting tubules, papillary duct	13–14	Medullary cystic disease, medullary sponge kidney
Number of lobes in mature kidney (14–16) established	16	
Demarcation of cortex and medulla, growth of nephron, 1/3 of nephrons formed	20–22	Renal hypoplasia, polycystic and medullary cystic kidney disease
Nephron induction ceases (≈ million nephrons per kidney)	32–36	

From Yared, A., Barakat, A.Y., & Ichikawa, I. (1990). Fetal nephrology. In R.D. Eden & F.H. Boehm (Eds.), *Assessment and care of the fetus* (p. 72). Norwalk, CT: Appleton & Lange.

weeks, and 27 ml at 40 weeks.[53, 70, 71] Urine flow rates are decreased in infants with intrauterine growth retardation.[15] Alterations in urine production or excretion can significantly alter amniotic fluid volume and alter development of other systems (see Chapter 2).

Fetal ability to concentrate urine and conserve sodium is limited, with a concentrating ability about 20 to 30% of adult values.[118] Fetal urine is hypotonic owing to greater tubular reabsorption of solute than water. The major solute in fetal urine is sodium.[143] The fetus is not dependent on the kidneys for sodium conservation since sodium is readily transported across the placenta. The expanded extracellular fluid compartment of the fetus may also stimulate decreased tubular reabsorption of sodium and water.[53] During the third trimester fetal urine may become isotonic with plasma during severe stress.[23] The fetal kidney is less sensitive to AVP, which is present by 11 weeks, possibly as a result of immaturity of AVP receptors or presence of antagonists such as prostaglandins.[119, 152] Osmoreceptors and volume receptors in the fetus stimulate prolonged secretion of AVP from about 26 weeks.[72]

The renin-angiotensin system is active in the fetus, with increased renal and extrarenal production of all components. This system is stimulated by prostaglandins, the levels of which are elevated in the fetus to promote patency of the ductus arteriosus.[152] The juxtamedullary cells produce increasing amounts of renin from the 3rd month of gestation.[67] Renal responsiveness to aldosterone is decreased in the fetus, which may

lead to increased sodium loss. Endothelial cells lining the villous capillaries and the cells of the trophoblast are rich in angiotensin converting enzyme (ACE); the fetal membranes and amniotic fluid contain large amounts of renin. The chorion produces renin and angiotensinogen.[141] The placental circulation is a major site for conversion of angiotensin I to angiotensin II (similar to processes in the pulmonary circulation after birth), which is involved in control of placental blood flow in the fetus.[3] The increased angiotensin II appears important in modulating fetal blood pressure and renal hemodynamics, especially at birth.[119]

During the last 20 weeks of gestation the weight of the kidney increases in a linear relationship to gestational age, body weight, and body surface area.[72] Prior to 5 months, renal growth occurs primarily in the inner medullary area, which contains mostly collecting ducts. From 5 to 9 months, major growth is in the cortex and outer medullary areas. After birth, nephron growth occurs primarily in the tubules and the loop of Henle. At birth, approximately 20% of the infant's loops of Henle are too short to reach into the medulla, which can lead to problems in concentrating urine.[81] The rate of tubular growth after birth is reflected in changes in glomerular-to-tubular surface area. This ratio is 27:1 at birth, 8:1 by 6 months, and 3:1 in adults.[57]

NEONATAL PHYSIOLOGY

The newborn's kidney differs from that of the older child and adult in glomerular and tubular function. The adult number of nephrons is achieved by 34 to 35 weeks, but the nephrons are shorter and less functionally mature. Alterations in renal function and fluid and electrolyte balance are heightened in preterm infants who have not yet achieved their full complement of nephrons. When evaluating postnatal renal function, both gestational age and postbirth age must be considered since postnatal renal maturation is more a function of postbirth than gestational age, that is, a preterm infant who is several weeks old may have more mature renal function than a newborn term infant.

Transitional Events

During intrauterine life the placenta is the major organ of excretion, handling many functions that are normally performed by the lungs and kidney. With birth the kidneys must rapidly take over control of fluid and electrolyte balance, excretion of metabolic wastes, and other renal functions. Activity of AVP and the renin-angiotensin system increases with birth, perhaps stimulated by catecholamines, prostaglandins, hypercarbia, and the kinin-kallikrein system.[133] As a result blood pressure increases, with peripheral vasoconstriction and redistribution of blood flow to the vital organs.[72, 111] Activity of the renin-angiotensin system increases further during the first few days after birth. Transient increases in GFR may occur during the first 2 hours after birth. These changes are variable, decreasing to previous levels by 4 hours.[15, 137]

Body Composition

Body composition changes with gestational age and is influenced by maternal fluid and electrolyte balance. Newborns have higher total body and extracellular water and less intracellular water than older individuals. With advancing gestation total body water content and extracellular water decrease, whereas intracellular water increases as cells proliferate and organs mature.[20] The fetus is 80% water at 32 weeks' gestation and 78% at term. Extracellular fluid decreases from 60% at 5 months' gestation to 45% at term, and intracellular water increases from 25 to 33% (Fig. 8–7).[32, 107] The relative interstitial volume of the newborn is three times greater than that of the adult.[133]

Electrolyte composition also changes with gestational age. Since the electrolyte composition of extracellular water is primarily Na^+ and Cl^-, the preterm infant with more extracellular water has more Na^+ and Cl^- and fewer intracellular ions (K^+, Mg^{2+}, PO_4) per unit weight. Protein, fat, and carbohydrate composition of the body also increases with age. Small for gestational age (SGA) infants have more water and less fat, whereas large for gestational age (LGA) infants have more fat and less water.

Shortly after birth extracellular fluid increases, possibly related to withdrawal of maternal hormones. Expansion of the extracellular fluid (ECF) volume peaks at about 3 days.[31, 32, 67] Infants may become slightly edematous during this time so that a transient mild edema in both term and preterm infants over the first 2 to 7 days is not unusual.[152] This increase in ECF volume is followed by a diuresis as fluid in the interstitial space is mobilized and eliminated and the extracellular space contracts. This change may be related to decreases in atrial natriuretic peptide (ANP), which is elevated in the fetus and for the first 3 days after birth.[19, 120, 131, 145] ANP is a recently discovered hormone that is important in regulating volume and sodium homeostasis and is released by atrial myocytes by factors such as atrial distention and vascular volume expansion.[19]

Loss of 5 to 10% of birth weight (10 to 15% in preterms) is usually seen during the 1st week following birth owing to these changes in body water compartments. Losses are higher in preterm infants because they produce a more dilute urine and have greater urine sodium (and therefore additional obligatory water) loss.[32] Fluid therapy during the 1st week must account for these changes, otherwise fluid overload, which is associated with a risk of congestive heart failure, necrotizing enterocolitis, and symptomatic patent ductus arteriosus, may occur.[107]

Urine Output

Urine output varies with fluid and solute intake, renal concentrating ability, perinatal events, and gestational age. Generally term infants excrete 15 to 60 ml/kg of urine/day and preterm infants 1 to 3 ml/kg/hour (24 to 48 ml/kg/day) during the first few days. Urine output less than 0.5 ml/kg/hour after 48 hours is considered oliguria. Output in-

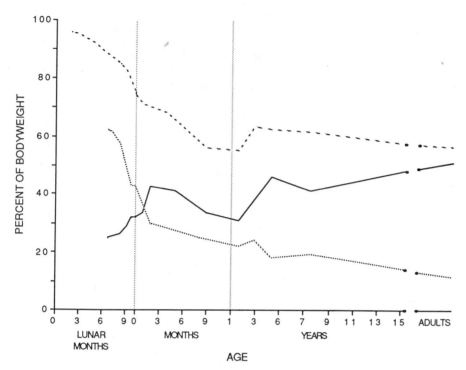

FIGURE 8–7. Changes in body fluid compartments as a function of age (total body water = dashed line; extracellular water = dotted line; intracellular water = solid line). (From Reed, M.D. & Besunder, J.B (1989). Developmental pharmacology: Ontogenic basis of drug disposition. *Pediatr Clin North Am, 36*, 1059. Modified by authors from Friis-Hansen, B. (1983). *Acta Paediatr Scand, 305* (Suppl.), 7.)

creases over the 1st month to 250 to 400 ml/day.[73]

The initial voiding after birth usually occurs within 24 hours but may be delayed. Approximately 66% of newborns void in the first 12 hours, 93% by 24 hours, and 99% by 48 hours.[132] About 23% urinate for the first time in the delivery room, where this event may be missed or not recorded. The force and direction of the urine stream are as important in assessing the urinary system as is the time of first voiding. A delay in spontaneous voiding, in the absence of renal anomalies, is usually due to inadequate perfusion with contraction of the intravascular compartment and temporary expansion of interstitial fluid volume.[101] Delayed voiding may occur in infants whose mothers received magnesium sulfate prior to delivery. Side effects of magnesium sulfate in the newborn include neuromuscular blockade with hypotonia and urine retention.[64]

Renal Blood Flow and Glomerular Filtration

Renal blood flow is reduced in both term and preterm infants at birth, primarily because the renal vascular resistance (RVR) is high. RVR is inverse to gestational age and falls after birth. RVR is normally high in the fetus, since renal function is not essential in utero (except for amniotic fluid production); therefore only a small percentage of the cardiac output perfuses the kidney. During the first 12 hours after birth 4 to 6% of the cardiac output perfuses the kidneys, increasing to 8 to 10% (versus 25% in adults) over the next few days.[15] In term infants there is a rapid decrease in RVR at birth with a concomitant increase in renal blood flow (RBF) and glomerular filtration rate (GFR). A similar pattern is seen in preterm infants greater than 34 to 35 weeks of gestational age, but the decrease in RVR is more gradual with a slower increase in GFR.[31, 67] The higher RVR and low blood flow to the outer cortex of the kidney in preterm infants may be due to the predominance of sympathetic tone in these infants.[67]

In all newborns the juxtamedullary nephrons are more mature than the outer cortical nephrons and a greater proportion of the blood perfuses the inner cortical and medullary nephrons versus the outer cortical nephrons. After birth perfusion of the outer cortex increases rapidly, perhaps in response to catecholamines and redistribution of placental blood flow.[137]

A major difference in renal function between the newborn and the adult is the lower GFR in the newborn, which is even lower when the infant's smaller size and surface area are considered. The GFR is approximately 20 ml/min/1.73 m^2 at term, 10 to 13 ml/min/1.73 m^2 in infants less than 28 weeks' gestational age, and as low as 2 ml/min/1.73 m^2 at 25 weeks (1.73 m^2 is a correction factor for differences in surface area that allows comparison of GFR between persons of different sizes). The GFR and RBF increase rapidly after birth, doubling by 2 weeks of age.[55, 70] The pattern of maturation is similar in preterm infants over 34 to 35 weeks' gestation and term infants, although the preterm infant may exhibit a slower increase, especially during the 1st week. The GFR is lower in preterm infants less than 34 to 35 weeks' gestational age and remains low until their full complement of nephrons has developed at about 35 weeks' conceptual age. After this point maturation of RBF and GFR follows a pattern similar to that of term infants.[2, 5]

The rapid increase in GFR after birth is due to redistribution of placental blood flow with increased RBF and perfusion pressure, decreased RVR, and increased systemic blood pressure, which increases glomerular capillary hydrostatic pressure, along with increasing glomerular surface area (initially glomerular surface area is about 10% of adult) and increased permeability of the glomerular membrane.[2, 64, 72, 137] GFR correlates with gestational age in infants prior to 35 weeks.[72] After 35 weeks GFR is more closely related to weight, length, and age. Maturation of GFR and other aspects of renal function may occur at varying rates in preterm infants, so infants must be evaluated individually in determining dosages of many pharmacologic agents.[130]

Tubular Function

Tubular function is also altered in the neonate. The decreased RBF and GFR reduce the volume of solutes per unit time that the tubules must handle. Tubular thresholds for reabsorption of many solutes are also reduced and neonates are more likely to lose sodium, glucose, and other solutes in urine.

Sodium

Rapidly growing infants are in positive sodium balance (sodium intake greater than output). Excretion of sodium is reduced in comparison to adults, possibly because of increased plasma renin activity and aldosterone levels as well as incorporation of sodium into the new tissue.[53] Renal tubular handling of sodium undergoes rapid changes after birth as the reabsorptive capacity for sodium and other solutes increases.

The pattern for renal reabsorption of sodium is different in the infant as compared with an older child or adult primarily because of the altered distribution of blood flow and changes in reabsorption in the proximal versus distal tubules. In infants a greater portion of RBF is to juxtamedullary nephrons, whereas in the adult the majority of RBF is to the cortical area and only about 10% goes to the medullary area. Since the juxtamedullary nephrons tend to be more involved in conservation than excretion of sodium, an infant's ability to excrete a sodium load is limited. This limitation increases the tendency toward sodium retention with increased ECF volume and edema formation.[133]

In addition, proximal tubule reabsorption of sodium in infants is decreased; distal tubule reabsorption is relatively increased, perhaps as a compensatory mechanism to reduce renal sodium loss.[67, 139] The increased distal tubule reabsorption is enhanced by elevated levels of aldosterone. Tubular reabsorption of sodium is greater in term than preterm infants who have increased urinary sodium losses and lower plasma sodium levels.

SODIUM BALANCE IN PRETERM INFANTS

Preterm infants are more likely to be in negative sodium balance (sodium intake less than output) during the first few weeks after birth.[137] Negative sodium balance has been observed in 100% of infants less than 30 weeks' gestation, 20% at 30 to 32 weeks, and 40% between 33 and 35 weeks.[2] Even though the GFR is lower in the preterm infant, so the kidneys have less sodium to handle, the altered tubular reabsorption with decreased proximal tubular reabsorption and increased distal tubule load results in increased fractional sodium excretion. Decreased proximal tubule reabsorption of sodium in preterm infants may be due to the shorter length of the tubules. As a result greater amounts of fluid and electrolytes such as Na$^+$ remain in the lumen and are sent to the distal tubule. The distal tubule is unable to increase its reabsorptive capacity to handle the additional sodium load despite elevated aldosterone levels, so more sodium is lost in the urine. The ability of the distal tubule to respond to aldosterone may be reduced or the distal tubule may already be under maximal aldosterone stimulation and thus unable to further increase its reabsorptive capacity.[137]

In the larger preterm infant fractional sodium excretion (FE_{Na}) is 1 to 5% versus 5 to 15% in very low birth weight (VLBW) and 0.5% in term infants.[72] Fractional sodium excretion is a measure of tubular function (as GFR is a measure of glomerular function) and calculated as

$$FE_{Na} = \frac{\text{urine sodium}}{\text{serum sodium}} \times \frac{\text{serum creatinine}}{\text{urine creatinine}} \times 100$$

Tubular reabsorption of sodium (T_{Na}) can be estimated by the formula $T_{Na} = 100\% - FE_{Na}$. The greater the FE_{Na}, the more sodium is lost in the urine. There is an inverse relationship between fractional sodium excretion and gestational age.[106] To determine if FE_{Na} is excessive, sodium and fluid intake must be considered.[53, 137] FE_{Na} generally decreases to less than 1% by 2 months.[152] By 2 to 3 weeks of age most preterm infants are in positive sodium balance as tubular function matures. Maturation takes longer in VLBW infants who are at risk for fluid and electrolyte disturbances for a longer period.[2]

Glucose

The ability of the tubules to reabsorb glucose is decreased in the preterm infant and increases to term.[67] Even at term the renal threshold for glucose (corrected for surface area) is lower in the infant. Even with this lower threshold most normoglycemic infants (unless very immature) are not glycosuric.[2] Although the glomerulotubular balance for glucose filtration and reabsorption can be demonstrated as early as 25 weeks' gestation, low renal thresholds for glucose (<100 to 150 mg/dl) have been reported in some VLBW infants.[69, 72] Urinary glucose levels are increased in the preterm infants with higher fractional glucose excretion, less reabsorption of glucose, and a tendency toward glycosuria.[15] VLBW infants are also at risk for hyperglycemia, as they are unable to readily excrete a glucose load. Since renal handling of glucose is interrelated with that of water, Na^+, K^+, and other solutes, attempts to excrete a glucose load may lead to hyponatremia, dehydration, and other abnormalities. Therefore VLBW infants with a glucose IV must be monitored for hyperglycemia, glycosuria, and fluid and electrolyte status.

Renal Handling of Other Solutes

In general renal excretion of solutes increases with gestation and postnatal age. Potassium excretion is low during gestation, and the newborn is less able to excrete a potassium load. With the lower GFR less sodium is delivered to and reabsorbed by the tubules. Since K^+ is exchanged for Na^+ in the distal tubule, less K^+ is secreted and subsequently excreted.[15] Healthy term and growing preterm infants are in positive potassium balance; stressed or ill infants may have a negative balance. Transient hyperkalemia (up to 5.5 to 6 mEq/L) occurs in some VLBW infants (less than 27 to 28 weeks of gestational age) probably owing to to their low GFR, decreased tubular response to aldosterone, and decreased renal adenosine triphosphatase (ATPase) activity.[68, 130] The turnover of potassium is related to that of nitrogen. Stressed infants have greater energy needs. After other energy sources (i.e., carbohydrate and fat stores) have been used, protein will be catabolized for energy with release of nitrogen. This leads to a negative nitrogen balance and increase in K^+ secretion and excretion. A negative potassium balance is also associated with the use of diuretics and parenteral fluid therapy.[53, 72]

Uric acid levels are higher in preterm than term infants (averaging 7.7 versus 5.2 ml/dl) and decrease with gestation. Serum levels are higher in infants owing to increased production of uric acid as a by-product of nucleotide breakdown.[152] Serum uric acid levels may also be elevated in hypoxic infants or following asphyxia.[72] Uric acid crystals may occasionally be seen as reddish staining of the diaper in normal newborns and can be misinterpreted as blood. Urea excretion is usually decreased in the neonate since they are using nitrogen for growth. Urinary protein excretion is greater at birth, gradually decreasing over the first few weeks.[136] Transient proteinuria may occur during the first 5 days.[2]

Renal excretion of phosphorus, calcium, and magnesium is interrelated with sodium reabsorption and excretion. During the 1st week calcium excretion varies inversely with gestational age and directly with urine flow and sodium excretion, thus increasing the risk for hypocalcemia in the VLBW infant.[15] Alterations in sodium intake and excretion alter renal handling of these solutes in ill infants, so liberal sodium supplementation may lead to development or exacerbation of hypocalcemia.[72] Phosphorus excretion is higher during the first weeks after birth and is related to gestational age and type of oral feeding. Calcium and phosphorus metabolism are discussed in Chapter 14.

Acid-Base Homeostasis

Serum bicarbonate levels and plasma pH are lower in neonates owing to a lower renal threshold for and reduced capacity to reabsorb bicarbonate. The lower threshold (serum level at which bicarbonaturia occurs) might be the result of altered transport capacity for bicarbonate or related to expansion of ECF volume.[15, 152] The more immature the infant, the lower the bicarbonate levels. Serum bicarbonate levels may be as low as 12 to 16 mEq/L in VLBW, 18 to 20 in LBW, and 20 to 22 in term infants (versus 24 to 28 in adults).[73, 137, 152] Serum bicarbonate levels in preterm infants increase to values greater than 20 mEq/L within the first 1 to 2 weeks. Urinary pH is 6 to 7 initially, with minimum values (4.5 to 5.3) reached by 1 to 2 weeks.[73] The occurrence of an alkaline urine along with a metabolic acidosis suggests renal tubular acidosis.[73]

Term and preterm infants are able to excrete an acid load, although the ability of the kidneys to respond to an acid load increases with gestational and postnatal age. The decreased response to an acid load in the VLBW infant may result from immaturity of the hydrogen ion secreting mechanism, decreased excretion of urinary buffers, or unresponsiveness of the distal tubule to aldosterone.[72] Normally most newborns are probably secreting near to their maximal ability with little reserve to cope with any disorders that produce acidosis. Thus any event that increases the potential for acidosis, such as cold stress or starvation, is more likely to produce alterations in acid-base status in the newborn.[64] The ability of term and preterm infants to excrete an acid load improves by 1 to 2 months.[15]

Water Balance

Regulation of water balance by the newborn is similar to that of adults but within a narrower range. The ability of the newborn to dilute and concentrate urine is limited. The ability to dilute is defined as the minimum amount of solute (electrolytes, protein) that can be excreted in a volume of urine, that is, there is an obligatory amount of solute that the body must lose in order to excrete water in urine. Since diluting segments of the distal tubule and ascending loop of Henle develop early, newborns can dilute their urine to osmolarities of 40 to 50 mOsm/L (similar to adult values) or lower, but cannot handle large or rapidly administered water loads owing to the low GFR.[32, 53, 136] Therefore the neonate is at risk for overhydration, water retention, and overload. The decreased ability to excrete a water load is related primarily to decreased GFR and perhaps decreased sensitivity of the tubules to arginine vasopressin. The ability to excrete water load increases after 3 to 4 days in term and more mature preterm infants.[152]

The ability to concentrate urine relates to the maximum amount of solute that can be excreted within a volume of urine, that is, the ability to excrete a solute load without becoming dehydrated. To excrete more solute, the body would have to increase the amount of urine water. The concentration of solutes in urine depends on a complex interaction of events called the countercurrent multiplier system (Fig. 8–8). The newborn can maximally concentrate urine to approximately half adult levels (600 to 800 mOsm/L versus 1200 to 1400 mOsm/L). This ability is further decreased in preterm infants, with maximum urinary concentration of 245 to 450 mOsm/kg/L in 1300- to 1500-g infants at 1 to 3 weeks of age and even lower levels in more immature infants.[72] The limitation in concentrating ability is due to several factors:

1. Decreased medullary osmotic gradient related to decreased accumulation of urea and other solutes and increased medullary blood flow.
2. Lower concentrations of blood urea. Urea is a solute that sets up the concentration gradient. Since urea is an end product of nitrogen metabolism, growing infants, who use nitrogen to make protein and new tissue, metabolize less nitrogen and produce less urea.

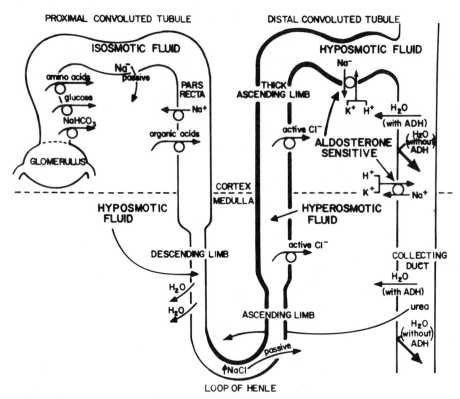

FIGURE 8–8. The countercurrent mechanism. The ability to concentrate urine is the maximum amount of solute that can be excreted within a volume of urine. Adults concentrate to a maximum of 1200 to 1400 mOsm/L; term newborns to 600 to 700 mOsm/L. To excrete more solute, the amount of urine water would have to be increased. Concentration of solutes in urine depends on the countercurrent system, which involves movement of Na$^+$, water, and other solutes between the tubular lumen, collecting ducts, and the surrounding interstitial fluid.

This system can be summarized as follows: Fluid entering the descending limb of the loop of Henle is hyposmotic owing to movement of solutes out of the proximal tubule. Since water but not Na$^+$ is reabsorbed in the descending limb, the fluid in the loop of Henle becomes hyperosmotic. As the filtrate moves through the ascending limb, Na$^+$ and Cl$^-$, but not water, move out of the lumen, so that the filtrate again becomes hyposmotic and the surrounding interstitial fluid becomes hyperosmotic. The longer the loops of Henle, the more concentrated the urine. As the filtrate passes through the distal tubule and collecting duct, Na$^+$ reabsorption is mediated by aldosterone and Na$^+$ is exchanged for secreted H$^+$ and K$^+$. There is little water movement in the distal tubule. In the collecting duct arginine vasopressin (AVP) controls water reabsorption. When AVP is present, water reabsorption increases, resulting in a hypertonic urine. (From Ramanathan, S. & Turndorf, H. (1988). Renal disease. In F.M. James, A.S. Wheeler, & D.M. Dewan (Eds.), *Obstetric anesthesia: The complicated patient* (2nd ed., p. 208). Philadelphia: FA Davis, 1988. Modified by authors from Petersdorf, R.G., et al. (1983). *Harrison's principles of internal medicine* (10th ed., p. 1602). New York: McGraw-Hill.)

3. Decreased solute levels for the concentration gradients in the interstitial space owing to decreased reabsorption and increased excretion of Na$^+$, Cl$^-$, glucose, and urea.

4. Decreased length of loops of Henle and collecting ducts.
5. Decreased response to circulating AVP.
6. Interference of prostaglandins with the hyposmotic action of AVP.[31, 32, 67, 72, 106, 140, 152]

Hormonal Regulation

Renin-Angiotensin-Aldosterone System

Plasma renin, angiotensin II, and aldosterone levels (see Fig. 8–4) are high in newborns and decrease gradually over the 1st month.[67, 73] Hyperfunction of this system may be due to the low systemic blood pressure and RBF, sodium wasting, and the normal decrease in ECF volume after birth.[152] The increased renin and aldosterone concentrations may be mediated by prostaglandins, which are also elevated at birth.[133] The aldosterone may increase sodium reabsorption by the distal tubules or, by influencing vasoconstriction, modulate changes in GFR to protect the renal tubules from overload with loss of electrolytes and other solutes in the urine.[5] Renin activity is higher in preterm than term infants, decreases in both groups by 30 minutes after birth, then increases again by 4 hours.[15, 152] In the VLBW infant adrenal production of aldosterone is decreased, as is distal tubule responsivity to aldosterone.[67] These changes increase the risk of hyponatremia and dehydration. The basis for the decreased response to aldosterone is uncertain but may relate to lack of receptors, the presence of an undetermined antagonist, or the deficiency of intracellular transport system enzymes.[2]

Arginine Vasopressin

Both the distal tubule and the collecting ducts of the infant respond to arginine vasopressin (AVP). AVP levels are not decreased in neonates, and sensitivity of volume and osmoreceptors is similar to that in adults. However, tubular response to circulating AVP is decreased, especially in preterm infants.[136, 143] Plasma and urinary AVP are increased in infants born vaginally (possibly stimulated by head compression), following perinatal asphyxia, and in infants with intracranial hemorrhage, respiratory distress syndrome, meconium aspiration, and pneumothorax. These findings may be due to decreased osmolarity in the medullary interstitium (from decreased tubular function and decreased reabsorption of solutes) or inhibition of AVP by increased levels of PGE_2.[53, 140] These infants are at greater risk for excessive water loss, early hyponatremia, and dehydration.

Factors regulating AVP secretion in neonates are not fully understood. Increased AVP and water retention may be important in the etiology of later hyponatremia in VLBW infants.[140] Chronically increased sodium excretion with contraction of the ECF compartment may stimulate the renin-angiotensin-aldosterone system and AVP secretion. AVP increases renal water reabsorption to restore ECF volume but may also decrease plasma sodium.

The Bladder

The neonate's bladder is almost entirely in the abdominal cavity and is cigar-shaped (as opposed to pyramidal shape in adults); therefore the ureters are short. As a result, distention of the bladder compresses the abdomen and increases pressure on the diaphragm. As the pelvic cavity increases in size during infancy and early childhood, the bladder gradually sinks into the pelvis and the ureters lengthen.[96]

CLINICAL IMPLICATIONS FOR NEONATAL CARE

The newborn infant is able to regulate sodium and water balance, but within a much narrower range than the older child or adult. As a result, the neonate is much more likely to develop fluid and electrolyte disturbances within a shorter period of time with a small margin between homeostasis and overload or underload. Careful calculation and monitoring of needs are essential to maintain homeostasis. Immaturity of renal function limits the ability of the infant, especially if preterm or ill, to cope with additional stress and increases the risk of renal dysfunction following pathophysiologic events such as perinatal asphyxia or with respiratory distress syndrome. In addition, alterations in renal function affect excretion of drugs and influence serum levels and drug half-life values, increasing the risks of side effects and toxicity.

Management of Fluid and Electrolyte Balance

Calculation of fluid needs for any infant involves consideration of maintenance needs, replacement of losses, and provision of allowances for growth. Maintenance needs include consideration of endogenous water produced by oxidative metabolism plus insensible water loss and loss of water in urine and stool. Usual values for these parameters are known and can be used to calculate fluid needs. In healthy term or large preterm infants individual variations from these values, unless major, are probably not crucial, since the infant's kidneys will adjust to ensure fluid and electrolyte homeostasis.[106] However, ill or VLBW infants may not be able to adjust, since their renal function is inefficient or compromised by illness. In addition, these infants are more likely to be in environments, such as an incubator or under a radiant warmer or phototherapy, that markedly alter insensible water loss.

Stool water loss is estimated at 5 to 10 ml/kg/day under basal conditions but can increase markedly with diarrhea. Stool water losses are considered to be minimal during the first few days after birth and thus are not included in calculation of initial fluid needs. Approximately 5 to 10 ml/kg/day of endogenous water is produced by oxidation. This water is often ignored in calculation of fluid requirements.[15] Water for growth varies with body water composition. For example, if an infant is assumed to have a water content of 70%, water needed for growth would be 0.70 ml per g of weight gain. Since body water composition is not static, water for growth is generally estimated at 10 to 20 ml/kg/day, with the higher values used for more immature infants who have a larger proportion of body water.[107] In the 1st week after birth during the period of physiologic weight loss, calculation of maintenance fluid needs does not include replacement of water for growth but is based primarily on calculation of insensible water loss and urine water loss.

Insensible Water Loss

Insensible water loss (IWL) is water loss from the skin (70%) and respiratory tract (30%).[16] Insensible water loss generally consists of about 32% of the total water requirement, unless IWL is markedly increased.[16] Basal levels of IWL in the neonate are 20 ml/kg/day or 0.7 to 1.6 g/kg/hour.[15] Insensible water loss is markedly increased in the preterm infant. Skin water loss is proportional to surface area, and these infants have greater surface area to weight. Preterm infants also have greater IWL because of increased permeability of their epidermis to water, greater percentage of body water, and increased skin blood flow in relation to metabolic rate.[16, 107] IWL can be significantly altered by conditions that increase the basal metabolic rate and by therapeutic modalities such as phototherapy, radiant warmers, heat shields, and incubators. Factors that increase or decrease IWL in neonates are summarized in Table 8–9.

Urine Water Loss

Urine water loss generally accounts for about 56% of total body water requirements (generally about 50 to 100 ml/kg/day).[16] The amount of water the infant must excrete in urine, maximum urine concentrating ability (urine osmolarity), and renal solute load are all interrelated (Fig. 8–9) and can be calculated using the following formula:

$$\text{urine volume (ml/kg)} = \frac{\text{solute load (mOsm/kg)}}{\text{urine osmolarity (mOsm/L)}} \times 1000$$

Variations in renal solute load can markedly alter obligatory urinary water losses. For example, a nongrowing infant who could concentrate to a maximum of 300 mOsm/L would have to excrete about 25 ml/urine/kg to get rid of a solute load of 7.5 mOsm/kg; the same infant would be obligated to lose 50 ml/urine/kg if receiving a solute load of 15 mOsm/kg (7.5/300 × 1000 = 25 ml/kg urine versus 15 ml/300 × 1000 = 50 ml/kg urine) and would be at greater risk for dehydration.

The renal solute load is the amount of solutes from metabolic end products, especially nitrogenous compounds and electrolytes, and exogenous sources that must be excreted by the kidneys. Endogenous solutes are produced from catabolism of tissues when caloric and protein intake is inadequate. Exogenous solutes are derived from parenteral solutions and enteral intake.[140] The solute load from exogenous sources can be calculated from the following formula:[153]

$$\frac{\text{solute load}}{\text{(mOsm/L)}} = 4 \text{ (g protein/dl)} + 1 \text{ (mEq Na + K + Cl)}$$

Renal solute load varies with the type of oral intake and whether or not the infant is receiving an intravenous solution with additional electrolytes and other solutes.

Daily solute excretion in most infants ranges from 7.5 to 30 mOsm/dl or more.[45] Renal solute load is lowest for growing infants fed human milk and highest for infants who are starved or receiving high osmolar parenteral fluids or a high protein formula.

TABLE 8–9
TABLE 8–9
Factors Influencing Insensible Water Loss (IWL) in the Neonate

INCREASE INSENSIBLE WATER LOSS	DECREASE INSENSIBLE WATER LOSS
Immaturity (50–300%)	Plastic heat shields (30–50%)
Radiant warmer (50–200%)	Double-wall incubator or heat shield (30–50%)
Forced convection incubator (30–50%)	Plastic banket under radiant warmer (30–50%)
Phototherapy (40–100%)	High humidity (50–100%)
Respiratory distress	Transport thermal blanket (70%)
Elevated body or ambient temperature*	Assisted ventilation with warmed and humidified air (20–30%)
Skin breakdown or injury	Increasing postnatal age
Congenital defects (omphalocele, gastroschisis, neural tube defect)	
Motor activity, crying (up to 70%)	
Other factors that increase metabolic rate	

*1° increase in body temperature = 30% increase in IWL.
Compiled from references 32, 57, 121, and 148.

Renal solute loads for commercial formulas can be found in the manufacturer's formula handbook. Renal solute loads for parenteral fluids average 10 to 20 mOsm of solute/100 kcal expended (in infants <10 kg, ml/kcal = cc/kg). For example, an intravenous line with a 10% glucose solution would average 10 mOsm/kg/day, and a maintenance IV with 3 mEq NaCl and 2 mEq KCl would yield an additional 10 mOsm/dl of solute from these electrolytes.[16]

Various factors can modify renal solute load and urine water excretion. In the grow-

ing preterm infant who is incorporating protein and other solutes into new tissue, each gram of weight gain decreases the renal solute load by about 1 mOsm. The decrease in solute load is reflected in decreased obligatory urine water loss. Urine water volume and thus fluid needs may be increased with glycosuria or furosemide therapy and decreased in infants on positive-pressure ventilation or with inappropriate ADH secretion or acute renal tubular necrosis.[16]

Estimating Fluid and Electrolyte Needs

During the first few days following birth maintenance fluid requirements are based on IWL and urine water loss. With increasing postbirth age fluid requirements increase owing to increased stool water losses and growth. There are many variations in specific recommendations for fluid and electrolyte needs (Table 8–10). Fluid needs for the first few days are generally calculated to account for the normal physiologic weight loss of 5 to 10% (10 to 15% in VLBW) of birth weight. If IWL is increased (see Table 8–9), fluid needs are also increased. On the other hand, fluid needs are reduced in infants with acute renal failure or congestive heart failure. Fluid needs are higher in infants less than 1000 g owing to markedly increased IWL and decreased renal concentrating ability (which increases obligatory urine water loss). These infants may need up to 200 to 300 ml/kg/day.[15]

Sodium Requirements of Preterm Infants

There are conflicting viewpoints on the management of fluid and electrolyte status in

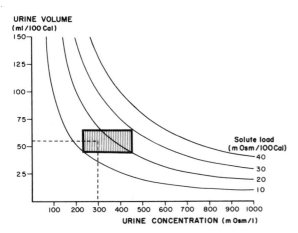

FIGURE 8–9. Interrelationships of urine volumes, concentrations, and renal solute loads in the neonate. Urine volume as a function of urine concentration for various solute loads, varying from high (40 mOsm/100 cal) to low (10 mOsm/100 cal). If urine volume were 55 ml/100 cal expended, both high and low solute loads could be excreted without taxing the minimum (about 50 mOsm/L) or maximum (about 1400 mOsm/L) concentrating power of the normal mature kidney. (From Winters, R.W. (1973). *The body fluids in pediatrics* (p. 123). Boston: Little, Brown.)

TABLE 8–10
Guidelines for Fluid (ml/kg/day) and Solute Provision by Patient Weight and Days of Age

WEIGHT	RANGE OF WATER LOSS		DAY 1*	DAY 2–3*	DAY 4–7*
<1250g	IWL†	40–130			
	Urine	50–100			
	Stool	5–10			
	TOTAL	95–230	120	150	175–200
1250–1750 g	IWL⁺	20–50			
	Urine	50–100			
	Stool	5–10			
	TOTAL	75–160	90	110	130–140
>1750 g	IWL⁺	15–40			
	Urine	50–100			
	Stool	5–10			
	TOTAL	70–150	80	90	100–120

Increment for phototherapy: 20–30 ml/kg/day
Increment for radiant warmer: 20–30 ml/kg/day
Maintenance solutes: Glucose: 7–12 g/kg (4–8 g/kg in VLBW infants)
                Na: 1–4 mEq/kg (2–8 mEq/kg in VLBW infants)
                K: 1–4 mEq/kg
                Cl: 1–4 mEq/kg
                Ca: 1 mEq/kg

*Adjustment based on a urine flow rate of 2 to 7 ml/kg/hr with a specific gravity of 1.003 to 1.010 and stable weight.
†May be reduced by 30% if infant is on a ventilator.
IWL, insensible water loss; VLBW, very low birth weight.
From Merenstein, G.B. & Gardner, S.L. (1989). *Handbook of neonatal care* (2nd ed., p. 211). St. Louis: CV Mosby.

preterm infants. Sodium intake is usually calculated at 1 to 3 mEq/kg/day. Preterm infants, particularly those less than 30 to 32 weeks' gestation, may be unable to maintain sodium balance on the standard sodium intake owing to increased urinary Na loss and require sodium intakes up to 4 to 8 mEq/kg/day.[1, 2] Others feel that these infants can be maintained on lower sodium intakes and that increasing fluid leads to increased sodium loss.[95]

Preterm infants are also at risk for hyperkalemia because of alterations in renal function. As a result, potassium needs must be carefully monitored and routine replacement may need to be decreased in the first few days.[32] Some infants less than 26 to 27 weeks have signs of dehydration at 24 to 48 hours, with elevated sodium, potassium, and glucose without oliguria, acidosis, or shock. This is thought to result from excessive evaporative losses (up to 100 to 200 ml/kg/day) due to the immature skin and greater surface area to body mass. These infants have an initial weight loss of up to 20% and high urine output.[32]

Various protocols have been recommended for management of fluids and electrolytes in VLBW infants. Lorenz and colleagues noted that preterm infants given increased fluid and sodium in the 1st week

actually had lower serum sodium values than infants who received less fluid.[95] Engle found that conservative fluid management during the first few weeks was associated with a positive sodium balance and fewer complications.[53] All infants have a reduction in ECF volume in the first few days, associated with increased excretion of fluid and sodium excretion. This in part accounts for the increased sodium losses in the 1st week.[106] Oh suggests that the high sodium excretion should not be corrected by increasing sodium intake in the 1st week, since this may impede the normal postbirth adjustments in body fluid compartment values.[106] After these adjustments have occurred sodium balance in the VLBW infant must be carefully evaluated and monitored. Some artificial formulas as well as human milk may not contain adequate sodium for the VLBW infant with immature renal function. These infants may require sodium supplementation until sodium balance is positive (see Chapter 9).

Risk of Overhydration and Dehydration

Although the infant can dilute urine to osmolarities of 30 to 50 mOsm/L, the usual diuretic response to a water load often diminishes before the entire load can be excreted.[53, 73] This decreased ability to excrete a water load makes the infant more susceptible to fluid overload. Term and larger preterm infants are more vulnerable to overhydration in the first 5 days following birth, since maximal dilution is not achieved until after that time.[107] GFR remains low in preterm infants until a conceptual age greater than 34 to 35 weeks is reached; thus these infants are at risk for volume overload for a longer period.[32] Fluid overload in preterm infants has been associated with an increased risk of necrotizing enterocolitis (NEC), bronchopulmonary dysplasia, and patent ductus arteriosus (PDA).[106] The expanded extracellular volume secondary to fluid overload may stimulate production of PGE_2, which maintains a patent ductus.[106] In infants with PDA and a large shunt, blood flow to the intestines is reduced, leading to hypoperfusion, ischemia, and NEC.

Owing to decreased concentrating ability, neonates, especially preterm infants, are at risk for dehydration, particularly if fluid intake is inadequate or extrarenal losses are elevated as with transepidermal loss in VLBW infants.[130] In evaluating dehydration in the 1st week, the usual postbirth weight loss must be considered so that infants do not become overhydrated.[107]

Electrolyte Imbalances

Limitations in renal function in preterm and ill neonates increase the risk of electrolyte disturbances from iatrogenic causes. Electrolyte imbalances can also arise from pathophysiologic problems, but these are not considered here.

HYPONATREMIA

Hyponatremia in preterm or sick infants can occur secondary to alterations in fluid (dilutional hyponatremia) or in sodium balance. Dilutional hyponatremia can arise from excess transfer of free water across the placenta because of rapid or excessive administration of fluids to the woman in labor. Excessive administration of a hypotonic solution overwhelms the limited fetal or neonatal renal capacity to deal with a water overload. This may occur if maintenance fluid requirements for the 1st week after birth do not allow for the physiologic weight loss, especially in VLBW infants. These events lead to rapid expansion of extracellular volume and reduced serum sodium and are associated with an increased incidence of patent ductus ar-

teriosus, congestive heart failure, necrotizing enterocolitis, intercranial hemorrhage, and bronchopulmonary dysplasia.[72]

Dilutional hyponatremia can also occur subsequent to water retention associated with the syndrome of inappropriate ADH (SIADH).[72] This syndrome is seen with a variety of pathophysiologic problems such as asphyxia, respiratory distress, sepsis, central nervous system problems, and following PDA ligation and other stressful situations. SIADH involves excessive secretion of arginine vasopressin (antidiuretic hormone) with normal fluid intake, serum hyponatremia and hyposmolality, increased urine osmolality and renal sodium excretion, absence of volume depletion and dehydration, and normal renal and adrenal function.[72]

Hyponatremia can also arise from negative sodium balance and excessive loss of sodium by immature kidneys of VLBW infants. In these infants the greater sodium loss increases water loss (renal excretion of sodium must be accompanied by excretion of water), leading to decreased ECF volume and hyponatremia.[72, 137] Renal sodium loss and subsequent hyponatremia in VLBW infants interfere with renal concentrating ability by changing the osmotic gradient and impairing ADH response. This further reduces water reabsorption and increases sodium loss and risk of hyponatremia.[140] Dilutional hyponatremia is an ever present risk for VLBW infants in the early postnatal period. This risk may be reduced by increasing sodium intake in VLBW infants during the first few weeks and careful monitoring of intake, output, electrolytes, weight, and fluid status.

HYPERNATREMIA

Hypernatremia related to immaturity of renal function may arise from dehydration caused by excessive sodium intake or increased IWL. The dehydration may be aggravated by limited concentrating ability of the immature kidney.[72] Hypernatremia can also follow intravenous administration of sodium bicarbonate, since the infant may not be able to rapidly excrete this sodium load.

LATE METABOLIC ACIDOSIS

Late metabolic acidosis can also occur owing to limitations in renal function, especially in VLBW infants. This disorder usually occurs at 2 to 3 weeks of age and is characterized by metabolic acidosis accompanied by an alkaline urine. Late metabolic acidosis is thought to be related to the amount of protein in the infant's diet, the amino acid composition of the protein, and the lower renal threshold for bicarbonate and often corrects with maturation of renal function.[73]

Measurement of Renal Function and Hydration Status

Parameters used to assess hydration status in the neonate include weight, fluid intake, urine specific gravity (1.002 to 1.010) and osmolarity (60 to 300 mOsm), urine output (minimum 1 to 3 ml/kg/hour) and electrolytes, and serum electrolytes and osmolarity. Changes in urine specific gravity are often an early response to alterations in hydration. Urine for this measurement can be obtained reliably from either collecting bags or aspirating several drops from the diaper.[98, 114] Urine output can be assessed by weighing diaper before and after use and noting the difference (1 g = 1 ml urine). Since urine rapidly evaporates from diapers of infants under radiant warmers, this assessment must be done soon after the infant voids.[29]

Serum osmolarity can be estimated by doubling the serum sodium value (since sodium and its anions are the major components of extracellular fluid) or more precisely by the following formula:[76]

$$\text{serum osmolality (mOsm/L)} = 2Na^+ + \frac{BUN\ (mg/dl)}{2.8} + \frac{Blood\ glucose\ (mg/dl)}{18}$$

(2.8 and 18 represent molecular weights divided by 10.) Measurement of renal function also involves assessment of GFR. Values for common parameters used to measure renal function and hydration status are listed in Table 8–11.

Plasma creatinine levels at birth reflect maternal values and increase shortly after birth (possibly because of a shift in extracellular fluid), followed by a decrease and stabilization at about 0.35 to 0.40 mg/dl (range, 0.14 to 0.70) by 1 to 2 weeks in term infants and later in preterm infants.[72, 129] Plasma creatinine levels are higher at birth in VLBW infants and inversely related to gestational age. Plasma creatinine measurement is often used to assess renal function for fluid and electrolyte management. This measure is somewhat limited in infants and children owing to the progressive changes in GFR and muscle mass.[129]

Creatinine clearance generally approximates GFR in term infants (as in adults) but is considerably more variable in preterm infants. At lower GFR values, creatinine clearance tends to overestimate GFR.[129] Creatinine clearance correlates with birth weight, length, and gestational age.[72] Plasma creatinine and creatinine clearance are useful measurements in stable infants but are less accurate in infants with renal failure or preterm infants whose renal function is rapidly changing with maturation.[129] The formula GFR (ml/min/1.73 m²) = KL/P$_{cr}$ (L = length in cm; P$_{cr}$ = plasma creatinine; K = estimate of muscle mass) is a better estimate of GFR than plasma creatinine alone, since it accounts for percentage of muscle mass. In this formula K = 0.27 for VLBW, 0.33 for appropriate for gestational age (AGA) preterm, 0.31 for SGA preterm, 0.45 for AGA term, and 0.33 for SGA term infants less than 1 year.[129] This formula can be used after the 1st week in term infants, and for preterm infants greater than 34 to 35 weeks' conceptual age, until 1 year of age.[135]

Renal Handling of Pharmacologic Agents

Alterations in renal function in neonate can markedly alter the infant's ability to excrete drugs and lead to an increased risk of toxic effects. The reduced GFR delays clearance of drugs that are eliminated by the kidneys, leading to prolonged half-lives. Plasma half-lives of many drugs used in the neonate including penicillin, aminoglycosides, furosemide, barbiturates, and digoxin vary inversely with creatinine clearance (which is a measure of GFR). Since GFR increases rapidly in the 1st week, dosages of these drugs often need to be increased at this point. Renal maturation progresses at variable rates after birth depending on gestation and conceptual ages. Therefore drug levels must be carefully and regularly monitored. Interactions between selected drugs and the immature kidney is summarized in Table 8–12.

Renal Function During Neonatal Illness

Immaturity in renal function in infants, especially preterm infants, limits their ability to

TABLE 8–11
Normal Values for Assessing Renal Function in the Neonate*

FUNCTION	PRETERM	FULL-TERM	2 WEEKS	8 WEEKS	1 YEAR
GFR (ml/min/1.73 m²)	12	20	50	75	120
Renal blood flow (ml/min)		120		300	425
Concentrating ability (mOsm/L)	482	800	900	1200	1400
Daily excretion of urine (ml/day)	1–3 ml/kg	15–60	250–400	250–400	500–600

*Kidney length is normally 5 to 7 cm, but it correlates best with the length of the infant rather than with gestational age. In preterm infants, plasma creatinine levels are 1.23 to 1.37 mg/100 ml, which is higher than in normal full-term infants. By 1 month of age, values return near normal (0.55 to 0.65 mg/100 ml).

From Cloherty, J.P. & Stark, A. (1981). *Manual of neonatal care* (p. 282). Boston: Little, Brown.

cope with additional stresses and can lead to significant alterations of renal function in association with specific pathologic problems such as respiratory distress syndrome, perinatal asphyxia, congestive heart failure, bronchopulmonary dysplasia, and patent ductus arteriosus. These disorders can also interfere with maturation of renal hemodynamics and tubular function.[70]

During perinatal asphyxia, severe respiratory distress syndrome, or other hypoxemic events, vascular resistance is increased, GFR decreased, and the renin-angiotensin-aldosterone system activated, further magnifying alterations that normally occur in normal newborns. In addition, cardiac output is redistributed, with increased blood flow to vital organs (heart, brain, adrenal glands) and reduced flow to less essential areas such as the renal and gastrointestinal systems. The percentage of decrease in flow to these nonessential systems is greater in immature animals and perhaps in human preterm infants as well.[106] The decreased blood flow increases the risk of renal and intestinal ischemia and disorders such as necrotizing enterocolitis and acute tubular necrosis. Following asphyxic episodes infants are at risk for SIADH, reduced urine output, impaired electrolyte reabsorption, hyperkalemia, and hyponatremia.[46] These infants require careful calculation and titration of fluid intake. Oliguria or anuria is most likely to develop within the first 24 hours. Initial fluid intake is limited to replacement of insensible and urinary water losses.

Infants with RDS and hypoxemia have marked changes in renal function with impairment of renal perfusion and reduced urine output by hypoxemia (Fig. 8–10). Oliguria is associated with renal tubular necrosis, decreased renal perfusion, and impaired diluting ability. These impairments can lead to a decreased ability to excrete water, water retention, and edema. The reduction in perfusion is due to vasoconstriction with increased renal vascular resistance possibly mediated by elevated activity of the renin-angiotensin system.[70] The decreased urine output is due to increased AVP and altered renal hemodynamics with a decreased GFR.[72] In hypoxemic infants an increase in urine output may occur prior to improvement in the alveolar-arterial oxygen gradient, suggesting that the improvement in respiratory function may be secondary to renal excretion of fluid sequestered in the lungs.[32, 72] Renal tubular function is also altered in these infants, with increased renal loss of protein, glucose, and sodium, decreased concentrating ability, and impairment of the ability to excrete acid (increasing the risk of renal tubular acidosis).

Positive pressure ventilation further alters renal function by decreasing cardiac output and renal perfusion, redistributing blood flow, and increasing intrathoracic and inferior vena caval pressure (Fig. 8–10). Positive-pressure ventilation and constant positive airway pressure alter renal function by decreasing GFR.[32, 72] Adequate hydration and careful monitoring of fluid and electrolyte status are especially critical for infants with respiratory problems and those on assisted ventilation.

MATURATIONAL CHANGES DURING INFANCY AND CHILDHOOD

Renal function undergoes rapid maturation during the first 2 years (increasing the risk of fluid and electrolyte alterations), when function comparable to that of adults is

TABLE 8–12
Effects of Selected Pharmacologic Agents on the Kidneys of the Neonate

DRUG	ACTION	RENAL EFFECTS	IMPLICATIONS
Aminoglycosides	Antibiotic	Excretion linked to GFR, which changes rapidly in first 1–2 weeks post birth May cause a transient decrease in GFR in term infants (not seen in preterm infants possibly owing to underperfusion of cortical nephrons) Serum half-lives inversely correlated with GFR, gestational age, birth weight, and postbirth age Toxic trough levels seen if dose not adapted to low GFR in VLBW infants	Monitor peak and trough serum levels and adjust dose as needed
β-Adrenergic agonists (ritodrine, terbutaline)	Treatment of preterm labor	Decreased GFR Increased plasma renin activity	Monitor renal function and fluid and electrolyte status in neonate
Captopril (and other ACE inhibitors)	Competitive inhibitor of ACE and may also interfere with bradykinin and prostaglandins Used to treat hypertension in adults	Rapidly crosses placenta, interfering with fetal renin-angiotensin system and prostaglandins Results in fetal oligohydramnios, hypotension, anuria, and cutaneous vasodilation	Avoid in pregnancy
Contrast agents	Hypertonic angiographic material	Markedly increases plasma osmolarity Associated with renal side effects (renal vein thrombosis, ischemia, medullary necrosis) Increases risk of intraventricular hemorrhage in preterm infants	Avoid use if possible, especially in preterm infant; use with adequate hydration Use nonionic agents with lower osmolalities (450 mOsm/kg H_2O) Monitor fluid and electrolyte status
Dopamine	Increases cardiac output and blood pressure in neonate Increases renal blood flow to mediate effects of indomethacin or tolazoline	Effects are dose related Some decrease in GFR in preterm infants with increased fluid and sodium loss	Monitor heart rate, blood pressure, urine output, hydration, and electrolyte status
Furosemide	Diuretic action Inhibits Na reabsorption in the thick ascending limb of loop of Henle Decreases K and Ca reabsorption and increases K secretion in distal tubule	Delayed onset of action in neonate with prolonged half-life Response related to urinary excretion rate (so effect decreased and weaker in VLBW and ill infant with decreased renal perfusion) Prolonged use associated with renal calcification, bone disease, ototoxicity (penetrates inner ear) Rapid fluid and electrolyte depletion with decreased cardiac output and altered tissue perfusion	Monitor fluid and electrolyte status Monitor for PDA Use with caution in VLBW and hypoxic infants Monitor for hypocalcemia Monitor for NEC Monitor renal function and output Monitor for metabolic acidosis
Indomethacin	Prostaglandin synthetase inhibitor Inhibit PDA closure	Transient decrease in GFR, urine output, urinary Na excretion, and renal blood flow, with increased BUN and creatinine Associated decrease in GFR can lead to significant peak and trough levels of aminoglycosides and digoxin	Monitor urine function, output, and fluid and electrolyte status Monitor peak and trough levels of aminoglycosides, digoxin, and other drugs
Tolazoline	α-Sympatholytic used as a pulmonary vasodilator	Associated with decreased systemic blood pressure and intense renal vasoconstriction and hypoperfusion with hematuria, transient renal failure, and oliguria	Monitor fluid and electrolyte status Maintain normal blood pressure during use with volume expanders, dopamine

Compiled from references 67, 69, 71, 72, and 152.

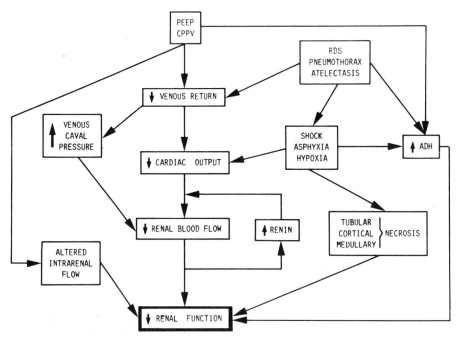

FIGURE 8–10. Physiopathology of renal changes during respiratory disturbances and mechanical ventilation. (From Guignard, J.-P. & John, E.G. (1986). Renal function in the tiny, premature infant. *Clin Perinatol, 13,* 377.)

achieved. RBF reaches 90% of adult values by 3 months and gradually increases to full adult levels by 12 to 24 months. GFR also increases rapidly during the first 3 months, then increases more slowly to reach adult values by 1 to 2 years.[81] Creatinine output per unit of body weight increases throughout childhood as muscle mass increases.[72] Plasma creatinine values are stable at values averaging 0.35 to 0.40 mg/dl until age 2 years, when they increase further until adolescence.[129]

By 2 months the infant is able to maximally excrete a water loss; concentrating ability does not approach adult levels until 6 to 12 months or later.[137] The ability to concentrate urine is probably related to increasing protein content in the diet, which increases urea levels in serum and tubular filtrate. This increase is important in creating the necessary gradient essential for maximizing renal concentrating mechanisms.[137] Plasma renin activity and aldosterone levels gradually decrease during early childhood.[109]

Anatomically the lobulation seen in the newborn kidney disappears and the glomerulus and tubules approach adult relationships by about 6 months.[15] The cuboidal epithelium of the newborn's glomerulus is gradually replaced by thin epithelium by age 1 year.[130] Total body water decreases to 60%, and ECF volume decreases to 27% by 12

months.[133] Urine output increases to 500 to 600 ml/24 hours by 1 year of age.[73] The bladder remains a cigar-shaped abdominal organ until early childhood, with achievement of the adult pelvic position and pyramidal shape by about 6 years.[96]

SUMMARY

The neonate is vulnerable to significant alterations in volume homeostasis and electrolyte balance owing to immaturity of renal function. This vulnerability is especially marked in the preterm infant, in which there is very little margin for errors in management of fluid and electrolyte status. These infants can rapidly become overhydrated or dehydrated or develop hyponatremia, hypernatremia, and other electrolyte disorders. By careful assessment and observation the nurse can prevent or minimize the effects of many of these disorders. Clinical recommendations for nurses working with neonates based on alterations, in the renal system and fluid and electrolyte balance are summarized in Table 8–13. By providing care to minimize these alterations, neonatal health can be enhanced with a reduction in the risks associated with pathophysiologic complications.

TABLE 8–13
**Summary of Recommendations for Clinical Practice Related to Changes in the
Renal System and Fluid and Electrolyte Homeostasis: Neonate**

Monitor fluid and electrolyte status of infants of mothers who received large volumes or rapidly administered intravenous fluids during labor or hypertonic IV solutions (pp. 349, 354).

Know normal values for parameters used to assess renal function and fluid and electrolyte status and recognize abnormalities (pp. 358–359, 370, Table 8–11).

Know expected patterns of weight loss following birth and monitor status (pp. 359, 369).

Carefully calculate fluid and electrolyte requirements (pp. 365–369, Table 8–10).

Record fluid intake and output and maintain within calculated limits (pp. 365–369).

Use infusion device to administer IV fluids, calculate intake hourly, and adjust as needed (pp. 363, 365, 368–370).

Assess hydration status of infants using weight, intake and output, urine specific gravity and osmolality, serum osmolality and electrolytes) (pp. 365–370, Table 8–11).

Observe for signs of overhydration, water retention, vascular overload, and dehydration (pp. 363–365, 368–369).

Know and monitor complications associated with excess fluid (pp. 363–365, 368–369).

Record time and character of first voiding (pp. 359–360).

Monitor voiding and fluid and electrolyte status in infants with perinatal asphyxia and those born to mothers on magnesium sulfate (pp. 360, 370–371).

Monitor infants on glucose IVs (especially VLBW) for glycosuria, hyperglycemia, and fluid and electrolyte status (pp. 362, 366–367).

Monitor potassium levels in infants with increased energy needs or who are stressed, or on diuretics or volume expanders (pp. 362–363).

Monitor calcium and magnesium levels in VLBW infants or those on sodium supplementation or with increased sodium excretion (pp. 362–363).

Monitor blood and urine pH values in LBW or ill infants (pp. 362–363).

Know risk factors for acidosis and observe for acid-base alterations in infants with cold stress, starvation, and fluid and electrolyte alterations (pp. 362–363).

Observe for renal sodium loss and hyponatremia especially in VLBW infants (pp. 361–362, 367–368).

Know effects of illness on renal function and monitor ill or stressed infants for problems such as hyponatremia and dehydration (pp. 361–371).

Recognize and monitor for drug side effects related to immature renal function (pp. 361, 370, 480–481, Table 8–12).

Monitor renal function and fluid and electrolytes in infants born to mothers who received beta adrenergic drugs (Table 8–12).

Know components (maintenance, replacement of loss, provision for growth) of usual fluid and electrolyte needs for infants and how these needs vary at different gestational ages (pp. 365–370, Table 8–10).

Calculate infant fluid and electrolyte needs and renal solute load (pp. 361–371).

Avoid use of high solute load formulas, especially in LBW infants (pp. 366–367).

Recognize factors influencing insensible water loss and act to minimize the effects of these losses (p. 366, Table 8–9).

Recognize and monitor for effects of neonatal pathophysiologic problems on renal function (pp. 361–371).

Recognize factors placing the infant at risk for overhydration, dehydration, and electrolyte imbalances and monitor infants for these problems (pp. 361–371).

Recognize parameters associated with SIADH and late metabolic acidosis (pp. 369–370).

Page numbers following each intervention refer to pages where rationale for intervention is discussed.

REFERENCES

1. Al-Dahhan, J., et al. (1984). Sodium homeostasis in term and preterm infants. III. The effects of salt supplementation. *Arch Dis Child, 59,* 945.
2. Al-Dahhan, J., et al. (1983). Sodium homeostasis in term and preterm infants. I. Renal aspects. *Arch Dis Child, 58,* 335.
3. Alhen-Gelas, F., et al. (1986). The renin-angiotensin system in pregnancy and parturition. *Adv Nephrol, 15,* 25.
4. Aperia, A., et al. (1975). Development of renal control of salt and fluid homeostasis in the first year of life. *Acta Paediatr Scand, 64,* 393.
5. Aperia, A., et al. (1981). Postnatal development of renal function in pre-term and full-term infants. *Acta Paediatr Scand, 70,* 183.
6. Arant, B.S. (1981). Nonrenal factors influencing renal function during the perinatal period. *Clin Perinatol, 8,* 225.
7. Arant, B.S. (1987). Postnatal development of renal function during the first year of life. *Pediatr Nephrol, 1,* 308.
8. Asrat, T. & Nageotte, M.P. (1990). Renal failure in pregnancy. *Semin Perinatol, 14,* 59.
9. Assali, N.S., Digman, W.J., & Dasgupta, K. (1979). Renal function in human pregnancy. II. Effects of venous pooling on renal hemodynamics and water, electrolyte, and aldosterone excretion during normal gestation. *J Lab Clin Med, 54,* 394.
10. Atherton, J.C. & Green, R. (1983). Renal function in pregnancy. *Clin Science, 65,* 449.
11. Bailey, R.R. & Rolleston, G.L. (1971). Kidney length and ureteric dilation in the puerperium. *J Obstet Gynaecol Br Comm, 78,* 55.
12. Barron, W.M. & Lindheimer, M.D. (1985). Renal function and volume homeostasis during pregnancy. In N. Gleicher N (Ed.), *Principles of medical therapy in pregnancy* (pp. 779–789). New York: Plenum Press.
13. Bay, W. & Ferris, T.F. (1979). Factors controlling plasma renin and aldosterone during pregnancy. *Hypertension, 1,* 410.
14. Baylis, C. (1987). The determinants of renal hemodynamics in pregnancy. *Am J Kidney Dis, IX,* 260.

15. Bell, E.F. & Oh, W. (1987). Fluid and electrolyte management. In G.B. Avery (Ed.), *Neonatology* (pp. 775–794). Philadelphia: JB Lippincott.

16. Bell, E.F. & Oh, W. (1979). Fluid and electrolyte balance in very low birth weight infants. *Clin Perinatol, 6*, 139.

17. Bellina, J.H., Dougherty, C.M., & Mickel, A. (1970). Pyeloureteral dilation and pregnancy. *Am J Obstet Gynecol, 108*, 356.

18. Beydoun, S.N. (1985). Morphologic changes in the renal tract in pregnancy. *Clin Obstet Gynecol, 28*, 249.

19. Bierd, T.M., et al. (1990). Interrelationships of atrial natriuretic peptide, atrial volume, and renal function in premature infants. *J Pediatr, 116*, 753.

20. Boineau, F.G. & Lewy, J.E. (1990). Estimation of parenteral fluid requirements. *Pediatr Clin North Am, 37*, 257.

21. Boonshaft, B., et al. (1968). Serum renin activity in pregnancy: Effect of alterations of posture and sodium intake. *J Clin Endocrinol Metabol, 28*, 1641.

22. Booth, G. (1980). Fetal homeostasis. In S. Aldjem, A.K. Brown, & C. Surreau (Eds.), *Clinical perinatology* (pp. 81–99). St. Louis: CV Mosby.

23. Brace, R.A. (1986). Amniotic fluid volume and its relationship to fetal fluid balance: Review of experimental data. *Semin Perinatol, 10*, 103.

24. Brans, Y. (1986). Fluid compartments in neonates weighing 1000 grams or less. *Clin Perinatol, 13*, 403.

25. Brinkman, C.R. & Meldrum, D. (1979). Physiology and pathophysiology of maternal adjustments to pregnancy. In S. Aldjem, A.K. Brown, & C. Surreau (Eds.), *Clinical perinatology* (2nd ed., pp. 1–31). St. Louis: CV Mosby.

26. Broughton, P.F., Oats, J.J.N., & Symonds, E.M. (1978). Sequential changes in the human renin-angiotensin system following delivery. *Br J Obstet Gynecol, 85*, 821.

27. Chesley, L.C. (1974). Renin, angiotensin, and aldosterone. *Obstet Gynecol Annu, 3*, 235.

28. Conrad, K.P. (1987). Possible mechanisms for changes in renal hemodynamics during pregnancy: Studies from animal models. *Am J Kidney Dis, IX*, 253.

29. Cooke, B.J., Werkman, S., & Watson, D. (1989). Urine output measurement in premature infants. *Pediatrics, 83*, 116.

30. Cosmi, E.V. & Caldeyro-Barcia, R. (1981). Fetal homeostasis. In E.V. Cosmi (Ed.), *Obstetric anesthesia and perinatology* (pp. 103–317). New York: Appleton-Century-Crofts.

31. Costarino, A. & Baumgart, S. (1986). Modern fluid and electrolyte management of the critically ill premature infant. *Pediatr Clin North Am, 33*, 153.

32. Costarino, A.T. & Baumgart, S. (1988). Controversies in fluid and electrolyte management for the preterm infant. *Clin Perinatol, 15*, 863.

33. Cotton, D.B., et al. (1984). Intrapartum to postpartum changes in colloid osmotic pressure. *Am J Obstet Gynecol, 149*, 174.

33a. Culpepper, L. & Jack, B. (1990). Prevention of urinary tract infection complications during pregnancy. In I.R. Merkatz & J.E. Thompson (Eds.), *New perspectives on prenatal care* (pp. 425–444). New York: Elsevier.

34. Dahlenburg, G.W., Burnell, R.H., & Braybrook, R. (1980). The relation between cord serum sodium levels in newborn infants and maternal intravenous therapy during labour. *Br J Obstet Gynaecol, 87*, 519.

35. Davison, J.M. (1983). The kidney in pregnancy: A review. *J R Soc Med, 76*, 485.

36. Davison, J.M. (1984). Renal haemodynamics and volume homeostasis in pregnancy. *Scand J Clin Lab Invest, 44*, 15.

37. Davison, J.M. (1985). The physiology of the renal tract in pregnancy. *Clin Obstet Gynecol, 28*, 257.

38. Davison, J.M. (1987). Overview: Kidney function in pregnant women. *Am J Kidney Dis, IX*, 248.

39. Davison, J.M. (1987). Renal transplantation and pregnancy. *Am J Kidney Dis, IX*, 374.

40. Davison, J.M. & Dunlop, W. (1980). Renal hemodynamics and tubular function in normal human pregnancy. *Kidney Int, 82*, 152.

41. Davison, J.M., Dunlop, W., & Ezimokhai, M. (1980). Twenty-four hour creatinine clearance during the third trimester of normal pregnancy. *Br J Obstet Gynaecol, 87*, 106.

42. Davison, J.M. & Hytten, F.E. (1974). Glomerular filtration during and after pregnancy. *J Obstet Gynaecol Br Comm, 81*, 588.

43. Davison, J.M., Katz, A.I., & Lindheimer, M.D. (1985). Kidney disease and pregnancy: Obstetric outcome and long-term prognosis. *Clin Perinatol, 12*, 497.

44. Davison, J.M. & Lovedale, C. (1974). The excretion of glucose during normal pregnancy and after delivery. *J Obstet Gynaecol Br Comm, 81*, 30.

45. De Curtis, M., Senterre, J., & Rigo, J. (1990). Renal solute load in preterm infants. *Arch Dis Child, 65*, 357.

46. Denson, S.E. (1989). Fetal asphyxia and its impact on the neonate. In M. Rathi (Ed.), *Current perinatology*. New York: Springer.

47. Devoe, S.J. & O'Shaughnessy, R. (1984). Clinical management and diagnosis of pregnancy induced hypertension. *Clin Obstet Gynecol, 27*, 836.

48. Dunlop, W. (1976). Investigations into the influence of posture on renal plasma flow and glomerular filtration rate in late pregnancy. *Br J Obstet Gynaecol, 17*, 17.

49. Dunlop, W. (1979). Renal physiology in pregnancy. *Postgrad Med, 55*, 329.

50. Dunlop, W. (1981). Serial changes in renal haemodynamics during normal human pregnancy. *Br J Obstet Gynaecol, 88*, 1.

51. Dunlop, W. & Davison, J.M. (1977). The effect of normal pregnancy upon renal handling of uric acid. *Am J Obstet Gynecol, 84*, 13.

52. Dure-Smith, P. (1970). Pregnancy dilation of the urinary tract. *Radiology, 96*, 545.

53. Engle, W.D. (1986). Development of fetal and neonatal renal function. *Semin Perinatol, 10*, 113.

54. El-Dahr, S.S. & Chevalier, R.L. (1990). Special needs of the newborn infant in fluid therapy. *Pediatr Clin North Am, 37*, 323.

55. Fawer, C.L., Torrado, A., & Guignard, J.P. (1979). Maturation of renal function in full-term and premature neonates. *Helv Paediatr Acta, 34*, 11.

56. Ferris, T.F. (1988). Renal diseases. In G.N. Burrow & T.F. Ferris (Eds.), *Medical complications during pregnancy* (pp. 277–302). Philadelphia: WB Saunders.

57. Fetterman, G.H., et al. (1965). The growth and maturation of human glomeruli and proximal convolutions from term to adulthood. *Pediatrics, 35*, 601.

58. Freed, S.Z. (1981). Hydronephrosis of pregnancy. In S.Z. Freed & N. Herzig (Eds.), *Urology in pregnancy*, (pp. 9–21). Baltimore: Williams & Wilkins.

59. Gabert, H.A. & Miller, J.M. (1985). Renal disease in pregnancy. *Obstetr Gynecol Surv, 40*, 449.

60. Gallery, E.D.M. & Brown, M.A. (1987). Control of sodium excretion in human pregnancy. *Am J Kidney Dis, IX*, 290.

61. Gant, N.F., et al. (1973). A study of angiotensin II pressor response throughout primigravid pregnancy. *J Clin Invest, 52*, 2682.

62. Gant, N.F., et al. (1987). Control of vascular reactivity in pregnancy. *Am J Kidney Dis, IX*, 303.

63. Gillerot, Y. & Koulischer, L. (1988). Major malformations of the urinary tract. *Biol Neonate, 53*, 186.

64. Gonzales, E.T. (1985). Urologic considerations in the newborn. *Urol Clin North Am, 12*, 43.

65. Gordin, D.B., Sachin, I.N., & Dodd, V.N. (1978). Low renin substrate levels in early pregnancy predict spontaneous abortion. *Clin Res, 26*, 306A.

66. Green, R. & Hatton, T.M. (1987). Renal tubular function in gestation. *Am J Kidney Dis, IX*, 265.

67. Green, T.P. (1987). The pharmacologic basis of diuretic therapy in the newborn. *Clin Perinatol, 14*, 951.

68. Gruskay, J.A., et al. (1988). Non-oliguric hyperkalemia in the premature infant <1000 gms. *J Pediatr, 113*, 381.

69. Guignard, J.P. (1982). Renal function in the newborn infant. *Pediatr Clin North Am, 29*, 777.

70. Guignard, J.P. (1982). Drugs and the neonatal kidney. *Dev Pharm Ther, 4*(Suppl. 1), 19.

71. Guignard, J.P. & Gouyon, J.B. (1988). Adverse effects of drugs on the immature kidney. *Biol Neonate, 53*, 243.

72. Guignard, J.P. & John, E.G. (1986). Renal function in the tiny, premature infant. *Clin Perinatol, 13*, 377.

73. Guignard, J.P. & Torrado, A. (1987). Neonatal renal function and disease. In L. Stern & P. Vert (Eds.), *Neonatal medicine* (pp. 941–974). New York: Masson Publishers.

74. Guyer, P.B. & Delaney, D.J. (1974). Over-distensibility of the female upper urinary tract. *Clin Radiol, 25*, 367.

75. Harrow, B.R., Sloane, J.A., & Salhanick, L. (1964). Etiology of hydronephrosis of pregnancy. *Surg Gynecol Obstet, 119*, 1042.

76. Hill, L.L. (1990). Body composition, normal electrolyte concentrations, and the maintenance of normal volume, tonicity, and acid-base metabolism. *Pediatr Clin North Am, 37*, 241.

76a. Henderson, P. & Little, G.A. (1990). The detection of pregnancy-induced hypertension. In I.R. Merkatz & J.E. Thompson (Eds.), *New perspectives on prenatal care* (pp. 479–500). New York: Elsevier.

77. Hutchinson, D.L., et al (1959). The role of the fetus in the water exchange of amniotic fluid in normal and hydramniotic patients. *J Clin Invest, 38*, 971.

78. Hytten, F.E. (1973). The renal excretion of nutrients in pregnancy. *Postgrad Med, 49*, 625

79. Hytten, F.E. & Leitch, I. (1971). In F.E. Hytten (Ed.), *The physiology of normal pregnancy* (2nd ed., pp. 132–164) Oxford: Blackwell Scientific Publications.

80. Jaffe, D.J. (1985). Postpartum evaluation of renal function. *Clin Obstet Gynecol, 28*, 298.

81. Jose, P.A. & Fildes, R.D. (1990). Postnatal development of renal function. In *The tiny baby* (pp. 71–76). Mead-Johnson Symposium on Perinatal and Developmental Medicine, No. 33. Evansville, IN: Mead Johnson.

82. Jose, P.A., et al (1987). Renal disease. In G.B. Avery (Ed.), *Neonatology* (pp. 795–849). Philadelphia: JB Lippincott.

83. Kauppila, A., Satuli, R., & Vuorinen, P. (1972). Ureteric dilation and renal cortical index after normal and pre-eclamptic pregnancies. *Acta Obstet Gynecol Scand, 51*, 14.

84. Kauppila, A., Ylostalo, P., & Litonius, U. (1972). Puerperal dilation of the upper urinary tract in realtion to the site of the placenta, parity and the birth weight of the infant. *Ann Chir Gynaecol Fenn, 61*, 318.

85. Keppler, A.B. (1988). The use of intravenous fluids during labor. *Birth, 15*(2), 75.

86. Lee, M.L.F. (1988). Infections and prematurity: Is there a relationship? *J Perinat Neonat Nurs, 2*, 10.

87. Lind, T. & Hytten, F.E. (1972). The excretion of glucose during normal pregnancy. *J Obstet Gynaecol Br Comm, 79*, 961.

88. Lind, T. (1983). Fluid balance during labour: A review. *J R Soc Med, 76*, 870.

89. Lindheimer, M.D. & Ehrlich, E.N. (1979). Postural effects on renal function and volume homeostasis during pregnancy. *J Reprod Med, 23*, 135.

90. Lindheimer, M.D. & Katz, A.D. (1975). Renal changes in pregnancy: Their relevance to volume homeostasis. *Clin Obstet Gynecol, 2*, 345.

91. Lindheimer, M.D. & Katz, A.D. (1986). The kidney in pregnancy. In B.M. Brenner & F.C. Rector (Eds.), *The Kidney* (3rd ed., pp. 1253–1295). Philadelphia: Ardmore Medical Books.

92. Lindheimer, M.D., et al. (1986). Water homeostasis and vasopressin secretion during gestation. *Adv Nephrol, 15*, 1.

93. Lindheimer, M.D., et al. (1987). Water homeostasis and vasopressin release during rodent and human gestation. *Am J Kidney Dis, IX*, 270.

94. Little, B. (1965). Water and electrolyte balance during pregnancy. *Anesthesiology, 26*, 400.

95. Lorenz, J.M., et al. (1982). Water balance in very low-birth-weight infants: Relationship to water and sodium intake and effect on outcome. *J Pediatr, 101*, 423.

96. Lowrey, G.H. (1986). *Growth and development of children.* Chicago: Year Book Medical Publishers.

97. Lumbers, E.R. (1983). A brief review of fetal renal function. *J Devel Physiol, 6*, 1.

98. Lybrand, M., Medoff-Cooper, B., & Munro, B.H. (1990). Periodic comparisons of urinary specific gravity using urine from a diaper and collecting bag. *MCN, 15*, 238.

99. Malinowski, J. (1978). Bladder assessment in the postpartum patient. *JOGN Nursing, 7*, 14.

100. Moore, K.L. (1982). *The developing human: Clinically oriented embryology* (3rd ed., pp. 255–270). Philadelphia: WB Saunders.

101. Moore, S. & Galvez, M.B. (1972). Delayed micturition in the newborn period. *J Pediatr, 80*, 867.

102. Moses, K.J. & Cotton, D.B. (1978). Colloid osmotic pressure and pregnancy. In S.L. Clark, J.P. Phelan, & D.B. Cotton (Eds.), *Critical care obstetrics* (pp. 71–90). Oradell, NJ: Medical Economics Books.

103. Munsick, R.A. (1970). Renal hemodynamic effects of oxytocin in antepartal and postpartal women. *Am J Obstet Gynecol, 108*, 729.

104. Nash, M.A. (1981). The management of fluid and electrolyte disorders in the neonate. *Clin Perinatol, 8*, 251.

105. Newton, N., Newton, M., & Broach, J. (1988). Psychologic, physical, nutritional and technologic aspects of intravenous infusion during labor. *Birth, 15*(2), 67.

106. Oh, W. (1988). Renal function and fluid therapy in high risk infants. *Biol Neonate, 53*, 230.

107. Oh, W. (1987). Water and electrolyte metabolism and therapy. In S. Stern & P. Vert (Eds.), *Neonatal medicine* (pp. 849–862). New York: Masson Publishers.

108. Pauerstein, C.J. (1987). *Clinical obstetrics* (pp. 65–82). New York: John Wiley & Sons.

109. Pelayo, J.C., Eisner, G.M., & Jose, P.A. (1981). The ontogeny of the renin-angiotensin system. *Clin Perinatol, 8*, 347.

110. Pitkin, R.M. (1985). Calcium metabolism in pregnancy and the perinatal period: A review. *Am J Obstet Gynecol, 151*, 99.

111. Pohjavuori, M. (1983). Obstetric determinants of plasma vasopressin concentrations and renin activity at birth. *J Pediatr, 103*, 966.

112. Ramanathan, S. & Turndorf, H. (1988). Renal disease. In F.M. James, A.S. Wheeler, & D.M. Dewan (Eds.), *Obstetric anesthesia: The complicated patient* (p. 207). Philadelphia: FA Davis.

113. Rasmussen, P.E. & Nielsen, F.R. (1988). Hydronephrosis during pregnancy: A literature survey. *Eur J Obstet Gynecol Reprod Biol, 27*, 249.

114. Reams, P.K. & Deane, D.M. (1988). Bagged versus diaper urine specimens and lab values. *Neonatal Network, 6*(6), 17.

115. Repke, J.T. (1986). Pharmacologic management of hypertension in pregnancy. In W.F. Rayburn & F.P. Zuspan (Eds.), *Drug therapy in obstetrics and gynecology* (pp. 55–65). Norwalk, CT: Appleton-Century-Crofts.

116. Resnick, L.M. & Laragh, J.H. (1983). The renin-angiotensin-aldosterone system in pregnancy. In F. Fuchs & A. Klopper (Eds.), *Endocrinology of pregnancy* (3rd ed., pp. 191–203). Philadelphia: Harper and Row.

117. Robertson, E.G. (1975). Water metabolism. *Clin Obstet Gynecol, 2*, 431.

118. Robillard, J.E., Nakamura, K.T., & Ayres, N.A. (1985). Control of fluid and electrolyte balance during fetal life. In C.T. Jones & P.W. Nathanielsz (Eds.), *The physiological development of the fetus and newborn* (pp. 527–532). New York: Academic Press.

119. Robillard, J.E. & Nakamura, K.T. (1988). Hormonal regulation of renal function during development. *Biol Neonate, 53*, 201.

120. Robillard, J.E. & Weiner, C.P. (1988). Atrial natriuretic factor in the human fetus. *J Pediatr, 113*, 552.

121. Robillard, J.E., et al. (1978). Maturation of the glucose transport processes by the fetal kidney. *Pediatr Res, 12*, 680.

122. Rowe, J.W., Brown, R.S., & Epstein, F.H. (1981). Physiology of the kidney in pregnancy. In S.Z. Freed & N. Herzig (Eds.), *Urology in pregnancy*, (pp. 1–8). Baltimore: Williams & Wilkins.

123. Roy, R.N. & Sinclair, J.C. (1975). Hydration of the low birth weight infant. *Clin Perinatol, 2*, 393.

124. Rubi, R.A. & Sala, N.L. (1968). Ureteral function in pregnant women. III. Effect of different positions and of fetal delivery upon ureteral tonus. *Am J Obstet Gynecol, 101*, 230.

125. Sadler, T.W. (1985). *Langman's medical embryology* (5th ed., pp. 247–280). Baltimore: Williams and Wilkins.

126. Sala, N.L. & Rubi, R.A. (1965). Ureteral function in pregnant women. *Am J Obstet Gynecol, 92*, 918.

127. Sala, N.L. & Rubi, R.A. (1967). Ureteral function in pregnant women. II. Ureteral contractility during normal pregnancy. *Am J Obstet Gynecol, 99*, 228.

128. Schulman, A. & Herlinger, H. (1975). Urinary tract dilation in pregnancy. *Br J Radiol, 96*, 638

129. Schwartz, G.J., Brion, L.P., & Spitzer, A. (1987). The use of plasma creatinine for estimating glomerular filtration rate in infants, children and adolescents. *Pediatr Clin North Am, 34*, 571.

130. Shaffer, S.E. & Norman, M.E. (1989). Renal function and renal failure in the newborn. *Clin Perinatol, 16*, 199.

131. Shaffer, S.G., et al. (1986). Elevated atrial natriuretic factor in neonates with respiratory distress syndrome. *J Pediatr, 109*, 1028.

132. Sherry, S.N. & Kramer, J.C. (1955). The time of passage of first stool and first urine. *J Pediatr, 46*, 158.

133. Siegel, S.R. (1982). Hormonal and renal interaction in body fluid regulation in the newborn infant. *Clin Perinatol, 9*, 535.

134. Sims, E.A. & Krantz, K.E. (1958). Serial studies of renal function during pregnancy and the puerperium in normal women. *J Clin Invest, 37*, 1764.

135. Springate, J.E., Fildes, R.D., & Feld, L.G. (1987). Assessment of renal function in newborn infants. *Pediatr Res, 9*, 51.

136. Sriwatanakul, K. & McCormick, K.L. (1984). Fluid and electrolyte disturbances. In M. Zia, T.A. Clarke, & T.A. Merritt (Eds.), *Assessment of the newborn* (pp. 343–347). Boston: Little, Brown.

137. Stewart, C.L. & Jose, P.A. (1985). Transitional nephrology. *Urol Clin North Am, 12*, 143.

138. Strauss, J., Daniel, S.S., & James, L.S. (1981). Postnatal adjustment in renal function. *Pediatrics, 68*, 802.

139. Sulyok, E. & Varga, F. (1983). Renal aspects of neonatal sodium homeostasis. *Acta Paediatr Acad Sci Hung, 24*, 23.

140. Sulyok, E. (1988). Renal response to vasopressin in premature infants: What is new? *Biol Neonate, 53*, 212.

141. Symonds, E.M. (1988). Renin and reproduction. *Am J Obstet Gynecol, 158*, 754.

142. Tarnow-Mordi, W.O., et al. (1982). Iatrogenic hyponatremia of the newborn due to maternal fluid overload: A prospective study. *Br Med J, 283*, 639.

143. Thomson, A.M., Hytten, F.E., & Billewicz, W.Z. (1967). The epidemiology of oedema during pregnancy. *J Obstet Gynaecol Br Comm, 74*, 1.

144. Vander, A.J. (1985). *Renal physiology*. New York: McGraw-Hill.

145. Weil, J., et al. (1986). Comparison of atrial natriuretic peptide levels in healthy children from birth to adolescence and in children with cardiac disease. *Pediatr Res, 20*, 1328.

146. Wilson, M., et al. (1980). Blood pressure, the renin aldosterone system and sex steroids throughout normal pregnancy. *Am J Med, 68*, 97.

147. Winston, J. & Levitt, M.F. (1985). Renal function, renal disease and pregnancy. In S.H. Cherry, R.L. Berkowitz, & N.G. Kase (Eds.), *Rovinsky and Gutt-*

macher's medical, surgical and gynecologic complications of pregnancy (pp. 142–173). Baltimore: Williams & Wilkins.

148. Winters, R.W. (1973). *The body fluids in pediatrics.* Boston: Little, Brown.

149. Worley, R.J., et al. (1979). Vascular responsiveness to pressor agents during human pregnancy. *J Reprod Med, 3*, 115.

150. Worley, R.J. (1984). Pathophysiology of pregnancy induced hypertension. *Clin Obstet Gynecol, 27*, 821.

151. Wright, A., et al. (1987). The urinary excretion of albumin in normal pregnancy. *Br J Obstet Gynaecol, 94*, 408.

152. Yared, A., Barakat, A.Y., & Ichikawa, I. (1990). Fetal nephrology. In R.D. Eden & F.H. Boehm (Eds.), *Assessment and care of the fetus.* Norwalk, CT: Appleton & Lange.

153. Ziegler, E.E. & Foman, S.J. (1971). Fluid intake, renal solute load and water balance in infancy. *J Pediatr, 78*, 561.

CHAPTER 9

The Gastrointestinal and Hepatic Systems and Perinatal Nutrition

Maternal Physiologic Adaptations
The Antepartum Period
  Mouth and Pharynx
  Esophagus
  Stomach
  Small and Large Intestines
  Pancreas
  Gallbladder
  Liver
  Weight Gain During Pregnancy
The Intrapartum Period
The Postpartum Period
Clinical Implications for the Pregnant Woman and Her Fetus
Nutritional Requirements of Pregnancy
Heartburn
Constipation
Hemorrhoids
Nausea and Vomiting
Food and Fluid Intake in Labor
Effects of Altered Maternal Nutrition
Pregnancy and Gastrointestinal Disorders
Pregnancy and Liver Disease
Drug Absorption and Metabolism
Development of the Gastrointestinal and Hepatic Systems in the Fetus
Anatomic Development
Functional Development
  Fetal Growth
Neonatal Physiology
Transitional Events
  Maturation of Gastrointestinal Function
  Initiation of Enteral Feeding
  Passage of Meconium
Functional and Anatomic Limitations
  Sucking and Swallowing
  Esophageal Motility and Lower Esophageal
    Sphincter Function

  Gastric Emptying
  Intestinal Motility
  Intestinal Surface Area
Physiologic Limitations
  Digestion and Absorption of Proteins
  Digestion and Absorption of Carbohydrates
  Digestion and Absorption of Fats
  Absorption of Other Substances
  Liver Function in the Neonate
Clinical Implications for Neonatal Care
Infant Growth
Nutritional Requirements of Full and Preterm
  Infants
Analysis of the Composition of Feedings
  Protein
  Carbohydrate
  Fat
  Vitamins, Minerals, and Trace Elements
  Calories and Renal Solute Load
  Use of Human Milk
  Components of Parenteral Nutrition Solutions
Feeding Infants with Various Health Problems
  Very Low Birth Weight Infants
  Infants with Respiratory Problems
  Infants with Cardiac Problems
  Infants with Short Bowel Syndrome
Considerations Related to Feeding Method
Monitoring Nutritional Status
Regurgitation and Reflux
Necrotizing Enterocolitis
Dehydration and Diarrhea
Drug Absorption and Metabolism
Maturational Changes During Infancy and Childhood
Introduction of Solid Foods

The gastrointestinal (GI) system consists of processes involved in intake, digestion, and absorption of nutrients and elimination of by-products in bile and stool.[236] Utilization of nutrients for production of energy and other vital functions is discussed in Chapters 13 and 14. This chapter focuses on the processes involved in preparing food substances for absorption of nutrients across the intestinal villi. These processes are summarized in Fig. 9–1; gastrointestinal enzymes are summarized in Table 9–1.

Maternal nutrition is one of the most important factors affecting pregnancy outcome. The maternal gastrointestinal tract must digest and absorb nutrients needed for fetal and placental growth and development and to meet the altered demands of maternal metabolism as well as eliminate unneeded by-products and waste materials from both the woman and the fetus. Structural and physiologic immaturity of the neonate's gastrointestinal tract can result in alterations in neonatal nutritional status and increase the risk of malabsorption and dehydration. This chapter reviews gastrointestinal and hepatic function in the pregnant woman, fetus, and neonate and implications for clinical practice.

MATERNAL PHYSIOLOGIC ADAPTATIONS

The gastrointestinal and hepatic systems during pregnancy are characterized by marked anatomic and physiologic alterations that are essential in supporting maternal and fetal nutrition. These changes are related to mechanical forces such as the pressure of the growing uterus and hormonal influences such as effects of progesterone on gastrointestinal smooth muscle and effects of estrogen on liver metabolism.

The Antepartum Period

The antepartum period is characterized by anatomic and physiologic changes in all the organs of the gastrointestinal system. These changes and their implications are summarized in Table 9–2. Pregnancy is associated with increased appetite, increased consumption of food, and alterations in the types of food desired including cravings, avoidance of certain foods, and pica (craving for non-nutrient substances). Specific changes in food consumption and the types of foods craved or avoided are strongly influenced by cultural and economic factors. Food consumption has been reported to increase 15 to 20% beginning in early pregnancy, peak at mid-gestation, and decrease near term.[198] Changes in maternal caloric intake do not parallel changes in basal metabolism or fetal growth (Fig. 9–2).

The basis for changes in patterns of food intake is unclear but may be a response to the drain of glucose and other nutrients by the fetus, alterations in taste threshold and acuity, or hormonal changes. Estrogen acts as an appetite suppressant and progesterone as an appetite stimulant. Influences of estrogen and progesterone on patterns of food intake are supported by similar changes during the menstrual cycle. Decreased appetite and food intake have been reported during the luteal phase of the menstrual cycle (when estrogen peaks), with increased appetite during the follicular phase (when progesterone peaks).[64, 236] During pregnancy alterations in insulin and glucagon combine with estrogen and progesterone to influence food intake.[235]

Mouth and Pharynx

Contrary to the old wives' tale regarding the loss of a tooth per baby, pregnancy does not result in demineralization of the woman's teeth. Fetal calcium needs are drawn from maternal body stores, not from the teeth. The major component of tooth enamel (hydroxyapatite crystals) is not reduced by the biochemical or hormonal changes of pregnancy.[266] As a result of gingival alterations the pregnant woman may become more aware of preexisting or newly developed dental caries. Calculus and debris deposits increase during pregnancy and are associated with gingivitis.[9, 52, 205]

Gingivitis occurs in 50 to 77% of pregnant women and is most severe during the second trimester.[9, 201, 205, 266] Estrogen increases blood flow to the oral cavity and accelerates turnover of gum epithelial lining cells. The gums become highly vascularized, with proliferation of small blood vessels and connective tissue, hyperplastic, and edematous.[68, 75, 87, 266] These changes along with the decreased thickness of the gingival epithelial surface result in friable gum tissues that may bleed easily or cause discomfort with chewing. Bleeding with brushing occurs more frequently during pregnancy.[9] The incidence of

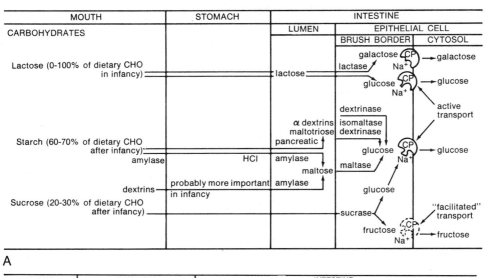

A

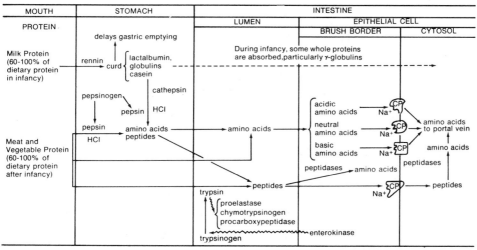

B

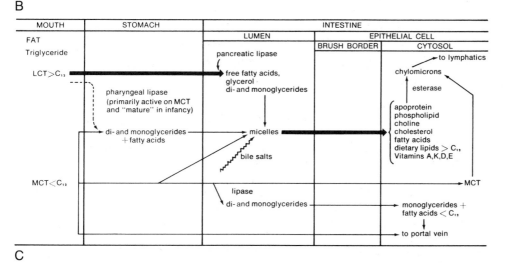

C

FIGURE 9–1.   Summary of digestion and absorption. *A*, Carbohydrate digestion. *B*, Protein digestion. *C*, Lipid digestion. (From Johnson, T.R., Moore, W.M., & Jeffries, J.E. (1978). *Children are different* (pp. 151–153). Columbus, OH: Ross Laboratories.)

TABLE 9–1
Gastrointestinal Enzymes

ENZYME	SOURCE	SUBSTRATE	SITE
Enzymes Involved in Fat Digestion			
Human milk lipase	Human milk	Triglyceride, lipovitamins	Small intestine
Lingual lipase	Oral glands (Ebner)	Triglyceride	Stomach
Gastric lipase	Gastric mucosa	Triglyceride	Stomach
Pancreatic lipase-colipase	Pancreas	Triglyceride	Small intestine
Phospholipase A$_2$	Pancreas	Phospholipid	Small intestine
Cholesterol esterase, nonspecific lipase	Pancreas	Cholesterol esterase, monoglyceride, lipovitamins	Small intestine
Intestinal lipase	Intestinal mucosa	Triglyceride	Small intestine
Alkaline lipases and phospholipases	Microbes	Triglyceride, other (?)	Colon, feces
Enzymes Involved in Protein Digestion			
Gelatinase	Gastric mucosa	Gelatin	Stomach
Pepsins	Gastric mucosa	Protein	Stomach
Enterokinase	Duodenal mucosa	Activates trypsinogen to trypsin	Duodenum
Trypsin	Pancreas	Peptides and basic amino acids (lysine, arginine)	Small intestine
Chymotrypsin	Pancreas	Peptides and aromatic amino acids (phenylalanine, leucine, tyrosine, tryptophan, methionine, glutamine)	Small intestine
Elastase	Pancreas	Peptides and aliphatic amino acids (valine, leucine, alanine, serine)	Small intestine
Carboxypeptidase A	Pancreas	Peptides, aliphatic and aromatic amino acids	Small intestine
Carboxypeptidase B	Pancreas	Peptides and basic amino acids	Small intestine
Intestinal peptidases	Small intestine	Di- and tripeptides	Small intestine
Oligopeptidases	Intestinal brush border	Larger peptides	Small intestine
Enzymes Involved in Carbohydrate Digestion			
Salivary amylase	Salivary glands	Starch	Mouth, stomach
Pancreatic amylase	Pancreas	Starch	Small intestine
Maltases	Small intestine brush border	Maltose, sucrose, dextrins	Small intestine
Lactase	Small intestine brush border	Lactose	Small intestine
Sucrase-isomaltase	Small intestine brush border	Sucrose, dextrins	Small intestine
Glucoamylase	Small intestine brush border	Glucose polymers	Small intestine
Mammary amylase	Human milk	Glucose polymers	Small intestine

Adapted from Watkins J. B. (1985). Lipid digestion and absorption. *Pediatrics, 75*(Suppl.), 151, as modified from Patton, J. S. (1983). Gastrointestinal lipid digestion. In Johnson, L. R. (Ed.), *Physiology of the gastrointestinal tract* (p. 1127). New York: Raven Press; and Sunshine, P. (1977). Digestion and absorption of carbohydrates. In *Selected aspects of perinatal gastroenterology* (pp. 17–21). Mead Johnson Symposium on Perinatal and Developmental Medicine, No. 11. Evansville, IN: Mead Johnson.

gingivitis is higher with increasing maternal age and parity, preexisting periodontal disease, and poor dentition.[201, 266]

In 0.5 to 2.7% of pregnant women, a specific tumor-like structure known as an epulis or pregnancy tumor develops.[236] With epulis formation the gingivitis is advanced and severe with a hyperplastic outgrowth generally found along the maxillary gingiva on the palatal side. This mass is very friable, bleeding easily and often interfering with chewing. Epulis usually regresses spontaneously after delivery. Occasionally these growths may need excising during pregnancy owing to bleeding, interference with chewing, or increasing periodontal disease.[266]

Saliva becomes more acidic during pregnancy with alterations in electrolyte content but generally does not increase in volume. Some women may experience a sense of increased saliva production due to difficulty in swallowing saliva during the period of nausea and vomiting in early pregnancy.[266] A few women do experience excessive salivation (ptyalism). This uncommon disorder begins as early as 2 to 3 weeks and ceases with delivery. The excessive salivation seems to occur primarily during the day.[65] The

TABLE 9–2
Summary of Alterations in the Gastrointestinal System During Pregnancy

ORGAN	ALTERATION	SIGNIFICANCE
Mouth and pharynx	Gingivitis	Friable gum tissue with bleeding and discomfort with chewing
		Increased periodontal disease
	Epulis formation	Bleeding and interference with chewing
	Increased saliva production	Annoyance
Esophagus	Decreased lower esophageal sphincter pressure and tone	Increased risk of heartburn
	Widening of hiatus with decreased tone	Increased risk of hiatal hernia
Stomach	Decreased tone and mobility with delayed gastric emptying time	Increased risk of gastroesophageal reflux and vomiting
		Increased risk of vomiting and aspiration with use of sedatives or anesthetics
	Incompetence of pyloric sphincter	Reflux of alkaline biliary material into stomach
	Decreased gastric acidity and histamine output	Improvement of peptic ulcer symptoms
Small and large intestines	Decreased intestinal tone and motility with prolonged transit time	Facilitate absorption of nutrients such as iron and calcium
		Increased water absorption in large intestine with tendency toward constipation
		Increased flatulence
	Increased height of duodenal villi	Increased absorption of calcium, amino acids, other substances
	Altered enzymatic transport across villi	Increased absorption of specific vitamins and other nutrients
	Displacement of cecum and appendix by uterus	Complicate diagnosis of appendicitis
Gallbladder	Decreased tone and motility	Alteration in measures of gallbladder function
		Increased risk of gallstones
Liver	Altered position	Mask mild to moderate hepatomegaly
	Altered production of liver enzymes, plasma proteins, bilirubin, and serum lipids	Some liver function tests less useful in evaluating liver disorders
		Early signs of liver dysfunction may be missed
	Presence of spider angiomata and palmar erythema	Alter early recognition of liver dysfunction
		Discomfort due to itching

pathogenesis of ptyalism is unknown, although improvement with ganglion-blocking drugs has been reported.[266]

Esophagus

Lower esophageal sphincter (LES) tone decreases primarily because of the smooth muscle relaxant activity of progesterone. The LES is a pressure barrier between the stomach and the esophagus, acting as a protective mechanism to prevent or minimize gastroesophageal reflux. LES pressure decreases during pregnancy with the magnitude of pressure change positively correlated with gestational length.[75, 139] At the beginning of the second trimester basal LES tone is unchanged, but a marked decrease in the normal rise in LES pressure in response to stimulation with a protein meal has been reported.[65, 78, 172] This suggests an inhibitory effect and may signal the loss of an important protective response, i.e., the ability to modify LES pressure in response to increased intragastric pressure so that reflux is prevented.[65]

Changes in the LES in pregnancy are similar to changes seen during the ovarian or menstrual cycle and in women on oral contraceptives, supporting the theory of a hormonal cause for this alteration. An increased incidence of acid reflux with heartburn, which is associated with decreased LES pressure, is seen in nonpregnant women during the luteal phase of the ovarian cycle when progesterone levels are highest.[235] Women on sequential oral contraceptives (as compared with agents that contain only an estrogen component) demonstrate similar decreases in

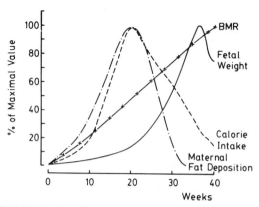

FIGURE 9–2. Changes in maternal caloric intake, maternal fat deposition, fetal weight, and basal metabolic rate (BMR) during pregnancy (values are expressed as percent of maximal change). (From Rosso, P. (1987). Regulation of food intake during pregnancy and lactation. *Ann NY Acad Sci, 499,* 191.)

LES pressure during the progesterone phase of the cycle. After delivery or discontinuance of oral contraceptives, LES function returns to normal.[18, 65, 78, 182, 236] Alterations in LES tone and pressure are major etiologic factors in the development of heartburn during pregnancy.

Other changes in the esophagus during pregnancy include an increase in secondary peristalsis and nonpropulsive peristalsis and increased incidence of hiatal hernia. Flattening of the hemidiaphragm causes a loss of the normal acute esophageal-gastric angle, which may also lead to reflux.[65]

Stomach

The stomach of the pregnant woman tends to be hypotonic with decreased motility due to actions of progesterone. Gastrointestinal motility is decreased with prolonged small intestinal transit time. Incompetence of the pyloric sphincter may result in alkaline reflux of duodenal contents into the stomach.[65]

The effects of pregnancy on gastric emptying time, particularly during early pregnancy, are unclear with contradictory findings due in part to use of different measurement techniques and study methodologies.[62, 66, 77, 139, 178, 267] As gestation advances, decreased smooth muscle tone and motility secondary to progesterone production tend to delay emptying time with a tendency toward reverse peristalsis. Gastric emptying time is especially prolonged following inges-

tion of solid foods. In this situation reduction in acid production and pepsin secretion due to progesterone action may slow digestion even further.[66]

The effect of pregnancy on gastric acid secretion is unclear. In several recent studies gastric volume was not increased nor was gastric pH decreased during early pregnancy.[139, 178, 241, 267] In general there seems to be a tendency for decreased gastric acidity in pregnancy, with small but statistically significant decreases in both basal and histamine-stimulated acid output.[65, 75, 170, 238] Production of hydrochloric acid is reduced during the first 6 months of pregnancy with a gradual return to nonpregnant levels during the third trimester.[75]

Secretion of pepsin parallels changes in gastric acid output.[75] Decreased gastric acidity is thought to result from hormonal influences (particularly estrogen) and increased levels of placental histaminase.[65, 201] Placental histaminase is thought to mediate acid and pepsin secretion by reducing parietal cell responsiveness to endogenous histamine.[65] Gastrin levels are normal during most of pregnancy with marked increases late in the third trimester, at delivery, and immediately post delivery.[197] The additional gastrin is probably of placental origin.[58]

Small and Large Intestines

The action of progesterone on smooth muscles also decreases intestinal tone and motility. The decreased motility observed in pregnancy may not necessarily be a direct effect of progesterone but rather due to inhibition by plasma motilin.[56] Decreased gastrointestinal tone leads to prolonged intestinal transit time, especially during the second and third trimesters.[139] Alterations in transit time increase with advancing gestation, paralleling the increase in progesterone.

Intestinal transit times during stages of pregnancy have been compared with phases of the ovarian cycle in nonpregnant women.[139, 241] Intestinal motility was altered and transit time prolonged during late pregnancy and the luteal phase of the ovarian cycle when progesterone secretion is elevated. The prolonged transit time in late pregnancy was due to an increase in small bowel transit secondary to inhibition of smooth muscle contraction and not to delayed gastric emptying time.[139, 207]

The height of the duodenal villi increases

(hypertrophies), which in turn increases their absorptive capacity.[147] This change along with the influences of progesterone on intestinal transit time increases the absorptive capacity for calcium, lysine, valine, glycine, proline, glucose, sodium, chloride, and water during pregnancy.[236] Progesterone also increases lactase and maltase activity. Absorption of other nutrients including niacin, riboflavin, and vitamin B_6 is reduced, perhaps owing to the influence of progesterone on enzymatic transport mechanisms.[236] Duodenal absorption of iron increases in late pregnancy, probably in response to depletion of maternal circulating iron stores by the placenta and fetus.[25] As a result of the decreased intestinal motility, nutrients and fluids tend to remain in the intestinal lumen for longer periods of time. This may facilitate absorption of nutrients such as iron and calcium.[24, 75]

Progesterone also enhances colonic absorption of calcium, sodium, and water and increases net secretion of potassium.[236] The reduced motility and prolonged transit time in the large intestine increase water absorption in the colon. Stools are smaller with a lower water content, which contributes to development of constipation during pregnancy. Increased flatulence may also occur owing to decreased motility along with compression of the bowel by the growing uterus. The appendix and cecum are displaced superiorly by the growing uterus so that by term the appendix tends to be located along the right costal margin.

Pancreas

The pancreas contains estrogen receptors, which in the rich estrogen environment of pregnancy may increase the risk of pancreatitis.[236] Serum amylase and lipase decrease during the first trimester. The significance of this change is unclear. Changes in the islet cells associated with increased production and secretion of insulin are discussed in Chapter 13.

Gallbladder

Muscle tone and motility of the gallbladder decrease during pregnancy probably owing to the effects of progesterone on smooth musculature. As a result, gallbladder volume is increased and emptying rate decreased.[40, 139] Most measures of gallbladder function are altered during pregnancy, especially after 14 weeks. Prior to 14 weeks decreased emptying time but normal residual and fasting volumes have been reported.[40] The residual gallbladder volume after emptying is nearly twice as large in the pregnant woman (2.5 to 16 ml versus 1.5 to 9 ml), with similar findings for fasting volume (15 to 30 ml versus 4 to 24 ml).[40] Increased fasting volume may be due to decreased water absorption by the mucosa of the gallbladder. This change results from reduced activity of the sodium pump in the mucosal epithelium secondary to estrogens.[30, 190] As a result, bile is more dilute with a decreased ability to solubilize cholesterol. The sequestered cholesterol may precipitate to form crystals and stones, increasing the tendency to form cholesterol-based gallstones in the second and third trimesters.[126, 190] Alterations in gallbladder tone also lead to a tendency to retain bile salts, which can lead to pruritus.

Liver

During pregnancy the liver is displaced superiorly, posteriorly, and anteriorly by the enlarging uterus. These changes may mask mild to moderate hepatomegaly during pregnancy. Hepatic blood flow per se is not significantly altered in spite of marked changes in total blood volume and cardiac output. This is because much of the increased cardiac output is sent to the intervillous spaces of the placenta. As a result there is a net decrease of 28 to 35% in the proportion of cardiac output delivered to the liver.[75, 131] Histologically only minor nonspecific changes such as increased fat and glycogen storage and variations in cell size have been reported.[113] The size of the liver does not increase.

Liver production of plasma proteins, bilirubin, serum enzymes, and serum lipids is altered. These changes arise primarily from estrogen and in some cases from hemodilution. Changes in liver products during pregnancy and their significance are summarized in Table 9–3. Although liver function is not impaired during pregnancy, most of the changes in liver function tests are in the same direction as seen in individuals with liver disorders. Some liver function tests are less useful in evaluating liver disorders during pregnancy; other tests such as aspartate aminotransferase (AST, serum glutamic oxaloacetic transaminase [SGOT]), alanine aminotransferase (ALT, serum glutamic-pyruvic

TABLE 9–3
Liver Function Tests in Normal Pregnancy and Post Partum

SUBSTANCE	PREGNANCY EFFECT	TRIMESTER OF MAXIMUM CHANGE	RETURN TO NONPREGNANT LEVEL
Albumin	↓ 20%	2	?
Gamma globulin	N to sl ↓	3	?
Alpha globulin	↑	3	?
Beta globulin	↑	3	?
Total protein	↓ 20%	2	?
Fibrinogen	↑ 50%	2	2 weeks
Ceruloplasmin	↑	3	?
Transferrin	↑	3	?
Bilirubin	N to sl ↑	3	?
BSP	N to sl ↑	3	Soon after delivery
AST (SGOT) and ALT (SGPT) in pregnancy	N	—	—
AST (SGOT) and ALT (SGPT) in labor	↑	In labor	By 2–3 weeks
GGTP	↑	3	?
Alkaline phosphatase	2–4 fold ↑	3	Usually by 3 weeks
Lactic dehydrogenase in pregnancy	sl ↑	3	?
Lactic dehydrogenase in labor	↑	In labor	By 2–3 weeks
Cholesterol	1½–2 fold ↑	2–3	Significant decrease within 24 hours

BSP, sulfobromophthalein; AST (previously referred to as SGOT), serum aspartate aminotransferase; ALT (previously referred to as SGPT), serum alanine aminotransferase; GGTP, serum gamma-glutamyl transpeptidase; N, normal; sl, slight.
Modified from Monheit, A. G., Cousins, L., & Resnik, R. (1980). The puerperium: Anatomic and physiologic adjustments. *Clin Obstet Gynecol, 23,* 973.

transaminase [SGPT]), and bilirubin are still reliable.

Spider angiomata and palmar erythema (common findings in many liver disorders) are seen in 70 to 90% of pregnant women owing to estrogens. These findings tend to develop during the 2nd month and disappear or diminish following delivery. Increases in the size of previously existing spider angiomata may also be noted.

Weight Gain During Pregnancy

Weight gain during pregnancy reflects increased maternal stores as well as those of the developing fetus and placenta. Approximately 62% of the gain is water, 30% fat, and 8% protein. About 25% of the total gain is attributable to the fetus, 11% to the placenta and amniotic fluid, and the remainder to the mother.[111] Optimal weight gain during pregnancy varies with maternal prepregnancy weight; greater weight gain is most important in women who are underweight, and a lower total weight gain is preferable for women who are obese. Results from the Collaborative Perinatal Project suggest that weight gains associated with lowest perinatal mortality rates were 30 lb in underweight women, 20 lb in normal

weight women, and 16 lb in overweight women (Fig. 9–3).[94]

The usual recommendation for weight gain in pregnancy in healthy women has been a gain of 24 to 28 lb (11 to 13 kg). Recently the Institute of Medicine issued new guidelines for weight gain and the pattern of gain based on prepregnancy weight for height (Table 9–4).[114] According to these guidelines the recommended gain for normal weight women is 25 to 35 lb (11.5 to 16 kg), with less for overweight women and more for underweight women, especially during the second and third trimesters. The target weight gain for twin pregnancies is 35 to 45 lb (16 to 20.5 kg).[114] The recommended pattern for normal weight women is approximately 8 lb during the first trimester followed by about 1 lb (0.4 kg)/week for the remainder of gestation, with higher gains (0.5 kg/wk) in underweight and less (0.3 kg) in overweight women.[94, 114]

This pattern results in the addition of approximately 8 lb of fat stores, acquired primarily during the first half of pregnancy. Weight gained during the second half of pregnancy goes toward growth of the fetus and maternal supportive tissues. Marked or persistent deviations from these patterns, including gains of less than 1 lb (0.5 kg)/month

TABLE 9–3
Liver Function Tests in Normal Pregnancy and Post Partum *Continued*

BASIS AND IMPLICATION

Due to hemodilution and increased catabolism; leads to decreased protein for binding and increased concentrations of
  free substances
Transfer of IgG to fetus in third trimester for protection of fetus from infection
Facilitate transport of lipids and carbohydrates to the placenta; transport of increased maternal thyroid hormones
Facilitate transport of lipids, carbohydrates, and iron to placenta; also transport of hormones
Due primarily to fall in albumin; decreases protein-bound substances, increases concentrations of free protein for
  transport across the placenta
Protection against excessive blood loss at delivery by facilitation clotting
Involved in the transport of most of the body copper needed by mother, fetus, and placenta
Involved in the binding and transport of iron to meet increased maternal and fetal needs
May be a slight increase in bilirubin clearance due to maternal clearance of bilirubin from fetus
Increased removal associated with decreased albumin; alterations may reflect the mild cholestasis seen in pregnancy
Do not change during pregnancy, so these enzymes can be used as indicators of liver or other organ damage during
  pregnancy. These enzymes increase during labor and delivery, perhaps reflecting the effects of the mechanical forces
  of labor
Enzyme important in synthesis of amino acids for maternal and fetal use
Much of increase is probably due to increased production by the placenta rather than the maternal liver
Enzyme associated with tissue injury that catalyzes lactic acid to pyruvic acid; increases further during labor, perhaps
  reflecting the effects of the mechanical forces of labor
Essential precursor for many lipid substances; needed for alterations in lipid metabolism and increased demands for lipids
  during pregnancy including production of estrogens and progesterone by the placenta

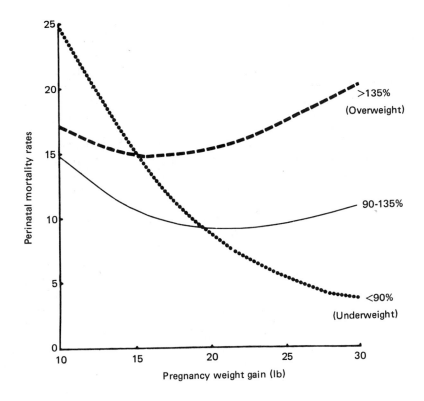

FIGURE 9–3. The relationship between weight gain in pregnancy and perinatal mortality. (From Naeye, R.L. (1979). Weight gain and the outcome in pregnancy. *Am J Obstet Gynecol, 135,* 3.

TABLE 9–4
Recommended Total Weight Gain Ranges for Pregnant Women by Prepregnant Body Mass Index (BMI)

WEIGHT-FOR-HEIGHT CATEGORY	RECOMMENDED TOTAL WEIGHT GAIN*	
	kg	lb
Low (BMI† <19.8)	12.5–18	28–40
Normal (BMI = 19.8–26.0)	11.5–16	25–35
High‡ (BMI >26.0–29.0)	7.0–11.5	15–25

*Young adolescents and black women should strive for gains at the upper end of the recommended range. Short women (<157 cm or 62 in) should strive for gains at the lower end of the range.
†BMI is calculated using metric units (BMI = kg/m² x 100).
‡The recommended target weight gain for obese women (BMI >29.0) is at least 6.0 kg (15 lb).
From Institute of Medicine. (1990). *Nutrition during pregnancy* (p. 10). Washington, DC: National Academy Press.

in an obese woman or less than 2 lb (1 kg)/ month in a woman of normal weight, necessitate evaluation and counseling.[114] Women whose weight gain significantly exceeds these limits or deviates from the expected pattern also require similar interventions. For example, if a woman gains 30 lb in the first 20 weeks of pregnancy, she has added approximately 25 lb of fat to her stores (and additional fat is often difficult to lose post partum). This woman will still need to gain approximately 20 lb during the second half of pregnancy to ensure adequate growth of the fetus and her own tissues.[301]

The Intrapartum Period

Gastric motility is further decreased during labor. This decrease is probably influenced by fear and pain as well as effects of narcotic administration.[58] The reduced competency of the LES along with decreased gastric motility and increased gastric acidity delay gastric emptying time and increase the risk of aspiration with sedatives or anesthesia.

Labor is accompanied by delays in gastric emptying times that differ (although perhaps not to the extent that was reported in earlier studies) from both third trimester and nonpregnant values.[70, 178, 255] The combination of gastric volumes greater than 25 ml and pH less than 2.5 is thought to increase the risk of chemical aspiration pneumonitis.[47] Roberts and Shirley reported that gastric volume at term tended to remain over 25 ml regardless of the time of the last meal or interval between the last meal and labor onset and 55% of woman had a gastric pH less than 2.5.[195] Narcotics also delay gastric emptying and increase the risk of aspiration if used in conjunction with general anesthesia.[174] Reduced use of general anesthesia for delivery has reduced the numbers of women at risk for intrapartum aspiration. However, any use

of general anesthesia with a pregnant woman whether for delivery or nonobstetric surgery requires careful monitoring and use of interventions to prevent vomiting and aspiration. Pharmacologic interventions include prophylactic use of antacids or H_2 receptor agonists.[47]

During labor alkaline phosphatase levels, which double during pregnancy, increase further. Serum aminotransferases (AST and ALT), which do not change in pregnancy, and lactic dehydrogenase increase up to twice normal values.[262] These enzymes are associated with tissue injury and may reflect the stresses of labor on the mother and placenta.

The Postpartum Period

During the postpartum period the anatomic and physiologic changes within the gastrointestinal and hepatic systems gradually return to their prepregnant state. Delivery results in an average weight loss of 12 lb.[191] Only 40% of postpartum women are reported to have further weight loss during the 1st week, with the remainder having no change or gaining weight.[210] Weight gain is most often seen during the first 3 days. The increased adrenocortical hormone and arginine vasopressin (ADH) activity associated with the stress of labor tends to lead to water and sodium retention that may prevent weight loss or lead to a gain. After 4 days most women begin to show some loss, especially if they are lactating. Drugs used to suppress lactation plus alterations in energy utilization may alter losses in nonlactating women.[42, 210] Most women lose weight steadily over the first 3 to 6 months, with the greatest loss in the first 3 months. Weight loss occurs sooner and to a greater degree in women of lower parity, age, and prepregnant weight.[42, 210] Lactation may facilitate postpartum weight and body fat loss as maternal tissue stores are catabolized to use as energy for milk production.[42]

LES pressure and tone return to normal levels by 6 weeks post partum.[238] Gallbladder contractility is enhanced post partum, enabling the previously atonic gallbladder to empty a larger proportion of its volume and expel microgallstones that developed during pregnancy.[236] Expulsion of these stones can lead to a gallstone pancreatitis.

Most of the liver enzymes return to nonpregnant levels shortly after delivery. Lipids and associated enzymes tend to reach normal levels by about 10 days.[166] AST, ALT, and lactic dehydrogenase, which rose during the intrapartum period, reach nonpregnant levels by 2 to 3 weeks. Alkaline phosphatase decreases after delivery but may remain elevated for up to 6 weeks.[262]

Gastrointestinal muscle tone and motility are decreased during the intrapartum and early postpartum periods. Decreased gastric motility along with relaxation of the abdominal musculature can result in gaseous distention 2 to 3 days post partum. Decreased intestinal motility can lead to postpartum ileus and constipation. Bowel movements usually resume 2 to 3 days post birth with resumption of normal bowel patterns by 8 to 14 days.

CLINICAL IMPLICATIONS FOR THE PREGNANT WOMAN AND HER FETUS

The normal alterations in gastrointestinal function and structure in the pregnant woman are responsible for some of the more common discomforts of pregnancy including heartburn and constipation. Alterations in the anatomic position of structures such as the appendix and liver and in concentrations of liver enzymes and other substances, as well as concerns about potential hazards with the use of radiographic contrast studies on the fetus, can lead to difficulty in assessing and diagnosing pathologic processes that arise. This section examines the basis for development of these problems and reviews the effect of pregnancy on selected chronic disorders such as peptic ulcer disease and cholelithiasis.

Nutritional Requirements of Pregnancy

The physical and physiologic demands of pregnancy on the mother along with fetal needs for nutrients significantly increase nutritional requirements during pregnancy. Nutrient needs are also altered post partum and during lactation (see Chapter 4). During pregnancy an additional 300 calories are needed during the second and third trimesters to meet energy and growth demands of the mother and fetus and to conserve protein for cell growth. Protein requirements increase to 60 g to provide nitrogen for maternal, fetal, and placental tissue synthesis and growth.[172a] Sources of protein should contain all the essential amino acids.

Maternal plasma levels of most vitamins and minerals gradually decline during gestation. This decline is probably due primarily to the effects of hemodilution rather than to greater fetal and maternal demands.[199a] Little is known about the effects of pregnancy on metabolism of most vitamins and minerals with the exception of vitamin D (see Chapter 14) and iron (see Chapter 5). Recommended dietary allowances (RDA) for childbearing-age, pregnant, and lactating women are available from the Food and Nutrition Board of the National Academy of Science.[172a]

Daily dietary allowances (RDA) for many vitamins are also increased, including vitamin E (10 mg), vitamin C (70 mg), thiamin (1.5 mg), riboflavin (1.6 mg), niacin (17 mg), vitamin B_6 (2.2 mg), and vitamin B_{12} (2.2 μg).[114, 172a] Vitamin E is essential during pregnancy for tissue growth and integrity of cell and red blood cell membranes. Vitamin C increases iron absorption and is needed for collagen formation and tissue formation and integrity. Thiamin, niacin, riboflavin, and vitamins B_6 and B_{12} serve as coenzymes for protein and energy metabolism, which are increased in the pregnant woman.[258] Requirements for minerals and other vitamins are discussed in Chapters 5 (iron and folate), 14 (calcium, phosphorus, magnesium, and vitamin D), and 16 (iodine). Excessive intake or marked deficiency of specific vitamins and minerals has been reported to be associated with adverse pregnancy outcome, although the number of observations is limited.[28a] The reader is referred to texts on nutrition during pregnancy for further discussion of nutritional assessment and requirements.[114, 199a, 258]

The Institute of Medicine recommends

that pregnant women with balanced diets do not need routine multivitamin/mineral supplementation, except for iron (see Chapter 5).[114] Additional multivitamin/mineral supplementation or supplementation of specific nutrients may be needed by women whose diet is inadequate or who have a multiple pregnancy, smoke, or are alcohol or drug abusers.

Fetal Nutritional Needs

The fetus is dependent on the mother and placenta for transfer of nutrients essential for normal fetal growth and development. (Fetal growth and alterations are discussed in the section on fetal development of the gastrointestinal system.) Nutritional needs of the fetus are met by three mechanisms depending on the stage of development. Prior to implantation, the blastocyst absorbs nutrients from its surrounding tissues and from fluids within the fallopian tube and uterus. Between implantation and placental development nutrients are absorbed via a sinusoidal space between maternal and fetal tissues. With formation of the placenta, nutrients are transferred across this structure from mother to fetus via a variety of mechanisms (see Chapter 2). The energy needs of the fetus near term are met through carbohydrates (80%) and amino acids (20%).[199a] Fat is not used as an energy source by the fetus owing to immaturity of fat metabolism (see Chapter 13). The major fetal energy source is glucose from the mother; free fatty acids are an alternative source as well as substrate for lipid formation.[193]

Amino acids are actively transported from mother to fetus, and imbalances in maternal plasma amino acid concentrations can result in excessive fetal concentrations and subsequent damage. For example, women with phenylketonuria (PKU) may be taken off a low phenylalanine diet by adolescence when the brain has matured to a point that the risk of mental retardation and neurologic damage is reduced. As a result, these women have elevated levels of phenylalanine in their blood. If they become pregnant, phenylalanine crosses the placenta and can damage the fetus. Infants born to mothers with elevated phenylalanine levels (regardless of whether the infant has PKU or not) are at high risk for intrauterine growth retardation, mental retardation, microcephaly, and congenital heart disease.[22, 155] Since fetal damage

often occurs before the woman is aware that she is pregnant, women with PKU are advised to return to a low phenylalanine diet prior to conception and remain on the diet during pregnancy (to keep maternal blood levels of phenylalanine <600 μmol/L).[155] These women require much support since the diet is restrictive and expensive and includes an unappealing low-phenylalanine protein supplement.

Fetal needs for most vitamins and minerals can be met if maternal intakes follow recommended dietary allowances.[114, 172a, 193] Lipid-soluble vitamins (A, D, E, and K) cross the placenta more readily than water soluble vitamins and with increasing ease with advancing gestation.[124] The vitamins most often associated with deficiencies during pregnancy are folate and B_6 (see Chapter 5).[193]

Calcium and phosphorus are actively transported across the placenta, which allows accumulation of calcium and calcification of the fetal skeleton (see Chapter 14). Trace elements such as zinc, copper, chromium, iodine, magnesium, and manganese are needed by the fetus. Maternal dietary intake of these elements is usually sufficient. Iron supplementation is recommended to prevent maternal iron deficiency anemia (see Chapter 5).

Heartburn

Heartburn (reflux esophagitis with retrosternal burning) arises from reflux of gastric acids into the lower esophagus. Heartburn has been reported in 30 to 70% of women at some time during pregnancy and daily in up to 25% in the latter half of pregnancy.[263] Heartburn usually begins during the second trimester, intensifies with advancing gestation, and disappears following delivery. Interventions are summarized in Table 9–5.

The pathogenesis of heartburn during pregnancy is multifactorial. The major etiologic factor is relaxation of the LES along with alterations in pressure gradients across the sphincter. In nonpregnant women LES tone increases in response to elevations in intragastric pressure as a protective mechanism to prevent or minimize reflux. Alterations in LES tone during pregnancy eliminate or significantly reduce this protective mechanism.[58] Pregnant women without heartburn tend to have LES pressures sufficient to maintain the normal pressure gradient across the gastroesophageal junction; whereas women

TABLE 9–5
**Nursing Recommendations for Common Problems During Pregnancy Related to the
Gastrointestinal System**

PROBLEM	NURSING RECOMMENDATIONS
Heartburn	Eat small, frequent meals.
	Eat bland foods.
	Avoid fatty or spicy foods.
	Avoid foods that reduce lower esophageal sphincter pressure (i.e., alcohol, chocolate, caffeine).
	Avoid lying down for 1 hour following meals.
	Chew gum.
	Sleep with torso elevated.
	Avoid lying flat or bending.
	Use antacids (aluminum and magnesium hydroxide combination is best since aluminum tends to cause diarrhea and magnesium constipation) after meals and at bedtime.
	Avoid use of antacids containing phosphorus (alter calcium-phosphorus balance, leading to leg cramps) or sodium (increase water retention).
	Monitor for side effects of chronic antacid use (alteration in muscle tone and deep tendon reflexes, electrolyte imbalance).
	Recognize potential effects of chronic antacid use on malabsorption of K, P, Ca, and drugs such as anticoagulants, salicylates, vitamin E.[79]
Constipation	Drink fluids.
	Drink hot or cold liquids (especially on an empty stomach).
	Eat high-fiber/bulk laxative foods such as fruits and raw vegetables.
	Encourage regular light exercise during pregnancy.
	Early ambulation post partum.
	Use stool softeners.
	Avoid use of mineral oil in pregnancy (absorbs fat-soluble vitamins including vitamin K).
	Monitor for side effects if laxatives are precribed (fluid accumulation, sodium retention and edema, cramping).
	Monitor for drug interactions if laxatives are prescribed (decreased serum K with diuretics, decreased effectiveness of anticoagulants and salicylates).[79]
Hemorrhoids	Use sitz bath.
	Eat bulk foods.
	Use astringents such as witch hazel (Tucks), lemon juice, or vinegar.
	Prevent constipation and straining (see above).
Nausea and Vomiting	Small, frequent high-carbohydrate meals and snacks (others suggest high-protein meals).
	Avoid strong odors, fatty or spicy foods, cold liquids.
	Consume dry crackers or toast prior to arising.
	Lie down when first experiencing symptoms.
	Teach relaxation techniques.
	Avoid factors and situations that precipitate symptoms.
	Monitor for side effects of pharmacologic agents (see text).

with heartburn do not demonstrate this compensatory mechanism.[151, 201] Pregnant women regardless of whether or not they experience heartburn have increased nonpropulsive esophageal motor activity with decreased wave amplitude and slower spread of peristaltic waves, with a 50% reduction in secondary peristalsis.[172, 201, 234] These findings are suggestive of reflux and are more prominent in women who experience symptoms of heartburn during pregnancy.[234]

Pressure from the growing uterus increases intragastric pressure and along with flattening of the hemidiaphragm causes anatomic distortion of the stomach and decreases the acuteness of the angle at the gastroesophageal junction.[58, 65] Elevations in intragastric and intraabdominal pressure are intensified by multiple pregnancy, hydramnios, obesity, lithotomy position, bending over, or application of fundal pressure.[58] The tendency toward reflux is increased by the decreased gastrointestinal tone and relaxation of the cardiac sphincter.[75] As a result of gastric stasis and pyloric incompetence, the refluxed material may be alkaline as well as acidic. Prolonged reflux of normal pH or alkaline duodenal material can lead to esophagitis.[65]

The frequency of hiatal hernia is also increased, occurring in 15 to 20% of pregnant women primarily after 7 to 8 months' gestation. This disorder arises from alterations in muscle tone and pressure with widening of the hiatus. Interventions are similar to those for heartburn (Table 9–5).

Constipation

In a retrospective study of bowel function in 1600 pregnant women, Levy and coworkers reported that 55% experienced no change, 35% experienced increased frequency, and 11% decreased frequency.[150] Others have reported that constipation occurs in approximately 30% of pregnant women.[90]

Constipation probably arises primarily from alterations in water transport and reabsorption in the large intestine. The smooth muscle relaxant effects of progesterone decrease intestinal motility and prolong transit time, which increases electrolyte and subsequently water absorption in the large intestine. Other predisposing factors are compression of the rectosigmoid area by the enlarging uterus and changes in dietary habits and activity and exercise patterns. Interventions for women with constipation are summarized in Table 9–5.

Hemorrhoids

Hemorrhoids arise more frequently during pregnancy and are aggravated by constipation. Factors that contribute to hemorrhoid formation during pregnancy include poor support for hemorrhoidal veins in the anorectal area, lack of valves in these vessels leading to reversal in the direction of blood flow and stasis, gravity, pressure of the expanding uterus, increased venous pressure in the pelvic veins, venous congestion and engorgement, and enlargement of the hemorrhoidal veins. Interventions for women with hemorrhoids are summarized in Table 9–5.

Nausea and Vomiting

Nausea with or without vomiting is a self-limiting event experienced by 50 to 88% of pregnant women in Western cultures.[76, 116, 160, 201] Nausea and vomiting in pregnancy (NVP) is seen most frequently between 5 and 12 weeks, but may occur as early as 2 to 3 weeks after the last menstrual period. NVP is experienced most prominently prior to rising in the morning and ingestion of food (hence the term "morning sickness"), but some women experience symptoms in the afternoon, evening, or throughout the day. NVP usually disappears by 10 to 12 weeks but persists to 14 weeks in 40% of women, 16 weeks in less than 20%, and 20 weeks in less than 10%.[201]

The exact cause of nausea and vomiting is unknown. Many theories have been proposed

TABLE 9–6
Proposed Causes for the Nausea and Vomiting of Pregnancy

Mechanical
  Congestion, inflammation, distention, displacement, or other conditions of the uterus or cervix
Endocrinologic
  Sensitivity to secretions of the corpus luteum of pregnancy
    Excessive estrogen or progesterone
  Excessive deportation of chorionic villi into maternal circulation
  Suppression of ovarian secretions
    Progesterone or estrogen deficiency
  Excessive hCG
  Relative adrenocortical insufficiency
  Secondary hypopituitarism
Allergic
  Allergy to secretions of corpus luteum or to placental proteins
  Allergy to antigens from father
  Isoagglutinins
  Histamine "poisoning"
Metabolic
  Intestinal toxins
  Gastric hypofunction
  Biochemical alterations such as decreased osmolality
  Carbohydrate deficiency
  Pyridoxine deficiency
  Alterations in serum lipids and lipoproteins
Genetic
Psychosomatic
  Unconscious repudiation or aversion to femininity, pregnancy, coitus, or the father of baby
  Ambivalence about the pregnancy
  Identity with the feminine role
  Self-punishment
  General psychological immaturity
  Hysteria
  Strong mother-dependence

Adapted from Niebyl, J. R. & Maxwell, K. D. (1982). Treatment of the nausea and vomiting of pregnancy. In J. R. Niebyl (Ed.), *Drug use in pregnancy* (pp. 9–19). Philadelphia: Lea & Febiger.

(Table 9–6), but none have substantial research support. The major schools of thought are that this phenomenon is physiologic-hormonal or psychogenic in origin.

The most common hormonal theories are related to rapidly increasing and high levels of estrogen and human chorionic gonadotropin (hCG). Support for a hormonal theory comes from studies documenting nausea in women on estrogen medications or combined oral contraceptive pills, the high correlation between women who experience nausea with both oral contraceptive use and pregnancy, and parallels between hCG patterns and the timing of symptom appearance and disappearance in NVP.[116, 160] Studies examining the correlation of hCG levels with symptom appearance and intensity in individual women have produced conflicting results.

Perhaps a combination of endocrine factors leads to NVP, and individual women may have different sensitivities to these substances. NVP has been associated with favorable pregnancy outcomes such as decreased miscarriage rates and perinatal mortality, although some researchers have found no differences.[76, 117, 118, 225, 249, 250]

Support for a psychological (although not necessarily pathologic) component to NVP comes from placebo studies in which over half of women with NVP experience dramatic improvement in their symptoms when given a placebo.[160] Some proponents of the psychogenic origin suggest that it may be related to emotional factors with ambivalence or unconscious rejection of the pregnancy. Few studies have been done to document this theory, and many available reports are case studies of women in psychotherapy. Studies that have been done on more representative populations present conflicting findings. Several investigators reported that women without NVP were more prone to psychological difficulties during pregnancy and post partum, felt less close to their mothers, and were less likely to breast-feed.[233, 257] Wolkind and Zajicek suggested that NVP is associated with greater identification with the maternal role.[257]

Interventions for women experiencing NVP are summarized in Table 9–5. Pharmacologic treatment may occasionally be required owing to severity of symptoms or interference with the woman's responsibilities. Use of pharmacologic agents is fraught with potential problems, since NVP and thus the administration of any drugs occur during the period of embryonic organogenesis. Until the early 1980s, Bendectin, which combined an antihistamine and pyridoxine, was commonly used to treat NVP. Litigation over the relationship of Bendectin and congenital defects resulted in removal of this drug from the market, although a causal relationship has never been documented.[63, 109, 160] Medications currently used include antihistamines (meclizine) and phenothiazines (Phenergan, Compazine, or Thorazine).[49, 160] As with any drug during pregnancy, these agents must be used with caution.

Hyperemesis gravidarum, an uncommon disorder seen in 1 to 2% of pregnant women, is intractable vomiting associated with alterations in nutritional status, dehydration, electrolyte imbalance, significant weight loss (>5%), ketosis, and acetonuria.[160] These women often require hospitalization.

Food and Fluid Intake in Labor

Food and beverage intake during labor is controversial. For many years most hospitals in the United States have not allowed women in active labor to eat or consume beverages other than ice chips or clear liquids. These prohibitions developed during the period when general anesthesia was commonly utilized during the second stage of labor with concerns regarding the risk of aspiration should the anesthetized woman vomit. These constraints are currently being questioned, with some practitioners advocating more liberal food and fluid policies during labor.[43, 44, 70]

Individuals opposed to a more liberal food and fluid policy in labor argue that, although rare, aspiration has devastating consequences and can still occur with an endotracheal tube in place or use of regional anesthesia. Pregnant women are at particular risk for pulmonary aspiration because of the delayed gastric emptying time, increased levels of gastrin (resulting in increased gastric volume and lowered gastric pH), and decreased LES tone (which allows stomach contents in an unconscious woman to passively move into the pharynx and into the lungs).[70] Antacids have been used to increase gastric pH and reduce the risk of damage to lung tissue should aspiration occur.[44, 47]

Those advocating relaxation of current restrictions note that (1) general anesthesia has been replaced by regional anesthesia; (2) the incidence of maternal mortality from aspiration of stomach contents in normal labor is rare; (3) gastric emptying may not be significantly altered in normal women who have not received narcotics; (4) use of intravenous fluid administration is increased; and (5) prolonged fasting during labor has physiologic and psychological effects.[43, 44] General anesthesia, if used, is safer than in the past as the result of changes in anesthetic agents and administrative techniques, such as the use of endotracheal tubes, which prevent aspiration of vomitus. Potential physiologic effects of fasting include increased ketones and fatty acids with decreased alanine, glucose, and insulin. Psychological effects include increased anxiety and stress.[44] Use of intravenous fluids has been associated with maternal and infant fluid and electrolyte problems (see Chapter 8). Low-risk women who deliver at home or in alternative settings and women in other cultures often consume food and beverages during labor with few complications.

Effects of Altered Maternal Nutrition

Weight gain during pregnancy is associated with improved infant growth and development. Most studies demonstrate a correlation between maternal weight gain and birth weight even when other variables that influence birth weight (gestational age, maternal height, birth order) are held constant. The relationship between weight gain during pregnancy and perinatal mortality varies with maternal prepregnancy weight and pregnancy weight gain (Fig. 9–3). Specific effects of altered maternal nutrition are listed in Table 9–7.

Undernutrition and Pregnancy

Women who are underweight have a higher incidence of pregnancy loss and small for gestational age (SGA) infants. These woman may fail to gain adequate weight during pregnancy, further increasing the risk of fetal growth retardation and maternal nutritional anemia and malnutrition. Kristal and Rush reviewed studies examining the effects of maternal undernutrition on fetal growth and concluded the following: (1) limitations in the overall amount of maternal food intake from either starvation or iatrogenic limitations lead to a consistent depression in birth weight (up to 550 g); (2) relief of acute undernutrition up to the beginning of the third trimester is associated with return of birth weight to previous levels; (3) results of supplementation studies with pregnant females at risk nutritionally (in developed and developing countries) are consistent, with increases in birth weight of 40 to 60 g; (4) there seems to be a limit in the amount of supplementation a given individual can tolerate and to the effect of these supplements; and (5) a consistent depression in birth weight is seen with use of high-density protein supplements in which more than 20% of calories supplied are protein.[134] High-density protein diets have also been associated with an increased incidence of prematurity and neonatal morbidity in some populations.[94, 259] These findings, and those from animal studies, suggest that restrictions in caloric intake have the most marked effects on fetal growth; protein deprivation may lead to alterations in later development.[94]

Maternal Obesity and Pregnancy

Maternal obesity is associated with an increased incidence of macrosomia, large for gestational age (LGA) infants, and perinatal

TABLE 9–7
Expected Consequences of Inadequate Nutrition in Women During a Reproductive Cycle

PREPREGNANCY	DEFICIENCY NUTRITION	
	Pregnancy	Postpregnancy
Low stature	Small placenta	Body weight deficient
Low body weight	Reduced duration of pregnancy	Poor lactation performance
Low adiposity	Risk of LBW, IUGR	Prolonged amenorrhea
Low lean body mass	Inadequate weight gain	Longer birth interval
Delayed menarche	Low deposition of fat	Nutrient deficiencies (Fe, Ca, Zn,
Low nutrient reserves (Ca, Fe, I, Zn,	Inadequate volume expansion	vitamin A, etc.)
vitamin A, etc.)	Inadequate hormonal response	Low discretionary activity
Low discretionary activity	Nutrient deficiencies (Fe, I, Zn,	Poorer prepregnancy nutrition
	vitamin A, folate, vitamin D, etc.)	
	Perinatal complications	
	Lower discretionary activity	
	RELATIVE EXCESS OF ENERGY (OBESITY)	
Poor health (higher prevalence of	Increased adiposity	Worsening of diabetes and health
hypertension, diabetes)	Risk of marcrosomic baby	consequences
Low discretionary activity	Perinatal complications	Low discretionary activity
	Risk of toxemia	
	Risk of diabetes	

IUGR, intrauterine growth retardation; LBW, low birth weight.
Adapted from Viteri, F.E., Schumacher, L., & Silliman, K. (1989). Maternal malnutrition and the fetus. *Semin Perinatol, 13,* 236.

mortality.[171] These LGA infants are usually larger than expected in weight but not length owing to increased deposition of adipose tissue.[94] The woman's excess adipose tissue reserves may be supplying some of the fuel needed for fetal growth. Cord blood triglyceride levels are elevated, reflecting enhanced fat synthesis by fetal liver and adipose tissue.[259] Since obese women tend to have LGA infants even when pregnancy weight gain is inadequate, it is difficult to determine if their infants are growth retarded.

Many of the metabolic changes seen in pregnancy (such as increased circulating insulin, insulin resistance) are similar to those seen in obese women.[94] Obese women tend to have more problems during delivery owing to increased fetal growth and macrosomia. The incidence of pregnancy-induced and chronic hypertension, thrombophlebitis, varicose veins, and diabetes mellitus is increased in obese woman.[259] These women may gain excess weight during pregnancy, which can be difficult to lose later.

Caloric restriction during pregnancy is generally not recommended because of potential adverse effects on the fetus. Severe caloric restriction can significantly reduce the availability of glucose (the major fetal energy substrate) and increase maternal serum amino acid and ketone levels. Maternal ketosis has been associated with poor neurologic development in offspring, although some studies have not confirmed this finding.[94] Caloric restriction may be indicated in the obese pregnant woman to maintain a weight gain that has been associated with an improved pregnancy outcome. Few studies have been reported, although carefully supervised restriction of carbohydrates leading to weight loss in one group of obese pregnant women did not result in elevation of serum or urinary ketones.[36]

Pregnancy and Gastrointestinal Disorders

The physiologic and anatomic changes of the gastrointestinal tract during pregnancy have varying effects on disorders of this system. The course of some disorders is minimally affected by pregnancy. For example, one of the more common gastrointestinal disorders occurring in the childbearing population, inflammatory bowel disease (IBD), which includes ulcerative colitis and Crohn's disease, is not adversely affected by pregnancy. If these disorders are quiescent at the time of pregnancy, outcome for both mother and fetus is normal. If the disorder is active at the time of conception there is a higher rate of spontaneous abortion. The risk of exacerbation of ulcerative colitis during pregnancy is similar to the risk in nonpregnant women. Risk of exacerbation is highest during the first trimester and post partum. Maternal immune tolerance or increases in corticosteroids during the second and third trimesters may have a protective effect.[33, 263]

Pregnancy and Acute Appendicitis

Appendicitis is two to three times more frequent in pregnant women.[178] The specific reason for this is unclear but may relate to delayed diagnosis. Diagnosis of appendicitis during pregnancy is complicated by anatomic and physiologic changes of pregnancy. Since the appendix is displaced upward and laterally to the right, the point of maximal tenderness may be as high as the right costal margin. By the second trimester, the appendix lies above the iliac crest. As a result, radiated pain associated with suppuration or perforation tends to be felt at the point where the appendix abuts the peritoneum, which becomes higher and more lateral as gestation progresses.[219a]

Guarding and rebound tenderness are often milder and less well localized, since the uterus is between the appendix and the parietal peritoneum.[24] Nausea is common in the first trimester, and changes in white blood cell (WBC) counts associated with appendicitis are similar to changes in pregnancy. Suidan and Young suggest that one way to differentiate uterine from appendiceal pain is to turn the woman onto her left side while pressing the point of maximal tenderness. If the pain decreases or ceases, the pain is probably uterine in origin; if not, appendicitis should be suspected.[219a]

Pregnancy in Women with Peptic Ulcer

Peptic ulcers in women are seen more often after menopause and are uncommon during the childbearing years.[83] In women of childbearing age estrogen may protect the gastric lining from ulcer formation, perhaps by increasing gastric and duodenal mucus secretion.[83, 236] Pregnancy has a further protective effect on the development and progression of peptic ulcer.[201] Up to 80% of women with peptic ulcers improve during pregnancy, although 50% experience recurrence of symptoms by 3 months post partum and almost all by 2 years after delivery.[57, 65, 201] Women with persistent symptoms during pregnancy usually have other problems such as hyperemesis gravidarum and albuminuria.[201]

The basis for improvement during pregnancy is still conjectural but thought to lie in the normal changes in gastric acidity that accompany pregnancy. Production of hydrochloric acid (both basal and in response to histamine) decreases in pregnancy, with a tendency to return to normal levels of acidity in the third trimester.[170] Decreased gastric acidity, increased serum histaminase (thought to mediate acid and pepsin secretion by reducing parietal cell responsiveness to endogenous histamine), and increased mucin secretion (which protects the gastric mucosa from the effects of acid) may all contribute to improvement in peptic ulcer symptoms.[65]

Gastrin levels are normal during most of pregnancy, with marked increases late in the third trimester, at delivery, and immediately post delivery.[197] Thus by late pregnancy gastric pH and pepsin output have returned to nonpregnant levels. It is at this time that peptic ulcer symptoms tend to recur.[57, 65, 201]

Cholelithiasis and Pregnancy

The incidence of cholelithiasis, which is more common in women, is increased further during pregnancy and in women taking oral contraceptive agents.[190, 209] A hormonal basis for the risk of gallstones in women has been suggested, since the increased risk is seen primarily between menarche and menopause. Elevated estrogen and progesterone levels during pregnancy may further aggravate the tendency toward cholelithiasis.

There are three forms of gallstones: cholesterol, pigment, and mixed (composed primarily of calcium bilirubinate). The increased incidence of gallstones associated with females and pregnancy is seen primarily with cholesterol gallstones. The process of gallstone development involves (1) production of bile supersaturated with cholesterol; (2) nucleation and crystallization of cholesterol, which initiates stone formation; and (3) growth of the stone.[77] Supersaturation of bile with cholesterol occurs when cholesterol secretion is high or bile acid secretion is low (concentrated bile is more likely to hold cho-

lesterol in solution). Cholesterol production increases during pregnancy. In addition, estrogens and progesterone increase biliary cholesterol saturation and estrogen decreases the proportion of chenodeoxycholic acid. This acid is a component of the bile acid pool that dissolves gallstones by decreasing biliary cholesterol secretion. Altered gallbladder tone during pregnancy, with incomplete emptying and increased fasting and residual volumes, may also increase the risk of gallstone formation by sequestering cholesterol crystals.[77, 190]

CHOLECYSTITIS AND PANCREATITIS

Acute cholecystitis is rare during pregnancy. Severe abdominal pain is more likely due to appendicitis, which occurs four to five times more often during pregnancy than does cholecystitis.[190] The incidence of pancreatitis increases in pregnancy and post partum. Pancreatitis in pregnancy is usually associated with gallstone formation and develops when gallstones traveling down the common bile duct collide with and traumatize the ampulla.[34, 77, 201]

Pregnancy and Liver Disease

Liver disease in pregnancy can be divided into two categories: (1) disorders seen only in pregnancy and associated with jaundice and abnormal liver tests (intrahepatic cholestasis, pregnancy-induced hypertension, and fatty liver of pregnancy) and (2) liver diseases that may occur during and are affected by pregnancy.[51] The most common liver disease seen in pregnant woman is hepatitis (see Chapter 10). Major effects of pregnancy on liver disorders are potential difficulties with diagnosis, increased fetal risk, and, especially with hepatitis B, transmission to the fetus. Alterations in some liver function tests during pregnancy can make diagnosis of liver disorders more difficult, although jaundice is always abnormal.[33]

Intrahepatic cholestasis is characterized by severe pruritus and jaundice. The risk of postpartum hemorrhage, gallstones, fetal distress, stillbirth, and prematurity is increased. The basis for this disorder is unclear, although it may have a genetic basis or hormonal cause, since a similar syndrome occurs with oral contraceptive use.[77] Fatty liver of pregnancy is a rare disorder of unknown cause that usually appears during the third trimester, often in association with pregnancy-induced hypertension (PIH), with high fetal and maternal mortality rates. Delivery of the infant results in rapid improvement.[77, 109]

Liver function and histologic changes are associated with PIH. The degree of liver abnormality tends to parallel the severity of PIH.[109] About 10% of women with PIH develop an additional group of findings (HELLP syndrome) that includes hemolysis (H), elevated serum levels of liver enzymes, especially SGOT and SGPT (EL), and low platelets (LP) (see Chapters 6 and 10).[77, 109]

Drug Absorption and Metabolism

The gastrointestinal and hepatic changes during pregnancy can alter absorption of drugs from the gastrointestinal system and biotransformation of drugs by the liver. Absorption of oral medications is influenced by gastric acidity, presence of bile acids or mucus, and intestinal transit time. During pregnancy there is decreased gastric acid (hydrochloric acid [HCl]) secretion, delayed gastric emptying time, and decreased intestinal motility. These factors tend to initially delay, then prolong absorption of oral medications. For example, decreased gastric pH decreases the rate at which weak acids (such as aspirin) are absorbed and increases absorption of weak bases (such as narcotic analgesics).[69]

Clearance and metabolism of drugs by the liver during pregnancy may be influenced by the increased steroid hormones. Some liver enzymatic processes may be slowed, delaying drug metabolism and degradation. Although hepatic blood flow is unaltered during pregnancy, the 35% decrease in the proportion of cardiac output delivered to the liver may slow clearance of drugs from the blood. In general, slowly metabolized drugs such as phenytoin (Dilantin) that are cleared primarily by the liver tend to be cleared more slowly in pregnancy owing to decreased enzymatic activity and the net decrease in liver blood flow. This may also increase the length of time potentially teratogenic intermediary metabolites remain in circulation.[69]

Drug distribution is also altered. The distribution of drugs within the body depends on many factors including the degree to which a drug is bound to plasma proteins (see Chapter 5) or body tissues. Tissue binding is a mechanism by which a drug is removed from circulation and stored in tissue such as hair, bone, teeth, and adipose tissue.

This mechanism can result in storage of significant quantities of a drug, since tissue storage sites may need to be saturated before there is sufficient free drug to be effective at receptor sites. When the drug is discontinued, tissue deposits may give up their stores slowly, resulting in persistent drug effects. Since lipid-soluble drugs are stored in adipose tissue, increased adipose tissue during pregnancy can lead to a slight decrease in the amount of free lipid-soluble drugs such as sedatives and hypnotics and persistence of drug effects ("hangover") after the drug has been discontinued.

SUMMARY

The pregnant woman experiences changes in gastrointestinal and hepatic function that enhance absorption of nutrients for herself and her fetus. These changes are associated with common experiences and discomforts of pregnancy such as heartburn, constipation, nausea, and vomiting. A major component of interconceptual and prenatal care is nutritional assessment and counseling. Maternal nutrition before and during pregnancy is critical for optimal growth and development of the fetus and prevention of maternal, fetal, and neonatal disorders. Table 9–8 summarizes recommendations for clinical practice related to the gastrointestinal system and perinatal nutrition.

DEVELOPMENT OF THE GASTROINTESTINAL AND HEPATIC SYSTEMS IN THE FETUS

The development of the gastrointestinal system can be divided into three phases. During early gestation anatomic development gives rise to the organs and other structures of the system. During mid- to late gestation functional components such as hormones, enzymes, and reflexes develop. Finally, after birth coordinated function develops with interaction of hormones and enzymes in the digestion of food substances along with maturation of suck-swallow coordination.[242] Characteristics and timing of common GI anomalies are listed in Table 9–9.

TABLE 9–8
Summary of Recommendations for Clinical Practice Related to Changes in the Gastrointestinal System:
Pregnant Woman

Counsel women regarding changes in appetite, food preferences, and intake during pregnancy (p. 380).

Counsel women regarding gingival changes during pregnancy and the need for dental hygiene (pp. 380–383).

Counsel women regarding common problems (heartburn, nausea and vomiting, constipation, hemorrhoids) associated with the gastrointestinal system (pp. 383, 385, 390–393, Table 9–2).

Implement interventions to reduce or relieve heartburn, nausea and vomiting, constipation, and hemorrhoids (pp. 390–393, Table 9–5).

Counsel women regarding the presence of spider angiomata and palmar erythema (p. 386).

Recognize usual parameters for liver function tests and patterns of change during pregnancy and the postpartum period (pp. 385–389, Table 9–3).

Know expected parameters for weight gain during pregnancy and monitor maternal patterns (pp. 386–388, Table 9–4).

Know recommended nutritional requirements during pregnancy (pp. 389–390).

Assess maternal nutritional status and provide nutritional counseling (pp. 389–390, 394–395).

Recognize potential maternal and fetal/neonatal complications associated with undernutrition and obesity during pregnancy (pp. 394–395, Table 9–7).

Counsel women regarding risk of caloric restriction during pregnancy (p. 395).

Recognize factors that increase the risk of vomiting and aspiration during labor and delivery (pp. 386, 393).

Monitor fluid, food, and caloric intake during labor and early postpartum period (pp. 386, 393–394).

Monitor women during labor for vomiting (pp. 386, 393–394).

Counsel women regarding weight loss patterns following delivery (pp. 388–389).

Recommend postpartal exercises to enhance weight loss and return of abdominal and perineal tone (pp. 388–389).

Evaluate gastrointestinal function post partum (pp. 388–389).

Recognize factors that increase the risk of gallstone formation and recognize signs of cholelithiasis (pp. 385, 389, 396).

Counsel women with gastrointestinal and liver problems regarding the impact of their disorder on pregnancy and of pregnancy on the disorder (pp. 395–397).

Recognize signs of appendicitis during pregnancy (p. 395).

Recognize signs of liver disorders that are unique to pregnancy (pp. 396–397).

Recognize the effects of altered gastrointestinal and hepatic function on drug absorption, distribution, and metabolism (p. 397).

Monitor and evaluate maternal responses to drugs (p. 397).

Know and counsel women regarding side effects of drugs and potential toxicity to mother, fetus, and neonate (pp. 393, 397).

Monitor for persistence of drug effects with the use of lipid-soluble agents (p. 397).

Counsel women with phenylketonuria and other metabolic disorders regarding risks to their infant and need for dietary restrictions (p. 390).

Provide support for women who must use special diets during pregnancy (p. 390).

Know fetal nutritional requirements and counsel women regarding fetal needs and growth patterns (pp. 390, 394, 406–408).

Know factors that can alter fetal growth and monitor fetal growth patterns (pp. 390, 394–395, 406–408, Table 9–7 and Figure 9–10).

Counsel women regarding changes in gastrointestinal function with use of oral contraceptive agents (pp. 383–384, 392, 396).

Page numbers in parentheses following each recommendation refer to pages in the text where rationale for that intervention is discussed.

Anatomic Development

Anatomic development of the gastrointestinal system begins during the 4th week with partitioning of the yolk sac into intra- and extraembryonic portions. Initially the cranial portion of the GI system develops concurrently with the respiratory system (see Chapter 7). The epithelium of the trachea, the bronchi, and the lungs and digestive tract arise from the primitive gut, a derivation of the yolk sac. The GI system develops in a cranial to caudal direction. The yolk sac arises at 8 days and by the 4th week has divided into two parts. The extraembryonic or secondary yolk sac provides for nutrition of the embryo, prior to development of the mature placenta, then is assimilated into the umbilical cord by 3 to 4 months. The intraembryonic portion is incorporated into the embryo as the primitive gut (Fig. 9–4).

The primitive gut is initially closed at both ends by membranes. The cranial (buccopharyngeal) membrane is reabsorbed during the 3rd week, and the caudal (cloacal) membrane during the 9th week. The midgut remains temporarily connected to the yolk sac by the vitelline duct. Development of the primitive gut and its derivatives can be divided into four sections: pharyngeal gut, foregut, midgut, and hindgut.[167]

Development of the Pharyngeal Gut

The pharyngeal gut extends from the buccopharyngeal membrane to the tracheobronchial diverticulum, forming the pharynx and its derivative, lower respiratory tract, and

TABLE 9–9
Incidence, Time of Occurrence, and Associated Defects of Various Gastrointestinal Anomalies

ANOMALY	INCIDENCE (Per Live Births)	FETAL AGE AT WHICH DEFECT OCCURS	PRESENCE OF HYDRAMNIOS	ASSOCIATED DEFECTS
Diaphragmatic hernia	1:4000	8th–10th week of fetal life	>75%	Lung hypoplasia, malrotation of bowel, patent ductus arteriosus (PDA), coarctation of aorta, neurologic malformations
Tracheoesophageal fistula and esophageal atresias	1:3000 1:4000	4th–5th week of fetal life	>60%	Encourage in more than 50% of patients and include GI, skeletal, and cardiac defects
Duodenal atresia	1:10,000– 1:40,000	8th–10th week of fetal life	Approx. 50%	Down syndrome, GI malformations, congenital heart disease
Jejunoileal atresia	1:330– 1:1500	During fetal life after embryogenesis (after 12th week of gestation)	35% jejunal 10–15% ileal	Infrequent, but may be associated with volvulus, malrotation, and meconium peritonitis
Colonic atresia	1:5000– 1:20,000	Vascular accidents in gestation	Rare	Occur in 30–40% and are associated with abdominal wall defects, vesicointestinal fistulae, and jejunal atresias
Anorectal anomalies	1:5000– 1:15,000	5th–8th week of fetal life	Rare	May be familial-associated anomalies in 30–70% and include cardiac, GI, and vertebral anomalies
Omphalocele	1:3000– 1:10,000	8th–11th week of fetal life	Common, but incidence unknown	Occur in 60%. Cardiac defects 15–20%. Tetralogy of Fallot, associated with specific syndromes, Beckwith's and trisomy D, E, and 21
Gastroschisis	1:6000	? 9th–11th week of fetal life	Incidence unknown	Foreshortened gut, intestinal atresias 15%; cardiac defects <10%
Duplications of GI tract	1:100– 1:4000	4th–6th week of fetal life	Unknown	Most common in ileum and esophagus
Meckel's diverticulum	1:150– 1:100	5th–7th week of fetal life	Rare	Usually occurs as isolated defect

From Sunshine, P. (1990). Fetal gastrointestinal physiology. In R.D. Eden & F.H. Boehm (Eds.), *Assessment and care of the fetus* (p. 99). Norwalk, CT: Appleton & Lange.

upper esophagus (Fig. 9–5). The pharyngeal area develops from bands of mesenchymal tissue (branchial or pharyngeal arches) separated by deep clefts (branchial or pharyngeal clefts) on the exterior of the embryo. A series of indentations (pharyngeal pouches) appear on the lateral walls of the pharyngeal gut and penetrate into the surrounding mesenchyme but do not communicate with the external clefts.[204] The pharyngeal arches form the muscular and skeletal components of the pharyngeal area, aortic arch, and nerve networks; mandible; dorsal portion of the maxillary process; hyoid bone; thyroid bone; laryngeal cartilage; and their associated vascular and nerve supplies. The pharyngeal pouches form the eustachian tube, tonsils, thymus, parathyroid, and part of the thyroid.[167, 204]

Development of the Foregut and Common Anomalies

The foregut extends from the tracheobronchial diverticulum to the upper part of the duodenum. Structures formed from the foregut (lower esophagus, stomach, liver, upper portion of the duodenum to the entry of the common bile duct, liver, biliary tree, and pancreas) are all supplied by the celiac artery.[167]

ESOPHAGUS

During the 4th week the tracheobronchial diverticulum appears along the ventral wall of the foregut, dividing the foregut into the ventral respiratory primordium and dorsal esophagus (Fig. 9–6A). The esophagus is initially short, but quickly elongates with ascent of the pharynx and cranial growth. The

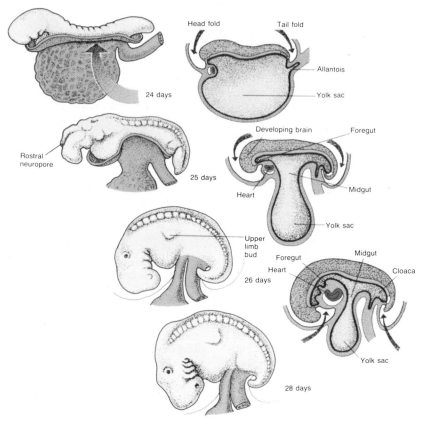

FIGURE 9–4. Development of the primitive gut and folding of the embryo from 24 to 28 days. (From Moore, K.L. (1988). *Essentials of human embryology* (p. 29). Philadelphia: BC Decker.)

rapidly growing endothelium temporarily obliterates the esophageal lumen, with recanalization of the lumen by 8 weeks.

Incomplete division of the foregut into respiratory and digestive portions at 4 to 5 weeks leads to tracheoesophageal fistula with or without esophageal atresia (Fig. 9–6*B* and Table 9–9). This malformation probably

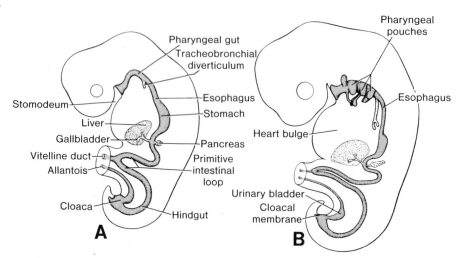

FIGURE 9–5. Formation of the gastrointestinal tract. *A*, 4th week. *B*, 5th week. (From Sadler, T.W. (1985). *Langman's medical embryology* (5th ed., p. 227). Baltimore: Williams & Wilkins.)

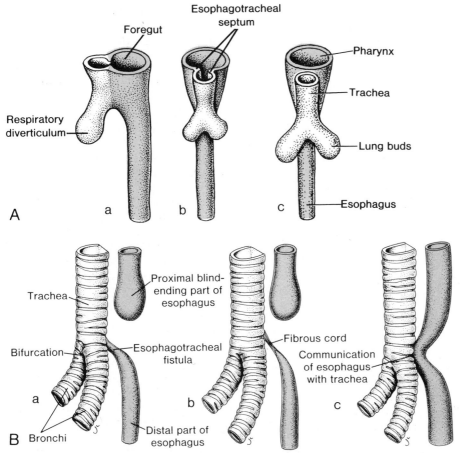

FIGURE 9–6. Development of the foregut and common anomalies. *A*, Partitioning of the foregut to form the respiratory diverticulum and esophagus during the 3rd (a) and 4th (b and c) weeks of development. *B*, Abnormalities of the esophagus. (a) Esophageal atresia and esophagotracheal fistula; (b) esophageal atresia with a connection between the distal part of the esophagus and trachea with a fibrous cord; (c) connection of the proximal and distal parts of the esophagus to the trachea by a narrow canal. (From Sadler, T.W. (1985). *Langman's medical embryology* (5th ed., pp. 226–227). Baltimore: Williams & Wilkins.)

arises from posterior deviation or unequal development of the septum developing between the primitive trachea and esophagus. Failure of the lumen to recanalize during the 8th week leads to esophageal stenosis or atresia.

STOMACH, DUODENUM, AND PANCREAS

The stomach arises during the 4th week as a spindle-shaped dilation in the caudal area of the foregut (see Fig. 9–5). The stomach dilates and enlarges, rotating around a longitudinal and an anteroposterior axis. During the longitudinal rotation the stomach rotates 90 degrees clockwise, ending with the left side facing anteriorly and the right posteriorly. The subsequent greater growth of the posterior wall in comparison with the anterior wall leads to the lesser and greater curvatures of the stomach. Initially the cephalic and caudal ends of the stomach are in midline. During the second or anteroposterior rotation of the stomach, the caudal (pyloric) portion moves right and upward, and the cephalic (cardiac) portion moves left and slightly downward.[167, 204] Embryonic anomalies of the stomach are rare, probably because stomach development is relatively simple. The most common stomach anomaly is pyloric stenosis, which is probably of genetic origin.

The duodenum arises from both the foregut and midgut. As the stomach rotates, the duodenum takes on a C-shaped form and rotates to the right. The lumen of the duodenum becomes obliterated by rapidly growing epithelium, with later recanalization. Failure to recanalize leads to duodenal atresia or stenosis.

The pancreas appears at about 5 weeks as dorsal and ventral buds in the duodenal area. As the duodenum rotates to the right and becomes C-shaped, the ventral pancreatic bud migrates toward the lower end of the common bile duct. The two pancreatic buds meet and fuse to form the final pancreas. In individuals with an annular pancreas, the ventral bud encircles the duodenum and may cause obstruction.[204]

LIVER AND GALLBLADDER

The liver appears during the 3rd week as a ventral thickening (liver bud or hepatic diverticulum) consisting of rapidly proliferating strands of cells at the distal end of the foregut. The hepatic diverticulum divides into a large cranial portion, which forms the hepatic parenchyma and main bile duct, and smaller caudal portion from which the gallbladder arises.[204] The liver initially grows into the septum transversum, a thick mesodermal plate separating the yolk sac and the thoracic cavity. The liver grows rapidly, eventually bulging into the caudal part of the abdominal cavity and stretching the mesoderm of the septum transversum until it becomes a thin membrane. The ventral portion of this membrane forms the falciform ligament; the dorsal portion forms the lesser omentum. The cranial portion of the septum transversum forms part of the diaphragm. Further growth of the liver promotes closure of the pleuroperitoneal canals (two large openings on either side of the foregut).

The lumina of the gallbladder, and the intra- and extrahepatic bile ducts are initially open, becoming temporarily obliterated by proliferating epithelium and later recanalizing. Biliary atresia can arise from failure of recanalization. With complete failure, the ducts are narrow nonfunctional fibrous cords. Failure of part of a bile duct to recanalize results in partial obstruction or atresia of that duct with distention of the gallbladder and hepatic duct proximal to the atretic area.[167, 204]

Development of the Midgut and Common Anomalies

Development of the midgut is characterized by rapid elongation of the gut and associated mesentery.[167] The midgut begins caudal to the liver and gives rise to the small intestine (except for the upper duodenum), cecum, appendix, ascending colon, and proximal portion of the transverse colon. These structures are supplied by the superior mesenteric artery.[167]

Initially midgut growth parallels the neural tube; however, the rapid growth of the midgut quickly exceeds that of the rest of the body, including the abdominal cavity. This occurs at a time when the liver and kidneys are relatively large, occupying much of the available space in the abdominal cavity. As a result, the midgut herniates into the extraembryonic coelom of the proximal umbilical cord. This physiologic herniation begins in the 6th week, with return of the midgut to the abdominal cavity during the 10th week.

Development of the midgut involves four steps: herniation, rotation, retraction, and fixation (Fig. 9–7).[167, 204] The midgut initially elongates and forms a U-shaped loop, which projects (herniates) into the proximal umbilical cord. The cranial limb of this loop grows rapidly, forming coils characteristic of the small intestine with little change in the caudal portion except for appearance of the cecal bud.

The midgut rotates a total of 270 degrees in a counterclockwise direction around an axis formed by the superior mesenteric artery. Midgut rotation occurs in two stages. The initial 90-degree rotation occurs while the midgut is in the umbilical cord; the second rotation (180 degrees) takes place as the gut returns to the abdomen at 10 weeks. The initial 90-degree rotation is in a counterclockwise direction. As a result, the cranial limb moves to the right and down and the caudal limb moves to the left and up (Fig. 9–7). The lumen of the intestines becomes temporarily obliterated by rapid epithelial growth with later recanalization.

Retraction or return of the midgut to the abdominal cavity occurs rapidly during the 10th week. The stimulus for this return is unknown, but it occurs as the rate of liver growth slows, the relative size of the kidneys decrease, and the abdominal cavity enlarges. As the midgut reenters the abdominal cavity, the gut rotates 180 degrees counterclockwise. The jejunum returns first and the area of the cecal bud last; the cecum and appendix end up near the liver in the right upper quadrant (Fig. 9–7).[204]

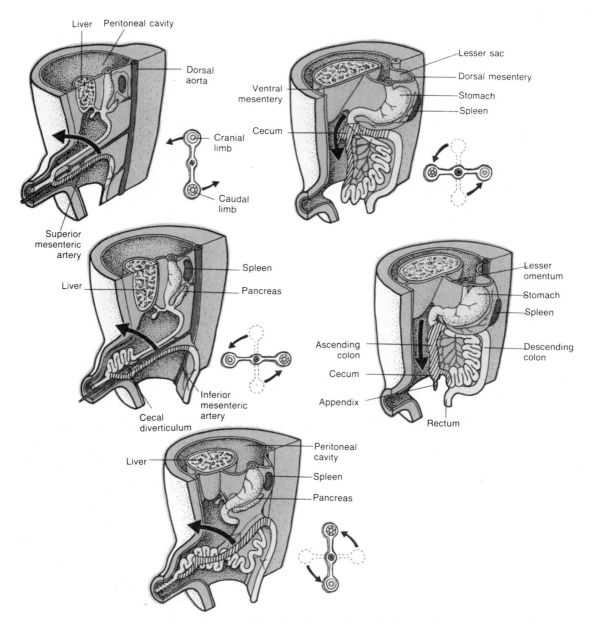

FIGURE 9–7. Development of the midgut from the 6th to 11th weeks (see text). Striped areas indicate future large intestine. (From Moore, K.L. (1988). *Essentials of human embryology* (p. 104). Philadelphia: BC Decker.)

The final step in development of the midgut is fixation. The cecum and appendix descend into the lower right quadrant. The proximal colon lengthens, becoming the ascending colon. The mesenteries are pressed against the posterior abdominal wall and fuse with the wall. In some regions of the midgut the mesenteries also fuse with the parietal peritoneum so that the ascending colon is rectoperitoneal.

CONGENITAL ANOMALIES OF THE MIDGUT

Congenital anomalies of the midgut include omphalocele, gastroschisis, umbilical hernia, intestinal stenosis and atresia, and malrotation (Table 9–9). Omphalocele arises at 8 to 11 weeks' gestation from a developmental arrest at the stage of herniation of the midgut into the umbilical cord with failure of all or part of the gut to return to the abdominal cavity. There is usually an associated defect in development of the abdominal musculature at the junction of the umbilical cord. This results from a primary failure in the formation of the lateral folds, which along with the cephalic and caudal folds form the abdominal wall.[167] The size of this defect influences the size of the omphalocele, which can range from a single loop of intestine to a mass containing most of the intestines and parts of the liver, bladder, and other organs. The omphalocele is covered by a thin, avascular membrane (derived from amnion), which may be ruptured. The umbilical cord generally inserts into the apex of the omphalocele sac.

In gastroschisis the extrusion of the intestines results from a defect in the anterior abdominal wall that probably arises between 9 and 11 weeks but may occur as early as 5 to 6 weeks.[154] This defect is usually to the right of, and not necessarily continuous with, the umbilical ring. Since there is usually no hernial sac present, the intestines extrude into the amniotic cavity and are embedded in a gelatinous mass. The embryonic basis for gastroschisis is not completely understood.[154] Omphalocele and gastroschisis have usually been considered to be different defects; some suggest that gastroschisis is an omphalocele that ruptured in utero and whose sac has been reabsorbed.[154, 176] Other theories regarding the cause of gastroschisis include: (1) failure of differentiation of the lateral fold somatopleure after the bowel has returned to the peritoneal cavity and the umbilical ring has formed; (2) failure in formation of the umbilical coelom with rupture of the amniotic membrane at the base of the umbilical cord; and (3) intrauterine rupture of an incarcerated hernia into the cord.[5, 96, 154]

An umbilical hernia is associated with an enlarged umbilical ring and failure of the rectus muscles to come together in midline. The protruding viscera are covered with normal skin.

Intestinal stenoses and atresias can arise as primary or secondary defects. Primary stenosis or atresia arises at 8 to 11 weeks, and perhaps as early as 6 to 7 weeks, as a result of partial or complete failure of the intestinal lumen to recanalize. Secondary stenosis or atresia is either due to fetal vascular accidents or infarction with interruption of blood supply to part of the intestines or secondary to twisting or inflammatory changes. Vascular accidents and infarction are common causes of jejunal and ileal atresias and probably occur after 12 weeks (Table 9–9).

Alterations in midgut development can also lead to malrotation. Three of the more common forms are nonrotation, mixed malrotation, and reverse rotation. With nonrotation the midgut rotates 90 degrees instead of 270 degrees, without the 180-degree rotation that normally occurs upon reentry of the gut into the abdominal cavity. As a result, the colon enters the abdomen first instead of last so that the colon ends up on the left and the small intestine on the right. This form of malrotation is sometimes referred to as left-sided colon. In mixed malrotation the midgut rotates only 180 degrees, so that the terminal ileum reenters first. The cecum is subpyloric and fixed to the abdominal wall, which may compress the duodenum. In reverse rotation the initial 90-degree rotation is clockwise instead of counterclockwise, resulting in placement of the transverse colon behind the duodenum. Malrotation increases the risk of volvulus, with twisting of the intestinal loops and abnormal fixation of the mesenteries resulting in excessive mobility of the bowel. This can lead to kinking of the bowel and blood vessels and necrosis.[167, 204]

Development of the Hindgut and Common Anomalies

Development of the hindgut and urogenital system is interrelated. The cloaca is the expanded terminal end of the gut and the hindgut ends at the cloacal membrane (Fig.

9–8). The hindgut gives rise to the distal transverse colon, descending and sigmoid colons, rectum, upper anal canal, bladder, and urethra, which are supplied by the inferior mesenteric artery.[167]

At 5 to 7 weeks the cloaca is divided into two parts by the urorectal septum, a wedge of downward-growing mesenchymal tissue. During 6 to 7 weeks the urorectal septum reaches and fuses with the cloacal membrane, forming the perineum. The area of fusion is the perineal body. The cloacal membrane has now been divided into two parts. The ventral urogenital membrane will be incorporated in the terminal portion of the urogenital system (see Chapters 1 and 8); the dorsal part becomes the anal membrane. A pit that develops in the anal membrane ruptures at 8 to 9 weeks, resulting in an open communication between the rectum and the body exterior. The lower portion of the anal canal develops around the site of the anal pit from ectodermal tissues.[204]

Imperforate anus and associated malformations arise from abnormal development of the urorectal septum. In the simplest form of imperforate anus, the anal membrane fails to rupture and the anal canal ends at the membrane. In more complex forms there may be a layer of connective tissue between the end of the rectum and the body surface. These forms can be caused by failure of the anal pit to develop or atresia of the end of the rectum. If the descent of the urorectal septum is arrested, the cloaca may remain, with abnormalities of the urogenital and lower GI systems.

Functional Development

Anatomically the fetal GI tract develops to the stage seen in the newborn by about 20 weeks.[145] Functional development begins during fetal life with development of diges-tive and liver enzyme systems and the absorptive surfaces of the intestine (Table 9–10). Although the placenta takes care of the nutrient needs of the fetus, function of the fetal GI tract is important in amniotic fluid homeostasis (see Chapter 2). Gut-regulating polypeptides appear by 6 to 16 weeks and act as local inducing agents regulating growth and development of the gut.[15, 17]

The intestinal villi begin to develop around 7 weeks and are present in the entire small intestine by 14 weeks, with well-developed villi and crypts seen by 19 weeks.[50] Intestinal motility and peristalsis develop gradually and mature during the third trimester.[50] Meconium begins to form at about 16 weeks.

Swallowing begins at 10 to 14 weeks, and by 16 weeks the fetus swallows 2 to 6 ml of amniotic fluid/day, increasing to 200 to 600 ml/day (average, 450 ml/day) by term.[98] Failure of the fetus to swallow amniotic fluid is associated with GI obstruction and polyhydramnios (see Chapter 2).

Most of the metabolic functions of the fetal liver are handles by the maternal liver. The fetal liver is primarily a hematopoietic organ until the latter part of gestation when bone marrow erythropoiesis and liver metabolic activity increase. Many liver enzyme systems are still immature at birth.[96]

Enzymes involved in protein digestion and absorption develop early in gestation and may be important in fetal life to prevent bowel obstruction by cellular debris.[12] Glucose from the mother is the major source of fetal energy (see Chapter 13). Disaccharidase enzymes are present by 9 to 10 weeks, increase rapidly after 20 weeks, and become very active after 27 to 28 weeks, except for lactase, which does not reach mature levels until 36 to 40 weeks.[8, 11, 89, 146, 220] Bile acids can be detected in the liver and gallbladder by 14 to 16 weeks and in the intestines by 22

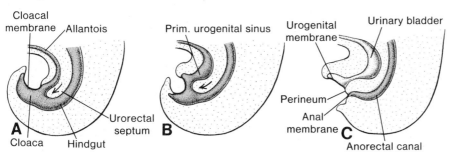

FIGURE 9–8. Development of the hindgut. (From Sadler, T.W. (1985). *Langman's medical embryology* (5th ed., p. 243). Baltimore: Williams & Wilkins.)

TABLE 9–10
Development of the Gastrointestinal Tract in the Fetus: First Appearance of Developmental Markers

ORGAN	SYSTEM MARKER	WEEKS GESTATION
Anatomic		
Esophagus	Superficial glands develop	20
	Squamous cells appear	28
Stomach	Gastric glands form	14
	Pylorus and fundus defined	14
Pancreas	Differentiation of exocrine and endocrine tissue	14
Liver	Lobules form	11
Small Intestine	Crypt and villi develop	14
	Lymph nodes appear	14
Colon	Diameter increases	20
	Villi appear	20
Functional		
Suck/swallow	Mouthing only	28
	Immature suck/swallow	33–36
Stomach	Gastric motility and secretion	20
Pancreas	Zymogen granules	20
Liver	Bile metabolism	11
	Bile secretion	22
Small Intestine	Active transport of amino acids	14
	Glucose transport	18
	Fatty acid absorption	24
Enzymes	α-glucosides	10
	Dipeptides	10
	Lactase	10
	Enterokinase	26

From Lebenthal, G. & Leung, Y.K. (1988). Feeding the premature and compromised infant: Gastrointestinal considerations. *Pediatr Clin North Am, 35*, 217.

weeks; however, the bile acid pool remains low even at term. The fetal jejunum and liver have decreased capacity for reabsorbing bile acids and poorer enterohepatic recirculation of taurine-conjugated bile acids, the major bile acid at birth.[96, 224] The appearance of gastrointestinal enzymes and concentrations of these substances at term are summarized in Table 9–11.

Fetal Growth

Fetal growth is dependent on factors such as genetic determinants, general maternal health and nutrition, availability of growth substrates, presence of fetal growth promoting hormones, and vascular support via changes in plasma volume during pregnancy and the maternal blood supply to the placenta. Availability of growth substrates depends on perfusion of the intervillous spaces and availability of glucose, amino acids, and fats in maternal blood (see Chapter 13). Fetal growth does not seem to be greatly dependent on hormones such as growth hormone, thyroid hormones, glucocorticoids, and sex steroids that are critical for postnatal growth. Hormones and peptide growth factors believed to be necessary for fetal growth include insulin, human placental lactogen (hPL), and insulin-like growth factor 1 (IGF1) or somatomedin. Insulin probably has a permissive rather than a direct effect on fetal growth by stimulating nutrient uptake and utilization.[81]

Initial growth is slow during the first 2 months (period of organ formation), then accelerates rapidly. Maximum growth rate is achieved at 4 to 6 months, then slows and remains constant to term.[93] At the cellular level growth occurs through hyperplasia (increased cell size) or hypertrophy (increased cell numbers). The human fetus undergoes primarily hyperplastic growth in early gestation (similar increases in deoxyribonucleic acid [DNA] and organ protein content), followed by a period of simultaneous hyperplasia and hypertrophy. From 34 to 35 weeks on, growth is predominantly hypertrophic.[93]

INTRAUTERINE GROWTH RETARDATION

Fetal growth retardation is defined as "the failure of a fetus to achieve its growth potential,"[115, p.360] which in practice is stated as measures of absolute (low birth weight) and relative (small for gestational age) size. Measures of relative size often vary (e.g., <3rd or <10th percentile or >2 standard deviations

TABLE 9–11
Neonatal Concentrations of Enzymes and Other Factors in Digestion and Absorption of Protein, Fat, and Carbohydrate

FACTOR	FIRST DETECTABLE (Weeks Gestation)	TERM NEONATE (% of Adult)
PROTEIN		
H$^+$	at birth	<30
Pepsin	16	<10
Trypsinogen	20	10–60
Chymotrypsinogen	20	10–60
Procarboxypeptidase	20	10–60
Enterokinase	26	10
Peptidases (brush border and cytosol)	<15	>100
Amino acid transport	?	>100
Macromolecular absorption	?	>100
FAT		
Lingual lipase	30	>100
Pancreatic lipase	20	5–10
Pancreatic colipase	?	?
Bile acids	22	50
Medium-chain triglyceride uptake	?	100
Long-chain triglyceride uptake	?	10–90
CARBOHYDRATE		
α-Amylases; pancreatic	22	0
α-Amylases; salivary	16	10
Lactase	10	>100
Sucrase-isomaltase	10	100
Glucoamylase	10	50–100
Monosaccharide absorption	11–19	<100 (?)

From Lebenthal, G., Lee, P.C., & Heitlinyer, L.A. (1983). Impact of development of the gastrointestinal tract on infant feeding. *J Pediatr, 102*, 1.

below mean), making comparisons between different centers difficult.[115] Fetal growth retardation is evaluated by serial ultrasonographic measurements.

Factors that cause alterations in growth, such as malnutrition during the period of hyperplasia, can decrease the rate of cell division and result in organs or a fetus that is smaller in size with fewer cells. This form of growth alteration is not reversible after the time when hyperplastic cell growth would normally have ceased. Malnutrition during the period of hypertrophy results in organs or a fetus that is smaller in size (due to reduction in cell size) but which has a normal number of cells. Hypertrophic growth alterations may be reversible with adequate nutrition. Since fetal tissues are undergoing hyperplastic growth throughout gestation, the fetus is especially vulnerable to irreversible changes at the cellular level.[237]

Factors altering fetal growth can be intrinsic or extrinsic (Fig. 9–9). Intrinsic factors are those within the fetus arising from chromosomal or genetic abnormalities or infectious agents that alter the normal process of cell division. Extrinsic factors include placen-

tal insufficiency and fetal malnutrition. Placental insufficiency due to maternal, fetal, or placental factors often results in caloric restriction to the fetus (inadequate glucose transported to meet fetal growth needs) and tends to occur later in gestation. Caloric restriction usually leads to an asymmetric growth failure in which brain growth is spared (Table 9–12). Fetal malnutrition due to maternal protein restriction (arising from maternal malnutrition or significantly protein reduced diets) results in symmetric fetal growth failure in which the brain is not spared (Table 9–12).[237]

Management of fetal growth retardation varies with the underlying cause. Strategies range from prepregnancy counseling and preventative interventions such as cessation of smoking and alcohol use, promotion of adequate nutrition, and early identification of and interventions for pathologic problems such as PIH to fetal therapies. Fetal therapies that have been proposed or implemented include providing nutrient supplements (glucose and amino acids) to the fetus via infusions into the maternal circulation, the amniotic fluid, or directly into the fetus (by

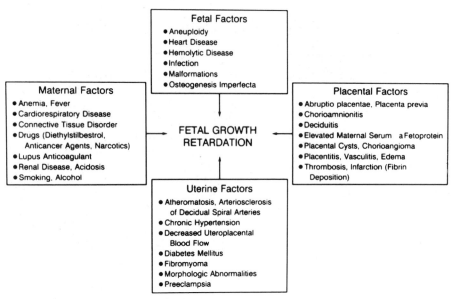

FIGURE 9–9.   Causes of growth retardation by compartment. (From Weiner, C.P. (1989). Pathogenesis, evaluation and potential treatments for severe, early onset growth retardation. *Semin Perinatol, 13,* 321.)

intraperitoneal catheter or cordocentesis) and improving uteroplacental blood flow (through maternal oxygen therapy, bed rest, and low-dose aspirin to reduce vasospasm).[93, 103, 115] The growth-retarded fetus and neonate are at risk for perinatal asphyxia, meconium aspiration, hypoglycemia, and other problems (Table 9–13).

NEONATAL PHYSIOLOGY

Gastrointestinal function in the neonate is characterized by functional, anatomic, and physiologic limitations, which are increased in the preterm infant. Provision of adequate nutritional support for growth and development is an ongoing challenge for nurses and other health care providers. As a result of the limitations in GI function, infants are at risk for dehydration, reflux, malabsorption, and electrolyte imbalance.

Transitional Events

Although the fetal GI system is involved with removal of amniotic fluid, digestive and ab-

TABLE 9–12
Effects of Intrinsic and Extrinsic Factors in Intrauterine Growth Failure

		EXTRINSIC	
	INTRINSIC	**Asymmetric (Placental Insufficiency)**	**Symmetric (Maternal Protein Restriction)**
Placenta			
Cellular growth	Normal	Reduced (20–30%)*	Reduced (20–30%)
Fetus			
Malformation	Multiple	Absent	Absent
Weight	Reduced	Reduced (20%)	Reduced (20%)
Head circumference	Variable	Normal	Reduced (20%)
Liver			
Cellular growth	—	Reduced (50%)	Reduced (20%)
Glycogen	—	Reduced (100%)	Reduced (20%)
Brain			
Cellular growth	—	Normal	Reduced (20%)

*Percentages are average figures and therefore only approximate.
Adapted from Van Thiel, D.H. & Schade, R.R. (1986). Pregnancy: Its physiologic course, nutrient cost and effects on gastrointestinal function. In V.K. Rustgi & J.N. Cooper (Eds.), *Gastrointestinal and hepatic complications in pregnancy* (p. 9). New York: Churchill Livingstone.

TABLE 9–13
Perinatal Adaptive Problems of Small for Gestational Age Infants

PROBLEM	PATHOGENESIS	PREVENTION
Perinatal asphyxia	↓ Placental reserve (insufficiency) ↓ Cardiac glycogen stores	Antepartum, intrapartum fetal heart rate monitoring
Meconium aspiration	Hypoxia/stress phenomenon	Oral-pharyngeal-tracheal suction
Fasting hypoglycemia	↓ Hepatic glycogen ↓ Gluconeogenesis	Early alimentation
Alimented hyperglycemia	"Starvation diabetes"	Avoid excessive carbohydrate loads
Polycythemia-hyperviscosity	Fetal hypoxia, ↑ erythropoietin Placental transfusion	Neonatal partial exchange transfusion
Temperature instability	↓ Adipose tissue ↑ Heat loss	Ensure neutral thermal environment
Pulmonary hemorrhage (rare)	Hypothermia, ↓ O_2, disseminated intravascular coagulation	Avoid cold stress, hypoxia
Immunodeficiency	"Malnutrition" effect	Unknown

Adapted from Kliegman, R.M. & Hulman, S.E. (1987). Intrauterine growth retardation: Determinants of aberrant fetal growth. In A.A. Fanaroff & R.J. Martin (Eds.), *Neonatal-perinatal medicine: Diseases of the fetus and infant* (p. 92). St. Louis: CV Mosby.

sorptive functions are performed by the placenta. With birth the infant's GI system, although still functionally immature, must assume responsibility for supplying the infant's energy, nutrient, and fluid needs. The intestinal mucosal barrier (glycocalyx) remains immature for 4 to 6 months. During this period antigens and other macromolecules can be transported across the intestinal epithelium into the systemic circulation, increasing the risk for both infection and the development of allergies.[13, 232] With maturation of the epithelium (gut closure) uptake of macromolecules decreases.[243] Gut closure and the development of intestinal flora are discussed in Chapter 10.

Maturation of Gastrointestinal Function

Postnatal development of GI function is influenced by the infant's genetic endowment, intrinsic timing mechanisms, initiation of feeding, composition of the diet, and hormonal regulatory mechanisms.[17, 50] Hormonal regulatory mechanisms have a critical role in mediating development of the gut after birth. Postnatal gut maturation is stimulated by increases in specific peptide hormones including enteroglucagon (growth of the intestinal mucosa), gastrin (growth of gastric mucosa and exocrine pancreas), motilin and neurotensin (development of gut motor activity), and gastric inhibitory peptide (initiation of enteroinsular axis and subsequent glucose tolerance).[154] A major stimulus for increases in these hormones is initiation of enteral feeding, which induces surges in plasma concentrations of the hormones listed above in both term and preterm infants. The

response is delayed in preterm infants.[153] Term infants with fetal distress have increased concentration of GI hormones, especially motilin, which may account for meconium passage. Increases in other hormones may cause redistribution of visceral blood flow in these infants.[17]

Term infants demonstrate marked changes in intermediary metabolites and secretions from the gut, pancreas, and pituitary within hours after birth. Marked differences are seen in hormonal secretion with human milk versus formula by 6 days, with a greater insulin response in formula-fed infants that lasts to at least 9 months. This suggests that early feeding practices may have prolonged and subtle effects on programming hormonal responses to feeding.[17] Similar changes in intermediary metabolites and secretions are not seen in infants who are being given nothing by mouth (NPO) or are on only parenteral or intravenous feedings.[17] These responses are delayed for several days in preterm infants on enteral feeding, reflecting immaturity of gut responses.[14, 15, 17, 152]

These surges seem to be triggered by small amounts of enteral feeding (as little as 0.5 to 1.0 cc/kg/hour or 12 cc/day) and are absent in unfed neonates.[15, 154] This finding has implications for gut maturation in infants fed from birth by total parenteral nutrition. Lucas and colleagues proposed the concept of "minimal enteral feeding,"[154] i.e., small amounts of enteral feeding may be important to induce surges in gut hormones and maturation of the gut rather than for nutritional reasons. Maturation of gut functions and enzymes is described in the next section and summarized in Tables 9–10 and 9–11.

Initiation of Enteral Feeding

In addition to stimulating release of hormones critical for maturation of gut function, enteral feedings are also important as a source of energy and fluid for the infant. A healthy infant can be breast-fed immediately after delivery. Colostrum is rich in antibodies, nonirritating, and easily swallowed, and it enhances meconium passage (see Chapter 4). Bottle-fed infants are usually fed within 6 to 8 hours, but can certainly be fed sooner, especially if at risk for hypoglycemia. The first feeding is usually sterile water. Animal studies suggest that D5W is as damaging to the lungs if aspirated as formula. D10W may be more damaging owing to its lower pH and higher glucose content.[180] Aspiration of regurgitated sterile water mixed with gastric acid can also be irritating to lung tissue. Early feeding and adequate fluid intake are associated with decreased bilirubin levels (see Chapter 15). Initiation of feeding in ill or preterm infants depends on infant health status, maturity, and ability to tolerate feeding.

Passage of Meconium

Passage of meconium is an essential step in initiation of intestinal function. Meconium consists of vernix caseosa, lanugo, squamous epithelial cells, occult blood, and bile and other intestinal secretions. Initially meconium is sterile, with bacteria appearing by 24 hours of age. Most infants pass meconium by 12 (69%) to 24 (94%) hours and almost all (99.8%) by 48 hours of age.[212] Although failure to pass meconium is a frequent sign of intestinal obstruction, infants with a high-level complete obstruction such as a duodenal atresia may occasionally pass meconium stool. Delayed passage of meconium is associated with elevated bilirubin levels, probably owing to continued action of the intestinal deconjugating enzyme, β-glucuronidase, with reabsorption of the unconjugated bilirubin and recirculation to the liver via the enterohepatic circulation (see Chapter 15).

Functional and Anatomic Limitations

Gastrointestinal function is still maturing at birth, especially in preterm infants, which increases the risk of malabsorption and malnutrition. Functional and anatomic maturation includes suck-swallow reflexes, esophageal motility, function of the lower esophageal sphincter, gastric emptying, intestinal motility, and development of absorptive surface area.

Sucking and Swallowing

Reflexes needed for food intake mature in the fetus during the third trimester. The swallow reflex is well developed by 28 to 30 weeks but easily exhausted. This reflex is complete by about 34 weeks. In newborns air enters the stomach via the nasal passages with swallowing. Since air can compete with milk for space in the infant's stomach and lead to regurgitation, burping is used to release this air. The gag reflex may be present by 18 weeks but is not complete until around 34 weeks.

Infants demonstrate nutritive and non-nutritive sucking. Nutritive sucking brings milk into the oral cavity by compression of the nipple and generation of negative pressure. Nonnutritive sucking occurs either with or without stimulation by a nipple, is more rapid than nutritive sucking, and has a regular burst-pause pattern.[98, 145] Fetuses at 13 to 15 weeks respond to oral stimulation with tongue protrusion, rooting, and sucking. Older fetuses have been noted on ultrasound to suck reflexively on their fingers.[7, 97] Nonnutritive sucking can be demonstrated in preterm infants by 26 weeks, and possibly earlier, but does not develop a rhythmic pattern until about 33 weeks.[97] The sucking reflex usually is not well enough developed for nutritive sucking until 32 to 34 weeks. Sucking can be affected by maternal medications and perinatal complications.

All components of sucking and swallowing are present by 28 weeks, but the infant is unable to coordinate these activities. Some suck-swallow synchrony is seen by 32 to 34 weeks; synchrony is complete by 36 to 38 weeks. Suck-swallow coordination has been demonstrated earlier for breast-feeding than for bottle feeding.[163a]

Gryboski and Walker described three stages in the development of suck-swallow patterns: (1) mouthing with no effective sucking; (2) an immature sucking pattern with short bursts of sucking not synchronized with swallowing; and (3) a mature pattern with long bursts of sucking accompanied by swallowing and associated with propulsive peristaltic waves in the esophagus.[96] Sucking is observed in term infants from birth; however, the mature suck-swallow pattern does not appear for several days. A transient immature suck-swallow pattern seen with the first few feedings is characterized by short bursts of three to five sucks followed by swallowing.[96] Within 24 to 48 hours a mature pattern emerges, characterized by a prolonged burst of 30 or more sucks with approximately 2 sucks/second. Swallowing occurs simultaneously with sucking one to four times during each burst.[145]

In contrast, preterm infants tend to have short bursts of sucking, followed by swallowing, often accompanied by a rest period (for breathing) before sucking resumes. Preterm infants are limited in their ability to suck by their weaker flexor control (important for firm lip and jaw closure) and immature musculature. Organization of sucking into a burst-pause pattern seems to occur earlier with breast-feeding than with bottle feeding. Meier reported than by 32 weeks breast-fed infants have an organized sucking pattern with bursts of two to three sucks followed by a pause.[163a] Assessment of an infant's suck-swallow-gag-breathing capabilities is important prior to enteral feeding.

Infants must also be able to coordinate breathing with sucking and swallowing. From 38 weeks to 6 months infants can easily coordinate these activities. After 6 months this ability is gradually lost. Until about 3 months of age solids placed in the infant's mouth will be forced up against the palate by the tongue and then either swallowed or flow out the mouth.[59] By 3 to 4 months of age the infant begins to be able to selectively transfer semisolid food to the back of the mouth for swallowing.

Esophageal Motility and Lower Esophageal Sphincter Function

Esophageal motility is decreased in the newborn, especially during the first 12 hours after birth. Esophageal peristalsis is increased and accompanied by simultaneous nonperistaltic contractions with poor coordination of esophageal motility and swallowing. (GI motility refers to oscillating contractions in small segments that mix food versus the large peristaltic waves that propel food along the tract.) Tone, pressure, and length of the lower esophageal sphincter (LES) are reduced. The LES in the neonate is primarily above the diaphragm and subjected to intrathoracic pressures.[105] As a result, esophageal reflux is common and can be seen on x-ray film in 38% of normal term infants in the 1st week after birth.[95] Alterations in the LES are related to incomplete development and possibly decreased responsiveness to gastrin (which enhances LES pressure) due to delayed maturation of hormonal receptors. LES tone develops rapidly during the 1st week; however, the sphincter remains small and potentially inadequate for 6 to 12 months.[242]

Gastric Emptying

Gastric motility and muscle tone are decreased and emptying time is delayed in the newborn. Gastric emptying may take 2 to 6 hours or longer.[12] The delay in gastric emptying may have a hormonal basis with delayed maturation of feedback control mechanisms. The elevated gastrin level in the newborn also delays emptying.[242]

Gastric emptying is influenced by other factors including muscle tone, mucus, pyloric sphincter tone, presence of amniotic fluid, hormones, and type of food. Carbohydrate increases emptying time, and fat decreases emptying time. Medium-chain triglycerides empty faster than long-chain ones.[214] Human milk empties more rapidly than formula or dextrose water, and D5W empties faster than D10W.[227] Higher caloric density formulas are retained in the stomach for longer periods (although these formulas are associated with emptying of more calories over comparative periods).[11, 213]

Mucus delays gastric emptying, especially during the first 24 hours after birth. The stomach empties more quickly if the infant is in a prone or right lateral position.[265] Upright or semi-upright positions decrease the likelihood of air passing from the stomach to the duodenum. The gastric capacity of an infant is approximately 6 ml per kilogram of body weight. In preterm infants large residual gastric volumes may develop, leading to gastric distention, compromised respiratory function, and interference with delivery of adequate nutrients.[242]

Intestinal Motility

Intestinal movement tends to be more disorganized and slower in newborns owing to immaturity of the intestinal musculature, poor coordination of peristaltic waves, and a tendency for segmentation of peristalsis.[12] Disorganized motility results in a decreased ability to clear the upper gut with impaired absorptive function, prolonged transit time in the upper intestine, and more rapid emptying of the ileum and colon. Prolonged transit time in the small intestine may also be an advantage by increasing chances for absorption of specific nutrients. However, faster emptying of the colon reduces the time for water and electrolyte absorption, increasing stool water content and the risk of dehydration and electrolyte imbalance. The gastrocolonic reflex is active in the neonate: entry of food into the beginning of the small intestine or colon causes reflexive propulsion of food toward the rectum.

The preterm infant experiences even more irregular and less predictable peristaltic waves along with antiperistaltic waves. These limitations further increase transit time and impair absorption. GI peristalsis develops gradually in the fetus from 33 to 40 weeks' gestation.[161] Immaturity of peristalsis in the preterm infant is one reason fetal passage of meconium is rarely seen prior to 34 weeks' gestation. Maturation of peristalsis in the fetus is delayed with hydramnios but accelerated with pregnancy-induced hypertension and erythroblastosis.[161, 242]

Intestinal Surface Area

The immature surface of the small intestine decreases absorptive area, especially in preterm infants. Numbers of intestinal villi and epithelial cells increase with gestation. In the mature intestine, epithelial cells in the crypts are undifferentiated and develop the ability to hydrolyze and transport nutrients as they migrate toward the top of the villus, replacing older cells. Turnover of intestinal epithelial cells is decreased in the newborn, impairing absorptive efficiency.

Alterations in the normal crypt–to–villous cell turnover rate lead to inadequate functional surface area along the brush border and glycocalyx and alter digestion, absorption, and host defense mechanisms. These changes are similar to those seen with malnutrition.[243] Enteric intake after birth induces epithelial hyperplasia, increasing cell turnover and stimulating production of microvillous enzymes such as pancreatic lipase, amylase, and trypsin.[153, 154, 242, 272] Gut regulatory peptides and hormones increase at birth and have a trophic effect on the intestine.[31]

Colostrum is thought to contain factors that stimulate epithelial cell turnover and maturation.[242] The surface area of the small intestine can be altered by anoxia and infection, further impeding absorption of nutrients.

Physiologic Limitations

Newborns are limited in their ability to digest and absorb certain nutrients owing to decreased activity of specific enzymes and other substances as well as functional and anatomic limitations. However, newborns, especially if fed human milk, have mechanisms available that partially compensate for these alterations, resulting in relatively proficient digestion in term and many preterm infants.

A prominent difference in digestive processes between the neonate and adult is immaturity of exocrine pancreatic function, which forces the infant to use compensatory mechanisms that rely on nonpancreatic enzymes found in the lingual area and salivary secretions, intestinal brush border, enterocyte, and human milk. Slow development of pancreatic exocrine function may be a protective mechanism to prevent degradation and loss of intestinal epithelial cells and brush border enzymes by the pancreatic proteolytic enzymes.[100] Limitations of the newborn related to digestion and absorption of protein, carbohydrate, and fat and compensatory mechanisms are summarized in Table 9–14.

Digestion and Absorption of Protein

In spite of limitations in amounts and function of proteolytic enzymes, term and many preterm infants digest and absorb proteins relatively well.[145, 221] The newborn's gastric pH is neutral or slightly alkaline.[144] Decreased secretion of gastric acid (HCl) and prolonged buffering by the stomach contents owing to delayed gastric emptying in newborns increase gastric pH. Amniotic fluid in the stomach further elevates gastric pH during the initial 24 hours. Acid secretion is further decreased and gastric pH increased in preterm infants.

Gastric acid secretion increases within 24 hours of birth, then falls rapidly and remains low for at least 3 weeks.[144] Pepsinogen production is less than 50% of adult levels (corrected for weight) for the first few months.[145] The elevated pH reduces pepsin activity and gastric peptic hydrolysis in both term and

TABLE 9–14
Physiologic Limitations in Digestion and Absorption of Protein, Carbohydrate, and Fat in the Neonate

FACTOR	LIMITATION IN NEONATE	IMPLICATION	COMPENSATORY MECHANISMS
Digestion and Absorption of Protein			
Gastric acid (HCl)	50% of adult values	Increased gastric pH Decreased pepsin activity Decreased gastric proteolysis	
Pepsinogen	50% of adult values	Decreased pepsin Decreased gastric proteolysis	
Trypsin	Near adult levels (but activity reduced)	Decreased proteolysis	
Enterokinase	10% of adult activity	Decreased activation of trypsin and other pancreatic peptidases	
Chymotrypsin	10–60% of adult activity	Decreased proteolysis	
Carboxypeptidases	10–60% of adult activity	Decreased proteolysis	
Intestinal mucosal dipeptidases	Adequate	Promotes protein digestion	
Amino acid absorption	Adequate	Adequate absorption of amino acids and some intact proteins	
Digestion and Absorption of Carbohydrate			
Salivary amylase	⅓ of adult levels	Decreased starch digestion (infants ingest little starch)	Increased gastric pH helps retain activity in stomach Used to digest glucose polymers
Pancreatic amylase	0.2–5% of adult levels	Decreased starch digestion	Mammary amylase
Sucrase, maltases, isomaltase Adequate	Adequate digestion of sucrose, maltose, isomaltose		
Glucoamylase	50–100% of adult levels	Enhances digestion of glucose polymers	
Lactase	Term: 2–4 times greater than older children Preterm: 30% of term by 28–30 weeks	Term infant able to digest lactose well; preterm infant has limited lactose digestion	Colonic salvage
Glucose absorption	Term: 50–60% of adult; lower in preterm	Adequate absorption at low levels; more problems in handling glucose load	
Digestion and Absorption of Fat			
Pancreatic lipase	10–20% of adult levels	Decreased fat digestion	Lingual and gastric lipase Human milk bile salt stimulated lipase
Bile acids	Synthesis and bile acid pool Term: ½ adult values Preterm: ⅙ adult values Decreased reabsorption through the enterohepatic circulation	Decreased fat digestion and absorption Steatorrhea in preterm infants	Human milk bile salt stimulated lipase

preterm infants.[144, 200] Although circulating levels of gastrin (which normally stimulates secretion of gastric acid and pepsin) are elevated, animal data suggest that receptors for this hormone may be immature.[145] The decreased gastric acidity and pepsinogen levels may enhance development of gut host defense mechanisms by promoting activity of immunoglobulins and antigen recognition by the gastrointestinal tract.[145]

Term and preterm infants have near adult levels of trypsin, but activity of trypsin and the other pancreatic proteolytic hormones is reduced. Chymotrypsin and carboxypeptidase B activity is 10 to 60% and enterokinase activity is 10% of adult values. Since enterokinase activates trypsin, which in turn activates the other pancreatic proteolytic enzymes, the level of enterokinase is the rate-limiting step for intestinal protein digestion.[145, 221] This limitation does not seem to have a major impact on infants over 26 to 28 weeks' gestation, who are usually able to digest and absorb 85% of the dietary protein in human milk and most formulas.[50] Preterm infants cannot handle excessive protein loads (>5 to 6 g/kg/day). Intestinal mucosal dipeptidase activity along with the ability to transport and absorb amino acids develops early in gestation. The newborn's intestine absorbs more intact proteins and macromolecules, which may increase the risk for development of allergies (see Chapter 10) and necrotizing enterocolitis.[13, 144]

Digestion and Absorption of Carbohydrates

Carbohydrate digestion in adults is dependent on salivary and pancreatic amylase and disaccharidases (Fig. 9–10A). Salivary amylase activity at birth is one-third that of adults. Levels increase after 3 to 6 months of age and may be related to the addition of starch (solid foods) to the infant's diet.[146, 165] Salivary amylase retains its activity in the infant's stomach and is effective in digestion of glucose polymers.

Pancreatic amylase activity is decreased in term and preterm infants to 0.2 to 5% of adult values. Adequate levels are achieved by 4 to 6 months.[100, 272] Cholecystokinin and secretin have little effect on pancreatic amylase secretion prior to 1 month. Amylase activity increases significantly after this time.[272]

Mammary amylase in human milk compensates for the decreased pancreatic amylase (Fig. 9–10A). Mammary amylase is highest in colostrum and retains high activity for 6 weeks after birth.[100] Buffers in human milk and the higher gastric pH in the neonate help maintain mammary amylase activity.[146]

The newborn has adequate levels of α-glucosidases such as sucrase, maltases, isomaltase, and glucoamylase. Sucrase and maltases attain maximal activity by 32 to 34 weeks' gestation or earlier. Glucoamylase is an intestinal brush border enzyme that digests glucose polymers found in many formulas.[50, 146] Levels of glucoamylase are 50 to 100% of adult values and increase rapidly after birth.[145] Glucoamylase is less susceptible

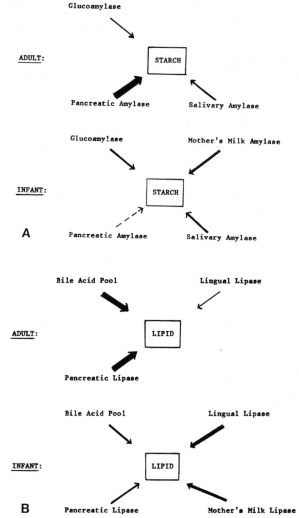

FIGURE 9–10. Relative importance of enzyme systems for carbohydrate and fat digestion in the adult versus the neonate. *A,* Amylolytic enzymes in infants and adults, indicating alternative pathways of starch digestion. *B,* Lipolytic enzymes in infants and adults indicating alternative pathways for the digestion of lipids. Thickness of arrows represents the relative importance of the pathway. (Redrawn from Lebenthal, G., Lee, P.C., & Heitlinyer, L.A. (1983). Impact of development of the gastrointestinal tract on infant feeding. *J Pediatr, 102,* 1.)

than disaccharidases to intestinal mucosal injury. This enzyme is evenly distributed along the small intestine, which along with the prolonged transit time seen in infants contributes to more efficient hydrolysis and mucosal uptake.[146] Digestion of glucose polymers depends on salivary amylase, glucoamylase, and human milk amylase. Neonates can effectively hydrolyze and absorb glucose polymers, especially those of short- to medium-chain length.

The major carbohydrate in human and cow's milk is lactose. Lactase activity increases rapidly in late gestation and is adequate after 36 weeks. At term lactase levels are two to four times higher than in older infants.[127, 165] Lactase activity at 28 to 34 weeks is only 30% of term values.[144] Activity of other disaccharidases is induced by exposure to appropriate substrate. This does not occur with lactase, so activity remains low in preterm infants.[200] In spite of low levels, many preterm infants digest lactose adequately.[127, 165] Lactose that is not absorbed in the small intestines is conserved by colonic salvage.

Colonic salvage involves bacterial fermentation of carbohydrate to hydrogen gas and short-chain fatty acids, which are absorbed by the colon, minimizing carbohydrate loss in stools.[35, 108, 127, 132, 165] In preterm infants two thirds of the ingested lactose may reach the colon. Changes in colonic bacterial flora following antibiotic use or surgery may alter the infant's ability to conserve energy via colonic salvage.[50] Lactase deficiency generally resolves when the preterm infant reaches a conceptual age of 36 to 40 weeks.[146] These infants need some lactose intake since lactose enhances calcium absorption.

Mechanisms for glucose, galactose, and fructose absorption develop early in gestation and are relatively mature. The capacity for mucosal glucose uptake at term is 50 to 60% of adult values.[145] Absorption of glucose is slower in preterm infants, with further reductions in SGA infants suggesting that intrauterine growth retardation may delay maturation of these processes.[163] Infants seem to absorb glucose as well as do adults at low glucose concentrations but have a maximal absorptive capacity about 20% that of the adult.[220] Glucose transport increases by 2 to 3 weeks of age.[146] Hypoxia and ischemia decrease intestinal perfusion, altering the ultrastructure of intestinal cells, which decreases active transport and uptake of glucose.[220]

Digestion and Absorption of Fats

Fat digestion in the adult relies on pancreatic lipase to break down triglycerides and bile acids to emulsify fat droplets prior to and during lipolysis. These processes are decreased in term and especially in preterm and SGA infants (Fig. 9–10B).[144, 246] Lipase

activity at term is 10 to 20% of that seen in older children, partly owing to minimal responsiveness by pancreatic acinar cells to secretin and cholecystokinin during the 1st month.[122, 175, 272] Term infants fail to absorb 10 to 15% and preterm infants 30% or more of ingested fat.[149] Steatorrhea is common in preterm infants with excretion of 10 to 20% (versus <10%) of dietary fat intake in their stools.[12]

Bile acid synthesis and pool size are one-half adult values in term infants and one-sixth adult and one-third term infant values in preterm infants.[144, 213] Since hepatic conjugation of bile acids in infants is taurine-dependent (versus glycine-dependent in the adult), adequate intake of taurine is essential in infancy.[145] The decreased bile acid pools are due to reduced hepatic synthesis and poorer recirculation and conservation of bile salts through enterohepatic shunting as a result of immaturity of liver and intestinal active transport processes.[145, 149, 248]

In preterm infants concentrations of bile acids in the duodenal lumen may be below critical levels necessary for micelle formation (water-soluble aggregates of lipids and lipid-soluble substances).[215, 247] Decreased micelle formation results in poor absorption of long-chain triglycerides, which are dependent on micelle formation for solubilization and subsequent hydrolysis (see Fig. 9–1C). Infants are better able to absorb medium- and short-chain triglycerides, which are not dependent on micelle formation.

Alternative pathways to compensate for the decreased levels of pancreatic lipase and bile acids include human milk bile salt stimulated lipase (mammary lipase) and lingual/gastric lipase (gastric lipase may be a separate entity or a form of lingual lipase), which have high activity at birth (Fig. 9–10B).[102] Lingual and gastric lipases hydrolyze 50 to 70% and mammary lipase 30 to 40% of dietary fat in infants.[100] Intragastric lipolysis by these extrapancreatic lipases breaks down triglycerides in the milk fat globule. As a result, the fat globule is a better substrate for the available pancreatic lipase and enhances action of bile salts. Extensive hydrolysis of fat in the stomach can be documented in preterm infants as young as 26 to 32 weeks' gestation.[100]

Sucking is a stimulus for secretion of lingual lipase. Since lingual lipase is decreased in some preterm infants, nonnutritive sucking with gavage feedings may stimulate secretion of this enzyme with subsequent improvement of fat digestion and absorption. This has been suggested as a basis for the improved weight gain reported with nonnutritive sucking.[7, 29, 48, 101]

Mammary lipase is present in the milk of term and preterm mothers. This enzyme is stable at low pH (and not inactivated in the stomach) and hydrolyzes triglycerides at low concentrations of bile salts.[100, 102] Mammary lipase works in the duodenum, and its activity is stimulated by bile salts at concentrations below those required for micelle formation such as are found in many preterm infants.[248] Temperatures above 55°C inactivate this enzyme; freezing (to −80° C) does not seem to affect its activity.[100] This lipase also produces monolauryl, a substance with antibacterial, antiviral, and antifungal activity.[102]

Absorption of Other Substances

Alterations in fat absorption affect absorption of fat-soluble vitamins, especially in preterm infants who may need supplementation with water-soluble analogues. Absorptive capacity for folate is also lower. Lower gastric secretion of intrinsic factor may interfere with absorption of vitamin B_{12}.[144] Neonates are less able to adapt to changes in osmotic load in the large intestine, increasing the risk of diarrhea and electrolyte imbalance.

Mechanisms for absorption of iron are relatively well developed in term and preterm infants, with a high rate of iron absorption for the first 10 weeks.[144] Iron in human milk is absorbed better than iron in formula, with absorption of up to 50% of the iron in human milk.[145] For the first few months preterm infants may not absorb large quantities of iron owing to saturation of transferrin with iron from turnover of red blood cells.[99]

Calcium absorption is influenced by vitamin D, calcium, and phosphorus concentrations; fatty acids; and lactose (see Chapter 14). The complex relationship between calcium and lipid intake makes determining calcium concentrations for formulas difficult. A high calcium intake alters absorption and retention of fatty acids; a high lipid intake can decrease calcium absorption.[144] Calcium absorption is lower in infants than in adults when calcium concentrations are low, but more efficient at higher levels.[145] Zinc and copper are well absorbed in term infants but not in preterm infants who may be in negative zinc or copper balance for several months.[145, 252, 267] Mechanisms for absorption of many nutrients have not been well studied in human neonates.

Liver Function in the Neonate

Portal blood flow is decreased in the fetus with shunting of blood flow away from the portal sinuses and liver parenchyma into the inferior vena cava via the ductus venosus. Many excretory and detoxification functions of the fetal liver are assumed by the placenta and maternal liver. With removal of the placenta, blood flow through the ductus venosus ceases, with anatomic closure by proliferation of connective tissue after 2 to 8 weeks.

The newborn liver accounts for about 5% of the infant's weight. This physiologic enlargement is due to (1) increased labile connective tissue (possibly in response to hypoxic stress with the abrupt shift in the oxygenation of blood supplying the liver at birth, i.e., from well-oxygenated blood from the placenta to systemic venous blood); (2) active liver hematopoiesis, which decreases in a few weeks as liver metabolic functions increase; (3) increased liver glycogen; and (4) hepatic congestion due to changes in blood flow with removal of the placenta.[96, 164]

Infants have a unique pathologic response to liver dysfunction, with active fibroblastic proliferation and early bile stasis that can alter the presentation of liver disorders. Decreased bile flow (cholestasis) often in association with a direct (conjugated) hyperbilirubinemia is seen with many liver disorders in infants. The cholestasis is due to disruption of the canalicular membrane, poor development of bile acid secretory mechanisms, and immaturity of bile acid synthesis.[96]

Liver enzyme systems necessary for metabolism of some drugs are depressed in the newborn. In the mature liver, oxidation and conjugation result in water-soluble drugs that are more readily excreted into bile. In the fetus, depression of these processes is an advantage, since lipid-soluble metabolites are more readily transferred across the placenta, where they can be handled by the maternal system. The liver smooth endoplastic reticulum (SER) is the location of many hepatic microsomal enzymes. The neonatal liver has little SER, and activities of microsomal enzymes are reduced or undetectable at birth, interfering with drug metabolism.[96]

CLINICAL IMPLICATIONS FOR NEONATAL CARE

Food and warmth are "two of the most important controllable factors in determining survival and normal development."[228, p.645] Limitations of GI function in term and preterm neonates have major implications for the infant's nutritional needs and the composition and method of feedings. The feeding of sick and preterm infants is associated with many controversies including when, what, and how to feed. Decisions regarding feeding can lead to other problems such as an increased risk of necrotizing enterocolitis and metabolic or nutritional alterations. This section reviews nutritional requirements of infants and implications of GI limitations for the selection of method and composition of feedings. Problems related to neonatal physiologic limitations such as reflux, dehydration, diarrhea, and necrotizing enterocolitis are also examined.

Infant Growth

Growth rates during the neonatal period are more rapid than at any other time. The method for growth assessment of term infants generally involves use of standardized charts from the National Center for Health and Statistics.[186] Expected patterns and assessment of growth for preterm infants are controversial, especially regarding whether these infants should be expected to follow intrauterine or extrauterine patterns. Both intrauterine and extrauterine growth standards are available.

The Committee on Nutrition of the American Academy of Pediatrics (AAP) recommends that postnatal growth of preterm infants follow the pattern for intrauterine growth of a fetus of the same gestation.[186] However, there is little evidence that intrauterine rates are appropriate or realistic for these infants.[186, 269] A variety of intrauterine growth charts are available, all of which have limitations in that they were developed from measurements of preterm infants at various gestations who may not represent a normal fetal population.[186] The growth chart used should be one that is most appropriate for the location and patient population (ethnic, socioeconomic, and demographic characteristics). Extrauterine growth charts are fewer in number and may not reflect current populations and care practices. These charts are probably not satisfactory for use with healthy preterm infants cared for using current feeding practices.[186]

Nutritional Requirements of Full and Preterm Infants

Nutritional requirements of infants vary with gestational age and health status. Requirements for healthy term infants are assumed to be those found in human milk (Table 9–15). For infants who are not breast-fed, commercial formulas are good alternatives for meeting nutritional needs. Whole cow's milk and evaporated milk do not meet current standards for infant nutrition.[193] Nutritional requirements for preterm infants are controversial. One problem is lack of knowledge and agreement on what is the optimal growth rate for the preterm infants and how closely this rate should parallel that of the fetus. Nutritional requirements for preterm infants are often estimated by assaying the body composition of fetuses at different gestational ages and examining fetal accretion of different nutrients. Water (see Chapter 8), energy, and caloric requirements are higher for preterm infants because of greater insensible water loss, increased exposure to stressors, and increased expectations for growth.

The caloric requirement for term infants averages 110 to 120 kcal/kg/day.[12] Most stable preterm infants achieve satisfactory growth on approximately 120 to 130 kcal/kg/day.[176, 252] Requirements for preterm infants on enteral feedings can range from 110 to 170 kcal/kg/day and occasionally higher, depending on the infant's basal metabolic rate (increased with health problems), activity level (decreased in infants on morphine or fentanyl), cold stress (increases metabolic rate), specific dynamic action (efficiency of nutrient absorption), fecal losses, and expected rate of growth (often 20 to 30 g/day). Caloric requirements for infants on parenteral feedings tend to be lower, averaging 85 to 95 kcal/kg/day.[12]

The AAP recommends a daily protein intake of 2.25 to 5 g/kg.[4] Fetal protein accretion is 3 to 4 g/kg/day. The type of dietary protein affects daily protein requirements. For example, infants can achieve adequate growth with 2 g/kg/day of a whey predominant feeding.[176] Inadequate protein leads to alterations in cardiorespiratory, liver, and

TABLE 9–15
Composition of Human Milk and Infant Formulas

	PROTEIN		CARBOHYDRATE		FAT		CALCIUM (mg/L)	PHOSPHORUS (mg/L)	RENAL (mOsm/L)	GASTROINTESTINAL (mOsm/kg H$_2$O)
CALORIC DENSITY	Whey/Casein	Total Calories (%)	Type	Total Calories (%)	Type	Total Calories (%)				
Human milk										
Mature										
20 kcal/oz (0.67 kcal/ml)	60:40	7	Lactose	38	Human milk fat	55	340	169	75	300
Premature										
22 kcal/oz (0.73 kcal/ml)	60:40		Lactose		Human milk fat		293	134		300
Premature infant formula										
Similac Special Care										
24 kcal/oz (0.81 kcal/ml)	60:40	11	Lactose/glucose polymers 50:50	42	MCT/soy/coconut 50:30:20	47	1462	731	162	300
Premature Enfamil										
24 kcal/oz	60:40	12	40:60	42	40:40:20	44	950	470	220	300
Premie SMA										
24 kcal/oz	60:40	10	50:50	42	Coconut/safflower/oleo/soy/MCT 27:25:20:18:10	48	750	400	175	300
Standard formula										
Similac										
20 kcal/oz	18:82	9	Lactose	43	Coconut and soy oils	48	510 520	390 438	110–120	285
SMA										
20 kcal/oz	60:40	9	Lactose	41–43	Corn coconut, and/or soy, oleo safflower oils	48–51	420	310	105	250
Enfamil										
20 kcal/oz	60:40	9	Lactose	41	Coconut and soy oils		460	345	97	285

From O'Leary, M. J. (1989). Nourishing the premature and low birth weight infant. In P. L. Pipes (Ed.), *Nutrition in infancy and childhood* (4th ed., pp. 301–360). St. Louis: Times Mirror/Mosby College Publishing; as modified from O'Leary, M. J. (1984). Nutritional care of the low birth weight infant. In M. V. Krause & L. K. Mahan (Eds.), *Food, nutrition and diet therapy* (7th ed.). Philadelphia: WB Saunders.

renal function; decreased immunocompetence; altered brain growth; and poor weight gain and somatic growth. Excessive intake (5 to 6 g/kg/day) results in a metabolic overload with irritability, late metabolic acidosis, azotemia, edema, fever, lethargy, diarrhea, elevated blood urea nitrogen (BUN), and possible lower IQ.[85, 96]

The major energy source in human milk and most formulas is fat, which accounts for 30 to 55% of the total calories (3.3 to 6 g/100 kcal).[4] Specific requirements include those for linoleic acid and possibly linolenic acid, essential fatty acids needed as precursors for synthesis of other fatty acids. The AAP recommends that 2.7% (300 mg linoleic acids/100 kcal) of the infant's energy intake be essential fatty acids.[4, 27] Inadequate fats or lack of essential fatty acids can lead to metabolic problems, skin disorders, and poor growth; excessive fats can lead to ketosis.

Carbohydrates should make up 30 to 50% of the caloric content. Inadequate carbohydrate can lead to hypoglycemia; excessive carbohydrate, to diarrhea. Infants, especially preterm infants who have poor stores and a higher growth rate, have increased needs for calcium, phosphorus, and vitamins to support growth and bone mineralization. Recommended intakes of specific nutrients for preterm infants are listed in Table 9–16.

Analysis of the Composition of Feedings

In order to maximize growth and reduce stress the limitations of the neonate's gastrointestinal, renal, and metabolic systems must be considered in selecting substances for feeding. This can be accomplished through analysis of the composition of human milk and commercial formulas and consideration of the advantages and disadvantages of each for that individual infant. This section discusses considerations in selecting feedings for term and preterm infants. Composition of mature and preterm milk and frequently used standard and preterm formulas is listed in Table 9–15.

Protein

Milk protein consists of casein and whey proteins. Whey forms soft, flocculent curds. Casein forms tougher, more rubbery curds; it requires a greater energy expenditure to digest and is more likely to be incompletely digested. Human milk has a whey-to-casein ratio of 60:40 (versus 20:80 in cow's milk). Whey is easier to digest in the presence of low levels of trypsin and pepsin. Whey protein contains a different mixture of amino acids than casein, with increased levels of cystine and decreased methionine. Human milk contains less protein than cow's milk but has higher levels of nonprotein nitrogen with an amino acid composition that is easy for the infant to use.[194]

The use of whey-dominant feedings reduces the risk of lactobezoar formation.[208] Lactobezoars are milk curd balls that develop within the stomach and are seen predominantly in preterm infants on whey-dominant, high caloric density formulas. This disorder may resolve spontaneously in asymptomatic infants. Symptomatic infants (abdominal distention, gastric residuals, and vomiting) may respond to discontinuation of feeding and gastric lavage, although about 11 to 14% develop gastric perforation.[96]

The amino acid composition of feedings is critical for optimal neonatal growth and development. Taurine is essential for central nervous system (CNS) growth, maintaining optimal retinal integrity and function, and bile acid synthesis. Intermediary metabolic pathways for synthesis of some amino acids are immature. For example, the last enzyme in transsulfuration is absent in the fetus and develops slowly in preterm infants. These infants cannot synthesize cystine and have limited tolerance for methionine (which is normally converted to cystine). Similar deficiencies exist in the ability of the infant to

TABLE 9–16
Daily Nutritional Intakes for Preterm Infants

NUTRIENT	ADVISABLE INTAKE (kg/day)		
	700–1000 g	1001–1500 g	1501–2000 g
Energy (kcal)	110	110	110
Protein (g)	3.6	3.5	2.9
Sodium (mmol)	3.5	3.1	2.6
Potassium (mmol)	2.4	2.2	2.1
Chloride (mmol)	3.2	2.6	2.2
Calcium (mg)	182	176	163
Phophorus (mg)	126	121	112
Magnesium (mg)	7.2	6.6	5.9
Iron (mg)	2.6	2.4	2.3
Zinc (mg)	1.6	1.4	1.3
Copper (mg)	0.2	0.2	0.2

From Bell, E. F. & Oh, W. (1988). Nutritional support. In J.P. Goldsmith & E.H. Karotkin (Eds.), *Assisted ventilation of the neonate* (pp. 307–327). Philadelphia: WB Saunders, as adapted from Ziegler, E. E. (1986). Feeding the low birth weight infant. In S.S. Gellis & B.M. Kagan (Eds.), *Current pediatric therapy* (12th ed., pp. 722–725). Philadelphia: WB Saunders.

oxidize tyrosine and phenylalanine. Transamination pathways are also not well developed so that histidine is an essential amino acid in the neonate but not in the adult.[145] Thus infants need a feeding that contains lower levels of methionine, phenylalanine, and tyrosine and adequate cystine, taurine, and histidine.[48, 219]

Phenylalanine and tyrosine can significantly increase net acid loads, which along with high protein feedings contributes to development of late metabolic acidosis. This disorder is seen in preterm infants usually at 2 to 3 weeks of age. Late metabolic acidosis is associated with the amount of protein in the diet, the amino acid composition of the diet, and the decreased ability of the immature kidney to conserve bicarbonate (see Chapter 8).

Carbohydrate

Immaturity of lactase activity in preterm infants may interfere with their ability to optimally use lactose-based formulas, although many infants have little difficulty digesting lactose. Carbohydrates other than lactose are often included in feedings if greater carbohydrate absorption is needed or if lactose is poorly tolerated.[145] Use of low-lactose feedings reduces the risk of overwhelming the infant's available lactase. Infants do require some lactose for calcium absorption.

Glucose polymers are often used as an alternative carbohydrate substrate in formulas. Preterm infants hydrolyze and absorb glucose polymers in a manner similar to lactose in term infants.[145] Glucose polymers have several advantages: (1) ready availability from natural sources including corn syrup solids; (2) high caloric density without significantly increasing the renal solute load (see Chapter 8); (3) incorporation into feedings without significantly increasing the osmotic load and risk of increased water loss and diarrhea; (4) more rapid emptying from the stomach of young infants than lactose or glucose; (5) independence from lactase and amylase; and (6) digestion by glucoamylase, which is present in adequate quantities in preterm infants and whose secretion is less likely to be altered by mucosal injury.[100, 145, 146, 214]

Fat

Fats are the primary source of energy in human milk and many formulas. Fats provide a higher caloric density without significantly increasing osmotic load. Limitations in neonatal fat digestion and absorption can reduce the usefulness of this energy source. High caloric density formulas tend to be retained in the stomach for longer periods, thus delaying gastric emptying.

Infants need both saturated and unsaturated fatty acids in their diet. Human milk and vegetable oils (corn, coconut, and soy) are absorbed better than saturated fat (cow's milk or butter fat).[48] Unsaturated fats in vegetable oils are a source of the essential fatty acid linoleic acid. Short- and medium-chain triglycerides (MCTs) can be absorbed intact across the gastric and intestinal mucosa and are not dependent on the reduced bile acid pools. MCTs are associated with more rapid gastric emptying and enhanced calcium, magnesium, and fat absorption.[214] MCTs may also increase the level of plasma ketones, which can be used as an alternative substrate to glucose for brain metabolism.[260] About 10 to 50% of the fat in preterm formulas is in the form of MCTs. Infants need some long-chain fatty acids for integrity of cell membranes and brain development.[218]

Vitamins, Minerals, and Trace Elements

Infants need adequate amounts of essential vitamins, minerals, and trace elements in their diet to support normal growth and development. Immature infants have decreased stores of most of these substances since stores accumulate late in gestation, and dietary supplementation may be needed. Specific requirements for many vitamins and trace elements in preterm infants are unknown. Increased quantities of fat-soluble vitamins (A, D, C, K) and their water-soluble analogues compensate for the inadequate bile acid pools and poorer absorption of fat, especially in preterm infants. Requirements for B vitamins (coenzymes for metabolic processes and energy production) and folic acid (a cofactor for DNA synthesis) may also be increased because of the infant's greater growth rate and decreased intestinal absorption.

VITAMIN A
Vitamin A enhances light perception and tissue integrity along with repair and growth of epithelial tissue. Vitamin A requirements range from 250 to 375 IU/100 kcal (or about 500 IU per day). Higher levels are needed

in preterm infants owing to poor absorption and stores. Decreased vitamin A has been reported in infants with bronchopulmonary dysplasia.[110, 211] It is unclear if this is due to lowered intake or consumption of vitamin A in the repair of damaged lung epithelial tissue.[255] Vitamin A levels should be monitored in infants on parenteral alimentation. Vitamin A in parenteral solutions decreases markedly over 24 hours as a result of adherence of the vitamin to IV tubing and photodegradation.[255]

VITAMIN C
Vitamin C is water soluble, readily absorbed, and not stored in significant amounts. It is important in amino acid metabolism (needed for growth) and intestinal iron absorption. Deficiencies are associated with scurvy (rare) and transient hypertyrosinemia. Recommended intake is 35 to 100 mg/day in infants, with an average of 60 mg in preterm and 20 mg in term infants.[187, 267]

VITAMIN D
Vitamin D facilitates intestinal calcium and phosphorus absorption, bone mineralization, and calcium reabsorption from bone. Infants at risk for rickets secondary to vitamin D deficiency are listed in Table 14–5. Preterm infants have lower serum concentrations of vitamin D and increased needs owing to more rapid growth and immaturity of enzymes involved in metabolism of dietary vitamin D to active substrates. Recommended intake for infants is 400 IU/day or up to 600 IU/day in preterm infants.[187, 267]

VITAMIN E
An important consideration related to both the fat and vitamin composition of feeding is the ratio of polyunsaturated fatty acid (especially linoleic acid) to vitamin E (see Chapter 5). The fat content of the red blood cell membrane is determined by dietary fat. Diets that contain high levels of polyunsaturated fatty acid (PUFA) or iron necessitate increased levels of vitamin E to protect red blood cells from oxidative injury and hemolysis. Recommended concentrations of vitamin E to PUFA are 1 IU vitamin E per g of linoleic acid.[4]

Preterm infants have lower vitamin E stores, poor absorption, and increased needs to protect cell membranes from peroxidative damage and prevent hemolytic anemia. Supplementation with 5 to 25 IU/dl/day in addition to amounts in feedings is recommended until the infant reaches a conceptual age of 36 to 40 weeks.[12] Elevated serum vitamin E levels have been associated with necrotizing enterocolitis and cerebral hemorrhage, so high doses must be avoided. Vitamin E levels can be monitored weekly or biweekly in vulnerable infants, and doses titrated to maintain serum levels of 1 to 3 g/dl.[187] Issues regarding the role of vitamin E in preventing retinopathy of prematurity, bronchopulmonary dysplasia, and intraventricular hemorrhage are discussed in Chapter 5.

FOLATE
Folate deficiency, which can lead to anemia, poor growth, and delayed CNS maturation, is seen more often in preterm infants. Folate needs are increased in very low birthweight (VLBW) infants, who have decreased stores and more rapid growth.[252] Supplementation with 50 to 70 μg/dl/day has been recommended for preterm infants during the first 2 to 3 months, when intake is limited.[267]

CALCIUM, PHOSPHORUS, AND MAGNESIUM
Calcium, phosphorus, and magnesium are essential in the neonate for bone mineralization and growth. The newborn with lower levels of parathyroid hormone (PTH) is less able to remove calcium from the bone, increasing the risk of hypocalcemia (see Chapter 14). Calcium levels in feedings may be increased to allow for calcium storage and support bone mineralization and growth. If calcium levels are altered, phosphorus intake also needs to be adjusted to maintain a homeostatic calcium-phosphorus balance. Vitamin D and magnesium are also needed for adequate bone mineralization and to prevent rickets.

IRON
Term and preterm infants develop a physiologic anemia during the first few months after birth because of postnatal suppression of erythropoiesis (see Chapter 5). During this period iron from destroyed red blood cells is stored for use when erythropoiesis resumes. Once the stored iron is used up the infant's hemoglobin will again fall if adequate iron is not available from dietary sources or supplementation. Iron supplementation is usually started prior to the point of depletion to maintain and build up stores. Supplementation is started earlier in preterm infants since their iron stores are lower at birth and often

further depleted by iatrogenic blood losses. Recommendations regarding iron supplementation are discussed in Chapter 5.

TRACE ELEMENTS

Stores of trace elements such as zinc, copper, iodine, chromium, selenium, and molybdenum are accumulated late in gestation. Requirements for trace elements are often also increased in preterm infants owing to poor stores and increased growth rates. Specific requirements and absorptive mechanisms for many of these elements are unknown. Concentrations in human milk are generally adequate, and commercial formulas are supplemented. Parenteral alimentation solutions must be supplemented with these elements or infants will rapidly become deficient.

Zinc. Zinc is an essential cofactor for over 70 enzymes. Zinc deficiencies inhibit uptake of fat-soluble vitamins and protein synthesis and can lead to growth retardation. Deficiencies have been reported in preterm infants fed human milk and infants on parenteral nutrition with inadequate supplementation. Excessive losses may occur in infants with ostomies or chronic diarrhea. Recommended intake is at least 0.5 mg/100 kcal.[187, 252]

Copper. Copper is also an enzyme component and essential for hemoglobin synthesis, myelinization, and formation of collagen. Copper deficiency (failure to thrive, iron-resistant anemia, pallor, edema, seborrheic dermatitis, and hypotonia) has been reported in preterm infants fed formulas with low levels of copper and in infants with ostomies or chronic diarrhea. Recommended intake is at least 90 μg/100 kcal.[187, 252]

ELECTROLYTES

Levels of potassium and sodium may be increased in preterm formulas to compensate for increased intestinal potassium and renal sodium losses and to support growth (sodium is coprecipitated in the bone during periods of active bone growth). Concentrations of specific electrolytes are also determined by fluid composition and levels of other electrolytes. For example, the AAP recommends that sodium-to-potassium ratios not exceed 1.0 mEq and potassium plus sodium–to–chloride ratios be 1.5 mEq or greater.[61]

Calories and Renal Solute Load

The caloric level of the formula should reflect the infant's energy needs, but at an osmolality that the infants's kidneys and other systems can handle. Caloric content of human milk is generally 20 kcal/oz but may vary. Preterm human milk has a caloric density of 22 kcal/oz. Standard formulas contain 20 kcal/oz and preterm formulas 24 kcal/oz. Higher calorie formulas may be used, but problems with osmotic and solute load often offset the advantages of extra calories. Osmolalities should be similar to those of physiologic fluids (250 to 300 mOm/kg water).

Caloric supplements such as Polycose (Ross Laboratories) and MCT Oil (Mead Johnson) may be used to increase the caloric density of feedings without significantly altering mineral content and solute load. These supplements may reduce the percentage of calories as protein (which may limit growth) and increase the percentage of calories as fat and carbohydrate (increasing the potential for ketosis and loose stools).[176] There is a risk of a lipoid pneumonia if MCT Oil is aspirated.

Use of Human Milk

Human milk is an ideal, nutritionally adequate feeding for term and mature preterm infants that meets the infant's unique nutritional needs and provides immunologic substances to protect the infant from infection and enhance gut maturation. Human milk contains substances such as human milk bile salt stimulated (mammary) lipase and mammary amylase and has a low renal solute load (see Chapter 8), which compensate for the neonate's physiologic limitations. Composition of human milk is described in Chapter 4 and Tables 4–3 and 9–15.

The use of human milk with very immature infants is still controversial. Milk from mothers of preterm infants is different from that of term mothers and more closely approximates what are thought to be the nutritional needs of these infants (Table 9–17). However, the composition of this milk changes gradually over the 1st month post birth and by 1 month is similar to term milk. Preterm human milk is low (in terms of the preterm infant's nutrient requirements) in protein, calcium, phosphorus, iron, vitamins, and sodium, even though nutrients such as protein, iron, and calcium are in forms that are more readily absorbed by the infant. For example, it has been estimated that preterm infants fed human milk retain calcium and phosphorus equivalent to 15 to 20% of the

TABLE 9–17
**Differences and Similarities Between Mature and Preterm Human Milk During Early Lactation
(0 to 4 Weeks)**

	MATURE MILK (Range per 100 ml)	PRETERM MILK (Range per 100 ml)	OVERALL CONSENSUS FROM MULTIPLE STUDIES
Energy (kcal)	70.2–73.6	73.0–76.0	Preterm > Mature
Protein (g)	1.3–1.8	1.5–2.1	Preterm > Mature
Fat (g)	2.9–3.4	3.2–3.6	Preterm ≥ Mature
Carbohydrate (g)	6.4–7.1	6.3–7.2	Preterm < Mature
Na (mg)	15.4–21.8	21.8–39.1	Preterm > Mature
Cl (mg)	36.4–58.8	38.5–63.0	Preterm > Mature
K (mg)	50.7–65.5	53.4–67.0	Preterm = Mature
Ca (mg)	26.7–29.3	26.6–31.4	Preterm ≤ Mature
P (mg)	13.8–16.9	12.9–13.8	Preterm ≥ Mature
Mg (mg)	2.7–3.1	3.0–3.6	Preterm ≥ Mature
Cu (μg)	57.0–73.0	63.0–83.0	Preterm = Mature
Fe (μg)	81.0–111.0	90.0–110.0	Preterm ≥ Mature
Zn (μg)	260.0–535.0	392.0–530.0	Preterm = Mature

From Pereira, G.R. & Barbosa, N.M.N. (1986). Controversies in neonatal nutrition. *Pediatr Clin North Am, 33,* 65.

calcium and 30 to 35% of the phosphorus accumulated by the fetus in utero.[252] Most preterm infants fed their own mother's milk gain at rates similar to intrauterine rates or those of infants fed whey formulas.[53, 92, 186, 121] VLBW infants fed human milk may need supplementation to promote growth and prevent deficiencies. Human milk fortifiers that contain protein, glucose polymers, calcium, phosphorus, fat-soluble vitamins, and sodium may be used.[121]

Components of Parenteral Nutrition Solutions

Total parenteral nutrition (TPN) is the intravenous administration of a hypertonic solution containing amino acids, carbohydrates, fats, electrolytes, vitamins, minerals, and trace elements (Table 9–18) in order to maintain positive nitrogen balance. Partial parenteral nutrition involves infusion of amino acids and carbohydrates with or without fats to supplement enteral feedings.[176] Infants generally cannot tolerate glucose loads over 6 to 8 mg/kg/min in the first 1 to 2 weeks. Parenteral alimentation has been associated with nitrogen retention and weight gain in low birth weight (LBW) infants.[104] Nutritional requirements of infants on parenteral feedings differ from those of infants on enteral feedings since these solutions are infused directly into the blood rather than the immature gut.

Problematic components of parenteral nutrition solutions have been amino acid mixtures and lipid emulsions. Abnormal plasma amino acid profiles have been reported in infants as well as older children and adults on parenteral nutrition.[104] These profiles are of particular concern in neonates with immature liver function and intermediary metabolic pathways for synthesis of some amino acids. Alternative mixtures and addition of specific amino acids have been used to try to normalize plasma values and approximate the amino acid pattern of human milk.[104]

Lipid emulsions are isotonic with a high caloric density and can be used to provide adequate caloric intake through a peripheral infusion. They are essential if the infant is on TPN for more than 1 week.[104] These solutions can lead to hyperlipidemia and hyperglycemia (reasons for alteration in glucose metabolism are unclear), especially with rates greater than 0.2 to 0.25 g/kg/hour or use in VLBW and SGA infants with little adipose tissue.[27, 218] Excess free fatty acids may compete with and displace bilirubin from albumin, increasing the risk of kernicterus (see Chapter 15). Fats may accumulate in pulmonary capillaries, arterioles, and alveolar macrophages, interfering with gas diffusion and oxygenation.[104] Effects on oxygenation may be minimized by prolonging the infusion period and using rates less than 0.2 g/kg/hour.[218]

Feeding Infants with Various Health Problems

Immature infants generally tolerate feeding with preterm formulas or preterm breast milk better than standard formulas. Considerations discussed below for selecting feedings for preterm infants are also important

TABLE 9–18
Suggested Composition for Intravenous Nutrition

COMPONENT	DAILY AMOUNT
Calories	
Dextrose, 3.4 kcal/g	10–20 g/kg
Lipids, 1.1 kcal/ml (10% solution)	1–4 g/kg
Nitrogen*	0.315 g/kg
Protein (6.4 g protein 1 g N₂)	2 g/kg
Electrolytes	
Sodium	3 mEq/kg
Potassium	2–3 mEq/kg
Chloride	3–4 mEq/kg
Phosphate	2mM/kg
Calcium	1 mEq (20 mg)/kg
Calcium gluconate, 10%	200 mg/kg
Magnesium	0.8 mEq (20 mg)/kg
Vitamins†	
Vitamin A	700 µg
Thiamine (B₁)	1.2 mg
Riboflavin (B₂)	1.4 mg
Niacin	17 mg
Pyridoxine (B₆)	1 mg
Ascorbic acid (C)	80 mg
Ergocalciferol (D)	400 IU
Vitamin E	7 IU
Pantothenic acid	5 mg
Cyanocobalamin	1 µg
Folate	140 µg
Vitamin K	200 µg
Trace elements	
Zinc (zinc sulfate)	300 g/kg
Copper (cupric sulfate)	20–30 µg/kg
Manganese sulfate	2–10 µg/kg
Chromium chloride	0.2 µg/kg
Selenium	1–2 µg/kg

*L-cysteine, 50 mEq/kg, should be added before administration.
†Or 1 packet of multivitamins such as MVI-Ped.
From Merenstein, G.B. & Gardner, S.L. (1989). *Handbook of neonatal intensive care* (2nd ed., p. 271). St. Louis: CV Mosby.

in planning nutritional support for infants with specific health problems. These infants have individualized nutritional needs that may require use of specialized formulas or feeding methods. For example, critically ill infants may need to be fed via total or partial parenteral nutrition because of their inability to digest and absorb enteral feedings or the risk of complications.

Very Low Birth Weight Infants

The considerations in selecting the feedings described above are even more critical in planning for nutritional support of VLBW infants, whose body systems are even more immature. Unique nutritional problems of these infants include

1. Limited protein and energy reserves (e.g., a 1000-g preterm has only 10 g of stored fat versus 400 g in a term neonate). En-

ergy needs may be increased by intermittent cold stress, infection, or stresses of the neonatal intensive care unit environment.
2. High ratio of surface area to body weight.
3. Small gastric capacity, which limits intake.
4. High water requirements due to increased insensible water losses and immature renal function. These factors limit the ability of the infant to tolerate high caloric density formulas owing to risks associated with hyperosmolar solutions.
5. Immature digestive and absorptive capacities for fats, carbohydrates, vitamins, and trace elements.
6. Immature brain and liver, which are vulnerable to damage from elevated plasma concentrations of amino acids such as tyrosine, methionine, and phenylalanine.[1, 48, 85]

Infants with Respiratory Problems

Infants with respiratory distress, including infants with bronchopulmonary dysplasia (BPD), may be unable to feed by bottle or breast owing to rapid respiratory rates, fatigue, and inability to coordinate sucking, swallowing, and breathing. These infants need to be fed by other enteral (intragastric or transpyloric) or parenteral methods. Fluid and caloric requirements are often increased because of the increased metabolic demands, respiratory work load, oxygen consumption, and insensible water losses. Energy needs may increase up to 20 to 40% above baseline in infants with BPD. Oxygen consumption, energy expenditure, and work load are higher for infants with respiratory problems who are breathing spontaneously than those on assisted ventilation.[27] Intestinal disaccharidases may be diminished in infants following shock or ischemia, with a temporary carbohydrate intolerance.[96] Infants recovering from respiratory distress syndrome have been reported to have decreased functional residual capacity, with increases in respiratory rate and minute ventilation during nasogastric feedings.[189] Feeding these infants in a prone position may improve their oxygenation during feeding.[96, 189]

Infants with Cardiac Problems

Infants with cardiac problems often grow poorly owing to increased metabolic demands and difficulty with feeding. Caloric requirements are increased because of hypermetabolism (higher metabolic rate and oxygen consumption secondary to increased cardiac and respiratory workload), tissue hypoxia, protein loss, increased frequency of infection, and poorer nutrient absorption due to decreased splanchnic blood flow.[88] Infants with cardiac problems may be fluid and sodium restricted. Feeding problems may limit intake since the infant may become fatigued, tachypneic, and stressed with feeding. Intervention strategies include use of higher caloric density and low-sodium formulas, frequent smaller feedings, feeding on demand and in an upright position, avoidance of feeding immediately after prolonged crying or when the infant is exhausted, and administration of oxygen with feeding as needed. Infants with cardiac or renal problems may need to be on low sodium or solute load formulas such as PM 60/40 and SMA.

Infants with Short Bowel Syndrome

Infants with reduction in the length of their small intestine, which usually results from surgical resection because of a congenital anomaly or necrotizing enterocolitis, are at very high risk for nutritional and growth problems owing to reduction in intestinal absorptive surface area. In addition, the remaining sections of bowel may have been ischemic with villous atrophy. Loss of intestinal surface area results in loss of brush border enzymes such as the disaccharidases, resulting in carbohydrate intolerance and a pool of unabsorbed sugars that act as a rich substrate for bacterial growth.[270] Infants who have less than 50 cm of residual small intestine (normal small intestinal length is 250 to 270 cm at term) are considered to be at the extreme of absorptive limitation.[96] During resection particular efforts are made to preserve the ileum, because of its critical role in bile acid and vitamin B_{12} absorption, and cecal valve.[96] Problems in digestion and absorption of nutrients resulting from small bowel resection are summarized in Table 9–19.

With adequate enteral nutrition, the remaining bowel usually undergoes villous hyperplasia with increased cell proliferation and migration.[96, 270] This response is similar to maturational responses seen in the newborn following initiation of enteral feedings and is related to exposure of the gut to

TABLE 9–19. Nutritional Limitations and Complications in Infants Following Small Bowel Resection

SITE	LIMITATION/COMPLICATION
Jejunum	Gastric hypersecretion
	Disaccharide intolerance
	Decreased secretin and cholecystokinin
	Decreased pancreatic secretions
	Decreased biliary secretions
	Impaired vitamin absorption (folate)
	Impaired calcium, iron, and magnesium absorption
	Protein malabsorption
	Zinc deficiency
	Steatorrhea
Ileum (distal)	Impaired vitamin B_{12} absorption
	Impaired bile salt absorption
	Bile salt depletion leads to fat malabsorption, vitamin malabsorption, cholelithiasis, colonic diarrhea and impaired water absorption, hyperoxaluria, and renal calculi
	Gastric hypersecretion

From Gryboski, J. & Walker, W.A. (1983). *Gastrointestinal problems in the infant* (2nd ed., p. 473). Philadelphia: WB Saunders.

enteral feedings and to the trophic effect of gastrointestinal hormones. Most infants receive parenteral nutrition immediately after surgery, but initiation of minimal enteral feedings as soon as the bowel has recovered is important in enhancing villous hyperplasia. Initial feedings may be with sterile water or D5W followed by gradual introduction of casein hydrolysate and fat-modified or elemental formulas or human milk diluted to 5 to 7 kcal/oz.[12, 189] Caloric density is increased slowly, with lactose and solids withheld for several months to allow regeneration of villi in the remaining bowel. Vitamin, mineral, and trace element supplementation is needed owing to increased intestinal loss.[96]

Considerations Related to Feeding Method

The healthy term infant is fed by breast or bottle depending on the parent's choice. The choice of feeding method for preterm or ill infants also depends on maturity, health status, growth pattern, and individual responses to specific methods. These infants can be fed by enteral or parenteral methods, each of which have specific advantages and disadvantages (Table 9–20). Clinically stable preterm infants can be breast-fed. Infants as young as 32 weeks and 1200 g have been reported to have an organized sucking pattern at the breast with two to three sucks per burst followed by a pause and stable transcutaneous oxygen pressures.[163a]

Infants who have not developed suck-swallow coordination, who fatigue easily, or for whom oral feeding is contraindicated owing to health status require an alternative feeding method. With preterm infants this method is usually gavage (transpyloric or intragastric) given either as a bolus or in a continuous drip.

No consistent advantages have been demonstrated for either intragastric or transpyloric feedings. Intragastric gavage permits normal digestive processes and hormonal responses to occur. Tube insertion is generally easy since most infants who require gavage do not have a well-developed gag reflex. Infants who are fed intragastrically are generally able to tolerate higher osmotic loads than those fed transpylorically, with less distention, vomiting, and diarrhea. Risks of intragastric gavage such as regurgitation, aspiration, and gastric distention, which may compromise respiratory function, are reduced with transpyloric feedings. Transpyloric feeding tubes are harder to insert, and this feeding method is associated with complications such as impaired fat absorption, intestinal perforation, and ileus (Table 9–20).

The enteral feeding–induced surge of gut hormones following birth is similar in infants fed by bolus and continuous drip methods.[15] Bolus feedings stimulate cyclic responses in the secretion of gut hormones, insulin, and glucagon that are not seen in infants fed by continuous drip, although which response is best at this age is unknown.[15] Use of mechanical pump infusion systems to deliver human milk by continuous infusion has been associated with loss of milk fat, decreased fat concentrations (especially at low infusion rates), and terminal delivery of a large fat load if fat in the tubing is recovered using an air infusion. Similar findings were not demonstrated with intermittent gavage or bolus feedings.[91, 138] The method and type of feeding influence gastric emptying. Increasing caloric density inhibits gastric emptying, supporting the practice of using diluted formula for the initial feedings.

Parenteral solutions may be given via central or peripheral lines, which have advantages and risks (Table 9–20). Infants on parenteral nutrition require careful monitoring since they are at greater risk for metabolic derangements, electrolyte imbalances, sepsis, anemia, and thromboembolytic complications.

Providing even small amounts of enteral feeding in the first weeks following birth is important to stimulate gut hormones and subsequent maturation of the intestine.[154] There is no postbirth rise in gut hormones

TABLE 9–20. Advantages and Risk of Various Feeding Methods

METHOD	ADVANTAGES	RISKS
Peripheral venous nutrition	Not dependent on GI function No danger of aspiration Low infection risk Few metabolic complications	Difficulty maintaining infusion sites Ischemic necrosis at extravasation sites Cold stress associated with restarting infusion repeatedly Water overload
Central venous nutrition	Higher concentrations of glucose can be given Possible when other methods fail Not dependent on GI function No danger of aspiration Once catheter inserted, less handling and cold stress than with peripheral IV	Surgical procedure (usually) Bacterial and fungal infections Thrombosis with superior vena cava syndrome Embolism Metabolic complications
Intermittent intragastric feeding	Promotes intestinal growth, gut hormone secretion, and bile flow Avoids risks associated with parenteral alimentation	Occasional aspiration Bypass salivary and lingual enzymes
Continuous intragastric feeding	Larger volumes may be tolerated	Not well studied
Transpyloric feeding	Larger volumes tolerated Less danger of aspiration	Intestinal perforation Intestinal perforation Intussusception Altered bacterial flora Impaired fat absorption

From Goldsmith, J.P. & Karotkin, E.H. (1988). *Assisted ventilation in the neonate* (2nd ed., p. 320). Philadelphia: WB Saunders.

in preterm infants on TPN, whereas infants fed orally demonstrate a marked increase in these hormones over the 1st week.[50] Surges of gut hormones still occur after up to 10 days (and perhaps longer) without oral feeding.[15] Avery and Fletcher recommend a gradual reintroduction of enteral feedings in infants managed with TPN.[12] Small volumes of dilute formula help build up mucosal bulk and stimulate development of brush border enzymes and pancreatic function and reduce the distention, vomiting, malabsorption, and diarrhea that often occur with resumption of enteral feeding.

Monitoring Nutritional Status

Nutritional needs are affected by age, weight, maturity, growth rate, and health status. Monitoring nutritional status includes assessment of physical status, tolerance of enteral or parenteral feeding, and growth. McLaren divides nutritional assessment into three areas: status (balance between intake and expenditures), process (how infant's growth has progressed over time and factors affecting this growth), and nonnutritional factors (genetics, psychosocial environment, stress).[263]

An indicator of health and nutritional status is growth. There is general consensus regarding growth rates for term infants. Although preterm infants are often expected to grow initially at a relatively faster rate than term infants, there is a lack of agreement on optimal growth rates and how closely this rate should approximate that of fetuses of similar gestations.

Growth is monitored by daily weight gain and loss and weekly monitoring of other anthropometric parameters (length, head circumference, mean arm circumference, and triceps skin fold thickness).[12, 148] There are problems with these measurements. Length is often measured inaccurately, and both length and head circumference are spared relative to weight in malnutrition. Mean arm circumference reflects muscle and fat deposition, and although sensitive to current protein and energy intake, few standards are available for preterm infants.[148] Triceps skin fold thickness estimates fat stores but values are difficult to interpret and standards are not available for preterm infants.[148]

The use of weight to monitor growth is particularly problematic in VLBW infants. The need for daily weights should be consid-

ered against the stress (and increased energy and caloric consumption) of this procedure. Weight gain may be due to water retention and not new tissue or influenced by the type of equipment attached to the infant.[148] As noted earlier, different growth charts exist, each reflecting the characteristics of the population from which the chart was developed.[186] These curves were not developed using many (or in some cases any) subjects fed human milk or human milk–like preterm formulas as is current practice. An awareness of the limitations of different charts and use of a chart based on a population with characteristics similar to those of the infant being assessed are important for their optimal use.

Nutritional status is also monitored by calculating daily caloric, fluid, and nutrient intake; physical assessment of the infant; biochemical monitoring; and assessment for signs of nutritional deficiencies. Biochemical monitoring to assess the adequacy of protein intake may involve evaluation of serum proteins with short half-lives such as prealbumin and retinol-binding protein. Assessment and monitoring of nutritional tolerance for infants on enteral feedings involve testing of stools for reducing substances and blood, measuring feeding residuals and abdominal girth, and observing for vomiting.[12, 148]

Regurgitation and Reflux

Newborns are more prone to regurgitation, vomiting, and gastroesophageal reflux (GER) owing to anatomic and functional immaturity of their GI system. Regurgitation is common in infants as a result of decreased LES tone and pressure, alterations in esophageal and gastric motility, delayed gastric emptying, entry of air into the stomach with swallowing, increased esophageal peristalsis, and a tendency toward reverse peristalsis. These limitations and the frequency of regurgitation are more marked in preterm infants. Interventions to reduce regurgitation include frequent burping; feeding slowly in a semi-upright position to reduce air swallowing and passage of swallowed air into the duodenum; using small, frequent feedings; and placing the infant in a prone or right lateral position after feeding to enhance gastric emptying.

GER is also seen more frequently in infants, particularly in preterm and ill neonates. GER is defined as the flow of gastric contents into the esophagus often accompanied by regurgitation.[96] Although this is a temporary phenomenon that generally resolves after 6 months, when LES tone increases, GER can be severe enough to result in failure to thrive, aspiration, esophagitis, and dysphagia. Infants with reflux may present with choking, gagging, apnea, or other respiratory symptoms.

Reflux in preterm infants is related to immaturity: decreased LES tone, pressure, and size; intrathoracic LES position; delayed gastric emptying; and impaired intestinal motility, with abdominal distention and higher pressure. Altered esophageal motility and peristalsis lead to poor clearance of refluxed material and increased risk of aspiration.[50, 105] Most infants with reflux respond to interventions such as positioning; small, frequent, or thickened feedings; or drugs (metoclopramide) that enhance gastric emptying. Some infants may require surgical correction.

Necrotizing Enterocolitis

Necrotizing enterocolitis (NEC) is a disorder seen primarily in preterm infants, with an incidence of 3 to 5% in infants admitted to intensive care units.[5, 130] Although the entire gut can be involved, NEC is most prominent in the jejunum, ileum, and colon. Clinical manifestations usually appear at 3 to 10 days and range from signs of feeding intolerance (abdominal distention, residuals, gross or occult blood in the stools, vomiting) or general systemic signs (lethargy, apnea, respiratory distress, thermal instability) to sepsis, shock, and peritonitis with intestinal perforation in about 30% of these infants.[12]

The cause of NEC is unclear with no single etiologic factor found in all infants. NEC is associated with prematurity, infection, hypertonic feedings, hypovolemia, perinatal asphyxia, and hypothermia. Although 90 to 95% of infants have had enteral feedings prior to the development of symptoms, significant mortality has been reported in VLBW infants before the first feeding.[72, 136] In addition early feeding does not necessarily predispose to an increased incidence of NEC.[71, 130, 216] LaGamma and coworkers suggest that small enteral feedings of dilute formula or human milk (along with parenteral feedings) may protect the bowel from NEC by stimulating gut maturation, promoting mucosal integrity, providing substrate for intestinal enzymes, reducing ileus, and increasing perfusion.[136]

Ischemia, feeding, and infection have been proposed as major etiologic events. With asphyxia blood is redistributed to the brain and heart. The bowel may become ischemic, with mucosal damage, ileus, and stasis. Initial gut colonization is followed by bacterial overgrowth and invasion of the injured mucosa. With initiation of enteral intake, feedings remain in the intestinal lumen for extended periods (owing to mucosal damage and limitations in absorptive function in immature infants) and serve as a substrate for further bacterial growth and intramural gas formation. The source of this gas is uncertain but it may arise from bacterial fermentation of carbohydrates.[12, 72]

The specific relationships between feeding and NEC are unclear. Excessive volume or rapid increases in feeding may be the critical factors rather than early feeding per se.[5, 127, 130] Rapid advances in feeding on top of impaired absorptive function secondary to immaturity or ischemia may result in intraluminal accumulation of fermentation products and bacteria derived peptides that lead to mucosal inflammation.[127] A large volume might further stress the mucosa (already injured from ischemia) and further impede blood flow by distention. This may lead to a local hypoxemia, vascular insufficiency, and accumulation of fermentation products due to impaired absorption.[5, 130] Finally, hyperosmolar feedings may overwhelm the immature or damaged mucosa.[232]

Dehydration and Diarrhea

Alterations in function of the GI system also increase the risk for dehydration and diarrhea. Increased transit time in the large intestine (the primary site for water and electrolyte absorption) limits the amount of these substances that can be absorbed. Infant stools tend to be smaller in volume and more frequent and have a higher water content. Infants may also lack an adaptive ability to conserve water and electrolytes when confronted with an osmotic load.[145]

Disruptions in water and electrolyte absorption can markedly increase fluid losses. Diarrhea can result from factors that send excess amounts of disaccharides to the colon that the colon cannot salvage (such as high caloric density diets with high osmotic loads, immaturity in carbohydrate digestive processes, or injury to the intestinal mucosa) or from lack of adequate intestinal flora for colonic salvage. Diarrhea can occur in VLBW or ill infants if large amounts of undigested lactose, a highly osmotic substance, reach the large intestine. The increased osmotic load will pull water into the intestinal lumen and deter water absorption. Additional water will be lost in stool along with electrolytes (potassium, bicarbonate) that are normally reabsorbed with water, with a risk of hypokalemia and metabolic acidosis.

Drug Absorption and Metabolism

Absorption of oral medications in the neonate is altered as follows: (1) decreased bile salts and pancreatic enzymes lead to poorer absorption of fat-soluble drugs; (2) slower gut transit time due to delayed gastric emptying and decreased motility initially delay then prolong absorption; (3) mucus in the stomach may delay absorption; and (4) the lower stomach pH may partially or totally inactivate some drugs. Intestinal absorption of drugs, gut transit time, and motility depend on perfusion and food intake. An ill infant who is NPO may have further impairment of gut function and erratic absorption of oral medications.

The reduced levels of hepatic microsomal enzymes extend the half-life of drugs dependent on them for metabolism and increase the risk of drug intolerance. Metabolic processes in the liver are divided into phase I reactions (oxidation, reduction, and hydrolysis) and phase II reactions (conjugation with glycine, glucuronic acid, and sulphate). Phase I reactions modify the activity of a compound; phase II reactions generally result in complete inactivation. Phase I reactions are reduced in the fetus and newborn, impairing degradation of drugs such as phenytoin, phenobarbital, diazepam, mepivacaine, lidocaine, phenylbutazone, salicylate, indomethacin, furosemide, and sulfa drugs.[168] After 2 weeks of age these enzyme systems mature at varying rates (with activity exceeding adult rates in some cases). As a result, drug metabolism may be markedly altered. Glucuronic acid conjugation is reduced at birth and does not reach adult levels until 24 to 30 months.[168] Other phase II reactions are similar to those in adults.

MATURATIONAL CHANGES DURING INFANCY AND CHILDHOOD

Digestive and absorptive capabilities gradually mature over the first 6 months to 2 years following birth. An important aspect of intestinal maturation is gut closure, which provides protection against the transport of macromolecules across the intestinal mucosa, reducing the risk of infection and allergy development (see Chapter 10). Lower esophageal sphincter (LES) pressure remains low for 1 to 2 months. This sphincter lengthens from 1 cm at birth to 2.5 cm by 6 months, with most of the increased length in the portion of the esophagus below the diaphragm.[96] LES tone increases after 6 months and is associated with resolution of reflux in most infants.[50]

Gastric acid and pepsinogen levels remain at 50% or less of adult levels for 1 to 3 months.[141, 145] Gastric acid production and pepsin activity do not reach adult levels until 2 years, limiting gastric proteolysis in infants.[55, 221] Levels of trypsin reach adult levels by 1 month.[145]

Pancreatic enzymes are minimal for the first 4 to 6 months, thus the infant is dependent on salivary and mammary amylase for initial digestion of carbohydrate. Pancreatic amylase activity increases after 4 to 6 months at about the time that starch (cereal) is introduced into the diet. Cereal is not efficiently digested prior to this time. Since hydrolysis of amylopectin (starch) is incomplete up to about 6 months, neonates given formula thickened with cereal may develop diarrhea.[141, 200]

Activity of maltase, isomaltase, and sucrase remains high into adulthood with some decrease seen in the elderly.[220] Retention of lactase activity is variable and genetically controlled. Lactase activity usually decreases after 3 to 5 years to very low levels.[220] Significant lactase activity is retained primarily in individuals of northern European descent. Mucosal glucose transport is reduced until about 12 months.[165]

Fat absorption does not approach adult efficiency until about 6 months. Lipase reaches adult levels by 2 years, so infants are dependent on lingual-gastric and mammary lipase.[145] Lipolysis and micelle activity are minimal until 4 to 6 months; liver uptake of bile acids is decreased until 6 months.[246, 248]

Introduction of Solid Foods

Maturation of the intestinal system in infancy may be stimulated by weaning and the introduction of solid foods in a manner somewhat similar to changes induced by enteral feed-

TABLE 9–21. Summary of Recommendations for Clinical Practice Related to the Gastrointestinal System and Perinatal Nutrition: Neonate

Assess feeding reflexes, suck-swallow coordination, cardiorespiratory and gastrointestinal function prior to initiating oral feedings (pp. 410–412).

Feed preterm infants slowly in a semi-upright position with frequent burping (pp. 411–412).

Offer nonnutritive sucking to preterm infants during gavage feeding (pp. 410–411, 415–416).

Observe for regurgitation and gastrointestinal reflux (pp. 411–412, 427–428).

Place in prone or right lateral position after feeding (pp. 411–412, 424–427).

Observe respiratory status after feeding (pp. 411–412, 425–427).

Monitor residuals and abdominal girth (pp. 411–412, 428).

Evaluate for signs of dehydration and electrolyte imbalance (pp. 411–412, 421–422).

Monitor stools for reducing substance, blood, and consistency (p. 428).

Record timing and appearance of first meconium stool (p. 410).

Know parameters used to measure growth and factors that alter accuracy of these parameters (pp. 417, 427).

Monitor growth parameters using appropriate curves (pp. 417, 427).

Counsel women regarding nutritional advantages of breast-feeding (pp. 414–415, 417–418, 422–423, Table 9–15).

Support breast-feeding in mothers of term and preterm infants (pp. 417–418, 422–423, 445–446).

Initiate early enteral feeding as appropriate (pp. 409–410, 426–428).

Promote early breast-feeding and colostrum intake (pp. 417–418, 422–423, 445–446, Chapter 4).

Know limitations of gastrointestinal function in term and preterm infants (pp. 410–416, Table 9–14).

Know the effects of health problems or surgery on digestion and absorption (pp. 423–425).

Monitor preterm, small for gestational age, and asphyxiated infants for hypoglycemia (pp. 408, 415, Chapter 13).

Evaluate composition of feedings (formula or human milk) in relationship to an individual infant's gastrointestinal system limitations (pp. 419–423, Table 9–15).

Avoid heating human milk above 55°C (p. 416).

Avoid use of high solute load and caloric density formulas in immature infants (pp. 366–367, 422, Chapter 8).

Evaluate renal function and fluid and electrolyte status in infants on high solute load or caloric density feedings (pp. 366–367, 422, Chapter 8).

Recognize signs of liver dysfunction in infants (p. 416).

Know nutritional requirements for preterm and term infants (pp. 417–418, Tables 9–15 and 9–16).

Monitor nutritional intake to ensure that nutritional requirements are met (pp. 417–418, 427).

Know caloric requirements and factors that alter these requirements (pp. 418–419, 423–425).

Monitor caloric intake of infants (pp. 417–418, 424–425).

Monitor neonates for signs of excessive or inadequate protein, carbohydrate, and fat intake (pp. 414, 417–420).

Monitor preterm infants for signs of late metabolic acidosis (pp. 369–370, 420).

Monitor intake and ratio of vitamin E and linoleic acid (pp. 419, 421, Chapter 5).

Ensure that term and preterm infants receive iron at recommended time points (pp. 421–422, Chapter 5).

Monitor intake of vitamins, minerals, and trace minerals (pp. 420–422, 416).

Provide dietary supplementation (vitamins, minerals, trace elements, calories) as required (pp. 420–422).

Monitor infants on caloric supplements for ketosis, diarrhea, regurgitation, and vomiting (pp. 418–419, 422).

Monitor infants for signs of vitamin, mineral, and trace element deficiencies (pp. 416, 420–422).

Monitor preterm infants for signs of hypocalcemia (pp. 421–422, 424).

Monitor VLBW infants for hyponatremia and hypokalemia (pp. 422–424).

Recognize the advantages and limitations of the use of human milk with preterm infants (pp. 422–423, Tables 9–15, 9–17).

Assist mothers of preterm and ill infants in providing breast milk for their infants (pp. 414–416, 422–423).

Recognize and monitor for signs of complications associated with parenteral nutrition (pp. 423–424, 426–427, Table 9–20).

Recognize potential problems of infants with IUGR and the basis for these problems (pp. 406–408, Table 9–13).

Know the effects of specific health problems on nutritional intake, feeding method, and gastrointestinal function (pp. 423–425).

Use feeding techniques that promote adequate intake and reduce stress in infants with cardiorespiratory problems (pp. 423–428).

Monitor infants following intestinal resection or with ostomies for adequacy of nutritional intake and excessive loss of nutrients (p. 425).

Know the advantages and disadvantages of different feeding methods and monitor infants for potential complications (pp. 425–428, Table 9–20).

Select feeding methods appropriate for an individual infants maturity, age, and health status (pp. 425–427, Table 9–20).

Use dilute formula for initial feedings in VLBW infants and for infants who have been on parenteral feedings (pp. 411, 426–427).

Identify infants at risk for necrotizing enterocolitis and monitor for signs (p. 428).

Recognize and monitor for increased half-life and drug side effects related to altered gastrointestinal and liver function (p. 429).

Avoid use of oral medications in infants who are NPO or following hypoxia (p. 429).

Recognize the effects of maturation of liver enzyme systems on drug metabolism and risks of side effects (pp. 416, 429).

Counsel parents regarding introduction of solids (pp. 429–431).

Page numbers in parentheses following each recommendation refer to pages in the text where rationale for that intervention is discussed.

ings after birth.[141] Timing for introduction of solids should be based on development of neuromuscular processes involved in the ability of the infant to handle solids. The infant's ability to handle foods can be divided into three physiologic stages: (1) nursing (birth to 6 months), when the infant has excellent suck-swallow coordination and does best if fed human milk or formula; (2) transitional (4 to 8 months), when neuromuscular processes needed to swallow pureed solids develop; and (3) modified adult (6 to 12 months), when chopped foods can be swallowed without choking.[20]

There are no particular advantages, and some disadvantages, to introducing solid foods prior to 3 to 4 months in formula-fed or before 5 to 6 months in breast-fed infants. Before 3 to 4 months an extrusion reflex is present (extrusion of material placed on the anterior tongue) and gastroesophageal reflux may still be present. Contrary to what many parents and professionals believe, feeding cereal prior to bedtime in young infants has not been demonstrated to reduce the incidence of night awakenings and may contribute to dental caries and obesity.[26, 156]

Introduction of solid foods is generally recommended at 4 to 6 months for formula-fed infants and after 6 months for breast-fed infants.[20] Infants fed foreign proteins prior to 6 months have a higher incidence of food allergies (see Chapter 10). Cereal is usually the initial solid food given to infants. Rice and barley cereals are of low antigenicity and contain iron in a relatively easy to digest form. Early introduction of high caloric density foods is associated with an increased risk of obesity.[20]

SUMMARY

Supporting nutritional needs and promoting nutritional status of infants are and continue to be a challenge, but one that is critical for optimal outcome. Management of nutritional needs must be based on understanding of the anatomic and physiologic limitations of the gastrointestinal system and the impact of these alterations on the infant's ability to consume, digest, and absorb various nutrients. Recommendations for clinical practice related to the gastrointestinal system and perinatal nutrition are summarized in Table 9–21.

References

1. Adamkin, D.H. (1986). Nutrition in very very low birth weight infants. *Clin Perinatol, 13*, 419.
2. Alemi, B., et al. (1981). Fat digestion in very low birth weight infants: Effect of addition of human milk to low birth weight formula. *Pediatrics, 68*, 484.
3. Allen, R.G. (1980). Omphalocele and gastroschisis. In T.M. Holder & J.W. Ashcraft (Eds.), *Pediatric surgery* (pp. 572–588). Philadelphia: WB Saunders.
4. American Academy of Pediatrics Committee on Nutrition. (1985). *Pediatric nutrition handbook* (2nd ed.). Evanston, IL: American Academy of Pediatrics.
5. Amspacher, K.A. (1989). Necrotizing enterocolitis: The never-ending challenge. *J Perinat Neonat Nurs, 3*(2), 58.
6. Anderson, A.G. (1990). Nutrient requirements of the premature infants. In N.M. van Gelder, R.F. Butterworth, & B.D. Drujan (Eds.), *(Mal)nutrition and the infant brain* (pp. 41–55). New York: Wiley-Liss.
7. Anderson, G. & Vidyasagar, D. (1979). Development of sucking in premature infants from 1 to 7 days postbirth. In G. Anderson & Raff, B. (Eds.), *Neonatal behavioral organization: Nursing research and implications.* New York: AR Liss.
8. Antonowicz, I., Chang, S.K., & Grand, R.J. (1974). Development and distribution of lysosomal enzymes and disaccharides in human fetal intestine. *Gastroenterology, 67*, 51.
9. Arafat, A. (1974). Periodontal states in pregnancy. *J Periodontol, 45*, 641.
10. Atlay, R.D., Gillison, E.W., & Horton, A.L. (1973). A fresh look at pregnancy heartburn. *J Obstet Gynecol Br Comm, 80*, 63.
11. Auricchio, S., Rubino, A., & Murset, G. (1965). Intestinal glycosidase activities in the human embryo, fetus and newborn. *Pediatrics, 35*, 944.
12. Avery, G.B. & Fletcher, A.B. (1987). Nutrition. In G.B. Avery (Ed.), *Neonatology: Pathophysiology and management of the newborn* (pp. 1173–1229). Philadelphia: JB Lippincott.
13. Axelson, I., et al. (1989). Macromolecular absorption in preterm and term infants. *Acta Paediatr Scand, 78*, 532.
14. Aynsley-Green, A. (1982). The control of the adaptation to postnatal nutrition. *Monogr Pediatr, 16*, 59.
15. Aynsley-Green, A. (1985). Metabolic and endocrine interrelations in the human fetus and neonate. *Am J Clin Nutr, 41*, 399.
16. Aynsley-Green, A., et al. (1977). Endocrine and metabolic responses in the human newborn to the first feed of breast milk. *Arch Dis Child, 52*, 291.
17. Aynsley-Green, A., et al. (1990). Gut hormones and regulatory peptides in relation to enteral feeding, gastroenteritis, and necrotizing enterocolitis in infancy. *J Pediatr, 117*, S24.
18. Baiocco, P.J. & Korelitzm B.I. (1985). Small and large bowel disease in pregnancy. In N. Gleicher (Ed.), *Principles of medical therapy in pregnancy* (pp. 820–825). New York: Plenum Press.
19. Barnes, L.W. (1957). Serum histaminase during pregnancy. *Obstet Gynecol, 9*, 730.
20. Barness, L.E. (1981). Introduction of supplemental foods to infants. In E. Lebenthal (Ed.), *Textbook of

gastroenterology and nutrition in infancy (pp. 287–291). New York: Raven Press.

21. Barness, L.A. & Gilbert-Barness, E.F. (1989). What lies ahead in infant nutrition. *Semin Perinatol, 13*, 112.

22. Barnico, L.M. & Cullinane, M.M. (1985). Maternal phenylketonuria: An unexpected challenge. *MCN, 10*, 108.

23. Barron, W.M. (1984). The pregnant surgical patient: Medical evaluation and management. *Ann Intern Med, 101*, 683.

24. Barron, W.M. (1985). Medical evaluation of the pregnant patient requiring nonobstetrical surgery. *Clin Perinatol, 12*, 481.

25. Batey, R.G. & Gallagher, N.D. (1977). Role of the placenta in intestinal absorption of iron in pregnant rats. *Gastroenterology, 72*, 255.

26. Beal, V. (1969). Termination of night feedings in infants. *J Pediatr, 75*, 690.

27. Bell, E.F. & Oh, W. (1988). Nutritional support. In J.P. Goldsmith & E.H. Karotkin (Eds.), *Assisted ventilation of the neonate* (pp. 307–327). Philadelphia: WB Saunders.

28. Bergstein, N.A.M. (1973). *Liver and pregnancy.* Amsterdam: Excerpta Medica.

29. Bernbaum, J.C., et al. (1983). Nonnutritive sucking during gavage feeding enhances growth and maturation in premature infants. *Pediatrics, 71*, 41.

30. Bernstein, L., et al. (1986). Higher maternal levels of free estradiol in first compared to second pregnancy: Early gestational differences. *JNCI, 76*, 1035.

31. Berseth, C.L., et al. (1990). Postpartum changes in patterns of GI regulatory peptides in human milk. *Am J Clin Nutr, 51*, 985.

32. Bitman, J., et al. (1983). Comparison of the lipid composition of breast milk from mothers of term and preterm infants. *Am J Clin Nutr, 38*, 300.

33. Bjorkmanm D.J., Burt, R.W., & Tolman, K.G. (1988). Primary care of women with gastrointestinal disorders. *Clin Obstet Gynecol, 31*, 974.

34. Block, P. & Kelly, T.R. (1989). Management of gallstone pancreatitis during pregnancy and the postpartum period. *Surg Gynecol Obstet, 168*, 426.

35. Bond, J.H., et al. (1980). Colonic conservation of malabsorbed carbohydrate. *Gastroenterology, 78*, 444.

36. Borberg, C., et al. (1980). Obesity in pregnancy: The effect of dietary advice. *Diabetes Care, 3*, 476.

37. Brady, M.S., et al. (1986). Specialized formulas and feedings for infants with malabsorption or formula intolerance. *J Am Diet Assoc, 86*, 191.

38. Brady, M.S., et al. (1982). Formulas and human milk for premature infants: A review and update. *J Am Diet Assoc, 81*, 191.

39. Brandes, J.M. (1967). First trimester nausea and vomiting as related to outcome of pregnancy. *Obstet Gynecol, 30*, 427.

40. Braverman, D.Z., Johnson, M.L., & Kern, F. (1980). Effects of pregnancy and contraceptive steroids on gall bladder. *N Engl J Med, 302*, 363.

41. Brennion, I.J. & Grundy, S.M. (1978). Risk factors for the development of cholelithiasis in man. *N Engl J Med, 299*, 1161.

42. Brewer, M.M., Bates, M.R., & Vannoy, L.P. (1989). Postpartum changes in maternal weight and body fat depots in lactating and nonlactating women. *Am J Clin Nutr, 49*, 259.

43. Broach, J. & Newton, N. (1988). Food and beverages in labor. Part I: Cross-cultural and historical practices. *Birth, 15*, 81.

44. Broach, J. & Newton, N. (1988). Food and beverages in labor. Part II: The effects of cessation of oral intake during labor. *Birth, 15*, 88.

45. Brock-Utne, J.G., et al. (1980). Effect of domperidone on lower esophageal sphincter tone in late pregnancy. *Anesthesiology, 53*, 321.

46. Brock-Utne, J.G., et al. (1981). Gastric and lower esophageal sphincter pressures in early pregnancy. *Br J Anaesth, 53*, 381.

47. Brock-Utne, J.G., et al. (1989). Influence of preoperative gastric aspiration on the volume and pH of gastric contents in obstetric patients undergoing caesarean section. *Br J Anaesth, 62*, 307.

48. Brooke, O.G. (1987). Nutritional requirements of low and very low birthweight infants. *Ann Rev Nutr, 7*, 91.

49. Brucker, M.C. (1988). Management of minor discomforts in pregnancy. III. Managing gastrointestinal problems in pregnancy. *J Nurse Midwifery, 33*, 67.

50. Bucuvalas, J.C. & Balistreri, W.F. (1987). The neonatal gastrointestinal tract: Development. In A. A. Fanaroff & R.J. Martin (Eds.), *Neonatal-perinatal medicine—Diseases of the fetus and infant* (pp. 894–899). St. Louis: CV Mosby.

51. Carlisle, W.R. (1987). The liver and pregnancy. *Ala Med, 57(3)*, 32.

52. Chenger, P. & Kovacik, A. (1987). Dental hygiene during pregnancy: A review. *MCN, 12*, 342.

53. Chessex, P., et al. (1983). Quality of growth in premature infants fed their own mother's milk. *J Pediatr, 102*, 107.

54. Chiles, C., et al. (1979). Lactose utilization in the newborn: Role of colonic flora. *Pediatr Res, 13*, 365.

55. Christie, D.L. (1981). Development of gastric function during the first month of life. In E. Lebenthal (Ed.), *Textbook of gastroenterology and nutrition in infancy* (pp. 109–120). New York: Raven Press.

56. Christofides, N.D., et al. (1982). Decreased plasmin motilin concentrations in pregnancy. *Br Med J, 285*, 1453.

57. Clark, D.H. (1953). Peptic ulcer in women. *Br Med J, 1*, 1254.

58. Cohen, S.E. & Masse, R.I. (1985). Physiology of pregnancy. In J.M. Baden & J.B. Brodsky (Eds.), *The pregnant surgical patient* (pp. 83–104). New York: Futura.

59. Colley, J.R. & Creamer, B. (1968). Sucking and swallowing in infants. *Br Med J, 2*, 422.

60. Combes, B., et al. (1963). Alterations in sulfobromophthalein sodium removal mechanisms from blood during normal pregnancy. *J Clin Invest, 42*, 1431.

61. Committee on Nutrition, American Academy of Pediatrics. (1979). *Pediatric nutrition handbook* (pp. 119–138). Evanston, IL: American Academy of Pediatrics.

62. Connon, J. (1988). Gastrointestinal complications. In G.N. Burrow & T.F. Ferris (Eds.), *Medical complications during pregnancy* (pp. 303–317). Philadelphia: WB Saunders.

63. Cordero, J.F., et al. (1981). Is Bendectin a teratogen? *JAMA, 245*, 2307.

64. Cripps, A.W. & Williams, V.J. (1975). The effect of pregnancy and lactation on food intake, gastrointestinal anatomy and the absorptive capacity

of the small intestine in the albino rat. *Br J Nutr, 33*, 17.

65. Cunningham, J.T. (1985). The esophagus and stomach. In N. Gleicher (Ed.), *Principles of medical therapy in pregnancy* (pp. 813–819). New York: Plenum Press.

66. Davison, J.S., Davison, M.C., & Hay, D.M. (1970). Gastric emptying time in late pregnancy and labour. *J Obstet Gynaecol Br Comm, 77*, 37.

67. DeCurtis, M., et al. (1986). Effect of nonnutritive sucking on nutrient retention in preterm infants. *J Pediatr, 109*, 888.

68. De Liefde, B. (1984). The dental care of pregnant women. *NZ Dent J, 80*, 40.

69. Dickason, E.J., Schult, M.O., & Morris, E.M. (1978). *Maternal and infant drugs and nursing interventions.* New York: McGraw-Hill.

70. Douglas, M.J. (1988). Commentary: The case against a more liberal food and fluid policy in labor. *Birth, 15*, 93.

71. Dunn, L., et al. (1988). Beneficial effects of early hypocaloric enteral feeding on neonatal gastrointestinal function: Preliminary report of a randomized trial. *J Pediatr, 112*, 622.

72. Egan, E.A. (1981). Neonatal necrotizing enterocolitis. In E. Lebenthal (Ed.), *Textbook of gastroenterology and nutrition in infancy* (pp. 979–986). New York: Raven Press.

73. Ehrenkranz, R.A. (1989). Mineral needs of the very-low-birthweight infant. *Semin Perinatol, 13*, 142.

74. Euler, A., et al. (1977). Increased serum gastrin concentrations and gastric acid hyposecretion in the immediate newborn period. *Gastroenterology, 72*, 1271.

75. Everson, G.T., et al. (1982). Gallbladder function in the human female: Effect of the ovulatory cycle, pregnancy and contraceptive steroids. *Gastroenterology, 82*, 711.

76. Fairweather, D.V.I. (1968). Nausea and vomiting in pregnancy. *Am J Obset Gynecol, 102*, 135.

77. Fallon, H.J. (1988). Liver diseases. In G.N. Burrow & T.F. Ferris (Eds.), *Medical complications during pregnancy* (pp. 318–344). Philadephia: WB Saunders.

78. Fisher, R.S., Roberts, G.S., & Grabowski, C.J. (1978). Altered lower esophageal sphincter function during early pregnancy. *Gastroenterology, 74*, 1233.

79. Forbes, G.B. (1981). Nutritional adequacy of human breast milk for premature infants. In E. Lebenthal (Ed.), *Textbook of gastroenterology and nutrition in infancy* (pp. 321–329). New York: Raven Press.

80. Forsyth, J.S., Donnet, L., & Ross, P.E. (1990). A study of the relationship between bile salts, bile-salt stimulated lipase, and free fatty acids in breast milk: Normal infants and those with breast milk jaundice. *J Pediatr Gastroenterol Nutr, 11*, 205.

81. Freemark, M. & Handwerger, S. (1989). The role of placental lactogen in the regulation of fetal metabolism and growth. *J Pediatr Gastroenterol Nutr, 8*, 281.

82. Frier, S. & Lebenthal, E. (1989). Neuroendocrine-immune interactions in the gut. *J Pediatr Gastroenterol Nutr, 9*, 4.

83. Fullman, H. & Ippoliti, A. (1986). Acid peptic disease in pregnancy. In V.K. Rustgi & J.N. Cooper (Eds.), *Gastrointestinal and hepatic complications in pregnancy* (pp. 87–103). New York: John Wiley & Sons.

84. Galbraith, R.M. (1985). Liver disease: General considerations. In N. Gleicher (Ed.), *Principles of medical therapy in pregnancy* (pp. 829–832). New York: Plenum Press.

85. Galeano, N.F. & Roy, C.C. (1985). Feeding of the premature infant. In F. Litshitz (Ed.), *Nutrition for special needs in infancy: Protein hydrolysates* (pp. 213–228). New York: Marcel Dekker.

86. Georgieff, M.K. & Gasnow, S.R. (1986). Nutritional assessment of the neonate. *Clin Perinatol, 13*, 73.

87. Gersch, I. & Catchpole, H.R. (1960). The nature of ground substance and connective tissue. *Perspect Biol Med, 3*, 282.

88. Gingell, R.L., Pieroni, D.R., & Hornung, M.G. (1981). Growth problems associated with congenital heart disease in infancy. In E. Lebenthal (Ed.), *Textbook of gastroenterology and nutrition in infancy* (pp. 853–860). New York: Raven Press.

89. Grand, R.J., Watkins, J.B., & Torti, F.M. (1976). Development of the human gastrointestinal tract: A review. *Gastroenterology, 70*, 790.

90. Greenhalf, J.O. & Leonard, H.S.D. (1973). Laxatives in the treatment of constipation in pregnant and breast feeding mothers. *Practitioner, 210*, 259.

91. Greer, F.D., McCormick, A., & Loker, J. (1984). Changes in the fat concentration of human milk during delivery by intermittent bolus and continuous mechanical pump infusion. *J Pediatr, 105*, 745.

92. Gross, S.J. (1983). Growth and biochemical response of preterm infants fed human milk or modified infant formula. *N Engl J Med, 308*, 237.

93. Gross, T.L. & Sokol, R.J. (1989). *Intrauterine growth retardation: A practical approach.* Chicago: Year Book Medical Publishers.

94. Gross, T.L. & Kazzi, G.M. (1985). Effects of maternal malnutrition and obesity on pregnancy outcome. In N. Gleicher (Ed.), *Principles of medical therapy in pregnancy* (pp. 332–351). New York: Plenum Press.

95. Gryboski, J.D., Thayer, W.R., & Spiro, H.M. (1963). Esophageal motility in infants and children. *Pediatrics, 31*, 382.

96. Gryboski, J.D. & Walker, W.A. (1983). *Gastrointestinal problems in the infant* (2nd ed.). Philadelphia: WB Saunders.

97. Hack, M., Estabrook, M., & Robertson, S. (1985). Development of sucking rhythm in preterm infants. *Early Hum Dev, 11*, 133.

98. Hack, M. (1987). The sensorimotor development of the preterm infant. In A.A. Fanaroff & R.J. Martin (Eds.), *Neonatal-perinatal medicine—Diseases of the fetus and infant* (pp. 473–494). St Louis: CV Mosby.

99. Halliday, H.L., Lappin, T.R.J., & McClure, G. (1984). Iron status of the preterm infant during the first year of life. *Biol Neonate, 45*, 228.

100. Hamosh, M. (1987). Compensatory enzymatic digestive mechanisms in the very-low-birthweight infant. In M. Xanthou (Ed.), *New aspects of nutrition in pregnancy, infancy and prematurity* (pp. 196–219). New York: Elsevier.

101. Hamosh, M., et al. (1978). Fat digestion in the stomach of premature infants. *J Pediatr, 93*, 674.

102. Hamosh, M., et al. (1984). Lipids in milk and the first steps in their digestion. *Pediatrics, 75* (Suppl.), 146.

103. Harding, J.E. & Charlton, V. (1989). Treatment of the growth-retarded fetus by augmentation of substrate supply. *Semin Perinatol, 13*, 211.

104. Heird, W.C. & Kashyap, S. (1988). Parenteral feeding during the neonatal period. In C.T. Jones (Ed.), *Research in perinatal medicine (VII): Fetal and neonatal development* (pp. 598–612). Ithaca, NY: Perinatology Press.

105. Herbst, J.J. & Mizell, L.L. (1985). Gastroesophageal reflux. In N.M. Nelson (Ed.), *Current therapy in neonatal-perinatal medicine 1985–1986* (pp. 183–186). Philadelphia: BC Decker.

106. Hey, V.M.H. & Ostick, D.G. (1978). Metaclopramide and the gastroesophageal sphincter: A study in pregnant women with heartburn. *Anesthesia, 33*, 462.

107. Hodge, C., et al. (1984). Salivary amylase and gastric amylase in premature infants: Their potential role in glucose polymer hydrolysis. *Pediatr Res, 18*, 998.

108. Hoverstad, T., Bohmer, T., & Fausa, O. (1982). Absorption of short-chain fatty acids from the human colon measured by the 14CO2 breath test. *Scand J Gastroenterol, 17*, 373.

109. Huff, P.S. (1980). Safety of drug therapy for nausea and vomiting of pregnancy. *J Fam Pract, 11*, 969.

110. Hustead, V.A., et al. (1984). Relationship of vitamin A (retinol) status to lung disease in the preterm infant. *J Pediatr, 105*, 610.

111. Hytten, F.E. & Chamberlain, G. (1980). *Clinical physiology in obstetrics* (pp. 193–223). Oxford: Blackwell Scientific Publications.

112. Hytten, F.E. & Leitch, I. (1971). *The physiology of human pregnancy* (2nd ed., 165–178). Oxford: Blackwell Scientific Publications.

113. Ingerslev, M. & Teilum, G. (1945). Biopsy studies on the liver in pregnancy. II. Liver biopsy in normal pregnant women. *Acta Obstet Gynecol Scand, 25*, 352.

114. Institute of Medicine. (1990). *Nutrition during pregnancy*. Washington, DC: National Academy Press.

115. James, D. (1990). Diagnosis and management of fetal growth retardation. *Arch Dis Child, 65*, 360.

116. Jarnfelt-Samsioe, A. (1987). Nausea and vomiting in pregnancy: A review. *Obstet Gynecol Surv, 41*, 422.

117. Jarnfelt-Samsioe, A., Samsioe, G., & Velinder, G.M. (1983). Nausea and vomiting in pregnancy—A contribution to its epidemiology. *Gynecol Obstet Invest, 16*, 221.

118. Jarnfelt-Samsioe, A., et al. (1985). Some new aspects of emesis gravidarum. *Gynecol Obstet Invest, 19*, 174.

119. Kabara, J.J. (1980). Lipids as host resistance factors of human milk. *Nutr Rev, 38*, 65.

120. Kappy, M.S. & Morrow, G. (1980). A diagnostic approach to metabolic acidosis in children. *Pediatrics, 65*, 351.

121. Kashyap, S., et al. (1990). Growth, nutrient retention and metabolic responses of LBW infants fed supplemented and unsupplemented preterm human milk. *Am J Clin Nutr, 52*, 254.

122. Katz, L. & Hamilton, J.R. (1974). Fat absorption in infants of birthweight less than 1300 g. *J Pediatr, 85*, 608.

123. Kauppila, A., Ylikorkala, O., & Jarrimen, P.A. (1976). The function of the anterior pituitary-adrenal cortex axis in hyperemesis gravidarum. *Br J Obstet Gynaecol, 83*, 11.

124. Kazzi, G.M. & Gross, T.L. (1985). Vitamins and minerals in pregnancy. In N. Gleicher (Ed.), *Principles of medical therapy in pregnancy* (pp. 315–320). New York: Plenum Press.

125. Kennedy, K.A. (1989). Dietary antioxidants in the prevention of oxygen-induced injury. *Semin Perinatol, 13*, 97.

126. Kern, F., et al. (1981). Biliary lipids, bile acids and gall bladder function in human females: Effects of pregnancy and the ovulatory cycle. *J Clin Invest, 68*, 1229.

127. Kien, C.L., et al. (1989). Digestion, absorption and fermentation of carbohydrates. *Semin Perinatol, 13*, 78.

128. Kien, C.L. (1990). Colonic fermentation of carbohydrate in the premature infant: Possible relevance to necrotizing enterocolitis. *J Pediatr, 117*, S52.

129. King, J.C. & Weininger, J. (1989). Nutrition during pregnancy. *Semin Perinatol, 13*, 162.

130. Kleigman, R.M. (1990). Models of the pathogenesis of necrotizing enterocolitis. *J Pediatr, 117*, S2.

131. Klion, F.M. & Wolke, A. (1985). The liver in normal pregnancy. In S.H. Cherry, R.L. Berkowitz, & N.G. Kase (Eds.), *Rovinsky and Guttmacher's medical, surgical, and gynecological complications of pregnancy* (pp. 207–214). Baltimore: Williams & Wilkins.

132. Kolacek, S., et al. (1990). Ontogeny of pancreatic endocrine function. *Arch Dis Child, 65*, 178.

133. Koldovsky, O. (1978). Digestion and absorption. In U. Stave (Ed.), *Perinatal physiology* (2nd ed., pp. 317–356). New York: Plenum Press.

134. Kristal, A.R. & Rush, D. (1984). Maternal nutrition and duration of gestation: A review. *Clin Obstet Gynecol, 27*, 553.

135. Kullander, S. & Kallen, B. (1976). A prospective study of drugs and pregnancy: II. Anti-emetic drugs. *Acta Obstet Gynecol Scand, 55*, 105.

136. LaGamma, E.F., Ostertag, S.G., & Birenbaum, H. (1985). Failure of delayed oral feeding to prevent necrotizing enterocolitis. *Am J Dis Child, 139*, 355.

137. Latham, P.S. (1985). Liver diseases of pregnancy. In N. Gleicher (Ed.), *Principles of medical therapy in pregnancy* (pp. 832–842). New York: Plenum Press.

138. Lavine, M. & Clark, R.M. (1989). The effect of short-term refrigeration of milk and addition of breast milk fortifier on the delivery of lipids during tube feeding. *J Pediatr Gastroenterol Nutr, 8*, 496.

139. Lawson, M., Kern, F., & Everson, G.T. (1985). Gastrointestinal transit time in human pregnancy: Prolongation in the second and third trimesters followed by postpartum normalization. *Gastroenterology, 89*, 996.

140. Lebenthal, E. (1982). Gastrointestinal ontogeny and its impact on infant feeding. *Monogr Pediatr, 16*, 17.

141. Lebenthal, E. (1983). Impact of digestion and absorption in the weaning period on infant feeding practices. *Pediatrics, 75* (Suppl.), 207.

142. Lebenthal, E. & Lee, P.C. (1980). Development of functional response in human exocrine pancreas. *Pediatrics, 66*, 556.

143. Lebenthal, E. & Lee, P.C. (1983). Interactions of determinants in the ontogeny of the gastrointestinal tract: A unified concept. *Pediatr Res, 17*, 19.

144. Lebenthal, G., Lee, P.C., & Heitlinyer, L.A. (1983).

Impact of development of the gastrointestinal tract on infant feeding. *J Pediatr, 102,* 1.

145. Lebenthal, E. & Leung, Y.K. (1988). Feeding the premature and compromised infant: Gastrointestinal considerations. *Pediatr Clin North Am, 35,* 215.

146. Lebenthal, E. & Tucker, N.T. (1986). Carbohydrate digestion: Development in early infancy. *Clin Perinatol, 13,* 37.

147. Lee, D.B. (1983). Unanticipated stimulatory action of glucocorticoids on epithelial calcium absorption: Effect of dexamethasone on rat distal colon. *J Clin Invest, 71,* 322.

148. Lefrak-Okikawa, L. (1988). Nutritional management of the very low birth weight infant. *J Perinat Neonat Nurs, 2,* 66.

149. Lester, R. (1977). The development of bile acid synthesis. In *Selected aspects of perinatal gastroenterology* (pp. 22–29). Mead Johnson Symposium on Perinatal and Developmental Medicine, No. 11. Evansville, IN: Mead Johnson.

150. Levy, N., Lemberg, E., & Sharf, M. (1971). Bowel habit in pregnancy. *Digestion, 4,* 216.

151. Lind, J.F., et al. (1968). Heartburn in pregnancy: A manometric study. *Can Med Assoc J, 98,* 571.

152. Lucas, A., Bloom, S.R., & Aynsley-Green, A. (1978). Metabolic and endocrine events at the time of the first feed of human milk in preterm and term infants. *Arch Dis Child, 53,* 731.

153. Lucas, A., Bloom, S.R., & Aynsley-Green, A. (1982). Postnatal surges in plasma gut hormones in term and preterm infants. *Biol Neonate, 41,* 63.

154. Lucas, A., Bloom, S.R., & Aynsley-Green, A. (1986). Gut hormones and "minimal enteral feeding." *Acta Paediatr Scand, 75,* 719.

155. Luder, A.S. & Greene, C.L. (1989). Maternal phenylketonuria and hyperphenylanemia: Implications for medical practice in the United States. *Am J Obstet Gynecol, 161,* 1102.

156. Mackin, M.L. (1990). Infant sleep and bedtime cereal. *Am J Dis Child, 143,* 1066.

157. MacLean, W.C. & Fink, B.B. (1980). Lactose malabsorption by premature infants: Magnitude and clinical significance. *J Pediatr, 97,* 383.

158. Martin, R.J., et al. (1979). Effect of supine and prone position on arterial oxygen tension in the preterm infant. *Pediatrics, 63,* 528.

159. Masson, G.M., Anthony, F., & Chau, E. (1985). Serum chorionic gonado-tropin (hCG), schwangerschaftsprotein 1 (SP1), progesterone and oestradiol levels in patients with nausea and vomiting in early pregnancy. *Br J Obstet Gynaecol, 92,* 211.

160. Maxwell, K.B. & Niebyl, J.R. (1982). Treatment of nausea and vomiting in pregnancy. In J.R. Niebyl (Ed.), *Drug use in pregnancy* (pp. 9–19). Philadelphia: Lea & Febiger.

161. McLain, C.R. (1963). Amniography studies of the gastrointestinal motility of the human fetus. *Am J Obstet Gynecol, 86,* 1079.

162. McLaren, D.S. (1982). Nutritional assessment. In D.S. McLaren & D. Burman (Eds.), *Textbook of paediatric nutrition* (2nd ed.). Edinburgh: Churchill Livingstone.

163. McNeish, A.S., Mayne, A., & Ducker, D.A. (1983). Development of D-glucose absorption in the perinatal period. *J Pediatr Gastroenterol Nutr, 2,* S222.

163a. Meier, P. (1990). Nursing management of breast feeding for preterm infants. In S.G. Funk, et al. (Eds.), *Key aspects of recovery: Improving nutrition, rest, and mobility* (pp. 77–82). New York: Springer.

164. Meyer, W.W. & Lind, J. (1966). Postnatal changes in portal circulation. *Arch Dis Child, 41,* 606.

165. Mobassaleh, M., et al. (1985). Development of carbohydrate absorption in the fetus and neonate. *Pediatrics, 75* (Suppl.), 160.

166. Monheit, A.G., Cousins, L., & Resnik, R. (1980). The puerperium: Anatomic and physiologic readjustments. *Clin Obstet Gynecol, 23,* 973.

167. Moore, K.L. (1988). *The developing human: Clinically oriented embryology* (4th ed., pp. 170–206; 217–245). Philadelphia: WB Saunders.

168. Morselli, P.L. & Thiercelin, J.F. (1987). Perinatal pharmacology. In L. Stern & P. Vert (Eds.), *Neonatal medcine* (pp. 192–205). New York: Masson Publishing.

169. Mueller, M.N. & Kappas, A. (1964). Estrogen pharmacology. I. The influence of estradiol and estriol on the hepatic disposal of sulfobromophthalein (BSP) in man. *J Clin Invest, 43,* 1905.

170. Murray, F.A. & Erskine, J. (1957). Gastric secretion in pregnancy. *J Obstet Gynaecol Br Comm, 64,* 373.

171. Naeye, R.L. (1990). Maternal body weight and pregnancy outcome. *Am J Clin Nutr, 52,* 273.

172. Nagler, R. & Spiro, H.M. (1961). Heartburn in late pregnancy: Manometric studies of esophageal motor function. *J Clin Invest, 40,* 954.

172a. Food and Nutrition Board. (1989). *Recommended Dietary Allowances* (10th ed.) Washington, DC: National Academy of Sciences, National Research Council.

173. Nebel, O.T., Fornes, M.F., & Castell, D.O. (1976). Symptomatic gastroesophageal reflux: Incidence and precipitating factors. *Am J Dig Dis, 21,* 953.

174. Nimmo, W.S., Wilson, J., & Prescott, L.F. (1975). Narcotic analgesia and delayed gastric emptying during labor. *Lancet, 1,* 890.

175. Norman, A., Strandvik, B., & Ojamae, O. (1972). Bile acids and pancreatic enzymes during absorption in the newborn. *Acta Paediatr Scand, 61,* 571.

176. O'Leary, M.J. (1983). Neonatal nutrition. In W.A. Hodson & W.E. Troug (Eds.), *Critical care of the newborn* (pp. 32–46). Philadelphia: WB Saunders.

177. O'Leary, M.J. (1988). Nourishing the premature and low birth weight infant. In P.L. Pipes (Ed.), *Nutrition in infancy and childhood* (4th ed., pp. 301–360). St. Louis: CV Mosby.

178. O'Sullivan, G.M., et al. (1987). Noninvasive measurement of gastric emptying in obstetric patients. *Anesth Analg, 66,* 505.

179. Okamoto, E., et al. (1982). Use of medium chain triglycerides in feeding low birth weight infants. *Am J Dis Child, 136,* 428.

180. Olson, M. (1970). The benign effects on rabbit's lungs of the aspiration of water compared with 5% glucose or milk. *Pediatrics, 46,* 538.

181. Page, E.W., Villee, C.A., & Villee, D.B. (1981). *Human reproduction: Essentials of reproductive and perinatal medicine.* Philadelphia: WB Saunders.

182. Palmer, R.L. (1973). A psychosomatic study of vomiting in early pregnancy. *J Psychosom Res, 17,* 303.

183. Parry, E., Shields, R., & Tumbull, A.C. (1970). Transit time in the small intestine in pregnancy. *J Obstet Gynaecol Br Comm, 77,* 900.

184. Parry, E., Shields, R., & Tumbull, A.C. (1970). The effect of pregnancy on colonic absorption of sodium, potassium and water. *Br J Obstet Gynaecol, 77,* 616.

185. Pauerstein, C. (1987). *Clinical obstetrics*. New York: John Wiley & Sons.

186. Pereira, G.R. & Barbosa, N.M. (1986). Controversies in neonatal nutrition. *Pediatr Clin North Am, 33*, 65.

187. Pereira, G.R. & Zucker, A. (1986). Nutritional deficiencies in the neonate. *Clin Perinatol, 13*, 175.

188. Pike, R.L. & Gursky, D.S. (1970). Further evidence of deleterious effects produced by sodium restriction during pregnancy. *Am J Clin Nutr, 23*, 883.

189. Pitcher-Wilmott, R., Shutack, J.G., & Fox, W.W. (1979). Decreased lung volume after nasogastric feeding of neonates recovering from respiratory disease. *J Pediatr, 95*, 119.

190. Present, D.H. (1985). Disorders of the biliary tract and pregnancy. In S.H. Cherry, R.L. Berkowtiz, & N.G. Kase (Eds.), *Rovinsky and Guttmacher's medical, surgical, and gynecological complications of pregnancy* (pp. 215–220). Baltimore: Williams & Wilkins.

191. Pritchard, J.A., MacDonald, P.C., & Gant, N. (1985). *Williams obstetrics* (16th ed.). New York: Appleton-Century-Crofts.

192. Raiha, N.C.R. (1985). Nutritional proteins in milk and the protein requirement of normal infants. *Pediatrics, 75*(Suppl.), 136.

193. Rassin, D. (1984). Nutritional requirements for the fetus and the neonate. In P.L. Ogra (Ed.), *Neonatal infections: Nutritional and immunologic aspects* (pp. 205–227). Orlando, FL: Grune & Stratton.

194. Rassin, D.K. (1990). Quality of human milk versus formulas: Protein composition. In N.M. van Gelder, R.F. Butterworth, & B.D. Drujan (Eds.), *(Mal)nutrition and the infant brain* (pp. 57–64). New York: Wiley-Liss.

195. Roberts, R.B. & Shirley, M.A. (1974). Reducing the risk of acid aspiration during cesarean section. *Anesth Analg, 53*, 859.

196. Rogers, I.M., et al. (1974). Neonatal secretion of gastrin and glucagon. *Arch Dis Child, 59*, 796.

197. Rooney, P.J., et al. (1975). Immunoreactive gastrin and gestation. *Am J Obstet Gynecol, 122*, 834.

198. Rosso, P. (1987). Regulation of food intake during pregnancy and lactation. *Ann NY Acad Sci, 499*, 191.

199. Rosso, P.R. (1990). Prenatal nutrition and brain growth. In N.M. van Gelder, R.F. Butterworth, & B.D. Drujan (Eds.), *(Mal)nutrition and the infant brain* (pp. 25–40). New York: Wiley-Liss.

199a. Rosso, P. (1990). *Nutrition and metabolism in pregnancy*. New York: Oxford University Press.

200. Roy, C. (1987). Intestinal adaptation, maturation and related disorders. In L. Stern & P. Vert (Eds.), *Neonatal medicine* (pp. 987–1011). New York: Masson Publishing.

201. Rubin, P.H. & Janowitz, H.D. (1985). The digestive tract and pregnancy. In S.H. Cherry, D.L. Berkowtiz, & N.G. Kase (Eds.), *Rovinsky and Guttmacher's medical, surgical, and gynecological complications of pregnancy* (pp. 196–206). Baltimore: Williams & Wilkins.

202. Rush, D., Johnstone, F.D., & King, J.C. (1988). Nutrition and pregnancy. In G.N. Burrow & T.F. Ferris (Eds.), *Medical complications during pregnancy* (pp. 117–135). Philadelphia: WB Saunders.

203. Rushton, C.H. (1990). Necrotizing enterocolitis: Part I. pathogenesis and diagnosis. *MCN, 15*, 296.

204. Sadler, T.W. (1985). *Langman's medical embryology* (5th ed., pp. 224–246). Baltimore: Williams & Wilkins.

205. Samant, A., et al. (1976). Gingivitis and periodontal disease during pregnancy. *J Periodontol, 47*, 415.

206. Schanler, R.J. (1989). Human milk for preterm infants: Nutritional and immune factors. *Semin Perinatol, 13*, 69.

207. Schrade, R.R., et al. (1986). Gastric emptying time during pregnancy. *Gastroenterology, 86*, 1234.

208. Schreiner, R.L., et al. (1982). Lack of lactobezoars in infants given predominantly whey protein formula. *Am J Dis Child, 136*, 437.

209. Scragg, R.K.R., McMichael, A.J., Seamark, R.F. (1984). Oral contraceptives, pregnancy and endogenous estrogen in gallstone disease. *Br Med J, 288*, 1795.

210. Sheikh, G.N. (1971). Observations of maternal weight behavior during the puerperium. *Am J Obstet Gynecol, 111*, 244.

211. Shenai, J.P., Chytil, F., & Stahlman, M.T. (1985). Vitamin A status of neonates with bronchopulmonary dysplasia. *Pediatr Res, 19*, 185.

212. Sherry, S.N. & Kramer, J.C. (1955). The time of passage of the first stool and first urine. *J Pediatr, 46*, 158.

213. Siegel, M., Lebenthal, E., & Krantz, B. (1984). Effect of caloric density on gastric emptying in premature infants. *J Pediatr, 102*, 118.

214. Siegel, M., Krantz, B., & Lebenthal, E. (1985). Effect of fat and carbohydrate composition on the gastric emptying of isocaloric feeding in premature infants. *Gastroenterology, 89*, 785.

215. Signer, E., et al. (1974). Role of bile salts in fat malabsorption in premature infants. *Arch Dis Child, 49*, 174.

216. Slagle, T.A. & Gross, S.J. (1988). Effect of early low-volume enteral substrate on subsequent feeding tolerance in very low birth-weight infants. *J Pediatr, 113*, 526.

217. Soules, M.R., et al. (1980). Nausea and vomiting of pregnancy: Role of human chorionic gonadotropin and 17-hydroxyprogesterone. *Obstet Gynecol, 55*, 696.

218. Stahl, G., Spear, M.L., & Hamosh, M. (1986). Intravenous administrations of lipid emulsions to premature infants. *Clin Perinatol, 13*, 133.

219. Stern, L. (1982). Early postnatal growth of low birth weight infants: What is optimal? *Acta Paediatr Scand, 296*, 6.

219a. Suidan, J.S. & Young, B.K. (1986). The acute abdomen in pregnancy. In V.K. Rustgi & J.N. Cooper (Eds.), *Gastrointestinal and hepatic complications in pregnancy* (p. 30). New York: John Wiley & Sons.

220. Sunshine, P. (1977). Absorption and malabsorption of carbohydrates. In *Selected aspects of perinatal gastroenterology* (pp. 11–16). Mead Johnson Symposium on Perinatal and Developmental Medicine, No. 11. Evansville, IN: Mead Johnson.

221. Sunshine, P. (1977). Digestion and absorption of proteins. In *Selected aspects of perinatal gastroenterology* (pp. 17–21). Mead Johnson Symposium on Perinatal and Developmental Medicine, No. 11. Evansville, IN: Mead Johnson.

222. Szabo, J.S., Hillemeier, A.C., & Oh, W. (1985). Effect of nonnutritive and nutritive suck on gastric emptying in premature infants. *J Pediatr Gastroenterol Nutr, 4*, 348.

223. Takeuchi, K. & Okabe, S. (1984). Factors related to gastric hypersecretion during pregnancy and lactation. *Dig Dis Sci, 29*, 248.

224. Thaler, M.M. (1981). Liver function and maturation in the perinatal period. In E. Lebenthal (Ed.), *Textbook of gastroenterology and nutrition in infancy* (pp. 177–184). New York: Raven Press.

225. Tierson, F.D., Olsen, C.L., & Hook, E.B. (1986). Nausea and vomiting of pregnancy and association with pregnancy outcome. *Am J Obstet Gynecol, 155,* 1017.

226. Tindall, V.R. (1965). The liver in pregnancy. *Clin Obstet Gynecol, 2,* 441.

227. Tomomasa, T., et al. (1987). Gasteroduodenal motility in neonates: Response to human milk compared with cow's milk formula. *Pediatrics, 80,* 434.

228. Topper, W.H. (1981). Enteral feeding methods for compromised neonates and infants. In E. Lebenthal (Ed.), *Textbook of gastroenterology and nutrition in infancy* (pp. 645–658). New York: Raven Press.

229. Torfs, C., Curry, C., & Roeper, P. (1990). Gastroschisis. *J Pediatr, 116,* 1.

230. Tsang, R. (1985). *Vitamin and mineral requirements in preterm infants.* New York: Marcel Dekker.

231. Uauy, R., Treen, M., & Hoffman, D.R. (1989). Essential fatty acid metabolism and requirements during development. *Semin Perinatol, 13,* 118.

232. Udall, J.N. (1990). Gastrointestinal tract host defense and necrotizing enterocolitis. *J Pediatr, 117,* S33.

233. Uddenberg, N., et al. (1971). Nausea in pregnancy: Psychological and psychosomatic aspects. *J Psychosom Res, 15,* 269.

234. Ulmsten, U. & Sundstrom, G. (1978). Esophageal manometry in pregnant and non-pregnant women. *Am J Obstet Gynecol, 132,* 260.

235. Van Thiel, D.H., Gavaler, J.S., & Stemple, J. (1976). Lower esophageal sphincter pressure in women using sequential oral contraceptives. *Gastroenterology, 71,* 232.

236. Van Thiel, D.H., Gavaler, J.S., & Stemple, J. (1979). Lower esophageal sphincter pressure during the normal menstrual cycle. *Am J Obstet Gynecol, 134,* 64.

237. Van Thiel, D.H. & Schade, R.R. (1986). Pregnancy: Its physiologic course, nutrient cost, and effects on gastrointestinal function. In V.K. Rustgi & J.N. Cooper (Eds.), *Gastrointestinal and hepatic complications in pregnancy* (pp. 1–29). New York: John Wiley & Sons.

238. Van Thiel, D.H., et al. (1977). Heartburn of pregnancy. *Gastroenterology, 72,* 666.

239. Vander, A.J., Sherman, J.H., & Luciano, D.S. (1980). *Human physiology: The mechanisms of body function.* New York: McGraw-Hill.

240. Viteri, F.E., Schumacher, L., & Silliman, K. (1989). Maternal malnutrition and the fetus. *Semin Perinatol, 13,* 236.

241. Wald, A., et al. (1982). Effect of pregnancy on gastrointestinal transit. *Dig Dis Sci, 27,* 1015.

242. Walker, W.A. (1977). Development of gastrointestinal function and selected dysfunctions. In *Selected aspects of perinatal gastroenterology* (pp. 3–10). Mead Johnson Symposium on Perinatal and Developmental Medicine., No. 11. Evansville, IN: Mead Johnson.

243. Walker W.A. (1981). Effect of colostrum on the maturation of infant host defense mechanisms. In E. Lebenthal (Ed.), *Textbook of gastroenterology and nutrition in infancy* (pp. 225–238). New York: Raven Press.

244. Walker, V., et al. (1989). Carbohydrate fermentation by gut microflora in preterm neonates. *Am J Dis Child, 64,* 1367.

245. Watkins, J.B., et al. (1975). Bile salt metabolism in the human premature infant. *Gastroenterology, 69,* 706.

246. Watkins, J.B. (1975). Mechanism of fat absorption and the development of gastrointestinal function. *Pediatr Clin North Am, 22,* 721.

247. Watkins, J.B. (1981). Role of bile acids in the development of enterohepatic circulation. In E. Lebenthal (Ed.), *Textbook of gastroenterology and nutrition in infancy* (pp. 167–176). New York: Raven Press.

248. Watkins, J.B. (1985). Lipid digestion and absorption. *Pediatrics, 75*(Suppl.), 151.

249. Weigel, M.M. & Weigel, R.M. (1989). Nausea and vomiting of early pregnancy and pregnancy outcome. An epidemiological study. *Br J Obstet Gynaecol, 96,* 1304.

250. Weigel, M.M. & Weigel, R.M. (1989). Nausea and vomiting of early pregnancy and pregnancy outcome. A meta-analytical review. *Br J Obstet Gynaecol, 96,* 1312.

251. Weiner, C.P. (1989). Pathogenesis, evaluation and potential treatments for severe, early onset growth retardation. *Semin Perinatol, 13,* 342.

252. Wharton, B.A. (1987). *Nutrition and feeding of preterm infants.* Oxford: Blackwell Scientific Publications.

253. Widdowson, E.M. (1974). Changes in body proportions and composition during growth. In J.A. Davis & J. Dobbing (Eds.), *Scientific foundations of paediatrics* (pp. 153–163). Philadelphia: WB Saunders.

254. Widstrom, A.M., et al.(1988). Non-nutritive sucking in tube-fed preterm infants: Effects on feeding time and gastric contents of gastrin and somatostatin. *J Pediatr Gastroenterol Nutr, 7,* 517.

255. Wilson, J. (1978). Gastric emptying in labour: Some recent findings and their clinical significance. *J Int Med Res, 6,* 54.

256. Wingate, M.B. & Chaudhuri, G. (1981). Nutritional and developmental determinants of intrauterine growth. In E. Lebenthal (Ed.), *Textbook of gastroenterology and nutrition in infancy* (pp. 9–18). New York: Raven Press.

257. Wolkind, S. & Zajicek, E. (1978). Psychosocial correlates of nausea and vomiting in pregnancy. *J Psychosom Res, 22,* 1.

258. Worthington-Roberts, B.S., Vermeersch, J., & Williams, S.R. (1985). *Nutrition in pregnancy and lactation* (3rd ed.). St. Louis: CV Mosby.

259. Worthington-Roberts, B. (1989). Obesity and nutrition during pregnancy. In S.A. Brody & K. Ueland (Eds.), *Endocrine disorders in pregnancy* (pp. 363–381). Norwalk CT: Appleton & Lange.

260. Wu, P.Y.K., et al. (1984). Variations in composition of infant formula and changes in plasma ketone bodies in preterm infants. *J Am Coll Nutr, 3,* 257.

261. Wyner, J. & Cohen, S.E. (1982). Gastric volume in early pregnancy: Effect of metoclopramide. *Anesthesiology, 37,* 209.

262. Yip, D.M. & Baker, A.L. (1985). Liver diseases in pregnancy. *Clin Perinatol, 12,* 683.

263. Ylikorkala, O., Kauppila, A., & Haapalaht, J. (1976). Follicle stimulating hormone, thyrotropin, human growth hormone and prolactin in hyperemesis gravidarum. *Br J Obstet Gynaecol, 83,* 518.

264. Younoszai, M.K. (1974). Jejunal absorption of hexose in infants and children. *J Pediatr, 85,* 446.

265. Yu, V.Y.H. (1975). Effect of body positioning on gastric emptying in the neonate. *Arch Dis Child, 60,* 500.

266. Zbella, E.A. & Gleicher, N. (1985). The oral cavity. In N. Gleicher (Ed.), *Principles of medical therapy in pregnancy* (pp. 811–813). New York: Plenum Press.

267. Zerzan, J.C. (1988). Nutritional needs of the premature infant. *NW Perinat Newsletter, 2*(4), 2.

268. Ziegler, E.E. (1985). Infants of low birth weight: Special needs and problems. *Am J Clin Nutr, 41,* 440.

269. Ziegler, E.E., Biga, R.L., & Fomon, S.J. (1981). Nutritional requirement of the premature infant. From R.M. Suskind (Ed.), *Textbook of pediatric nutrition* (pp. 29–39). New York: Raven Press.

270. Ziegler, M.M. (1986). Short bowel syndrome in infancy: Etiology and management. *Clin Perinatol, 13,* 163.

271. Ziskin, D.E. & Nesse, G.J. (1946). Pregnancy gingivitis: History, classification and etiology. *Am J Orthodont Oral Surg, 32,* 390.

272. Zoppi, G., et al. (1972). Exocrine pancreas function in premature and fullterm neonates. *Pediatr Res, 6,* 880.

CHAPTER 10

The Immune System and Host Defense Mechanisms

Maternal Physiologic Adaptations
    The Antepartum Period
    The Intrapartum Period
    The Postpartum Period
Clinical Implications for the Pregnant Woman and Her Fetus
    Maternal Tolerance of the Fetus
    Risk of Maternal Infection
    Infection and Preterm Labor
    Perinatal HIV Infection
    Antibiotic Use During Pregnancy
    Immunization and the Pregnant Woman
    Malignancy and Pregnancy
    Immunologic Aspects of Pregnancy-Induced Hypertension
    Pregnancy-Induced Immune States
    The Pregnant Woman with an Autoimmune Disease
    Transplacental Passage of Maternal Antibodies
    Rho(D) Isoimmunization and ABO Incompatibility
    Protection of the Fetus from Infection

Development of Host Defense Mechanisms in the Fetus
Neonatal Physiology
    Transitional Events
    Alterations in Primary Host Defense Mechanisms
    Alterations in Specific Immune Responses
    Alterations in Gut Host Defense Mechanisms
Clinical Implications for Neonatal Care
    Risk of Specific Infectious Processes
        Immune Responses to Bacterial Infections
        Immune Responses to Viral Infections
    Diagnosis of Neonatal Infection
    Antibiotic Use in the Neonate
    Immunotherapy for Neonatal Sepsis
Maturational Changes During Infancy and Childhood
    Maturation of Host Defense Factors
    Physiologic Hypogammaglobulinemia
    Immunizations
    Development of Allergies

Host defense mechanisms consist of immunologic and nonimmunologic factors. Nonimmunologic factors include genetic susceptibility, skin and mucosal barriers, digestive enzymes, pH, temperature, proteins, and enzymes such as lysozyme, transferrin, and interferon. Immunologic factors consist of primary, secondary, and tertiary defense mechanisms and nonspecific responses such as the inflammatory response and phagocytosis, and specific immune responses such as antibody- and cell-mediated immunity. The immune system and host defense mechanisms in the pregnant woman and neonate are altered so that each is to some extent an immunocompromised host. The interaction between the mother's host defense mechanisms and the fetus, who is antigenically unique from the mother, presents one of the more challenging questions in immunology:

Why doesn't the mother reject the fetus? Current theories regarding this question, along with alterations in host defense mechanisms in the mother and neonate and implications for clinical practice, are examined in this chapter. Host defense mechanisms and terminology are summarized in Figure 10–1 and Table 10–1.

MATERNAL PHYSIOLOGIC ADAPTATIONS

Alterations in the immune system during pregnancy affect primary and specific host defense mechanisms. These alterations help the mother's host defense system tolerate the fetus, but may also increase the severity of maternal infections and influence the course of chronic disorders such as autoimmune diseases.

The Antepartum Period

Adaptations in the maternal immune system during pregnancy include alterations in the inflammatory response, phagocytosis, and in B- and T-lymphocyte function. In addition a variety of nonimmunologic hormonal and serum factors modulate various aspects of maternal host defense mechanisms. These alterations and their implications are summarized in Table 10–2.

Alterations in Primary Host Defense Mechanisms

White blood cell (WBC) count increases during pregnancy beginning at 2 months and reaches a plateau during the second and third trimesters at a mean level of 10,350/mm^3 with a usual range of 6000 to 12,000/mm^3.[51, 119] The increase is primarily due to increased polymorphonuclear neutrophils (PMNs). Functional alterations in the PMNs have also been reported.[15, 47, 163] Altered metabolic activity of maternal leukocytes along with both increased and decreased (especially in response to gram-negative organisms) phagocytic and bacteriocidal activity has been reported by different investigators.[15, 47] Chemotaxis (movement of neutrophils toward the site of infection) is decreased during pregnancy, which may delay initial maternal responses to infection.[48, 151]

A lysosomal stabilizer, which in conjunc-tion with alterations in the leukocytes may alter the inflammatory response, has been found in the serum of pregnant women.[163] The decreased numbers of natural killer (NK) cells may assist in maternal tolerance of the fetus by protecting the trophoblast from destruction.[2, 47] Fibronectin, a glycoprotein with opsonic and clot-stabilizing properties, increases about 2.5 times. Further increases are seen in women with pregnancy-induced hypertension (PIH). The increased fibronectin is reported to precede clinical signs of PIH, supporting vascular endothelial injury as a primary event in the development of this disorder (see Chapter 6).[126]

Alterations in Cell-Mediated Immunity

Cell-mediated immunity is altered during pregnancy by changes in the function and efficiency of the T lymphocytes. Most investigators report that the total number of lymphocytes does not change significantly during pregnancy.[47, 51, 153] Others have found no change in the relative number but a reduction in the absolute number of T lymphocytes.[145] Some investigators have reported an inversion of the usual B lymphocyte–to–T lymphocyte ratio of 1:3 at 10 to 13 weeks' gestation with a return to a normal ratio by 20 weeks.[47, 158, 159]

The number of T-helper (T4) cells decreases progressively to 700 to 800 cells/µl by 7 months then increases to about 1000/µl by term.[7, 82] T-suppressor cells (T8) remain relatively unchanged.[47, 86] Thus, the T4-to-T8 ratio falls to 0.9 to 1.92 during pregnancy (versus the normal 1.7 to 2.3).[48] Since T-helper cells normally augment the cytotoxic responses involved in graft rejection, the decreased number of these cells may help protect the fetus from rejection by the mother. T-suppressor cell function may increase in late pregnancy and suppresses or decreases B-lymphocyte function.[163] Decreased T-lymphocyte function and efficiency may increase the risk of viral and mycotic infections. The maternal reaction to the tuberculin test is depressed during the second half of pregnancy. As a result, diagnosis of tuberculosis in the pregnant woman may be more difficult.[47]

Alterations in Humoral (Antibody)-Mediated Immunity

Humoral (antibody)-mediated immunity is not significantly altered during pregnancy,

TABLE 10–1
Definitions of Terms

TERM	DEFINITION
Active immunity	Exposure to antigen (attenuated or inactivated/killed virus or bacterium) that leads to formation of antibodies and memory cells against that antigen.
Allograft	Graft taken from an organism that is the same species as the recipient but not genetically identical.
Antibody	Proteins that react with specific antigens.
Antibody (humoral)-mediated immunity	Specific host defense mechanisms mediated by B cells that provide protection against most bacteria and some viruses through production of antibodies.
Antigen	Substances perceived by one's host defense mechanisms as "foreign" (may include bacteria, viruses, pollutants, dust, certain foods, etc.).
Blocking antibody	Antibody that inhibits immune responses by binding to antigens, antigenic sites, or T lymphocytes.
Cell-mediated immunity	Specific host defense mechanisms, mediated by T-helper, T-suppressor, and cytotoxic cells, that provide protection against certain organisms, regulate B-cell function, defend against cancer, and mediate graft rejection.
Chemotaxis	Movement of neutrophils and other phagocytes in an organized fashion toward a site of antigenic invasion.
Complement	Sequential series of discrete plasma proteins and their fragments that when activated enhance other aspects of the immune system. Actions include attraction of various cell types to the initial site of invasion, promotion of chemotaxis and phagocytosis, enhancement of opsonization and the inflammatory response, and direct destruction of antigens by lysis of cell membranes.
Cytotoxic/killer T cell	Type of T lymphocyte acting directly on specific antigens or target cells with specific antigen resulting in cell lysis.
Fibronectin	Nonspecific opsonin, inhibitor of bacterial adherence to epithelial cells, and clot-stabilizing protein found in plasma and endothelial tissue.
Helper T (T4) cell	Type of T lymphocyte that acts to enhance the activity of B lymphocytes (by interleukin-2), other T cells, and macrophages (by γ-interferon).
HLA	Abbreviation for "human leukocyte antigens," the major forms of specific tissue antigens found on tissue surfaces that are unique to each person (includes HLA-A, HLA-B, HLA-C, and HLA-D).
Immunoglobulin	Antibodies produced by B lymphocytes (includes IgG, IgM, IgA, IgD, and IgE).
Interleukin-2	Protein mediator (lymphokine) released by T-helper cells that stimulates production of immunoglobulins by B cells.
Lymphokine	Chemical mediators released by T lymphocytes that enhance the actions of other immune system components including B cells, macrophage migration and activity, and phagocytosis.
Memory cell	Form of lymphocytes sensitized to specific antigens; with subsequent stimulation by the specific antigen, an exaggerated and accelerated response usually occurs.
MHC (major histocompatibility complex)	Specific antigens found on tissue surfaces divided into 3 groups: MHC I (HLA-A, HLA-B, and HLA-C, which are found on most of a person's cells); MHC II (found on surface of immune cells such as T and B lymphocytes); and MHC III (includes some components of complement).
NK cells	Natural killer (NK) cells or a subpopulation of lymphoid cells that attack without previous immunization and independent of antibodies, phagocytosis, and complement; form a first line of defense against antigens until other defense mechanisms can be mobilized.
Opsonization	Processing and marking or altering the cell surface of an antigen by actions of immunoglobulin or complement; substances acting in this manner are called opsonins; this process is critical in allowing phagocytosis of organisms with a capsular polysaccharide coat such as group B streptococci.
Passive immunity	Transfer of antibodies from an actively immunized to a nonimmunized person.
Plasma cell	Form of B lymphocyte able to secrete immunoglobulins.
Primary host defense responses	Nonimmune responses, the inflammatory response and phagocytosis, which result in either elimination of the foreign substance or antigen with cessation of the response or formation of a "processed antigen" while stimulating secondary mechanisms.
Secondary host defense responses	Involve antibody (humoral)- and cell-mediated immunity, which are mediated by B (antibody-mediated) and T (cell-mediated) lymphocytes.
Suppressor T (T8) cell	Suppresses B-lymphocyte function including production of antibodies to autoantigens; may help to slow or terminate immune response once the antigens are destroyed.
Tertiary host defense responses	Involve immune responses to overwhelming infection or responses such as allergy, malignancy, and autoimmune disease.

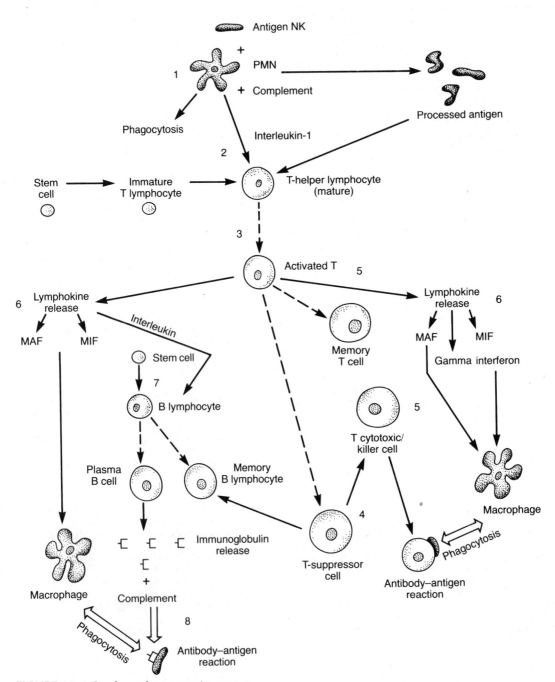

FIGURE 10–1 *See legend on opposite page*

TABLE 10–2
Alterations in Host Defense Mechanisms During Pregnancy

ALTERATION	RESULT	IMPLICATION
Primary Host Defense Mechanisms		
Increased PMNs	Increased available phagocytes	Protection of mother and fetus from infection
Altered metabolic activity and chemotaxis of PMN	Delay initial response to infection	Increase risk of colonization Protect fetus and trophoblast from rejection
Decreased NK cells	Delay initial response to infection	Increase risk of colonization Protect fetus and trophoblast from rejection
Cell-Mediated Immunity		
Decreased T-helper cells	Suppress B-cell function Alter cell-mediated immunity	Increase risk of mycotic, fungal, other opportunistic infections
Increased T-suppressor cells	Decrease graft rejection	Protect fetus from rejection
Altered T-cell function and efficiency	Depress reaction to tuberculin test	Confuse diagnosis of infection in second half of pregnancy
Antibody-Mediated Immunity		
Suppression of B-cell function	Due to decreased T-helper cells	Increased risk of colonization with streptococci, staphylococci, other organisms
Decreased IgG	Due to transfer to fetus and hemodilution	Increased risk of colonization
Complement		
Increased total complement and C2, C3, C3 split products	Enhance chemotaxis and action of immunoglobulins through opsonization	Augment maternal defenses against bacterial infection Protect fetus from infection
Decreased C1, C1a, B, D	Delay initial activation of complement system	Protect fetus and trophoblast from rejection

FIGURE 10–1. The immune system. *1,* Nonspecific mechanisms (NK cells, inflammatory response, phagocytosis) eliminate antigen or form "processed antigen." *2,* Processed antigen and interleukin-1 activate T4 (helper) cells, which stimulate immunoglobulin (Ig) production by B cells. *3,* T4 cells enhance activity of B and other T cells, produce γ-interferon (activates macrophages), and stimulate Ig production by B cells. *4,* T8 (suppressor) cells suppress B cells and help to terminate the immune response once the antigen has been destroyed. *5,* Activated T cells react by direct cytotoxicity (binding antigen to antibodies on the T-cell membrane); release nonspecific toxins that destroy the target antigen; release lymphokines; and form memory cells. *6,* Lymphokines include a factor that transfers sensitivity to a specific antigen to unsensitized T cells; macrophage migration-inhibiting factor (MIF), which helps keep macrophages concentrated at the site; macrophage-activating factor (MAF), which increases activity and aggressiveness of macrophages; chemotaxic factors, which attract neutrophils and macrophages; interferon (inhibits viral replication and transfer); and interleukin-2, which stimulates B-lymphocyte function. *7,* Stimulation of B cells by antigen, interleukins, or other mediators produced by T4 cells transforms the B cell into a plasma (Ig-producing) or memory cell (rapidly differentiates into plasma cells after subsequent exposure to a specific antigen). *8,* Ingestion and digestion of antigen–antibody complexes by phagocytes and macrophages. Bacteria with a capsular polysaccharide must first undergo opsonization (processing of an organism by coating it with Ig and complement).

probably because production of blocking antibodies is essential for shielding fetal and placental antigens from detection by the maternal cell-mediated immunity. Changes in the humoral system are reflected primarily through changes in immunoglobulin G (IgG) and complement. Levels of maternal IgG fall as gestation progresses with decreases ranging from 15 to 32% reported.[43, 47] Others have found relatively little change.[4, 160] The fall in IgG has been attributed to hemodilution, loss of IgG in the urine, and transfer of maternal IgG to the fetus in the last trimester. Higher maternal IgG levels have been noted in pregnancies complicated by intrauterine death and severe intrauterine growth retardation. Maternal and cord blood IgG levels are lower in women with PIH.[47] The decrease in IgG along with alterations in WBCs may increase the risk of streptococcal colonization.

Immunoglobulin A (IgA) decreases or remains stable during gestation, immunoglobulin M (IgM) and immunoglobulin E (IgE) change little, and immunoglobulin D (IgD) increases to term.[163] The slight decrease in serum IgA may reflect increased levels of IgA found in saliva and other mucosal fluids.[47] The specific role of IgD is unknown.

Alterations in the Complement System

Alterations in the complement system during pregnancy begin at 11 weeks with an increase (due to greater hepatic synthesis) in both total serum complement and specific proteins of the complement system, including C2, C3, and C3 split products.[47, 72] These components enhance chemotaxis and actions of immunoglobulins through opsonization, thereby augmenting maternal defenses against bacterial infection. Other proteins of the complement system such as C1, C1a, B, and D are decreased.[51] Since these proteins are involved in activation of the complement system through either the classical or the alternative pathway, activity of the complement system early in the immune response may be delayed. This may afford additional protection for the trophoblast and fetus.

Influences of Nonimmunologic Serum and Hormonal Factors

Host defense mechanisms during pregnancy are also influenced by changes in nonimmunologic hormonal and serum factors that may modulate lymphocyte and macrophage synthesis, activation, or function.[48, 156, 167] Elevated levels of specific hormones in pregnancy depress various aspects of cell-mediated immunity. Estradiol inhibits graft rejection and enhances maternal tolerance of the fetus and placenta. Corticosteroids suppress activation of T-cell lymphokines, phagocytic activity, and lymphokine responsiveness of the macrophages.[69, 86, 167] Progesterone may enhance local immunosuppression of lymphocytes in the placenta.[47] The role of human chorionic gonadotropin (hCG) in the maternal immune system is controversial. A localized function at the trophoblast site to prevent maternal rejection of the fetus has been proposed.[47, 167] Prostaglandins (especially PGE_1 and PGE_2), human placental lactogen (hPL), and alphafetoprotein (AFP) also appear to have an immunosuppressive role during pregnancy. AFP may act by inducing production of suppressor T lymphocytes.[47, 74]

Alterations in defense mechanisms may be mediated by a serum protein known as pregnancy zone protein (PZP), which increases during pregnancy and has an inhibitory effect on the inflammatory process.[163] An immunologic regulatory role has also been proposed for a unique group of pregnancy-associated plasma proteins (PAPPs) produced by the syncytiotrophoblast. The exact functions of the PAPPs are still being determined. Alterations in levels of specific PAPPs have been associated with pregnancies complicated by PIH, diabetes, and multiple gestation.[47]

The Intrapartum Period

The WBC count increases during labor and in the early postpartum period to values up to 25,000 to 30,000/mm³. This increase is primarily due to an increase in neutrophils and may represent a normal response to physiologic stress.[119] The rise in absolute numbers of WBCs and in neutrophils may complicate the diagnosis of infection during this time. Impairment in the functional activity of peripheral blood lymphocytes and a decrease in the absolute number of total, helper, and suppressor T lymphocytes immediately after delivery have been reported.[145]

The Postpartum Period

The WBC count, which increased in labor and immediately after birth, gradually returns to normal values by 4 to 7 days. Ratios of T-helper to T-suppressor cells remain altered for 2 to 3 months with an ongoing reduction in the number of T-helper cells.[167]

Immunologic Properties of Human Milk

Human milk contains many immunologic components including leukocytes, immunoglobulins, and other proteins (Table 10–3). Colostrum is especially rich in immunologic factors. Leukocytes in colostrum consist of 40 to 50% monocytic macrophages, 40 to 50% PMN neutrophils, and 5 to 10% lymphocytes.[175] Later in lactation the leukocytes in human milk are 85 to 90% monocytic macrophages and 10 to 15% lymphocytes, with some neutrophils and epithelial cells.

Monocytic macrophages in human milk synthesize complement, lysozyme, and lactoferrin; transport immunoglobulin; and protect against necrotizing enterocolitis. These cells also have phagocytic activity against *Staphylococcus aureus*, *Escherichia coli*, and *Candida albicans* and may help to regulate T-cell function.[108] Since the macrophages adhere to glass, plastic containers should be used for collection and storage of human milk.[108, 175]

Similar concentrations of B and T lym-phocytes are found. B lymphocytes in human milk produce IgA, IgG, and IgM. T lymphocytes produce interferon, macrophage migration-inhibiting factor (MIF), and other lymphokines. Human milk T cells respond to antigenic stimulation in a manner similar to those from an immunologically competent person, especially in response to *E. coli*. Since the neonate's own T cells are functionally immature, human milk may provide significant protection against gram-negative organisms. Human milk often contains antibodies against the O and K antigens of several *E. coli* serotypes including K1, which has been associated with neonatal meningitis.[33]

The immunoglobulins in human milk are predominately secretory IgA (sIgA). The secretory component attached to the IgA monomer protects the IgA molecule from proteolytic digestion in the gastrointestinal tract. The sIgA does not enter the circulation from the gut but provides localized gut barrier protection by attaching to the mucosal epithelium and preventing attachment and invasion by specific infectious agents.[49] Secretory IgA also neutralizes certain viruses and bacterial enterotoxins and inhibits intestinal absorption of proteins and other macromolecules found in foods.[23] The latter function may provide protection against the development of allergies. Levels of sIgA are highest in colostrum, fall gradually until 12 weeks, then remain stable for the next 2 years of lactation.[49]

sIgA action is enhanced by complement. Human milk contains C3 and C4 and produces complement by the alternative pathway, which can be activated by factors such as bacterial products and circulating proteins. IgM and IgG are also present in human milk but in much lower concentrations than sIgA.

Most of the immunoglobulins in human milk are produced by sensitized plasma cells in the breast that have been transported to that site from maternal intestinal (gut) and bronchotracheal associated lymphatic tissue (GALT and BALT). Specific sIgA against a wide variety of respiratory and enteric bacterial and viral organisms can be found in human milk.[49, 122, 167] The specificity in any woman is related to her previous antigenic exposure. Depending on the mother's immunologic experience, the immunoglobulins in human milk may provide the infant with protection against diphtheria, pertussis, shigella, salmonella, polio virus, and echoviruses.

TABLE 10–3
Immunologic Properties of Human Milk

Parameter	Immunologic Factors
Cellular components	PMN neutrophils
	Lymphocytes (T-cell and B-cell)
	Monocytic macrophages
Immunoglobulins	Secretory IgA (major immunoglobulin)
	IgM
	IgG
Complement	C3 and C4
Antibacterial factors	Lactoferrin
	Folic acid– and vitamin B_{12}–binding proteins
	Lysozyme
	Lactoperidase
	Bifidus factor
	Antistaphylococcal factor
Antiviral factors	Interferon
	Lipase
Anti-inflammatory factors	Histaminase
	Vitamins C and E
	Prostaglandins (PGE$_2$ and PGF$_2$)
	Oligosaccharides and other factors that inhibit microbial attachment
Nonspecific factors	Low pH
	Lactose
	Low protein

Human milk contains other nonspecific protective factors that act synergistically with each other and sIgA and include:

1. Lactoferrin (an iron-binding protein that restricts the availability of iron needed for growth by certain fungi and bacteria such as staphylococcus and *E. coli*). Lactoferrin, α-lactalbumin, and sIgA form the major whey proteins in human milk and constitute 60 to 80% of total human milk protein. Levels of lactoferrin decrease gradually to 12 weeks then remain stable over the next 2 years of lactation.

2. Folic acid and vitamin B_{12}-binding protein (restricts available folate and vitamin B_{12} for bacterial and fungal growth).

3. Lysozyme (bacteriocidal enzyme that lyses cell walls of many bacteria and enhances lactobacillus growth). Lysozyme falls in the first 2 to 4 months post partum then rises gradually to 6 months with stable levels to 2 years.

4. Lactoperidase (inhibits bacterial growth).

5. Bifidus factor (nitrogen-containing polysaccharide that promotes growth of anaerobic lactobacilli that compete with invasive gram-negative organisms). Other factors in human milk that promote lactobacilli growth include lactose, low pH, and buffers.

6. Interferon (prevents viral replication).

7. Lipase (increases levels of free fatty acids and monoglycerides that may act against certain viruses).[21, 49, 74, 115, 170]

Other components of human milk include macrophage-inhibiting factor and antiviral and antistaphylococcal factors.

Human milk produces acetic and lactic acid in the gut. These acids decrease stool pH and inhibit growth of shigella and *E. coli*. In addition to the intrinsic protective factors inherent in it, human milk may also induce the production of immune factors such as sIgA by the infant, although this remains controversial.[49]

Human milk may provide protection against infection and the development of allergies in the preterm infant. The preterm infant's gastrointestinal (GI) tract lacks many intrinsic local host defense factors including sIgA, lysozyme, and gastric acid, and there is immaturity of the intestinal mucosal barrier function.[23] As a result, the preterm infant is especially at risk for bacterial penetration through the intestines and development of sepsis and necrotizing enterocolitis. The lack of sIgA and immaturity of the intestinal mucosa increase the likelihood of foreign macromolecules entering the circulation, which may increase the risk of allergies in genetically susceptible infants.[23] Human milk may enhance maturation of the intestinal mucosal barrier, thereby reducing the risk of both infections and allergies. Increased levels of sIgA, lactoferrin, and lysozyme have been found in milk from mothers of preterm infants.[55, 108] Thus, mothers of preterm infants may have an important adaptation that provides additional protection from infection to their infants.

CLINICAL IMPLICATIONS FOR THE PREGNANT WOMAN AND HER FETUS

The maternal-fetal immunologic relationship is unique. Not only must the fetus be protected against a variety of potentially pathogenic organisms, but the fetus must also be protected from rejection as foreign tissue by the mother. Maternal adaptations also have the potential to interact with disorders of the immune system or other underlying alterations in host defense mechanisms that may complicate pregnancy such as human immunodeficiency virus (HIV), acquired immunodeficiency syndrome (AIDS), and other infections; autoimmune disorders; and malignancy. Pregnancy is also associated with several pregnancy-specific immune states that can increase the risk of pregnancy loss or lead to severe maternal disease. Interactions between the normal pregnancy-induced changes in host defense mechanisms and pregnancy complications affecting these mechanisms are reviewed in this section along with issues and concerns related to maternal-fetal relationships, immunization and antibiotic use during pregnancy, and interactions between infection and preterm labor.

Maternal Tolerance of the Fetus

The fetus is an allograft, that is, foreign tissue from the same species but with a different antigenic makeup. Since the fetus has maternal, paternal, and embryonic antigens, major antigenic differences may exist between the fetus and mother, including blood group antigens and tissue antigens such as human lymphocyte antigen (HLA). Yet in most pregnancies the mother does not reject the fetus. Thus, the major immunologic question regarding pregnancy is "How does the pregnant mother continue to nourish within itself, for many weeks or months, a fetus that is an antigenically foreign body?"[14, p. 256] The answer to this question is uncertain, although many theories exist. To understand the mechanisms currently proposed to explain why the pregnant woman's host defense mechanisms tolerate the fetus, it is helpful to briefly examine general aspects of graft rejection.

Specific antigenic characteristics of tissues are classified by major histocompatibility complex (MHC) antigens on the tissue surface. The MHC antigens in humans are HLA-A, HLA-B, HLA-C, and HLA-D/DR. HLA-A, HLA-B, and HLA-C (class I antigens) are found on most adult cells and are actively involved in graft rejection. HLA-D/DR (class II antigens) is associated with antibody-mediated immunity and found primarily on immune cells such as lymphocytes or macrophages.

Graft rejection processes involve (allogeneic) recognition by the host that donor cell surface (MHC) antigens are antigenically different from its own. This recognition is mediated by T lymphocytes in cooperation with macrophages. Initially (afferent limb) T lymphocytes move into the lymph nodes, where they divide or recruit other lymphocytes capable of recognizing foreign MHC antigens. This recognition and proliferation is stimulated by class II MHC antigens. These effector limb or activated T lymphocytes accumulate in the graft and either lyse cells directly or release factors such as lymphokines that cause cell destruction. The cytotoxic activity of the T lymphocytes is directed toward the foreign MHC antigens on the graft.[86, 123]

Many theories have been proposed to explain maternal tolerance of the fetal allograft (Table 10–4). Although the woman's immune system is altered during pregnancy, her system is still capable of responding to and rejecting tissue transplants from the father and the fetus grafted onto areas other than the uterus.[69] Therefore protection of the fetus from rejection seems to be predominantly a localized uterine response. Proposed mechanisms currently under investigation include formation of blocking antibodies, reduced antigenicity of the tro-

phoblast, production by the fetus of immunosuppressor cells or factors, suppression of the maternal immune system by hormonal or other factors such as PAPPs, and intrinsic alterations in the maternal immune system.[47] The last two mechanisms were discussed under maternal physiologic alterations. The other mechanisms are described below.

The first direct contact between maternal and fetal tissues occurs 6 to 7 days after conception at the time of implantation. The trophoblast cells invade the maternal endometrial lining and erode endothelial tissue of the maternal spiral arteries (see Chapter 2). After the placenta is established, the two points of contact between maternal and fetal tissues are the syncytiotrophoblast lining the intervillous spaces, which is in direct contact with maternal blood, and the extravillous trophoblast (primarily cytotrophoblast), which is in direct contact with maternal decidual tissue. Beginning in early pregnancy, small quantities of trophoblast cells detach and enter maternal blood through the uterine veins. These cells form minute emboli that eventually lodge in pulmonary capillaries and are cleared by proteolysis. This appears to be a normal process that does not lead to a maternal inflammatory response or other problems.[123]

The trophoblast has a fibrinoid sialomucin glycoprotein coating with an alpha globulin of the IgG class that may act as an antigenic barrier. Electromagnetic properties of the coating are thought to block stimulation of maternal lymphocytes by fetal antigens and decrease cell-mediated immune responses. This coating is produced by the maternal liver and appears within 48 hours after implantation. Before implantation the zona pellucida mucoprotein coat provides a barrier between maternal and fetal tissues.[111]

Another mechanism proposed to reduce antigenicity of the trophoblast by masking of its surface antigens is the binding of masking agents.[47, 111] Potential masking substances are transferrin, antibodies, and antibody–antigen (immune) complexes. Recent evidence suggests that reduced antigenicity of the trophoblast has a minor role in maternal tolerance of the fetus.[14]

Blocking antibodies prevent recognition of fetoplacental antigens by maternal cells. An early phase of cytotoxic reactions with graft rejection involves allogeneic recognition by the host. Blocking of this recognition by an-

TABLE 10–4
Mechanisms or Factors Proposed to Explain the Nonrejection of Allogeneic Fetoplacental Units

Complete separation of maternal and fetal blood circulations.
Afferent blockade of the immunologic reflex arc:
    Impairment of lymphatic drainage from placenta by decidual tissue.
    Avoidance of lymphatic vessels and lymph nodes by invading trophoblast.
Immunologic barrier or buffer zone at maternal-fetal tissue interface resulting from:
    Adaptive failure of trophoblast to synthesize or express alloantigens in immunogenetically effective manner
      (intrinsically determined privileged tissue).
    Modulation of antigenic expression by trophoblast in response to maternal antibodies (extrinsically determined
      privileged tissue).
Masking by surface alloantigens on the trophoblast cells:
    By own synthesis of sialomucin coat that discourages or prevents interaction with maternal lymphocytes.
    As a consequence of the passive acquisition or absorption of agents that result in "masking":
      By transferrin that binds to specific receptors on the trophoblast cells.
      By antibodies or antibody–antigen complexes that bind specifically or nonspecifically (by Fc receptors) to
        trophoblast surface.
Specific binding, internalization, and inactivation (digestion of maternal immunologic effector agents by trophoblast).
Synthesis by syncytial trophoblast, and maintenance in high local concentration, of hormones and other agents that
    fulfill an immunosuppressive role, e.g., progesterone, estrogen, chorionic gonadotropin, cortisol-binding globulin.
Production by fetus of immunosuppressive agents that enter maternal circulation, e.g., alpha-fetoprotein, factor released
    from stimulated fetal lymphocytes.
Production by the mother of immunoregulatory agents that confer protection on the fetoplacental unit:
    Increased synthesis of adrenal corticosteroids, special plasma proteins (pregnancy-zone or PZ proteins), early
      pregnancy factor, alpha-2-globulins.
    Synthesis of "blocking" antibodies.
    Generation of suppressor cells.
    Inversion of T- and B-cell number in bloodstream.

From Beer, A.E., et al. (1981). Major histocompatibility complex antigens, maternal and parental immune responses and chronic habitual abortion in humans. *Am J Obstet Gynecol, 141,* 988.

tibodies from B lymphocytes can inhibit subsequent activation of T lymphocytes and the succeeding steps in graft rejection.[95] The presence of blocking antibodies in maternal blood during pregnancy specific for paternal antigens has been demonstrated.[95] Blocking antibodies are thought to be IgG molecules and may be formed by binding of the Fc fragment of the IgG molecule to receptors on B lymphocytes.[111] Blocking antibodies may protect the fetus by:

1. Binding to fetal or trophoblast cells that enter the maternal circulation so that fetal and trophoblast cell antigens and maternal T lymphocytes do not interact.

2. Crossing the placenta (if blocking antibodies are of the IgG class, which are the only immunoglobulins to cross the placenta in significant amounts) and binding to antigenic sites on fetal cells to protect fetal tissue from maternal lymphocytes that cross the placenta.

3. Binding with fetal antigens to produce antigen–antibody (or immune) complexes that bind to receptor sites on maternal T lymphocytes and interfere with maternal T-cell recognition of fetal cells as antigenic material.[69, 111]

The potential actions of blocking antibodies

in protecting the fetal allograft are illustrated in Figure 10–2.

For the mother to form blocking antibodies, she must first recognize the antigens on the trophoblast as foreign. The occurrence of recognition responses has been demonstrated by maternal host defense responses (i.e., the initial release of cytotoxic maternal antibody from B lymphocytes and lymphokines from T lymphocytes).[95] In animal models maternal recognition depends on incompatible MHC antigens on the trophoblast. The trophoblast surface and basement membrane have been reported to be lacking in MHC antigens, although HLA antigens are found in the mesenchymal stroma of the villi and on placental and endothelial tissues.[95, 123] The trophoblast appears to have other antigens that stimulate the maternal immune system, however.

Two groups of trophoblast antigens have been described. The first group (TA1 antigens) elicits formation of specific blocking antibodies by B lymphocytes. Failure to form blocking antibodies or formation of cytotoxic instead of protective antibodies results in pregnancy loss and has been associated with habitual abortion.[72, 95] The role of the second group of trophoblast antigens is to identify the tissue of the trophoblast as foreign to the

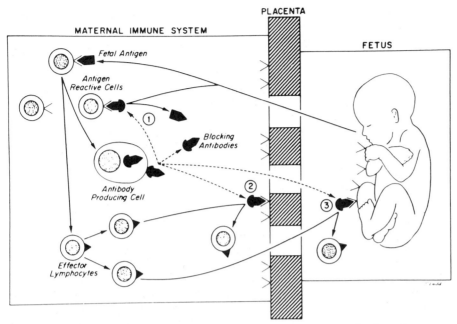

FIGURE 10–2. Potential roles of blocking antibodies in protecting the fetus from rejection. *1*, Binding with fetal antigens producing antibody–antigen complexes. *2*, Binding to trophoblast or fetal cells entering maternal circulation. *3*, Crossing the placenta and binding to antigenic sites on fetus (see text). (From Pattilo, R. [1981]. Immunology of gestation. In L. Iffy & H. Kaminetzky [Eds.], *Obstetrics and Perinatology* [Vol. 1, pp. 101–125]. New York: John Wiley & Sons.)

mother. This second group of antigens alerts the mother's system to the need to protect the blastocyst from rejection and stimulates formation of blocking antibodies.[14, 72, 123] These antigens are known as trophoblast lymphocyte cross-reactive (TLX) antigens and are closely related to HLA antigens.[161] The exact nature of the TLX antigens is still under investigation.

Failure of or incomplete recognition can lead to failed or faulty implantation and pregnancy loss.[72, 95] Contrary to experience with organ transplants, in which the best outcome is seen when patients receive HLA-matched organs, survival of the fetal allograft does not seem to depend on maternal-paternal antigenic similarity. This is demonstrated by the success of surrogate mothers in carrying infants conceived by in vitro fertilization from another woman and her partner. In fact, couples with similar HLA antigens have a higher rate of pregnancy loss, probably because of lack of stimulation of the maternal immune system. As a result, her system fails to recognize the fetus as foreign and to develop appropriate protective mechanisms.[48, 95, 96, 123] This implies that ". . . the mother must be clearly able to distinguish self from nonself,

and produce the appropriate blocking antibodies to nonself fetoplacental tissue in order to prevent rejection."[48, p. 212]

The fetus may play a more direct role in suppression of maternal immune responses. Fetal WBCs enter maternal circulation, with fetal lymphocytes actively crossing the placenta beginning as early as 14 to 15 weeks. Approximately 0.1 to 0.5% of the lymphocytes in the peripheral blood of pregnant women are of fetal origin.[47] Fetal lymphocytes have been shown to inhibit mitosis of stimulated lymphocytes in both the mother and other unrelated women. Fetal suppressor T lymphocytes may adhere to maternal lymphocytes or affect maternal B lymphocytes by suppressing immunoglobulin production. The fetus produces cytotoxic antibody that may suppress maternal T-cell activity.[47, 69, 123, 145]

Risk of Maternal Infection

In spite of alterations in host defense mechanisms, most women are not significantly immunocompromised during pregnancy. Suppression of maternal cell-mediated immunity is associated with an increased incidence of certain infections, however, especially viruses and certain opportunistic pathogens, including *C. albicans, Pneumocystis carinii, Toxoplasma gondii, Listeria monocytogenes, Streptococcus pneumoniae, Neisseria gonorrhoeae, Myobacterium tuberculosis,* polio, rubella, influenza, varicella, cytomegalovirus, and herpes simplex virus (HSV). As a result, viral infections are seen more frequently during pregnancy, especially during the second and third trimesters, tend to be more severe and take longer to resolve, with reactivation of subclinical infections.[47, 167, 172] Alterations in neutrophil chemotaxis and function also contribute to the greater severity and persistence of infections during pregnancy.[48] Changes in the frequency of infections during pregnancy are also due to other reasons. For example, the increased incidence of urinary tract infections and pyelonephritis during pregnancy is primarily due to anatomic alterations in the urinary tract that result in stasis (see Chapter 8).

The incidence of infection with protozoal (e.g., malaria and amebiasis) and helminthic (intestinal parasites) organisms is increased, particularly in Third World countries. During pregnancy malaria is more frequent and more severe, with an increased risk of sequelae. In some endemic areas malaria is the most common cause of maternal death.[167] The malaria parasite has an affinity for placental tissue, leading to stillbirth and preterm birth. Latent malaria can be reactivated by iron overload during pregnancy.

Infection and Preterm Labor

Both acute and chronic maternal infections are associated with preterm labor. Urinary tract infections have long been associated with preterm labor (see Chapter 8). Recently there has been increasing evidence of the role of vaginal and cervical organisms and chorioamnionitis in the initiation of preterm labor and premature rupture of membranes.[50, 127] Unrecognized infection may be an important etiologic factor when no apparent cause for preterm labor can be identified. In women with acute infections, high fever along with other stressors may lead to the release of catecholamines and increase uterine irritability. The link between bacterial infections and preterm labor may relate to the action of bacterial endotoxin on prostaglandin synthesis.

Current understanding of the initiation of labor in humans suggests that a primary mechanism is production of prostaglandins from precursors in the fetal membranes and decidua that stimulate cervical dilation and uterine contractions (see Chapter 3). Prostaglandins are synthesized in decidual and myometrial tissue. Arachidonic acid, an obligatory precursor for prostaglandin synthesis, is stored in the fetal membranes and decidua in an esterified inactivated form as glycerophospholipids. Conversion of the glycerophospholipids to active arachidonic acid is dependent on the enzyme phospholipase A_2, which is contained in small organelles or lysosomes in the fetal membranes (see Figs. 3–5 and 3–6). Release of this enzyme from the organelles is stimulated by decreased progesterone and probably factors such as disruption or stretching of the fetal membranes.

Bacteria may play a role in initiation of labor by either disrupting fetal membranes or producing enzymes or other mediators that activate arachidonic acid and increase prostaglandin biosynthesis.[127] Many of the bacteria that colonize the female urogenital tract (*Bacteroides fragilis, Streptococcus viridans, Peptostreptococcus,* and *Fusobacterium*), as well as other organisms associated with preterm delivery (*N. gonorrhoeae, Trichomonas vaginalis, Chlamydia trachomatis,* and group B streptococcus [GBS]), also produce phospholipase A_2.[9, 50, 92] Bacterial phospholipase A_2 activity is higher than fetal membrane phospholipase A_2 activity, which potentiates the likelihood of labor initiation. Alternatively or in conjunction with production of phospholipase A_2, these organisms may ascend into the fetal compartment and interfere with the integrity of the fetal membranes, leading to membrane rupture or release of prostaglandin from lysosomes in the fetal membranes.

Other factors that may stimulate prostaglandin production and increase the risk of labor onset include bacterial products such as endotoxin that increase maternal production of interleukin-1 (IL-1). IL-1 is an endogenous pyrogen that stimulates PGE_2 production in the hypothalamus. Maternal immune responses to infection involving release of lymphokines from activated T lymphocytes may also initiate or potentiate labor-initiating mechanisms.[93, 127] Labor may also be triggered by premature rupture of the membranes. Bacteria, either directly or indirectly through the action of IL-1 or other lymphokines on the mother's phagocytes, induce proteolytic enzymes such as collagenase and elastase. These enzymes break down the fetal membranes by causing focal impairment and weakening of the amnion and chorion.[93, 94, 127]

Perinatal HIV Infection

Acquired immunodeficiency syndrome (AIDS) is an infectious disorder caused by the human immunodeficiency virus (HIV). HIV is a retrovirus that invades and eventually destroys T4 helper lymphocytes. Since T4 cells are the "conductors of the immune orchestra,"[144, p. 139] this disrupts the entire immune system resulting in a severely immunocompromised host.[144]

The genome (genetic information) of retroviruses such as HIV consists of ribonucleic acid (RNA) that is transcribed into a deoxyribonucleic acid (DNA) copy by an enzyme called reverse transcriptase. The newly synthesized viral DNA (the provirus) can be integrated into the chromosomes of the host cell (T lymphocyte or monocytic macrophage) and serve as a template for replication of the virus in the host cell (Fig. 10–3).[132] Once activated (by an event not yet known), the proviral DNA makes viral RNA, which produces viral proteins using the host cell's cellular enzyme systems. Viral particles are released from the host cell and spread the virus either through production of additional viruses or fusion with and infection of other cells.

HIV proviral DNA may lie dormant in cells for months or years before it begins to divide and cause overt disease. In the latent stage little or no viral RNA is produced and the virus will often not be recognized by the person's immune system.[87, 99] During this period, infected cells can be transferred to other people through blood, semen, vaginal secretions, and breast milk.

Immunologic alterations found in people with HIV infection include decreased numbers of total and T lymphocytes (especially T-helper cells), reversed T-helper–to–T-suppressor (T4-to-T8) cell ratio, decreased T-cell suppressor and cytotoxic function, decreased NK activity, and increased levels of immunoglobulins. Decreased T-killer (cytotoxic) cells reduce the levels of interleukin-2 and interferon (proteins that stimulate NK cells and macrophages). Thus, the activity of NK cells and macrophages is further reduced and the overall risk of infection increased.[19]

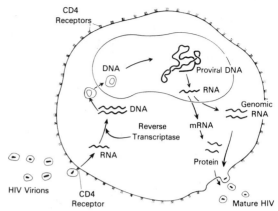

FIGURE 10–3. HIV replication. HIV contains glycoproteins that bind to specific CD4 receptors, which allows the virus to enter the cell. The CD4 receptors are found most often on membranes of T4 lymphocytes and monocytes. HIV is a retrovirus. Normally genetic information is stored as DNA and transcribed by RNA for use in protein synthesis. In a retrovirus the genetic information is stored as RNA and must first be transcribed back into DNA (retrograde step) by reverse transcriptase (azidothymidine [AZT] targets this enzyme). The viral DNA can be integrated into the nucleus of the host cell and act as a template for transcription of viral RNA in the host cell. The viral RNA is translated in the ribosome of the host cell into viral proteins, which are then released. (Modified from Sever, J. L. [1989]. HIV: Biology and immunology. *Clin Obstet Gynecol, 32,* 423.)

The inflammatory response is also altered in HIV infection, possibly because of decreased lymphokine production and alterations in monocyte chemotaxis.[37]

In the absence of adequate T-helper activity, B lymphocytes produce inadequate amounts of specific antibody to HIV and other organisms. This change, in conjunction with changes in T-lymphocyte (especially cytotoxic and suppressor) function, increases the risk of opportunistic and other infections. The B lymphocytes do respond to HIV, but this response involves secretion of large amounts of nonspecific immunoglobulins that are not useful in preventing infection. The result is hypergammaglobulinemia with elevated levels of immunoglobulins (increased levels of IgG with or without elevations of IgM and IgA) characteristic of HIV infection.[110] Although levels of immunoglobulins are elevated, there is a functional hypogammaglobulinemia. Elevated levels of nonspecific immunoglobulins are particularly characteristic of people with asymptomatic HIV infection. With development of symptoms, they may have decreased immunoglobulin levels.[37]

The impact of changes in the immune system during pregnancy on the progression of AIDS is still unclear. Pregnancy is associated with alterations in cell-mediated immunity, such as decreased lymphocyte function and decreased levels of T-helper cells, that increase the risk of infection with viruses and opportunistic pathogens. Since AIDS is a viral disorder and is associated with an increased risk of opportunistic infections, there is the potential for and some evidence that AIDS may have a more fulminant course during pregnancy.[30, 82, 154] Asymptomatic women whose infants develop HIV infection have a high rate of symptom development in the first 6 months after delivery.[30, 99]

Pregnancy can mask the symptoms of HIV infection since many nonspecific symptoms (fatigue, dyspnea, anemia) associated with this disorder can also occur with pregnancy. Immunologic changes seen with HIV infection such as decreased T4 (helper) cells and a reversed T4-to-T8 ratio also occur in healthy pregnant women. T4 levels in HIV-seropositive pregnant women are reported to be 10 to 20% lower than those in seronegative controls, however.[82] Careful assessments must be performed throughout pregnancy on women who are in high-risk categories for developing AIDS or are HIV positive.

HIV can be transmitted to the fetus and neonate by transplacental passage of the virus, contact with maternal blood or vaginal secretions at delivery, or through breast milk. The specific method of transmission is uncertain, but it most probably occurs through transplacental passage of the virus.[88, 110, 112] Currently most infants with perinatal AIDS are born to women who are intravenous drug abusers, although the number of women infected through sexual contact is increasing. The incidence of transmission from mother to fetus is currently estimated to range from 25 to 35%, although higher rates have been reported.[109, 110] Approximately half of the mothers of infected infants are asymptomatic.

Women who are seropositive for HIV need counseling about transmission to the fetus and neonate so they can make an informed choice regarding continuation of the pregnancy and need to receive information on ways to reduce the risk of transmitting the virus to others. HIV is excreted in breast milk, so infected women should be counseled regarding the potential risks of breast-feeding. The Centers for Disease Control currently recommends that HIV-infected women in the United States do not breast-feed, since alternatives are available.[24] Conversely, the World Health Organization recommends that infected women in Third World countries continue to breast-feed since breast milk is usually the only source of calories and protein for the infant and the risk of death from malnutrition outweighs the risk of acquiring HIV.[174]

Maternal HIV infection is currently not an indication for cesarean section since perinatal transmission is thought to occur primarily through transplacental passage of the virus. In addition, there is inadequate evidence to support the use of cesarean section as a way to decrease infection, and the risks of surgery in a potentially immunocompromised host are significant.[58, 82, 109, 112]

Antibiotic Use During Pregnancy

Antibiotics are some of the more frequently prescribed drugs during pregnancy. The effect of maternal physiologic adaptations on pharmacokinetics of antibiotics, achievement of therapeutic dosages, and development of toxic effects in both the mother and fetus are not well understood. Antibiotics act by interfering with the structural integrity or metabolic function of bacteria. Bacteriocidal antibiotics produce changes in bacterial cell walls or membranes that result in cell lysis. Bacteriostatic drugs alter the organism's metabolism by interfering with protein or nucleic acid synthesis. This leads to a suspension in bacterial growth but is not immediately lethal to the organism. Antibiotics are potentially dangerous to the fetus since agents that are not specific for bacterial cells may also disrupt fetal cells.[81]

Maternal physiologic adaptations that may alter the pharmacokinetics of antibiotics include changes in the hepatic, GI, renal, and hematologic systems (see Chapters 5, 8, and 9).[27, 81] Decreased GI motility and delayed gastric emptying alter initial absorption of oral antibiotics and lead to unpredictable patterns of intestinal absorption. The reduction in plasma proteins may increase plasma levels of free (active) drug. (Drugs are carried in the blood either bound to plasma proteins or as free drug. Protein-bound drugs provide a reservoir for future use, whereas free drug is the active component available to interact with target bacteria.)

Elevated blood and plasma volumes during pregnancy increase the volume for distribution, which may reduce serum levels of drugs and necessitate larger loading doses. Alterations in hepatic metabolism can increase the rate of biotransformation and clearance of drugs from maternal serum. The increased glomerular filtration rate augments renal clearance of antibiotics, thus further reducing serum levels. Most antibiotics are lipid soluble and readily cross the placenta. Thus, a portion of the drug may be sequestered in the fetal compartment and unavailable for maternal use. With increased placental efficiency as gestation advances, a larger proportion of the drug may be transferred to the fetus, increasing the maternal-fetal gradient. Factors reducing maternal serum levels increase the risk of subtherapeutic drug levels.[27, 103] Decreases in maternal serum antibiotic levels of 10 to 50% have been reported.[27]

As a result of these alterations, dosages of some antibiotics may need to be increased or the dosing interval reduced.[27, 103, 138] Maternal antibiotic levels must be carefully monitored to ensure that the mother is receiving an adequate therapeutic dose and to avoid maternal or fetal toxicity. With most local infections the reduction in maternal serum concentrations probably does not alter therapeutic efficacy of the antibiotic. Pregnant women with acute infections or who need high serum concentrations require much higher doses than nonpregnant women.[103] During the immediate postpartum period the pattern of pharmacokinetics and drug distribution is similar to that of late pregnancy and remains so until the pregnancy-induced physiologic alterations of each system return to nonpregnant status.[27]

Since antibiotics cross the placenta primarily by simple diffusion, rate-limiting factors include maternal-fetal concentration gradients, molecular weight and other physicochemical characteristics of the drug, placental surface area, diffusing distance, and the degree to which the drug is bound to maternal plasma proteins (see Table 2–6). A general pattern of antibiotic distribution to the fetus has been described.[23, 62] After an IV dose, peak maternal serum concentrations are seen within 15 minutes then fall exponentially.

Peak umbilical cord values are seen in 30 to 60 minutes followed by an exponential fall. Peak amniotic fluid levels are seen in 4 to 5 hours. This lag results from slow excretion in fetal urine due to fetal renal immaturity.[27, 81, 103]

Administration of antibiotics to the mother with the purpose of protecting the fetus is probably reasonably effective for protection of the GI (swallowing of amniotic fluid) and renal (adequate blood flow) systems. The fetal circulation shunts blood away from the lungs, however, which limits delivery of antibiotics to the respiratory tract for protection against congenital pneumonia in the presence of chorioamnionitis. Since amniotic fluid levels of antibiotics are dependent on excretion of the drug in fetal urine, therapeutic levels of antibiotics in amniotic fluid are attained only with a live fetus. This limits the effectiveness of this treatment for chorioamnionitis after intrauterine death.[27, 81, 138]

Schwartz divided fetal risks from maternal antibiotic use into three groups: (1) no known contraindications or low risk (i.e., penicillin and cephalosporin, which although bacteriocidal are specific to bacterial cell walls and theoretically are not harmful to the fetus); (2) relative risk that is not peculiar to the fetus (i.e., the risk of nephrotoxicity and ototoxicity seen with aminoglycosides at any age); and (3) absolute contraindications during at least some part of gestation due to well-documented adverse fetal and neonatal effects (i.e., tetracycline and chloramphenicol).[138] Adverse effects associated with these and other antibiotics and their proposed mechanisms are summarized in Table 10–5. The overall incidence of maternal adverse effects from antibiotics is not increased during pregnancy except for an increased risk of hepatotoxicity with erythromycin estolate (other forms of this drug are generally safe), tetracycline, and isoniazid (Table 10–5).

The impact of maternal physiologic alterations and fetal drug transfer can be illustrated by examining pharmacokinetics and distribution of several antibiotics. Only about 20% of ampicillin is protein bound, increasing the level of free drug that readily crosses into the fetal compartment. As a result, fetal and amniotic fluid levels are elevated and maternal serum and plasma levels decreased. The volume of distribution and renal clearance are increased and the half-life of ampi-

TABLE 10–5
Toxicity of Selected Antibiotics in the Pregnant Woman, Fetus, and Neonate

DRUG GROUP OR AGENT	PLACENTAL TRANSFER	PHARMACOKINETICS: MATERNAL	PHARMACOKINETICS: FETAL/NEONATAL
Contraindicated			
Chloramphenicol	High	Unchanged	↓ Hepatic conjugation ↓ Renal excretion ↑ Half-life
Tetracycline	High	Probably unchanged	Probably unchanged
Erythromycin estolate	Low	↓ Serum level ↓ Absorption	Low penetration
Trimethoprim	High	Serum level unchanged ↓ Half-life	Serum level unchanged ↓ Half-life
Use With Caution			
Aminoglycosides	Low to moderate	↓ Serum level ↑ Volume of distribution ↑ Excretion	↑ Volume of distribution ↓ Excretion
Clindamycin and lincomycin	Moderate	Serum level unchanged ↓ Half-life	Unchanged
Nitrofurantoin	High	↓ Serum level ↑ Excretion	↓ Excretion
Metronidazole	High	Probably unchanged	Probably unchanged
Sulfonamides	High	Serum level unchanged ↓ Half-life	Unchanged
Isoniazid	Yes	Serum level unchanged	Unchanged
Considered Safe			
Penicillins	Moderate to high	↓ Serum level ↑ Excretion ↑ Volume of distribution ↓ Half-life	Probably unchanged
Ampicillin	High	Similar to above	10% protein bound
Cephalosporins	Moderate to high	↓ Serum level ↑ Excretion ↑ Volume of distribution ↓ Half-life	Probably unchanged

Adapted from Chow, A.W. & Jewesson, P.J. (1985). Pharmacokinetics and safety of antimicrobial agents during pregnancy. *Rev Infect Dis, 7,* 287.

cillin reduced in the pregnant woman.[27, 81, 113] Ampicillin alters intestinal flora and reduces urinary estriol excretion.

Decreased maternal serum and plasma levels of aminoglycosides are also found, increasing the likelihood of subtherapeutic levels. For example, Weinstein and associates reported that 40% of pregnant women required twice the recommended dose of gentamicin to achieve therapeutic levels.[168] Cord blood levels of gentamicin are about half of maternal levels and are often subtherapeutic.[81] If aminoglycosides are used, blood levels (risk of subtherapeutic levels) and maternal renal function (risk of nephrotoxicity) require careful monitoring.

Higher maternal serum levels and lower fetal and amniotic fluid levels are seen with the use of antibiotics with increased protein binding such as methicillin (40%) and dicloxacillin (96%). As a result, a drug such as dicloxacillin would be appropriate for treating a maternal infection but not effective in treating an intrauterine infection.[27] Dicloxacillin and erythromycin have limited placental transfer so fetal levels are low. Maternal absorption, serum levels, and tissue levels of erythromycin tend to be erratic and unpredictable.[81] Higher concentrations of antibiotics are found in the fetus and amniotic fluid after bolus versus continuous drip infusion to the mother and after multiple versus single doses.[27]

The transfer of antibiotics in human milk is influenced by factors similar to those affecting placental transfer. Although most antibiotics can be detected in human milk, the concentration of drug to which the infant is exposed is usually low and rarely toxic. The pH of human milk (average, 6.8 to 7.0; range, 6.4 to 7.6) tends to be lower than plasma pH, so antibiotics that are weak bases

TABLE 10–5
Toxicity of Selected Antibiotics in the Pregnant Woman, Fetus, and Neonate *Continued*

MATERNAL TOXICITY	FETAL/NEONATAL TOXICITY	EXCRETION IN BREAST MILK/TOXICITY	
Bone marrow depression; aplastic anemia	Aplastic anemia; gray baby syndrome; cardiovascular collapse	Yes	Avoid, similar to neonatal effects
Hepatotoxicity; renal failure	Tooth discoloration and dysplasia; inhibition of bone growth	Yes	Low bioavailability (chelated with Ca)
Cholestatic hepatitis	None known	Yes	Probably safe
Allergic reactions; vasculitis	Folate antagonism; anomalies; hemolysis (G6PD deficiency)	Yes	Use with caution
Ototoxicity and nephrotoxicity	Eighth nerve toxicity; possible alterations in intestinal flora	Low	Poorly absorbed from GI tract
Allergic reactions; diarrhea; pseudomembranous colitis	None known	Trace	10 to 20% of serum levels
Neuropathy; hemolysis (G6PD deficiency)	Hemolysis (G6PD deficiency)	Trace	
Blood dyscrasia, neuropathy	None documented	Yes	100% of serum levels
Allergic reactions	Kernicterus; hemolysis (G6PD deficiency)	Yes	Use with extreme caution during 1st week
Hepatotoxicity	Possible neuropathy and seizures	Yes	
Allergic reactions	None known, risk of allergic reactions	Trace	
Decreases urinary estriol excretion	Diarrhea, candidiasis	Trace	
Allergic reactions	Allergic reactions	Trace	Small amounts safe

tend to be found in higher concentrations in human milk than in maternal serum. Lipid-soluble antibiotics reach higher peak levels in human milk in a shorter period of time than do less lipid-soluble agents.[27, 81] Some antibiotics may be excreted in human milk as inactive metabolites, remain unabsorbed, or be destroyed in the infant's digestive tract after ingestion. Excretion of antibiotics in human milk and potential adverse effects are summarized in Table 10–5.

Immunization and the Pregnant Woman

Ideally immunization of women of childbearing age should occur at least 3 months before conception (or immediately post partum) to reduce the risk of infection and fetal malformations.[130] At times immunizations may need to be given during pregnancy after accidental or potential exposure to a preventable transmissible organism associated with significant maternal or fetal risks.[42] Alterations in the immune system during pregnancy do not seem to significantly alter the woman's responses to immunization.[42, 43] Potential risks of immunization during pregnancy include fetal viremia, teratogenesis, interference with development of the infant's response to immunizations during childhood, and maternal side effects that might compromise uteroplacental function.[42]

Immunity can be achieved by either passive or active means. Passive immunity involves transfer of antibodies from an actively immunized to a nonimmunized person. Passive immunity provides short-term protection until the antibodies are catabolized by the nonimmunized person's system. Transfer of antibodies from mother to fetus during the third trimester and injection of gamma globulin are examples of passive immunity. Active immunity involves exposure to some form of the antigen (attenuated or live organisms rendered noninfectious, inactivated or killed organisms, inactivated exotoxins or toxoids) and the formation of antibodies and memory cells against that antigen by the nonimmunized person. Active immunization may take weeks or months for adequate protection to develop, but long-lasting or permanent immune responses are induced.[42, 130]

Immunization of pregnant women with active viruses or bacteria is dangerous because of the risk of transfer of the antigen to the fetus. Immunization with measles (rubeola), mumps, and rubella vaccines is specifically contraindicated because of potential adverse fetal consequences. This risk appears to be primarily theoretical at least with rubella. If a women is accidentally vaccinated early in pregnancy with live rubella vaccine, the risk of adverse fetal effects appears to be low, based on several series of women accidentally vaccinated before they realized they were pregnant.[22, 42, 117] Passive immunization of nonimmunized women exposed to rubella in the first trimester has been recommended as a method to reduce the risk of congenital infection and fetal anomalies. The use of this therapy is controversial since it may prevent clinical disease but not necessarily infection and transmission of the virus to the fetus.[11] Pregnant women who discover that they are pregnant after being immunized, especially with a live virus, must be counseled about possible risks and alternatives.

Oral polio viruses (using inactivated [killed] viruses) appear to be safe if given during pregnancy and provide protection to both the fetus and mother.[42, 117] This immunization is not recommended for routine protection but only if an unvaccinated woman is traveling to an area where polio is endemic.[130] Other immunizations may occasionally be required during pregnancy. The risk of fetal and maternal infection must be compared with the risks of vaccination; passive immunization or an inactivated (killed) vaccine or toxoid should be used if available; and, if possible, vaccination should be delayed until the second trimester or later (i.e., after the period of organogenesis).[130] Faix and Shope recommend use of both passive and active immunization (to provide immediate protection while the woman's endogenous protection is developing), if safe and effective forms of both types of immunization are available.[42]

Administration of immunizations during the first few days post partum is often recommended. If live virus vaccines are used, the woman should be counseled to use methods to prevent conception for 3 months. Blood and blood products given within 14 days of active immunization may interfere with the vaccine's effectiveness since blood may contain antibodies against the antigens in the vaccine and therefore interfere with the woman's own immune response.[42] Rho(D) immune globulin (RhIG) does not seem to interfere with immunizations given at this time, probably because doses of RhIG are relatively small. Faix and Shope note that although there is a small theoretical risk of transfer of antigens through breast milk or nasopharyngeal secretions from a recently immunized woman to her infant, this is a rare event without significant morbidity.[42] Current recommendations regarding specific immunizations during pregnancy can be found in several reviews.[42, 130]

Malignancy and Pregnancy

Theoretically, alterations in the maternal immune system could increase the risk of malignancy since cell-mediated immunity, which is suppressed in the pregnant woman, normally protects against virally-induced tumors. This finding is not supported by most reviewers, however.[34, 68, 102] Some investigators have specifically suggested an increase in rate and decreased survival for women with breast and cervical cancer during pregnancy, but this has generally not been supported.[68] Melanoma may intensify during pregnancy, then recede or disappear after delivery.[167] The basis for this change has been attributed to increased levels of melanocyte-stimulating hormone during pregnancy (see Chapter 11) and hormonal stimulation of estrogen receptors found on melanoma cells.[78, 97]

Immunologic Aspects of Pregnancy-Induced Hypertension

Pregnancy-induced hypertension is a complex, multifaceted disorder involving alterations in many major body systems. There is increasing evidence that vascular endothelial cell injury is an early event in the pathogenesis of PIH.[121] The exact cause of this damage is unclear but an immunologic role has been suggested. Factors that support an immunologic basis for PIH include an increased incidence of the disorder in primigravidas, first pregnancies with a different father, and pregnancies with a large placental mass or hydatidiform mole; a decreased incidence in repeat pregnancies (even if the previous pregnancy ended in a miscarriage) with the same father and consanguineous marriages; and pathologic changes in the uterine vessels near the placental site, similar to those with allograft rejection.[141, 161] In addition, specific alterations in the immune system have been observed in women with PIH. Many of these changes are exaggerations of the changes normally found during pregnancy. Women with PIH have a further reduction of NK cell activity, more T8 suppressor cells, decreased T4-to-T8 cell ratio, increased immune (antibody–antigen) complexes and fibronectin, and alterations in complement.[90, 121, 133, 161]

Several mechanisms have been proposed to explain the immunologic basis of PIH. Women with PIH may have an inadequate antibody response to the fetal allograft with a deficiency in either blocking antibody or suppressor cell function. As a result, the mother rejects the fetus as she would any foreign tissue graft. PIH might be an immune complex disorder with inadequate clearance of these complexes by the mother's reticuloendothelial system due to an inadequate maternal antibody response or to an excess of fetal antigen (i.e., with a large placental mass as is seen with multiple pregnancies or hydatidiform mole). These circulating complexes then become trapped in structures such as the glomerulus of the kidney, leading to organ damage and dysfunction.[47, 141, 161] In addition, the presence of antibodies to human vascular endothelial cells has been reported in many women with PIH.[121]

Pregnancy-Induced Immune States

Specific immune states complicating pregnancy in the absence of overt autoimmune disease have been described. These immune states seem to occur primarily at two points. Early in gestation a "reproductive autoimmunity" with failure of the mother to appropriately recognize the fetal allograft can lead to interference in normal fetoplacental growth and development and pregnancy loss. Recently, several clinical syndromes have been reported in the latter part of pregnancy and the early postpartum period. These syndromes include many findings characteristic of autoimmune disorders but are not associated with any documented autoimmune disease in the pregnant woman. Gleicher described these disorders as "pregnancy-induced autoimmunity" and compared them with pregnancy-induced gestational diabetes.[53] There has been little long-term follow-up to determine if these disorders are transient or precede the development of autoimmune disease.

The characteristics of these syndromes include a sudden onset of symptoms in the third trimester or early postpartum period, frequent single organ preponderance of clinical manifestations but always multiorgan involvement, and passive transfer of the disease to the fetus. Disorders that might be examples of altered immune states during pregnancy include postpartum hemolytic uremic syndrome, idiopathic thrombocytopenia with multiple organ failure, acute respiratory distress with other organ system failure, and the HELLP syndrome (see later). Termination of pregnancy usually results in rapid improvement although these disorders can recur, often with increased severity, with subsequent pregnancies.[53]

Gleicher proposed that pregnancy-induced immune states may arise during the third trimester or early postpartum period as a response of the maternal immune system to the increasing number of fetal cells entering her circulation as pregnancy progresses.[53] If maternal tolerance of the fetus is a localized (uterine) phenomenon and enough fetal cells enter the general maternal circulation, or if the mother's host defense system is particularly sensitive, an immune response may be triggered. The higher risk of transfer of fetal cells into the maternal circulation with placental separation would account for the high incidence of these disorders post partum.

HELLP Syndrome

The HELLP syndrome (see Chapter 6) is characterized by findings similar to those of severe preeclampsia along with hemolysis (H), elevated liver enzymes (EL), and low platelet counts (LP) that may represent an acute autoimmune state.[147, 169] The cause of this syndrome is poorly understood and there is much speculation and debate.[147] The HELLP syndrome seems to involve a group of clinical and pathologic manifestations resulting from some type of insult that leads to platelet activation and release of thromboxane and serotonin. These vasoconstrictors lead to vasospasm with further platelet aggregation and endothelial damage.[147] Gleicher suggests that although the HELLP syndrome is often diagnosed as PIH, it is actually a specific pregnancy-induced immune syndrome.[53] Others believe that this disorder is a severe form of preeclampsia.[121, 161] The HELLP syndrome is also associated with transient fetal hematologic alterations including thrombocytopenia, passive transfer from the mother to the fetus of an antiplatelet antibody of the IgG class, an abnormal peripheral smear, and an increased incidence of hyperbilirubinemia.[53, 169]

The Pregnant Woman with an Autoimmune Disease

The effect of pregnancy on autoimmune disorders is varied; individual women experience improvement, exacerbation, or no change depending on the disorder. Autoimmune disorders are thought to impair T-suppressor cell activity, resulting in hyperactive B-lymphocyte response and production of autoantibodies that form immune (antibody–antigen) complexes with their target antigens. These immune complexes activate the complement cascade, which in turn mediates phagocytosis and an inflammatory response.

Since the usual changes in the immune system during pregnancy are the exact opposite of these events, women with autoimmune disorders may experience an improvement.[163] For example, most women with rheumatoid arthritis experience improvement during pregnancy, generally beginning in the first trimester; 90% relapse between 6 weeks and 6 months post partum.[75, 163] Specific mechanisms underlying this improvement are unclear, but these changes are reported to parallel the rise in pregnancy zone protein, which has a suppressive effect on the inflammatory process.[163] Other changes during pregnancy that might lead to the amelioration include changes in maternal humoral factors, depression of cell-mediated immunity, and suppression of inflammatory reactions.[75]

Conversely, systemic lupus erythematosus (SLE) has been associated with exacerbation, particularly in women with renal involvement. Women with mild involvement whose disease is under control before and during pregnancy often experience no exacerbation and a few may improve. Exacerbation has been reported to be more frequent in early pregnancy and during the first 6 to 8 weeks post partum. Postpartum exacerbation may represent a rebound phenomenon as suppression of cell-mediated activity is terminated.[53] Several recent series have reported exacerbation rates of only 10 to 15% during pregnancy and no increase in flareups post partum.[35, 100]

SLE is associated with an increased frequency of stillbirth, abortion, preterm birth, and intrauterine growth retardation that may result from the presence of a lupus anticoagulant factor.[163] This factor is an immunoglobulin that binds to prothrombin-activating complexes and predisposes the woman to recurrent thrombosis in the spiral arteries and placental infarction.[123] SLE and other maternal autoimmune disorders are associated with passively-acquired, transient fetal autoimmune manifestations.

Transplacental Passage of Maternal Antibodies

Both protective and potentially damaging antibodies cross the placenta. Maternal IgG antibodies, predominantly in the IgG1 and IgG3 subclasses, are the only ones to cross in significant amounts, primarily because of the size of the molecules and the presence of an IgG-specific carrier for active placental transport. Fetal levels of IgG are low until 20 to 22 weeks' gestation, when passive and active transfer of IgG across the placenta increase. Although fetal IgG levels increase from that point to term, significant transfer of IgG probably does not occur until after 32 to 34 weeks and is greatest during the last 4 to 6 weeks of term gestation.[102]

Active transfer of IgG across the placenta through pinocytosis (see Chapter 2) is mediated by a carrier attached to a trophoblast surface receptor that is specific for the Fc fragment of IgG and does not bind other immunoglobulins. Active transfer allows for transfer of IgG even when maternal levels are low.[23] Placental dysfunction seems to limit transfer of maternal IgG as lower levels are seen in small for gestational age (SGA) infants and in infants born after 44 weeks' gestation.[26] Maternal IgA does not cross the placenta in significant amounts; IgM is not transferred.

The fact that only IgG crosses the placenta is both an advantage and disadvantage to the fetus. Passage of IgG provides passive immunity against many disorders through passage of antibodies acquired by the mother from previous infection or immunization. Depending on maternal antibody complement, passive immunity against tetanus, diphtheria, polio, measles, mumps, group B streptococcus, *E. coli*, hepatitis B, salmonella, and other disorders may be acquired by the fetus. Conversely, damaging antibodies in the IgG class, such as in Rh incompatibility, also cross the placenta.

Potentially damaging antibodies in other immunoglobulin classes, such as the ABO antigens, which are primarily IgM, and allergy-producing IgE antigen generally do not cross, so the fetus is protected. Conversely, transplacental passage of IgM would be an advantage in enhancing protection of the fetus and newborn from gram-negative bacteria and the TORCH organisms. (TORCH stands for *T*oxoplasmosis, *O*ther viruses, *R*ubella, *C*ytomegalovirus, *H*erpes simplex.)

Potentially damaging maternal IgG antibodies may cross the placenta with several maternal chronic diseases as well as Rh incompatibility and lead to transient disorders in some neonates. Neonatal effects range from mild to severe. In general, if the disorder is not fatal during the perinatal period, manifestations are transient and regress as maternal antibody is catabolized.

Graves' disease involves transplacental passage of a thyroid-stimulating immunoglobulin that leads to neonatal hyperthyroidism in a few infants. Myasthenia gravis is associated with passage of a maternal antibody against the acetylcholine receptors, resulting in transient myasthenia gravis in 10 to 20% of offspring. Symptoms last from a few hours to weeks. Since symptoms usually develop at 1 to 2 days of age, infants who appear healthy at birth may later develop respiratory failure.[11, 105, 139]

Maternal antiplatelet antibodies induce fetal thrombocytopenia in up to 50% of the offspring of women with immune thrombocytopenia purpura. The greatest neonatal risk is for severe hemorrhage in the perinatal period. In most infants platelet levels reach lowest levels at 4 to 6 days after birth and return to normal by 1 to 2 months.[10, 11, 139]

In women with SLE, a maternal autoantibody to blood elements may result in fetal neutropenia, thrombocytopenia, and congenital heart block. Recent reports indicate that many infants with congenital heart block have mothers with IgG antibodies to fetal heart tissue ribonucleoprotein. It is unclear if the antibodies are responsible for pathologic changes within the heart conduction system such as atrioventricular (AV) node absence, AV bundle lesions, or absent connections between the AV node and the atrial conduction system.[139] All mothers with these antibodies do not have infants with heart block. Congenital heart block is associated with viral infections such as cytomegalovirus (CMV) and with latent or overt maternal connective tissue disorders. About 30 to 60% of mothers of infants with congenital heart block either have or eventually develop SLE.[8, 53, 123, 139]

Rho(D) Isoimmunization and ABO Incompatibility

Rho(D) isoimmunization can be used as a model to examine the application of immunologic principles and to illustrate how the interaction of maternal and fetal host defense mechanisms can result in pathophysiologic processes during the perinatal period. Isoimmune hemolytic disease, hemolytic disease of the newborn, and erythroblastosis fetalis are all terms for a disorder caused by transplacental passage of maternal IgG antibody that reacts with antigens on the fetal red blood cell (RBC) and leads to cell lysis. The fetal-neonatal effects may be minimal or may include severe anemia, congestive heart failure, and death. Because maternal antibody remains in the infant's circulation, the hemolytic process continues after birth.

The Rh system involves a group of over 30 known antigens controlled by three pairs of genes (Cc, Dd, Ee). Antigens of the D group are the ones usually involved in incompatibility between mother and fetus. Rho(D) isoimmunization occurs when a Rho(D)-negative mother carrying a Rho(D)-positive fetus produces antibody against the D antigen on the fetal RBC. Isoimmunization can occur with other RBC antigens such as Kell, Duffy, Kidd, MNS, and ABO.

Factors that influence whether a reaction between maternal antibody and fetal antigens will occur, and the intensity of that reaction, include the presence of antigens on fetal tissue that are not found on maternal tissue, distribution of the antigen in fetal tissue (if the antigen is widely distributed, competition for antibody is greater and the risk of tissue injury to specific body systems is reduced), strength and quantity of the antigen, efficacy of the maternal immune response, presence or absence of previous exposure and sensitization to the antigen, and the type of antibody produced by the mother.[83, 128] In terms of Rho(D) isoimmunization, the D antigen is a powerful antigen, present in large amounts on the fetal RBC, and stimulates formation of IgG-type antibody and memory cells in the mother. The amount of antigen necessary to trigger an immune response in the mother varies for each person, as does the intensity of the response by the mother's immune system. The incidence of Rho(D) isoimmunization is actually relatively low, ranging from 10 to 14% (if Rho(D) immune globulin [RhIG] is not given post partum) to less than 2% if RhIG is given.[16]

Rho(D)-negative women are unlikely to have antibodies against the D antigen unless they have been immunized during a previous pregnancy or from a mismatched blood transfusion. As a result isoimmunization is rare in first pregnancies. Normally during pregnancy the small amounts of fetal blood (<0.05 ml) that cross the placenta and enter the maternal circulation are too small to trigger production of antibodies by the mother's immune system. In a few women, however, as little as 0.01 ml of fetal blood has been reported to cause maternal immunization (sensitization).[83, 128] Approximately 1 to 2% of Rho(D)-negative women develop anti-D antibodies during their first pregnancy.[16]

With delivery and placental separation or with other traumatic events larger quantities of fetal blood (0.5 ml or more) may enter the maternal circulation. This amount of fetal blood (if the fetus is Rho(D) positive) is sufficient to stimulate formation of both anti-D antibody and memory cells in many women (Fig. 10–4A). Formation of memory cells results in immunization. Once a woman is immunized, she is immunized for life. During subsequent pregnancies even a very small amount of blood from a Rho(D)-positive fetus entering her system may be enough to trigger memory cells to produce antibodies against the D antigen on the fetal RBC. The antibodies that are produced in this second-

ary response are predominantly of the IgG class and are thus able to cross the placenta to the fetal circulation and hemolyze fetal RBCs (Fig. 10–4B). With each subsequent exposure to this same antigen, the maternal immune system's response is as intense as previous responses, and it often responds more rapidly and intensely with each succeeding pregnancy.[16, 83]

Intrauterine transfusions (IUTs) into the fetal abdominal cavity have been used for many years as in utero therapy for the affected fetus. Currently IUTs are performed directly into the vascular compartment through cordocentesis (see Chapter 2). More recently several other techniques involving alterations in the maternal and or fetal immune mechanisms have been tried to improve fetal outcome for Rho(D)-immunized women. These techniques include: (1) decreasing or removing maternal anti-D antibodies using plasmapheresis; (2) interfering with fetal destruction of its RBC through the use of promethazine, which reduces coating of fetal cells by maternal anti-D antibody and interferes with phagocytosis; (3) oral administration of antigen to the mother to desensitize her system (similar to the process used with allergies); and (4) intrauterine fetal exchange transfusions to replace fetal antigen-coated RBCs with nonantigen-containing donor cells.[76, 83] Results for the first three techniques have been equivocal; use of intrauterine exchange transfusions appears to be a more promising therapy.

With development of RhIG, a human gamma globulin concentrate of anti-D, initial immunization of most women can be prevented. RhIG is given in the postpartum period, prophylactically at 28 to 29 weeks (to prevent sensitization during pregnancy), or after any potentially sensitizing event such as an abortion, ectopic pregnancy, amniocentesis, or significant antepartal bleeding. RhIG acts by destroying fetal RBCs in the mother's system before the foreign D antigen on these cells can be recognized by her immune system and can trigger formation of antibodies and, more importantly, memory cells (Fig. 10–4C). RhIG is generally given within 72 hours of a potentially sensitizing event such as birth. Since in the absence of previous sensitization development of an adequate antibody response to a specific antigen can take days or weeks, RhIG can probably be given up to 3 to 4 weeks later if omitted earlier for some

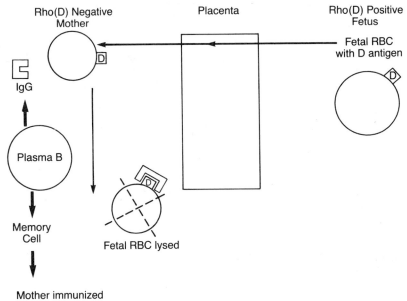

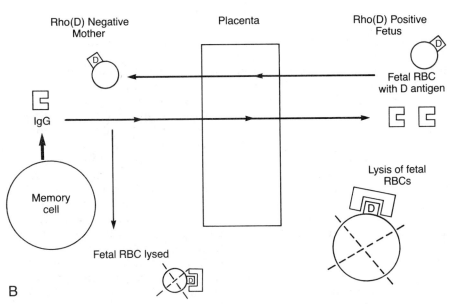

FIGURE 10–4. Rh isoimmunization. *A,* Process of immunization if RhIG is not given to previously unsensitized woman. *B,* Action of maternal immune system in subsequent pregnancies once the mother has been immunized.

Illustration continued on following page

reason. After administration of RhIG during the antepartum period some women may develop a low (1:4 or less) anti-D serum antibody titer. This positive titer reflects a passive immunity from the RhIG. The infant of a mother who received RhIG prophylaxis may have a weakly positive direct Coombs' test owing to placental transfer of RhIG an-tibodies. Neither of these responses indicates maternal sensitization and postpartum RhIG administration is indicated.[16, 76, 83]

Three potential mechanisms have been suggested for the action of RhIG: (1) clearance of antigen from the mother's system; (2) antigen-blocking by attaching to antigenic sites on the fetal cells, preventing interaction

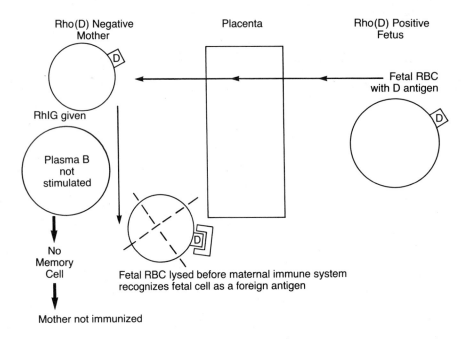

C

FIGURE 10–4 *Continued C,* Role of RhIG in prevention of maternal immunization.

with maternal lymphocytes; or (3) central inhibition of antibody production.[76] The last theory suggests that RhIG forms immune complexes with the Rho(D) antigen. Immune complexes suppress the stimulating effect of helper T lymphocytes, which in turn suppresses antibody formation by B lymphocytes.[76]

The potential for isoimmunization also exists with ABO incompatibility, although severe hemolytic disease in the fetus and newborn is rare. ABO incompatibility is three times as common as Rho(D) incompatibility. Previous exposure and immunization are not necessary with ABO incompatibility since the mother already has naturally occurring antibodies against fetal RBC antigens. The most common situation in which ABO incompatibility occurs is with a type O mother and a type A (Fig. 10–5A) or, less frequently, a type B infant (the A antigen seems to be more antigenic than B). The type O mother has naturally occurring anti-A and anti-B antibodies in her serum that can react against the A or B antigens on the fetal RBCs. ABO incompatibility could also occur with a type AB, but never with a type O infant (type O RBCs have neither A nor B antigens for maternal anti-A or anti-B antibodies to react against).

Since the mother already has antibodies against fetal RBC antigens, why is ABO incompatibility a relatively mild disorder compared with Rho(D) isoimmunization? The major reason is that the primary antibodies of the ABO system are IgM, which does not cross the placenta. Some of these antibodies may be of the IgG type. IgG antibodies of the ABO system are more common in those with type O blood, hence ABO isoimmunization occurs most frequently with type O mothers. Since A and B antigens also appear on somatic cells and are secreted into body fluids in most people, there is a large quantity of antigen to compete with the fetal RBCs for any maternal antibody.[83] In addition, the fetus may have its own anti-A or anti-B antibodies that can neutralize maternal antibody; there are fewer A and B antigens on the fetal RBC (resulting in only a weakly positive Coombs' test); and these antigens are relatively weak.[175] ABO isoimmunization, and probably Rho(D) isoimmunization, do not occur in the opposite direction (i.e., from baby to mother) because fetal antibodies tend to be in a macroglobulin form that cannot cross the placenta.

The simultaneous occurrence of Rho(D) and ABO isoimmunization has a protective effect that reduces the likelihood of maternal Rho(D) sensitization. This is illustrated in a Rho(D)-negative, type O (naturally occurring

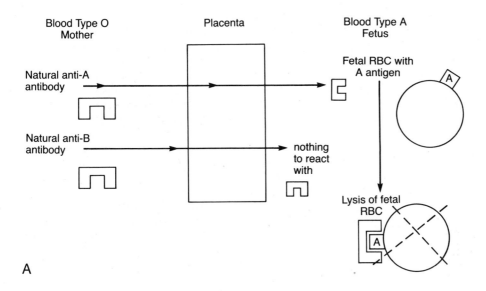

A

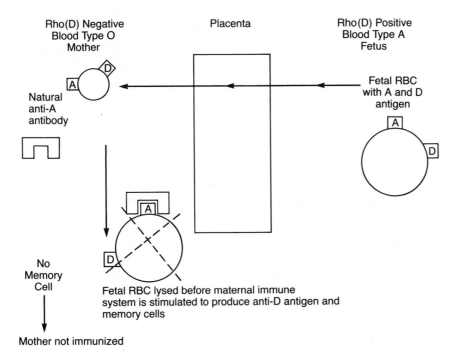

B

FIGURE 10–5. ABO incompatibility. *A,* Mechanisms of ABO incompatibility. *B,* Mechanism by which ABO and Rh incompatibility occurring simultaneously reduce the severity of Rh incompatibility.

anti-A and anti-B serum antibodies) woman with a Rho(D)-positive, type A (with A and D RBC antigens) fetus. Fetal cells entering maternal circulation (during pregnancy or at delivery) are destroyed by the naturally-occurring maternal anti-A antibody before they can trigger the mother's immune system to produce anti-D antibodies and memory cells (Fig. 10–5B). If anti-D antibodies and memory cells are not formed, the woman remains unsensitized.[16]

Protection of the Fetus from Infection

The fetus is a compromised host at increased risk for infection throughout gestation because of developmental limitations in the infant's host defense mechanisms. During gestation the potential for fetal exposure to pathogenic organisms from maternal bacterial colonization of the genital tract or primary or recurrent maternal viral infection and sexually transmitted diseases is an ongoing risk. Maternal, fetal, and placental factors play a role in protecting the fetus from infection.

Maternal factors include anatomic barriers such as maternal skin, respiratory mucosa, intestinal epithelium, and genitourinary tract surfaces. Maternal IgA enhances barrier function, whereas mucosal macrophages provide protection through phagocytic activity. The placenta acts as a barrier to the passage of bacteria that are too large to be transferred from maternal to fetal blood, although most viruses and some bacteria are able to be transferred. Organisms may occasionally reach the fetus by directly infecting placental tissue. The placenta allows transfer of maternal antibody to the fetus primarily through pinocytosis. The placenta also contains phagocytes and lymphocytes, and produces enzymes such as interferon.[64, 111]

Amniotic fluid contains antibacterial and other protective substances similar to many of those found in human milk. These substances include transferrin, beta-lysin, peroxidase, fatty acids, immunoglobulins, and lysozyme.[135] The antibacterial capacity of amniotic fluid improves with advancing gestation.[64] The fetal membranes provide barrier protection against ascending infection, although some organisms can penetrate intact membranes.[84, 111]

Premature rupture of the membranes is associated with a significant increase in perinatal mortality from intrauterine infection as the length of time between rupture of the membranes and delivery increases. This is particularly apparent after 24 hours. The usual cause of infection is chorioamnionitis due to an ascending infection from the vagina and cervix. In pregnancies in which rupture occurs before term, the risks associated with prematurity may significantly exceed the risk of fetal infection.[33, 50]

Maternal responses to infection, in particular fever, may have a damaging effect on the fetus. Fever due to either maternal infection or hyperthermia secondary to sauna use or intense exercise may result in fetal anomalies (see Chapter 17). Maternal fever can increase uterine activity, which, along with elaboration of prostaglandins, may result in initiation of labor.[116, 151]

SUMMARY

Alterations in maternal host defense mechanisms are critical for maintenance of the pregnancy, ensuring that the mother does not reject the fetus and protecting the fetus against infection. Yet these same mechanisms may increase the risk of infection and other immune system disorders in the pregnant woman. Transplacental passage of maternal immunoglobulins provides protection against specific pathogens but can also lead to fetal disease. Concerns related to organisms that colonize the maternal genital tract and sexually transmitted diseases such as herpes, hepatitis B, and AIDS have increased interest in host defense mechanisms and maternal-fetal interrelationships in recent years and altered practice in many settings. Clinical recommendations for nurses working with pregnant women based on changes in host defense mechanisms are summarized in Table 10–6. By recognizing the changes in maternal host defense mechanisms the nurse can identify women and infants at risk and initiate appropriate interventions and counseling.

DEVELOPMENT OF HOST DEFENSE MECHANISMS IN THE FETUS

Cellular components of the immune system arise from precursor cells within blood is-

TABLE 10–6
Summary of Recommendations for Clinical Practice Related to Changes in Host Defense Mechanisms:
Pregnant Woman

Recognize normal parameters for immune system components and patterns of change during pregnancy and the postpartum period (pp. 440–445, Table 10–2).

Obtain and evaluate complete history for possible exposure to infectious organisms or potential for current illness (pp. 440–444, 449–451).

Recognize risk factors for development of specific infections (pp. 440–444, 449–452, Table 10–2).

Monitor and counsel women regarding early signs and symptoms of infection and risk of prolonged hyperthermia (pp. 449–450, 464, 679).

Recognize clinical and laboratory changes during labor and delivery and post partum that may mask signs of infection (pp. 444–445).

Monitor women with infections during the second and third trimesters for signs of initiation of labor (pp. 450–451).

Teach women regarding methods to prevent or reduce the risk of infection while pregnant (pp. 449–452).

Recognize that pregnancy may depress reactions to tuberculin tests (especially in the second half of pregnancy) (p. 440).

Counsel woman regarding the immunologic advantages of human milk and its potential role in preventing gastrointestinal infections and allergies (pp. 445–446, 472–474, Table 10–3).

Monitor iron intake and serum ferritin levels in women at risk for or with a history of malaria (p. 450).

Recognize the effects of maternal physiologic adaptations on the pharmacokinetics of antibiotics (pp. 452–455).

Know or verify usual doses for antibiotics given during pregnancy or post partum (pp. 452–455).

Know and counsel women regarding side effects of antibiotics and potential toxicity to mother, fetus, and neonate (pp. 452–455, Table 10–5).

Know antibiotics not recommended during pregnancy and lactation (pp. 453–454, Table 10–5).

Monitor and evaluate maternal responses to antibiotics (pp. 452–455).

Recognize that ampicillin may decrease maternal urinary estriol excretion (p. 454).

Counsel women regarding risks of immunizations during pregnancy and to avoid pregnancy for 3 months after immunization (pp. 455–456).

Avoid giving immunizations within 14 days of administration of blood or blood products (except RhIG) (p. 456).

Give RhIG to unsensitized Rho(D)-negative women prophylactically at 28 weeks' gestation and after potentially immunizing events (pp. 459–462).

Understand implications of low antibody titers in some women who have received RhIG during the prenatal period and need for RhIG post partum (pp. 460–461).

Understand the implications of a weakly positive direct Coombs' test in some infants of women who have received RhIG during the prenatal period and the need for RhIG post partum (pp. 460–461).

Give RhIG post partum to unsensitized Rho(D)-negative women with a Rho(D)-positive fetus (pp. 459–469).

Counsel women with autoimmune disorders regarding potential effects of pregnancy (pp. 458–459).

Use universal precautions for blood and body fluids during the perinatal period (pp. 451–452, 479–480).

Counsel HIV-positive women regarding risks of transmission of the virus to their fetus and infant and their options (pp. 451–452, 479–480).

Counsel HIV-positive women regarding potential risks of breast-feeding (pp. 451–452).

Monitor HIV-positive women for signs of AIDS and AIDS-related complex (ARC) and of other infections (pp. 451–452).

Counsel women regarding safe sexual practices (pp. 451–452, 479–480).

Recognize that women who are HBeAg or HBsAg positive are infectious and institute hepatitis precautions (pp. 477–479, Table 10–11).

Counsel women with HBV, HSV, and other viral infections regarding long-term effects on infant (including shedding of virus) and use of precautions to prevent spread of the infection (pp. 451–452, 479–480).

Recognize women at risk to develop the HELPP syndrome and signs and symptoms of this syndrome (pp. 457–458, Chapter 6).

Counsel women with chronic disorders associated with transplacental passage of antibodies regarding the potential impact on their fetus and neonate (pp. 458–459).

Page numbers in parentheses following each intervention refer to the page(s) in the text where the rationale for that intervention is discussed.

lands of the yolk sac. Multipotential stem cells arise in these islands and migrate into the liver and spleen and later to the bone marrow and thymus. Table 10–7 summarizes development of fetal host defense mechanisms.

Pre-B cells are seen in the liver by 7 to 8 weeks; immature B lymphocytes with surface IgM receptors are found by 10 to 11 weeks in the fetal liver. By 12 weeks B lymphocytes are found in peripheral blood and bone marrow, with numbers reaching adult proportions by 15 to 18 weeks. Few of these B lymphocytes are plasma cells capable of secreting immunoglobulins. Synthesis of IgG, IgM, and IgE begins by 12 to 15 weeks; synthesis of IgA begins by 30 weeks, and sIgA is not seen until after birth.[12, 15, 23, 85]

TABLE 10–7
Development of Host Defense Mechanisms in the Fetus

	ANATOMIC DEVELOPMENT	FUNCTIONAL DEVELOPMENT
T cells	Early development 　7 to 9 wks First T lymphocytes 　thymus: 10 to 12 wks 　spleen: 13 to 15 wks 　blood: 14 wks	Antigen recognition: 12 wks Antigen binding: 13 wks Cell-mediated lympholysis: 7 months Antibody-dependent cytotoxicity: cord blood Graft-versus-host reactivity: 13 wks Mitogenic stimulation: 12–22 wks Antigenic stimulation: newborns Lymphotoxin production: cord blood
B cells	Fetal liver 　Pre-B cells (precursors of immature B 　　lymphocytes): 8 wks 　B lymphocytes with surface IgG, IgD, 　　IgM: 10 to 12 wks Peripheral blood 　B lymphocytes with surface antigen: 12 to 　　15 wks	IgG, IgM, IgE synthesis demonstrable at 10 to 23 wks; IgA at 30 wks Secretory IgA absent in neonate Very little antibody production by fetus, IgG actively transported 　across the placenta in third trimester
Complement	Complement synthesis identifiable in fetal 　tissue by 6 wks	Complement function not assessed in fetus but suspected to be 　diminished because of decreased concentrations of complement 　components
Neutrophils	Identifiable in 7-wk embryo	Most studies in term infants 　Chemotaxis decreased 　Phagocytosis, inconclusive data; subtle defects with serum 　　concentrations of less than 10% or in stressed neonates 　Bacteriocidal capacity 　　Nitroblue tetrazolium reduction, inconclusive data 　　Glycolytic enzymes reduced 　　Myeloperoxidase normal 　　Stressed neonates may have decreased bacteriocidal activity
Monocytes	Identifiable in 7-wk embryo	Most studies in term infants 　Chemotaxis, inconclusive data 　Phagocytosis, normal 　Bacteriocidal capacity, normal 　Antigen processing decreased in experimental animals, not 　　studied in humans

Modified from Yoder, M.C. & Polin, R.A. (1986). Immunotherapy of neonatal septicemia. *Pediatr Clin North Am, 33*, 481.

Levels of fetal immunoglobulins produced by the fetus normally remain low throughout gestation. Fetal serum IgG levels rise in the second and third trimesters with transplacental passage from the mother, with transfer highest during the last 4 to 6 weeks before term.[139] Elevated IgM levels in cord blood (>20 mg/dl) suggest intrauterine infection and are seen with pathogens such as cytomegalovirus, rubella, and toxoplasmosis. This IgM is of fetal origin since IgM does not cross from the mother.

Differentiation of the thymus begins at 6 weeks. Stem cells from the liver and spleen migrate to the thymus to form thymocytes. T lymphocytes appear in the thymus by 7 to 9 weeks. T lymphocytes with surface receptors are detected in lymphoid tissue by 11 to 12 weeks and in peripheral blood and spleen after 12 to 14 weeks, and they reach nearly adult proportions by 20 to 22 weeks. Concurrently, T cells begin to express characteristic surface markers that will later distinguish them as helper or suppressor cells. Cell-mediated cytotoxicity is deficient in the fetus.[102] Transplantation responses develop relatively early. Antigen recognition can be demonstrated by 12 weeks and graft-versus-host reactions by 13 weeks. Thus, one potential form of fetal and neonatal therapy, transplantation of normal tissue into an infant with a specific congenital anomaly or inherited disorder, is difficult. Cell-mediated lympholysis can be detected by 18 to 20 weeks.[12, 23, 85, 102, 175]

WBCs also arise from yolk-sac stem cells. Granulocytic cells from which neutrophils arise can be found in the liver by 8 weeks. After 5 months neutrophils are produced primarily in the bone marrow. Myelopoiesis is 10 times more active in the fetus than in the adult. Few granulocytes are found in peripheral blood during the first half of gestation, but by term numbers are similar to those in adults.[175] NK cells, which have a major role in surveillance against viral infection, are found in the liver by 8 to 9 weeks and in the spleen by 19 weeks but basal activity of these cells is almost undetectable until after 20 weeks and does not increase significantly until after 32 weeks.[102] Complement synthesis by the fetal liver begins as early as 4 to 6 weeks but individual components develop gradually; serum complement is seen after 20 to 22 weeks and increases rapidly after 26 to 28 weeks.[12, 23, 31]

In summary, a nonspecific immune response can be identified in the fetus early in gestation but specific immune functions remain immature to term. In terms of the functional development of the immune system, 32 to 33 weeks' gestation seems to be a critical time. Before this point the fetus or infant is significantly compromised in comparison with the term neonate in terms of neutrophil, macrophage, and NK cell function and concentrations of complement and immunoglobulins.[104] After this time the preterm infant's immune system rapidly approaches that of the term infant.

NEONATAL PHYSIOLOGY

The increased rate and severity of infection in the fetus and neonate are well documented. The fetus and newborn are "compromised hosts" and thus vulnerable to infection for two major reasons. The first reason is the immaturity-associated limitations of their host defense mechanisms. The second reason is lack of experience and exposure to many common organisms, resulting in delayed or diminished responses to foreign antigens. Limitations in neonatal host defense mechanisms are found in the inflammatory response as well as in humoral and cell-mediated immunity and the complement system (see Fig. 10–1). The newborn is also at increased risk for entry of pathogenic organisms owing to the breaks in mucosal or cutaneous barriers that may occur during delivery. Finally, the neonate is at increased risk for gastrointestinal infections and for later development of allergies owing to immaturity of the gut host defense mechanism.

Although these limitations are found in both term and preterm infants, the preterm infant (especially less than 33 to 34 weeks' gestation) is more vulnerable to pathogenic organisms because of further immaturity of all aspects of the immune system and decreased levels of protective IgG from the mother. The risk of infection in the preterm and ill neonate is also increased secondary to disruption of skin barriers because of the need for invasive procedures and tape and monitor lead abrasions, which create portals of entry for pathogenic organisms.

Transitional Events

With the transition to extrauterine life newborns move from the generally sterile, protected environment of the uterus into an environment filled with potentially pathogenic organisms and other antigens that challenge their still immature host defense mechanisms. During the initial days after birth the newborn's mucosal surfaces (skin, respiratory system, and gastrointestinal tract) must develop normal microorganism flora and respond to bacterial colonization by potential pathogens, exposure to dietary proteins that are potential allergens, and exposure to other ingested or inhaled environmental agents.[89]

Newborns are initially colonized with organisms from the maternal genital tract acquired during the birth process. This is followed by colonization with maternal skin flora and other organisms in the environment. The maternal genital tract flora at delivery normally includes *Lactobacillus*, *E. coli*, and protective anaerobes, but may contain potentially dangerous organisms such as group B streptococcus and *Chlamydia trachomatis*.[33] Colonization occurs initially on the skin, umbilical cord, and genitalia, followed by mucous membranes of the eyes, throat, and nares.[40, 124]

The newborn's skin is usually sterile immediately after a cesarean birth; after a vaginal birth the skin flora reflects the organisms of the maternal genital tract. Skin flora is increased in infants with little or no vernix caseosa, which normally acts as a protective mechanical barrier. With the use of common antiseptic preparations (triple dye, neomycin sulfate), colonization is reduced and the umbilicus remains sterile in most infants during the first week.[33]

Colonization of the gastrointestinal system occurs in two stages. Before birth the gut is sterile. During the first stage (birth to 1 week) the infant is inoculated with organisms that he or she comes into contact with during and after birth. In the second stage (1 to 4 weeks) the infant's diet significantly influences the pattern of bacterial flora.[89] The normal gut flora provides an important protective mechanism against gastrointestinal infections by occupying potential pathogen-binding sites on intestinal mucosa. The upper small intestine is usually sterile or sparsely colonized, probably owing to the gastric pH, or possibly the antibacterial properties of bile, secreted immunoglobulins, and normal intestinal motility. Coliform colonization of the upper small intestine is increased in very low birth weight (VLBW) infants and infants who are intubated or fed by transpyloric tube.[33]

Meconium is usually sterile at birth, except perhaps after prolonged ruptured membranes. Bacteria can be found in meconium within a few hours of birth and increase rapidly over the next few days. Use of antimicrobial drugs from birth partially suppresses but does not prevent colonization and may result in a shift in the dominant gut flora and an increase in resistant flora.[33]

In the first few days after birth the neonate may be further protected from potentially pathogenic gut organisms by the acidity of gastric secretions (which inhibits growth of gram-positive and gram-negative bacteria) and by immaturity of the gut epithelium (which mediates attachment of pathogenic organisms). Infants for whom oral feedings are delayed are more likely to have no bacterial growth in fecal samples. The intestines of these infants are similar to the germ-free state. This state is associated with a slower mucosal cell turnover (which allows toxins to have a more profound effect), fewer lymphoid cells in the gut, and alterations in gut immune responses that may increase the risk of infection.[114]

Breast-fed infants develop different colonization patterns than formula-fed infants. These different patterns may reflect physicochemical differences or the influence of antimicrobial factors in human milk. The lower buffering capacity of human milk (due to lower concentrations of proteins and minerals) allows acids from bacterial metabolic end-products to increase. The resulting acidic environment is one in which *Lactobacillus* and *Bifidobacterium* thrive, preventing growth of acid-sensitive organisms. The low protein and phosphate and high lactose contents of human milk also promote growth of this flora. Formula feedings buffer the acid produced by gut bacteria. This leads to an alkaline environment in which the bifidobacteria cannot compete with gut enterobacteria. Gram-negative enterococci become the dominant gut organism. As formulas become more similar to human milk, differences in

colonization, although present, are less apparent.[33, 124]

Antimicrobial factors found in human milk may also alter gut colonization patterns. For example, lactoferrin is an iron-binding protein that is only 9% saturated in human milk. As a result, lactoferrin can bind iron entering the gut that is not absorbed and reduce the availability of iron for bacteria metabolism.[124]

Alterations in Primary Host Defense Mechanisms

The inflammatory response and phagocytosis are altered in the newborn primarily because of functional limitations of the infant's polymorphonuclear neutrophils (PMNs) that affect leukocyte metabolic activities, mobilization, chemotaxis, opsonization, phagocytic activity, and intracellular killing. The neonate's PMNs are more rigid and less deformable and have a poorer response to chemotaxic stimulators and impaired receptor mobilization. These limitations alter movement kinetics and orientation of the PMNs. The neonate's PMNs are less able to leave the blood vessel to reach the site of pathogen invasion because of the decreased deformability. These limitations may decrease adherence of the PMNs to the vascular epithelium, leading to poorer aggregation of PMNs along the vessel wall near the site of injury.[3, 62]

Chemotaxis is altered in the neonate, resulting in slower movement of neutrophils to the site of antigenic invasion. The decreased chemotaxis results from the structural and functional limitations of neonatal PMNs and from deficiency of chemotaxis-stimulating substances in the blood. Newborns and particularly preterm infants have decreased serum opsonic activity, resulting from low levels of immunoglobulins and complement components. (Opsonization is a process by which immunoglobulin or complement coats microorganisms. This enhances recognition of the antigen by PMNs and monocytes, leading to increased phagocytosis.)[3, 62]

There are conflicting findings regarding phagocytic activity in the newborn.[22, 23, 33, 137, 152] Phagocytosis is altered to some extent by the decreased availability of neutrophils (the primary circulating phagocyte) at the invasion site due to altered chemotaxis. Macrophage (the primary tissue phagocyte) activity in response to lymphokines from T cells is also decreased. In general, however, the newborn's neutrophils seem to be as effective in killing bacteria as adult neutrophils when numbers of bacteria are relatively low or when numbers of bacteria and neutrophils are similar and the infant is not stressed.[23] Therefore phagocytic activity and intracellular bacteriocidal activity of PMNs are probably not significantly altered in most healthy infants.

Infants who are stressed either in utero or after birth (e.g., by perinatal asphyxia, respiratory distress, meconium aspiration, premature rupture of the membranes, sepsis, or hyperbilirubinemia) demonstrate significantly decreased bacteriocidal activity for both gram-positive and gram-negative organisms. Phagocytosis has been found to be normal in most stressed neonates, although decreased phagocytosis for some gram-negative bacteria has been reported. Bacteriocidal activity may be reduced even further in VLBW infants who weigh less than 600 grams.[23, 33, 137]

The cause of these alterations in stressed infants is unclear but may relate to intrinsic alterations or defects in leukocyte metabolic activity or result from perioxidative damage to the cell.[23, 62] Changes in cellular metabolism associated with phagocytosis (such as increased oxygen consumption, hexose monophosphate [HMP] shunt [involved with glycolysis] activity, and production of toxic oxygen metabolites necessary for bacteriocidal activity) are reduced in stressed and SGA infants.[152]

The number of monocytes in infants is similar to that in adults but monocyte chemotaxis may be altered, although studies have yielded conflicting results, with decreased delivery of these macrophages to the infection site.[85, 173] Production of interferon by monocytic macrophages is reduced. Monocytic bacteriocidal activity and processing of antigens are generally considered to be adequate. Phagocytic activity may be reduced and correlates with gestational age.[85]

Fibronectin, a glycoprotein found in plasma and tissues, inhibits bacterial adherence to epithelial cells, enhances antibody binding of bacteria such as staphylococci and group B streptococci, and is involved in opsonization and clearance of fibrin, immune complexes, and platelets. Levels of plasma fibronectin average 50% of adult values, with the lowest levels seen in preterm infants and those with perinatal asphyxia or respiratory

distress.[23, 173, 175] Numbers of NK cells, which provide protection against tumors or virus-infected cells before the initiation of specific immune responses, are similar to those in adults, but activity is decreased 15 to 60% and averages 50% of adult activity.[69] Neonatal NK cells are especially deficient in binding to target cells and have decreased lytic ability.[173] The altered activity is probably due to decreased levels of lymphokines, especially immune interferon, which augments NK cell function.[23]

The number of neutrophils varies during the first few days after birth, with an increase after birth to peak at 12 to 14 hours, followed by a fall to adult values by 72 hours.[173] Lower levels are seen in preterm infants.[157] In general, the total number of circulating lymphocytes is similar to adult levels at birth but falls during the first 3 days, then plateaus by 10 days. The ratio of T lymphocytes to B lymphocytes is lower in cord blood than in adult blood.[41] Numbers of neutrophil precursors in the blood and marrow are increased. In neonates, especially preterm infants, the marrow is probably functioning at or near capacity for neutrophil proliferation. Therefore, these infants are less able to increase production much further with infection.[173]

These alterations decrease the ability of neonates to localize infection. As a result, neonates are much more likely to develop generalized septicemia with spread of the pathogenic organism to the blood and cerebrospinal fluid. The major factor in this inability to localize infection is impaired chemotaxis. Sacchi and associates found that chemotaxis was altered in term and preterm infants at birth; chemotaxis was similar to that in adults in term infants by 15 to 17 days after birth and in preterm infants born after 34 weeks' gestation by the time they reached 42 weeks' of gestational age.[131] Achievement of adult chemotaxis was delayed in more immature preterm infants, with fewer than two thirds of them achieving adult values by 42 weeks. Thus, these infants remained at higher risk for infection even after reaching their due date. Adequate phagocytosis and killing of many pathogenic organisms such as group B streptococci depend on complement (especially C3) and opsonic activity. Serum concentrations of C3 and thus opsonic activity are proportional to gestational age, further increasing the risk of sepsis in preterm infants.[31, 38]

The inability to localize infection can delay

the diagnosis of sepsis by altering the clinical manifestations of infection. As a result, signs of sepsis in the neonate are often subtle and nonspecific, involving changes in activity, tone, color, or feeding. Neonates have a poor hypothalamic response to pyrogens, therefore fever is not a reliable indicator of infection in the neonate.

Alterations in Specific Immune Responses

Preterm and term neonates experience significant alterations in humoral (antibody)- and cell-mediated immunity and in the complement system. These developmental limitations increase the frequency and severity of neonatal infection.

Humoral (Antibody)-Mediated Immunity

Alterations in humoral immunity are primarily due to reductions in many of the immunoglobulins and to the suppressor effects of T lymphocytes on B-lymphocyte function. The total amount of immunoglobulin at birth is 55 to 80% of adult values and reflects IgG acquired from the mother.[98] Levels of serum immunoglobulins from birth to adulthood are presented in Table 10–8. Mean IgG levels at birth correlate with birth weight and gestational age, whereas levels of IgA and IgM do not. Immunoglobulin levels in the fetus and infant are illustrated in Figure 10–6.

IgG, especially IgG1 and IgG2, crosses the placenta from mother to fetus beginning in the 3rd month and increases progressively to term (Fig. 10–6). Neonatal values depend on gestational age since placental transfer of IgG increases during the third trimester. Thus, preterm infants may have inadequate protection. For example, cord blood values average 400 mg/dl at 32 weeks and 600 to 1670 mg/ dl at term.[63] Term IgG levels are 90 to 95% of adult values and similar to or up to 5 to 10% higher than maternal values.[23, 131, 175] As a result of IgG transfer, the neonate has antibodies against infectious agents for which the mother has circulating antibodies because of previous exposure or immunization. Levels of IgG are lower in SGA infants, possibly owing to impaired placental transport.[173] After birth levels fall gradually as maternal IgG is catabolized. Since significant production of IgG by the infant does not occur until after 6 months, all infants experience a transient "physiologic hypogammaglobulinemia" in the first 6 months.

IgA does not cross the placenta in significant amounts. Neonatal (term and preterm) values are low (0.1 to 5 mg/dl, or less than 2% of adult values). Elevated IgA is found in cord blood after maternal-fetal transfusion. IgA occurs as a monomer or is attached to a secretory component in saliva, tears, colostrum, and human milk, which provides resistance to pH changes and protects the IgA molecule from proteolytic digestion in the gastrointestinal tract. Secretory IgA is not found at birth but can be detected in saliva and tears by 2 to 5 weeks.[175]

IgM also does not cross the placenta. Neonatal values are low (5 to 15 mg/dl) with

TABLE 10–8
Levels of Serum Immunoglobulins from Birth to Adulthood

AGE	LEVEL OF IgG* mg/100 ml (range)	% of Adult Level	LEVEL OF IgM* mg/100 ml (range)	% of Adult Level	LEVEL OF IgA* mg/100 ml (range)	% of Adult Level	LEVEL OF TOTAL IMMUNOGLOBULIN* mg/100 ml (range)	% of Adult Level
Newborn	1031 ± 200	89 ± 17	11 ± 5	11 ± 5	2 ± 3	1 ± 2	1044 ± 201	67 ± 13
1–3 mo	430 ± 119	37 ± 10	30 ± 11	30 ± 11	21 ± 13	11 ± 7	481 ± 127	31 ± 9
4–6 mo	427 ± 186	37 ± 16	43 ± 17	43 ± 17	28 ± 18	14 ± 9	498 ± 204	32 ± 13
7–12 mo	661 ± 219	58 ± 19	54 ± 23	55 ± 23	37 ± 18	19 ± 9	752 ± 242	48 ± 15
13–24 mo	762 ± 209	66 ± 18	58 ± 23	59 ± 23	50 ± 24	25 ± 12	870 ± 258	56 ± 16
25–36 mo	892 ± 183	77 ± 16	61 ± 19	62 ± 19	71 ± 37	36 ± 19	1024 ± 205	65 ± 14
3–5 yr	929 ± 228	80 ± 20	56 ± 18	57 ± 18	93 ± 27	47 ± 14	1078 ± 245	69 ± 17
6–8 yr	923 ± 256	80 ± 22	65 ± 25	66 ± 25	124 ± 45	62 ± 23	1112 ± 293	71 ± 20
9–11 yr	1124 ± 235	97 ± 20	79 ± 33	80 ± 33	131 ± 60	66 ± 30	1334 ± 254	85 ± 17
12–16 yr	946 ± 124	82 ± 11	59 ± 20	60 ± 20	148 ± 63	74 ± 32	1153 ± 169	74 ± 12
Adult	1158 ± 305	100 ± 26	99 ± 27	100 ± 27	200 ± 61	100 ± 31	1457 ± 353	100 ± 24

*Mean is ± 1 S.D.

Adapted from Stiehm, E.R. & Fudenberg, H.H. (1966). Serum levels of immune globulins in health and disease: A survey. *Pediatrics, 37,* 715.

FIGURE 10–6. Immunoglobulin levels in the fetus, newborn, and infant. (From Stiehm, E. R. & Fulginiti, V. A. [1989]. *Immunologic disorders in infants and children* [3rd ed., p. 63]. Philadelphia: WB Saunders.)

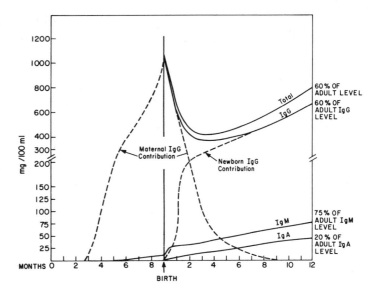

means of 6 mg/dl at 28 weeks and 11 mg/dl or about 11% of adult values at term.[173] The fetus is capable of producing significant IgM in response to exposure to certain antigens, such as the TORCH organisms, after 19 to 20 weeks' gestation. (TORCH stands for *Tox*oplasmosis, *O*ther viruses, *R*ubella, *C*ytomegalovirus, *H*erpes simplex.) Neonatal B lymphocytes secrete primarily IgM; IgM is the major immunoglobulin synthesized in the 1st month of life. Neonatal IgM has less specificity than adult IgM in responding to specific antigens, which may limit the initial recognition of pathogenic organisms. IgM levels increase rapidly after 2 to 4 days probably secondary to stimulation from environmental antigens. IgE and IgD do not cross the placenta in significant amounts and newborn values are less than 10% of adult values.[23, 98, 175]

In addition to alterations in immunoglobulin concentration, neonatal B lymphocytes are hyporesponsive, possibly owing to the suppressor effects of T lymphocytes (see Fig. 10–1). These B cells also lack experience and exposure to many common organisms and thus have few memory cells. This delays the initial response of the immune system in producing antibodies to specific organisms.

Cell-Mediated Immunity

T-lymphocyte cell-mediated immunity is also significantly altered in the neonate. Absolute numbers of T lymphocytes in the newborn are relatively comparable with adults, but the functional ability of newborn T cells is decreased, as is the diversity of specific T-cell receptors, which delays the response to specific organisms.[173] Cytotoxic activity of neonatal T cells is 30 to 60% less than in adults.[173] Lymphokine production is reduced to about 40% of adult values. Specific lymphokines that are reduced include lymphotoxin, migration inhibiting factor (MIF), which may be 10% of adult values, and immune interferon. T-suppressor activity tends to dominate in the newborn.[102] T cells generally do not cross the placenta. The newborn's T cells are "virginal," that is, they have had no previous experience with most antigens until exposed and sensitized after birth, and it probably takes 4 to 6 weeks for the newborn to achieve minimal protection.[11, 23, 98, 175]

Cell-mediated immunity is further depressed in SGA infants. These infants have a smaller proportion of T lymphocytes and altered lymphocyte function, perhaps secondary to alterations in thymic activity. The thymus of SGA infants is smaller in weight and volume and demonstrates histologic alterations and decreased activity of thymic inductive factors.[25]

The Complement System

Total complement in the newborn is about 50 to 60% of maternal and 70 to 90% of adult values. Serum levels of both classical and alternative pathway components (Fig. 10–7) are decreased. Levels of several key complement proteins (C1, C3, C4, C7, C9) are 55 to 75% of adult values in term infants (10 to 30% in 28-week preterm infants), leading to decreased opsonization, decreased chemotactic activity, and decreased cell lysis.

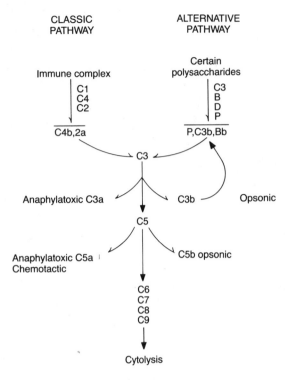

FIGURE 10–7. The complement system. The complement system involves a sequential series of discrete plasma proteins and their fragments that, when activated, enhance other parts of the immune system. Actions of complement include attraction of various cell types to the initial site of antigen invasion, promotion of chemotaxis and phagocytosis, enhancement of opsonization and other immunoglobulin functions, enhancement of histamine release and the inflammatory response, and direct destruction of antigens. Proteins of the complement system circulate in the plasma in an inactive state. Complement is activated through a sequential cascade. Activated molecules either act as enzymes to activate other proteins or fragments in the complement system or enhance actions of other parts of the immune system. There are two activation sequences. The classical pathway requires antibody or antigen–antibody complexes for activation, which occurs by C1 through C3. Complement activation and fixation are important for IgG and IgM function. Early in the immune response and during the initial inflammatory response antibody may not be present, so an alternative activation sequence is needed. The alternative or properdin pathway is activated by factors B through C3 by substances such as bacterial products and circulating proteins. (From McLean, R. H. & Winkelstein, J. A. [1984]. Genetically determined variations in complement synthesis: Relationship to disease. *J. Pediatr 105*, 179.)

Deficient activity of the alternative pathway is seen in two thirds of newborns. Concentrations of properdin and factor B are 35 to 70% and 35 to 60% of adult values, respectively; properdin levels are markedly lower in preterm infants.[11, 23, 98, 175] The classical and alternative pathways are further depressed in infants with documented sepsis.[38]

Alterations in Gut Host Defense Mechanisms

Host defense mechanisms in the gut involve both nonimmune and immune factors. Many of these factors are initially altered in the neonate, reducing the effectiveness of the gut mucosal barrier and increasing the risk of GI disorders, entry of pathogenic organisms into systemic circulation, and development of allergic reactions (Table 10–9). As defense mechanisms mature, GI barriers become more impermeable, offering greater protection against uptake of antigenic substances. The development of gut defense mechanisms is called "gut closure." A major task of the neonate is development of the mucosal barrier and other defense mechanisms to maintain the gut epithelial surfaces

as an impermeable barrier against the uptake of antigens and antigenic fragments.[67, 165] Gut closure is delayed in preterm and SGA infants, who may absorb macromolecules across their intestinal epithelium for up to 8 to 12 months.[26] Nonimmune factors include gastric acid, intestinal motility and peristalsis, intraluminal proteolytic activity, and the mechanical barrier properties of the gut mucosal surface. Integrity of the intestinal epithelial lining is further compromised by hypoxia or hypotension.

The major specific immune factors are sIgA and cell-mediated immunity. Changes in cell-mediated immunity, especially a localized depression of T-lymphocyte suppressor activity, and the decreased IgA alter the response of the infant to antigens that can cross the intestinal barrier. This increases the incidence of antigen-induced disorders such as GI infection and allergies in infants.

The mature response to the presence of antigens in the gut is immune tolerance. With immune tolerance, the absorbed antigen elicits a localized IgA response that destroys most of the antigen. As a result there is less antigen available to enter the systemic system. T-suppressor cell activity is also triggered,

TABLE 10–9
Alterations in Gut Host Defense Mechanisms in the Newborn

DEFENSE MECHANISM	MODE OF ACTION	ALTERATION IN NEWBORN
	Nonimmune Factors	
Gastric acid	Decreased number of organisms entering intestines	Decreased in term and preterm infants until 4 weeks' postnatal age
Intestinal motility and peristalsis	Remove organisms and antigen	Decreased to 29 to 32 weeks postconceptual age
Intraluminal proteolysis	Determines amount of macromolecular transport across intestinal epithelium	Decreased pancreatic enzyme function in preterm infant; some decrease in response in both term and preterm infants to 2 years; result: increased absorption of intact proteins across small intestine
Mucosal surface		
Mucous coat	Provides physical barrier to attachment, uptake, and penetration of organisms and other antigens CHO moieties act as receptor inhibitors to protect against antigen penetration	Decreased and altered CHO content and lack of mucus-specific receptor inhibition may interfere with surface defenses against organisms, toxins, and other antigens
Microvillous membrane	CHO composition influences specific adherence of organisms and other antigens to intestinal surface and prevents penetration	Altered membrane composition and incompletely developed surface leading to abnormal colonization, increased antigen penetration, and disease susceptibility
	Immunologic Factors	
Secretory IgA (sIgA)	Complexes with antigens to impede absorption from intestinal lumen Interferes with antigen attachment and uptake at mucosal surface	Low levels of IgA and especially sIgA resulting in increased transport of organisms, antigens, and other macromolecules across intestinal epithelium
Gut-associated lymphoid tissue (GALT)	Composed of Peyer's patches (aggregates of lymphoid tissue), plasma cells that are predominantly IgA producing, B and T lymphocytes, and specialized M epithelial cells. M cells bind and transport antigens to macrophages in lymphoid tissue	GALT develops more slowly than other lymphoid tissue and in newborns contains primarily T cells with few B cells Paucity of IgA-producing plasma cells (requires weeks to months to establish protective levels) Low levels of IgA Delayed response time to antigen penetration
Cell-mediated immunity	Includes activated T lymphocytes, mast cells, and macrophages along the intestinal lamina along with intraepithelial lymphocytes (cytotoxic T cells)	Immature and virginal T lymphocytes, altered T-suppressor function, and depression of responsiveness to specific antigens Decreased intestinal and intraepithelial lymphocytes in SGA and nutritionally-deprived infants Respond to antigens with priming response versus tolerance

CHO = carbohydrate.
Compiled from references 33, 67, 89, 124, and 165.

which interferes with and inhibits systemic responses to these antigens.[26, 67] Immune tolerance appears to be enhanced by the presence of partially digested polypeptide fragments. These fragments may not be formed in the neonate with immature proteolysis. In the infant the absorbed antigens may actually prime the immune system and enhance rather than inhibit specific responses. With decreased IgA greater amounts of antigen are absorbed. Decreased T-suppressor response can enhance systemic immune responses and lead to inflammatory or allergic responses.

Immaturity of gut defense mechanisms may have an etiologic role in the development of necrotizing enterocolitis (NEC). Lake and Walker describe NEC as a disorder of the immature intestinal barrier in the preterm infant.[80] NEC is a multifactorial disorder that results in focal or diffuse ulceration and necrosis in the lower small intestine and colon (see Chapter 9). Factors involved in the development of NEC include intestinal ischemia, bacterial proliferation, and enteral feedings.[67] These factors may interact with the immature intestinal barrier to further increase mucosal permeability to enteric bacteria, toxins, and antigens.[67, 80]

Human milk, particularly colostrum, facilitates gut closure by enhancing maturation of the mucosal epithelial cells and development of brush border enzymes such as lactase, sucrase, and alkaline phosphatase; reducing antigen penetration; and providing sIgA.[165] Other factors contributing to the lower rate of GI infection in breast-fed infants include antibacterial factors in human milk, stimulation of IgA, and the presence of ingested maternal antigen, which tends to promote immune tolerance responses.[67]

CLINICAL IMPLICATIONS FOR NEONATAL CARE

Alterations in host defense mechanisms in neonates and their inexperience as hosts place them at increased risk for sepsis and meningitis (owing to the inability to localize infection) and for the development of infections due to specific bacterial and viral organisms. These risks are examined in this section along with consideration of the physiologic basis for specific laboratory findings used in the diagnosis of neonatal sepsis, immunotherapy techniques, and neonatal AIDS. Immunodeficiency diseases are rarely seen in newborns since the effects of these disorders are usually masked by maternally-acquired IgG and sIgA in breast milk.

Risk of Specific Infectious Processes

When examining limitations of the neonate's host defense system, the basis for an increased risk of infection with certain organisms becomes apparent (Table 10–10). The inability to localize infection increases the risk of sepsis from gram-positive cocci such as group B streptococci (GBS) that often colonize the birth canal and can be transferred to the infant during delivery. The risk of sepsis from gram-negative rods is increased since protection against these organisms is provided by IgM, IgA (against enteropathic *E. coli*), and T lymphocytes, which have decreased levels or altered activity in the neonate. Similarly, markedly low values of IgA and the lack of sIgA increase the risk of respiratory and GI infections, whereas low IgM levels increase the risk of rubella, toxoplasmosis, CMV, and syphilis. The risk of GI infections is increased because of immaturity of the intestinal mucosal barrier and lack of gut closure.

Decreased complement activity, particularly in relation to the alternative pathway, leads to decreased opsonic activity. This may be critical if the infant also lacks type-specific antibodies for organisms with a capsular polysaccharide coating, such as GBS or K1 *E. coli*. In this situation, the infant's immune system is dependent on the (deficient) alternative pathway for opsonization of the organism in preparation for phagocytosis.

Altered activity of T lymphocytes along with their lack of antigen exposure increases the risk of infection due to herpes simplex virus, CMV, and *Candida*. Decreased production of immune interferon (which inhibits viral replication) by the lymphocytes increases the risk of viral infection. In addition, immune interferon is an important macrophage-activating factor that has an important role in destruction of intracellular pathogens such as *Toxoplasma* and *L. monocytogenes*.

Wilson examined the impact of altered neonatal host defense mechanisms on groups of infectious organisms including GBS and the herpes simplex virus (HSV).[172, 173] The response of the neonate to these organisms provides a model for examining the vulnerability of the newborn to bacterial and viral infections.

Immune Responses to Bacterial Infections

GBS and *E. coli* are currently the most common pathogens causing neonatal sepsis in North America. Neonatal infection generally occurs after exposure to organisms from the birth canal. Usually only a few infants exposed to these pathogens become infected. Both GBS and *E. coli* sepsis are more common with certain strains that contain specific capsular polysaccharide.

GBS can be divided into five serotypes based on either their bacterial capsular polysaccharide (Ia, Ib, II, and III) or surface protein (Ibc). Type III accounts for two thirds of all GBS infection in infants, 90% of GBS meningitis, and 90% of late-onset GBS sepsis. One third of early-onset sepsis without meningitis is caused by types Ia, Ib, and Ic.[52] Similarly, infection with *E. coli* that results in neonatal meningitis occurs most often with organisms that have the K1 polysaccharide capsule. Capsular polysaccharide protects the organism from destruction unless it is opsonized. Opsonization and phagocytosis of type III and perhaps other GBS types require

TABLE 10–10
Alterations in Host Defense Mechanisms in the Neonate

ALTERATION	RESULT	IMPLICATION
Primary Host Defense Mechanisms		
Structural alterations of PMNs: more rigid, less deformable	Altered movement kinetics and orientation of PMNs	Delayed initial response to invasion by pathogenic organisms
Altered chemotaxis	Slower movement to site of antigenic invasion	Less able to localize infection
Reduced bacteriocidal activity in stressed neonates	Delayed initial response to injection	Increased risk of severe infection
Reduced monocyte phagocytic activity	Delayed initial response to infection	Less able to localize infection Increased risk of generalized sepsis
Decreased fibronectin	Delayed initial response to infection	Less able to localize infection Increased risk of generalized sepsis
Decreased NK cells	Delayed initial response to infection	Less able to localize infection Increased risk of generalized sepsis
Poor hypothalamic response to pyrogens	Fever is not a reliable sign of sepsis	Signs of sepsis often subtle and nonspecific
Humoral (Antibody)-Mediated Immunity		
Decreased IgG in preterm infant	Due to lack of transfer from mother Reduced defense against many bacteria	Increased risk of bacterial sepsis, especially from gram-positive cocci
Decreased IgA and absent sIgA	Reduced defense against GI and respiratory infections; increased in breast-fed infants	Increased risk of respiratory and GI infections
Decreased IgM	Reduced defense against viral and gram-negative organisms	Increased risk of *E.coli* sepsis and rubella, syphilis, toxoplasmosis, CMV, and other viral infection
Suppression of B-cell function	Due to increased T-suppressor (versus helper) function	Increased risk of severe infection
Lack of previous exposure of B cells to many organisms, with lack of development of memory cells	Delayed specific responses to pathogenic organisms	Increased risk of severe or overwhelming infection
Cell-Mediated Immunity		
Decreased T-cell function (reduced lymphokine production, cytotoxic activity)	Reduced defenses against viral and fungal infections	Increased risk and severity of infection from herpes, CMV, other TORCH organisms
Increased T-suppressor activity	Alteration in B-lymphocyte function	Increased risk and severity of bacterial infection
"Virginal" T cells	Delayed responses to specific pathogenic organisms	Increased risk of viral and fungal infections
Complement		
Decreased total complement	Decreased opsonization	Decreased ability to localize infection
Deficient activity of alternative pathway	Decreased chemotaxis Decreased cell lysis	Decreased ability to opsonize and eliminate organisms with capsular polysaccharide such as GBS Increased risk and severity of bacterial sepsis

both type-specific immunoglobulins and complement.

The risk of neonatal sepsis from GBS is increased because of limitations in mucocutaneous barriers and humoral and cell-mediated defense mechanisms (Fig. 10–8). The ability of organisms to penetrate human mucocutaneous barriers is facilitated by epithelial adherence, exposure to a high density of bacteria, and disruption of the skin or mucosal membranes. Neonates whose mothers are colonized with GBS are likely to be exposed to dense concentrations of the organism. In addition, bacterial adherence to the epithelium may be altered by decreased levels of sIgA and fibronectin. Type III organisms tend to adhere better to neonatal buccal epithelium, particularly in infected infants.[166]

GBS sepsis tends to occur only in infants deficient in type-specific IgG antibody. Neonates may lack these antibodies if their mother does not have the type-specific antibody to transfer to her infant, if the mother's antibody is in an immunoglobulin class that does not cross the placenta, or if the infant is born prematurely before maternal antibody is normally transferred to the fetus.[28] In the neonate GBS antibody is acquired

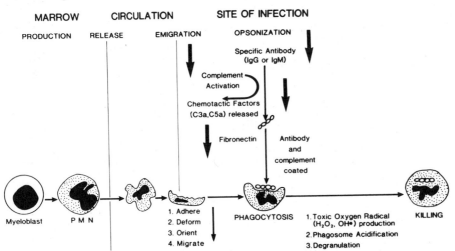

FIGURE 10–8. Limitations in neonatal defense mechanisms against group B streptococci. Limitations in the neonate are denoted by arrows. (Adapted from Wilson, C. B. [1986]. Immunologic basis for increased susceptibility of the neonate to infection. *J Pediatr, 108,* 1.)

primarily from the mother (through transplacental transfer) if the mother has developed antibodies to specific GBS strains by previous exposure. Many women do have antibodies against type III GBS as well as types Ia, Ib, and II, and thus many term infants are protected.[5] This may partially explain why women who are colonized can have healthy infants even after prolonged ruptured membranes.

Preterm infants are more vulnerable to GBS infection since these antibodies, like other IgG antibodies, do not cross the placenta in significant amounts until the latter part of the third trimester. A prenatal vaccination to develop type-specific GBS antibodies in the mother, which could then be passively transferred to the fetus, is being tested.[52] Anti-K1 *E. coli* IgG antibodies are much rarer in the adult population so the mother is less likely to provide protection to her fetus against this organism.[5]

Once infected, the neonate is often unable to mount an appropriate response to GBS. Optimal destruction of GBS depends on type-specific antibody, complement, and functional phagocytes.[177] In infected neonates who do not have type-specific antibody, an increase in the time required for neutrophil migration to the invading organisms has been noted, along with a delay of 4 to 6 hours between the onset of infection and release of neutrophils from bone marrow storage pools (versus 2 hours in infants with type-specific antibodies).[28] This results in decreased complement activation (and thus opsonization and phagocytosis) and inability to localize the infection and increases the risk of a rapidly progressing overwhelming septicemia. When exposed to GBS, the B lymphocytes of most neonates do not produce adequate quantities of type-specific antibody critical for opsonization and phagocytosis. Lower levels of complement in newborns, especially in preterm infants, further reduce opsonization of GBS and interfere with the phagocytotic ability of the PMNs. In infants with GBS sepsis the number of lymphocytes is reduced. Factor B is also reduced by 30 to 35% and C3 by 40 to 60% from cord blood levels.[173, 175]

Because of functional and structural alterations in PMNs that decrease chemotaxis, neonates are unable to rapidly deliver adequate numbers of phagocytes to the site of initial infection. Neutropenia, rarely seen in infected adults, is a frequent finding in neonatal septicemia. The reasons for this neutropenia include a small marrow storage pool of neutrophils and their precursors that is rapidly depleted with sepsis, inability of the marrow to increase production of neutrophils (stem-cell proliferation rate is already at maximal activity), failure of the marrow to release additional neutrophils, sequestration of neutrophils along vessel walls (margination), and the short circulating half-life (4 to 7 hours) of neutrophils in the neonate.[177]

PMNs of ill and stressed infants have decreased chemotaxis as well as decreased phagocytic and bacteriocidal activity. Neonates may also be deficient in local defense mechanisms in the lungs because of decreased numbers (and possibly altered function) of lung macrophages.[172] This deficit may predispose the infant to GBS pneumonia. In summary, the increased susceptibility of the neonate to bacterial pathogens results primarily from lack of type-specific antibody, alterations in the functional ability of PMNs (especially decreased chemotaxis), poor bone marrow response to maintain adequate numbers of neutrophils, and decreased complement leading to ineffective opsonic activity necessary for phagocytosis and bacteriocidal activity (Fig. 10–8).[173]

Immune Responses to Viral Infections

Viral infections tend to be more serious and devastating disorders in neonates than in adults because of limitations in the infant's host defense mechanisms and lack of previous exposure to many organisms. The major defense mechanisms against viral infections (cell-mediated immunity, NK cells, IgM, and the ability to localize infection) are all altered in the neonate. In addition most neonates have T lymphocytes that are not yet sensitized. This section examines immunologic aspects of neonatal herpes simplex, hepatitis B, and HIV infection.

HERPES SIMPLEX VIRUS INFECTION

Neonatal HSV infection is a rapidly progressing disorder usually involving multiple body systems with high morbidity and mortality rates. Severe systemic HSV infection is an age-related phenomenon, with the morbidity, mortality, and severity of illness decreasing after the first 4 weeks of life.[77]

Susceptibility of neonates to severe HSV infection is due to immaturity of the immune system, alterations in neutrophil function, and the inability of the neonate to generate a fever (HSV is a thermolabile organism). Alterations in the neonate's immune system that increase the risk of HSV infection include decreased NK-cell cytotoxicity, reduced ability of lymphocytes and monocytes to lyse HSV, decreased antibody-dependent cell-mediated toxicity, decreased or delayed production of and response to interferon, decreased diversity of specific receptors for HSV, and delayed lymphocyte proliferation in response to antigens.[77, 172, 173]

Lack of maternal antibody may also increase the risk of neonatal HSV infection. Maternal antibodies to HSV, which are capable of neutralizing the virus and mediating antibody-dependent cell-mediated cytotoxicity, are of the IgG class and can cross the placenta. These antibodies do not provide immunity to the neonate but do reduce severity of the disease. Women with primary HSV genital infection produce little IgG and their offspring are more likely to develop severe infection. There are several reports of a dose-dependent relationship between the amount of maternal anti-HSV antibody and the severity of neonatal infection, in which increasing levels of maternal antibody were associated with milder neonatal infection and a decreased incidence of disseminated infection or central nervous system involvement.[77]

HEPATITIS B VIRUS INFECTION

Another virus that has become increasingly prevalent in perinatal care is hepatitis B virus (HBV). HBV can be transmitted from the mother to the fetus and newborn by infected vaginal secretions, amniotic fluid, maternal blood, saliva, and possibly breast milk. Most infants who develop HBV infection acquire the organism late in the third trimester or at delivery. Up to 40 to 60% of infants of mothers with active, untreated infections late in the third trimester develop HBV infection.[74] Although many newborns who are exposed to HBV do not develop clinical infection, others develop a fulminant neonatal disease. In addition, infants may be at risk for later disorders since HBV can cause acute and chronic hepatitis, cirrhosis, and hepatocellular carcinoma.[60]

HBV is a DNA virus associated with three distinct antigen forms (surface, core, and e) and their respective antibodies (anti-HBs, anti-HBc, and anti-HBe). The outer protein surface contains a surface antigen (HBsAg), whereas the inner core of the virus contains the DNA genome (circular DNA form) and the core antigen (HBcAg). The third antigen (HBeAg) is a soluble serum antigen usually seen in association with HBsAg. Table 10–11 summarizes characteristics of these antigens and antibodies.

HBeAg is a marker of infectivity and reflects ongoing viral replication. This antigen is usually seen in people with active disease and HBsAg-positive serum. HBsAg and HBeAg are detectable 1 to 3 weeks after HBV exposure but before onset of clinical

TABLE 10–11
Interpretation of the Presence of Combinations of Serologic Markers of HBV

HBsAg	HBeAg	Anti-HBe	Anti-HBc	Anti-HBs	INTERPRETATION	INFECTIVITY*
+	+	−	−	−	Incubation period for early acute HB	High
+	+	−	+	−	Acute HB or chronic carrier	High
+	−	+	+	−	Late during HB or chronic carrier	Low
−	−	+	+	+	Convalescent from acute HB infection	Low
−	−	−	+	+	Recovered from past HB infection	None
−	−	−	−	+	Immunized without infection; repeated exposure to HBsAg without infection; recovered from past infection	None
−	−	−	+	−	Recovered from past HB infection with undetectable anti-HBs; early convalescence or chronic carrier	??

*Infectivity of blood.
HBV, hepatitis B virus; HB, hepatitis B.
From Hanshaw, J.B., Dudgeon, J.A., & Marshall, W.C. (1985). *Viral diseases of the fetus and newborn* (p. 187). Philadelphia: WB Saunders, using data from Deinhurst, F. & Gust, I.P. (1982). *Bull World Health Organ, 60*, 661.

symptoms.[39, 74] HBeAg may also be present after the active disease subsides, indicating either chronic disease or a carrier state. Women with HBeAg are usually infectious and appropriate blood and body-fluid precautions should be taken.[73]

HBcAg is found only in hepatocytes and thus is not detectable in serum. Antibodies to this antigen (anti-HBc) are seen during both acute infection and convalescence, however, making anti-HBc a reliable indicator of HBV infection.[39] Anti-HBc during an acute infection is primarily IgM-type antibody, which may persist for 4 to 6 months and indicate recent infection. Anti-HBc antibodies, which are primarily IgG type, are also found in the carrier state.[60, 74] Anti-HBc in HbsAg-positive serum indicates low infectivity.

HBsAg can be found in the serum of people who have acute or chronic HBV infections or are carriers for the virus. Infants who acquire the virus during birth are seronegative initially, but develop elevated serum HBsAG within 2 to 4 months.[74] The woman who is HBsAg positive, regardless of whether she is a carrier or actively infected, can transmit the virus to her fetus and neonate and to others with whom she comes in contact. Therefore, blood and body-fluid precautions are recommended for health care personnel caring for the woman and her infant. The appearance of antibody against HBsAg (anti-HBs), in response to either active infection or immunization, reflects immunity to HBV.[39, 60, 73, 74]

The risk of maternal transmission to the neonate depends on the types of antigens and antibodies present. If the mother is positive for both HBsAg and HBeAg, there is a high likelihood of transmission to the fetus. Most of these infants will become HBV carriers.[73] Maternal anti-HBs antibodies do not provide significant protection of the infant from HBV infection since the amount of antibody transferred provides only transient protection.[74] Women who are chronic carriers of HBsAg can transmit HBV to their infants after birth especially if the woman's serum is both HBsAg and HBeAg positive (indicating high infectivity), versus HBsAg and anti-HBe positive (indicating lower infectivity) or anti-HBe positive (indicating minimal likelihood of transfer).[74] Patterns of antigens and antibodies in acute HBV are illustrated in Figure 10–9.

A combination of active and passive immunization is recommended for prevention of HBV infection in the neonate.[60, 73] Thus, HBV immune globulin (HBIG) and HBV vaccine are administered to infants of HBsAg-positive women. HBIG provides passive immunity by supplying antibodies to destroy HBV antigen that the infant may have

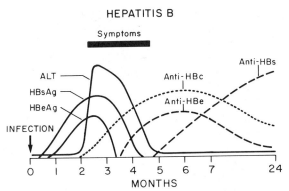

HEPATITIS B

FIGURE 10–9. The course of acute hepatitis B infection (HBsAg, hepatitis B surface antigen; anti-HBs, antibody to HBsAg; HBeAg, heptitis B e antigen; anti-HBe, antibody to HBeAg; anti-HBc, antibody to hepatitis B core antigen; ALT, alanine transferase). (From Klion, F. M. & Wolke, A. [1986]. Liver in normal pregnancy. In S. H. Cherry, R. L. Berkowitz, & N. G. Kase [Eds.], *Rovinsky and Guttmacher's medical, surgical, and gynecological complications of pregnancy* [pp. 207–214]. Baltimore: Williams & Wilkins.)

acquired from the mother during the birth process. HBIG provides initial protection for the infant, although passive immunization may not completely suppress HBV infection.[60] Since infants of carrier mothers are at constant risk of reinfection, HBV vaccine is administered to provide immunization by stimulating the infant's system to produce its own antibodies against HBV.

HIV INFECTION IN THE NEONATE

Perinatal HIV infection is increasing in frequency. General aspects (see Fig. 10–3) and maternal infection were reviewed earlier. Neonates can acquire HIV perinatally through transplacental transmission, from exposure to HIV-contaminated secretions during birth, or, less commonly, from breast milk. Transplacental transmission is believed to be the most frequent mechanism. Women who are HIV seropositive, whether symptomatic or asymptomatic, can transmit the virus to their offspring. Although the number of neonates with this disorder is still relatively small, HIV infection and AIDS appear to have a more fulminant course in infants than in adults. The mean age at diagnosis is 12 months.[109, 140] Initial clinical signs in infants include failure to thrive, hepatosplenomegaly, lymphadenopathy, chronic or recurrent diarrhea, bacterial infections, and oral candidiasis. The average life span of infants with AIDS is 1 year after diagnosis.[91] Microceph-

aly and craniofacial dysmorphism (AIDS embryopathy) have been noted in some infants with congenital infections.[110]

Immaturity of the neonate's immune system, especially the limitations in cell-mediated immunity, interferes with the ability of the infant to mount an effective response to HIV. As a result, infants develop clinical manifestations and overt disease more frequently than adults and have a shorter latency period between acquisition of HIV and the development of clinical signs, and an increased mortality rate.

Immunologic alterations found in infants and children with HIV infection are generally similar to those found in adults and reflect significant defects in cell-mediated immunity (i.e., dysfunction and reduction in T-helper cells, reversed T helper–to–T suppressor ratio, decreased T-suppressor and cytotoxic function, and decreased NK-cell activity).[58] Infants and children with AIDS frequently have an additional and severe defect in humoral (antibody)-mediated immunity with increased vulnerability to bacterial infections.[37] Adults are often protected from these infections since before becoming infected with HIV they developed memory B cells that respond rapidly with specific antibodies to infection from many common bacterial pathogens.

Infants have few memory cells and, especially if infected in utero, have impaired development of memory B cells after birth owing to decreased numbers of T4-helper cells. These T cells are important in the maturation and differentiation of B lymphocytes into plasma or memory cells (see Fig. 10–1).[37] Hypergammaglobulinemia (especially of IgG but also of IgA and IgM) is seen in many children with AIDS; severe hypogammaglobulinemia has been reported in some infants, especially preterm infants, or late in the course of this disease.[44, 58, 110]

The diagnosis of HIV infection in the neonate is difficult. Antibodies to HIV are primarily of the IgG class and therefore cross the placenta from mother to fetus. As a result, infants born to infected woman generally acquire antibodies to HIV regardless of whether or not the infant is actually infected with the virus.[110] Maternally-acquired HIV antibodies usually persist in the neonate for 6 to 9 months, but may remain for up to 15 months. Thus positive antibody tests such as the screening enzyme-linked immunosorbent assay (ELISA) test or the more specific

Western blot or immunofluorescent assays to confirm the diagnosis have less diagnostic value in the neonate and young infant. Diagnosis can be confirmed by culturing the HIV virus from peripheral cells but this assay is only available at a few centers.[52] Recent findings that specific antibody subclasses produced by HIV-infected infants may be different from those produced by HIV-infected adults may be useful in diagnosing this infection in infants.[91]

Persistence of HIV antibodies after 9 to 12 months of age generally indicates HIV infection. After maternal HIV antibodies disappear, however, some children, although infected with HIV (and virus positive), may be antibody negative. This response can be transient, with reappearance of HIV antibody as the child's immune system eventually produces antibody. Other children are so severely hypogammaglobulinemic that they are unable to produce an antibody response to HIV.[110] Preterm infants infected with HIV may have negative antibody tests at birth, especially VLBW infants born before transfer of significant quantities of maternal IgG.[110] Since the infection status of most neonates is unknown, infection control procedures (universal precautions) are appropriate whenever there is a chance of exposure to blood or body fluids.

Diagnosis of Neonatal Infection

Although microbiologic techniques are the basic tools used in the diagnosis of infection, other parameters that reflect changes in components of the immune system can be useful. Newborns usually have low serum levels of IgM at birth. Thus, elevated IgM levels (over 20 mg/dl) in cord blood or in the 1st week are suggestive of an intrauterine or intrapartally-acquired nonbacterial (fungal, viral, or parasitic) infection. Elevated IgM levels are not diagnostic of infection because an infant with an intrauterine infection may have normal IgM levels, whereas a healthy infant may have elevated levels, especially if there was maternal bleeding into the fetal circulation. Generally IgM levels continue to rise in infected infants but remain stable or decrease in noninfected infants.

The total number of WBCs or percentages of individual WBC cell types are often not useful in diagnosing neonatal sepsis, but may provide evidence suggestive of infection. At birth the WBC count averages 15,000/mm^3 (range, 9000 to 25,000, although some healthy infants may have lower or higher values) falling to about 12,000 by the end of the 1st week. Total WBC counts less than 3000 to 4000/mm^3 or more than 25,000 to 30,000/mm^3 suggest infection.

The neutrophil count varies significantly in normal newborns during the first few days, with lower counts seen in preterm infants. A transient neutrophilia usually occurs during this period, so moderately elevated neutrophil counts of 10,000 to 25,0000/µl are not suggestive of infection. Neutropenia, however, can be a useful sign of sepsis in some neonates. Strauss suggests that infants with absolute neutrophil counts of less than 3000/µl in the first 5 to 7 days should be suspected of having sepsis.[157]

The differential count can also be useful in the recognition of neonatal sepsis. Normally in the first few days after birth the majority of WBCs are PMN neutrophils (60%) with 20 to 40% of these neutrophils being band forms. Findings associated with infection include a relative absence of PMNs, an increased "shift to the left," that is, a predominance of immature forms of PMNs (bands, metamyelocytes, occasional myelocytes) due to an outpouring of immature cells from the bone marrow, an increase in toxic granulations in the PMNs, and an increase in the absolute number of bands or metamyelocytes (even with normal total neutrophil counts). In some septic infants there is a marked decrease in the bone marrow neutrophil storage pool (NSP). Christensen notes that the decreased NSP probably arises from the release of stored neutrophils in response to sepsis, the increased need for phagocytes, and an inability of the bone marrow to significantly increase production of neutrophils since production is already near maximum capacity in the neonate.[28] Infants with neutropenia and a markedly decreased NSP (less than 10%) or marked shift to the left (>75% of the circulating neutrophils are immature) are reported to be much more likely to die from sepsis if treated only with antibiotics and may be candidates for granulocyte transfusions.[28]

Antibiotic Use in the Neonate

The functional immaturity of the neonate's body systems alters drug distribution and pharmacokinetics and renders the infant more susceptible to adverse reactions. The ability to metabolize and excrete a given agent varies with gestational age, health status, and postbirth age. Individual infants often have unique responses to drugs so infants with similar gestational and postbirth ages may vary in their ability to metabolize and excrete a specific drug.

Specific physiologic alterations that influence handling of antibiotics by the neonate include changes in the volume of distribution, liver and renal function, and protein binding (see Chapters 5, 8, and 9).[176] The volume of distribution is altered in the neonate because of an increased proportion of extracellular water. As a result, peak volumes of drugs are reduced and excretion delayed. Immaturity of liver enzyme systems can delay metabolism and clearance of drugs. For example, chloramphenicol is eliminated by the kidney after conjugation in the liver. The hepatic glucuronyl transferase system responsible for conjugation is immature in the neonate (especially in preterm infants), and free (unconjugated) drug is eliminated by glomerular filtration, which is reduced in neonates. The result is higher and prolonged peak serum chloramphenicol concentrations and an increased risk of toxicity ("gray baby syndrome") with aplastic anemia, shock, and cardiovascular collapse.[103, 176]

The reduced glomerular filtration rate (GFR) seen in neonates increases serum concentrations and prolongs the half-life of many antibiotics. Serum half-lives of antibiotics change rapidly over the first few weeks after birth as renal function matures.[176] As a result, antibiotics such as penicillin or ampicillin are usually given every 8 hours in term and more mature preterm infants from birth to 7 days, and every 6 hours after 1 week of age.[68a] Maturation of renal function may be delayed in VLBW infants who have not yet developed the mature number of nephrons (see Chapter 8). Since renal handling of drugs is altered, antibiotics are given less frequently to VLBW infants. For example, penicillin and ampicillin are often given to VLBW infants (and sometimes to other neonates as well) every 12 hours during the first 7 days and every 8 hours after 7 days of age. Similar changes in timing of doses are seen with other antibiotics.[68a] In older children and adults tubular secretion is the most important mechanism for penicillin excretion (versus GFR in neonates). As a result, penicillin clearance is one fifth of that of adults,

and penicillin blood levels may persist for three times as long.

Reduced concentrations of plasma proteins, especially albumin, interfere with neonatal handling of antibiotics and other drugs. Reduction in albumin or competition for albumin-binding sites can lead to increased serum levels of free drug. Drugs such as the sulfonamides compete successfully with indirect (unconjugated) bilirubin for albumin-binding sites, often displacing bilirubin. As a result, sulfonamide use during the 1st week after birth is associated with hyperbilirubinemia and an increased risk of bilirubin encephalopathy (see Chapter 15).

Because of these physiologic limitations, peak and trough levels and serum concentrations of antibiotics, along with drug dosages, must be carefully monitored. Monitoring of peak and trough levels of aminoglycosides (e.g., kanamycin, gentamicin) is particularly important, since levels associated with toxicity are close to therapeutic levels. Peak (highest drug concentration) plasma levels are measured approximately 30 minutes after administration, whereas trough (lowest drug concentration) levels are measured immediately before an ordered dose. If peak levels are not within therapeutic ranges (i.e., subtherapeutic or in the toxic range), the dose should be altered. Trough levels can be used to determine how frequently the antibiotic should be given. Drug doses cannot be determined on infant size only but must also take into account postbirth age, maturity, and health status. Absorption of drugs through the GI system or after intramuscular injection is slow and erratic in hypoxic infants. Adverse effects associated with selected antibiotics are summarized in Table 10–5.

Immunotherapy for Neonatal Sepsis

As understanding of limitations in the neonate's immune responses has evolved, and in particular recognition of the significant limitations in the ability of VLBW infants to respond to pathogenic organisms, new therapies have been developed to augment the infant's defense mechanisms. Immunotherapy or immunoprophylactic techniques include granulocyte exchange, immunoglobulin and fibronectin transfusions and immunization using serum type-specific antibodies against GBS. These therapies are still experimental, with few or no prospective randomized clinical trials. The most frequently used type of immunotherapy in the neonate, and the therapy that has been the subject of the most investigations is intravenous administration of human immune globulin (IVIG). The general purpose of immunotherapy techniques is to improve opsonic activity and phagocytosis of bacteria by providing the infant with functional neutrophils and other cells, complement, fibronectin, or type-specific antibody.[28, 45, 52, 164, 177] Another form of immunotherapy, gamma globulin, which is often given to older people to prevent or treat certain disorders, is not practical in neonates since it must be given intramuscularly. In the neonate only a small volume can be given this way and, because of slow absorption, peak serum levels may not be achieved for 2 to 4 days.[45, 52] The use of immunotherapy has been associated with clinical improvement and reduced mortality; however, some of these therapies are associated with serious potential side effects. The benefits of IVIG therapy in preventing and treating neonatal infections have not yet been clearly documented.[72a] Table 10–12 summarizes rationales, uses, and side effects for these therapies.

Immunoprophylaxis is another technique that has been proposed as a mechanism for protecting against GBS. The purpose of this therapy is to provide the fetus or newborn with serum type-specific antibodies. Since GBS sepsis occurs primarily in neonates who lack type-specific antibodies, immunoprophylaxis might reduce the incidence of neonatal GBS infection and associated mortality. Immunoprophylaxis could be achieved by active or passive immunization of the pregnant woman (with transplacental passage of antibody to the fetus) or passive immunization of the neonate.[52, 164] Immunization of pregnant women offers little potential protection against GBS in VLBW infants since transport of IgG antibody is limited until 32 to 34 weeks.

MATURATIONAL CHANGES DURING INFANCY AND CHILDHOOD

Infants and children remain at greater risk for infection because of decreased levels of immunoglobulins. This risk is most marked during the first 6 months because of low levels of IgG associated with a physiologic hypogammaglobulinemia. Infancy is a time when hypersensitivity to food substances may develop because of immaturity of gut defense mechanisms. In this section maturation of components of the host defense system is described followed by discussion of the physiologic hypogammaglobulinemia of infancy, immunizations, and the development of allergies.

Maturation of Host Defense Factors

By 1 year of life total levels of immunoglobulins are 60% of adult values.[98] IgG production by the infant is minimal during the first few months but increases significantly after 6 months of age, with a gradual increase toward adult levels by 5 to 6 years. The increase in IgG and other immunoglobulins is probably stimulated by exposure to environmental antigens. Maternally-derived IgG has generally disappeared by 9 months of age. IgG1 and IgG3 reach 50% of adult values by 1 year and 100% by 8 years; IgG2 and IgG4 are 50% by 2 to 3 years and 100% by 10 to 12 years. As a result, infants and toddlers are more susceptible to disorders such as infection with *Haemophilus influenzae* type b, which is dependent on IgG2 antibodies for opsonization of its capsular coating.[33, 173]

IgA levels increase after birth and reach 20% of adult levels by 1 year.[98] Levels of sIgA reach adult values by 6 to 8 years; serum IgA levels attain adult values during adolescence.[173] Since IgA protects against many respiratory and GI infections, young children are more predisposed toward developing these disorders. IgM reaches 50% of adult values by 6 months and 75 to 80% by 1 year in both term and preterm infants. During the 1st year of life the infant's B cells secrete primarily IgM.

Serum complement levels gradually increase to adult values by 6 to 12 months.[12, 31, 38] T-cell function is relatively mature by 3 to 6 months. Chemotaxis of neutrophils is decreased until 2 years, and monocyte chemotaxis is decreased until 6 to 12 years.[173] Responses to bacteria with capsular polysaccharide do not reach adult capabilities until 2 years.[102] Fibronectin reaches low adult levels by 1 year.[173] The exact age at which other components of the immune system reach maturity is unknown, although the risk of infection with many of the pathogens associ-

TABLE 10–12
Immunotherapy for Neonatal Infections

THERAPY	RATIONALE	USES/OUTCOME	SIDE EFFECTS
Granulocyte transfusion	Increase number of neutrophils to replace depleted marrow pool (NSP). Provide adult neutrophils with improved chemotaxis and other functional abilities.	Uses: infants with neutropenia (<3000/μl in first week, <1000 later) especially if NSP depleted; possibly infants with antibiotic-resistant organisms. Outcome: most studies report improved survival, some no difference.	Graft-versus-host disease Hepatitis, CMV, or other infection Respiratory distress due to pulmonary sequestration of WBCs Sensitization to WBC alloantigens
Exchange transfusion	Remove bacteria and toxins. Improve circulation and tissue oxygenation. Enhance immune system function by transfusion of adult lymphocytes and immune system components.	Uses: septic infants especially with associated acidosis, shock, coagulopathy. Outcome: improved clinical status and survival reported. No prospective randomized controlled studies.	Fresh blood (<12 hr) required, stored blood associated with transient decrease in neutrophils. Risks/benefits similar to any exchange: Volume overload. Thromboembolic complications. Graft-versus-host disease. Electrolyte imbalances, hypoglycemia. Acidosis.
Immunoglobulin transfusion	Provide adequate blood titers of antibacterial antibody. Improve serum opsonization capabilities and neutrophil accumulation (may be ineffective in absence of neutrophils and complement). Types tested include IV immune globulin (IVIG) and monoclonal antibodies.* Recent IVIG preparations include antibodies for CMV, HBV, HSV, other viruses plus antibodies to GBS, *E.coli*, *Klebsiella*, and *Pseudomonas*.	Uses: infants with documented bacterial sepsis (especially GBS or *E.coli*) or prophylactically to infants at risk. IVIG has been given to pregnant women in last trimester with passage of antibody to the fetus (not useful if delivery before 32 to 33 weeks due to poor transfer). Outcome: still experimental, although used with increasing frequency in some centers. Few clinical or randomized controlled studies on humans. Reduction of infection rate and improved survival have been reported by some but not all.	Problem has been variability in amount and effectiveness of type-specific antibody in preparations of IVIG. Side effects have been reported in adults, but less often in infants.
Fibronectin transfusion	Enhance neutrophil activity at inflammation site. Improve opsonization and phagocytosis. Activate monocytes. Improve reticuloactivating system clearance of bacteria and tissue debris.	Experimental	Not yet determined

*Monoclonal antibodies are antibodies that are secreted by a single clone of cells within a tissue cluster and thus have similar properties and specificity.
    Compiled from references 28, 29, 45, 52, 79, 106, 157, 164, and 177.

ated with neonatal infection decreases after 2 to 3 months of age.[172]

Physiologic Hypogammaglobulinemia

At term IgG is 90 to 95% of adult values because of placental transfer of maternal IgG. After birth IgG levels fall gradually as maternal IgG is catabolized with minimal production of new IgG by the infant. This results in a "physiologic hypogammaglobulinemia" during the 1st year of life. Lowest levels of IgG occur at 2 to 4 months and remain low until at least 6 months (see Fig. 10–6).

The initial 6 to 12 months is therefore a period of heightened vulnerability to infection in all infants, with a higher risk in preterm infants. These infants have lower IgG levels at birth, reach lowest levels of IgG sooner, and remain at low levels longer since the ability to synthesize IgG is more closely related to conceptual age than to postbirth age. Sasidharan found that 42.8% (18 of 42) of VLBW infants had IgG levels lower than 100 mg/dl by 2 to 3 months of age, with values of 22 mg/dl in one infant.[134] The lowest IgG levels during the first few months were directly proportional to gestational age and inversely proportional to postbirth age. The period of hypogammaglobulinemia is also exaggerated in SGA infants. These infants often have lower levels of maternal antibody, probably owing to placental dysfunction.

Immunizations

Although immunizations have been part of well-baby care for many years, there is still controversy regarding timing, dosage, and side effects. Bernbaum and associates identified several related areas of controversy including the ability of the preterm infant to form antibodies to different antigens and the effect of passively transferred maternal antibody on the ability of the neonate to respond to immunization.[12] The American Academy of Pediatrics has recommended that diphtheria–pertussis–tetanus (DPT) and oral polio vaccine (OPV) immunizations be given to preterm infants at the same chronologic age as term infants (Table 10–13).[12, 23] If infants are still hospitalized at this time, only DPT is recommended, with OPV immunization delayed until discharge. (OPV is a live virus vaccine with a risk of nosocomial transmis-

sion.) Hospitalized infants may be receiving blood or blood products. Vaccinations should not be given within 14 days of these treatments since blood or blood products may contain specific antibodies against the vaccine's antigen and interfere with the development of an appropriate immune response.[42]

The ability to respond to antigens with production of specific antibodies improves with age and is influenced more by exposure to antigens than by maturation of the immune system per se.[12] Both preterm and term infants respond similarly to OPV immunization, attaining adequate titers after two doses. Infant responses are not dependent on either birth weight or gestational age.[18] Bernbaum and associates examined antibody responses of term and preterm infants to DPT injections at 2, 4, and 6 months after birth.[12] Before the first immunization 84% of preterm and 100% of term infants had adequate antibody levels to diphtheria and tetanus (but only 16% of preterm infants and 86% of term infants to pertussis) from transplacental passage of maternal IgG. Thus, the preterm infants would have had fewer antibodies to protect them if they were exposed to organisms that cause these disorders before immunization. Adequate immune responses to diphtheria and tetanus were noted in term infants after one dose and in preterm infants after two doses. Both groups required two doses of DPT to mount adequate responses to pertussis. Preterm infants have fewer febrile or local reactions to DPT injections, probably owing to immature primary host defense mechanisms.[12, 13]

Use of half-dose DPT for preterm infants in an effort to reduce immunization risks is not recommended.[13] Bernbaum and associates found that fewer than half of preterm infants who received half-dose immunizations were able to mount an appropriate serologic response after three doses and required a fourth full dose to achieve this response.[13] Thus use of half-dose immunizations with preterm infants leaves about half of these infants unprotected.

Pertussis vaccination is contraindicated in infants with progressive neurologic disorders or a history of severe reactions to earlier doses. Nonprogressive neurologic disorders such as cerebral palsy or a history of neonatal seizures that occurred months earlier or that are well controlled is not a contraindication

TABLE 10–13
Schedule of Recommended Immunizations

TIME	IMMUNIZATION				
	DPT	TVOPV	MMR	HIB	Td
2 months	X	X		X	
4 months	X	X	X		
6 months	X			X	
15 months			X	X*	
15 to 18 months	X	X			
4 to 6 years	X	X			
11 to 12 years			X		
14 to 16 years					X
Every 10 years					X

*Booster.
DPT, diphtheria, pertussis, tetanus; TVOPV, trivalent oral poliovirus vaccine; MMR, measles, mumps, rubella; HIB, *Haemophilus influenzae* type b; Td, adult form of tetanus and diphtheria.[178]

to this vaccination, nor is the use of pertussis with preterm infants who have had a severe intracranial hemorrhage or prolonged frequency of apnea of prematurity, although concerns have been raised.[12, 23, 150]

Passively-acquired maternal antibody generally does not interfere with DPT or OPV immunization, perhaps because maternal antibody levels to these organisms are relatively low because of the length of time since vaccination. Term or preterm infants do not respond well to vaccination, except with tetanus, before 1 month.[23] After that time infants respond adequately to tetanus and diphtheria at any age and to pertussis after 3 months, which is why several doses of pertussis may be required before an adequate antibody response is observed.

IgG acquired through placental transfer from the mother can interfere with live virus immunizations by neutralizing the viruses and preventing successful vaccination. The predominance of T-suppressor versus T-helper cells in the neonate may also interfere with the ability of the infant to respond appropriately. Therefore, vaccination with live viruses other than OPV is usually delayed until after the 1st year. Vaccination with HBV vaccine is effective early in infancy because this is an inactivated protein antigen. Live virus vaccines have been contraindicated in infants and children seropositive for HIV, although the effects of the acquired disorder on the child versus the risk for developing systemic disease from the immunization is currently being reevaluated. Inactivated vaccines (DPT, inactivated poliovirus, *Haemophilus influenzae* type B [HIB], and HBV) are

TABLE 10–14
Summary of Recommendations for Clinical Practice Related to Host Defense Mechanisms: Neonate

Recognize normal parameters for immune system components and patterns of change during the neonatal period (pp. 468–472).

Obtain and evaluate maternal history of possible exposure to infectious organisms or potential for current illness (pp. 464, 467–468, 474–480).

Recognize risk factors for development and clinical manifestations of specific infections (pp. 474–480, Table 10–10).

Recognize the subtle signs of infection in the neonate and that hyperthermia is rarely a sign of infection (pp. 469–470).

Recognize laboratory findings associated with an increased likelihood of neonatal infection (p. 480).

Monitor neonates for signs of infection, especially infants with disruption of their skin barrier, who are preterm, ill, SGA, stressed, or with delayed oral feedings (pp. 467–468, 470–477, 484, Tables 10–9 and 10–10).

Monitor for signs of necrotizing enterocolitis (pp. 468, 473–474).

Monitor for signs of GBS and *E. coli* sepsis and meningitis in infants of mothers colonized with these organisms who do not have type-specific antibody (pp. 474–477, Fig. 10–8, Table 10–10).

Use careful hand-washing and other aseptic techniques (pp. 467, 469–470, Table 10–10).

Recognize the effects of neonatal physiologic adaptations on the pharmacokinetics of antibiotics (pp. 480–481, Table 10–5).

Know or verify usual doses for antibiotics given during the neonatal period (pp. 480–481).

Recognize side effects of antibiotics and potential toxicity to the neonate (pp. 480–481, Table 10–5).

Know antibiotics not recommended during the neonatal period (pp. 480–481, Table 10–5).

Monitor and evaluate neonatal responses to antibiotics, including peak and trough and serum levels (p. 481).

Know types of immunotherapy and associated side effects (pp. 481–482, Table 10–12).

Teach parents regarding methods to prevent or reduce the risk of infection in their infant (pp. 469–470, 482–484, Table 10–10).

Monitor infants of women with chronic disorders associated with transplacental passage of antibodies for antibody-related clinical problems (pp. 458–459).

Monitor Rho(D)-positive infants of Rho(D)-negative women and A, B, or AB infants of type O mothers for hyperbilirubinemia (pp. 459–464).

Recognize antigens and antibodies associated with HBV infection and institute hepatitis precautions for infants born to mothers who are HBsAg or HBeAg positive (pp. 477–479, Table 10–11, Fig. 10–9).

Give HBIG and HBV to infants of mothers who are HBsAg positive (pp. 478–479).

Recognize that neonates who are HIV-antibody positive at birth are not necessarily infected with HIV (pp. 479–480).

Know that the VLBW newborn of an HIV-positive mother may not be antibody-positive even though infected with the virus at birth (pp. 479–480).

Use universal precautions for blood and body fluids during the perinatal period (pp. 478–480).

Avoid use of DeLee mucus traps in infants at risk for HIV infection (pp. 479–480).

Know recommended schedule of immunizations (pp. 484–485, Table 10–13).

Monitor infants to ensure that they receive immunizations as scheduled, especially preterm infants and infants with chronic problems (pp. 484–485).

Avoid use of live virus vaccines in infants who are hospitalized and in infants who are HIV positive (pp. 484–485).

Avoid giving immunizations within 14 days of administration of blood or blood products (p. 484).

Counsel parents regarding practices to reduce risks of allergies (p. 486).

Page numbers in parentheses following each intervention refer to the pages in the text where the rationale for that intervention is discussed.

preferred for these children.[58, 66, 72a] Inactivated OPV should also be given to family members due for immunizations to reduce the risk of nosocomial infection.[44, 140]

Development of Allergies

Hypersensitivity to cow's milk and foods is more frequent in infants than in older children. By 1 to 2 years many children can tolerate substances to which they were "allergic" earlier.[67] Exposure to potentially allergic substances in early infancy may sensitize susceptible infants to specific ingested proteins, however (similar to the process described earlier for Rh isoimmunization). Later exposure to even small quantities of that protein may invoke an allergic response. Therefore, food substances known to have strong antigenic potential, such as egg white, are usually not recommended for young infants.

Young infants are more likely to develop food allergies because of immaturity of gut defense mechanisms, lack of gut closure, and the ability of the immature gut to absorb intact protein macromolecules. Most infants fed cow's milk early develop IgG and IgA antibodies to cow's milk antigens. These antibodies are found from 3 to 9 months, then gradually decrease but may return (at lower levels) with later ingestion of cow's milk. Breast-feeding may reduce the risk of allergy by limiting ingestion of foreign antigens or, with early development of the IgA barrier in the gut, by binding foreign proteins with specific antibodies to prevent their absorption.[67, 108] The American Academy of Pediatrics recommends delaying introduction of solids until 4 to 6 months in all children and until 6 months if there is a history of allergies in the family.[67]

SUMMARY

The fetus and neonate are immunocompromised hosts because of alterations in their host defense mechanisms that increase their risk of infection. This risk is particularly evident in relation to organisms that colonize the maternal genital tract such as GBS and sexually transmitted diseases such as herpes, hepatitis B, and AIDS. Clinical recommendations for nurses working with neonates based on changes in host defense mechanisms are summarized in Table 10–14. By understanding the limitations of the immune system in the neonate and infant, nurses can appreciate the vulnerabilities to infection from specific organisms and the risk for developing sepsis, develop increased understanding of the rationales behind specific infection control policies, and provide appropriate parent teaching.

REFERENCES

1. Agatsuma, Y., et al. (1981). Cell mediated immunity to cytomegalovirus in pregnant women. *Am J Reprod Immunol, 1,* 174.
2. Alanen, A. & Lassila, O. (1982). Deficient natural killer cell function in pre-eclampsia. *Obstet Gynecol, 60,* 631.
3. Ambruso, D.R., Altenburger, K.M., & Johnston, R.B. (1979). Defective oxidative metabolism in newborn neutrophils: Discrepancy between superoxide anion and hydroxyl radical generation. *Pediatrics, 64*(Suppl.), 722.
4. Amino, N., et al. (1978). Changes in serum immunoglobulins IgG, IgA, IgM and IgE during pregnancy. *Obstet Gynecol, 52,* 415.
5. Anthony, B.F. (1986). The role of specific antibody in neonatal bacterial infections. *Pediatr Infect Dis, 5,* S164.
6. Baker, C.J., et al. (1989). Multicenter trial of intravenous immunoglobulin (IVIG) to prevent late-onset infection in preterm infants: Preliminary results. *Pediatr Res, 25,* 275A.
7. Barnett, M.A., et al. (1983). T helper lymphocyte depression in early human pregnancy. *J Reprod Immunol, 5,* 55.
8. Beer, A.E. & Billingham, R.E. (1976). *The immunobiology of mammalian reproduction.* Englewood Cliffs, NJ: Prentice Hall.
9. Bejar, R., et al. (1981). Premature labor: Bacterial sources of phospholipidase. *Obstet Gynecol, 57,* 479.
10. Bellanti, J.A. (1978). *Immunology II.* Philadelphia: WB Saunders.
11. Bellanti, J.A., Boner, A.L., & Valletta, E. (1987). Immunology of the fetus and newborn. In G.B. Avery (Ed.), *Neonatology: Pathophysiology and management of the newborn* (pp. 850–873). Philadelphia: JB Lippincott.
12. Bernbaum, J., et al. (1984). Development of the premature infant's host defense mechanisms and its relationship to routine immunizations. *Clin Perinatol, 11,* 73.
13. Bernbaum, J., et al. (1989). Half-dose immunization for diphtheria, tetanus, pertussis: Response of preterm infants. *Pediatrics, 83,* 471.
14. Billingham, R.E. & Head, J. (1981). Current trends in reproductive immunology: An overview. *J Reprod Immunol, 3,* 253.
15. Bjorkstein, B., et al. (1978). Polymorphonuclear leukocyte function during pregnancy. *Scand J Immunol, 8,* 257.
16. Blackburn, S. (1985). Rho(D) isoimmunization: Implications for the mother, fetus, and newborn. NAACOG Update Series, Volume III. Princeton, NJ: Continuing Professional Education Center.
17. Blaise, R.M., Poplak, D.G., & Mulclimade, A.V.

(1979). The mononuclear phagocyte system: Role in expression of immunocompetence in neonatal and adult life. *Pediatrics, 64*(Suppl.), 829.

18. Bland, R.S., et al. (1983). Antibody responses of preterm infants to oral polio vaccine. *Pediatr Res, 17*, 265A.

19. Boue, A. & Malbrunot, C. (1987). Fetal and neonatal viral infections. In L. Stern & P. Vert (Eds.), *Neonatal medicine* (pp. 637–663). New York: Masson Publishing.

20. Boxer, L.A. (1978). Immunological function and leucocyte disorders in newborn infants. *Clin Haematol, 7*, 123.

21. Butler, J.E. (1979). Immunologic aspects of breast-feeding: Antiinfectious activity of breast milk. *Semin Perinatol, 3*, 255.

22. Calame, A. & Vaudaux, B. (1987). Bacterial infections in the newborn. In L Stern & P. Vert (Eds.), *Neonatal medicine* (pp. 587–621). New York: Masson Publishing.

23. Cates, K.L., Rowe, J.C., & Ballow, M. (1983). The premature infant as a compromised host. *Curr Prob Pediatr, 13*, 1.

24. C.D.C. (1985). Recommendations for assisting in the prevention of perinatal transmission of human T-lymphotropic virus type III/lymphadenopathy-associated virus and acquired immunodeficiency syndrome. *MMWR, 34*, 721.

25. Chandra, R.K. (1981). Serum thymic hormone activity and cell mediated immunity in healthy neonates, preterm infants, and small for gestational age infants. *Pediatrics, 67*, 407.

26. Chandra, R.K. (1984). Influence of the nutritional-immunity axis on perinatal infections. In P.L. Ogra (Ed.), *Neonatal infections: Nutritional and immunologic interactions* (pp. 229–245). Orlando, FL: Grune & Stratton.

27. Chow, A.W. & Jewesson, P.J. (1985). Pharmacokinetics and safety of antimicrobial agents during pregnancy. *Rev Infect Dis, 7*, 287.

28. Christensen, R.D. (1987). Intravenous immunoglobulin for prophylaxis or treatment of bacterial infections in neonates. *J Perinatol, 7*, 58.

29. Clapp, D.W. (1989). Use of intravenously administered immune globulin to prevent nosocomial sepsis in low birth weight infants: Report of a pilot study. *J Pediatr, 115*, 973.

30. Cohn, J.A. (1989). Virology, immunology, and natural history of HIV infection. *J Nurs Midwifery, 34*, 242.

31. Cole, F.S. & Colton, H.R. (1984). Complement. In P.L. Ogra (Ed.), *Neonatal infections: Nutritional and immunologic interactions* (pp. 37–45). Orlando, FL: Grune & Stratton.

32. Davies, M. & Browne, C.M. (1985). Antitrophoblast antibody responses during normal human pregnancy. *J Reprod Immunol, 7*, 285.

33. Davies, P.A. & Gothefors, L.A. (1984). *Bacterial infections in the fetus and newborn infant.* Philadelphia: WB Saunders.

34. DiSaia, P.J. & Berman, M.L. (1984). Cancer in pregnancy. In R.K. Creasy & R. Resnik (Eds.), *Maternal-fetal medicine* (pp. 1063–1089). Philadelphia: WB Saunders.

35. Dombroski, R.A. (1989). Autoimmune disease in pregnancy. *Med Clin North Am, 73*, 605.

36. Durandy, A., et al. (1982). Respective roles and interactions of T lymphocytes and PGE–2 mediated monocyte suppressive activities in human

newborns and mothers at the time of delivery. *Am J Reprod Immunol, 2*, 12.

37. Eales, L.J. & Parkin, J.M. (1988). Current concepts in the immunopathogenesis of AIDS and HIV infection. *Br Med Bull, 44*, 38.

38. Edwards, M.S. (1986). Complement in neonatal infections: An overview. *Pediatr Infect Dis, 5*, S168.

39. Edwards, M.S. (1988). Hepatitis B serology–Help in interpretation. *Pediatr Clin North Am, 35*, 503.

40. Edwards, M.S. & Baker, C.J. (1984). Bacterial infections. In P.L. Ogra (Ed.), *Neonatal infections: Nutritional and immunologic interactions* (pp. 91–108). Orlando, FL: Grune & Stratton.

41. Faden, H. & Rosales, S. (1984). Infections in the compromised host. In P.L. Ogra (Ed.), *Neonatal infections: Nutritional and immunologic interactions* (pp. 185–202). Orlando, FL: Grune & Stratton.

42. Faix, R.G. & Shope, T.C. (1986). Immunization during pregnancy. In W.F. Rayburn & F.P. Zuspan (Eds.), *Drug therapy in obstetrics and gynecology* (pp. 147–161). Norwalk, CT: Appleton-Century-Crofts.

43. Falkoff, R. (1987). Maternal immunologic changes during pregnancy: A critical appraisal. *Clin Rev Allergy, 5*, 287.

44. Falloon, J. & Pizza, P.A. (1990). Acquired immunodeficiency syndrome in the infant. In J.S. Remington & J.O. Klein (Eds.), *Infectious diseases of the fetus and newborn infant* (pp. 306–324). Philadelphia: WB Saunders.

45. Fischer, G.W. (1988). Therapeutic uses of intravenous gammaglobulin for pediatric infections. *Pediatr Clin North Am, 35*, 517.

46. Gall, S.A. (1977). The maternal immune system during human gestation. *Semin Perinatol, 1*, 119.

47. Gall, S.A. (1983). Maternal adjustments in the immune system in normal pregnancy. *Clin Obstet Gynecol, 26*, 521.

48. Gall, S.A. & Wenstrom, K.D. (1990). Maternal-fetal immunology. In R.D. Eden & F.H. Boehm (Eds.), *Assessment and care of the fetus* (pp. 207–214). Norwalk, CT: Appleton & Lange.

49. Garza, C., et al. (1987). Special properties of human milk. *Clin Perinatol, 14*, 11.

50. Gazaway, P. & Mullins, C.L. (1986). Prevention of preterm labor and premature rupture of the membranes. *Clin Obstet Gynecol, 29*, 835.

51. Gibbs, R.S. & Sweet, R.L. (1984). Maternal and fetal infections. In R.K. Creasy & R. Resnik (Eds.), *Maternal-fetal medicine* (pp. 603–678). Philadelphia: WB Saunders.

52. Givner, L.B. & Baker, C.J. (1988). The prevention and treatment of neonatal group B streptococcal infections. *Adv Pediatr Infect Dis, 3*, 65.

53. Gleicher, N. (1986). Pregnancy and autoimmunity. *Acta Haematol, 76*, 68.

54. Gleicher, N., Deppe, G., & Cohen, C. (1979). Common aspects of immunologic tolerance in pregnancy and malignancy. *Obstet Gynecol, 54*, 335.

55. Goldman, A.S., et al. (1982). Effects of prematurity on the immunologic system in human milk. *J Pediatr, 101*, 901.

56. Gonzales, L.A. & Hill, H.R. (1989). The current status of intravenous gamma globulin use in neonates. *Pediatr Infect Dis, 8*, 315.

57. Grady, C. (1989). The immune system and AIDS/HIV infection. In J. Flaskerud (Ed.), *AIDS/HIV infection* (pp. 37–57). Philadelphia: WB Saunders.

58. Grossman, M. (1988). Children with AIDS. *Infect Dis Clin North Am, 2*, 533.

59. Hamosh, M. & Hamosh, P. (1988). Mother to infant biochemical transfer through breast milk. In G.H. Wiknjosastro, W.H. Prakoso, & K. Maeda (Eds.), *Perinatology* (pp. 155–159). Amsterdam: Elsevier.

60. Hanshaw, J.B., Dudgeon, J.A., & Marshall, W.C. (1985). *Viral diseases of the fetus and newborn*. Philadelphia: WB Saunders.

61. Head, J.R. & Billingham, R.E. (1986). Concerning the immunology of the uterus. *Am J Reprod Immunol, 10*, 76.

62. Hill, H.R. (1987). Biochemical, structural, and functional abnormalities of polymorphonuclear leukocytes in the neonate. *Pediatr Res, 22*, 375.

63. Hobbs, J.R. & Davis, J.A. (1967). Serum G-globulin levels and gestational age in premature babies. *Lancet, 1*, 757.

64. Honkonen, E. & Erkkola, R. (1987). Antibacterial capacity in amniotic fluid in normal and complicated pregnancies. *Ann Chir Gynecol, 76*(Suppl. 202), 14.

65. Howie, P.W., et al. (1990). Protective effect of breast feeding against infection. *Br Med J, 300*, 11.

66. Ippolito, C. & Gibes, R.M. (1988). AIDS and the newborn. *J Perinat Neonat Nurs, 1*(4), 78.

67. Israel, E.J. & Walker, W.A. (1988). Host defense development in gut and related disorders. *Pediatr Clin North Am, 35*, 1.

68. Jacob, J.H. & Stringer, C.A. (1990). Diagnosis and management of cancer during pregnancy. *Semin Perinatol, 14*, 79.

68a. Jacobs, N.M. (1991). Antibacterial therapy. In T.F. Yeh (Ed.), *Neonatal therapeutics* (2nd ed., pp. 180–204). St. Louis: Mosby-Year Book.

69. Jacoby, D.R., Olding, L.B., & Oldstone, M.B. (1984). Immunologic regulation of fetal-maternal balance. *Adv Immunol, 35*, 157.

70. Jones, L.C. & Bennett, M. (1990). Human immunodeficiency virus (HIV) during pregnancy. *Int J Childbirth Education, 5*, 21.

71. Johnson, U. & Gustavil, B. (1987). Complement components in normal pregnancy. *Acta Pathol Microbiol Immunol Scand, 95*, 97.

72. Kim, I.C. & Sabourin, C.L.K. (1987). Antigenic analysis of human trophoblast membrane: Detection of a lymphocyte crossreactive antigen. *Am J Reprod Immunol Microbiol, 13*, 44.

72a. Kim, K.S. (1991). Immune therapy in neonates and small infants. In T.F. Yeh (Ed.), *Neonatal therapeutics* (2nd ed., pp. 229–238). St. Louis: Mosby-Year Book.

73. Klein, M.E. (1988). Hepatitis B virus: Perinatal management. *J Perinat Neonat Nurs, 1*(4), 12.

74. Klion, F.M. & Wolke, A. (1985). Liver in normal pregnancy. In S.H. Cherry, R.L. Berkowitz, & N.G. Kase (Eds.), *Rovinsky and Guttmacher's medical, surgical, and gynecological complications of pregnancy* (pp. 207–214). Baltimore: Williams & Wilkins.

75. Klipple, G.L. & Cecere, F.A. (1989). Rheumatoid arthritis and pregnancy. *Rheum Dis Clin North Am, 15*, 213.

76. Kochenour, N.K. & Scott, J.R. (1985). Rh isoimmunization in pregnancy. In J.R. Scott & N.S. Rote (Eds.), *Immunology in obstetrics and gynecology* (pp. 141–164). Norwalk, CT: Appleton-Century-Crofts.

77. Kohl, S. (1984). Neonatal herpes. In P.L. Ogra (Ed.), Neonatal infections: Nutritional and immunologic interactions (pp. 147–172). Orlando, FL: Grune & Stratton.

78. Koren, G., et al. (1990). Cancer in pregnancy. *Obstet Gynecol Surv, 45*, 509.

79. Kyllonen, K.S., et al. (1989). Dosage of intravenously administered immune globulin and dosing interval required to maintain target levels of immunoglobulin G in low birth weight infants. *J Pediatr, 115*, 1013.

80. Lake, A.M. & Walker, W.A. (1977). Neonatal necrotizing enterocolitis: A disease of altered host defense. *Clin Gastroenterol, 6*,463.

81. Landers, D.V., Green, J.R., & Sweet, R.L. (1983). Antibiotic use during pregnancy and the postpartum period. *Clin Obstet Gynecol, 26*, 391.

82. Landesman, S. (1989). Human immunodeficiency virus infection in women: A overview. *Semin Perinatol, 13*, 2.

83. Laros, R.K. (1986). Erythroblastosis fetalis. In R.K. Laros (Ed.), *Blood disorders in pregnancy* (pp. 103–120). Philadelphia: Lea & Febiger.

84. Larsen, B. & Galask, R.P. (1977). Protection of the fetus against infection. *Semin Perinatol, 1*, 183.

85. Lawton, A.R. (1984). Ontogeny of the immune system. In P.L. Ogra (Ed.), *Neonatal infections: Nutritional and immunologic interactions* (pp. 3–20). Orlando, FL: Grune & Stratton.

86. Lederman, M.M. (1984). Cell mediated immunity and pregnancy. *Chest, 86*(Suppl.), 6s.

87. Levy, J.A. (1988). The human immunodeficiency virus and its pathogenesis. *Infect Dis Clin North Am, 2*, 285.

88. Lockshin, M.D. (1990). Pregnancy associated with systemic lupus erythematosus. *Semin Perinatol, 14*, 130.

89. Losonsky, G.A. & Ogra, P.L. (1984). Mucosal immune system. In P.L. Ogra (Ed.), *Neonatal infections: Nutritional and immunologic interactions* (pp. 51–66). Orlando, FL: Grune & Stratton.

90. Massobrio, M., et al. (1985). Immune complexes in preeclampsia and normal pregnancy. *Am J Obstet Gynecol, 152*, 578.

91. Mayock, D.E. (1988). Detecting HIV infection in the neonate. *Northwest Perinatal Newsletter, 2*(2), 3.

92. McGregor, J.A. (1985). Microorganisms and arachidonic acid metabolites in preterm birth. *Semin Reprod Endocrinol, 3*, 273.

93. McGregor, J.A. (1988). Prevention of preterm birth: New initiatives based on microbial-host interactions. *Obstet Gynecol Surv, 43*, 1.

94. McGregor, J.A., et al. (1990). Antibiotic inhibition of bacterially induced fetal membrane weakening. *Obstet Gynecol, 76*, 124.

95. McIntyre, J.A. & Faulk, W.P. (1986). Trophoblast antigens in normal and abnormal human pregnancy. *Clin Obstet Gynecol, 29*, 976.

96. McIntyre, J.A., et al. (1986). Immunologic testing and immunotherapy in recurrent spontaneous abortion. *Obstet Gynecol, 67*, 169.

97. McManamny, D.S., et al. (1989). Melanoma and pregnancy: A long term followup. *Br J Obstet Gynaecol, 96*, 1419.

98. Miller, M.M. & Stiehm, E.R. (1983). Immunology and resistance to infection. In J.S. Remington & J.O. Klein (Eds.), *Infectious diseases of the fetus and newborn infant* (pp. 27–68). Philadelphia: WB Saunders.

99. Minkoff, H.L. (1987). Care of the pregnant woman

infected with human immunodeficiency virus. *JAMA, 258*, 2714.

100. Mintz, G. & Rodriguez-Alvarez, E. (1989). Systemic lupus erythematosus. *Rheum Dis Clin North Am, 15*, 255.

101. Mitchell, G.W., Jacobs, A.A., & Haddad, V. (1970). The role of the phagocyte in host-parasite interaction: Metabolic and bacteriocidal activities of leukocytes in pregnant women. *Am J Obstet Gynecol, 108*, 805.

102. Mitchell, M.S. & Capizzi, R.L. (1988). Neoplastic diseases. In G.N. Burrow & T.F. Ferris (Eds.), *Medical complications during pregnancy* (pp. 540–569). Philadelphia: WB Saunders.

103. Moellering, R.C. (1979). Special consideration of the use of antimicrobial agents during pregnancy, postpartum and in the newborn. *Clin Obstet Gynecol, 22*, 373.

104. Moriyama, I., et al. (1987). Infection and the functional immaturity of the fetal immune system. In K. Maeda (Ed.), *The fetus as patient '87* (pp. 247–257). Proceedings of the Third International Symposium. Amsterdam: Excerpta Medica.

105. Namba, T., Brown, S.B., & Grob, D. (1970). Neonatal myasthenia gravis: Report of two cases and review of the literature. *Pediatrics, 45*, 488.

106. Noya, F.J.D. & Baker, C.J. (1989). Intravenously administered immune globulin for premature infants: A time to wait. *J Pediatr, 115*, 969.

107. Ogra, P.L. & Dhar, R. (1984). Viral infections. In P.L. Ogra (Ed.), *Neonatal infections: Nutritional and immunologic interactions* (pp. 125–146). Orlando, FL: Grune & Stratton.

108. Ogra, P.L. & Fishaut, M. (1990). Human breast milk. In J.S. Remington & J.O. Klein (Eds.), *Infectious diseases of the fetus and newborn infants* (pp. 68–88). Philadelphia: WB Saunders.

109. Oxtoby, M.J. (1990). Perinatally acquired human immunodeficiency virus infection. *Pediatr Infect Dis J, 9*, 609.

110. Pahwa, S. (1988). Human immunodeficiency virus infection in children: Nature of immunodeficiency, clinical spectrum and management. *Pediatr Infect Dis J, 7*, S61.

111. Pattillo, R. (1981). Immunology of gestation. In L. Iffy & H. Kaminetzky (Eds.), *Obstetrics and perinatology* (Vol. I, pp. 101–125). New York: John Wiley & Sons.

112. Peckham, C.S., Senturia, Y.D., & Ades, A.E. (1987). Obstetric and perinatal consequences of human immunodeficiency virus (HIV) infection: A review. *Br J Obstet Gynaecol, 94*, 403.

113. Philipson, A. (1977). Pharmacokinetics of ampicillin during pregnancy. *J Infect Dis, 136*, 370.

114. Pitt, J. (1984). Necrotizing enterocolitis: A model for infection-immunity interaction. In P.L. Ogra (Ed.), *Neonatal infections: Nutritional and immunologic interactions* (pp. 173–184). Orlando, FL: Grune & Stratton.

115. Pittard, W.B. (1979). Breast milk immunology. *Am J Dis Child, 133*, 83.

116. Pleet, H.B., et al. (1980). Patterns of malformations resulting from the teratogenic effects of first trimester hyperthermia. *Pediatr Res, 14*, 587.

117. Preblad, S. & William, N. (1985). Fetal risks associated with rubella vaccine: Implications for vaccination of susceptible women. *Obstet Gynecol, 66*, 211.

118. Prindall, G. (1974). Maturation of cellular and humoral immunity during human embryologic development. *Acta Pediatr Scand, 63*, 607.

119. Pritchard, J.A., MacDonald, P.C., & Gant, N. (1985). *Williams obstetrics* (16th ed.). New York: Appleton-Century-Crofts.

120. Pullen, C.R. & Hull, D. (1989). Routine immunization of preterm infants. *Am J Dis Child, 64*, 1438.

121. Rappaport, V.J., et al. (1990). Anti-vascular endothelial cell antibodies in severe preeclampsia. *Am J Obstet Gynecol, 162*, 138.

122. Redman, C.W.G. (1986). Immunology of the placenta. *Clin Obstet Gynecol, 13*, 469.

123. Redman, C.W.G. & Sargent, S.I.L. (1986). Immunological disorders of human pregnancy. *Oxford Rev Reprod Biol, 8*, 223.

124. Roberts, A.K. (1987). Factors influencing bacterial growth in the neonatal large intestine. In M. Xanthou (Ed.), *New aspects of nutrition in pregnancy, infancy and prematurity* (pp. 171–179). New York: Elsevier Science Publishers.

125. Rodeck, C.H. & Letsky, E. (1989). How the management of erythroblastosis fetalis has changed. *Br J Obstet Gynaecol 96*, 759.

126. Rodriguez, C., et al. (1989).. Comparative functional study of colostral macrophages from mothers delivering preterm and at term. *Acta Paediatr Scand, 78*, 337.

127. Romero, R. & Mazor, M. (1988). Infection and preterm labor. *Clin Obstet Gynecol, 31*, 553.

128. Rote, N.S. (1982). Pathophysiology of Rh isoimmunization. *Clin Obstet Gynecol, 25*, 243.

129. Rote, N.S. (1985). Maternal-fetal immunology. In J.R. Scott & N.S. Rote (Eds.), *Immunology in obstetrics and gynecology* (pp. 55–76). Norwalk, CT: Appleton-Century-Crofts.

130. Saballus, M.K., Lake, K.D., & Wager, G.P. (1987). Immunizing the pregnant woman: Risks versus benefits. *Postgrad Med, 81*, 103.

131. Sacchi, F., et al. (1982). Differential maturation of neutrophil chemotaxis in term and preterm newborn infants. *J Pediatr, 101*, 273.

132. Salahuddin, S.Z. & Markham, P.D. (1988). Retroviruses: New viral infections in man. *Pediatr J Infect Dis, 7*, S107.

133. Samuels, P., et al. (1987). Abnormalities in platelet antiglobulin tests in preeclamptic mothers and their neonates. *Am J Obstet Gynecol, 157*, 109.

134. Sasidharan, P. (1988). Postnatal IgG levels in very-low-birth-weight infants. *Clin Pediatr, 27*, 271.

135. Schlievert, P., Johnson, W., & Galask, R.P. (1977). Amniotic fluid antibacterial mechanisms. *Semin Perinatol, 1*, 59.

136. Schroeder, J. & de la Chapelle, A. (1972). Fetal lymphocytes in maternal blood. *Blood, 39*, 153.

137. Schuit, K.E. & Powell, D.A. (1980). Phagocytic dysfunction in monocytes of normal newborn infants. *Pediatrics, 65*, 501.

138. Schwartz, R.H. (1981). Considerations of antibiotic therapy during pregnancy. *Obstet Gynecol, 58*(Suppl.), 95s.

139. Scott, J.R. (1985). Immunologic diseases in pregnancy. In J.R. Scott & N.S. Rote (Eds.), *Immunology in obstetrics and gynecology* (pp. 165–196). Norwalk, CT: Appleton-Century-Crofts.

140. Scott, G.B. (1989). Perinatal HIV–1 infection: Diagnosis and management. *Clin Obstet Gynecol, 32*, 477.

141. Scott, J.R. & Beer, A.A. (1976). Immunologic as-

pects of preeclampsia. *Am J Obstetr Gynecol, 125,* 418.

142. Semenzato, G., et al. (1980). T cell immune function in newborn infants. *Biol Neonate, 37,* 8.

143. Sever, J.L. (1982). Infections in pregnancy: Highlights from the collaborative perinatal project. *Teratology, 25,* 227.

144. Sever, J.L. (1989). HIV: Biology and immunology. *Clin Obstet Gynecol, 32,* 423.

145. Shohat, B., et al. (1986). Cellular immune aspects of the human fetal-maternal relationship. *Am J Reprod Immunol Microbiol, 11,* 125.

146. Shore, S.L., et al. (1977). Antibody-dependent cellular cytotoxicity to target cells in infants with herpes simplex virus: Functional adequacy of the neonate. *Pediatrics, 59,* 22.

147. Sibai, B.M. (1990). The HELLP syndrome (hemolysis, elevated liver enzymes, and low platelets): Much ado about nothing? *Am J Obstet Gynecol, 162,* 311.

148. Siiteri, P.K. & Stites, D.P. (1982). Immunologic and endocrinologic interrelationships in pregnancy. *Biol Reprod, 26,* 1.

149. Simpson, M.L., et al. (1988). Bacterial infections during pregnancy. In G.N. Burrow & T.F. Ferris (Eds.), *Medical complications during pregnancy* (pp. 345–371). Philadelphia: WB Saunders.

150. Sixby, J. (1987). Routine immunization and the immunosuppressed child. *Adv Pediatr Infect Dis, 2,* 79.

151. Smith, D.W., Clause, S.K., & Harvey, M.A.S. (1978). Hyperthermia as a possible teratogenic agent. *J Pediatr, 92,* 878.

152. Speer, C.P. & Johnson, R.B. (1984). Phagocyte function. In P.L. Ogra (Ed.), *Neonatal infections: Nutritional and immunologic interactions* (pp. 21–36). Orlando, FL: Grune & Stratton.

153. Sridama, V., et al. (1982). Decreased levels of helper T cells. *N Engl J Med, 307,* 352.

154. Stear, L.A. & Elinger, S.S. (1988). Understanding acquired immunodeficiency syndrome: Implications for pregnancy. *J Perinat Neonat Nurs, 1*(4), 33.

155. Stiehm, E.R. (1975). Fetal defense mechanisms. *Am J Dis Child, 129,* 438.

156. Stites, D.P. & Siiteri, P.K. (1983). Steroids as immunosuppressants in pregnancy. *Immunol Rev, 75,* 117.

157. Strauss, R.G. (1986). Current issues in neonatal transfusions. *Vox Sang, 51,* 1.

158. Strelkaukas, A.J., et al. (1975). Inversion of human T and B cells in early pregnancy. *Nature, 258,* 331.

159. Strelkaukas, A.J., Wilson, B.S., & Dray, S. (1978). Longitudinal studies showing alterations in levels and functional responses of T and B lymphocytes in human pregnancy. *Clin Exp Immunol, 32,* 531.

160. Studd, J.W.W. (1971). Immunoglobulins in normal pregnancy, pre-eclampsia and pregnancy complicated by nephrotic syndrome. *J Obstet Gynaecol Br Comm, 78,* 786.

161. Thurnau, G.R. (1985). Hypertension in pregnancy. In J.R. Scott & N.S. Rote (Eds.), *Immunology in obstetrics and gynecology* (pp. 107–140). Norwalk, CT: Appleton-Century-Crofts.

162. Trofatter, K.F., et al. (1990). Fetal immunology. In R.D. Eden & F.H. Boehm (Eds.), *Assessment and care of the fetus* (pp. 135–149). Norwalk, CT: Appleton & Lange.

163. Urowitz, M.B. & Gladman, D.D. (1988). Rheumatic disease during pregnancy. In G.N. Burrow & T.F. Ferris (Eds.), *Medical complications during pregnancy* (pp. 499–525). Philadelphia: WB Saunders.

164. Von Muralt, G. & Sidiropoulos, D. (1988). Prenatal and postnatal prophylaxis of infections in preterm infants. *Pediatr Infect Dis J, 7,* S72.

165. Walker, W.A. (1987). Macromolecular transport in the neonatal gut: Its role in milk allergy. In M. Xanthou (Ed.), *New aspects of nutrition in pregnancy, infancy and prematurity* (pp. 181–205). New York: Elsevier Science Publishers.

166. Wara, D.W. & Barrett, D.J. (1979). Cell-mediated immunity in the newborn: Clinical aspects. *Pediatrics, 64*(Suppl.), 822.

167. Weinberg, E.D. (1984). Pregnancy associated depression of cell-mediated immunity. *Rev Infect Dis, 6,* 814.

168. Weinstein, A.J., Gibbs, R.S., & Gallager, M. (1976). Placental transfer of clindamycin and gentamicin in term pregnancy. *Am J Obstet Gynecol, 124,* 688.

169. Weinstein, L. (1982). Syndrome of hemolysis, elevated liver enzymes and low platelets: A severe consequence of hypertension in pregnancy. *Am J Obstet Gynecol, 142,* 159.

170. Welsh, J.K. & May, J.T. (1979). Antiinfective properties of breast milk. *J Pediatr, 94,* 1.

171. Wenstrom, K.D. & Gall, S.A. (1989). HIV infection in women. *Obstet Gynecol Clin North Am, 16,* 627.

172. Wilson, C.B. (1986). Immunologic basis for increased susceptibility of the neonate to infection. *J Pediatr, 108,* 1.

173. Wilson, C.B. (1990). Developmental immunology and role of host defenses in neonatal susceptibility. In J.S. Remington & J.O. Klein (Eds.), *Infectious diseases of the fetus and newborn infants* (pp. 17–67). Philadelphia: WB Saunders.

174. World Health Organization (1987). Breast feeding/breast milk and human immunodeficiency virus (HIV). *Weekly Epidemiol Rev, 33,* 245.

175. Xanthou, M. (1987). Neonatal immunity. In L. Stern & P. Vert (Eds.), *Neonatal medicine* (pp. 555–586). New York: Masson Publishing.

176. Yaffe, S.J. (1981). Antimicrobial therapy and the neonate. *Obstet Gynecol, 58*(Suppl.), 85S.

177. Yoder, M.C. & Polin, R.A. (1986). Immunotherapy of neonatal septicemia. *Pediatr Clin North Am, 33,* 481.

178. AAP. (1991). *Report of committee on infectious diseases.* Elk Grove, IL: American Academy of Pediatrics.

CHAPTER 11

The Integumentary System

Maternal Physiologic Processes
   The Antepartum Period
      Alterations in Pigmentation
      Changes in Connective Tissue
      Vascular and Hematologic Changes
      Alterations in Cutaneous Tissue and Mucous
         Membranes
      Alterations in Secretory Glands
      Alterations in Hair Growth
      Alterations in the Nails
      Pruritus
   The Postpartum Period
      Hair Loss
**Clinical Implications for the Pregnant Woman and
   Her Fetus**
   Dermatoses Associated with Pregnancy
   Effects of Pregnancy on Preexisting Skin
      Disorders
   Pharmacologic Treatment of Skin Disorders
      During Pregnancy
**Development of the Integumentary System
in the Fetus**
   Anatomic Development
      Epidermis
      Dermis
      Adipose Tissue
      Cutaneous Innervation
      Epidermal Appendages

Functional Development
   Amniotic Fluid
   Permeability
   Vernix Caseosa
Transitional Events
Neonatal Physiology
   Barrier Properties
   Permeability
   Transepidermal Water Loss
   Thermal Environment
   Cohesion Between Epidermis and Dermis
   Collagen and Elastin Instability
   Protective Mechanisms
   Tactile Perception
Clinical Implications for Neonatal Care
   Skin Care
   Adhesives
   Protection from Infection
   Transepidermal Absorption
   Limitations in Specific Infant Groups
**Maturational Changes During Infancy and
   Childhood**

The integumentary system consists of the skin and its appendages: eccrine, apocrine, apoeccrine, and sebaceous glands; hair; and nails. Functions of the skin include protection from physical and chemical injury, infection, and ultraviolet radiation; prevention of fluid loss; and thermoregulation. The skin is also important in sensation (pain, pressure, touch, and temperature), contributes to maintenance of blood pressure by dilation or con- striction of the peripheral capillaries, and con- tains precursor molecules for vitamin D.[19, 142]

The skin and its associated structures are markedly altered during pregnancy. These changes are seen in most pregnant women, and while the changes themselves are seldom associated with serious physiologic conse- quences, they are of concern to most women because of the subsequent cosmetic altera- tions that may persist following delivery. In addition, there are several dermatologic disorders that are seen almost exclusively in pregnant women that can cause severe physical discomfort and may be associated with increased fetal morbidity.

The skin is also an organ of considerable significance in the neonate. There are a variety of common nonpathologic variations in the neonate involving the skin (Table 11–1). In addition, immaturity of the skin alters its permeability, immunologic capacity, bonding of the epidermis to the dermis, and role in thermoregulation and fluid balance. As a result, neonates, especially preterm and ill infants, are at risk for toxicity from topical substances, infection, skin excoriation, fluid loss, and thermal instability.

MATERNAL PHYSIOLOGIC PROCESSES

Physiologic changes in the skin and its appendages during pregnancy and the postpartum period include alterations in pigmentation, connective and cutaneous tissue, integumentary vascular system, hair, nails, and secretory glands, and pruritus. Some of integumentary alterations regress completely during the postpartum period; others recede but never completely disappear.

The Antepartum Period

The basis for changes in the skin, hair, and secretory glands during pregnancy is generally believed to be hormonal, in particular the effects of estrogen and adrenocortical steroids. Similar alterations are often seen in women using oral contraceptives. There also seems to be a familial tendency or genetic predisposition for many of the cutaneous and vascular changes.[78, 109, 132, 166, 190, 192]

Alterations in Pigmentation

Alterations in pigmentation are common during pregnancy and include hyperpigmentation of specific areas of the body, melasma (chloasma), and development of pigmentary demarcation lines. For many years pigmentary alterations were thought to be due to increased production of melanocyte stimulating hormone (MSH) by the pituitary gland. More recent studies using immunologic methods have documented only slight changes in MSH, primarily during late pregnancy (whereas pigmentary changes tend to occur early in pregnancy). Thus pigmentary changes are currently believed to be primarily due to estrogens and possibly progesterone (which are strong melanogenic stimulants). This is also consistent with reports of alterations in pigmentation associated with use of oral contraceptives.[30, 109, 190, 132, 158, 166, 167, 175]

HYPERPIGMENTATION

Hyperpigmentation is the most frequent integumentary alteration during pregnancy. Changes in pigmentation are seen in 90% of pregnant women and tend to be more frequent in women with dark hair or complexions. Most women experience a mild, generalized increase in pigmentation that is especially prominent in areas of the body that tend to be naturally more intensely pigmented. These areas include the areolae, genital skin, axillae, inner aspects of the thighs, and linea alba. The pigmentary changes in these specific areas may be due to an increased number of melanocytes or an increased sensitivity to hormones.[21, 109, 132, 137, 154, 192]

The linea alba is a tendinous median line that extends along the anterior of the abdomen from the umbilicus to the symphysis pubis and occasionally superiorly to the xiphoid process. Hyperpigmentation during pregnancy causes the linea alba to darken and become the linea nigra. Up to one-third of women on oral contraceptives also develop a linea nigra. Pigmentary changes tend to fade during the postpartum period in fair skinned women, but some pigmentary changes may remain in women with darker skin and hair. Hyperpigmentation may be exacerbated by sun exposure.[21, 109, 132, 137, 192]

Freckles, nevi, and recent scars may darken during pregnancy. Existing melanocytic nevi may also increase in size or new nevi may form with an increase in development of dendritic processes and in junctional activity of nevus cells. These changes may be similar to early melanoma but generally revert to their previous state following pregnancy. Prophylactic removal of these nevi following pregnancy may be considered.[21, 48, 109, 132, 190, 192]

MELASMA (CHLOASMA)

Melasma (also known as chloasma or the "mask of pregnancy") occurs in 50 to 75% of pregnant women. Melasma is characterized

TABLE 11–1
Normal Neonatal Skin Variations

CONDITION	CHARACTERISTICS
Milia	1-mm yellow-white cysts
	Appear on cheeks, forehead, nose, and nasolabial folds
	Frequently occur in clusters
	Affect 40% of all infants
Miliaria	Develops within the first 12 hours
	Caused by obstructed eccrine sweat ducts
	Appears on forehead and skin folds
	Superficial, thin-walled grouped vesicles (m. crystallina) or deep, grouped red papules (m. rubra)
Erythema toxicum	Most common transient lesion
	Irregular erythematous macules or patches with yellow or white central papule
	Can affect any area of body except plams and soles
	Appears between and 24 and 72 hours after birth; continued eruption up to 3 weeks; dissipates in a few days
	More often affects full-term infants (30–70%)
Mongolian spots	Macular, gray-blue
	Most frequently occur in lumbosacral region
	Cover an area 10 cm or greater
	Caused by infiltrate of melanocytes deep in dermis
	Affect 70% of black, Asian, American Indian infants and 10% of Caucasian infants
	Gradually disappear over first few years of life
Petechiae	Discrete blue-black pinpoint macules
	Fade in 3 to 4 days
	Do not blanch to pressure
Ecchymoses	Subcutaneous hemorrhage
	Localized
	Usually seen over presenting part
Café au lait spots	Brown macules or patches
	Less than 3 cm in diameter
	May occur occasionally in newborns
	With larger than usual spots (4–6 cm) or more than 6 spots, infant may develop underlying neurofibromatosis
Junctional nevi	Flat, pigmented lesions
	Brown to black
	Less than 1 cm
	Affect 15% of black infants
	Large number present at birth associated with tuberous sclerosis, xeroderma pigmentosum, and generalized neurofibromatosis
Hemangiomas	Relatively common
	Developmental vascular anomaly
	Capillary hemangiomas: dilated vessels
	Cavernous hemangiomas: large, dilated, blood-filled cavities
	65% are superficial; 15% are subcutaneous; 20% are mixed
Salmon patch hemangioma	Occurs in 30–50% of normal newborns
	Flat macular hemangioma
	Appears on nape of neck, eyelids, glabella
	Indistinct borders
	Blanches with pressure
	Facial lesions disappear by 1 year of age
Nevus flammeus	Port-wine stain hemangioma
	Sharply delineated
	Blanches only slightly
	Purple to red, or jet black
	Does not involute
	If distributed over trigeminal territory of face, angiomatous malformation of the brain may occur
Strawberry hemangioma	Raised capillary lesion
	Bright red vascular tumor
	Sharply demarcated borders
	Blanches with pressure
Cavernous hemangioma	Deeper, less common
	Margins obscured by overlying epidermal tissue
	Reddish-blue
	Somewhat compressible
	Increases in size after birth
Cradle cap	Seborrheic eczema
	Reactive response to irritant
	Scaling lesions
	Greasy feeling

by irregular, blotchy areas of pigmentation on the face. The areas of altered pigmentation are not elevated and can range in color from light to dark brown. Three distribution patterns have been described: centrofacial (63%), involving the cheeks, forehead, upper lip, nose, and chin; malar (21%), over the cheeks and nose; and mandibular (16%), over the ramus of the mandible. Two histologic patterns have also been identified: epidermal (increased deposition of melanin in the melanocytes of the basal and suprabasal layers) and dermal (macrophages with large amounts of melanin can be found in both the papillary and reticular layers of the dermis). The pigmentary changes tend to fade completely within 1 year following pregnancy but may persist for years especially in dark-haired individuals.[109, 132, 146, 192]

There seems to be a genetic predisposition toward development of melasma. Melasma is seen most frequently in women with dark hair and complexions, is exacerbated by the sun, and tends to recur (often with increased intensity) in subsequent pregnancies or with use of oral contraceptives. Of women using oral contraceptives, 5 to 30% develop melasma. Melasma has also been reported occasionally in nonpregnant individuals who are not on oral contraceptives or other hormonal medications.[21, 109, 132, 146, 192]

Avoidance of suntanning during pregnancy and use of sun screens may reduce the severity of melasma (Table 11–2). Since melasma often fades spontaneously following pregnancy, treatment is generally limited to individuals with persistent pigmentation. Various depigmenting formulas have been developed to treat persistent melasma with varying success. These formulas tend to be relatively effective on epidermal type melasma but have little effect on the dermal type. Treatment may need to be continued for 5 to 7 weeks before satisfactory results are achieved. Topical 2 to 5% hydroquinone has also been used, again with varying success. This treatment can result in complications such as hypopigmentation, hyperpigmentation, and contact dermatitis.[21, 146, 192]

PIGMENTARY DEMARCATION LINES

Pigmentary demarcation lines occur normally in many individuals especially Japanese, black, and Hispanic persons. These lines mark abrupt transitions between deeply pigmented skin and lighter skin and are most common along the anterior brachial surface of the arms.[77] Five patterns of pigmentary demarcation lines have been identified: type A, upper arms across the pectoral area; type B, lower limbs on posteromedial surface; type C, medially paired lines on chest in the sternal area with occasional midline extension onto the abdomen; type D, posteromedian demarcation along the spine; and type E, bilateral symmetric markings along the chest from the middle third of the clavicle to the periareolar area. There have been several reports of the development of (in Caucasian women) or increase in (in Japanese, black, and Hispanic women) type B pigmentary demarcation lines during pregnancy. This pigmentary change seems to be relatively rare.[4, 50, 77]

Changes in Connective Tissue

Striae gravidarum (often called linear striae, striae distensae, or linear "stretch marks") are linear tears in dermal collagen that are commonly seen during pregnancy. These markings initially appear as irregular, pink or purple wrinkled linear streaks that gradually become white. Striae are most prominent by 6 to 7 months. They appear initially over the abdomen oriented in opposition to skin tension lines, then are found on the breasts, thighs and inguinal area. Striae are seen more frequently in Caucasian women and there appears to be a familial tendency.[21, 38, 109, 132, 165, 192]

Striae gravidarum usually fade following pregnancy but never completely disappear, remaining as depressed, irregular white bands. Some women report striae itching, although since both pruritus and striae formation are prominent over the abdominal area during pregnancy, these two phenomena may not be related. There is no effective treatment to prevent striae formation. Topical emollients and antipruritics may be used (Table 11–2). Use of olive oil and massage to prevent striae formation is controversial and unsubstantiated.[21, 38, 98, 132, 137, 192]

The cause of striae is unclear. Previous explanations of collagen disruption by mechanical stretching are no longer widely accepted. Currently, striae gravidarum are believed to arise from hormonal alterations or a combination of hormonal changes and stretching. It has been suggested that increased levels of estrogens, corticosteroids, and relaxin relax the adhesiveness between collagen fibers and foster formation of mu-

TABLE 11–2
Nursing Management for Common Problems During Pregnancy Related to the Integumentary System

ALTERATION	INTERVENTION
All alterations	Provide anticipatory teaching regarding appearance of alteration.
	Counsel regarding basis for alteration and course.
	Evaluate impact on body image and relationship with partner and provide counseling.
Hyperpigmentation	Avoid suntanning during pregnancy and use broad spectrum sunscreen.
	Use nonallergenic cover-ups.
Melasma	Avoid suntanning during pregnancy or when using oral contraceptives.
	Use broad spectrum sunscreen (rating of 15 or greater).
	Use nonallergenic cover-ups.
	Counsel regarding risk of similar changes with oral contraceptives.
	Counsel regarding alternative methods of birth control.
	Avoid use of topical 2–5% hydroquinone during pregnancy.
	Counsel regarding use of sun screen and protection from sun with use following pregnancy.
Striae gravidarum	Use topical emollients or antipruritics as required.
	Use supportive garments for breasts and abdomen.
Spider nevi	Reassure that most fade following pregnancy.
	Use cosmetic cover-up creams.
	Suggest considering electrocauterization if of great concern to patient.
Nonpitting edema	Elevate legs when sitting or lying down; sleep in Trendelenburg position.
	Avoid prolonged standing or sitting.
	Rest in left lateral decubitus position.
	Exercise.
	Avoid excessive added salt.
	Avoid tight clothing and girdles.
	Try elastic stockings (although effectiveness is controversial).
Varicosities	Elevate legs when sitting or lying down; sleep in Trendelenburg position.
	Avoid prolonged standing or sitting.
	Rest in left lateral decubitus position.
	Exercise.
	Avoid tight clothing and girdles.
	Wear elastic stockings or support hose.
Increased eccrine gland activity	Wear light, loose clothing.
	Increase fluid intake.
	Regular bathing/showering.
Pruritus	Wear loose nonsynthetic clothing.
	Use cool compresses, baths/showers.
	Use oatmeal baths.
	Consider topical antipruritics and emollients.

copolysaccharide ground substance, which causes separation of the fibers and striae formation. Others suggest that the hormonal changes lead to rupture of elastic fibers or intradermal tears in the collagen.[36, 192] The degree of distention has been shown to be unrelated to striae formation. There are reports that striae formation is more strongly correlated to adrenocortical activity than abdominal girth and that obese women with striae have increased corticosteroid excretion.[131, 163] Braverman suggests that striae formation depends on both skin stretching and the presence of a "striae factor" that lead to weakening and rupture of dermal collagen and elastic fibers.[21] The most frequently proposed "striae factor" is increased adrenocortical activity.[21, 102, 109, 130, 132, 137, 163, 192]

Vascular and Hematologic Changes

Vascular and hematologic changes during pregnancy related to the integumentary system include development of spider nevi or angiomas, palmar erythema, nonpitting edema, cutis marmorata, purpura, hemangiomas, and varicosities. Other alterations in the vascular and hematologic systems are described in Chapters 5 and 16.

Cutis marmorata is a transient bluish mottling of the legs on exposure to cold that arises from vasomotor instability secondary to elevated estrogens. Persistence postpartally is abnormal and may suggest underlying pathology such as blood dyscrasia, collagen vascular disorder, or neoplasm. Other changes due to vasomotor instability during pregnancy include pallor, facial flushing, and heat and cold sensations. Purpura secondary to increased capillary fragility and permeability occurs during the last months of pregnancy in many women.[109, 190, 192]

SPIDER NEVI

Spider nevi (or spider angiomas) are found in 10 to 15% of normal adults, in individuals with liver dysfunction, and in up to two thirds of pregnant women. These nevi are more common in Caucasian (67%) than black (11.5%) pregnant women. Spider nevi consist of a central dilated arteriole that is flat or slightly raised with extensive radiating capillary branches. They are most prominent in areas of the skin drained by the superior vena cava (i.e., around the eyes, neck, throat, and arms). The basis for formation has been related to increased estrogen, since these structures are seen more frequently both during pregnancy and with use of oral contraceptives. However, many individuals with spider nevi associated with liver disorders do not have elevated estrogen levels.[78, 109, 132, 192]

Spider nevi generally appear between months 2 and 5 of pregnancy and may increase in size and number as pregnancy progresses. These structures tend to regress spontaneously and fade within the first 7 weeks to 3 months following delivery, although they rarely completely disappear. They may recur or enlarge during subsequent pregnancies. Unresolved spider nevi can be treated by electrocauterization.[109, 132, 192]

PALMAR ERYTHEMA

Two patterns of palmar erythema are seen during pregnancy: erythema of hypothenar and thenar eminences, palms, and fleshy portions of the finger tips; and diffuse mottling of the entire palm. The latter form is more common and similar to changes seen with hyperthyroidism and cirrhosis. Palmar erythema generally appears during the first two trimesters and disappears by 1 week post delivery. This phenomenon has a familial tendency and is seen in approximately two thirds of Caucasian and one third of black pregnant women. Spider nevi and palmar erythema often occur together suggesting a common etiology generally believed to be elevated estrogen levels with increased skin blood flow.[14, 109, 132, 192,]

NONPITTING EDEMA

Increased vascular permeability and sodium retention due to the effects of estrogen result in transient nonpitting edema of the face, hands, and feet during late pregnancy. In the lower extremities this is aggravated by pressure from the growing uterus. This form of edema occurs in the face in approximately 50% of women and lower extremities in 70% and is not associated with pregnancy-induced hypertension.[132, 192] Although generally pres-

ent in the morning, it usually improves during the day (Table 11–2).

CAPILLARY HEMANGIOMAS

Preexisting capillary hemangiomas may increase in size during pregnancy.[21, 98] In about 5% of pregnant women new hemangiomas appear by the end of the first trimester with slight enlargement during the remaining trimesters.[192] New hemangiomas usually appear on the head and neck and are unusual elsewhere.[21] Enlarged existing hemangiomas and new hemangiomas regress post partum but may not completely disappear. Hemangioma development in pregnancy is related to elevated estrogen.[36, 192]

VARICOSITIES

Varicosities develop in approximately 40% of pregnant women. Varicosities occur most commonly in the legs but may also appear in the pelvic vessels, vulva, and anal area with hemorrhoid formation. Varicosities arise from estrogen-induced elastic tissue fragility, increased venous pressure in the lower extremities and pelvis from pressure of the gravid uterus, and familial tendency for valvular incompetence. Varicosities generally regress postpartum but do not completely disappear. Thrombi are rare with leg varicosities, but are more frequent with hemorrhoids. Hemorrhoids are discussed in Chapter 9.[21, 132, 192]

Alterations in Cutaneous Tissue and Mucous Membranes

The most common mucous membrane alterations are changes in the vagina and cervix (see Chapter 2), which are seen in all pregnant women, and gingivitis, which is seen in the majority of women. A less common oral finding is a cutaneous lesion of the gums known as pregnancy tumor or epulis. Epulis and gingivitis are discussed in Chapter 9.

Another relatively common cutaneous change during pregnancy is the development of skin tags called fibromata molle or molluscum fibrosum gravidarum.[132, 154, 192] These are soft, flesh colored or pigmented skin tags, which are small (usually 1 to 5 mm), pedunculated fibromas that appear during the second half of pregnancy primarily on the lateral aspects of the face and neck, upper axillae, groin, and between and underneath the breasts. The cause of fibromata molle is unknown but thought to be hormonal. These growths may regress or clear spontaneously following delivery, although many remain. Remaining skin tags can be removed by electrocoagulation or clipping with sterile scissors.[132, 137, 192]

Alterations in Secretory Glands

Activity of the sebaceous, apocrine, and eccrine glands of the skin is altered during pregnancy. Sebaceous gland activity is generally reported to increase during pregnancy.[132, 190, 192] Many pregnant women report that their skin, especially on the face, feels "greasy." Montgomery's tubercles (small sebaceous glands on the areola) enlarge beginning as early as 6 weeks' gestation. Changes in Montgomery's tubercles and in the breasts are described in Chapter 4.

Apocrine sweat gland activity decreases during pregnancy, possibly as a result of hormonal changes.[192] Eccrine sweat gland activity increases gradually during pregnancy, possibly because of increased thyroid activity along with increased body weight and metabolic activity.[132, 190, 192] Since eccrine glands are important along with the cutaneous blood vessels in thermoregulation at the skin surface (see Chapter 17), their increased activity reflects dissipation of excess heat produced by the increased metabolic activity of the pregnant woman and her fetus. Increased eccrine activity during pregnancy can lead to miliaria (prickly heat) or dyshidrotic eczema.[192] Palmar sweating is decreased in pregnancy even though this is an area where eccrine glands are highly concentrated. The basis for this is unclear but may be related to increased adrenocortical activity. Interventions are listed in Table 11–2.[107]

Alterations in Hair Growth

Estrogen increases the length of the anagen (growth) phase of hair follicles during pregnancy. This results in increased hair loss post partum. A mild hirsutism may develop early in pregnancy with increased growth of hair on the upper lip, chin, and cheeks and in the suprapubic midline. Fine new hairs tend to disappear by 6 weeks post partum, but the coarser hairs tend to remain. During late pregnancy some women develop hair loss with frontoparietal recession of the hairline similar to changes seen in male-pattern baldness. This loss is rare, and is usually associated with complete regrowth and not with later development of female-pattern alopecia.[21, 106, 192]

Alterations in the Nails

Changes in fingernails and toenails during pregnancy are uncommon and of unknown pathogenesis. Nail changes occur as early as 6 weeks and include transverse grooves, increased brittleness, distal separation of the nail bed (onycholysis), and subungual keratosis.[109, 132, 192]

Pruritus

Pruritus is the most common cutaneous symptom during pregnancy, occurring in approximately 20% of pregnant women. The itching may be localized, especially over the abdomen during the third trimester, or generalized. Abdominal pruritus at the end of the first trimester may be an isolated finding or an early sign of pruritus gravidarum (intrahepatic cholestasis of pregnancy) with or without associated jaundice or one of the other specific dermatoses of pregnancy (see Table 11–3). Pruritus always clears post partum. Pregnant women with pruritus should also be assessed for other skin disorders including pregnancy dermatoses, contact dermatitis, and drug reactions.[51, 109, 113, 153, 192]

The Postpartum Period

As noted earlier, some of the changes in the integumentary system and its associated structures clear spontaneously following delivery; other alterations may regress or fade but do not disappear completely. The alterations in hair growth during pregnancy result in an increased hair loss during the postpartum period in many women.

Hair Loss

The scalp contains approximately 100,000 hair follicles. Hair fibers in each follicle independently cycle through three growth stages: anagen, catagen, and telogen. The anagen or growth stage lasts for 4 to 6 years and is characterized by intense metabolic activity. In this stage hair grows an average of 0.34 mm/day. Catagen is a transitional stage lasting several weeks. During this stage metabolic activity and growth slow as the hair bulb is retracted upward into the follicle. Growth of the hair fiber stops during telogen (resting stage). Eventually a new hair bulb begins growing, which ejects the previous hair.[141] Normally about 80% of hair follicles are in the anagen stage and 15 to 20% of hair fibers are in the telogen stage, with about 100 hairs shed per day.[137]

Under the influence of estrogen during pregnancy, the rate of hair growth slows and the anagen stage is prolonged. This results in an increased number of anagen hairs and a decrease in telogen hairs to less than 10% during the second and third trimesters. During the postpartum period these anagen hairs enter catagen and then telogen and are shed. Since there are more anagen hairs (and thus telogen hairs) than usual, most postpartum women experience a increased hair loss beginning 4 to 20 weeks following delivery. During this time 30 to 35% of the hairs may enter telogen. Generally, complete regrowth occurs by 6 to 15 months, although the hair may be less abundant than prior to pregnancy. "Telogen effluvium" is the term used to describe the rapid transition of hair follicles into the telogen stage following delivery, surgery or severe emotional or physical stress.[87, 106, 152, 190, 192]

CLINICAL IMPLICATIONS FOR THE PREGNANT WOMAN AND HER FETUS

The physiologic changes in the integumentary system during pregnancy and post partum are common experiences for many women. These changes seldom significantly alter the function or structure of the integumentary system and are considered by some to be minor nuisances.[21] However, these changes may have significant psychological and cosmetic implications for the pregnant woman and can contribute to alterations in body image. General interventions include anticipatory counseling, education, and reassurance. For example, the hair loss post partum can be devastating to the primipara who is unprepared for this event (Table 11–2).

Dermatoses Associated with Pregnancy

In addition to the normal physiologic skin changes associated with pregnancy, there are several integumentary disorders that are unique to pregnancy. Specific dermatoses seen only during pregnancy include herpes gestationis, impetigo herpetiformis, (Spangler's) papular dermatitis of pregnancy, prurigo gestationis of Besnier (similar to Nurse's prurigo of late pregnancy), pruritic urticarial papules and plaques of pregnancy (PUPPP), and pruritus gravidarum.[21, 36, 76, 137, 147, 179, 190] Several of these disorders have been associated with increased fetal morbidity and mortality (Table 11–3).

The etiology for many of these disorders is unclear, although some may have a hormonal or immunologic basis.[190] There has often been confusion in classifying some of the rarer dermatoses since much of the literature regarding these disorders involves reports of small numbers of women, which may represent different variations of the same disorder.[132] Treatment involves use of topical emollients, antipruritics, cold compresses, oatmeal baths (for relief of itching), and topical steroids. In women with moderate to severe eruptions, systemic steroids and antihistamines may be used.

Effects of Pregnancy on Preexisting Skin Disorders

The effects of pregnancy on preexisting skin disorders varies from no effect to marked improvement or worsening.[21, 109, 137, 189, 190, 192] With disorders such as psoriasis, eczema, contact dermatitis, and acne vulgaris this range of effects during pregnancy has been described within the same disease in different women.[21, 109, 137, 189] Neurofibromas increase in size during pregnancy and new tumors may appear.[173, 190] The effect of pregnancy on malignant melanoma is controversial.[190] Shiu and colleagues suggest that pregnancy may have no effect on stage I melanoma, with an increased incidence of stage II and decreased survival.[157] Effects of pregnancy on other integumentary disorders are reviewed in depth in the literature.[21, 137, 189]

Pharmacologic Treatment of Skin Disorders During Pregnancy

The dermatoses associated with pregnancy and other skin disorders are often treated with topical steroids and antihistamines. Antihistamines such as chlorpheniramine, tripelennamine, pheniramine, and diphenhydramine are reported to be safe in pregnancy; there are insufficient data available on other agents.[57, 192] Use of topical steroids during pregnancy is reported to be safe, except for application of potent fluorinated creams to large areas of vasodilated skin, which may result in secondary adrenal suppression.[21]

Systemic corticosteroids such as prednisone and prednisolone are often required for treatment of severe skin disorders. The use of these drugs for treatment of skin disorders during pregnancy is controversial.[9, 69, 91, 119, 132, 147, 190] Animal studies (often using doses per weight higher than recommended human doses) demonstrate an increased incidence of abortion, placental insufficiency, intrauterine growth retardation, and cleft palate.[9, 69, 91, 147] There is no clear evidence of teratogenic effects in humans, although avoidance during the first trimester is recommended.[9, 69, 91]

The effects of these corticosteroids on placental function and fetal growth is less clear since corticosteroids cross the placenta and also suppress placental estriol production.[69, 190] Holmes and Black note, however, that use of systemic steroids to treat severe herpes gestationis and Spangler's papular dermatitis of pregnancy has significantly reduced fetal mortality and morbidity.[76] Systemic corticosteroids are also associated with maternal side effects that may interact with changes in other body systems during pregnancy. These side effects include gastrointestinal irritation, nausea and vomiting, increased excretion of calcium, hyperlipidemia, increased susceptibility to bacterial and viral infection, and sodium retention with elevation of blood pressure and edema formation.[68]

Women who are pregnant and nonpregnant women of childbearing age often seek treatment for acne. Several available agents useful for acne therapy are contraindicated during pregnancy because of their teratogenic effects or maternal side effects. The use of oral and topical agents for acne in pregnancy was recently reviewed by Rothman and Pochi.[143] Oral tetracycline during pregnancy is associated with maternal liver toxicity (acute fatty liver of pregnancy) and, when given during the second or third trimester, with fetal tooth staining, tooth abnormalities, and possibly alterations in bone growth.[32, 52, 183] Tetracycline binds to calcium

in the mineralizing zones of the teeth, and use during pregnancy is associated with staining of the primary teeth. The permanent teeth are protected since calcium deposition does not begin until 4 to 6 months after birth. Topical erythromycin and tetracycline appear to be safe for short term use during pregnancy.[143]

Retinoic acids (analogues of vitamin A) such as oral isotretinoin (Accutane) are teratogenic and contraindicated during pregnancy and in sexually active women not using a highly effective method of birth control for at least 1 month prior to, during, and following therapy and who have a negative pregnancy test (treatment is started with the next menstrual cycle).[143] Use of oral isotretinoin during pregnancy results in a characteristic pattern of fetal anomalies involving the craniofacial structure, central nervous system, and heart.[93] Topical retinoic acid (tretinoin) has not been associated with congenital anomalies.[143]

SUMMARY

The effects of pregnancy on the integumentary system include physiologic changes in the skin and its appendages that are experienced by most pregnant women, skin disorders that are unique to pregnancy, and possible changes in preexisting skin disorders. Nursing management of the pregnant woman in relation to these effects includes preparation for the physiologic changes and their sequelae, and reassurance and support, as well as assessment for the specific dermatoses of pregnancy that are associated with maternal systemic symptoms and, if severe and untreated, with increased fetal mortality and morbidity. Clinical recommendations related to changes in the integumentary system during pregnancy are summarized in Table 11–4.

DEVELOPMENT OF THE INTEGUMENTARY SYSTEM IN THE FETUS

For the neonate the skin is the most sophisticated and the major sensory organ for obtaining and receiving information about the environment. Since the neonate is an immunologically compromised host, the integrity

TABLE 11–3
Dermatoses of Pregnancy

DISORDER*	INCIDENCE	ONSET AND ETIOLOGY	CHARACTERISTICS
Herpes gestationis (36,76,80,81,89,96,136, 147,150,159,190)	Reports vary from 1/3000–10,000 to recent estimates of 1/50,000–60,000 Seen most often in Caucasian women Has a familial tendency	Usually 4–5 months Can appear as early as 2 weeks' gestation or up to 2 weeks post partum May clear toward the end of pregnancy, then exacerbate post partum Etiology unknown; may have an immunologic basis or be an autoimmune disorder Associated with an IgG autoantibody ("HG factor")	Generalized, intense pruritus with erythematous urticarial plaques initially, followed by crops of fluid-filled vesicles and/or tense serum-filled bullae
Impetigo herpetiformis (12,16,36,76,103,125, 147,150,190)	About 100 cases have been reported	First to third trimesters with peak incidence in third trimester Etiology unknown, associated with hypocalcemia May be a form of pustular psoriasis	Small (1–2 mm), sterile, white pustules on irregular erythematous plaques; central pustules become crusted as new pustules develop in periphery of plaque
Papular dermatitis of pregnancy (Spangler) (36,76,114,147,170,190)	1/2000	Any trimester May be due to hypersensitivity to placental antigens	Severe pruritus with 3–5 mm papules that are not in crops or grouped; primary papules may be destroyed by scratching, leaving excoriated crusts as initial presentation
Prurigo gestationis of Besnier (Nurse's prurigo of late pregnancy) (34,36,76,121,147,190)	1/120–2/100	Second or third trimester Etiology unknown	Small groups of pruritic papules, often with excoriation due to scratching
Pruritic urticarial papules and plaques of pregnancy (PUPPP) (2,4,5,27,36,76,95,118, 147,176,190)	0.5% of pregnant women (primarily primiparas)	Third trimester (usually after 35 weeks) Etiology unknown	Erythematous papules and urticarial plaques with excoriation usually absent
Pruritus gravidarum (intrahepatic cholestasis of pregnancy) (36,39,51,76,113,140,147, 153,190)	0.02–2.4% of pregnant women	Third trimester Cholestasis	Severe generalized pruritus without any skin lesions, although excoriation may result from scratching

*Numbers in parentheses refer to citations in reference list.

of the skin as a barrier to that same environment is essential to the survival and well-being of the infant. In order to understand the importance of this system to the infant, an overview of anatomic and functional development is needed.

Anatomic Development

The epidermis consists of two parts: the stratum corneum and the living basal layer. The basal layer is divided into four layers, which contain melanocytes (pigment-producing cells) or keratinocytes that cornify the outer layer (Fig. 11–1).[22, 44, 110]

Underneath the epidermis lies the dermis, which is 2 to 4 mm thick at birth.[22, 110] Fibrous protein, collagen, and elastin fibers are woven together to form this layer.[40] It contains the nerves and blood vessels that nourish the skin cells and carry sensations from the skin to the brain (Figs. 11–1 and 11–2).[22]

TABLE 11–3
Dermatoses of Pregnancy Continued

LOCATION OF ERUPTIONS	COURSE	OTHER MATERNAL FINDINGS	EFFECT ON FETUS/ NEONATE
Initially around umbilicus, then spreads over abdomen to chest, back and extremities, palms and soles	Spontaneous resolution, usually within 1st month post partum Often recurs in subsequent pregnancies (with earlier onset and increased severity) May reappear with menstrual cycle or with use of oral contraceptives	Pruritus, fatigue, fever, nausea, headache, and secondary infections May involve cyclic remissions and exacerbations	Severe forms have been associated with increased incidence of stillbirth, preterm birth, small for gestational age infants, and transient neonatal skin lesions Use of systemic steroids has reduced fetal risk
Often appears initially in femoral or perineal areas; spreads to lower abdomen, to medial aspects of the thighs, and around the umbilicus; occasionally involves hands, feet, under nails, and tongue	Spontaneous resolution post partum Tends to recur in subsequent pregnancies, appearing earlier	Variable pruritus, associated with hypocalcemia, fever, lethargy, nausea and vomiting, and diarrhea	Increased incidence of abortion and stillbirth and possible placental insufficiency
Trunk (usually initial presentation) and/or extremities	Spontaneous resolution within 3–4 weeks after delivery Often recurs in subsequent pregnancies	Intense itching Urinary chorionic gonadotropin and plasma cortisol, urinary estriols	Earlier studies reported increased abortion and stillbirth, but this has not been confirmed in later reports
Abdomen, trunk, and extremities (especially extensor surfaces)	Spontaneous resolution with delivery Little tendency to recur	Pruritus	None
Often appear initially in abdominal striae, then spread across abdomen to thighs, arms, and buttocks; rarely found above midthorax on chest	Spontaneous clearing within 2–3 weeks after delivery Little tendency to recur	May have mild pruritus	None
Pruritus usually begins on abdomen, then spreads to other areas	Clears rapidly after delivery May recur with subsequent pregnancy or use of estrogen medications such as oral contraceptives	May occur with or without jaundice If jaundice occurs, serum alkaline phosphatase, SGOT and serum bilirubin are elevated	If jaundice occurs, associated with decreased birth weight, increased incidence of meconium staining

Epidermis

The epidermis initially consists of a single layer of cuboidal cells that develop from the outer germinal stratum (surface ectoderm) and can be identified during the 3rd week of gestation. During the 4th week a second layer called the periderm develops.[40, 44, 117] At the end of 11 weeks the epidermis has three layers: the basal layer, an intermediate layer, and the superficial layer (periderm). The intermediate layer becomes more complex by the end of the 4th month, and the four characteristic layers of the skin have differentiated. They are the stratum germinativum; the stratum granulosum, which contains small keratohyalin granules; the stratum spinosum, which is made up of large polyhedral cells connected by tonofibrils; and stratum corneum, which is made up of dead

TABLE 11–4
**Summary of Recommendations for Clinical Practice Related to Changes in the Integumentary System:
Pregnant Woman**

Recognize usual changes involving the skin, hair, nails, and sebaceous and sweat glands during pregnancy and the post-partum period (pp. 492–498).
Provide anticipatory teaching regarding usual alterations in the skin and its appendages during pregnancy (pp. 492–498).
Counsel the pregnant woman regarding the basis for integumentary alteration and their usual course, including whether or not the change will regress post partum (pp. 492–498).
Evaluate the impact of integumentary changes on the woman's body image and relationship with her partner and provide counseling (pp. 492–498).
Counsel women regarding potential for integumentary alterations during subsequent pregnancies or with use of oral contraceptives (pp. 492–498).
Recommend specific interventions to reduce or ameliorate the effects of integumentary changes (Table 11–2).
Recognize the specific dermatoses associated with pregnancy (pp. 498–499, Table 11–3).
Recognize and monitor for the potential side effects associated with the use of systemic steroids (pp. 498–499).
Recognize and counsel women regarding the risks associated with the use of oral tetracycline and isotretinoin during pregnancy (p. 499).
Avoid use of isotretinoin in pregnant women or sexually active women of childbearing age who are not using a reliable, highly effective form of birth control (p. 499).
Counsel women with chronic integumentary disorders regarding the impact of pregnancy on their disorder (pp. 498–500).

Page numbers in parentheses following each intervention refer to pages where rationale for that intervention is discussed.

cells packed full of keratin.[1, 94, 126, 168] Peridermal cells are replaced continuously until the 21st week of gestation. After this the periderm gradually disappears and the stratum corneum develops.[44]

The periderm serves as the protective barrier for the embryo. Until the underlying layers develop, active transport occurs across the periderm between the amniotic fluid and the embryo. The outer border of the cells have microvillous projections, which are coated with very fine filaments.[44, 67]

As the cells in the stratum germinativum proliferate, they develop down growths (epidermal ridges) that extend into the dermis and become permanent by 17 weeks. Ridge pattern is genetically determined and can be seen on the surface of the hands and soles of the feet.[117] Certain chromosomal abnormalities modify the ridge pattern (e.g., Down syndrome).

Protoplasmic fibers and cellular bridges begin to form during this time. These make up the prickle cell layer (stratum spinosum), eventually protecting the neonate from dehydration and reducing permeability to noxious substances.[150] From 11 to 18 weeks, this layer has an abundance of glycogen to provide energy for growth.[40]

Glycogen reserves decrease around 18 weeks. Keratogenic structures are now evident, leading to regional differences in epidermal thickness. By 24 weeks, the skin has largely concluded its period of histogenesis and moves into a time of structural and functional maturation.[74]

Keratinocytes are derived from the stratum germinativum and are arranged in columnar fashion adjacent to the dermis.[40] The first signs of keratinization are seen at the end of the 4th month.[53]

As replacement keratinocytes mature, they rise and move through the stratum granulosum. Here they acquire an undefined matrix in the form of keratohyalin. As they continue to travel upward the keratinocytes lose 85% of their water content and their organelles, which are replaced by keratin.[47, 85]

As the keratinocytes dehydrate and flatten, they adhere to each other to form a tough, resilient, and relatively impermeable membrane, the stratum corneum.[86] Transit time for a keratinocyte from the basal layer to the uppermost stratum takes approximately 28 days.[40, 117, 181] It is at this time (5 months) that the periderm is completely shed, mixing with secretions from the sebaceous glands to form the vernix caseosa.[94, 126, 168]

During the 13th week the epidermis is invaded by cells from the neural crest. These are termed the melanoblast and have long processes much like dendrites. They come to lie adjacent to keratinocytes at the dermal-epidermal junction. During the 4th month the melanoblasts are converted to melanocytes and transport melanin along their dendrites, from which it is taken up by the basal cells.[83, 84, 126, 134]

Melanin is responsible for skin color; variations are due to the amount and color of the melanin.[127] Prenatal pigmentation is seen in the nipples, axillae, and genitalia and around the anus.[40] Melanin protects deoxyribonucleic acid (DNA) from ultraviolet radiation damage.[75]

Langerhans cells are distinctive melano-

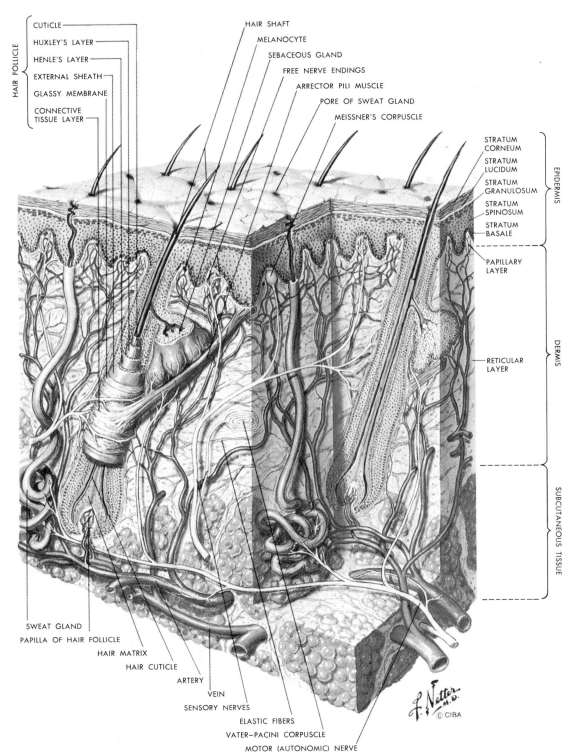

FIGURE 11–1. Structural components of the epidermis, dermis, and subcutaneous tissue. (© Copyright 1967, CIBA Pharmaceutical Company, Division of CIBA-GEIGY Corporation. Reprinted with permission from Clinical Symposia illustrated by Frank H. Netter, M.D. All rights reserved.)

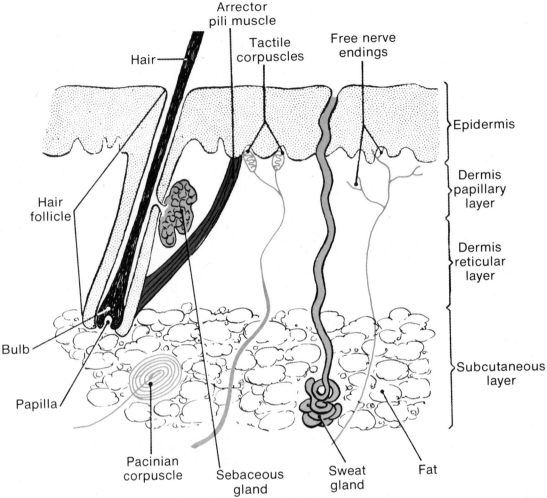

FIGURE 11–2.   Diagrammatic section of the skin and sebaceous layer. (From Wilson, D.B. & Wilson, W.J. (1983). *Human anatomy* (2nd ed., p. 78). New York: Oxford Press.)

cytes that have special organelles. Although their function is not entirely known, they do have phagocytic activity and are involved in skin host defense mechanisms.[174]

Dermis

Lying below the epidermis is the metabolically active dermis, which exerts a symbiotic and controlling influence on the epidermis. It consists of three types of connective tissue, amorphous ground substance, free cells, nerves, blood vessels, and lymphatic vessels. The connective tissue consists of collagen (90%) and elastic and reticular fibers.[169] The fibroblasts are the most numerous cells, producing collagen and mucopolysaccharides.

Mast cells, histiocytes, macrophages, lymphocytes, and neutrophils are all present in the dermis (Figs. 11–1 and 11–2).

The dermis originates from the somatopleuric mesenchyme and the somites which migrate ventrally.[44, 60, 117] The dermis in the 8-week embryo has undifferentiated cells, appears myxedema-like (similar to the umbilical cord), and contains no fibrils.[40, 44] Eventually two layers form: the corium is the superficial layer, and the subcorium is the deep layer of subcutaneous tissue (Fig. 11–1).

Between 8 and 12 weeks the fibroblasts form, leading to differentiation of the connective tissues. During this time fibrillae appear between dermal cells, which continue to grow, developing a network of collagenous and elastic fibers.[22, 60, 94, 117, 126, 168] Capillaries and lymph vessels form simultaneously. Initially the blood vessels are simple endothelium-lined structures from which new capillaries grow.

The subcapillary vascular network is disorganized at birth. During the next 17 weeks the adult structures form, and vasomotor tone control is refined. Vasomotor tone is achieved through a complex series of nervous and chemical control mechanisms. These involve the sympathetic nervous system, norepinephrine, acetylcholine, and histamine. Other possible chemical influences include serotonin, vasoactive polypeptides, corticosteroids, and prostaglandins.[169]

Over the rest of gestation the dermal layer moves from an organ abundant in water, sugars, and hyaluronidase to one enriched with collagen and sulfated polysaccharides.[40] Neonatal skin is often edematous, a sign of the excess water and sodium contained within it and the continued immaturity of the system.

During the 3rd and 4th months the corium proliferates to form papillary projections that extend into the epidermis. These irregular structures are called the dermal papillae. Some contain capillary loops that nourish the epidermis, and others have sensory nerve endings.[60, 126]

Fat appears in the deeper portion of the dermis, becoming the subcorium (subcutaneous tissue). The major portion of the fat is laid down during the last trimester of pregnancy, to act as a heat insulator, shock absorber, and calorie storage area.[85, 110]

Adipose Tissue

The hypodermis or subcutaneous tissue is a passive tissue that forms from mesenchymal cells. It has a lobar structure that is surrounded by connective tissue and has its own blood supply.[40]

The first cells can be seen around 14 weeks; initially they are cytoplasmic and contain no fat droplets. With maturation single or multiple fat granules develop.[40, 117]

Brown fat is deposited in fetuses after 28 weeks' gestation, accumulating in the neck, underneath the scapulae, and in the axillae, mediastinum, and perirenal tissues. It differentiates from the hypodermal primitive cells between 26 and 30 weeks. Development of brown adipose tissue continues after delivery,

increasing by another 150% in the 3rd to 5th week after delivery. Brown fat allows for nonshivering thermogenesis when the neonate is cold stressed (i.e., upon delivery; see Chapter 17).[40, 164]

Cutaneous Innervation

In the 3rd month of gestation free nerve endings connect with the papillary ridges of the finger and toe pads. By term these nerve endings are exceptionally well developed around the lips, sucking pad, and perioral zone.[40] Specialized nerve endings are less well developed and continue their maturation throughout infancy.

The glands and muscles of the skin are innervated, and some are functional at birth; however, refinement of these responses continues after delivery. The arrector pili muscles, arterioles, and eccrine glands are innervated by the sympathetic nervous system in varying degrees. The sensory nerves may carry parasympathetic fibers to the vessel walls at birth; however, the vasodilation abilities are reduced until further innervation takes place. The axon reflex (stimulus in one branch of a nerve cell that is transmitted to an effector organ down another branch of the cell) is poorly developed in the full-term infants so that sweating is an unusual occurrence.[169]

Epidermal Appendages

The structures that result from either the downward growth of the epidermis into the dermis or the epidermis itself are the epidermal appendages. These include the eccrine sweat, sebaceous, and apocrine sweat glands, the lanugo and hair, and the nails.[1]

HAIR

The hair originates from deep in the dermis. Initially the hairs develop from solid epidermal proliferations, cylindrical downward growths of the stratum germinativum into the dermis. The base of these growths becomes the club-shaped hair bulb. The epithelial cells of the hair bulb form the germinal matrix, which later gives rise to the hair itself. The lower part of the hair bulb becomes rapidly invaginated by the mesoderm, in which vessels and nerve endings develop. This is the pilary complex.[60, 94, 110, 117, 126, 168]

The central cells of each downgrowth (germinal matrix) form the hair shaft. As the epithelial cells continue to proliferate the hair shaft is pushed upward toward the epidermal surface. The peripheral cells (epithelial hair sheath) become cuboidal and form the wall of the hair follicle.[60, 94]

At the end of the 3rd month, extensive fine hairs have developed. Hair on the eyebrows, upper lip, and chin regions develops first. Lanugo is shed before or after delivery and replaced by shorter coarser hairs (vellus hairs) from new follicles.[60, 126]

Melanoblasts migrate into the hair bulb and differentiate into melanocytes. During the second half of pregnancy melanogenesis is active in the fetal hair follicle.[60]

SEBACEOUS GLANDS

The sebaceous glands form within the epithelial wall of the hair follicle, usually as a small outbudding of ectodermal cells that penetrate the surrounding mesoderm at the hair follicle neck. The outgrowths branch to form the primordia of the glandular alveoli and ducts. The center cells degenerate to form a fat-like substance (sebum), which is secreted into the hair follicle or directly onto the skin. The sebum mixes with the desquamated peridermal cells to help form the vernix caseosa.[94, 126, 168]

Most of the sebaceous glands differentiate at 13 to 15 weeks' gestation, immediately producing sebum in all hairy areas. Each gland usually consists of several lobules filled with disintegrated cells that dump into an excretory duct. The rapid growth during gestation and immediately post birth is due to circulating maternal androgens and, possibly, endogenous steroid production by the fetus.

ARRECTOR PILI MUSCLE

Some of the surrounding mesenchymal cells differentiate to form the arrector pili muscle, which is made up of smooth muscle fibers that attach to the connective tissue sheath of the hair follicle and dermal papillary layer. These muscles are located a short distance from the follicular wall in a region where the ground substance is metachromatic. The connection of the muscle root sheath is a secondary event with innervation occurring later.[60, 94, 126, 168]

The sweat glands are also appendages of the epidermal layer. There are three types of sweat glands. Only two will be discussed here; very little is known about the third type

(apoeccrine), which develop in adolescence and are found only in adult axillae.

SWEAT GLANDS

The eccrine glands develop first and are distributed throughout the cutaneous barrier. The apocrine glands develop later and are more specialized. Both are downgrowths of solid cylindrical epidermal tissue that invade the dermal layer.

The eccrine glands appear in the 6th week of embryogenesis and are innervated by the sympathetic nervous system. The epidermal tissue for this gland is more compact than that of the hair primordia, and it does not develop mesenchymal papillae. Once the bud reaches the dermis, it elongates and coils, developing a lumen at around 16 weeks.[60, 126]

Eccrine glands retain two layers of cells once the lumen is formed. The inner layer is made up of the lining and gland cells; the outer layer is specialized ectodermal smooth muscle cells that aid in the expulsion of secretions.

The apocrine glands are large organs that develop after the eccrine glands. They are confined to the axillae, pubic area, and areola of the mammary glands. Apocrine glands originate from and empty into the hair follicles, just above the sebaceous glands. At 7 to 8 months' gestation, they start to produce a milky white fluid containing water, lipids, protein, reducing sugars, ferric iron, and ammonia.[60, 169] Decomposition of this fluid by skin bacteria produces a characteristic odor.

Functional Development

The skin is one of the organ systems in the fetus that begins to function prior to delivery. Intrauterine physiologic functioning of the skin is dependent upon the growth, development, and maturation of the fetus. The fluid environment of the uterus also has an impact on cutaneous functioning.

Amniotic Fluid

The amniotic environment ensures an even distribution of temperature and protection from trauma and injury, allowing for symmetric development of the fetus, and providing a medium in which the fetus can move. In the beginning of pregnancy, the amniotic fluid is a dialysate of maternal plasma, fetal plasma, or both.[82] As pregnancy progresses the electrolyte content changes as the fetus contributes larger volumes of urine, and respiratory tract and upper alimentary canal secretions (see Chapter 2).

The longer the gestation, the more the skin contributes to the amniotic environment. As the fetus approaches 38 weeks, there is increased sloughing of anucleated cells and keratinized lipid-containing skin flakes. These changes can be used to assess fetal maturity. Increased numbers of lipid-laden cells are an indication of fetal maturity and can be used in developing the biophysical profile of the fetus.[10, 17, 40]

Permeability

The periderm provides the embryo with a barrier to the amniotic environment but does not eliminate the exchange of water and electrolytes between the amniotic fluid and the embryo. Fetal skin permeability is dependent upon morphologic changes and maturation in the epidermis related to sulfhydrylation and keratinization. Permeability therefore does not decrease until the third trimester. Vernix caseosa contributes to this change.[40, 101, 127]

The decrease in permeability is also associated with a decrease in skin water content. A 22-week fetus has a skin water content close to 100%, which reduces to 92% in the full-term infant and 77% in adults. This decrease in water is associated with an increase in connective tissue, especially collagen.[40]

Vernix Caseosa

Vernix caseosa forms as a superficial fatty film after the 5th month. It is made up of sebaceous gland secretions and peridermal cells or stratum corneum cells and is rich in triglycerides, cholesterol, and unsaponified fats. At term, the heaviest layers are found on the face, ears, shoulders, sacral region, and inguinal folds. It has a tendency to accumulate at sites of dense lanugo growth.

Vernix covers the fetus until birth and provides protection from amniotic fluid maceration. In utero it also prevents the loss of water and electrolytes from the skin to the amniotic fluid. In addition to providing insulation for the skin during gestation, vernix also minimizes friction at delivery.

TRANSITIONAL EVENTS

During the birth process the skin is subjected to the mechanical stress of the delivery process, changes in blood circulation, and the bacterial flora of the maternal genital tract.[40] The skin also serves as a diagnostic barometer for systemic phenomena, especially those related to transition.

Mechanical stresses include pressure from contractions, which alters blood flow to various regions and results in edema formation. Maternal structures (bony pelvis and musculature) can exert pressure on the presenting part, causing further edema and hematoma formation. Exertion of enough pressure may result in abrasions or cellular ischemia and tissue sloughing, threatening the integrity of the cutaneous barrier.

In addition to natural forces, epidermal breaks can also be caused by obstetric interventions such as internal fetal monitoring, fetal scalp sampling, and amnihook scratches. Use of vacuum extraction and forceps can result in bruising, edema, tissue ischemia, tissue sloughing, subcutaneous fat necrosis, and nerve damage.

In the first hours following delivery, the infant develops an intense red color, which is characteristic of the newborn. This may remain for several hours; however, exposure to the cooler environment usually leads to a bluish mottling, which dissipates quickly upon warming.

Neonatal skin is relatively transparent and smooth looking and is soft and velvety to touch. This appearance is due to the lack of large skin folds and skin texture. There is localized edema, especially over the pubis and the dorsa of the hands and the feet. Initially the skin is covered with the greasy yellow-white vernix caseosa. This insulating layer is lost with the bathing that occurs in the nursery. Removal results in exposure of the stratum corneum to the much dryer postnatal environment. Desquamation of the upper layers of the stratum corneum results, leaving the skin with a grayish-white or yellowish cast. After the 1st week, visible desquamation gives way to normal proliferation and flaking, signaling adaptation. Common neonatal skin variations are summarized in Table 11–1.

Once these initial stages are complete the skin takes on the adult protective functions by providing the needed environmental barrier. This development includes the discharge of water and electrolytes, an acid mantle, resorptive capacities, generalized pigmentation, and regulation of blood circulation and nerve supply.[24, 40, 169]

NEONATAL PHYSIOLOGY

The physiology of the integumentary system in the neonate includes the barrier properties of the skin, permeability, transepidermal water loss, heat exchange between the environment and the infant, collagen instability, and the protective mechanisms of the skin. Along with these functions, the skin is the major source of information about the environment for the infant, providing tactile perceptions of the immediate environment.

Barrier Properties

The barrier properties of the skin are located almost entirely in the stratum corneum. As skin matures, the thickness of the stratum corneum increases. In the full-term infant this is a relatively well-developed barrier. However, in the preterm infant (especially those less than 30 weeks) the barrier is immature.

One measurement of maturation is the thickness of the epidermal layer. Evans and Rutter found that epidermal thickness does not increase until 24 weeks. From that point until term there is progressive thickening, which is seen in dermoepidermal undulations. This characteristic is barely perceptible in the 34-week fetus.[47]

In the full-term neonate, the epidermis has marked regional variations in thickness, color, permeability, and surface chemical composition. In the preterm infant, the stratum corneum is very thin, averaging five cell layers in thickness. This is one-third the thickness of the stratum corneum of the term neonate and adult. The thinness of this layer leaves the preterm neonate with an increased transepidermal loss, an increased skin permeability to chemical substances and microbes, and a decreased ability to withstand mechanical forces of friction (Table 11–5).

For both the full-term and preterm infant there are two consequences of barrier immaturity: increased permeability and increased transepidermal water loss (TEWL). Both are a function of gestational and postnatal age. For example, a 31-week-gestation

TABLE 11–5
Skin Appearance by Gestational Age

GESTATIONAL AGE	SKIN APPEARANCE
27 weeks	Translucent and shiny
28–33 weeks	Red
34–37 weeks	Pink to red
38–41 weeks	Pinkish-white
42 weeks or more	Thicker and white, desquamated

infant who is more than 7 days old has had striking epidermal development in the first 2 weeks of postnatal life. This infant may be better able to cope with the extrauterine environment at this age than the newly delivered full-term infant. By 14 postnatal days, the permeability of the skin of preterm infants of all gestational ages resembles that of the term infant. In all cases, the optimal skin condition is one that is dry and flaking but without cracks and fissures.[47, 64, 111, 117]

Permeability

Skin permeability correlates with gestational age in the first few weeks of life. With decreasing gestational age there is increasing permeability. This was demonstrated by Nachman and Esterly, who evaluated blanching of the skin in infants exposed to a 10% Neo-Synephrine solution.[120] For those infants of 28 to 34 weeks gestational age there was more blanching and it lasted longer (anywhere from 30 minutes to 8 hours). Infants of more than 35 weeks gestational age, however, showed minimal to no blanching. The rapid blanching is an indication of the immature epidermal barrier.

Beyond this, these researchers noted that postnatal age also affected the degree of blanching. Of the infants tested, not one experienced blanching by the time they were 21 days old.

Creased, scaly, and opaque skin does not blanch, and drying out of the skin is part of the natural maturational process. Any interference in this keratinization (e.g., use of emollients) only delays the development of an effective barrier and prolongs the difficulties associated with a defective cutaneous surface, such as increased water loss and thermal instability.[120, 193]

Transepidermal Water Loss

Due to the thinner stratum corneum, the higher water content, and the increased permeability, TEWL in the preterm infant is greatly increased.[186] In infants less than 1500 g, Wu and Hodgman found extremely high TEWL during the first days of life.[186] They attributed this to the characteristic skin factors that predispose infants to water loss; these include a larger surface area in relation to body weight, thinner epidermis, increased water content, increased permeability, and increased blood supply that is closer to the skin surface.[43, 55, 162, 185]

These water losses can have a significant effect on fluid balance and the management and treatment of both preterm and full-term neonates (see Chapter 8). In the 28- to 30-week infant, water loss may be as much as 15 times greater than in their full-term counterpart.[61, 155] This may be compounded by environmental (e.g., radiant warmers) and therapeutic (e.g., phototherapy) modalities.

The degree of TEWL is dependent upon the hydration of the stratum corneum, the skin surface temperature, ambient humidity, and the neural capability for control of sweating. Factors that may contribute to these losses include basal metabolic rate, body temperature, activity, and phototherapy.[55, 71, 99, 122, 123] Initially the losses are high, but they fall to mature levels by the end of 10 days, as accelerated maturational processes of the skin occur.[63]

According to Rutter and Hull, skin water loss at the age of 13 days is about half of what it is on the first day of life for both term and preterm infants.[145] In premature infants, the postnatal decline in TEWL may be related to the change in balance between postnatal maturation of the skin and postnatal rise in basal metabolic rate. For term infants, the postnatal rise in TEWL may be secondary to an increase in activity and basal metabolic rate during the 2nd week of life.[72]

Reduction of TEWL losses can be achieved through the use of a thermal blanket, plastic blanket, or plastic hood (see Chapter 17). The mechanisms by which blanketing works appear to be a complex interaction of metabolic activity changes and a modified physical environment.[13, 108] The blanket alters the air flow around the infant, creating an insulating layer of saturated air that reduces the vaporization of water and heat loss from the skin.[108]

Thermal Environment

Heat exchange between infant skin and the environment is dependent on the thermal gradient between the body surface and environment. Studies found minimal O_2 consumption when the body surface and environmental temperature gradient did not exceed 1.5°C. Use of incubators, radiant warmers, and phototherapy modifies the environment, either reducing or accelerating oxygen consumption. The rate of thermal exchange between infant and environment is dependent upon relative humidity, wind velocity, radiant surfaces, and ambient air temperatures.[25, 70, 187] Fifty to 75% of heat loss in the neonate occurs through radiation and therefore is dependent upon both ambient (incubator) and environmental (room) temperature (see Chapter 17).[18, 25, 70, 187]

Phototherapy is an added radiant heat source. Infants receiving phototherapy have demonstrated increases in insensible water losses (IWL), respiratory rate, peripheral blood flow, and heel skin temperature. Absorption of the infrared bands increased kinetic, energy producing a degradation of the radiant energy to heat and leading to the clinical changes noted. The increased IWL is a compensatory mechanism to dissipate heat through hyperpnea and peripheral vasodilatation.[123, 124, 187] Careful temperature control can reduce some of these effects.

The differences observed between term and preterm infants (term infants were found to have greater water losses when exposed to phototherapy) are explained by a mature sweating response and an ability to respond in greater magnitude to alterations in skin temperature. This has also been used to explain the differences seen in infants weighing more than 1500 g when exposed to changes in environmental temperatures.[71]

Transepidermal water loss and heat loss via the skin are intimately tied together (increased environmental temperature increases TEWL). Sweating is an important mechanism for heat regulation when thermal stress occurs and is a source of IWL.[24] However, the ability to sweat in response to thermal or emotional stressors is dependent upon gestational and postnatal age.[64]

Infants 36 weeks of gestational age or older are able to generate sweat.[64] The onset of sweating is delayed in preterm infants more than 30 weeks' gestation; sweating is minimal or nonexistent in infants less than 30 weeks' gestation, owing to inadequate sweat gland development. For many infants less than 36 weeks' gestation, crying had to accompany thermal stimulus to yield sweating, and rectal temperatures had to be higher before sweating was induced.[24, 64]

Research indicates that sweating appears first on the forehead, and that may be the only place where it does occur. There is a correlation between gestational age and the number of sites where sweating is found during the 1st week of life.[64] After that period this correlation disappears. The amount of water loss varies with the state of arousal, the site of sweating, and the ambient and body temperatures, with the highest loss occurring from the forehead and then from the chest and the upper arms.[46, 64]

The development of the sweat response is accelerated after birth, although adult function is not achieved until 2 to 3 years of age.[110] The ability to respond to thermal stress matures between 21 and 33 days in more mature preterm infants and by 5 days in term infants. The actual water loss due to perspiration in the term infant is low, and although the preterm infant has greater losses, most are due not to perspiration but to direct TEWL.[99]

Maturation of the sweat response may be a function of gland development (anatomic and functional) or maturation of the nervous system. In the 28-week fetus, the full complement of sweat glands is in place, many having formed lumina. The cholinergic fibers of the sympathetic nervous system are also in place. Chemical maturation, however, has not occurred, contributing to the absence of the sweat response in these infants.[64]

Cohesion Between Epidermis and Dermis

Increased fluid losses may occur owing to stripping of the corneum stratum through the repeated removal of tape. This problem is due to decreased cohesion between the epidermis and dermis. The epidermis firmly adheres to the underlying dermis in the adult at the dermoepidermal junction. The basal layer is anchored to the basement membrane by hemidesmosomes, anchoring filaments, and fibers that protrude from the undersurface of the basal cells. The undulations encountered in its structure enhance resistance to shearing stress at the junction.[169]

In the preterm infant there is a combination of decreased anchoring structures, higher water content, and widely spaced collagen fiber bundles in the dermis. This structural liability makes the skin integrity fragile and more susceptible to skin trauma from shearing and frictional or adhesive forces.[85, 180] For the preterm infant cutaneous injury may occur with very little manipulation. Denuded and damaged skin increases TEWL and may be a site of entry for bacterial infection until healing occurs. Therefore, extreme care when applying and removing tape or monitoring devices is warranted, especially in the very low birth weight infant.[26, 65, 104, 110, 111, 180]

Collagen and Elastin Instability

Collagen is the connective tissue of the dermis that is composed of fibrocytes. Collagen makes up more than 90% of the connective tissue, with fibroblasts being the most numerous cells of the dermal tissue. Just like epidermal-dermal cohesion, collagen stability also increases with gestational and postnatal age.[1, 110, 111]

Collagen maintains the tensile properties of skin while the elastic fibers allow elastic recoil of the stretched skin. Because the elastin fibers are finer and less mature in the neonate, the skin stretches less and is more susceptible to damage from shearing forces. These liabilities are compounded in preterm infants.[161, 180]

Large amounts of glycosaminoglycans, proteoglycans, and glycoproteins in newborn skin bind large amounts of water. This provides a gel-like composition, which increases the compressibility of the newborn skin and decreases the potential for skin breakdown in the full-term infant.

Lack of connective tissue can result in increased trauma to the cutaneous layers in the very low birth weight infant. In addition to this, decreased collagen may contribute to edema formation in the dermal layer with concomitant increases in fluid loss due to increased fluid availability. This tendency toward water fixation decreases with gestational age as collagen stability increases. Heat loss may be enhanced, with thermal stability jeopardized, owing to the decreased insulative capabilities of the fibrous elements of the dermal layer.

Protective Mechanisms

Although there are many immaturities to the cutaneous system, the accelerated maturation along with the pH of the infant's skin results in a protective barrier to the environment as long as the skin stays intact. Dietel noted that an acid skin surface with a pH lower than 5.0 has bacteriostatic properties.[40] The acid mantle is formed from the uppermost layer of the epidermis, sweat, superficial fat, metabolic by-products, and external substances (i.e., amniotic fluid and microorganisms). Immediately after birth the pH is 6.34, but within 4 days it drops to 4.95. The mechanism for this change remains unclear.[15] Dietel suggests that it may be due to changes in the composition of the surface lipids and the activity of the eccrine glands.[40]

Immediately following delivery microbial colonization also begins. These bacteria grow in a state of equilibrium, providing protection against invading pathogenic organisms.[7] A rise in pH toward neutral causes an increase in the total number of bacteria and a change in the species present.[156] See Chapter 10 for more information regarding this function of the skin.

Along with its physiologic functions, the skin is the most sophisticated sensory organ system in the neonate. The neonate obtains the vast majority of its information about the environment through the skin. Montague believes that the quality of touch and cutaneous stimulation is responsible for the infant's later responses to other people and the environment.[116]

Tactile Perception

Weiss explains that receptors triggered at the skin surface provide the afferent impulses that construct the activity of the central nervous system (CNS). The specialization of neuronal pathways allows for selective responses to stimuli with various types of feedback.[182]

In infants tactile and kinesthetic sensory pathways are the first to be myelinated, followed by auditory and visual pathways.[88] The earlier a function develops the more fundamental it appears to be, indicating the importance of tactile experiences for the neonate.[92]

CLINICAL IMPLICATIONS FOR NEONATAL CARE

There are numerous clinical implications for the neonate owing to the limitations of the integumentary system. These implications include skin care, absorption of substances through the skin, and the use of adhesives. Some nursing practices need to be reevaluated in light of the current knowledge regarding neonatal skin.

Skin Care

Washing infants with alkaline soap (e.g., Ivory) destroys the acid mantle by neutralizing the pH. For the full-term infant it takes 1 hour for the pH to return to baseline; for preterm infants this takes even longer.[40] McManus Kuller and coworkers discourage the use of alkaline substances during the 1st week of life for all neonates.[111] Warm water baths are adequate, and warm sterile water should be used on delicate or excoriated areas.[172] Bathing is recommended only two to three times per week with less alkaline soaps (e.g., Neutrogena, Basis, Aveeno).[111]

Creams, emollients, and lotions should not be used routinely. Not only do these substances affect the acid mantle, but they may also be absorbed percutaneously.[40] As stated previously, the optimal skin condition for the neonate is dry and flaking, without cracks and fissures. If cracking does occur, a thin application of nonperfumed emollient can be used.[111]

In order to facilitate rapid epidermal maturation following delivery, manipulation (handling) should be minimized, especially with preterm infants. No routine use of lubricants and dry skin care practices should be instituted.[171] Dry skin care includes the use of cotton sponges and water to remove blood from the face and head as well as meconium from the perineum. The remainder of the skin should be left untouched unless grossly soiled.[8]

Adhesives

The epidermis is pulled off when adhesives are removed. The denuded areas not only are a potential source of infection but are also uncomfortable and are areas of increased fluid loss. Use of pectin-based barriers, transparent dressings, and minimal tape to secure monitoring equipment and intravenous lines is recommended. Pectin-based barriers prevent tape from being applied directly to the skin. They are soft and pliable and can be removed without excoriation of the skin.[66, 105]

Transparent dressings are impermeable to water and bacteria, while providing protection to abrasions and skin irritations, or can be used for dressings to cover line insertion sites or incision sites for invasive procedures. The advantages to this type of dressing include providing an optimal moist environment for healing, allowing serous exudate to form over the wound, facilitating migration of new cells across the wound area, and preventing cellular dehydration.[3, 29, 49, 111]

Transparent dressings also allow for continual observation because of their transparent nature while conforming to the body shape. Because of their impermeability to water, bathing can be accomplished without difficulty.[111]

The use of benzoin to promote adhesion is not recommended owing to the already significant cohesion that occurs with tape. Benzoin improves tape-epidermis adhesion and potentiates epidermal stripping upon tape removal. In addition, benzoin is absorbed through the skin, allowing acids to be released into the bloodstream.

Protection from Infection

Protection from infection requires that the skin, as the first line of defense against infection, stay intact.[6, 110] Current monitoring modalities require manipulation and attachment of equipment to the infant's epidermal layer. Careful handling can reduce shear damage and epidermal sloughing. Application of noninvasive monitoring equipment needs to be done such that pressure or constriction of blood flow does not occur. Use of heated electrodes can lead to local hyperthermia and erythema.[20] Crater formation may occur in preterm infants with very thin skin.[56]

In order to combat erythema and crater formation, Golden recommends keeping the temperature of the transcutaneous electrode under 44°C, using the lowest temperature necessary for adequate readings.[56] Increasing the frequency of site changes may also reduce skin damage; either use extreme care in removing the adherent ring or use equipment that allows for electrode site changes without moving the ring each time.

Transepidermal Absorption

Percutaneous absorption of substances can occur through two pathways via the cells of the stratum corneum, termed the transepidermal route, and via the hair–follicle–sebaceous gland complex, the transappendageal route.[120] The major pathway is most likely transepidermally, with diffusion of a substance through the stratum corneum and epidermis into the dermis and microcirculation. In addition, the subepidermal circulation is readily accessible, enhancing rapid absorption.

Neonates are at increased risk for toxic reactions from absorption of topically applied substances for the reasons listed in Table 11–6. Along with these differences, skin metabolization is different in neonates, so drugs applied topically may result in the release of metabolites different from those that would occur if the drugs were given by other routes. This increases the risk of toxicity.[184] Occlusion of the skin (e.g., placement against the mattress) permits more complete absorption, with longer contact enhancing absorption of the substance. Kopelman notes that for the preterm infant percutaneous absorption occurs even more rapidly and completely as a result of the increased permeability.[90]

History of neonatal practice demonstrates the problems with the use of topical agents (Table 11–7). For example, central nervous system damage was encountered with the use of hexachlorophene to prevent coagulase-positive staphylococci colonization.[23, 37] Eventually the Food and Drug Administration modified the allowable uses of hexachlorophene.

Current practices also can lead to detrimental effects if not monitored carefully. Topical application of povidone-iodine (Betadine) yields significantly elevated levels of

TABLE 11–6
Factors Placing Neonates at Risk for Toxic Reactions Secondary to Absorption of Topically Applied Substances

Increased permeability of the skin
Increased surface area–to–body weight ratio
Lower blood pressure
Variable skin blood flow patterns
Greater proportion of body weight being made up of brain and liver
Incomplete kidney development resulting in changes in drug excretion
Body compartment ratios are different
Total body water content is larger
Ratio of intracellular to extracellular water is elevated
Decreased adipose tissue

From West, D., Worobec, S., & Solomon, L. (1981). Pharmacology and toxicology of infant skin. *J Invest Dermatol, 76*, 147.

TABLE 11–7
Neonatal Cutaneous Absorption

YEAR	SAMPLE	AGE OF INFANTS	ROUTE	AGENT	SIGNS OF INTOXICATION	COURSE
1946 (Scott)	32	Neonates	Transepidermal	Aniline oil on diapers stamped in 6 places; clothes; washcloths; bed linen	Cyanosis Diarrhea with excoriated buttocks	3 died
1949 (Kagan)	9	Neonates 3–64 days (mean = 19) weight 1000–2015 g (mean = 1272)	Transepidermal ? volatilized in incubator–inhalation	Aniline dye used to stamp diapers	Peculiar, gray cyanosis Methemoglobinemia Anorexia, vomiting	All recovered; mild to severe bronchopneumonia between 2–4 weeks after poisoning
1961 (Fisch)	18	Neonates 1–9 days 12 <1250 g	Transepidermal	Laundry rinse containing trichlorocarbanilide	Methemoglobinemia Cyanosis	All survived
1969 (Armstrong)	20	Neonates younger than 5 days (awaiting adoption)	Transepidermal	Sodium pentachlorophenol Laundry neutralizer used in diapers, linen clothes	Profuse, generalized diaphoresis Fever Tachycardia Hepatomegaly Acidosis Phenol derivatives in urine and serum	9 severely ill 2 died Attack rates: 19% April 24% May 3% July–August
1969 (Robson)	9	6–12 days	Transepidermal	Sodium pentachlorophenol used in laundering infant's diapers	Excessive sweating Tachycardia Tachypnea Respiratory distress Hepatic enlargement ↓ BUN Proteinuria Ketonuria	2 died 11 additional affected with similar but milder illness Exchange transfusions used 1 infant died within 3 hours of onset of symptoms
1972 (Martin-Bouyer)	204	126 neonates 78 >1 month	Transepidermal	"Bebe Talc Morhange" Baby powder that contained 6.3% hexachlorophene (manufacturing error)	Low grade fever Severe diaper rash Ulcerative skin lesions Encephalopathy (irritability with hypertonicity)	36 died Spongiform changes in spinal tract

On September 22, 1972, the FDA restricted all over-the-counter products with hexachlorophene.

YEAR	SAMPLE	AGE OF INFANTS	ROUTE	AGENT	SIGNS OF INTOXICATION	COURSE
1973 (Powell)	7	Ill Neonates 1100–1300 grams	Transepidermal	pHisoHex containing 3% hexachlorophene Daily exposure (4) Alternate days (3) 7 had >9 exposures	Acidosis Hyperbilirubinemia	All died Spongiform changes in nervous tissue
1974 (Shuman)	248 coming to autopsy. Investigated neonatal deaths from 1966–1972	The lesion occurred only in neonates hospitalized at least 4 or more days	Transepidermal	pHisoHex containing 3% hexachlorophene		17 cases with vacuolar encephalopathy along myelin tracts
1977 (Pyati)	Study involving 4 groups of infants receiving povidone-iodine applied to the umbilical cord (1 control group)	Term healthy newborns	Transepidermal	Povidone-iodine (pH = 2.43)		Cord total plasma iodine comparable in all 4 groups Plasma iodine levels significantly higher than controls and related to the number of applications The corresponding urine iodine values were high

Table continued on following page

TABLE 11–7
Neonatal Cutaneous Absorption *Continued*

YEAR	SAMPLE	AGE	ROUTE	AGENT	SIGNS OF INTOXICATION	COURSE
1982 (Harpin)	2	27-week gestation twins	Transepidermal (need to absorb only 0.3 ml to reach dangerous blood levels)	Alcohol (95% ethanol, 5% wood naphtha) Solution used to prep umbilicus; it dripped down to soak surface upon which baby was lying	Extensive skin damage Severe hemorrhage Skin necrosis on back and buttocks Blood ethanol levels	1 died
1982 (UC Neonatology)	2	756 g 850 g	Transepidermal De-esterified skin with tissue destruction	Isopropyl alcohol (70%) solution was used to prep umbilicus	3rd degree burns with blister formation Skin sloughing and eschar formation	1 died

Cavanagh, E. (1988). Postnatal preterm skin development and the efficacy of skin care practices. Unpublished manuscript. University of Washington, Seattle. (Compiled from references 10a, 23, 37, 49a, 68, 83, 106a, 131, 135, 141a, 154a, and 161.)

iodine in blood plasma if not removed completely from the skin after completion of invasive procedures (e.g., chest tube insertion, percutaneous line insertion).[135] Gentle cleansing of the skin with water reduces this risk. Benzoin contains many different acids, all of which can be absorbed, causing either immediate or delayed reactions.[54]

Isopropyl alcohol is also absorbed through the skin. Alcohol use can result in dry skin, skin irritation, and skin burns. The concentration of the solution, duration of exposure, and condition of the exposed skin determine the effects of alcohol use. Tissue destruction occurs with the de-esterifying of the skin and the disruption of the cell structure. Exposure, pressure, and decreased perfusion can contribute to the development of burns from alcohol, complicating fluid management and providing portals for infection.[28, 151]

Limitations in Specific Infant Groups

For specific infant groups there are special conditions and circumstances that make integumentary integrity more difficult to maintain. For these infants attention to preventive measures and careful monitoring and handling must be incorporated into nursing care activities.

The Extremely Immature Infant

The very low birth weight infant has edematous and shiny skin, covered with abundant vernix and lanugo. These infants have decreased subcutaneous tissue and an increased water content. This is compounded by a greater ratio of surface area to body weight. All of these characteristics create difficulties in fluid balance and temperature control due to the high IWL.[145] The use of heat shields and plastic or thermal blankets to reduce TEWL and promote thermal stability is recommended (see Chapter 17).

The premature infant's skin is exceedingly sensitive because skin permeability and collagen instability decrease with gestational age. Cohesion at the dermoepidermal junction is also markedly reduced, which can cause stratum corneum and epidermal stripping with handling and attachment of monitoring devices. Careful handling and policies about skin adhesive practices should be employed. The maintenance of skin integrity should be the goal. Denuded areas may benefit from transparent dressings, thereby reducing further damage, providing protection from microbial invasion, and reducing fluid losses.

The stratum corneum is extremely thin; therefore cutaneous permeability is greater, providing little protection against topical substances.[120] Percutaneous absorption occurs more rapidly and completely, placing these infants at greater risk for toxic reactions.[90, 110] The use of harsh de-esterifying substances (soaps and alcohol) should be kept to an absolute minimum. The acid mantle is easily disrupted, and cellular destruction is possible.

Collagen instability and incomplete dermal structures result in increased cutaneous edema and decreased resiliency. This may result in skin necrosis due to edema pressure within the dermis. The use of waterbeds, gentle handling with little compression force or friction, careful regular turning, and range of motion exercises may help to reduce this tendency.[110, 112]

Postmature Infants

There are different categories of postmature infants, and the skin characteristics of these infants are unique, dictating distinctive care practices. For the postmature infant who is also dysmature, weight loss has occurred in utero secondary to placental insufficiency. This results in a loss of subcutaneous tissue, scaling, and parchment-like skin. There may also be a decrease in muscle mass, and bile staining of the skin may have occurred as the result of meconium passage.[129]

Those infants who do not experience placental insufficiency continue to gain weight and may be quite large at the time of delivery. These infants have skin characteristics typical of the term neonate. However, owing to their size the possibility of cutaneous injury during passage through the birth canal or as the result of mechanical intervention (e.g., forceps or vacuum placement) to facilitate delivery is increased.[187] The need to assess skin integrity and protect the infant from infection is high in the postmature infant.

The postmature-dysmature infant has special skin needs due to the loss of the protective covering of vernix caseosa in utero. This is accompanied by a change in skin turgor and consistency. Osmotic damage from the amniotic fluid occurs leading to the development of abnormal skin folds, shedding of large patches of the stratum corneum, and formation of areas of maceration.[40]

Following delivery the skin shrinks and becomes wrinkled, almost parchment-like. There is general desquamation over the first few days. Cracks and fissures may develop in the joint areas, especially the joints of the fingers, toes, and ankle.

Special care to promote the maturation of the underlying epidermal tissue is warranted. Scrubbing and peeling of the sloughing skin are to be avoided since damage to the underlying tissue is possible. Routine lubrication should not be used. Emollients may also interfere with the needed maturation of the "new" epidermis, while altering the desired pH of the acid mantle. A nonperfumed cream or a thin layer of antibiotic ointment may be used to moisten fissured skin and reduce discomfort in these areas. Allowing the normal desquamation, which is followed by epidermal and stratum corneum maturation, is recommended.

Infants Receiving Phototherapy

There are several side effects associated with phototherapy that impact on the integumentary system. The increased radiant heat from the ultraviolet lights results in an increase in environmental and body temperature, depending on the neonate's thermoregulatory abilities. Clinically this can be seen in an increase in respiratory rate and an increase in skin and muscle blood flow leading to erythema. Sweating may be seen, especially if the infant is irritable and crying. The change in core temperature results in an increase in oxygen consumption and metabolic rate (see Chapter 15).[194]

The erythema is due to the vasodilatation and increased peripheral blood flow that the radiant heat causes. There is also a dramatic increase in IWL. A 30 to 40% increase is seen in full-term infants; premature infants may encounter fluid losses of 80 to 190% in non–Servo-controlled incubators (42 to 113% in Servo-controlled). These losses are the result of evaporative loss from the skin, an increase in metabolic rate, and an increase in respiratory rate.[11, 31, 45, 124, 193, 194]

Factors affecting the degree of IWL include the air flow, humidity and temperature of the nursery, type of incubator, type of radiant warmer, respiratory rate, and metabolic rate. Whether the phototherapy unit is equipped to dissipate heat and the distance it is positioned from the incubator hood determine the amount of radiant energy focused on the infant.[194] Meticulous evaluation of hydration status is necessary in order to compensate appropriately for these higher than normal fluid losses (see Chapter 8). The use of Servocontrol may also help.[194]

Perineal and buttock skin integrity may be compromised owing to the increased frequency of stools. Gentle warm water washing after each stool should help to reduce this risk. Decreased activity levels may result in increased compression pressure with decreased perfusion and edema formation. Turning the infant every couple of hours maintains skin integrity and exposes new skin areas to the phototherapy lights.[42, 194]

Transient rashes are relatively common, occurring in 9.5 to 12% of neonates. This scattered pinpoint red rash is due to injury of the skin mast cells with histamine release. It is unrelated to the length of therapy and disappears following the discontinuance of treatment.[47, 79] Burning is not common, but may occur when excessive exposure to short light-wave emission occurs.[194]

Dark brown or greenish-toned skin discoloration can occur in infants with cholestatic jaundice and a high direct bilirubin. This is termed the "bronze baby" syndrome and usually disappears after phototherapy is discontinued (see Chapter 15).

MATURATIONAL CHANGES DURING INFANCY AND CHILDHOOD

Although the full-term infant's skin is functionally comparable to the adult's, loss of water content, desquamation, and drying of the stratum corneum bring the skin to maturation within the first few days.[188] For the premature infant, this may take longer because the water content is higher. The initial edema decreases within the first few days of life, after which the skin lies loosely over the entire body.[62]

Transfer from the intrauterine amniotic fluid environment to the external air environment results in accelerated maturation of skin function in the preterm infant. By 10 days postnatal age the integrity of the skin improves, approaching that of the term infant.[73] As the water content decreases, integrity and barrier function also improve.

Collagen stability results in a decreased ability to retain fluid within the dermis. This improves with increasing gestational age and in the early postnatal period. Most of the other components of the dermis are not formed until after birth and may not be mature until age 3. Resiliency is therefore affected; it is low in full-term infants and even lower in premature infants.[156]

Melanin production and pigmentation are low during neonatal life, although high circulating maternal and placental hormones can lead to deep pigmentation of certain areas (i.e., linea alba, areola, and scrotum). This decrease in production is even greater in the preterm infant. Given that melanin protects the skin from the ultraviolet rays of the sun by absorbing their radiant energy, neonates have an increased sensitivity to sunlight.[1] Sunburn can damage the barrier ef-fectiveness of the skin by causing dehydration and desquamation and can promote the development of skin cancer.[33]

Although the sweat glands are functional within a short time of birth, activating influences are different in the infant than in the adult. For the first 2½ years of life the sweat glands function irregularly and the total number of glands that are active is small.[178] Emotionally induced eccrine sweating is much less marked in the prepubertal individual than in the adult.[139] The sebaceous glands are also somewhat dormant until puberty.

Although the sebaceous glands are large and active in utero, contributing to the lipid content of the vernix caseosa, they rapidly decrease in size and remain so until puberty. At puberty, they once again become active structures.[115] The free fatty acids in the gland secretions have a fungistatic effect and provide immunity against scalp infections from these pathogens.[144]

Lastly, the vasculature also changes over the first few months of life. Initially the cutaneous capillary network is imperfectly developed, and a progression to an orderly mature pattern occurs during infancy.[129]

SUMMARY

It is apparent that the skin plays a major role in the protection of neonates from the atmospheric environment to which they are born. The development of the acid mantle and microbial colonization provide protection against pathogenic organisms. The thickness of the stratum corneum determines the effectiveness of this protection as well as reducing permeability to the loss of fluids and absorption of topical substances.

Gestational age is the major determinant of collagen and elastin stability, the thickness of the stratum corneum barrier, and thermal regulatory abilities. Delivery results in a rapid proliferation of the stratum corneum in the preterm infant in an attempt to compensate for some of the liabilities these infants must cope with. The fragility of the premature infant's skin results in denuded areas due to friction and shearing forces, as well as separation of the epidermis through adhesive stripping.

Understanding the normal developmental processes that the integumentary system undergoes as well as the goal of each of these processes provides the basis for nursing ther-

TABLE 11–8
Summary of Recommendations for Clinical Practice Related to the Integumentary System in the Neonate

General Considerations in Skin Care
Develop knowledge of normal development of the neonatal integumentary system (pp. 500–507).
Know the normal integumentary variations encountered in the neonate (Table 11–1) (pp. 507–508).
Monitor skin integrity on a routine basis (pp. 507–508).
Maintain a neutral thermal environment (pp. 509–510).
Evaluate intake, output, and hydration status (pp. 508–510).
Avoid routine lubrication (pp. 507–508, 511, 515).
Implement infrequent bathing using plain water or less alkaline soaps (pp. 510–511).
Counsel parents to gradually expose infant to sunlight, especially fair-skinned infant (p. 516).

Fluid and Heat Loss
Use thermal or plastic wrap blankets or plastic heat shields (pp. 508–509).
Protect from drafts (pp. 508–510).
Utilize phototherapy equipment that dissipates radiant heat to the environment (pp. 509–510, 515–516).
Position phototherapy lights a few inches above incubator hood (pp. 515–516).
Utilize Op-Site over denuded areas (pp. 511–512).
Monitor environmental and body temperature regularly (pp. 509–510).
Avoid removing vernix (pp. 507–508).
Assess skin for stratum corneum stripping and institute measures to reduce it (pp. 510–511, 514–515).
Recognize potential thermal and emotional stress situations (pp. 508–510).
Maintain appropriate humidity levels within nursery (pp. 509–510).

Barrier Maintenance
Implement minimal tape use policies (pp. 510–512).
Avoid using adhesive bandages such as Band-aids (pp. 510–512, 514–515).
Remove tape carefully, using warm water to facilitate process (pp. 511–512).
Use pectin-based or hydrogel-backed electrodes (pp. 511–512).
Apply pectin-based barriers between skin and tape (pp. 510–512, 514–515).
Avoid benzoin preparations (pp. 512–514, Table 11–7).
Implement dry skin care practices for the first 2 weeks of postnatal life (p. 511).
Avoid the use of gauze pads on premature skin (pp. 514–515).
Implement plain water bathing of premature infants (pp. 511, 514).
Initiate position changes every 2 hours (pp. 508–509, 515–516).
Ensure appropriate positioning, avoiding pressure on bony prominences (pp. 510, 514–515).
Recognize friction stress points and cover them with Op-Site (pp. 514–515).
Use alcohol sparingly (pp. 512–514, Table 11–7).
Observe for cracking and apply a nonperfumed emollient (p. 515).
Promote careful handling of preterm infants (pp. 510, 514–515).
Recognize activities that produce friction, shearing, or stress, and implement interventions to reduce them (pp. 510, 514–515).

Permeability
Avoid routine lubrication (pp. 507–508, 511, 515).
Know the factors that place neonates at risk for toxic responses to topically applied substances (pp. 512–514, Table 11–6).
Practice conservative treatment of integumentary disruptions (pp. 510–511).
Counsel parents regarding the use of topical emollients and powders (pp. 507–508, 511, 515).
Avoid the use of benzoin (pp. 512–514, Table 11–7).
Ensure cleansing of skin prepped with Betadine following invasive procedures (pp. 512–514, Table 11–7).
Use alcohol sparingly (pp. 514–515, Table 11–7).

Page numbers in parentheses following each intervention refer to pages where rationale for that intervention is discussed.

apeutics. Careful assessment of skin integrity, knowledge of normal neonatal variations, and conservative therapeutics can result in appropriate and timely interventions. The care of the skin can enhance integumentary capabilities and contribute to the infant's ability to assimilate information from the environment. Clinical implications for nursing practice are summarized in Table 11–8.

REFERENCES

1. Ackerman, A. (1975). Structure and function of the skin. In S.L. Moschella, D.M. Pillsbury, & H.J. Hurley (Eds.), *Dermatology* (Vol. 2). Philadelphia: WB Saunders.
2. Ahmed, A.R. & Kaplan, R. (1981). Pruritic urticarial papules and plaques of pregnancy. *J Am Acad Dermatol, 4,* 679.
3. Ahmed, M.C. (1982). Op-site for decubitis care. *Am J Nurs, 82,* 61.
4. Alcalay, J., et al. (1988). Hormonal evaluation and autoimmune background in pruritic urticarial papules and plaques of pregnancy. *Am J Obstet Gynecol, 158,* 417.
5. Alcalay, J., et al. (1987). Pruritic urticarial papules and plaques of pregnancy: A review of 21 cases. *J Reprod Med, 32,* 315.
6. Aly, R. & Marbach, L. (1981). Factors controling skin bacteria flora. In L. Marbach and R. Aly (Eds.), *Skin microbiology: Relevance to clinical infection.* New York: Springer-Verlag.
7. American Academy of Pediatrics. (1974). Skin care of newborns. *Pediatrics, 54,* 682.

8. American Academy of Pediatrics. (1988). *Guidelines for Perinatal Care* (2nd ed., p. 127). Elk Grove, IL: AAP.

9. Amon, I. (1984). Adrenal corticoid hormones. In H.P. Kuemmerle & K. Brendel (Eds.), *Clinical pharmacology in pregnancy. Fundamentals and rational pharmacotherapy*. New York: Thieme-Stratton.

10. Andrews, B.F. (1970). Amniotic fluid studies to determine maturity. *Pediatr Clin North Am, 17,* 9.

10a. Armstrong, R.W., et al. (1969). Pentachlorophenol poisoning in a nursery for newborn infants. *J. Pediatr. 75,* 317.

11. Bacham, A. (1955). Time factors of erythema and pigmentation by ultraviolet rays of different wavelength. *J Invest Dermatol, 25,* 215.

12. Baker, H. & Ryan, T.J. (1968). Generalized pustular psoriasis: A clnical and epidemiological study of 104 cases. *Br J Dermatol, 80,* 771.

13. Baumgart, S., Fox, W.W., & Polin, R.A. (1982). Physiologic implications of two different heat shields for infants under radiant warmers. *J Pediatr, 100,* 787.

14. Bean, W.B., et al. (1949). Vascular changes of the skin in pregnancy. *Surg Gynecol Obstet, 88,* 739.

15. Behrendt, H. & Green, M. (1971). *Patterns of skin pH from birth through adolescence*. Springfield, IL: Charles C Thomas.

16. Beveridge, G.W., Harkness, R.A. & Livingstone, J.R.B. (1966). Impetigo herpetiformis in two successive pregnancies. *Br J Dermatol, 78,* 106.

17. Bishop, E.H. & Corson, S. (1968). Estimation of fetal maturity by cytologic examination of amniotic fluid. *Am J Obstet Gynecol, 102,* 654.

18. Blijham, A.O., Franz, W., & Bohn, E. (1982). Effects of forced convection of heated air on insensible water loss and heat loss in preterm infants in incubators. *J Pediatr, 101,* 108.

19. Borysenko, M. & Beringer, T. (1984). *Functional histology*. Boston: Little, Brown.

20. Boyle, R.J. & Oh, W. (1980). Erythema following transcutaneous PO$_2$ monitoring. *Pediatrics, 65,* 332.

21. Braverman, I.M. (1988). The skin in pregnancy. In G.N. Burrow & T.F. Ferris (Eds.). *Medical complications during pregnancy*. Philadephia: WB Saunders.

22. Breathnach, A.S. (1971). Embryology of the human skin. *J Invest Dermatol, 57,* 133.

23. Bressler, R. et al. (1977). Hexacholorophene in the newborn nursery. A risk-benefit analysis and review. *Clin Pediatr, 16,* 342.

24. Brown, M.S. & Alexander, M.M. (1973). Physical examination: Part 3. Examining the skin. *Nursing '73,* 39.

25. Bruck, K. (1961). Temperature regulation in the newborn infant. *Biol Neonate, 3,* 65.

26. Bryant, R.A. (1988). Saving the skin from tape injuries. *Am J Nurs, 88,* 189.

27. Callen, J.P. & Hanno, R. (1981). Pruritic urticarial papules and plaques of pregnancy (PUPPP). A clinicopathologic study. *J Am Acad Dermatol, 5,* 401.

28. Champagne, S., Fussell, S. & Scheifele, D. (1984). Evaluation of skin antisepsis prior to blood culture in neonates. *Infection Control, 5,* 489.

29. Chrisp, M. (1977). New treatment for pressure sores. *Nursing Times, 73,* 1202.

30. Clark, D., et al. (1978). Immunoreactive alpha-MSH in human plasma in pregnancy. *Nature, 273,* 163.

31. Clyman, R.I. & Rudolph, A.M. (1978). Patent ductus arteriosus: A new light on an old problem. *Pediatr Res, 12,* 92.

32. Cohlan, S.Q. (1977). Tetracycline staining of teeth. *Teratology, 15,* 127.

33. Coody, D. (1987). There is no such thing as a good tan. *J Pediatr Health Care, 1,* 125.

34. Cooper, A.J. & Fryer, J.A. (1980). Prurigo of late pregnancy. *Aust J Dermatol, 21,* 79.

35. Costello, M.J. (1941). Eruptions of pregnancy. *NY State J Med, 41,* 849.

36. Cummings, K. & Derbes, V.J. (1967). Dermatoses associated with pregnancy. *Cutis, 3,* 120.

37. Curley, A., et al. (1971). Dermal absorption of hexochorophene in infants. *Lancet, 2,* 296.

38. Davey, C.M.H. (1972). Factors associated with the occurrence of striae gravidarum. *J Obstet Gynaecol Br Comm, 79,* 1113.

39. Denman, S.T. (1986). A review of pruritus. *J Am Acad Dermatol, 14,* 375.

40. Dietel, K. (1978). Morphological and functional development of the skin. In U. Stave (Ed.), *Perinatal physiology*. New York: Plenum Press.

41. Downing, J.W. & Bees, L.T. (1976). The influence of lateral tilt on limb blood flow in advanced pregnancy. *S Afr Med J, 50,* 728.

42. Drew, J.H., et al. (1976). Phototherapy: Short- and long-term complications. *Arch Dis Child, 51,* 454.

43. Dubowitz, L., Dubowitz, V., & Goldberg, C. (1970). Clinical assessment of gestational age in the newborn infant. *J Pediatr, 77,* 1.

44. Ebling, F.G. (1970). The embryology of the skin. In R.T. Champion, et al. (Eds.), *An introduction to the biology of the skin*. Philadelphia: FA Davis.

45. Engle, W., et al. (1974). Insensible water loss in the critically ill neonate. *Am J Dis Child, 135,* 516.

46. Esterly, N.B. & Solomon, L.M. (1987). The skin. In A.A. Fanaroff & R.J. Martin (Eds.). *Neonatal-perinatal medicine, Diseases of the fetus and infant*. St Louis: CV Mosby.

47. Evans, N.J. & Rutter, N. (1986). Development of the epidermis in the newborn. *Biol Neonate, 49,* 74.

48. Foucar, E., et al. (1985). A histopathologic evaluation of nevocellular nevi in pregnancy. *Arch Dermaol, 121,* 350.

49. Freeman, P. & Boyer, J. (1982). How to get the most out of Opsite. *RN, 43,* 37.

49a. Fisch, R.O., et al. (1963). Methemoglobinemia in a hospital nursery. *JAMA, 185,* 760.

50. Fulk, C.S. (1984). Primary disorders of hyperpigmentation. *J Am Acad Dermatol, 10,* 1.

51. Furhoff, A.K. (1974). Itching in pregnancy. *Acta Med Scand, 196,* 403.

52. Genot, M.T., et al. (1970). Effect of administration of tetracycline in pregnancy on the primary dentition of the offspring. *J Oral Med, 25,* 75.

53. Gerstein, W. (1971). Cell proliferation in human fetal epidermis. *J Invest Dermatol, 57,* 262.

54. Gill, N.N. (1982). Benzoin contains many acids (letter to editor). *Am J Nurs, 82,* 244.

55. Gleiss, J. & Stuttgen, G. (1970). Morphologic and functional development of the skin. In U. Stave (Ed.), *Physiology of the perinatal period* (Vol. 2). New York: Appleton-Century-Crofts.

56. Golden, S.M. (1981) Skin craters—a complication of transcutaneous oxygen monitoring. *Pediatrics, 67,* 514.

57. Greenberger, P. & Patterson, R. (1978). Safety of therapy for allergic symptoms during pregnancy. *Ann Intern Med, 89,* 234.

58. Habif, T.P. (1985). *Clinical dermatology. A color guide to diagnosis and therapy.* St Louis: CV Mosby.

59. Hale, P.A. & Ebling, F.J. (1975). The effects of epilation and hormones on the activity of rate hair follicles. *J Exp Zool, 191,* 49.

60. Hamilton, W.J. & Mossman, H.W. (1972). *Human embryology: Prenatal development of form and function.* Baltimore: Williams & Wilkins.

61. Hammarlund, K. & Sedin, G. (1979). Transepidermal water loss in newborn infants. Relation to gestational age. *Acta Dis Child, 54,* 477.

62. Harmon, J. & Steele, S. (1975). *Nursing care of the skin: Structure and function.* New York: Appleton-Century-Crofts.

63. Harpin, V. & Rutter, N. (1985). Humidification of incubators. *Arch Dis Child, 60,* 219.

64. Harpin, V.A. & Rutter, N. (1982). Sweating in preterm babies. *J Pediatr, 100,* 614.

65. Harpin, V. & Rutter, N. (1983). Barrier properties of the newborn infant's skin. *J Pediatr, 102,* 419.

66. Harrell-Bean, H.A. & Klell, C.A. (1983). Neonatal ostomies. *J Obstet Gynecol Neonatal Nurs, 12* (Suppl.), 69s.

67. Hashimoto, K, et al. (1966). The ultrastructure of the skin of human embryos. *J Invest Dermatol, 47,* 317.

68. Harpin, V.A. & Rutter, N. (1982). Percutaneous alcohol absorption and skin necrosis in a premature infant. *Arch Dis Child, 57,* 477.

69. Hays, P.M. & Cruikshank, D.P. (1985). Hormonal therapy during pregnancy. In T.A.B. Eskes & M. Finster (Eds.), *Drug therapy during pregnancy.* London: Butterworths.

70. Hey, E. & Mount, L. (1966). Temperature control in incubators. *Lancet, 1,* 202.

71. Hey, E. N. & Katz, G. (1969). Evaporative water in the newborn baby. *J Physiol, 200,* 605.

72. Hill, J.R. & Rahimtulla, K.A. (1965). Heat balance and the matabolic rate of newborn babies in relation to environmental temperature, and the effect of age and of weight on basal metabolic rate. *J Physiol, 180,* 239.

73. Holbrook, K.A. (1982). A histological comparison of infant and adult skin. In H.I. Maibach & E.K. Boisits (Eds.), *Neonatal skin: Structure and function.* New York: Marcel Dekker.

74. Holbrook, K.A. & Sybert, V. (1988). Basic Science. In L.A. Schachner and R.C. Hansen (Eds.), *Pediatric dermatology* (Vol. 1). New York: Churchill Livingstone.

75. Holbrook, K. & Odland, G. (1980). Regional development of the human epidermis in the first trimester embryo and the second trimester fetus. *J Invest Dermatol, 74,* 161.

76. Holmes, R.C. & Black, M.M. (1983). The specific dermatoses of pregnancy. *J Am Acad Dermatol, 8,* 405.

77. James, W.D., et al. (1984). Pigmentary demarcation lines associated with pregnancy. *J Am Acad Dermatol, 11,* 438.

78. Jelinek, J.E. (1970). Cutaneous side effects of oral contraceptives. *Arch Dermatol, 101,* 181.

79. John, E. (1975). Complications of phototherapy in neonatal hyperbilirubinemia. *Aust Paediatr J, 11,* 53.

80. Jordon, R.E., et al. (1976). The immunopathology of herpes gestationis. Immunofluorescence studies and characteristics of "HG factor." *J Clin Invest, 57,* 1426.

81. Katz, S.I., Hertz, K.C. & Yaoita, H. (1976). Herpes gestationis. Immunopathology and characterization of the HG factor. *J Clin Invest, 57,* 1434.

82. Kerpel-Fronius, E. (1970). Electrolyte and water meabolism. In U. Stave (Ed.), *Physiology of the perinatal period.* New York: Appleton-Century-Crofts.

83. Kagan, B.M., et al. (1949). Cyanosis in premature infants due to aniline dye intoxication. *J Pediatr, 34,* 574.

84. Klaus, S.N. (1969). Pigment transfer in mammalian epidermis. *Arch Dermatol, 100,* 756.

85. Klein, L. (1988). Maintenance of healthy skin. *J Enterostom Ther, 15,* 227.

86. Kligman, A.M. (1964). The biology of the stratum corneum. In W. Montagna & W. Lobitz (Eds.), *The epidermis.* New York: Academic Press.

87. Kligman, A.M. (1961). Pathologic dynamics of human hair loss. I. Telogen effluvium. *Arch Dermatol, 83,* 175.

88. Kolb, L. (1959). Disturbances of the body image. In S. Arieti (Ed.), *American handbook of psychiatry* (Vol. 1). New York: Basic Books.

89. Kolodny, K.C. (1969). Herpes gestationis: A new assessment of incidence, diagnosis and fetal prognosis. *Am J Obstet Gynecol, 104,* 39.

90. Kopelman, A.E. (1973). Cutaneous absorption of hexacholorophene in low-birth-weight infants. *J Pediatr, 82,* 972.

91. Koppe, J.G., Smolders de Haas, H. & Kloosterman, G.J. (1977). Effects of glucocorticoids during pregnancy on the outcome of the children directly after birth and in the long run. *Eur J Obstet Gynecol Reprod Biol, 7,* 293.

92. Krieger, D. (1975). Therapeutic touch: The imprimatur of nursing. *Am J Nurs, 75,* 784.

93. Lammer, E.J., et al. (1985). Retinoic acid embryopathy. *N Eng J Med, 313,* 837.

94. Langman, J. (1981). *Medical embryology* (4th ed.). Baltimore: Williams & Wilkins.

95. Lawley, T.G., et al. (1979). Pruritic urticarial papules and plaques of pregnancy. *JAMA, 241,* 1696.

96. Lawley, T.J., Stingl, G. & Katz, S.I. (1978). Fetal and maternal risk factors in herpes gestationis. *Arch Dermatol, 114,* 552.

97. Leeson, C.R., Leeson, T.S. & Paparo, A.A. (1985). *Atlas of histology* (2nd ed.). Philadelphia: WB Saunders.

98. Letterman, G. & Schwiter, M. (1962). Cutaneous hemangiomas of the face in pregnancy. *Plast Reconstr Surg, 29,* 293.

99. Levine, S.Z. & Marples, E. (1930). The insensible perspiration in infancy and in childhood: III. Basal metabolism and basal insensible perspiration of the normal infant: A statistical study of reliability and of correlation. *Am J Dis Child, 40,* 269.

100. Liley, A.W. (1972). Disorders of amniotic fluid. In N.S. Assali (Ed.), *Pathophysiology of gestation.* Orlando: Academic Press.

101. Lind, T., Kendall, A., & Hytten, F.E. (1973). The role of the fetus in the formation of amniotic fluid. *J Obstet Gynaecol Br Comm, 79,* 289.

102. Liu, D.T. (1974). Striae gravidarum. *Lancet, 1,* 625.

103. Lotem, M., et al. (1989). Impetigo herpetiformis: A variant of pustular psoriasis or a separate entity. *J Am Acad Dermatol, 20,* 338.

104. Lund, C., et al. (1984). Evaluation of the pectin-based barrier under tape to protect neonatal skin. *J Obstet Gynecol Neonatal Nurs, 152,* 668.

105. Lund, C. & Alterescu, V. (1984). Skin care in the intensive care nursery: Part III Stoma care. *Neonat Netw, 3*, 28.

106. Lynfield, Y.L. (1960). Effect of pregnancy on the human hair cycle. *J Invest Dermatol, 35*, 323.

106a. Martin-Bouyer, G., et al. (1972). Outbreaks of accidental hexachlorophene poisoning in France. *Lancet, 1*, 91.

107. MacKinnon, P.C.B. & MacKinnon, I.L. (1955). Palmar sweating in pregnancy. *J Obstet Gynaecol Br Comm, 62*, 298.

108. Marks, K.H., Friedman, Z., & Maisels, M.J. (1977). A simple device for reducing insensible water loss in low-birth-weight infants. *Pediatrics, 60*, 223.

109. McKensie, A.W. (1971). Skin disorders in pregnancy. *Practitioner, 206*, 773.

110. McManus Kuller, J. (1984). Part I: Skin development and function. *Neonat Netw, 3*, 18.

111. McManus Kuller, J., Lund, C., & Tobin, C. (1983). Improved skin care for premature infants. *MCN, 8*, 200.

112. Mechanic, H.F. & Perkins, B.A. (1988). Preventing tissue trauma. *Dimens Crit Care Nurs, 7*, 210.

113. Medline, A., et al. (1976). Pruritus of pregnancy and jaundice induced by oral contraceptives. *Am J Gastroenterol, 65*, 156.

114. Michaud, R.M., Jacobsen, D. & Dahl, M.C. (1982). Papular dermatitis of pregnancy. *Arch Dermatol, 118*, 1003.

115. Montagna, W. (1956). *The structure and function of the skin.* New York: Academic Press.

116. Montague, A. (1971). *Touching: The human significance of the skin.* New York: Columbia University Press.

117. Moore, K.L. (1988). *The developing human: Clinically oriented embryology* (4th ed.) Philadelphia: WB Saunders.

118. Moreno, A., Noguera, J. & DeMoragas, J.M. (1985). Polymorphic eruptions of pregnancy: A histopathologic study. *Acta Derm Venereol* (Stockh), *65*, 313.

119. Murphy, J.F. (1984). Drugs and pregnancy. *Ir Med J, 77*, 52.

120. Nachman, R.L. & Esterly, N.B. (1971). Increase skin permeability in preterm infants. *J Pediatr, 79*, 628.

121. Nurse, D.S. (1968). Prurigo of pregnancy. *Aust J Dermatol, 9*, 258.

122. O'Brien, D., Hansen, J., & Smith, C. (1954). Effect of supersaturated atmosphere on insensible water loss in the newborn infant. *Pediatrics, 13*, 126.

123. Oh, W. & Karecki, H. (1972). Phototherapy and insensible water loss in the newborn infant. *Am J Dis Child, 124*, 230.

124. Oh, W, et al. (1973). Peripheral circulatory response to phototherapy in newborn infants. *Acta Paediatr Scand, 62*, 49.

125. Oosterling, J., et al. (1978). Impetigo herpetiformis or generalized pustular psoriasis? *Arch Dermatol, 114*, 1527.

126. Pansky, B. (1982). *Medical embryology.* New York: Macmillan.

127. Parmley, T.H. & Seeds, A.E. (1970). Fetal skin permeability to isotopic water (DHO) in early pregnancy. *Am J Obstet Gynecol, 108*, 128.

128. Perera, P., Kurban, A.K. & Ryan, T.J. (1970). The development of the cutaneous microvascular system in the newborn. *Br J Dermatol, 83*, 186.

129. Pernoll, M.L., Benda, G.I. & Babson, S.G. (1986). *Diagnosis and management of the fetus and neonate at risk: A guide for team care.* St. Louis: CV Mosby.

130. Poidevin, L.O.S. (1959). Striae gravidarum: Their relation to adrenocortical hyperfunction. *Lancet, 2*, 436.

131. Powell, H., et al. (1973). Hexachlorophene myelinopathy in premature infants. *J Pediatr, 82*, 976.

132. Powell, F. & Powell, B. (1987). Cutaneous changes during pregnancy. *Ir Med J, 80*, 50.

133. Pritchard, J.A. & Macdonald, P.C. (1980). *Williams obstetrics* (16th ed.). New York: Appleton-Century-Crofts.

134. Prunieras, M. (1969). Interactions between keratinocytes and dendritic cells. *J Invest Dermatol, 52*, 1.

135. Pyati, SP, et al. (1977). Absorption of iodine in the neonate following topical use of providone iodine. *J Pediatr, 91*, 825.

136. Quinby, S.R., Xenias, S.J. & Perry, H.O. (1982). Herpes gestationis. *Mayo Clin Proc, 57*, 520.

137. Rapini, R.P. & Jordon, R.E. (1989). The skin and pregnancy. In R.K. Creasy & R. Resnik (Eds.), *Maternal-fetal medicine: Principles and practice* (2nd ed., pp. 1110–1121). Philadelphia: WB Saunders.

138. Rassner, G. (1983). *Atlas of dermatology* (2nd ed.). Baltimore-Munich: Urban & Schwarzenberg.

139. Rebell, G. & Kirk, D. (1962). In W. Montagna, R.A. Ellis, & A.F. Silver (Eds.), *Advances in biology of skin* (Vol 3). London: Pergamon Press.

140. Rencoret, S. & Aste, H. (1973). Jaundice during pregnancy. *Med J Aust, 1*, 167.

141. Robbins, C.R. (1988). *Chemical and physical behavior of human hair* (2nd ed.). New York: Springer-Verlag.

141a. Robson, A.M., et al. (1969). Pentachlorophenol poisoning in a nursery for newborn infants. *J Pediatr, 75*, 309.

142. Ross, M.H. & Reith, E.J. (1985). *Histology.* New York: Harper & Row.

143. Rothman, K.F. & Pochi, P. (1988). Use of oral and topical agents for acne in pregnancy. *J Am Acad Dermatol, 19*, 431.

144. Rothman, S. (1954). *Physiology and biochemistry of the skin.* Chicago: The University of Chicago Press.

145. Rutter, N. & Hull, D. (1979). Water loss from the skin of term and preterm babies. *Arch Dis Child, 54*, 858.

146. Sanchez, N.P., et al. (1981). Melasma: A clinical, light microscopic, ultrastructual and immunofluorescence study. *J Am Acad Dermatol, 4*, 698.

147. Sasseville, D., Wilinson, R.D. & Schnader, J.Y. (1981). Dermatoses of pregnancy. *Int J Dermatol, 5*, 215.

148. Sato, K, et al. (1989). Biology of sweat glands and their disorders. I. Normal sweat gland function. *J Am Acad Dermatol, 20*, 537.

149. Sauer, G.C. & Geha, B.J. (1961). Impetigo herpetiformis. *Arch Dermatol, 83*, 119.

150. Sauer, G.C. (1985). *Manual of skin diseases* (5th ed.) Philadelphia: JB Lippincott.

151. Schick, J.B. & Milstein, J.M. (1981). Burn hazard of isopropyl alcohol in the neonate. *Pediatrics, 68*. 587.

152. Schiff, B.L. & Kern, A.B. (1963). A study of postpartum alopecia. *Arch Dermatol, 87*, 609.

153. Schoenfield, L.J. (1969). The relationship of bile acids in pruritis in hepatobiliary disease. In L. Schiff, J.B. Carey, & J. Dietschy (Eds.), *Bile salt metabolism.* Springfield, IL: Charles C Thomas.

154. Scroggins, R.B. (1979). Skin changes and diseases

in pregnancy. In T.B. Fitzpatrick, et al. (Eds.), *Dermatology in general medicine* (2nd ed.). New York: McGraw-Hill.

154a. Scott, E.P., et al. (1946). Dye poisoning in infancy. *J Pediatr, 28*, 713.

155. Sedin, G., et al. (1981). Water transport though the skin of newborn infants. *Ups J Med Sci, 86*, 27.

156. Shalita, A. (1981). *Principles of infant skin care.* Skillman, N.J.: Johnson & Johnson Baby Products.

157. Shiu, M.H., et al. (1976). Adverse effect of pregnancy on melanoma. *Cancer, 37*, 181.

158. Shizuma, K. & Lerner, A.B. (1954). Determination of melanocyte-stimulating hormone in urine and blood. *J Clin Endocrinol, 14*, 1491.

159. Shornick, J.K. (1987). Herpes gestationis. *J Am Acad Dermatol, 17*, 539.

160. Shornick, J.K., et al. (1983). Herpes gestationis: Clinical and histologic features of twenty-eight cases. *J Am Acad Dermatol, 8*, 214.

161. Shuman, R.M., Leech, R.W., & Alvord, E.C. (1974). Neurotoxicity of hexachlorophene in the human: I. A clinicopathologic study of 248 children. *Pediatrics, 54*, 689.

162. Silverman, W.A. (1964). General considerations, relationship between length, weight, surface area and fetal age. In W.A. Silverman, *Dunham's premature infants* (3rd. ed.), New York: Harper & Row.

163. Simkin, B. & Arce, R. (1962). Steroid excretion in obese patients with colored abdominal striae. *N Engl J Med, 266*, 1031.

164. Sinclair, J.C. (1976). Metabolic rate and temperature control. In C.A. Smith & N.M. Nelson (Eds.), *The physiology of the newborn infant* (4th ed.). Springfield, IL: Charles C Thomas.

165. Sisson, W.R. (1954). Colored striae in adolescent children. *J Pediatr, 45*, 520.

166. Snell, R.S. & Bischitz, P.G. (1960). The effect of large doses of estrogen and progesterone on melanin pigmentation. *J Invest Dermatol, 35*, 73.

167. Snell, R.S. (1964). The pigmentary changes occurring in the breast skin during pregnancy and following estrogen treatment. *J Invest Dermatol, 43*, 181.

168. Snell, R.S. (1983). *Clinical embryology for medical students* (3rd ed.). Boston: Little, Brown.

169. Solomon, L.M. & Esterly, N.B. (1970). Neonatal dermatology. I. The newborn skin. *J Pediatr, 77*, 888.

170. Spangler, A.S., et al. (1962). Papular dermatitis of pregnancy: A new clinical entity. *JAMA, 181*, 577.

171. Stanford University Hospital, Department of Nursing Services. (1984). Policies and procedures: Skin care guidelines for the extremely premature infant (26 weeks gestation or less). *Neonat Netw, 3*, 48.

172. Storer, J. & Hawk, R. (1988). Neonatal skin disorders. In L.A. Schachner & R.C. Hansen (Eds.), *Pediatric dermatology* (Vol. 1). New York: Churchill Livingstone.

173. Swapp, G.H. & Main, R.A. (1973). Neurofibromatosis in pregnancy. *Br J Dermatol, 88*, 431.

174. Tarnowski, W.M. & Hashimoto, K. (1967). Langerhans cell granules in histiocytosis. *Arch Dermatol, 96*, 298.

175. Thody, A.J., Plummer, N.A. & Buron, J.L. (1974). Plasma beta melanocyte stimulating hormone levels in pregnancy. *J Obstet Gynaecol Br Comm, 81*, 875.

176. Uhlin, S.R. (1981). Pruritic urticarial papules and plaques of pregnancy. Involvement in mother and infant. *Arch Dermatol, 117*, 238.

177. Vasquez, M., Ibanez, M.I. & Sanchez, J.L. (1986). Pigmentary demarcation lines during pregnancy. *Cutis, 22*, 263.

178. Vorbu, J. & Baxter, J. (1974). Onset of palmar sweating in newborn infants. *Br J Dermatol, 90*, 269.

179. Wade, T.R., Wade, S.L. & Jones, H.E. (1978). Skin changes and diseases associated with pregnancy. *Obstet Gynecol, 52*, 233.

180. Weber, B.B. & Stone, K.S. (1988). Application and removal of adhesive tapes: Does it make a difference in skin repair? *Focus Crit Care, 15*, 50.

181. Weinstein, G.D. & Frost, P. (1971). Replacement kinetics. In T.B. Fitzpatrick, et al.(Eds.), *Dermatology in general medicine.* New York: McGraw, Hill, & Blakiston.

182. Weiss, S. (1979). The language of touch. *Nurs Res, 28*, 76.

183. Wenk, R.E., et al. (1981). Tetracycline-associated fatty liver of pregnancy, including possible pregnancy risk after chronic dermatologic use of tetracycline. *J Reprod Med, 26*, 135.

184. West, D., Worobec, S., & Solomon, L. (1981). Pharmacology and toxicology of infant skin. *J Invest Dermatol, 76*, 147.

185. Widdowson, E. (1968). Growth and composition of the fetus and newborn. In N. Assali (Ed.), *Biology of gestation* (Vol. 2). New York: Academic Press.

186. Wildnauer, R.H. & Kennedy, R. (1970). Transepidermal water loss of human newborns. *J Invest Dermatol, 54*, 483.

187. Williams, P.R. & Oh, W. (1974). Effects of radiant warmer on insensible water loss in newborn infants. *Am J Dis Child, 128*, 511.

188. Wilson, D.R. & Maibach, H. (1982). An in vitro comparison of skin barrier function. In H.I. Maibach & E.K. Boisits (Eds.), *Neonatal skin: Structure and function.* New York: Marcel Dekker.

189. Winton, G.B. (1989). Skin diseases aggrevated by pregnancy. *J Am Acad Dermatol, 20*, 1.

190. Winton, G.B. & Lewis, C.W. (1982). Dermatoses of pregnancy. *J Am Acad Dermatol, 6*, 977.

191. Wolff, L., Weitzel, M.H. & Fuerst, E.V. (1989). *Fundamentals of nursing* (6th ed.). New York: JB Lippincott.

192. Wong, R.C. & Ellis, C.N. (1984). Physiologic skin changes in pregnancy. *J Am Acad Dermatol, 10*, 929.

193. Wu, P.Y.K. & Hodgman, J.E. (1974). Insensible water loss in preterm infants: Change with postnatal development and non-ionizing radiant energy. *Pediatrics, 54*, 704.

194. Wu, P.Y.K. (1982). Phototherapy: In vivo side effects. *Perinatol Neonatol, 6*, 21.

195. Zweymuller, E. & Preining, O. (1970). The insensible water loss of the newborn infant. *Acta Paediatr Scand* (Suppl.), *205*, 7.

CHAPTER 12

The Neuromuscular and Sensory Systems

Maternal Physiologic Adaptations
   The Antepartum Period
      Ocular Changes
      Otolaryngeal Changes
      Musculoskeletal Changes
      Sleep
   The Intrapartum Period
   The Postpartum Period
Clinical Implications for the Pregnant Woman and Her Fetus
   Ocular Adaptations
   Musculoskeletal Discomforts
   Headache
   The Pregnant Woman with a Chronic Neurologic Disorder
      The Pregnant Woman with Epilepsy
   Peripheral Neuropathies
   The Woman with a Spinal Cord Transection
   The Woman with a Brain or Spinal Cord Tumor
   Cerebral Vascular Disorders
   Pregnancy-Induced Hypertension
Development of the Neuromuscular and Sensory Systems in the Fetus
   Anatomic Development
      Embryonic Development
      Common Anomalies of the Central Nervous System

      Fetal Neurodevelopment
      Development of Specific Systems
   Functional Development
Neonatal Physiology
   Transitional Events
   Neural Connections and Conduction of Impulses
   Circulation in the Neonatal Brain
   Neonatal Sensory Function
   Neonatal Motor Function
   Sleep-Wake Pattern
   Neurobehavioral Organization
Clinical Implications For Neonatal Care
   Risks Posed by the Caregiving Environment
   Vulnerability to Hypoxia and Pressure-Related Injury
      Intraventricular and Periventricular Hemorrhage
      Periventricular Leukomalacia
      Hypoxic-Ischemic Encephalopathy
   Neonatal Seizures
   Neonatal Pain
   Effects of Drug Exposure In Utero
Maturational Changes During Infancy and Childhood

The neuromuscular and sensory systems are two of the most complex systems in the human body. Normal function of the central nervous system (CNS) is critical for functioning of individual organs and integration of organ systems to achieve coordinated physiologic and neurobehavioral processes. Alterations in neuromuscular and sensory processes during pregnancy give rise to common experiences such as musculoskeletal discomforts, sleep disturbances, and alterations in sensation. Discomforts and pain during the antepartum, intrapartum, and postpartum periods influence maternal adaptations and the course of labor. Newborn and particularly preterm infants must respond to the extrauterine environment with neuromuscular and sensory systems that are still immature. Neurologic dysfunction during the neonatal period due to insults before, during, or after birth can affect the infant's ability to survive the perinatal and neonatal periods and has implications for later developmental and cognitive outcome. This chapter first examines physiologic adaptations in the mother and implications for healthy pregnant women and those with chronic health problems, and then discusses neurodevelopmental processes and clinical implications for the fetus and newborn.

MATERNAL PHYSIOLOGIC ADAPTATIONS

During pregnancy the neurologic and sensory systems are influenced by the altered hormonal milieu and by alterations in other systems. The effects of these changes on the sensory system are well documented. Many of the hormones of pregnancy have CNS activity, although their specific effects on neurologic function are not as well understood as their effects on other body systems. As a result, there is little known about specific changes in the function of the neurologic system, other than effects on endocrine glands (see Chapters 1 and 4 and Unit III), during pregnancy. During the intrapartum period maternal physiologic and psychological responses are altered by the discomfort and pain of labor. These responses can have a significant impact on fetus homeostasis in addition to having important implications for management of the woman in labor.

The Antepartum Period

This section examines specific alterations during pregnancy in ocular and otolaryngeal function, sleep, and the musculoskeletal system. The hormonal changes of early pregnancy may also play a role in the mood swings and emotional lability characteristic of this period.

Ocular Changes

The eyes of the pregnant woman undergo several alterations throughout gestation that result from physiologic and hormonal adaptations. The pregnant woman develops a mild corneal edema, particularly during the third trimester. The cornea becomes slightly thicker, which along with the fluid retention, changes its topography and may slightly alter the refractory power of the eye. Corneal hyposensitivity also develops during this period, probably because of the increased thickness and fluid retention.[124, 126, 135, 191] A few women experience an increase in corneal epithelia pigmentation (known as Krukenberg's spindles), possibly secondary to increases in estrogens, progesterone, adrenocorticotropic hormone (ACTH), and melanocyte stimulating hormone.[191] The composition of tears changes slightly with an increase in secretion of lysozyme.[126]

Intraocular pressure falls, especially during the second half of gestation.[12, 87] This change is believed to be due to the effects of progesterone, relaxin, and human chorionic gonadotropin combined with an increase in aqueous outflow and decreased episcleral pressure.[178, 191] Similar findings have been reported for women on oral contraceptives.[96] Changes in intraocular pressure are independent of changes in systemic blood pressure.[148]

Ptosis occasionally develops for unknown reasons.[126] Ptosis may also occur as a complication of lumbar anesthesia, either as an isolated finding or as part of Horner's syndrome. Horner's syndrome is characterized by ptosis, miosis, and anhidrosis secondary to interruption of sympathetic innervation.[159, 191] Some women experience an increased pigmentation of the face and lids known as chloasma (see Chapter 11).

During pregnancy there is a progressive decrease in blood flow to the conjunctiva that is most marked in women with pregnancy-induced hypertension, with spasm and ischemia.[10] In these women changes in the conjunctival vessels may occur earlier than in the retinal vessels.[104, 191] Subconjunctival hemorrhages may occur spontaneously during pregnancy or in labor with spontaneous resolution.

Otolaryngeal Changes

Changes in the ear, nose, and larynx are related to modifications in fluid dynamics and vascular permeability, increased protein synthesis, vasomotor alterations of the autonomic nervous system, and increased vascularity, along with hormonal (especially estrogen) influences.[109] As a result of these alterations the nasal mucosa becomes congested and hyperemic. The pregnant woman experiences nasal stuffiness and obstruction associated with serous rhinorrhea or postnasal discharge. These symptoms usually begin in the second trimester and parallel increasing estrogen levels.[82] The symptoms may interfere with sleep and the sense of smell. Vascular congestion may result in epistaxis from rupture of superficial blood vessels. Prolonged use of topical sympathomimetic nasal sprays should be avoided because they cause rebound congestion.[109]

The pregnant woman may also complain of ear stuffiness or blocked ears unrelieved by swallowing. This change is believed to result from estrogen-induced changes in mucous membranes of the eustachian tube, edema of the nasopharynx, and alterations in fluid dynamics and pressures of the middle ear.[82, 109] There may be a transient, mild hearing loss and an increased risk of serous effusion. Management is usually supportive.

Laryngeal changes during pregnancy are hormonally induced and include erythema and edema of the vocal cords accompanied by vascular dilation and small submucosal hemorrhages.[82] The woman may note hoarseness, deepening, or cracking of the voice, persistent cough, or other vocal changes. Laryngeal changes can complicate administration of endotracheal anesthesia (see Chapter 7). Similar changes are reported in women premenstrually and with progesterone-dominated oral contraceptives.[82]

Musculoskeletal Changes

Pregnancy is characterized by changes in posture and gait. Relaxin and progesterone affect the cartilage and connective tissue of the sacroiliac joints and the symphysis pubis. This increases the mobility of these joints and leads to the characteristic "waddle" gait of pregnancy. Distention of the abdomen with growth of the infant tilts the pelvis forward, shifting the center of gravity. The woman compensates by developing an increased curvature (lordosis) of the spine that may strain muscles and ligaments of the back. Stretching and decreased tone of the abdominal muscles also contribute to the lordosis. Diastasis of the rectus abdominis muscles in the third trimester may persist after delivery. Breast tenderness, heaviness, tingling, and occasionally pain occur by 6 weeks. These changes are due to estrogens, progesterone, human placental lactogen (hPL), increased blood volume, and venous stasis.

Sleep

Sleep patterns are altered during pregnancy and the postpartum period. Sleep is divided into rapid eye movement (REM) and non-rapid eye movement (NREM) sleep, which is subdivided into four stages. The pregnant woman has increased REM sleep from 25 weeks, peaking at 33 to 36 weeks, then decreasing to nonpregnant levels by term.[21] Alterations in NREM sleep with an increase in stage I (sleep latency or transition between wakefulness and sleep) and a decrease in stage IV (delta sleep or deep sleep stage) during late pregnancy have also been noted.[94] The decrease in stage IV NREM sleep has implications for the pregnant woman's functioning, since this stage is important for basic biologic processes such as tissue repair and recovery from fatigue.[111a] During the first trimester total sleep time increases as does napping. By second half of gestation pregnant women had less overall sleep time and more night awakenings than nonpregnant women. During pregnancy night awakenings are often associated with nocturia, dyspnea, heartburn, nasal congestion, muscle aches, stress, and anxiety and can lead to sleep disturbances and insomnia. Sleep medications should be avoided because these drugs alter the physiologic mechanisms of sleep by suppressing REM and NREM stages 3 and 4 and may cross the placenta to the fetus.

The Intrapartum Period
Pain and Discomfort During Labor

The woman in labor experiences two types of pain: visceral pain and somatic pain. Visceral pain is related to contraction of the uterus and dilation and stretching of the cervix. Uterine pain during the first stage of labor results from ischemia caused by constriction and contraction of the arteries supplying the myometrium. Somatic pain is caused by pressure of the presenting part on the birth canal, vulva, and perineum. Visceral pain is experienced primarily during the first stage of labor, somatic pain is experienced during transition and the second stage.

Pain from uterine contractions and dilation of the cervix during the first stage of labor is transmitted by afferent fibers to the sympathetic chain of the posterior spinal cord at T10, T11 to T12, and L1. In early labor, pain is transmitted primarily to T11 to T12.[57, 177] As activation of peripheral A delta and C nerve fibers of these nerve terminals by kinin-like substances released from the uterine and cervical tissues intensifies, transmission spreads to T10 and L1. Pain during the first stage may be referred; that is, the nerve impulses from the uterus and cervix stimulate spinal cord neurons innervating both the uterus and the abdominal wall. As a result the woman experiences pain over the abdominal wall between the umbilicus and symphysis pubis, around the iliac crests to the gluteal area, radiating down the thighs, and in the lumbar and sacral regions.[177] During transition and the second stage pain impulses from distention of the birth canal, vulva, and perineum by the presenting part are transmitted by the pudendal nerves through posterior roots of the parasympathetic chain at S2, S3, and S4.

As the A delta and C nerve fibers enter the spinal cord, they synapse and ascend to the brain stem by the spinothalamic system. The pain impulses entering the brain stimulate a variety of neurons including cortical neurons and those of the reticular formation and the thalamic nuclei of the brain stem. The result is a the conscious sensation of pain as well as a variety of ventilatory, circulatory, and metabolic responses.[1, 177] These responses, which include increases in ventilation, cardiac output, peripheral resistance, gastric acid secretion, metabolic rate, oxygen consumption, and catecholamine release, are discussed further in Chapters 6, 7, and 9 and Unit III.

The perception of pain is influenced by physiologic, psychological, and cultural factors. Pain can lead to anxiety and influence maternal physiologic responses and the course of labor. For example, physical manifestations of anxiety may include muscular tension, hyperventilation, increased sympathetic activity, and norepinephrine release, which can lead to increased cardiac output, blood pressure, metabolic rate, and oxygen consumption, and impaired uterine contractility (Fig. 12–1).[92a] Anxiety can also increase fear and tension, reducing pain tolerance which further decreases uterine contractility.[92a] Relaxation techniques such as progressive muscle relaxation, touch, breathing, imagery, and autosuggestion help reduce anxiety and prevent or stop this cycle.[92a]

The gate control theory postulates that nervous stimuli can be inhibited at the level

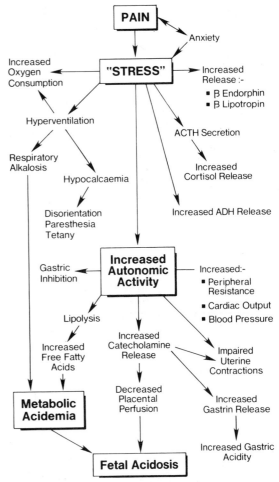

FIGURE 12–1. Physiologic changes secondary to pain in labor. (From Brownridge, P. & Cohen, S. (1988). Neural blockade for obstetric and gynecologic surgery. In M.J. Cousins & P.O. Bridenbaugh (Eds.), *Neural blockade* (2nd ed., p. 600). Philadelphia: J.B. Lippincott.)

of the substantia gelatinosa and dorsal horn of the spinal cord from reaching the thalamus and cerebral cortex (Fig. 12–2):

> ... the theory proposes that a neural mechanism in the dorsal horns of the spinal cord acts like a gate which can increase or decrease the flow of nerve impulses from peripheral fibres to the central nervous system. Somatic input is therefore subjected to the modulating influence of the gate before it evokes pain perception and response. The degree to which the gate increases or decreases sensory transmission is determined by the relative activity in large-diameter (A-beta) and small diameter (A-delta and C) fibres and by descending influences from the brain. When the amount of information that passes through the gate exceeds a critical level, it activates the neural areas responsible for pain experience and response.[125, p.222]

Techniques to close the gate (inhibit) include stimulation of large nerve fibers to block impulses from the smaller pain fibers. This provides a basis for use of massage and effleurage during labor. With continued use of these techniques, the large nerve fibers become habituated and stimuli from smaller fibers are no longer blocked. Thus, as labor progresses the woman needs to stimulate other fibers (heat, pressure with change of position, massage of other areas). Since descending fibers may also inhibit transmission to the brain, concentration techniques may also be useful.[92a]

Endorphins

Pain during the intrapartum period may be modulated by endogenous opiate peptides such as β-endorphin and enkephalins. These substances alter the release of neurotransmitters from afferent nerves and interfere with efferent pathways from the spinal cord to the brain.[57] Thus, within the spinal cord pain signals may be blocked at the level of the dorsal horns and never transmitted to the brain. Maternal plasma β-endorphin levels increase during pregnancy and are significantly elevated during late pregnancy and labor in both humans and animals.[57, 64, 173] Maximum levels are found during parturition and decrease post partum. Endorphin release may be stimulated by stress as an adaptive response. Endorphins may increase the pain threshold, are associated with feelings of euphoria and analgesia, and may enable the woman to tolerate the pain of labor and delivery. Experimental intrathecal administration of β-endorphin to women during the intrapartum period has been associated with pain relief.[64] The specific role of β-endorphins in the pregnant woman and during labor and delivery is unknown.

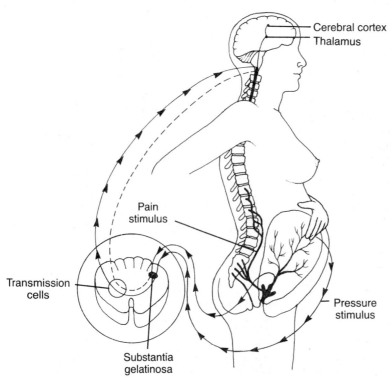

FIGURE 12–2. Schematic diagram of the gate-control theory. The diagram shows the route of the uterine pain impulse as it travels to the spinal cord where, in the substantia gelatinosa (see insert of enlarged vertebra), it is blocked by the large-fiber stimulation provided by the woman's hand massaging her abdomen. The dotted line indicates the path the pain impulse would have taken had the gate been open. (From Jimenez, S.L.M. (1983). Application of the body's natural pain relief mechanisms to reduce discomfort in labor and delivery. *NAACOG Update Series, 1*(1), 3. The NAACOG Update Series is a program sponsored by NAACOG and published by CPEC, Inc.)

Cerebral cortex
Thalamus
Pain stimulus
Transmission cells
Pressure stimulus
Substantia gelatinosa

The increased levels of β-endorphins during labor may contribute to the decreased doses of anesthetic drugs required in pregnancy.[57] The variable decreased in dose of local anesthetics for epidural and spinal blocks are also caused by vascular congestion within the spinal canal and progesterone as well as the altered neuronal sensitivity.[57] Increased progesterone levels also contribute to the decreased doses of inhalation anesthetics through their impact on the respiratory system (see Chapter 7).

The Postpartum Period

During the postpartum period the ocular and otolaryngeal changes resolve as the physiologic and hormonal adaptations of pregnancy are reversed. Sensitivity of the cornea returns to usual parameters by 6 to 8 weeks post partum.[124, 126, 135, 191] Intraocular pressure returns to prepregnancy levels by 2 months post partum.[12, 87] Both ptosis and subconjunctival hemorrhages disappear spontaneously.[126] Nasal congestion, ear stuffiness, and laryngeal changes and related discomforts also disappear within a few days after delivery.[132]

Headaches, generally bilateral and frontal, are a common discomfort in the first week after delivery. Postpartum headaches tend to begin around the time of postpartum weight loss and have been attributed to alterations in fluid and electrolyte balance.[61, 172]

Sleep During the Postpartum Period

Sleep is also altered during the immediate postpartum period. Most of these changes normalize by 2 weeks post partum.[21] Stage I NREM sleep is longer immediately after birth. Stage IV NREM sleep is longer immediately after birth than before birth, with a gradual increase to normal levels by about 2 weeks. REM sleep is decreased and awake time increased on the 1st postpartum night, with a reversal of these findings by 3 days.[94, 95] These changes are probably related to the initial euphoria and discomfort after childbirth, followed by fatigue and restoration. Postpartum women have less overall sleep time and more night awakenings than nonpregnant women. These night awakenings are often associated with urination, discomfort, activity by roommates or nursing staff, and infant feeding. Opportunities for restorative sleep after delivery and during the first postpartum night are often impeded by the environment and interruptions for nursing care activities.[111a] Sleep medications alter sleep physiology, suppress REM sleep and NREM stages 3 and 4 and thus should be avoided.

Newborn rooming-in does not appear to significantly alter the total amount of maternal sleep. Keefe[97] found that mothers whose babies were in the nursery slept slightly less than mothers whose infants roomed in. The mothers in the rooming-in group also reported a slightly better quality of sleep.

Postpartum Discomfort

During the first few days to week of the postpartum period the woman may experience considerable discomfort. The discomfort and pain can arise from a variety of sources, including the episiotomy, lacerations, perineal trauma, incisions, uterine contractions after delivery (afterpains), hemorrhoids, breast engorgement, and nipple tenderness. Breast engorgement initially occurs in both the lactating and nonlactating woman because of stasis and distention of the vascular and lymphatic circulations. In the breast-feeding woman, secondary engorgement occurs because of distention of the breast with milk as lactation is established. Alterations in comfort not only cause physical and emotional stress but can also interfere with the ability of the woman to interact with and care for her infant.

Postpartum Blues

Many women experience a transient, mild depression in the first few days to weeks post partum commonly known as the "postpartum blues" or "baby blues." The postpartum blues are characterized by mild to moderate depression and labile emotions, with feelings of anxiety, tearfulness, irritability, restlessness, headaches, forgetfulness, fatigue, loneliness, mood swings, sleep disturbances, and an inability to concentrate. These feelings are experienced by 50 to 80% of women during the first 2 weeks after delivery and are not indicative of underlying pathologic processes.[80] It is important that the mother's feelings be recognized, however, and needed support be provided. The "blues" are generally self-limiting and transient. They most often begin on the 3rd or 4th day after delivery and usually peak by 5 to 10 days.[92b] Similar feelings are seen across different cultures.[61, 78]

The cause of postpartum blues is unknown. The rapid physiologic and hormonal alterations after birth, such as the decrease in estrogen, progesterone, and alterations in blood electrolytes and monamines such as tryptophan and other chemistries; increased cortisol; changes in fluid dynamics and body weight; transient thyroid dysfunction (see Chapter 16) and a transient mild hyperparathyroidism with a slight change in serum calcium levels are believed to have an effect on maternal affect.[61] In addition, cyclic adenosine monophosphate (cAMP), a second messenger in many hormonal interactions, is elevated post partum.[13] Others suggest that postpartum blues is a response to the stress of childbirth or a normal developmental process to release anxiety and tension associated with childbirth and mothering. Postpartum blues have also been related to a variety of background, social, environmental; and psychological factors.[92b] Postpartum depression occurs in a smaller percentage of women (3 to 28%); postpartum psychosis is rare (1.1 to 4 per 1000 deliveries).[92b] These disorders are more serious complications with potentially long term consequences.

CLINICAL IMPLICATIONS FOR THE PREGNANT WOMAN AND HER FETUS

Changes in the neurologic, sensory, and musculoskeletal systems may result in common alterations and discomforts of pregnancy such as backache and contact lens intolerance. In addition, the physiologic and hormonal changes of pregnancy, along with mechanical forces during pregnancy, labor, and delivery can lead to specific neurologic disorders in the pregnant woman. These disorders are primarily peripheral neuropathies and compression/entrapment disorders that arise late in gestation or during the intrapartum and postpartum periods. The usual physiologic and hormonal changes of pregnancy can also alter the course of preexisting neurologic disorders such as epilepsy, myasthenia gravis, and migraine headaches. Finally, pregnancy may occasionally be associated with development of a disorder

(multiple sclerosis) or the initial presentation of symptoms (brain tumors, arteriovenous malformations) that can affect both the woman and her infant.

Ocular Adaptations

Although ocular alterations during pregnancy generally do not have major clinical significance, they can result in minor discomforts, particularly for women who wear contact lenses. These women may be unable to tolerate their lenses and may occasionally develop corneal edema. The basis for this intolerance is believed to be retention of water by the cornea, changes in the composition of tears, and alterations in corneal topography.[191] Changes in tear composition can make the contact lenses feel greasy shortly after insertion and cause blurring of vision.[126] Alterations in refractory power along with occasional transient insufficiency of accommodation can cause difficulty in reading and in near vision or blurred vision in someone who is farsighted.[126, 178] These alterations resolve in the postpartum period. New prescriptions for glasses or contact lenses should be delayed until several weeks after delivery. Cycloplegic and mydriatic agents used for routine eye examinations should be avoided unless they are needed to evaluate retinal disease. These agents can cross the placenta or have systemic effects in the mother that affect the fetus.[178]

Women with specific disorders such as pregnancy-induced hypertension (PIH) and diabetes mellitus may have ocular complications associated with their disease process. PIH is associated with vasospasm of the conjunctival vessels and narrowing of the retinal arterioles. The latter may progress to severe arteriolar spasm, multiple retinal hemorrhages, retinal hemorrhage, and in severe disease, retinal detachment. Mild to moderate visual disturbances are most common; severe or complete loss of vision is rare.[178]

For many years it was believed that pregnancy significantly influenced the onset and progression of diabetic retinopathy, and pregnancy was discouraged for these women. It now appears that development and progression of retinopathy in both pregnant and nonpregnant women is more closely correlated with the duration of the disorder, severity of the diabetes, and degree of glycemic control. The pregnant diabetic, particularly those with proliferative retinopathy, demonstrates deterioration related to the metabolic and hormonal changes of pregnancy. Although remission usually occurs over the first 6 months post partum, many women, especially those with preexisting retinopathy, do not experience complete return to their prepregnant status.[50, 127, 161]

Since intraocular pressure falls during pregnancy, the pregnant women with glaucoma may experience an improvement with a decreased need for medications.[87, 178, 191] This has an additional advantage of reducing fetal exposure to these agents.[101] Many ocular inflammatory disorders improve during pregnancy, possibly because of increased cortisol and other glucocorticosteriods, with exacerbation post partum.[191]

Any symptoms of eye infections in the pregnant woman must be assessed, since some sexually transmitted organisms, including herpes simplex virus and chlamydia, may cause concurrent ocular infections. The presence of these organisms can have adverse consequences for the neonate if the mother also has an genital infection. For example, chlamydia can cause conjunctivitis and pneumonia in the newborn. Treatment of maternal ocular disorders during pregnancy should be done cautiously and with attention paid to the possible effects of the medication on the fetus. Even topical eye ointments must be used with caution because they can be absorbed systemically and cross the placenta to the fetus.[178] If these agents must be used, nasolacrimal occlusion after instillation may reduce systemic absorption.[101]

Musculoskeletal Discomforts

The pregnant woman may experience discomfort or pain associated with breast changes or stretching of the round ligament with growth of the uterus, pressure of the uterus nerve roots, or pressure of the presenting part on the perineum. The latter type of pain is most prominent close to the onset of labor and is aggravated by vascular engorgement of these tissues. Increased joint mobility can result in muscle and ligament strain and discomfort.

Many pregnant women experience backache during pregnancy caused by exaggeration of the lumbar lordotic curve due to shifting of the center of gravity, weight gain, and relaxation of ligaments, or from muscle spasm due to pressure on nerve roots.[12] Backache occurs most commonly after the 5th

month of pregnancy, although high backache earlier may result from breast alterations.[47, 115] Approximately 15% of these women experience severe back pain, peaking in intensity during the evening and night, and localized to the lower back or sacroiliac region. Recommendations include avoiding anything that increases the lordosis (e.g., high-heeled shoes), application of local heat, use of a firm mattress or bed board, pelvic tilt exercise, aerobic exercise such as swimming, and conditioning before subsequent pregnancies.[12, 47] Backache, round ligament pain, or other discomfort should be assessed to distinguish "normal" discomfort from other processes such as preterm labor.

The incidence of prolapsed intervertebral disc is increased during pregnancy and the immediate postpartum period, probably because of postural changes and an increase in mechanical stress.[10] The most frequently affected areas are the fifth lumbar and first sacral nerve roots. Management usually involves bed rest.[12]

During the third trimester, the woman may experience numbness and tingling of the arms, fingers, legs, and toes. Paresthesia of the upper extremities may be caused by marked lordosis along with anterior flexion of the neck and slumping of the shoulders, placing traction on the brachial, ulnar, and median nerves. In the legs and toes paresthesia may be caused by pressure of the uterus on the blood vessels and nerves supplying the lower extremities.[129] Painful legs are experienced by many pregnant women and arise either from the mechanical effects of the uterus or secondary to systemic alterations (Table 12–1).[110] These causes must be differentiated from thromboembolitic disorders, which are also more prevalent during pregnancy (see Chapter 5). Leg cramps during the last few months of gestation are common. These cramps may be related to alterations in calcium and phosphorus metabolism (see Chapter 14) or to pressure of the enlarged uterus on pelvic blood vessels or nerves supplying the lower extremities.

Restless Legs Syndrome

Restless legs syndrome is an idiopathic disorder seen in 10 to 11% of pregnant women.[52, 119] This syndrome is often mistaken for leg cramps, and neuromuscular findings may be similar to those associated with excess caffeine consumption.[47] Restless legs syn-

TABLE 12–1
Effects of Pregnancy on the Legs: Factors That May Result in Painful Legs

Mechanical effects of the gravid uterus
    Compression of the inferior vena cava and iliac veins, especially when supine
    Altered gait and posture
Systemic effects of pregnancy
    Relaxation of cartilage and collagen; reduced pelvic girdle stability; altered gait and posture
    Reduced concentration of serum albumin causing increased colloid osmotic pressure and dependent edema
    Increased concentrations of clotting factors VII, VIII, IX, X*
    Diminished activity of antithrombin III*
    Alterations in endocrine mileau: does estrogen decrease production of tissue plasminogen factor?*
    Physiologic hyperventilation and hypocapnia
    Alteration in calcium and phosphorus metabolism and diet
Iatrogenic effects of pregnancy
    Lithotomy position with pressure problems secondary to stirrups
    Operative delivery

*Increases risk of thromboembolitic disorders.
From Lee, R.V., McComb, L.E., & Mezzardi, F.C. (1990). Pregnant patients, painful legs: The obstetrician's dilemma. *Obstet Gynecol Surv, 45,* 290.

drome usually occurs 10 to 20 minutes after the woman gets into bed. It is characterized by a ". . . creeping, wormy, burning ache [that] develops within their legs. The more the urge to allow the legs to fidget is resisted, the greater the urge becomes until it can no longer be withstood."[47, p.485] This transient disorder generally appears after 20 weeks and disappears shortly after delivery.[52, 119] The neurologic examination is negative.

The cause of restless legs syndrome is unknown. It may be related to the hormonal changes of pregnancy. If the woman is iron deficient, improvement in the symptoms of restless legs syndrome may occur with treatment of the anemia. Women who are supplemented with folic acid have been reported to be less likely to develop this disorder.[19] Restless legs syndrome may also be associated with polyneuropathy and vascular insufficiency. Usually no treatment is indicated, although if the disorder is severe, low doses of clonazepam may be used.[47] Walking may relieve some symptoms.

Chorea Gravidarum

Chorea gravidarum is a disorder involving rapid, brief, nonrhythmical, involuntary, jerky movements of the limbs and nonpatterned facial grimacing.[44] Mild cases may involve only persistent restlessness and clumsiness.[10] This disorder is seen both in pregnancy (incidence of 1 in 139,000) and in women on oral contraceptives.[10, 44, 47] Symptoms are most prominent in primiparas and during early pregnancy, late in the third trimester, and immediately post partum. Approximately 30% of women with this disorder become asymptomatic by term; the remainder become symptomatic shortly after delivery.[44] About one-third of women with this disorder are asymptomatic in the third trimester. The reason for this is unknown. A recurrence rate of 20% has been reported with subsequent pregnancies.[10]

The cause of chorea gravidarum is unknown, although it is related to streptococcal infection and is most common in woman with a history of rheumatic fever or heart disease.[10] This disorder has also been related to hormonal changes during pregnancy or contraceptive use, since estrogen can stimulate postsynaptic dopamine receptors (inhibitory transmitters with effects in the motor cortex and basal ganglia).[47] Chorea gravidarum may have a hematologic or immunologic basis. Changes in these systems during pregnancy may exacerbate a preexisting basal ganglia disturbance.[10] There are no fetal effects reported.

Headache

The most common form of headache during pregnancy is caused by muscular contraction or tension.[12] This type of headache is characterized by a persistent band-like or vise-like pain extending from the base of the neck to the forehead. The woman often notices the headache on awakening, with worsening of symptoms during the evening.[10, 12] The discomfort may be aggravated by postural changes or stress. Headaches during pregnancy may also be due to hormonal influences, eye strain secondary to ocular changes, nasal congestion, emotional tension, muscle spasm, fatigue, altered cerebral fluid dynamics, or mild respiratory alkalosis. Since headaches may also be a symptom of disorders such as PIH, however, any pregnant woman complaining of headaches must be carefully evaluated. Management includes massaging neck and shoulder muscles, application of heat or ice to the neck, rest, warm baths, and minimal use of simple analgesics.[44, 47] Sedatives and hypnotics are not recommended for routine use in pregnant or lactating women since they are ineffective and metabolites cross the placenta and the blood–milk barrier and are slowly excreted by the fetus.[12]

Migraine Headaches

Migraine headaches occur in 5 to 10% of the general population.[62] Migraines are more common in women and often occur with menses, with the initial development of migraine headaches associated with onset of menses. Migraines may also occur for the first time during the first 2 to 3 months post partum. Although the frequency of headaches decreases with age, migraines may flare up or start with menopause.[44, 117] Headaches are also more frequent and severe in women on oral contraceptives, especially pills with higher estrogen content.[10]

Both classic and common migrane are both vascular headaches caused by cerebral vasodilation and cranial artery dilation. The severe throbbing during the initial phases is attributed to intense cerebral vasoconstriction with subsequent vasodilation.[44] Classic migraine is seen most frequently and is characterized by 20 to 30 minutes of sensorimotor prodromal symptoms followed by a severe unilateral headache accompanied by nausea. The prodromal symptoms usually involve visual phenomena, but may also include aphasia, hemiplegia, and paresthesia. Common migraine is unilateral less often and not associated with prodromal symptoms.

During pregnancy approximately 80% of women with a history of migraine headaches experience complete remission or decreased frequency.[12] This change is particularly notable in women with a history of menstrual migraine (i.e., migraine associated with estrogen withdrawal).[62, 167] A small number of women will experience their first migraine during pregnancy, however, usually during the first trimester.[44] Remission during pregnancy is most prominent during the second half of pregnancy. Migraines usually return within a few hours or days after delivery or with the first postpregnancy menses.[117]

The basis for remission of migraine headaches during pregnancy is unclear. Migraines are associated with periods of estrogen withdrawal such as menses or menopause and pregnancy, which involves changes in estrogen and progesterone levels and patterns of circulating estrogens.[10] Although the cause of migraines is unknown, migraines have been attributed to estrogen deficiency, excessive gonadotropins, fluid and salt retention, and increased red blood cell (RBC) mass.[117] Thus, migraine remission during pregnancy may be related to changes in estrogen, progesterone, and aldosterone or to hematologic and cardiovascular alterations.

Classic migraine headaches are often treated with ergot alkaloids. Since these compounds have oxytocic properties, they are generally not used during pregnancy because of the risk of preterm labor. Analgesics and antiemetic suppositories are used for symptomatic relief. Propranolol has been used as a prophylactic treatment for frequent migraines, but its use is controversial since this drug has been associated with altered fetal growth and fetal and neonatal β-adrenergic blockade and subsequent decreased responsiveness to stress during asphyxia.[10, 47, 117]

The Pregnant Woman with a Chronic Neurologic Disorder

The physiologic and hormonal changes of pregnancy can influence the course of chronic neurologic and neuromuscular disorders such as epilepsy, myasthenia gravis, and multiple sclerosis. These disorders also have ramifications for the health and well-being of the mother and her infant. The pregnant woman with epilepsy is discussed below. The implications of selected neurologic and neuromuscular disorders during pregnancy are summarized in Table 12–2.

The Pregnant Woman with Epilepsy

Epilepsy is one of the most common neurologic disorders seen in pregnant women. The incidence of epilepsy in pregnancy is 0.3 to 0.6%.[16] Donaldson states that the goal in managing the pregnant epileptic is to keep the mother free of seizures and to minimize the effects of epilepsy on both the pregnant woman and fetus, including fetal teratogenic effects.[47]

EFFECTS OF PREGNANCY ON EPILEPSY
The effect of pregnancy on the course of epilepsy is variable and unpredictable.[10] The frequency of seizures may increase (40%), decrease (10%) or stay the same (50%).[37] Epilepsy may appear for the first time during pregnancy or reappear after many seizure-free years.[10] In general, the longer the woman has been seizure-free before preg-

TABLE 12–2
Implications for the Pregnant Woman and Her Infant of Selected Neurologic and Neuromuscular Disorders

DISORDER/BASIS	IMPLICATIONS FOR THE PREGNANT WOMAN	IMPLICATIONS FOR THE FETUS/ NEONATE
Myasthenia Gravis Autoimmune disorder involving IgG antibody against acetylcholine receptors on striated muscle. Reduction of available acetylcholine postsynaptic receptors at the neuromuscular junction. Results in muscular weakness and fatigue.	May improve, worsen, stay the same (and effects are variable with each pregnancy). Most often exacerbates in first trimester, improves in second and third trimesters possibly due to effects of blocking of IgG antibodies by immunologic changes of pregnancy (see Chapter 10) or alpha–fetoprotein. Increased frequency of exacerbation in first few months post partum. No effect on smooth muscle/ myometrium so labor is not prolonged, although the woman may have difficulty with expulsive efforts. Avoid use of muscle relaxants; magnesium sulfate for PIH (can lead to apnea as hypermagnesemia inhibits release of acetylcholine); inhalation anesthetics and narcotics (since these pregnant women tend to hypoventilate if they have a bulbar muscle weakness); procaine and congeners if on pyridostigmine or neostigmine, which inhibit hydrolysis of the former drugs and can result in seizures (can use lidocaine); extensive regional blocks (may compromise respiration); and azathioprine owing to potential teratogenic effects.	Fetal myasthenia gravis does not occur, possibly due to blocking of the IgG antibody by alpha– fetoprotein 10 to 12% of neonates develop transient myasthenia gravis due to passage of maternal IgG antibody against the acetylcholine receptors of striated muscle (see Chapter 10). Symptoms appear within 72 hours of birth and resolve spontaneously in 2 to 6 weeks. Often feed poorly, are hypotonic, and are at risk for respiratory difficulty and aspiration. Many infants require anticholinesterase therapy and some will need assisted ventilation.
Myotonic Dystrophy Progressive autosomal dominant disorder that appears as a congenital form (possibly requiring an additional maternally transmitted factor) or, more commonly, with onset in young adulthood. Muscular weakness and myotonia affecting both striated and smooth muscle including the myometrium.	Muscular weakness and myotonia may worsen, often in the second half of pregnancy (possibly due to effects of progesterone on cell membranes). Delayed gut motility with increased constipation in pregnancy. Increased risk of spontaneous and habitual abortion, and preterm labor. Abnormal uterine contractions, prolonged first stage, poor voluntary expulsive efforts in second stage, poor involution with postpartum hemorrhage. Avoid use of inhalation anesthetics (often hypoventilate with chronic respiratory acidosis) and depolarizing muscle relaxants (succinylcholine) that can cause myotonic spasms and hyperthermia.	Presence of maternal disorder does not affect infant per se. If fetus has inherited myotonic muscular dystrophy, severe fetal and neonatal myotonia may occur. Fetal effects may include poor swallowing with hydramnios and arthrogryposis from inactivity; neonates may have respiratory distress and feeding problems.

TABLE 12–2
Implications for the Pregnant Woman and Her Infant of Selected Neurologic and
Neuromuscular Disorders Continued

DISORDER/BASIS	IMPLICATIONS FOR THE PREGNANT WOMAN	IMPLICATIONS FOR THE FETUS/ NEONATE
Multiple Sclerosis Multifocal CNS demyelinating disorder of unknown cause. Onset in early adulthood with unpredictable exacerbations and remissions over many years with increasing disability.	Rate of relapses decreases with each trimester, possibly owing to immunosuppressant effects of alpha-fetoprotein. 3-fold increase in relapses in first 3 to 6 months post partum. Usually minimal effect on course of pregnancy or incidence of complications. May experience worsening of bowel and bladder problems and urinary tract infection; for paraplegic or quadriplegic, care and risks similar to those for woman with spinal cord transection.	None reported

Compiled from references 10, 12, 15, 16, 17, 44, 47, 90, 99, 102, 131, 149, 179, 190, and 195.

nancy, the greater the likelihood that she will not develop seizures during pregnancy.[16, 38, 47] The risk of seizures during pregnancy is also increased with women who are noncompliant with their medical therapy.[160] Although the effect of pregnancy on the epilepsy may vary with each pregnancy, the woman usually returns to her prepregnant pattern after delivery.[146]

The course of epilepsy is affected by the hormonal and physiologic changes of pregnancy, as well as psychological stress. Estrogens and progesterone alter seizure thresholds, estrogens by activating seizure foci and progesterone by dampening activity. These responses may account for the exacerbation of seizure activity with menses in many women with severe epilepsy.[47] Increases in estrogens and progesterone during pregnancy may therefore alter the seizure threshold.[146] Seizure activity or susceptibility to seizures may also be affected by water and sodium retention, sleep alterations, and the mild respiratory alkalosis of pregnancy.[91, 92, 146, 160]

A major factor affecting the pregnant epileptic is the effect of the usual physiologic changes of pregnancy on the metabolism of anticonvulsant drugs. These changes are summarized in Table 12–3. As a result of these changes, the apparent plasma clearance of anticonvulsant drugs decreases with subtherapeutic plasma concentrations and increased risk of seizures. In general the pregnant epileptic woman on anticonvulsants needs to have the dosages of her medica-

tion(s) increased 30 to 50% above prepregnant levels.[12] These changes occur predominantly during the second half of pregnancy and reverse by 6 weeks post partum.[47] As the physiologic alterations of pregnancy are reversed post partum, drug levels may fluctuate rapidly, leading to toxicity. Monitoring of drug levels must include evaluation of free (unbound) drug since this parameter is better correlated with seizure activity than total drug levels.[12] Drug levels are monitored regularly during pregnancy to ensure therapeutic dosages, with monitoring continuing after delivery until drug levels have stabilized.[146]

TABLE 12–3
Effects of Pregnancy on Metabolism of
Anticonvulsant Drugs

PREGNANCY CHANGE	EFFECT
Hemodilution	Increased volume of distribution
Decreased protein binding and concentrations of serum proteins/unit of volume	Increased unbound (free) drug Increased availability of drugs for placental transfer
Placental transfer	Similar cord and maternal blood levels of drugs
Impaired gastrointestinal absorption	Decreased absorption of phenytoin
Altered hepatic metabolism	Increased metabolism of primidone, carbamazepine, and phenytoin
Altered renal function	Increased renal excretion of phenobarbital

Compiled from references 12, 16, 37, 47, 91, 92, and 146.

EFFECTS OF EPILEPSY ON PREGNANCY

Epileptic women have a higher incidence of stillbirth and possibly preterm labor, but risks of spontaneous abortion, abruptio placentae, hyperemesis gravidarum, PIH, or other complications are not increased.[12, 37, 47, 146, 155, 196] Women who have seizures during the third trimester must be evaluated for eclampsia, however. Maternal bleeding may occur secondary to deficiency of vitamin K–dependent clotting factors, and is usually associated with phenytoin or phenobarbital use.[146] The epileptic woman on anticonvulsants is also at risk for folate deficiency due to competitive malabsorption and increased hepatic clearance. Some investigators have suggested that folate supplements during pregnancy may decrease the risk of fetal anomalies; however, use of these supplements is also associated with decreased anticonvulsant levels and an increased risk of seizures.[12] Enhancement of hepatic metabolism in women treated with anticonvulsants and taking oral contraceptives increases the risk of breakthrough bleeding and contraceptive failure.[146]

EFFECTS OF EPILEPSY AND ANTICONVULSANTS ON THE FETUS AND NEONATE

The major risks to the fetus and neonate of an epileptic woman are from pathophysiologic consequences of maternal seizures and the use of anticonvulsants. Grand mal seizures are associated with maternal apnea that can cause transient fetal hypoxia and acidosis. Each of the available anticonvulsant drugs has potential fetal and neonatal risks (Table 12–4). These risks include congenital anomalies, hemorrhagic disease of the newborn, folic acid deficiency, and neonatal addiction and withdrawal. In comparison with the general population, congenital anomalies occur more frequently among both epileptic women who are not on anticonvulsants and those who are.[146, 155, 197]

The teratogenicity of specific anticonvulsant drugs, especially phenytoin and phenobarbital, is controversial and the evidence is contradictory.[91, 92] The most common anomalies are cleft lip and palate, limb deformities, and congenital heart defects. The classic "fetal hydantoin syndrome" (microcephaly, poor growth, dysmorphic facies, and mental retardation) is not specific for any of the anticonvulsant either alone or in combination.[47] Although the risk of congenital malformations is higher for epileptic women on anticonvul-

sant drugs, this effect may be due either to the effects of the epilepsy per se or to the effects of epilepsy in interaction with these drugs, folate deficiency, or a genetic predisposition, such as an inherited metabolic defect, that predisposes to fetal anomalies. For example, many anticonvulsant drugs are metabolized by the epoxide metabolic pathway. Infants with a familial defect in epoxide metabolic detoxification are more likely to develop congenital anomalies with exposure to phenytoin and other anticonvulsant drugs.[175a] The incidence of congenital anomalies is highest in offspring of epileptic women on anticonvulsants, followed by infants of epileptic fathers on anticonvulsants, and then by epileptic women who do not require anticonvulsant therapy.[12] The incidence in all these groups is higher than that in the general population. In addition hypoxia and acidosis secondary to seizures may cause anomalies or disorders such as cerebral palsy and mental retardation and increase the risk of stillbirth.[146]

Dalessio[37] recommends the following regarding management of epileptic women:

1. If possible, attempt to withdraw anticonvulsant medication from who wish to become pregnant and who have been seizure-free for at least 2 years. This should be done slowly, tapering the drug or drugs over a period of 60 to 90 days, *before* pregnancy occurs. Do not attempt to withdraw anticonvulsants from an epileptic woman with a long history of seizures who clearly requires medication. [For these women and their infants, the risks and effects of seizures outweigh the risk of anticonvulsants.]

2. When possible, attempt to obtain seizure control using a single drug (monotherapy).

3. Monitor plasma levels of anticonvulsants frequently during pregnant.

4. Try to ensure medication compliance and good health habits during pregnancy.

5. Informed consent of the pregnant epileptic is mandatory. The patient must understand the relative risks of epilepsy and its treatment for the developing fetus.[37]

These recommendations are consistent with those from the American Academy of Pediatrics on management of epileptic women.[8]

Hemorrhagic disease of the newborn (HDN) can occur in offspring of mothers on phenytoin, phenobarbital, or primidone. This disorder is due to a deficiency of vitamin

TABLE 12–4
Effects of Anticonvulsants on the Fetus and Neonate

ANTICONVULSANT	CLASS*	FETAL AND NEONATAL EFFECTS
Phenytoin	D	Hemorrhagic disease of the newborn secondary to deficiency of vitamin K–dependent clotting factors Folic acid deficiency Implicated in craniofacial and limb malformations but evidence is contradictory
Primidone	D	Hemorrhagic disease of the newborn secondary to deficiency of vitamin K–dependent clotting factors Folic acid deficiency
Trimethadione	D	Reported high incidence of cluster malformations (craniofacial, limb and cardiac), developmental delay and mental retardation Avoid in pregnancy if possible and use ethosuximide for petit mal[22]
Carbamazepine	C	Anomalies associated with fetal hydantoin syndrome have been reported Minimal experience with pregnancy use to date, but considered by some the drug of choice[22]
Valproic acid	D	Associated with neural tube defects (1% risk with first trimester exposure) and possible other anomalies; teratogenic in animals Avoid in pregnancy if possible
Phenobarbital	D	Hemorrhagic disease of the newborn secondary to deficiency of vitamin K–dependent clotting factors Implicated in craniofacial and limb malformations but evidence is contradictory; similar malformations not reported in women who are not epileptic and on this drug Neonatal addiction and withdrawal
Clonazepam	C	Neonatal depression and apnea

*Drug classifications are as follows:
   C: These drugs should be used only if the potential risk is justified by the potential benefit. Class C drugs are those for which ". . . either studies in animals have revealed adverse effects on the fetus (teratogenic, embryocidal, or other); or there are no controlled studies in women, or studies in women and animals are not available."[146, p.663]
   D: Drugs in this category have had positive evidence of fetal risk; however, the benefits may be acceptable ". . . when the drug is needed in a life-threatening situation or for a serious disease for which safer drugs cannot be used or are ineffective."[146, p.663]
Compiled from references 10, 12, 22, 24, 47, 91, 92, 132, 135, 146, 163, 168, and 174.

K–dependent clotting factors secondary to competitive inhibition of the formation of precursor molecules (see Chapter 5).[12, 38, 170] Neonatal bleeding can usually be prevented by administration of vitamin K_1 after birth, although some infants may require fresh-frozen plasma to control the bleeding initially. Fetal bleeding with subsequent stillbirth has been reported.[168] Vitamin K_1 administered to the mother during the last few weeks of pregnancy has been used to reduce the risk of maternal, fetal, and neonatal bleeding.[47, 146]

BREAST FEEDING IN EPILEPTIC WOMEN

Women with epilepsy, including those on anticonvulsants, can successfully breast-feed. Although anticonvulsant drugs pass into breast milk, levels are much lower than in the mother and generally do not pose a significant risk to the infant.[123] These infants may be sedated and drowsy initially because of residual effects from in utero exposure to maternal anticonvulsants, especially phenobarbital and primidone. This may interfere with suckling and lead to undernutrition in the infant and inadequate stimulation of the mother's milk supply. Supplementation of the infant and maternal breast pumping may be necessary.[108] Kaneko and associates found that the duration of poor sucking correlated with both the specific drug and drug levels.[93] They recommend feeding these infants with a combination of breast milk and formula during the early postpartum period (along with maternal pumping). This reduces infant serum levels of the drug and allows the infant's hepatic enzyme systems to mature and clear residual drugs more effectively.

Peripheral Neuropathies

Pregnancy, labor and delivery, and lactation are associated with an increased incidence of a variety of peripheral neuropathies. Most of these disorders, although uncomfortable, do not alter the course of pregnancy, nor are they associated with maternal or fetal and neonatal complications. Other peripheral neuropathies develop secondary to trauma or pressure injury during the intrapartum or postpartum periods. Table 12–5 summarizes these disorders and their implications.

The Woman with a Spinal Cord Transection

Successful pregnancies are not uncommon for women who are paraplegic or quadriplegic. The usual physiologic changes of pregnancy place the woman with a spinal cord transection at increased risk for certain problems, however, including increased urinary incontinence, urinary tract and other infections, constipation, and pressure sores. Most of these problems can be prevented or minimized with good care. Management of the paralyzed pregnant women usually includes careful attention to bladder and skin care, high bulk diet, adequate fluid intake, prevention of anemia, stool softeners, and acidification of the urine with vitamin C supplements.[10, 47, 73]

Labor and Delivery

Labor and delivery present unique challenges and risks. Since contraction of the myometrium is relatively independent of neuronal influence (see Chapter 3), uterine contractions are usually normal. The level of the lesion influences the woman's perception of contractions, however. Sacral anesthesia is present in all of these women. Women with cauda equina lesions have relaxed perineal muscles. Women with lesions below T10 to T11, the level at which the uterine sensory nerves enter the spinal cord, experience labor pain.[47]

If the lesion is above T11, labor will be painless, the onset of contractions will not be felt, and delivery may be precipitous.[12] These women need careful monitoring of the cervix and contractions from about 24 weeks' gestation since preterm labor is common.[10, 154] If the woman also has spasticity, local somatic reflex arcs may be activated by labor contractions. This may result in painful extensor and flexor muscle spasms and sustained ankle clonus.[10, 47]

Autonomic hyperreflexia or dysreflexia (also called the autonomic stress syndrome) may occur during labor in women with complete cord lesions above T5 to T6 (above the outflow of the splanchnic autonomic nerves). This syndrome is characterized by hyperstimulation of the autonomic system with brief periods of severe hypertension, throbbing headaches, reflex bradycardia, sweating, nasal congestion, cutaneous vasodilation with flushed skin, and piloerection above the level of the lesion.[10, 47, 73] Symptoms generally occur with uterine contractions and are most prominent immediately before to delivery. Symptoms may be mistaken for preeclampsia.[10, 47] Autonomic hyperreflexia occurs because of the sudden release of large amounts of catecholamines during uterine contractions. This syndrome can result in life-threatening complications including intercranial hemorrhage and cardiac arrhythmias. Treatment includes regional anesthesia and perhaps use of beta blockers.[47]

Forceps may be required during delivery if the muscles used for expulsion during the second stage are paralyzed or if severe hyperreflexia occurs.[47] During the postpartum period care involves prevention of complications of the elimination and integumentary systems. Poor wound healing is a concern and may be aggravated by anemia. Paraplegic and quadriplegic women have let-down reflexes and can successfully breast-feed.[154]

The Woman with a Brain or Spinal Cord Tumor

Brain tumors usually enlarge during pregnancy because of stimulation of tumor estrogen receptors that stimulate growth of neoplastic cells, increased vascularity and blood volume, and increased extracellular volume.[195] As a result of these changes, many tumors become symptomatic during the second half of pregnancy. Tumors may temporarily regress post partum. About one third of women with brain tumors die during pregnancy, usually during the second half. Brain tumors account for nearly 10% of maternal deaths.[10, 12, 44, 47, 87]

Spinal cord tumors tend to exacerbate with pregnancy and menstruation. The most common spinal cord lesions in pregnant woman are arteriovascular malformations (AVM) and angiomas. An AVM is characterized by rapid shunting of blood between an artery and vein without any intervening capillaries, thus depriving adjacent areas of oxygen and nutrients. Exacerbations during pregnancy may be related to: (1) mechanical pressure of the gravid uterus on the vena cava, causing partial outflow obstruction with shifting of blood flow to vertebral and epidural veins

TABLE 12–5
Peripheral Neuropathies During Pregnancy and Lactation

DISORDER	DESCRIPTION	IMPLICATIONS
Neuropathies Associated with Pregnancy		
Bell's palsy	Acute unilateral neuropathy of the seventh cranial nerve leading to facial paralysis with weakness of the forehead and lower face.	Three times more frequent during pregnancy, possibly owing to compression of facial nerve as it traverses the facial canal. Most often occurs in the third trimester or first 2 weeks post partum. Onset late in pregnancy is usually associated with full recovery and generally requires no treatment if partial or mild.
Transient carpal tunnel syndrome	Entrapment and compression of the medial nerve at the wrist, more prominent in dominant hand.	May develop in pregnancy because of excessive fluid retention. Nocturnal hand pain reported by 20 to 40% of pregnant women with electromyographic (EMG) evidence of this syndrome in about 5%. Supportive treatment (splinting of wrist at night); few may require surgery. Most resolve by 3 months post partum; may recur with later pregnancies.
Meralgia paresthesia	Unilateral or bilateral entrapment and compression of lateral femoral cutaneous nerve as it passes beneath the inguinal ligament.	Associated with obesity and rapid weight gain in pregnancy; also related to trauma and stretch injury. Lumbar lordosis in pregnancy may make nerve more vulnerable to compression. Develops in third trimester, resolves spontaneously over first 3 months post partum.
Neuropathies Occurring in the Intrapartum and Postpartum Periods		
Postpartum foot drop	Compression of the lumbosacral trunk against the sacral ala by the fetal head or of the common peroneal nerve between leg braces and the fibular head.	Most common intrapartum nerve injury. Seen most often in women of short stature with large infants. Clinical manifestations may not appear until 24 to 48 hours post partum. Prognosis is good if only the myelin sheath had been distorted with improvement in 2 to 3 months.
Other traumatic neuropathies	Compression of the lumbosacral plexus or obturator, femoral, or peroneal nerves against the pelvic wall leading to muscular weakness and palsy.	Associated with obstetric practices including use of lithotomy position, application of forceps, prolonged pressure from the fetal head, or trauma or hematomas from cesarean delivery. Prognosis is good if only the myelin sheath had been distorted with improvement in 2 to 3 months.
Neuropathies associated with breastfeeding	Pressure on the nerves of the axilla.	Occurs during engorgement with numbness and tingling of flexor surface of arms to ulnar distribution of hands that abates as the infant sucks. Disappears as engorgement resolves.
	Pain and tingling with flexion of the elbow.	Seen in women using a hand pump.
	Transient carpal tunnel syndrome.	Develops about 1 month after delivery and resolves within a month of weaning.

Compiled from references 10, 12, 16, 44, 47, 83, 87, 108, 119, 179, and 195.

and engorgement of the venous side of the malformation; (2) increased vascularity and blood volume; or (3) dilation of the shunt by estrogen.[44, 47, 195]

Cerebral Vascular Disorders

The physiologic and hormonal changes of pregnancy also increase the risk of certain cerebral vascular disorders with life-threatening consequences. Although most individual disorders are relatively rare, cerebral vascular disorders as a group are not uncommon during pregnancy.[10] The basis for and risks of subarachnoid hemorrhage, cerebral ischemia, and cerebral venous thrombosis during pregnancy are summarized in Table 12–6.

Pregnancy-Induced Hypertension

PIH is associated with CNS changes in both preeclamptic and eclamptic women. The more severe changes markedly increase the risk of fetal and maternal mortality. CNS manifestations of PIH may include cerebral irritability (hyperreflexia, headache, clonus, altered consciousness, and convulsions [eclampsia]), visual disturbances, cerebral edema, cerebral hemorrhage, or convulsions. These events are the result of arteriolar vasospasm and vasoconstriction, fluid shifts from the vascular to intravascular space, and possibly a failure of cerebral autoregulation with localized capillary rupture.[47]

Eclampsia is the development of seizures in a pregnant woman with signs and symptoms of preeclampsia. The criteria for diagnosis of eclampsia are "the development of convulsions in a patient with hypertension, proteinuria or edema after the 20th week of gestation or within 48 hours postpartum."[187, p.357] Convulsions may be focal, multifocal, or generalized. Potential etiologic factors for seizures and coma in these woman include cerebral vasospasm, hemorrhage, ischemia, edema, and hypertensive or metabolic encephalopathy.[187]

Donaldson[47] suggests that the cerebral manifestations of eclampsia are primarily due to severe vasoconstriction in association with failure of cerebral autoregulation. This leads to a pressure-induced rupture of thin-walled capillaries with vasogenic edema and hemorrhage. "In physiologic terms the upper limit of the autoregulation of cerebral perfusion by blood pressure has been exceeded. The upper limit of autoregulation is proportional to mean arterial blood pressure [and thus not standard diastolic or systolic values]. Cerebral eclampsia is hypertensive encephalopathy in previously normotensive women."[47, p.495]

Magnesium sulfate has long been the drug of choice for treatment of severe preeclampsia or eclampsia. This drug has an anticonvulsant effect, slowing transmission of nerve impulses at neuromuscular junctions and decreasing CNS irritability, and decreases smooth muscle contractility (see Chapter 14). Phenytoin has been used as an alternative to magnesium sulfate, but recent data suggest this drug is less effective.[43, 164]

SUMMARY

The neurologic system and mediation of discomfort and pain are often of major concern for women during the intrapartum period. This system is probably the one about which least is known regarding specific effects of pregnancy. The pregnant woman experiences alterations in her neuromuscular and sensory systems related to the hormonal and physiologic adaptations of gestation. These changes may result in common experiences and discomforts of pregnancy, including back and headaches, ocular and voice changes, nasal stuffiness, epistaxis, sleep disturbances, postpartum blues, and peripheral neuropathies, and alter the course of neurologic disorders. Recommendations for clinical practice related to the neuromuscular and sensory systems during pregnancy are summarized in Table 12–7.

DEVELOPMENT OF THE NEUROMUSCULAR AND SENSORY SYSTEMS IN THE FETUS

The neuromuscular and sensory system undergo a series of complex structural and functional changes to reach maturation. The CNS is one of the earliest systems to begin development and the latest to completely mature. Table 12–8 summarizes CNS development and timing of origin of specific anomalies. This section will examine anatomic and functional development of the nervous system, sensory abilities, and motor abilities.

TABLE 12–6
Cerebrovascular Disorders: Possible Basis for Increased Risk During Pregnancy

DISORDER	RISK	BASIS
Subarachnoid hemorrhage (SAH)	1 to 2 in 10,000 deliveries. Accounts for about 10% of all maternal deaths usually due to arteriovenous malformation (AVM) or berry aneurysm. Risk due to aneurysm increases with each trimester and post partum. AVMs most often bleed in second trimester or in intrapartum period. One-third of SAHS occur with bearing down and Valsalva maneuvers.	Bleeding during pregnancy may be associated with enlargement or increased shunting during pregnancy related to altered hemodynamics, increased CBF, changes in coagulation, or hormonal influences altering integrity of blood vessels. Bleeding during labor in women with these anomalies may be initiated by rapid pressure and flow changes associated with Valsalva maneuver.
Cerebral ischemia	5- to 10-fold increase during pregnancy (similar to increase noted with oral contraceptives). Most occur in second and third trimesters and during the first week post partum.	Hormonal changes, anemia, and altered blood coagulation during pregnancy may be factors predisposing to emboli formation. Often occurs secondary to other disorders such as mitral valve prolapse, hypertension, subacute bacterial endocarditis, hypotension, sickle cell anemia, or use of anticoagulants.
Cerebal venous thrombosis	1 in 10,000 deliveries. Most occur from 3 days to 1 month post partum.	Hematologic changes and alterations in blood coagulation in pregnancy may increase risk.

Compiled from references 10, 12, 44, 45, 47, 120, 186, 192, and 195.

Anatomic Development

Embryonic Development

After fertilization and implantation, the early development of the nervous system begins at approximately 18 days after fertilization.[128] The process by which the beginnings of the nervous system are laid down is called neurulation and includes formation of the neural plate, neural folds, and neural tube (Fig. 12–3). The processes occurring on the dorsal surface of the embryo leading to formation of the brain and spinal cord are called dorsal induction.[189] Ventral induction refers to processes occurring on the ventral portion leading to the formation of the face and forebrain, including eye formation, olfactory formation, and forebrain structures. Thus, errors of ventral induction origin may produce both facial and nervous system anomalies.[189]

The neural plate develops an invagination in its center, called the neural groove, beginning 22 to 23 days after fertilization. Bulging on both sides of the neural tube groove, called the neural folds, accompanies the invagination process. The neural folds continue to enlarge, enveloping the neural groove, and at approximately 28 days fuse to form the neural tube, an entity separate from the overlying ectodermal layer.[128] The neural tube forms the CNS with the rostral portion becoming the brain and the caudal portion the spinal cord. The ventricles and canal of the cord are derived from the lumen of the neural tube.[128] Closure of the neural tube begins in the area of the future lower medulla at about 22 days and proceeds in cephalic and caudal directions. The rostral opening (neuropore) closes at 24 to 25 days; the caudal neuropore (at L1 to L2) closes 2 days later at 26 to 27 days.[128] Failure of these neuropores to close gives rise to neural tube defects.

As the neural tube is forming, neuroectodermal cells migrate into the neural folds located on both sides of the developing neural groove, forming the neural crest. The neural crest develops into the peripheral nervous system, including the cranial and spinal nerve sensory ganglia, the autonomic nervous system, Schwann cells, the pia and arachnoid layers of the meninges, and the peripheral nerves.[128]

After closure of the rostral portion of the neural tube, three vesicles form that are the precursors of the brain. The forebrain (prosencephalon), midbrain (mesencephalon), and hindbrain (rhombencephalon) develop in the 4th week. With further differentiation the

TABLE 12–7
Summary of Recommendations for Clinical Practice Related to the Neuromuscular and Sensory Systems During Pregnancy

Recognize usual ocular, otolaryngeal, and neuromuscular changes during pregnancy (pp. 523–524).

Provide anticipatory teaching regarding usual ocular, otolaryngeal, and neuromuscular changes during pregnancy (pp. 523–524, 527–529).

Counsel women regarding intervention strategies for common problems related to ocular changes (pp. 523, 528–529).

Counsel women, when possible, to delay getting new prescriptions for glasses or contact lenses until several weeks post partum (p. 528).

Counsel women to avoid cycloplegic or mydriatic agents and topical ophthalmic ointments during pregnancy or, if necessary, to use nasolacrimal occlusion after use (pp. 528–529).

Counsel women regarding intervention strategies for common problems related to otolaryngeal changes (p. 524).

Counsel women regarding intervention strategies for common problems related to musculoskeletal changes (pp. 524, 529).

Assess posture and lifting techniques used by pregnant women (pp. 524, 529).

Teach pregnant women relaxation techniques and exercises to reduce muscle strain and tension (pp. 524, 529).

Recognize and assess for factors associated with painful legs during pregnancy (pp. 529–530, Table 12–1).

Assess sleep patterns of pregnant and postpartum woman and implement interventions to enhance rest and sleep (pp. 524, 527).

Avoid use of sleep medications during pregnancy (pp. 524, 527).

Assess women complaining of backache, headache, round ligament pain, or other discomfort for signs of other disorders (pp. 524, 529–531).

Understand the basis for maternal feelings of pain and discomfort during labor and delivery and implement appropriate interventions (pp. 524–527, Fig. 12–1).

Counsel women during the postpartum period regarding alterations in comfort and implement appropriate interventions (pp. 527, 529).

Counsel women during the postpartum period regarding postpartum blues and implement appropriate interventions (pp. 527–528).

Assess and counsel women with diabetes mellitus and PIH regarding potential ocular complications (pp. 528–529).

Assess eye infections in pregnant women and evaluate for pathogenesis by organisms implicated with sexually transmitted disorders (p. 529).

Counsel women with migraine headaches regarding effects of pregnancy on their disorder and remission post partum (pp. 530–531).

Know and counsel women regarding the side effects of drugs, including anticonvulsants, used to treat specific neurologic disorders and potential toxicity to the woman and fetus (pp. 531–535, Tables 12–2 and 12–3).

Counsel women with chronic neurologic disorders, including epilepsy, regarding the impact of their disorder on pregnancy and of pregnancy on the disorder (pp. 531–535, Tables 12–2 and 12–6).

Know the effects of physiologic alterations during pregnancy on metabolism of anticonvulsants (pp. 531–534, Table 12–2).

Monitor epileptic women during pregnancy and post partum for levels of and responses to anticonvulsant (pp. 531–534, Table 12–2).

Monitor nutritional status of the pregnant epileptic woman (pp. 533–534).

Evaluate the infant of an epileptic woman for congenital anomalies, folate deficiency, drug withdrawal, bleeding, and feeding behavior (pp. 534–535, Table 12–5).

Ensure that vitamin K is administered to newborns of epileptic women who are on anticonvulsants (pp. 534–535, Table 12–5).

Provide support for women with epilepsy and other neurologic disorders who choose to breast-feed (p. 535, Table 12–4).

Recognize signs and symptoms of peripheral neuropathies and implement appropriate preventative and intervention strategies (pp. 535–536, Table 12–5).

Evaluate the woman with a spinal cord transection for bowel, bladder and integumentary complications and implement appropriate interventions (p. 536).

Monitor the woman with a spinal cord lesion for initiation of contractions, progression of labor, and autonomic hyperreflexia (p. 536).

Recognize the cerebral manifestations of preeclampsia and eclampsia and implement appropriate interventions (p. 538).

Page numbers in parentheses following each recommendation refer to the pages in the text where the rationale for that intervention is discussed.

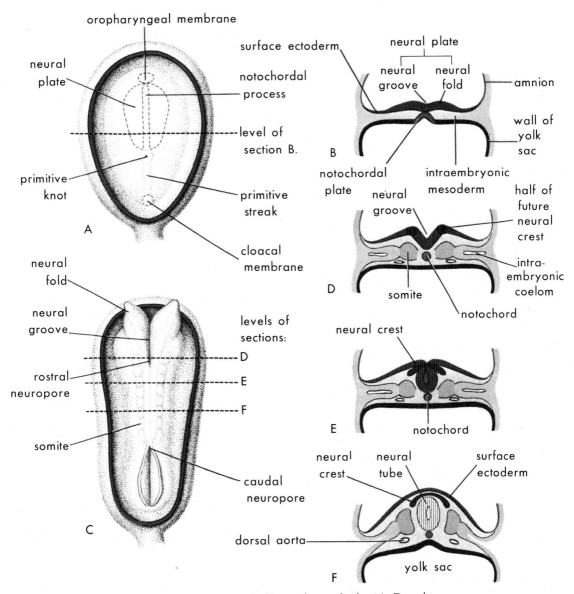

FIGURE 12–3. Embryonic formation of neural plate and neural tube. *A,* Dorsal view of an embryo of about 18 days, exposed by removing the amnion. *B,* Transverse section of this embryo, showing the neural plate and early development of the neural groove. The developing notochord is also shown. *C,* Dorsal view of an embryo of about 22 days. The neural folds have fused opposite the somites but are widely spread out at both ends of the embryo. The rostral and caudal neuropores are indicated. Closure of the neural tube occurs initially in the region corresponding to the future junction of the brain and spinal cord. *D* to *F,* Transverse sections of this embryo at the levels shown in *C,* illustrating formation of the neural tube and its detachment from the surface ectoderm. (From Moore, K.L. (1988). *The developing human* (4th ed., p. 365). Philadelphia: WB Saunders.)

forebrain becomes the telencephalon and diencephalon, while the hindbrain becomes the metencephalon and myelencephalon, creating five vesicles. Adult derivatives of the vesicles are shown in Fig. 12–4. The primitive brain structures go through a series of flexures or foldings (Fig. 12–5).

In the caudal portion of the neural tube, the alar (dorsal) and basal (ventral) plates develop (Fig. 12–6). These structures are the

TABLE 12–8
The Major Stages of Human Brain Development and Related Defects

TIME OF OCCURRENCE (WEEKS)	STAGE OF HUMAN DEVELOPMENT	MAJOR EVENTS
3 to 4	Neurulation	Notochord
4 to 7	Caudal neural tube formation	Canalization followed by regressive differentiation
5 to 6	Ventral induction	Precordal mesoderm Prosencephalon
8 to 16	Neuronal proliferation	Cellular proliferation in the ventricular and subventricular zones Proliferation of vascular tree, particularly venous Interkinetic nuclear migration Neuroblasts Glioblasts
12 to 20	Migration	Radial migration in cerebrum Radial tangential migration in the cerebellum
24 to postnatal	Organization	Late neuronal migration in cerebrum and cerebellum Alignment, orientation, and layering of cortical neurons Synaptic contacts Proliferation of glia and differentiation
Peak at birth to years postnatal	Myelinization	Bulbospinal tracts Motor roots Medial lemniscus Pyramidal tract Frontopontine tract Corpus callosum

Adapted from Hill, A. & Volpe, J.J. (1989). *Fetal neurology* (p. 271). New York: Raven Press.

beginning formation of the motor and sensory tracts that form in the ventral and dorsal areas, respectively, of the cord.[128] In conjunction with formation of the spinal cord from the caudal neural tube, cells from the neural crest break into groups along the length of the cord, forming spinal and cranial ganglia, in addition to the ganglia of the autonomic nervous system. Further differentiation and migration of neural crest cells and their fibers form the peripheral nerves (somatic and visceral, sensory and motor) and their connections (Fig. 12–6).

Common Anomalies of the Central Nervous System

The most common CNS anomalies arise during the period of dorsal induction as a result of failure of neural tube closure. Neural tube defects (NTDs) are usually accompanied by alterations in vertebral, meningeal, vascular, and dermal structures and arise from environmental or genetic factors. These anomalies include anencephaly, myelomeningocele, encephalocele, and spina bifida occulta. The cellular basis for these defects is uncertain but one theory suggests that they result from damage to the ectoderm, resulting in a bleb of fluid in the neural cleft that leads to embryonic scarring that prevents neural tube fusion.

Anencephaly is due to failure of the neural tube to fuse in the cranial area. Since this area forms the forebrain, anencephalic infants have minimal development of brain tissue above the midbrain. Tissue that does develop is poorly differentiated and becomes

TABLE 12–8
The Major Stages of Human Brain Development and Related Defects *Continued*

MAJOR EVENTS (Continued)		MAJOR ANOMALIES DURING STAGE
Neural plate	Neural tube	Anencephaly
	Neural crest cells	Exencephaly
Neural tube	Brain differentiation of prosencephalon, mesencephalon, and rhombencephalon at 20 days	Meningocele
		Meningomyelocele
		Myeloschisis
	Spinal cord	Arnold-Chiari malformation
	Dura	
Neural crest cells	Dorsal root ganglia	
	Pia and arachnoid	
	Schwann cells	
	Autonomic ganglia, etc.	
		Spina bifida occulta
		Dermal sinus
Face and forebrain		Faciotelencephalic malformations
Cleavage of prosencephalon into cerebral vesicles to form 2 cerebral hemispheres at 33 days		
Differentiation of the hypothalamus		Microencephaly "vera"
Optic vesicles		Macrencephaly
Olfactory bulbs and tracts		
First fibers in internal capsule at 41 days		
Thalamus and basal ganglia		
Cortical lamination		Schizencephaly
Neuronal migration in the cerebral cortex is completed at about 5 months		Agenesis of the corpus callosum
		Hirschsprung's disease
Neuronal migration in the cerebellum is completed at about 1 year postnatally		
		Mental retardation
		Down syndrome
		Perinatal insults
24 to postnatal		Cerebral white matter hypoplasia
24 to postnatal		
24 to postnatal		
38 to 2 years postnatally		
7 to 8 months to postnatal to 2 years		
4 months postnatal to 16 years		

necrotic with exposure to amniotic fluid. This results in a mass of vascular tissue with neuronal and glial elements and a choroid plexus with partial absence of the skull bones.[180] Since anencephaly arises from failure of the neural tube to close cranially, the insult must occur at or before 24 to 25 days.

Encephaloceles also arise from failure of closure of a portion of the caudal portion of the neural tube. About 75% of these defects occur in the occipital region with the sac protruding from the back of the head or base of the neck.[18a] Hydrocephalus occurs with 60 to 70% of occipital encephaloceles due to alterations in the posterior fossa. Hydrocephalus may be present at birth or develop after repair of the defect. Encephaloceles may occur in association with meningomyelocele. The protruding sac varies considerably in

size but the size does not correlate with the presence of neural elements.

Spina bifida is a general term used to describe defects in closure of the neural tube associated with malformations of the spinal cord and vertebrae that usually arise from defects in closure of the caudal neuropore. Approximately 80% occur in the lumbar area, which is the final area of neural tube fusion. Thus, spina bifida must occur at or before 26 to 27 days. Defects range from minor malformations to disorders that result in paraplegia or quadriplegia and loss of bladder and bowel control. The degree of sensory and motor neurologic deficit depends on the level and severity of the defect. The two major forms of spina bifida are spina bifida occulta and spina bifida cystica.

Spina bifida occulta is a vertebral defect at

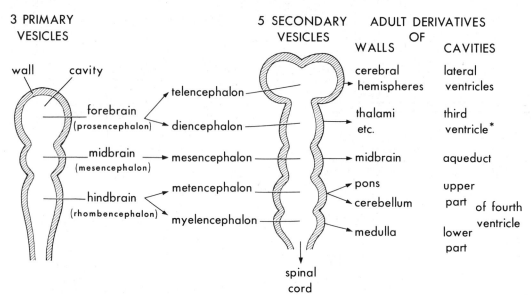

FIGURE 12–4. Embryonic development of the brain vesicles. (From Moore, K.L. (1988). *The developing human* (4th ed., p. 380). Philadelphia: WB Saunders.)

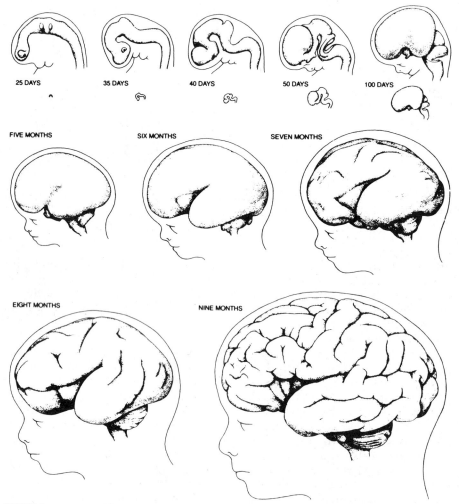

FIGURE 12–5. Folding of embryonic brain and formation of gyri. (From Cowan, W. M. (1979). The development of the brain. *Sci Am, 241,* 116.)

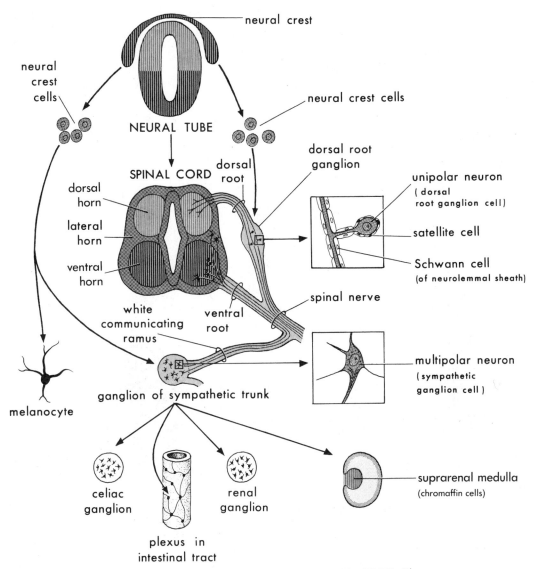

FIGURE 12–6.   Derivatives of the neural crest. (From Moore, K.L. (1988). *The developing human* (4th ed., p. 372). Philadelphia: WB Saunders.)

L5 or S1 that arises from failure of the vertebral arch to grow and fuse.[18a] It is a defect in formation of the caudal portion of the spinal cord (Fig. 12–7A). Most people with this defect have no problems and the defect may be unrecognized. A few have underlying abnormalities of the spinal cord or nerve roots, which are manifested externally by a hemangioma, dimple, tuft of hair, or lipoma in the lower lumbar or sacral area.

Spina bifida cystica describes neural tube defects characterized by a cystic sac, containing meninges or spinal cord elements, along with vertebral defects, covered by epithelium or a thin membrane, and usually occurring in the lumbar or lumbosacral area. The three

main forms of spina bifida cystica are meningocele, meningomyelocele, and myeloschisis (Fig. 12–7). Meningocele involves a sac containing meninges and cerebrospinal fluid (CSF) but with the spinal cord and nerve roots in their normal position. These infants usually have minimal residual neurologic deficit if the defect is covered with skin and is managed appropriately.

With a meningomyelocele, the most common form of spina bifida cystica, the sac contains spinal cord or nerve roots in addition to meninges and CSF. During development nerve tissues become incorporated into the wall of the sac, impairing differentiation of nerve fibers.[18a] These infants have a neu-

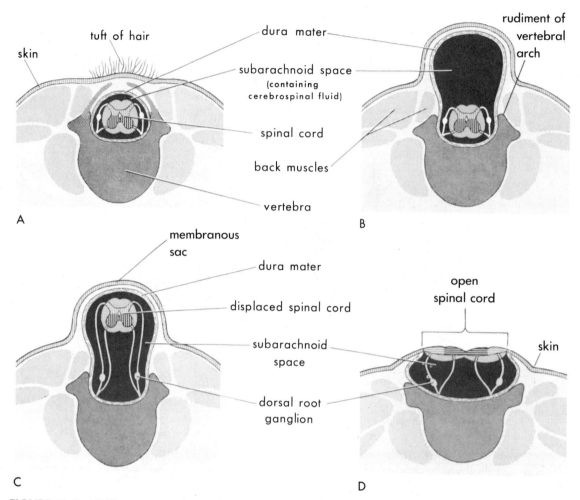

FIGURE 12–7.   Different types of spina bifida: *A,* spina bifida occulta; *B,* spina bifida cystica: meningocele; *C,* spina bifida cystica: meningomyelocele; *D,* spina bifida cystica: myeloschisis. (From Moore, K.L. (1988). *The developing human* (4th ed., p. 375). Philadelphia: WB Saunders.)

rologic deficit below the level of the sac. Myeloschisis is a severe defect in which there is no cystic covering; the spinal cord is an open, exposed, flattened mass of neural tissue. These infants have significant neurologic deficits and are at great risk for infection. This defect can involve the entire length of the spinal cord and can occur in association with anencephaly.[18a]

Fetal Neurodevelopment

In the nervous system, structures continue to be elaborated beyond the fetal period. The earliest growth of brain occurs in the lower level structures, such as basal ganglia, thalamus, midbrain, and brain stem, whereas higher level structures, such as the cerebrum

and cerebellum, form somewhat later.[193] Once the embryologic formations are established, CNS development is characterized by overlapping processes: neuronal proliferation, migration, organization, myelinization, and formation of synapses.

NEURONAL PROLIFERATION

Neuronal proliferation is a period of massive production of neurons or their precursors. The maximal rate of neuronal proliferation occurs between 12 and 18 weeks of gestational age, although neurons continue to proliferate until term and beyond.[42] Cerebellar neurons, in particular, proliferate after birth. During proliferation the walls of the neural tube thicken, forming layers. The ependyma is the lining of the neural tube interior that later becomes the lining of the ventricles and the central canal of the spinal cord. In the subependymal layer, the neurons and glial cells of the CNS are formed in the ventricular and subventricular zones of the germinal layer.[189] Neuronal proliferation thus occurs in the subependymal layer, producing neurons that become situated in the gray areas of the CNS.[128] In conjunction with the proliferation of neurons, glial cells also increase in number, however, the peak in glial cell numbers occurs roughly from 5 months' gestational age through the 1st year of life.[189] Thus, a large proportion of the neuronal compliment is formed early in fetal life, but a few areas, notably the cerebellum, continue to acquire neurons during the early months after birth. This pattern of neuronal formation produces a particular vulnerability at time of birth since the cerebellar neurons may be damaged by asphyxia and anoxia.

MIGRATION

Once formed, neurons travel from the germinal layer, near the ventricles in the subependymal layer, to the areas of the nervous system where they will further differentiate and take on unique and individual functions.[189] Neurons migrate from the ventricular area to the areas where gray matter is located. The bulk of migration occurs at 3 to 5 months' gestational age.[189] Studies of the development of the cortical plate have found that neuron migration is assisted by specialized glial cells, called the radial glia.[189]

Processes extending from the glial cell guide the neuron to its respective site. The early neurons migrate to areas deep within the cortex whereas later neurons migrate further to the surface of the cortex. As a result, neurons formed early come to lie in deeper layers of cortex and subcortex; those formed later end at more superficial layers.[151] Most cortical neurons have reached their sites by 20 to 24 weeks' gestation.[189] The cortex generally has a complete component of neurons by 33 weeks' gestation.[151] The radial glial cells later develop into astrocytes.[189] Radial glial-assisted migration is also known to occur in the cerebellum.

ORGANIZATION

Organization refers to the processes by which the nervous system takes on the capacity to operate as an integrated whole. This phase of neurodevelopment begins at approximately 6 months' gestational age and extends many years after birth, and is believed to continue into adulthood. During the period of organization five processes occur.[189] First, cortical neurons become arranged in layers. Second, the dendrites and axons undergo extensive branching, called arborization. The increase in cellular processes is prerequisite for communication throughout the nervous system (Fig. 12–8). This increase in the size of the neuronal field is followed by the formation of connections or synapses between neurons, the third component of organization. Additionally the intracellular structures and enzymes that will produce neurotransmitter also develop at this time. Connections between cells are critical for integration across all areas of the nervous system. Throughout development synapses continue to restructure; this process is believed to be the basis for memory and learning.

The fourth organizational process entails reduction in the number of neurons and their connections through the death of many neurons as well as regression of a number of dendrites and synapses.[152] Approximately half of neurons die.[189] Neuronal survival has been likened to survival of the fittest, because neurons compete for resources such as nutrients, electrical impulses, or synapses.[20] Neuronal death assists in elimination of errors within the nervous system. The appropriate number of neurons and their connections is sustained and, in addition, neurons that are improperly located or fail to achieve adequate connections are eliminated. Finally, glial cells differentiate from the general precursor cell into specific types and proliferate (see Fig. 12–6). Within the CNS astrocytes provide support for neurons, and oligodendroglial cells produce myelin.[189] The increase in glial cells begins at approximately 30 weeks' gestational age and continues into the 2nd year.

MYELINIZATION

Myelinization refers to the laying down of myelin, the lipoprotein insulating covering of nerve fibers. This process occurs in both the central and peripheral nerve systems. Glial cells migrate to locations along the developing nerve fibers. Myelin is formed as the glial cell (either Schwann cells in the peripheral nervous system or oligodendroglial cells in the CNS) wraps itself around the fiber. The glial cell's cellular membrane, once wrapped around the fiber, fuses to become myelin. Myelinization begins during the second

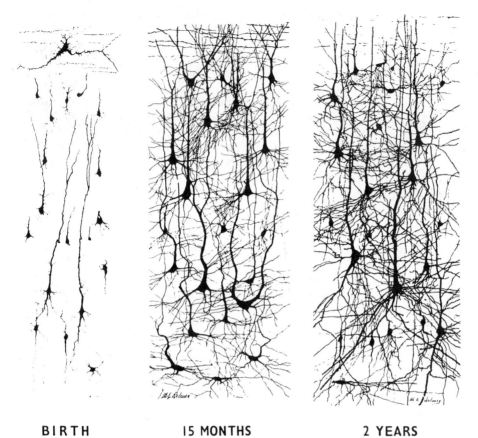

| BIRTH | 15 MONTHS | 2 YEARS |

FIGURE 12–8. Dendritic growth. (From Dobbing, J. (1975). Human brain development and its vulnerability. In *Biologic and clinical aspects of brain development* (p. 7). Mead Johnson Symposium on Perinatal and Developmental Medicine, No. 6. Evansville, IN: Mead Johnson.)

trimester and continues into adulthood.[189] The process of myelinization occurs at differing times in areas throughout the nervous system. Although incomplete myelinization does not prevent function, incomplete myelinization, because it affects nerve conduction, does alter the speed of impulse conduction. Generally, myelinization precedes mature function.[128] Myelinization first begins in the peripheral nervous system, with motor fibers becoming myelinated before sensory fibers. In the CNS, myelinization of sensory areas precedes that of motor areas, with the primary sensory areas becoming myelinated relatively early in development. The order of myelinization parallels overall nervous system functional development. Areas of the brain that support higher level functions, such as cognition and learning, myelinate later in life.[189] Several brain areas continue to lay down myelin well into adulthood. Since myelin is a lipoprotein, dietary adequacy of fats

and protein is important for normal myelinization.

ELECTRICAL ACTIVITY AND IMPULSE CONDUCTION

The earliest synapses appear at about 8 to 9 weeks' gestational age, whereas cortical synapses are present at about 23 weeks' gestational age.[151] Impulse conduction provides for functional validation of connections. Evidence suggests that use of conduction pathways may increase or alter connections.[189] Characteristics of early neuronal activity include poor spontaneous neuronal activity, slow conduction velocity, slow synaptic potentials, and synaptic transmission uncertainty.[31]

Development of Specific Systems

AUTONOMIC NERVOUS SYSTEM

The autonomic nervous system has both central and peripheral components. Peripheral portions form from neural crest cells (see Fig. 12–6). Ganglia are formed from neural crest cells that migrate beyond the neural tube. Sympathetic ganglia are derived from neural crest cells that collect along either side of the developing spinal cord at about 5 weeks' gestational age.[128] The ganglia of the parasympathetic ganglia and plexi also form by migration.[128] Once they reach their respective sites, neurons in the autonomic ganglia continue to differentiate. Nerve fibers, originating in the cord, grow out and make connections with the ganglia. The autonomic nervous system regulates many endocrine functions through nerve impulses. The embryonic origins of some autonomic end organs demonstrate a structural basis for these regulatory actions. The pituitary, a primary source of autonomic regulation, is derived from two forms of tissue. The adenohypophysis is formed from ectoderm and the neurohypophysis is formed from neuroectoderm. Similarly, the adrenal gland is derived from two types of tissue. The adrenal cortex is derived from mesoderm, whereas the medulla, which secretes catecholamines, is derived from neuroectoderm, specifically neural crest cells, and is controlled by the sympathetic nervous system.

PERIPHERAL NERVOUS SYSTEM

The peripheral nervous system is derived from the neural crest (see Fig. 12–6). Through migration and specialization, cells of the neural crest develop into cranial, spinal, and visceral nerves and ganglia. Neural crest cells are precursors of the adrenal medulla chromaffin cells.[128] Support cells of the peripheral nervous system also derive from the neural crest. Nerve fibers, which eventually innervate skeletal motor fibers, emerge from the spinal basal plate, combine into bundles to form the ventral root, and migrate to the developing motor fibers.[128] Similarly, sensory fibers form the dorsal root.

Functional Development

Studies of fetal neural activity in utero are limited to external monitoring of CNS electrical activity or noninvasive detection of fetal responses using measures of fetal movement or ultrasonography. The knowledge of fetal neural capabilities has been augmented by an accident of nature—premature birth. Studies of preterm infants have greatly increased

information concerning operation of the fetal nervous system. In the following section, the neural function of the fetus, defined as gestational age less than 38 weeks, is described. In many instances information pertains to the "fetal infant" or preterm infant. Appreciation of fetal neural development provides a basis for anticipation of the many capabilities of the preterm and term infant.

Sensory Abilities

Generally the somatic sensory and special sensory systems develop in the following order chronologically: touch, smell, vestibular, taste, hearing, and vision.[71, 76] As noted in the previous section on myelinization, in the periphery motor fibers myelinate before sensory fibers whereas in the central nervous system sensory fibers myelinate before motor fibers. Thus, in terms of rate of impulse transmission, differences in myelinization are one basis for limited integration of sensory and motor actions in the fetus.

The early fetus has been shown to respond to touch around the mouth at around 2 months of gestational age.[76] Responsivity to touch is generally present before 32 weeks' gestation.[76] Touch in utero entails contact with amniotic fluid that is approximately at body temperature and contact with body parts or the wall of the uterus. Maternal movement and buoyant amniotic fluid provide rich vestibular stimulation for the fetus in utero.

Since odors must be airborne to stimulate the olfactory bulbs, it is unreasonable to assume that the fetus, in utero, experiences the sense of smell. Responsivity to odors is observed in preterm infants beginning at approximately 26 weeks, however, and is readily documented by 32 weeks' gestation in most infants.

The fetus is known to ingest amniotic fluid (see Chapter 2). Although slight variations occur in the composition of the amniotic fluid, it is unknown to what extent the fetus experiences taste. Research with term infants, however, has documented the ability of infants to discriminate tastes.[33]

The structures of the auditory system, including the inner ear and cochlea, mature at approximately 20 weeks' gestation.[63] Auditory evoked potentials can be recorded as early as 25 weeks' gestation.[74] Responses to sound are observed in preterm infants at approximately 25 to 28 weeks.[74, 145, 171] The preterm infant can be observed to orient to sound, turning the head in the direction of auditory stimulus and showing evidence of arousal and attention.[71] The hearing threshold decreases with gestational age. In infants of 28 to 34 weeks' gestation, the hearing threshold is approximately 40 decibels, whereas in term infants the hearing threshold is approximately 20 decibels.[106] Intrauterine recordings have revealed that sounds in the external environment are audible to the fetus; high frequency sounds are attenuated, but low frequency sounds are not.[63] The intrauterine auditory environment includes sounds within the mother such as breathing, heart beat, and intestinal peristalsis.

Formation of the eyes begins in embryonic development. By 22 weeks the layers of the retina have formed.[74] Rods and cones are present by 23 weeks' gestational age and myelinization of the optic nerve begins at 24 weeks. The neurons forming the visual cortex are in place at 26 weeks, and between 28 and 34 weeks' gestation visual neuronal connections and processes undergo rapid development.[74] Visual evoked potentials can be recorded between 25 and 30 weeks.[74, 151] Visual attention is observed in preterm infants at about 30 to 32 weeks' gestational age.[74]

The natural sensory environment of the uterus is developmentally appropriate for the fetus. This environment provides stimuli that are rich, varied, and rhythmical. Intrauterine sensory stimulation programs have not been studied extensively and cannot be assumed to be beneficial or without risk. Since the normal uterine sensory environment is already rich, the benefits of programs to supplement intrauterine stimulation are unclear at the present time.

Motor Abilities

The development of motor activity in the fetus is a function of both neural and muscle maturation. Muscle cells develop from mesoderm. Innervation during development is critical for muscle fiber development.[189] Muscle cells, as well as neurons, undergo migration and differentiation during development. Mature myocytes are present at approximately 38 weeks; muscle cells increase in size postnatally.[189] Gross motor movement appears as early as 7 weeks' gestation, whereas limb movement occurs at 9 weeks.[74]

The pattern of fetal motor development

includes differences in both emergence of muscle tone and the amount of movement over time.[74] Development of muscle tone follows a caudocephalad and distal–proximal pattern; that is, lower extremities precede upper extremities and extremities precede axial or truncal muscle tone.[2] Motor development is associated with increased flexor tone with lower extremities demonstrating flexion before upper extremities. In the lower extremities passive flexor tone is noticed at 29 weeks' gestation and active flexor tone becomes apparent at 31 weeks.[2] Tone in the upper extremities develops later with flexor tone demonstrated in the upper extremities by 34 weeks.[63] Active tone develops before passive tone, that is, muscle tone is seen during movement or action before resting muscle tone. Both tone and flexion increase with gestational age. Motor movement also shows increasing coordination with gestational age, with less tremor, smoother movement, and more coordination.[74] Complex motor movements are observed after 24 weeks' gestation.[74] Muscle tone is used as one criteria in scoring gestational age.

Muscle tone is limited at 28 weeks' gestation. By 32 weeks flexor tone can be observed in the lower extremities, and is observable in the upper extremities by 36 weeks. The term gestation infant demonstrates flexion.[189] Movement changes with development. At 28 to 32 weeks' gestation, movement is slow, writhing or twisting, and uncoordinated, resembling flailing or flapping.[189] By 32 weeks' gestation flexion movements are somewhat more coordinated.[189] Neonates of this age can turn their head, but head control is lacking. With continued development there is increasing strength, alternating movements may be seen in lower extremities, and head control improves.[189]

During pregnancy the pattern of fetal movements is one of increasing frequency of movements, followed by a reduction in movement close to term. Spontaneous movements begin at 8 weeks' gestation followed by discrete limb movements at 9 weeks. The development of movement involves twitching type movement before 10 weeks, followed by independent limb movement (10 to 12 weeks); limb, head, and torso movement (12 to 16 weeks); and increasingly complex hand, face, and respiratory movements after 24 weeks.[189] Maternal perception of fetal movement occurs at approximately 16 weeks' gestation in multiparas, and slightly later in primiparas. Before this time fetal movements are too fine to be noticed. Fetal movements increase during gestation, reaching a maximum between 26 and 32 weeks; after this time the constraints of the uterine environment reduce fetal movement. Movements are largely spontaneous but can be stimulated.

The motor activity of the fetus reflects integration of nervous system activity as well as general fetal well-being. Changes in fetal movement may reflect placental insufficiency, hypoxemia, or other evidence of fetal distress. Daily fetal movement monitoring has been used as a screening tool for fetal well-being during the third trimester. In addition to changes in tone and frequency of movement during pregnancy, fetal movements provide evidence of fetal sleep–wake or state patterns.

Fetal State Patterns

Although the constancy of the uterine environment may suggest similar consistency in fetal behavior, this assumption is untrue. Fetal behaviors exhibit regular patterns of occurrence, particularly sleep–wake behaviors or behavioral states.[137] In the adult sleep–wake behaviors demonstrate a diurnal pattern of activity and sleep. Sleep in the fetus and infant does not follow this pattern. Sleep changes with maturation of the central nervous system. Because sleep is qualitatively and quantitatively different in the young compared with adults, fetal and infant sleep–wake patterns are more commonly described as states. In the infant, state is determined by characteristics of heart and respiratory regularity, eyes open or closed, motor activity, and presence or absence of rapid eye movements (REM). Although not all of these parameters can be observed in the fetus, fetal state can be determined by regularity of heart rate, presence of eye movements, and fetal movement.[137]

In the fetus as well as the infant, motor activity and irregular heart rate occur during REM sleep. Motor movement also occurs during awake periods. During quiet sleep, regular heart rate and minimal motor movement are noted. Alteration of quiet and active periods in fetal movement have been reported as early as 21 weeks' gestation; however, there is little evidence of regular, rhythmic pattern and limited coordination among state parameters.[174] Fetal movement

is largely continuous in early pregnancy, but with increasing maturation, quiet periods emerge. At 24 to 26 weeks' gestation there is almost continual motor activity of the fetal extremities.[49] By 32 weeks' gestation, alteration of activity and quiet periods becomes more regular and rhythmic. By 32 weeks' gestation patterns of fetal heart rate, eye movement, and gross body movements also begin to show coordination.[188] This periodic function is credited with being a prenatal version of the alteration of REM and quiet sleep, representing a underlying rest–activity cycle.[174] The fetal state cycle is approximately 40 minutes long.[174] With continuing development the length of quiet periods and the integration among state behaviors increase.[143] These changes continue after birth.

NEONATAL PHYSIOLOGY

Much of our understanding of fetal function comes from the study of preterm infants who, technically, are not fetal. The behaviors of these infants provide one means of appreciating fetal behavior at various gestational ages, however. This section on neonatal neural physiology discusses both preterm and term infants. Areas of neural function that are particularly effected by maturation are emphasized.

Transitional Events

At birth, the transition from intrauterine to extrauterine life entails a number of changes in the nervous system. The nervous system does not "turn on" at birth; rather, nervous system activity has increased steadily during pregnancy, producing a term gestation infant whose nervous system is prepared to receive and process information and respond in ways suited to neonatal development. In examining transition, it is useful to identify the behavioral abilities of the neonate, experiences of the fetus in the intrauterine environment, and differences between the intrauterine and extrauterine environments. The change in environment is the major challenge for the neonate's nervous system. The transitional characteristics of four areas of nervous system function will be examined: autonomic, motor, sensory, and state regulation.

Autonomic Regulation

During fetal life, placental circulation provided a steady flow of oxygen and nutrients supporting metabolic needs of the fetus. At birth, the first challenge faced by the neonate is initiating and sustaining respiration (see Chapters 6 and 7). In addition to an intact pulmonary and cardiovascular system, nervous system control of the respiration and heart activity are required. Although fetal respiratory movements are preparation for this action, the fetus has no experience breathing independently or in regulating cardiac and pulmonary functions to produce stable blood oxygen requirements in ambient air. The fetus has had experience monitoring autonomic functions and, to a degree, regulating vegetative behaviors. These capabilities are evidenced by fetal responses to hypoxemia or hypoglycemia, such as changes in activity, heart rate, and blood pressure.

In extrauterine life, nutrient intake must be derived independently from an outside source. Two primary changes in feeding occur: route of intake and pattern of intake. The neonate must switch to oral intake, which is achieved through sucking. In the uterus the fetus has had sucking and feeding experiences in which amniotic fluid has been ingested, but the fetus has not needed to coordinate breathing during sucking and swallowing. Second, neonatal feeding is periodic, rather than the continuous supply of nutrients provided the fetus. Hunger, thirst, and satiety centers must regulate food intake and the neonate must exhibit appropriate hunger cues to elicit feeding from the caregiver and must also be able to end feeding with cues indicating satiety.

In the uterus the fetal temperature varied little. Thus, a major challenge at the time of birth is initiation of thermoregulation. Although thermoregulatory abilities begin at approximately 30 weeks' gestation, the fetus has not been required to independently monitor body temperature and adjust metabolic rate to meet thermal needs (see Chapter 17).

Motor Functions

Beginning early in fetal development, skeletal muscles are involved in movement. These experiences with motor activities provide a means of promoting motor development as well as an opportunity to test out motor innervation. Within the uterus, however, motor activities are enacted in an environment that reduces the effects of gravity and provides confinement. The buoyant amniotic fluid and uterine walls are replaced by the extrauterine environment in which motion is not confined and gravity has a greater effect. Although movements of the fetus may have been smooth and limited in scale, movements of the neonate are often erratic, weak, or flailing. The neonate must exert energy to maintain body position against the pull of gravity.

Sensory Functions

The sensory input provided by the extrauterine environment is markedly different from that of the uterus. Before looking at these differences, however, it is important to recognize the sensory experience of birth itself. Although the fetus has experienced Braxton-Hicks contractions, the steady, rhythmic contractions of the uterus and resultant pressure changes are a new experience. The continuous flow of oxygen and nutrients through the placenta may be altered during contractions, providing intense autonomic input. The descent into the birth canal, given a vaginal birth, increases pressure, perhaps to the degree of being uncomfortable. During labor the mother's activity pattern may change and the sounds from the mother's body may be altered, such as rapid or heavy breathing or heart rate increase. Concurrent with the experiences of labor, changes in the extrauterine environment may be sensed by the infant, including noise. It would seem that the process of birth is one of being bombarded with stimuli. After birth a number of new sensory experiences await. In general sensations in the extrauterine environment are different in nature, more intense, and lack the pattern experienced in the intrauterine environment.

Whereas the uterus is dark, the extrauterine environment provides more light, often intense light in the immediate postbirth period. In the uterus, the fetus was bathed in amniotic fluid that exhibited rare temperature variation, but the extrauterine environment is much cooler and can exhibit great variability. Until birth the fetus has never experienced cold stimulation. In the intrauterine environment, the sounds of the mother's heart and other internal organs were constant and rhythmical. Sounds from the mother's environment did reach the fetus, but were muted to a degree by body tissue and the amniotic fluid. The sounds in the external environment vary from silence to an overwhelming din and include many new sounds the neonate has not previously experienced. For the fetus, touch consisted of warm amniotic fluid and the smooth wall of the uterus. After birth, for the first time the newborn infant has dry skin. Forms of touch increase dramatically after birth, including input from handling, stroking, rubbing, and possibly pain. The newborn has never worn clothing; even the touch of fabric against the skin is a new sensation. Taste sensations had been limited to amniotic fluid ingested in utero, and breast milk, formula, and possibly oral medications provide new taste experiences. Since odors are conducted by air, it is unlikely that the transitional infant has experienced olfactory input.

Sleep–Wake Pattern

After birth the neonate must manage sleep and activity patterns. Caregivers are important timekeepers for the neonate, but neonates and their mothers are frequently separated. In animals, the mother has an important influence on establishing biorhythms in her offspring. There is evidence that state organization is disturbed in the first few days after birth—there may be increased alertness in the first few days, followed by the infant beginning to establish his or her own individual pattern.[74]

Neural Connections and Conduction of Impulses

Gestational age determines the level of brain maturation including acquisition of neuronal component, dendritic and axonal branching, formation of connections between neurons, and myelinization. Although at term gestation most all neurons have formed and migrated to their respective sites, a number of cerebellar neurons are completing this process and are at particular risk in terms of neonatal asphyxia or hypoxia. For the preterm infant, depending on the degree of prematurity, formation and migration of neurons bears even greater risk.

Although the elaboration of dendritic and axonal branches and connections between neurons begins in fetal life, these processes continue into adulthood. The ability of a neuron to change structure and function has been called plasticity. The more immature the infant at birth the greater the impact of CNS plasticity. There is considerable evidence in animal studies that sensory input influences later neuronal structure and function; for instance, an enriched environment improves developmental outcome by maximizing brain potential.[40] This plasticity is both an advantage and a liability. Although sensory input may increase cellular processes and interconnections, the sensory environment may also produce undesired changes in structure and function.[193]

Myelinization occurs predominantly in fetal and infant life but continues through the 4th decade and beyond. Brain areas governing high-level functions myelinate late in life. In the fetus and infant myelinization involves both sensory and motor fibers and pathways. The primary effect of myelinization is on speed of transmission or conduction, since the presence of myelin insulates the nerve fiber, increasing conduction rate. Since myelin is being laid down at varying rates throughout the central and peripheral nervous system, rate of conduction potentially effects the integration of sensory information and effector response. In terms of sensory perception, the difference in conduction speed (msec) is not appreciable at the conscious level; however, even seemingly minor differences in transmission have an impact on integration of information. Speed of transmission is important in spatial (number of impulses coming into the CNS from various sites) and temporal (rapidity with which impulses are being sent) summation. Thus systems in which summation is required for neuronal firing may react less quickly. Conduction rate is inversely related to postconceptual age, becoming similar to that in adults by 3 to 4 years.[189]

Circulation in the Neonatal Brain

The brain of the neonate demonstrates differences in circulation compared with that of the adult. These differences produce vulnerability to damage by hypoxemia and pressure.

Brain Barriers

Early in embryonic life, circulation is conducted by a capillary network.[193] Development is accompanied by proliferation of blood vessels, increasing the blood supply to meet the increasing metabolic demands of the growing CNS. The complexity of the brain's vascular system increases in the last trimester.[193] Sources of the brain barrier include the tight junctions between endothelial cells forming the capillaries, which limit diffusion of substances into the brain tissue, the basement membrane of the endothelial cells, and the astrocyte foot processes surrounding the capillary.[69] In the fetus and neonate, the tight junction between the capillary endothelial cells is not as well formed as that of the adult. Endothelial tight junctions can be altered by hypo-osmolar conditions, hypercarbia, asphyxia, and intracranial infection leading to vasculitis with increased permeability and potential for rupture.[189] A second component of the blood–brain barrier is the basement membrane supporting capillary endothelial cells. In the neonate and infant this basement membrane is not fully developed.[69] Additionally, the astrocyte feet, which normally surround the capillary, are not completely developed in the neonate.[69] These three alterations in the blood–brain barrier predispose to capillary leakage and hemorrhage. Since cellular junctions are not well formed, the brain capillaries are sensitive to osmolar, and hence volume, changes of the blood.[69]

Cerebral Autoregulation

Cerebral autoregulation refers to the local control of brain blood flow, modifying resistance to compensate for changes in pressure, thus sustaining consistent flow (Fig. 12–9A). The autoregulatory capabilities of the fetal and neonatal brain are limited. In utero this is not a severe limitation, since metabolic demands of the brain are less and the cardiovascular system is not required to act independently. In the neonate, however, restriction of autoregulation predisposes the neonate to inadequate or excess pressure, resulting in too little or too much blood flow. Consequences are risk of bleeding from vascular rupture, increased intracranial pressure, and hypoxia/ischemia.

Cerebral perfusion pressure is a function of gestational age and cerebral blood flow (CBF) increases with maturation.[184, 189] Compared with the adult, however, cerebral perfusion pressure is low in the term and even lower in the preterm infant (Fig. 12–9B). Preterm infants have an extremely narrow range of autoregulation. In the preterm infant CBF is close to the level at which oxygen and nutrient delivery is potentially compromised.[189] Normal blood pressure in the preterm infant is slightly above the lower limit of autoregulation.[189]

Since autoregulation in the neonate is not fully mature, CBF tends to be more pressure-passive (i.e., dependent on blood pressure).[189] Thus, in the neonate and especially in the preterm infant, a rise in blood pressure results in an increase in CBF and a drop in blood pressure results in a reduction in blood flow. Low CBF and limited autoregulation combine to place the neonate in a position where there is a fine balance between cerebral ischemia and potential rupture of vessels or increased intracranial pressure. The lower the gestational age, the greater the vulnerability.[189] Autoregulation additionally exhibits a lag in responsiveness. A sudden intense rise or drop in cerebral blood pressure or flow may not be immediately controlled through autoregulatory efforts.[184]

By itself, autoregulation of CBF creates a high risk situation magnified by the influence of hypoxemia. Hypoxemia (including asphyxia) abolishes autoregulation.[189] Thus during hypoxemia, CBF becomes pressure passive. Autoregulation is further influenced by hypercarbia and acidosis, conditions that frequently occur in conjunction with hypoxemia.[184] The nature of respiration in preterm infants predisposes to hypoxemia, hypercarbia, and acidosis. Because autoregulation exhibits a lag, even transient alterations in O_2 and CO_2 can have deleterious results as autoregulation is compromised.

Effects of autoregulation are a consequence of alterations in cerebral blood pressure and flow. Pressure, resistance, and flow are related physical processes. When blood flow is pressure-passive, a rise in blood pressure produces an increase in flow. The fragile capillaries of the immature brain possess neither tight junctions between endothelial cells or a strong basement membrane, therefore increased blood pressure and flow increase intracranial pressure.[68, 69] This increased pressure and flow may rupture the delicate capillaries, leading to bleeding.

Impairment of autoregulation may also produce damage through inability to respond to low blood pressure. Under normal circumstances cerebral perfusion in the neonate is marginally adequate. Given any reduction in blood pressure, autoregulatory abilities do

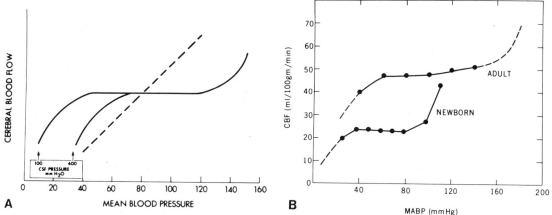

FIGURE 12–9. CBF and autoregulation in the neonate. *A*, Relationship of CBF and blood pressure. (From Goldstein, G.W. (1981). Special features of the brain microcirculation: Role in brain edema formation. In *Perinatal brain insult* (p. 43). Mead Johnson Symposium on Perinatal and Developmental Medicine, No. 17. Evansville, IN: Mead Johnson.) *B*, Cerebral autoregulation. (From Vannucci, R.C. & Hernandes, M.J. (1981). Perinatal cerebral blood flow. In *Perinatal brain insult* (p. 22). Mead Johnson Symposium on Perinatal and Developmental Medicine, No. 17. Evansville, IN: Mead Johnson.)

not support maintenance of blood flow. As a result, reduction in blood pressure may reduce cerebral perfusion, producing ischemia and hypoxia. Thus, hypoxic damage of brain tissue may ensue. Hypoxia, therefore, is a critical concern since brain tissue may be injured by lack of oxygen as well as a reduction in cerebral blood flow.

Certain areas of the brain are more sensitive than others to changes in blood flow. The nature of the distribution of the vascular system in the brain and the type of tissue (white or gray matter) are associated with risk for hypoxic damage. Vessels supplying blood to the brain have little overlap. The area defining margins between two vascular beds is called a boundary (or watershed) area. Boundary areas are particularly prone to disruptions of circulation and hypoxia because blood supply is limited.[184] The subependymal germinal matrix layer, located in ventricular and subventricular areas, is one such area.[69]

Blood flow is linked to metabolism. Gray matter has a higher metabolic rate than that of white matter and consequently perfusion of gray matter exceeds that of white matter.[189] The lower blood flow in white matter predisposes this form of nervous tissue to the effects of limited autoregulation and hypoxemia.[184, 189] One area particularly vulnerable to pressure- and hypoxia-related injury is the periventricular white matter.

Neonatal Sensory Function

In general the rate of nerve transmission continues to increase with postconceptual age. Evidence from animal experiments suggests that active use of sensory receptors and pathways is required for further development. Sensory deprivation results in degeneration of neural structures, leading to permanent damage and long-term implications for sensory function.[130] Thus, sensory·development follows the "use it or lose it" principle. In most circumstances, however, sensory deprivation does not occur. Rather, as discussed in later sections, sensory stimulation is more often excessive and the quality and pattern of stimulation may be inappropriate for the neonate.

A second consideration is the need for attention as a prerequisite for sensory input. The neonate's level of alertness and arousal determines attention to sensory stimulation. Thus, any condition affecting neurologic control of alertness interferes with reception and processing of sensory input. The autonomic nervous system mediates responsivity to external environment.[71] Alertness and arousal are functions of the infant's sleep–wake patterns or state, as well as the infant's physiologic status. Sensory input must always be considered in light of the infant's state.

Sensory Modalities

The term neonate can detect odors and respond to noxious odors. Neonates and infants can differentiate breast pads soaked with their mother's breast milk from those soaked with water or other substances.[114] Term neonates exhibit a preference for sweet taste, showing aversion to sour or salty tastes,[188] and can differentiate tastes.[32]

Although vision in the term neonate is qualitatively different than that of the adult, the visual abilities of these infants are adept. Vision is functional at birth, but massive changes occur in the first 6 months of life.[76] The retina continues to mature after birth. The fovea, the most sensitive area of the retina associated with high level discrimination, is not as sensitive in the neonate as in adults.[76] The neonate's limited accommodation ability decreases the ability to focus on objects that are extremely close to or far from the face. Accommodation improves during the first 3 months of life.[76] Infants can best perceive objects that are within 8 to 9 inches from their eyes and have high contrast or contours.[71, 76] Neonates can follow movement of an object.

Preterm infants demonstrate pupillary light responses and blinking to light by 29 weeks' gestation with awake visual attention by 30 weeks. These infants fix on simple patterns by 30 weeks' gestation and demonstrate pattern preferences by 31 to 32 weeks. Visual scanning with cessation of sucking is seen from 30 weeks and is active after 36 weeks.[74, 189] Preterm infants take longer to fixate on an object and are less responsive to visual stimuli than term infants and have poorer visual acuity and ability to accommodate. Most of the visual stimuli to which very low birth weight (VLBW) infants are exposed to during their brief periods of awake are probably inappropriate to the infants visual capabilities.[74]

Term neonates can hear and discriminate sounds. Hearing acuity is best in the low and mid-range frequencies with high frequency hearing developing in later infancy.[71] Additionally, hearing sensitivity increases with development and hearing threshold decreases.[71] Neonates differentiate sounds, attending to sounds of interest and showing aversion to noxious sounds. Neonates can distinguish their mothers' voices and readily turn toward the direction of the mother's voice.[39] Neonates and infants demonstrate a preference for high intonation and the rhythmic, sing-song vocalization that is called "motherese." Auditory capabilities and other sensory abilities of VLBW infants were discussed in the section on fetal development (pp. 549–550).

Neonates possess well-developed sensitivity to vestibular and kinesthetic stimulation. Rocking motions produce soothing and quieting of the neonate and infant. Use of vestibular stimulation with preterm infants has been associated with increased rhythmicity and organization, decreased apnea, improved weight gain, sleep promotion, and increased alertness and attention.[111]

Sensory Processing

The neonate is readily capable of receiving sensory information. The neonate also demonstrates the ability to discriminate sensory information and to attend to sensory input. Knowledge of the neonate's sensory reception abilities must be balanced with appreciation of sensory processing abilities, since in this area the neonate demonstrates developmental differences of the nervous system that have implications for long-term outcomes. Although reception of sensory input is grossly intact, the ability to process information and respond in an organized fashion is limited. Adaptation, habituation, and inhibition limit responsiveness to stimuli; without these processes people would be bombarded with input. In the brain of the neonate the structures and processes that underlie the ability to modulate sensory input are not well developed.

The neonate's brain continues to develop connections between neurons and lay down myelin. The degree of connectedness between neurons and speed of electrical conduction affect integration and organization of overall nervous system function. Behaviors of the neonate reflect these underlying maturational differences in the CNS. Neonates may exhibit differences in arousability, the extensiveness of responses, attention, tolerance to stimulation, soothability, regularity of state, motor tone, activity, synchrony, and rhythmicity.[5, 22, 49, 88] Although stimulation is required for normal development, the neonate can also be overwhelmed by sensory input because of the level of brain development. Just as environmental temperature for the neonate must be neither too warm or too cool, so too the sensory input for a neonate must be balanced to the infant's individual needs and tolerance.

Neonatal Motor Function

Movement may be reflexive or volitional in nature. In adults, as in neonates, volitional motor activity entails movement under the control of the cortex and other higher level control. In the neonate, however, control of motor function is emerging and demonstrates increasing integration and organization of the CNS. Reflexes in the neonates are somewhat different from those seen in the adult. Some of the reflexes exhibited by the neonate reflect both development of the muscles themselves as well as CNS control. Additionally, some reflexes normally observed only in the neonate and infant indicate the effects of development in motor control mechanisms. In general motor activities include muscle tone, motor abilities, the quality of movement, and presence and strength of reflexes.[70] Motor control is critical to further development. Through movement and reflexes, infants are capable of expressing needs, eliciting care, taking in oral nutrients, and experiencing and manipulating the environment.

Muscle Development

The motor abilities of the neonate demonstrate a characteristic pattern of development that reflects underlying changes in both nervous system control and maturation of the muscle cells themselves. Muscle is derived from mesoderm. During embryonic development formation of muscle cells is dependent on innervation by the nervous system. The full complement of muscle cells is generally achieved at approximately 38 weeks' gestational age, with formation of few muscle cells after this time. After birth, muscle cells increase in size by increasing the diameter of the muscle fibers and also grow in length.[128] Muscle strength is partially an outcome of muscle enlargement and growth.

Developmental changes in the innervation of muscle include myelinization of afferent fibers and pathways, increasing activity in the motor cortex, and increasing coordination of system-modifying motor actions such as the cerebellum, basal ganglia, and reticular activating system. Myelinization improves the speed of motor nerve conduction. Matura-

tion of the motor cortex allows conscious control of motor activities. The increasing integration of all levels of motor control results in smooth, coordinated movements, balance, and appropriate motor tone. Neonates exhibit a characteristic pattern of tone and flexion that undergoes predictable change throughout development. Muscle tone in the fetus shows caudal-cephalic progression. The term neonate demonstrates strong muscle tone, which is largely passive.[189] After birth, active motor tone, which is the tone during use of muscles, increases and passive tone decreases (Figs. 12–10 and 12–11). Alterations in muscle tone interfere with motor activities. Hypertonicity (excessive muscle tone) and hypotonicity (inadequate muscle tone) affect the underlying muscle tension that normally supports motor function. The predominant flexed position of the neonate shows innervation of flexor muscles and reciprocal relaxation of extensor muscles. The flexed position is not only protective but also assists in conservation of energy by reducing motor movements and assists in thermoregulation by reducing the surface area for heat loss. Motor development entails inhibition of flexion and increasing extensor activity. These changes occur in part because of increasing control by the motor cortex. When cortical innervation is interrupted, as in many pathologic conditions, loss of extensor innervation results in flexion. Increasing sophistication of control by the CNS improves coordination of movement, control and accuracy of movement, and synchrony and rhythmicity of movement. These capabilities support ongoing motor development including head control, turning over, reaching, and grasping.

Neonatal Reflexes

Reflexes are automatic, built-in motor behaviors occurring at the spinal level. Reflexes therefore provide information about muscle tone and lower level motor function. In the neonate the presence of "built-in" behaviors is critical, since at birth the neonate has no experience in the extrauterine environment. Reflexes serve many neonatal needs and also provide valuable information regarding the neonate's motor and neural status. Although reflexes are automatic rather than volitional, the reflexive responses of the neonate provide evidence to parents and other caregivers of the neonate's motor capabilities, respon-

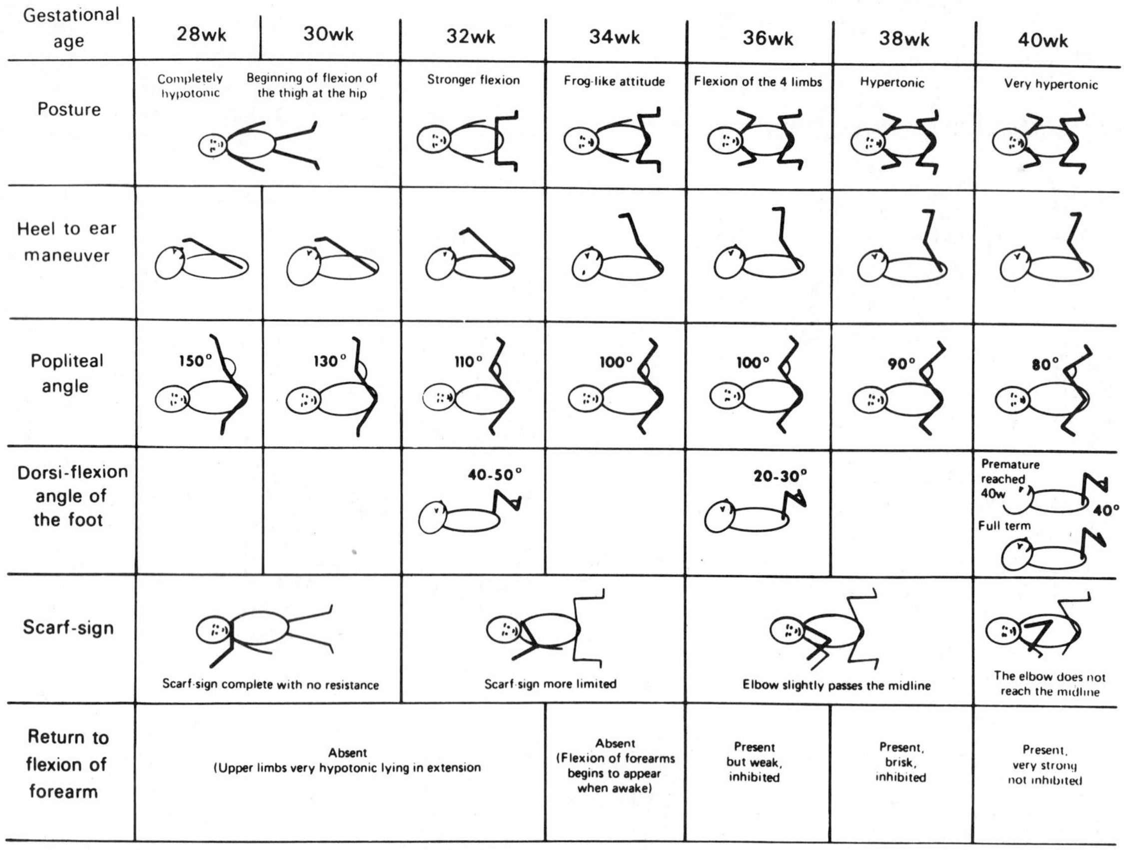

Gestational age	28wk	30wk	32wk	34wk	36wk	38wk	40wk
Posture	Completely hypotonic	Beginning of flexion of the thigh at the hip	Stronger flexion	Frog-like attitude	Flexion of the 4 limbs	Hypertonic	Very hypertonic
Heel to ear maneuver							
Popliteal angle	150°	130°	110°	100°	100°	90°	80°
Dorsi-flexion angle of the foot			40-50°		20-30°		Premature reached 40w 40° Full term
Scarf-sign	Scarf-sign complete with no resistance		Scarf-sign more limited		Elbow slightly passes the midline		The elbow does not reach the midline
Return to flexion of forearm	Absent (Upper limbs very hypotonic lying in extension			Absent (Flexion of forearms begins to appear when awake)	Present but weak, inhibited	Present, brisk, inhibited	Present, very strong not inhibited

Heel-to-ear: With the infant lying flat, the examiner lifts the legs as far as possible in an attempt to reach the ear with the feet without lifting the pelvis. The amplitude of the arc transversed by the legs is recorded.

Popliteal angle: The examiner flexes the infant's thighs laterally beside the abdomen, then extends the knees. The angle formed between the leg and the thigh, the popliteal angle, is recorded.

Dorsiflexion angle: The examiner dorsiflexes the ankle with the knee extended by applying pressure with the thumb to the sole of the foot. The angle formed by the dorsum of the foot and the anterior aspect of the leg is observed. This movement should be done twice, first slowly, then quickly. A difference of 10° or more between the slow and rapid movement is abnormal. The rapid maneuver will stimulate the stretch reflex; a phasic or jerky response is suspicious, while a sustained resistance to rapid flexion is abnormal.

Scarf sign: The infant is supported in a semi-reclining position with the examiner's hand, keeping the head straight. The infant's hand is pulled across the chest toward the opposite shoulder. Three positions are described: the elbow does not reach the midline; the elbow passes the midline; or the arm encircles the neck.

Forearm recoil: This can be elicited only when the infant is in a spontaneously flexed position. With the infant supine, the examiner extends the infant's arms by pulling on the hands, and, on release of the hands, observes how quickly the forearms return to the position of flexion. If recoil is observed, the arms are again extended for 20 to 30 sec, then released to determine if prolonged extension inhibits recoil.

FIGURE 12–10. Posture and passive tone from 28 to 40 weeks' gestational age. (Reprinted with permission from Rudolph, A., et al. (1991). *Rudolph's pediatrics* (19th ed., p. 178). Norwalk, CT: Appleton & Lange.)

siveness, and individual needs. The development and strength of reflexes varies with gestational age (Table 12–9).

Many reflexes characteristic to the neonate seemingly disappear with development. Some reflexes (such as the Babinski reflex) are masked by higher order functions but are observed in the adult when pathologic conditions interfere with higher level control. Other reflexes considered abnormal in the adult are seen in the neonate. For instance, clonus of the knee and ankle is commonly observed in the neonate, as is the Babinski reflex.[2]

The Moro reflex involves abduction of the arms at the shoulder with the elbows in

FIGURE 12–11. Active tone from 32 to 40 weeks' gestational age. (Reprinted with permission from Rudolph, A., et al. (1991). *Rudolph's pediatrics* (19th ed., p. 179). Norwalk, CT: Appleton & Lange.)

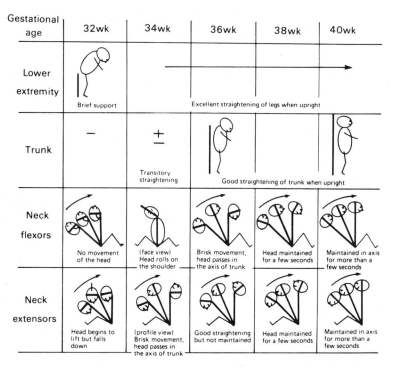

Gestational age	32wk	34wk	36wk	38wk	40wk
Lower extremity	Brief support	Excellent straightening of legs when upright			
Trunk	−	± Transitory straightening	Good straightening of trunk when upright		
Neck flexors	No movement of the head	(face view) Head rolls on the shoulder	Brisk movement, head passes in the axis of trunk	Head maintained for a few seconds	Maintained in axis for more than a few seconds
Neck extensors	Head begins to lift but falls down	(profile view) Brisk movement, head passes in the axis of trunk	Good straightening but not maintained	Head maintained for a few seconds	Maintained in axis for more than a few seconds

Righting reaction: The examiner holds the infant in a standing position (place the hands in the axillae to support the chest). Contraction of extensor muscles of the legs and trunk, allowing the infant to support some of his or her weight, is observed.

Neck flexors: The examiner grasps the infant's shoulder and pulls the infant from the supine to the sitting position. The position of the head in relation to the trunk is noted as the neck flexor muscles contract to raise the head to the vertical position.

Neck extensors: With the infant sitting and leaning forward and the head hanging down on the chest, the examiner moves the infant backward and observes the action of the neck extensors, which lift the head before the vertical position is reached.

extension and the hands open, followed by adduction of the arms at the shoulder into an embrace position with flexion of the elbows. Crying often accompanies the Moro reflex. Portions of the Moro reflex can be observed as early as 28 weeks' gestational age with a mature reflex seen at approximately 36 to 37 weeks.[9]

Neonates exhibit a strong palmar grasp reflex with fingers tightly flexed and curled into the palm. The palmar grasp reflex is so strong that infants can grasp, although not consciously, items placed in the hand. In addition, the palmar grasp is assessed in the pull-to-sit maneuver. Although the palmar grasp is first observed at approximately 28 weeks' gestational age, full strength is achieved at approximately 32 weeks.[9]

The tonic neck reflex is also termed the fencing position and is stimulated by rotation of the head to the side. The reflex movements include extension of the arm and leg on the side to which the head is turned, and flexion of the arm and leg on the side opposite to which the head is turned. The movements of the extremities are similar to the crossed extensor reflex (see Table 12–9). Portions of the tonic neck reflex appear during later fetal development, but the reflex is often not well established until 1 month after birth.[189] Like the Moro reflex, the tonic neck reflex stabilizes position, preventing rolling.

Neonates demonstrate a rhythmic stepping motion of their lower extremities. When the neonate is held upright with the feet touching a solid surface, and alternating stepping motion is observed. There is some evidence that coordination exhibited in the stepping reflex may be predictive of later developmental outcomes.

The sucking and rooting reflexes are essential for oral intake of nutrients by the neonate. Rooting assists the neonate in locating and latching on to the nipple and occurs

TABLE 12–9
Strength of Six Reflexes for Infants Between 28 and 40 Weeks' Gestation

	28	30	32	34	36	38	40
Sucking[a]	Weak, not really synchronized with swallowing		Stronger and better synchronized with swallowing		Perfect		
Palmar grasp[b]	Present but weak			Stronger		Excellent	
Response to traction[b]	Absent		Begins to appear	Strong enough to lift part of body weight		Strong enough to lift all of body weight	
Moro reflex[c]	Weak, obtained just once, incomplete		Complete reflex				
Crossed extension[d]	Flexion and extension in random pattern, purposeless reaction		Good extension but no tendency to adduction		Tendency to adduction but imperfect	Complete response with extension, adduction, fanning of toes	
Automatic walking[e]	—	—	Begins tiptoeing with good support on sole and righting reaction of legs for a few seconds	Pretty good; very fast tiptoeing	A premature who reaches 40 wk walks in toe-heel progression or tiptoes. A full-term newborn of 40 wk walks in heel-toe progression on whole sole of foot		

[a]**Sucking reflex:** The examiner evaluates the sucking reflex by introducing a finger into the infant's mouth to observe the strength and rhythm of sucking. The synchrony of sucking and swallowing is observed during feeding.

[b]**Palmar grasp and response to traction:** The examiner inserts the index finger into the infant's hand from the ulnar side and gently presses against the palmar surface. The infant's fingers flex around the finger. When the hands are drawn upward, the response to traction spreads to the flexor muscles of the arm. The term infant can support his or her entire weight by this traction response.

[c]**Moro reflex:** The examiner grasps the infant's hands and lifts the shoulders a few centimeters while keeping the back of the head on the bed, then suddenly releases the hands. The normal reflex is a brisk abduction of the arms at the shoulder and extension of the forearms at the elbow, followed by adduction of the arms and flexion of the forearms. Complete opening of the hands occurs in the first phase.

[d]**Crossed extension reflex:** The examiner holds one of the infant's feet in extension and rubs the sole. The complete response has three components: (1) the opposite leg rapidly flexes or "retreats" followed by extension; then (2) the opposite leg adducts; and (3) the toes of the opposite foot fan.

[e]**Automatic walking:** The examiner holds the infant by the trunk and lifts him or her slightly forward. The infant steps forward as each foot contacts the surface.

Reprinted with permission from Rudolph A., et al. (1987). *Pediatrics* (18th ed., p. 123). Norwalk, CT: Appleton & Lange.

at about 32 weeks' gestation.[2] Stimulation of the perioral region result in turning of the head in the direction of the stimulus and mouthing actions in search of the nipple. The sucking reflex is present at 28 weeks' gestation, but is weak and uncoordinated with swallowing. Sucking and swallowing are weakly coordinated at 32 weeks. By 34 to 36 weeks sucking is strong and coordinated with swallowing (see Table 12–9).[9]

Sleep–Wake Pattern

Fetal activity records document fluctuating periods of activity and quiescence, seen as early as 21 weeks' gestation.[174] After birth the infant exhibits alternating periods of sleep and wakefulness. Sleep in neonates and infants exhibits developmental differences from that of the adult. As a result, sleep is not as well defined and definitions are less precise than in the adult. Consequently, neonatal and infant sleep is described in terms of state, that is, a group of physiologic and behavioral characteristics that regularly recur together.[18]

Neonates and infants spend a large portion of the 24-hour day sleeping. Sleep therefore does not follow a light-dark pattern and is not diurnal, as in the adult. A major accomplishment in the development of the infant is the ability to sleep through the night and adapt to the diurnal pattern of activity and sleep–wake behaviors of the family. The sleep–wake pattern is an indicator of neurologic status and the neonate's ability to organize behavior.

Definition of Infant States

A number of systems have been developed to code or score neonatal and infant sleep–wake states. The major difference between conventional definitions of infant states is the number of types of states and therefore the specificity and precision of the various states. Generally, the more immature the neonate according to gestational and postconceptional age, the grosser or less precise the definitions of state, since the quality of state and consistency among indicators improve with age (Table 12–10). The six categories of infant state described by Wolff[194] will be discussed. Each state is complete unto itself, representing a particular form of neural control.[74] The six sleep–wake states include: quiet (deep) sleep, active (light) sleep, drowsy, awake (quiet) alert, active alert, and crying (Table 12–11). The ability to clearly differentiate these states is dependent on the infant's postconceptional age. The proportion of time spent in each of these states also varies with postconceptional age.

Quiet (NREM) sleep is deep, restful sleep with the eyes closed, little body or facial movement, except for an occasional startle or twitch, regular respiration and heart rate, and no movement of the eyes.[143] Quiet sleep is restorative and anabolic. An increase in cell mitosis and replication occurs during this state. Oxygen consumption reaches the lowest levels during quiet sleep. In addition, the release of growth hormone is associated with quiet sleep, as are high levels of serotonin and low levels of glucocorticoid.

During active sleep the eyes are closed but there are movements of the extremities and face, mouthing, grimacing, and sucking movements. Respiration and heart rate are irregular and penile erections occur. Active bouts of REM occur in association with dreaming; the fine, rapid movement of the eyes can be observed beneath the lid. Active sleep is also called paradoxical sleep or REM sleep and has been likened to "wide awake asleep" because the level of brain activity is similar to the awake state. Information is processed during active sleep and entered into memory; thus, active sleep has been linked to learning and restructuring of synapses and changes in protein synthesis increase during active sleep.

During the drowsy state, the neonate or infant seems partially awake and partially asleep. Drowsiness usually indicates a state transition between awake and sleep states. In the awake or quiet alert state the neonate or infant is awake, the eyes are open, and there is little motor movement. The neonate or infant is alert and shows interest or attention by focusing on visual stimulation. The infant appears to be "drinking in" information from the surrounding environment and processing this information. The awake alert state is sometimes referred to as quiet alert, emphasizing the limited motion and activity associated with the infant attending to sensory information.

The neonate or infant's motor activity escalates in the active awake state. The eyes may have a hyperalert appearance. There may be spitting up or hiccoughing. Respiration often becomes increased and irregular and skin color changes may occur. The active alert state often precedes crying. In healthy infants crying is easily recognizable. Crying behaviors include closed eyes with facial characteristics and the vocalization of cry sounds. In preterm infants the motor actions associated with cry sounds are evident, but because of the infant's immaturity and weakness, the sounds may not be produced.

Sleep–Wake States Related to Brain Maturation

Sleep–wake patterns change with CNS maturation; and sleep is required for brain development. Postnatal development of sleep–wake state pattern reflects the underlying maturation of the reticular activating system, brain stem, and related circadian rhythms. The developmental changes in state include both alterations in temporal pattern and the

---

TABLE 12–10
Infant State Parameters by Gestational Age

	WEEKS GESTATIONAL AGE					MONTHS PAST TERM	
	24	28	32	36	40	3	8
Body movements	+ −	+	+ +	+ + +	+ + + +	+ + + +	+ + + +
Eye movements		+	+ +	+ + +	+ + + +	+ + + +	+ + + +
Respiration pattern			+ −	+ +	+ + +	+ + + +	+ + + +
EEG			+ −	+ +	+ + +	+ + + +	+ + + +
Chin EMG*				+	+ + +	+ + + +	+ + + +

*EMG, electromyelograph.

From Parmelee, A.H. & Stern, E. (1972). Development of states in infants. In C.D. Clemente, D.P. Purpura, & F.E. Mayer (Eds.), *Sleep and the maturing nervous system* (pp. 199). New York: Academic Press.

TABLE 12–11
Infant State Chart (Sleep and Awake States)

STATE	BODY ACTIVITY	EYE MOVEMENTS	FACIAL MOVEMENTS
Sleep States			
Deep (Quiet) Sleep	Nearly still, except for occasional startle or twitch.	None.	Without facial movements, except for occasional sucking movement at regular intervals.
Light (Active) Sleep	Some body movements.	Rapid eye movements (REM), fluttering of eyes beneath closed eyelids.	May smile and make brief fussy or crying sounds.
Awake States			
Drowsy	Activity level variable, with mild startles interspersed from time to time. Movements usually smooth.	Eyes open and close occasionally, are heavy-lidded with dull, glazed appearance.	May have some facial movements. Often there are none, and the face appears still.
Quiet Alert	Minimal.	Brightening and widening of eyes.	Faces have bright, shining, sparkling looks.
Active Alert	Much body activity. May have periods of fussiness.	Eyes open with less brightening.	Much facial movement. Faces not as bright as in quiet alert state.
Crying	Increased motor activity with color changes.	Eyes may be tightly closed or open.	Grimaces.

State is a group of characteristics that regularly occur together: body activity, eye movements, facial movements, breathing pattern, and level of response to external stimuli (e.g., handling) and internal stimuli (e.g., hunger).
From Blackburn, S. & Kang, R. (in press). *Early Parent-Infant Relationships* (2nd ed.). Series 1: The First Six Hours After Birth, Module 3. White Plains, New York: March of Dimes Birth Defects Foundation.

integration of variables within the state. Inhibitory ability increases with CNS maturation. Increased inhibitory ability results in smoother muscle movements, reduces global responses, improves habituation and adaptation, and generally acts to improve the infant's attentional abilities as well as bring about specific changes in sleep. These sleep changes include increasing duration of sleep periods, consolidation of sleep into nighttime hours, and maturation of the sleep states themselves.[30] Within each state, synchrony among the state variables increases.

Infant development entails increasing amounts of quiet sleep as well as increasing periods of quiet alertness. Both of these states reflect sophisticated neural control. Sustaining a state consistently or making a transition from one state to another requires tremendous neural organization. Thus, sleep–wake patterns are an excellent window to the infant's neurologic status. Alterations in sleep–wake patterns are observed in infants with Down syndrome, biochemical disturbances,

brain malformations, and following asphyxia.[74]

Sleep is necessary for somatic and brain growth and development. As described earlier, during quiet sleep restorative and growth processes are facilitated. REM sleep is important for learning and memory. Attention behavior development parallels development of quiet sleep, indicating both inhibition and maturity.[143] The amount of quiet awake time parallels quiet sleep, and both increase with development.[74]

Development of Infant State

Before 28 to 30 weeks of gestational age the preterm infant shows minimal pattern of state activity either by behavioral or electroencephalographic (EEG) characteristics. Active sleep or REM appears at 28 to 30 weeks' gestation with evidence of cycling of states at 32 weeks.[48, 74] Quiet sleep appears much later in postconceptual development, initially becoming apparent at approximately 36 weeks

TABLE 12–11
Infant State Chart (Sleep and Awake States) Continued

BREATHING PATTERN	LEVEL OF RESPONSE	IMPLICATIONS FOR CAREGIVING
Smooth and regular.	Threshold to stimuli is very high so that only very intense and disturbing stimuli will arouse infants.	Caregivers trying to feed infants in deep sleep will probably find the experience frustrating. Infants will be unresponsive, even if caregivers use disturbing stimuli (flicking feet) to arouse infants. Infants may arouse only briefly and then become unresponsive as they return to deep sleep. If caregivers wait until infants move to a higher, more responsive state, feeding or caregiving will be much pleasanter.
Irregular.	More responsive to internal and external stimuli. When these stimuli occur, infants may remain in light sleep, return to deep sleep, or arouse to drowsy.	Light sleep makes up the highest proportion of newborn sleep and usually precedes awakening. Because of brief fussy or crying sounds made during this state, caregivers who are not aware that these sounds occur normally may think it is time for feeding and may try to feed infants before they are ready to eat.
Irregular.	Infants react to sensory stimuli although responses are delayed. State change after stimulation frequently noted.	From the drowsy state, infants may return to sleep or awaken further. To awaken, caregivers can provide something for infants to see, hear, or suck, as this may arouse them to a quiet alert state, a more responsive state. Infants who are left alone without stimuli may return to a sleep state.
Regular.	Infants attend most to environment, focusing attention on any stimuli that are present.	Infants in this state provide much pleasure and positive feedback for caregivers. Providing something for infants to see, hear, or suck will often maintain a quiet alert state. In the first few hours after birth, most newborns commonly experience a period of intense alertness before going into a long sleep period.
Irregular.	Increasingly sensitive to disturbing stimuli (hunger, fatigue, noise, excessive handling).	Caregivers may intervene at this state to console and bring the infant to a lower state.
More irregular.	Extremely responsive to unpleasant external or internal stimuli.	Crying is the infant's communication signal. It is a response to unpleasant stimuli from the environment or within infants (fatigue, hunger, discomfort). Crying tells us infants' limits have been reached. Sometimes infants can console themselves and return to lower states. At other times, they need help from caregivers.

of gestational age.[143] With maturation, transitional sleep decreases.[189] General trends in sleep development include increasing quiet sleep, decreasing active sleep, and chaining sleep cycles together, which yields longer sleep periods.[86]

The EEG of the infant is not always consistent with the behavioral expression of state. State is evidenced behaviorally before it is apparent on the EEG. Before 30 weeks' gestation, EEG activity is present but is discontinuous and of low amplitude. At 30 to 36 weeks of gestational age active sleep can be determined by EEG.[189] Between 36 to 40 weeks of gestational age both active and quiet sleep can be determined by EEG. Maturation of EEG activity includes differentiation of discontinuous activity into mature EEG wave forms and an increase in the amplitude of EEG waves.[53] The EEG of the newborn frequently shows paroxysmal activity, asymmetry of the left and right portions of the brain, and considerable individual variation.[75]

Continued development of sleep–wake patterns after birth also involves changes in the temporal pattern of sleep and the integration of variables within states. Neonates sleep an average of 16 to 17 hours per day. Periods of sleep occur around the clock. Periods of sleep are short, typically not extending beyond 3 or 4 hours. The sleep cycle is roughly 50 minutes, compared with the 90-minute adult sleep cycle, and sleep is predominantly active in nature, with 50 to 90% of sleep time in active sleep depending on postconceptional age.

State Modulation

Some infants seem to "sleep like babies," whereas some are difficult to soothe, awaken easily, and sleep for short intervals and at unpredictable times. Other infants are overly drowsy, difficult to arouse, and sleep excessive periods of time. Differences in sleep–wake patterns reflect differences in neurologic development and the infant's ability to modulate state. State modulation refers to the infant's ability to make smooth transitions between states, arouse when appropriate, and sustain sleep states. By modulating or regulating state, the infant can control sensory input to some extent and the response to the environment.[23, 71] In addition, the infant can use state behaviors to guide caregiving and to modify social interactions. Problems with state modulation, therefore, entail problems regulating sensory input and responses. Infants who cannot use state changes to turn stimulation on or off may be either missing important input or sensorily overloaded. State modulation is therefore an asset in the infant's adaptation to the environment. Problems with state modulation may emanate from the infant or environment. Infant factors influencing state modulation include immaturity, pain, stress, maternal substance abuse, and illness. Environmental factors that affect state regulation and interfere with the infant's sleep–wake pattern include noise, light, temperature, and caregiver actions.

Neurobehavioral Organization

The concept of neurobehavioral organization is a means of holistically viewing the infant's response capabilities. The connectedness between elements of the nervous system is the basis for integration and organization of overall function. Neurobehavioral organization captures the essence of neonatal and infant function in the extrauterine environment and determines the infant's interaction with the surrounding physical and social environment.

What does neurobehavioral organization encompass? Als' Synactive Theory of Development defines five subsystems governing the infant's interaction with the environment: autonomic/physiologic, motor, state organizational, attentional/interactive, and self-regulatory capacity.[3] These subsystems are interdependent and hierarchical, that is, the order of development begins with autonomic/physiologic stability, followed in succession by motor, state, and attentional/interactive, and finally development of self-regulatory capacity. The level of organization is determined by development and is largely dependent on postconceptional age; however, illness or injury may alter neurologic function and therefore neurobehavioral organization. In addition, organization at any level is determined by the previous levels. Thus, state organization is dependent on organization and stability of the motor and autonomic/physiologic subsystems; attentional/interactive behaviors require organization of the state, motor, and autonomic/physiologic subsystems. An infant's behavioral responses or cues are indicative of the level of organization.

Autonomic organization entails regulation of cardiorespiratory activity, gastrointestinal peristalsis, and peripheral skin blood flow. Motor organization includes skeletal muscle tone, posture, and quality of movement. State organization involves orderly progression of sleep–wake states, the ability to sustain a state, and smooth state transitions. The culmination of neurobehavioral organization is the infant's attentional/interactive and self-regulatory abilities. The attentional/interactive subsystem involves the infant's ability to orient and focus on stimuli and achieve well-defined periods of alertness. Self-regulatory capacity is the ability of the infant to maintain integrity and balance between the other subsystems, integrate all the subsystems, and modulate state.

Neurobehavioral organization refers to the ability to modulate state, control internal reactions, control motor responses, self-regulate, respond to people and events in the external stressors, and maintain an appropriate degree of alertness.[23] Thus, neurobehavioral organization is critical to energy consumption, oxygen and calorie requirements, and growth, as well as the foundation for development and interactions with parents and other caregivers. Examples of neurobehavioral organization include the ability to regulate sensory input, feed efficiently and effectively, coordinate sucking and swallowing, self-console, exhibit smooth coordinated movement, maintain muscle tone, and elicit caregiving through appropriate cues. Tools to asses neurobehavioral organization rely on observation of the infant in interaction with both the physical and social environments. The Brazelton Newborn Behavioral Assessment Scale (BNBAS) is an assessment of the infant's ability to organize and modulate states, habituate to external stimulation, regulate motor activity in the face of increasing sensory input, respond to reflexive testing, alert and orient to visual and auditory stimuli, interact with a caregiver, and self-console.[23] The Assessment of Preterm Infants' Behavior (APIB) is a neurobehavioral tool based on Als' Synactive Theory of Development and geared to the assessment of the preterm infant and high risk term infants. The purpose of the APIB assessment is to determine how the infant is coping with the intense environment of the neonatal intensive care unit (NICU) and the degree of CNS organization.[6]

CLINICAL IMPLICATIONS FOR NEONATAL CARE

During the neonatal period, glial proliferation, myelinization, cell differentiation, dendrite expansion, and synapse formation and remodeling are occurring. The developing CNS is vulnerable to a number of influences, including the effects of the environment, handling, and caregiving. In addition, the immature CNS produces variations in seizure activity and influences the diagnosis and treatment of pain. These concerns are particularly important when considering the infant born prematurely since development of the nervous system is not consistent with demands posed by the extrauterine environment.[41] The preterm infant is usually a third trimester fetus, and, with the increasing survival of extremely premature infants, viability is extending into the second trimester.

Risks Posed by the Caregiving Environment

Healthy, term gestation infants are well equipped to adapt to life outside the uterus. When neonates are compromised by illness or prematurity, adaptive abilities are challenged. The extrauterine environment is a critical factor in the development of the immature CNS and may alter developmental outcomes.[182] The hospital care environment has been viewed as providing a deficient sensory environment. Studies of infant stimulation have produced variable results in terms of improved growth and developmental outcome.[79] The rich background provided by stimulation research has led to caregiving based on recognition of infant cues (Table 12–12).[3] Emphasis has been placed on controlling the physical environment, including noise and light, and pacing caregiving to fit the infant's level of neurobehavioral maturation.[3, 7, 18, 107]

Stability or engagement cues (sometimes referred to as approach cues) demonstrate organization and reflect the infant's readiness for interaction (Table 12–12). Distress or disengagement cues (Table 12–12) indicate disorganization and signal the caregiver to provide supportive measures and time for recuperation. Supportive measures include interventions such as positioning, providing boundaries, swaddling, and reducing handling.[18a, 25, 107, 185] The Neonatal Individualized

TABLE 12–12
Infant Neurobehavioral Cues

DISTRESS/DISENGAGEMENT CUES	STABILITY/ENGAGEMENT CUES
Bradycardia, apnea	Facial gaze
Rapid heart or respiration rate	Smiling
Grunting	Vocalization
Stooling	Feeding posture
Mottled skin	Flexion of arms, legs
Dusky color	Eyes alert
Cyanosis	Stable heart rate
Tremor	Stable respiratory rate
Finger splay	Smooth movements
Fingers interlaced	Hand-to-mouth
Arching	Finger folding
Hyperalert face	Smooth state transitions
Facial grimace	Sucking, mouthing
Limb extension	Consolable
Gaze aversion	"Ooh" face
Eyes closed	Alert
Slack jaw	Eye-to-eye contact
Open mouth	Grasping
Tongue thrusting	
Sighing	
Regurgitation	
Jittery	
Flaccid	
Vomiting	
Hand-to-ear	
Worried face	
Rapid state change	
Eyes floating	
Staring	
Hyperextension	
Glassy eyed	
Tongue protrusion	
Flushed	
Hiccough	
Startle	
Yawn	
Flaccidity	
Sneezing	

Compiled from references 14, 18, 72, 107, 112, and 134.

Developmental Care and Assessment Program (NIDCAP) is a specialized training program for high-risk infant care providers that focuses on sensitive recognition of infant behavioral cues and intervention strategies to promote and support neurobehavioral organization.[4]

Vulnerability to Hypoxic and Pressure-Related Injury

Systemic hypoxemia and decreased cerebral perfusion leading to ischemia can lead to hypoxic-ischemic damage to the brain with hemorrhage and edema (Fig. 12–12). The site of injury varies with maturational changes in the vascular anatomy and metabolic activity of the brain. In preterm infants

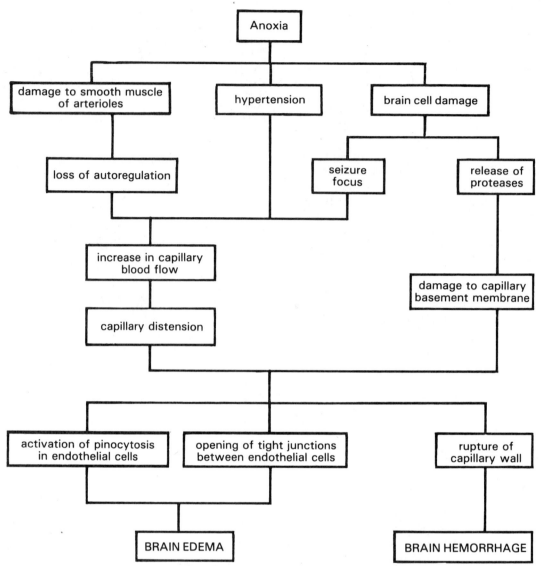

FIGURE 12–12. Relationship of anoxia and brain edema and hemorrhage. (From Goldstein, G.W. (1981). Special features of the brain microcirculation: Role in brain edema formation. In *Perinatal brain insult* (p. 47). Mead Johnson Symposium on Perinatal and Developmental Medicine, No. 17. Evansville, IN: Mead Johnson.)

of less than 32 to 34 weeks' gestation, injury is usually associated with periventricular–intraventricular hemorrhage. In older preterm and term infants, insults of this type result in hypoxic-ischemic encephalopathy.

Intraventricular and Periventricular Hemorrhage

Intraventricular hemorrhage (IVH) and periventricular hemorrhage (PVH) are common forms of intracranial hemorrhage in the neonate.[189] The consequences of intracranial hemorrhage include direct neuronal damage due to pressure and inflammation and potential hydrocephalus; severe hemorrhage often results in death.[103] Long-term outcomes are variable but include motor and sensory disabilities as well as cognitive delay.

The occurrence of IVH and PVH is related to structural and functional differences in the immature CNS including the nature of the subependymal germinal matrix, differences in regulation of CBF, and venous pressure. The hemorrhage usually begins as microvascular event that spreads, presumably due to overperfusion of the area.[193] The site of IVH/PVH is developmentally related. In term infants the hemorrhage is predominantly in the ventricular choroid plexus and trauma is more often a precipitating factor.[189] In preterm infants bleeding occurs more often in the subependymal germinal matrix located adjacent the lateral ventricles in the subependymal layer.[69, 193] PVH occurs most often in the area of the caudate nucleus and foramen of Monro.[103] The highest risk of IVH and PVH is during the period of germinal matrix involution in the third trimester and neonatal periods.[69] Thus, the more immature the neonate, the greater the risk of IVH and PVH [193]

The germinal matrix is a highly cellular, high metabolic area characterized as gelatinous in structure.[189] The germinal matrix receives a rich blood supply chiefly through a large bed of capillaries that are fragile in nature and prone to disruption.[103] In addition, the venous drainage in the area of the germinal matrix entails a distinctive U-shaped curve, and venous tributaries merge and flow into the vein of Galen, which is predisposed to stasis and increased venous pressure.

The physical characteristics of the germinal matrix, along with its highly vascular nature and potential limits in venous drainage, predispose to bleeding. These characteristics interact with autoregulation and the effects of hypoxia on autoregulation. During episodes of hypoxemia, autoregulation is abolished and blood flow becomes pressure-passive. Hypercarbia and acidosis also disrupt autoregulation. Thus, any condition that reduces blood oxygen levels may alter autoregulation and contribute to the development of IVH and PVH (Fig. 12–12). Although cardiorespiratory problems are easily recognized as sources of hypoxia, any factor that increases oxygen demand beyond the supply capabilities (i.e., increased metabolic rate) is also suspect in producing hypoxia, altered autoregulation, and IVH/PVH. Examples include thermoregulatory requirements, effects of handling, environmental disruptions, pain, or motor activity. During periods of pressure-passive flow, fragile capillaries of the germinal matrix may rupture if CBF or pressure increase. Once capillary disruption occurs, alterations in coagulation, thought to accompany perinatal complications, potentially perpetuate the hemorrhage. Evidence suggests excess fibrinolytic activity in the area of germinal matrix.[189]

Factors that produce fluctuating, decreased, or increased CBF contribute to IVH and PVH.[189] Since autoregulation of CBF is often compromised, alterations in systemic blood pressure are also causative factors. Examples of conditions thought to contribute to IVH/PVH include the pressure effects of ventilatory assistance, infusion of volume expanding fluids, hypercarbia and other causes of cerebral vasodilation, increase in central venous pressure, or respiratory distress.[189]

Many of the health care procedures experienced by preterm infants alter oxygen level and blood pressure, such as handling or suctioning. Research on the effects of procedures has shown that blood pressure initially drops, followed by a rise; the more intensive the care the greater the initial drop and the greater the rebound.[141] Prevention of PVH and IVH requires sensitivity regarding the fragile nature of the capillaries within the CNS and recognition of the effects of hypoxemia on autoregulation, as well as the role of autoregulation and pressure in cerebral perfusion.[34]

Periventricular Leukomalacia

Periventricular leukomalacia (PVL) is a condition in which necrotic changes subsequent to ischemia occur in the white matter in the area of the ventricles.[193] Blood flow is typically impaired by hypotension. As in IVH and PVH, vascular structure and factors influencing CBF place the preterm infant at risk for PVL. Marginal areas of blood flow occur near the lateral ventricles because of inadequate overlap in circulation.[193] Underperfusion of these areas leads to ischemia and necrosis. Conditions that produce hypoxemia effect PVL in two ways. First, reduction of blood oxygen decreases delivery of oxygen to such vulnerable regions. Second, hypoxia reduces autoregulation. Loss of autoregulation in the presence of low system blood pressure results in low CBF, since flow is pressure passive. Clinical implications for IVH, PVH, and PVL entail recognition of the role of energy demands and oxygen level as well as regulation of both systemic blood pressure and cerebral flow.

Hypoxic-Ischemic Encephalopathy

After 33 to 34 weeks' gestation blood flow and brain metabolic activity are less prominent in the periventricular area and shift to the cortical area. As a result hypoxia and ischemia in older preterm and term infants is more likely to damage areas of the peripheral and dorsal cerebral cortex. The primary lesion in hypoxic injury is necrosis of neurons in the cortices of the cerebrum and cerebellum, and possibly the brain stem. The primary ischemic injury occurs in the posterior (boundary area) portion of the parasagittal region. This area is farthest from the original blood supply of the major cerebral vessels and with systemic hypotension or hypoperfusion receives the least blood. With asphyxia and systemic hypotension cerebral perfusion is maintained at first by cerebral vasodilation and redistribution of blood flow to the brain from other organs. If the asphyxia continues, brain water balance and cerebral blood flow are altered and ischemia and edema develop (Fig. 12–12).

Neonatal Seizures

Seizure activity is the most frequent sign of neurologic problems in the neonate and infant.[189] Seizures result from an abnormal neuronal electrical discharge. Thus, seizures are caused by a number of conditions in which the environment of neurons, which support normal electrical activity, is altered. These conditions include hypoxemia, ischemia, hypoglycemia, hypocalcemia, hyperkalemia, hypomagnesemia, hypo- or hypernatremia, acidosis, and meningitis.[189] In general seizure activity may entail eye movements, oral movements, changes in posture, motor movements such as bicycling or rowing actions, and apnea. Types of seizures and their description are provided in Table 12–13. The timing of seizure onset is related to pathology and gestational age.[189]

Seizure activity is determined by brain maturation. Thus, seizures are expressed differently based on gestational age and postmenstrual age and do not resemble the seizure activity of adults.[180] These differences in seizure activity result from the structural and functional differences in the immature CNS. Lower rate of nerve conduction, limited myelinization, and reduced connectivity between neurons effect the propagation of the seizure.[189] Consequently, the signs of seizure in the neonate are often subtle and more localized than in the adult. Neonatal seizures contain elements of jitteriness, but the two can be differentiated (Table 12–14).

TABLE 12–13
Types of Neonatal Seizures

SUBTLE SEIZURES
Premature and full-term infants
Ocular–tonic horizontal deviation of the eyes ± jerking; and sustained eye opening with ocular fixation
Eyelid blinking or fluttering
Sucking, smacking, drooling, or other oral–buccal–lingual movements
"Swimming," "rowing," and "pedaling" movements
Apneic spell

GENERALIZED TONIC SEIZURES
Primarily premature infants
Tonic extension of upper and lower limbs (mimics decerebrate posturing)
Tonic flexion of upper limbs and extension of lower limbs (mimics decorticate posturing)

MULTIFOCAL CLONIC SEIZURES
Primarily full-term infants
Multifocal clonic movements: simultaneous or in sequence
Nonordered ("non-Jacksonian") migration

FOCAL CLONIC SEIZURES
Full term more than premature infants
Well-localized clonic jerking
Infant usually not unconscious

From Volpe, J.J. (1987). *Neurology of the newborn* (2nd ed., pp. 134–135). Philadelphia: WB Saunders.

Since seizures involve massive discharge of neurons, a seizure is associated with an intense increase in energy consumption by the neurons. Additionally, the seizure activity may interfere with adequate oxygenation of the blood. Hypoxia as well as hypoglycemia and other metabolic changes may occur within the CNS during seizures.[189] Seizures are related to developmental problems, particularly the effects of repeated seizures on the developing nervous system.[165]

Neonatal Pain

That pain occurs in the neonate and infant is unequivocal. In the history of infant care, the understanding of pain in infants was determined largely by conceptualization of brain function at this age. Since the infant's central nervous function was believed to be similar to a laboratory brain stem preparation, that is, no function above the level of the brain stem, the infant's ability to perceive and respond to pain was ignored. It was also believed that the infant's level of myelinization prevented reception of pain and therefore attenuated the effects of pain. Finally, discrediting of pain was further rationalized because it was assumed that the infant had

TABLE 12–14
Differentiation of Jitteriness and Seizure Activity

CLINICAL FEATURE	JITTERINESS	SEIZURE
Abnormality of gaze or eye deviation	0	+
Movements exquisitely stimulus-sensitive	+	0
Predominant movement	Tremor	Clonic jerking
Movements cease with passive flexion	+	0

From Volpe, J.J. (1987). *Neurology of the newborn* (2nd ed., p. 135). Philadelphia: WB Saunders.

no memory for painful experiences. Although a mass of data confirms the occurrence of pain in neonates and infants, many practices in the care of infants continue to be colored by previous thinking. In addition, the difficulty in objectively assessing pain in infants as well as appropriate management are still challenges to neonatal care.

Pain Reception in Neonates and Infants

A number of excellent reviews summarize studies that document the presence of pain in neonates and infants.[11, 144, 162] Because of the neurologic development of the neonate, pain may be qualitatively different from that experienced later in life, but it does exists. Pain receptors are in place and in fact the density of pain receptors or nociceptors is greater in the neonate.[67] The fibers that conduct pain stimuli to the spinal cord are in place early in fetal life. Nociceptive receptors are among the first fibers to grow into the spinal cord in the fetus. The density of nociceptive nerve endings in the skin is similar to that in adults until 28 weeks' gestation and then increases to exceed adult density until approximately 2 years of age.[11] Pain fibers are unmyelinated; therefore, myelinization occurring with development does not alter transmission of pain messages to the cord. In the spinal cord, the pathways that carry pain stimuli to the brain (anterolateral pathways) are undergoing myelinization. The pain pathways are myelinated by 30 weeks' gestation and thalamic fibers that relay information to the cortex are myelinated by 37 weeks' gestation.[65] Thus, the rate of transmission may be altered (slower), but offset by the shorter distance impulses must travel to reach the brain. These factors may be particularly important in temporal and spatial summation. Myelinization may have an effect on central processing and integration of pain information. Neonates have all the anatomic and functional requirements for pain perception.[11] Neonates possess the ability to produce

endogenous opiates; increased levels of these substances are found after birth and levels increase with difficult births and during times of stress.[11, 144] These increased opiate levels are still lower than needed to produce analgesia.[11]

Consequences of Pain in the Neonate

There is ample evidence to show that the physiologic response to pain is similar in the adult and the neonate.[11] Neonates and infants feel pain, and pain may have severe consequences in terms of health status and outcomes.[144] Although the infant's inability to verbally describe pain is limited, physiologic responses evidence distress. In general, responses to pain include release of catecholamines and cortisol. Heart rate changes and respiratory rate are linked to increased oxygen consumption. Blood glucose levels rise and the increase in metabolic rate increases energy requirements. A rise in blood pressure produces an elevation in intracranial pressure. Each of these responses may have adverse effects for the neonate, including increased oxygen and ventilatory requirements and changes in blood osmolarity.[144] Hypoxia and the risk of intracranial hemorrhage increase. Furthermore, the energy demands of the stress response to pain have implications for growth and wound healing. Of great concern are the long-term effects of early pain experiences on personality development and psychological outcomes. Although this area has not been thoroughly studied, evidence of memory capacities in the neonate augment this concern.

It is well established that neonates and infants exhibit stress in response to pain. There is further evidence that infants may be more vulnerable to the effects of pain because of their level of neurobehavioral organization and limited coping skills.[144] Neonates have virtually no control over the pain experience and cannot cognitively appreciate what is happening or why.

Assessment of Pain

Identification of pain in neonates and infants requires recognition that the expression of pain is different than that in the mature person. Developmental differences in the CNS as well as other body system alters the expression of pain. Responses to pain are both behavioral and physiologic (Table 12–15) and assessment is based on these expressions.[36, 60] Although many investigators have compiled lists of variables to be assessed, development of a clinically reliable tool for the assessment of pain in neonates and infants continues. Documentation of pain is complicated by the many expressions of pain exhibited by neonates and infants as well as the fact that many behavioral expressions are dependent on gestational age and, consequently, development. Pain expression appears to be a highly individual process. Ad-

TABLE 12–15
Pain Responses of Neonates and Infants

MOTOR RESPONSES	
Generalized motor activity	Reflexive withdrawal from
Swiping movements	pain
Increase/decrease of motor	Positioning
tone	Fist clenching
Kicking	Wiggling
Guarding	Thrashing
Pulling away	

FACIAL EXPRESSIONS	
Grimace	Furrowed brow
Chin quiver	Wincing
Frowning	Cry face
Tears in eyes	Gazing

VOCALIZATIONS	
Cry	Whimper
Groan	

SLEEP–WAKE/ACTIVITY DISTURBANCE	
Rapid state changes	Inability to sustain state
Increased or decreased	Fussiness
activity	Irritability
Decreased consolability	Restlessness
Agitation	
Lethargy	

AUTONOMIC RESPONSES	
Pallor	Flushing
Diaphoresis	Palmar sweating
Dilated pupils	Hyperglycemia
Increased/decreased heart	Shallow respirations
rate	Apnea
Increased/decreased	Increased ventilatory needs
respiratory rate	Increase/decrease CO_2 level
Decreased O_2 level	Increase in intracranial
Increase in blood pressure	pressure
Cyanosis	Increase in serum cortisol
Palmar sweating	

Compiled from references 11, 35, 60, 81, 89, 116, 144, 149, and 162.

ditionally, it is particularly difficult to assess pain in intubated infants and those receiving muscle-paralyzing medications.[59] Furthermore, one of the few coping abilities of the neonate is withdrawal. Thus, passivity, flaccid motor tone, or increased sleep, signs that may not be linked with pain, actually represent the infant's attempt to cope by withdrawing.

Management of Pain

Neonates and infants often are not consistently medicated for pain, even surgical pain. These practices reflect both an ambivalence regarding pain in neonates and problems with the use of analgesia and anesthetics. In one study pacifiers were found to be the most commonly used intervention for pain; medication ranked sixth.[59] Many times analgesia is not ordered, even when the infant's circumstances suggest that pain is occurring. When ordered, medication may be administered in partial doses or at uneven intervals. Medication is more commonly used for pain when other comforting measures have failed, if the infant is dying, or in the early postoperative period.[59] The balance of risks versus benefits and the appropriate dosages for anesthesia and analgesia are not clearly established.[144] Treatment of pain raises concerns of drug overdose and the long-term effects of medication on the developing brain.

Although therapies other than drugs may prove useful in the treatment of infant pain, many therapies rely on mechanisms not yet developed in the infant. For instance, in one study music and audiotapes of intrauterine sounds did not alter pain experienced during circumcision.[116] Nonpharmacologic interventions such as swaddling or containment, decreasing environmental stimulation, positioning, holding, and soothing techniques may enhance the therapeutic effects of pharmacologic agents and modulate mild or moderate pain.

ANALGESICS/NARCOTICS/NEUROMUSCULAR BLOCKING AGENTS

As in the administration of any medication, the use of medications to control discomfort entails appreciation of pharmacokinetics in infants. Absorption, distribution, metabolism, and excretion of drugs are developmentally different in infants and adults.[183] Absorption of oral analgesics or narcotics is unpredictable and slowed by variable pH, irregular peristalsis, and decreased bile and enzyme production (see Chapter 9). Intramuscular medications are influenced by the infant's small muscle mass and alterations in peripheral perfusion. Topical analgesic agents are easily absorbed because of increased skin permeability, increasing the risk of toxicity (see Chapter 11).

The distribution of analgesics and narcotics is influenced by the infant's large extracellular fluid space and increased total body water as well as decreased plasma protein binding. The brain barriers described earlier are less well developed, which may result in increased medication reaching the CNS. The large surface-to-mass ratio and high metabolic rate of the neonate and infant affect drug metabolism. Neonates and infants have immature organ systems, especially the lungs (see Chapter 7), kidney (see Chapter 8), and liver (see Chapter 9), which are typical routes for drug excretion.

Nonnarcotic analgesics are usually limited to acetaminophen in the neonate and infant. Although effective for minor discomfort, such analgesia is inappropriate for invasive procedures or moderate or severe pain. Narcotics, both natural and synthetic, are more commonly used for the treatment of moderate and severe pain, including morphine, meperidine, codeine, and fentanyl.[162] Whether narcotic use in the neonate produces or predisposes to narcotic addiction is unknown. One of the characteristics of narcotics is respiratory depression. Fear of respiratory depression is not a valid reason for withholding pain relief; but neonates and infants receiving narcotics must be closely monitored, a task simplified by cardiorespiratory monitors, and antinarcotic drugs must be on hand for the emergency treatment of respiratory depression. Often the fear of overdose leads nurses to give narcotics infrequently or at uneven intervals, but the analgesic effect of the narcotic is maximized when doses are given at regular intervals.[162]

Specific narcotics entail consideration of individual characteristics. Morphine causes the release of histamine and the possibility of lowering blood pressure leading to circulatory compromise.[157] The potential effect on CBF must be recognized. In addition, the half-life of morphine in the neonate and early infant is longer than in the adult.[113] Although evidence is limited to one study, neonates treated with fentanyl appear to have more difficulty with withdrawal compared with infants receiving morphine for comparable periods of time. In infants administered fentanyl there was a greater percentage of withdrawal signs, longer duration of withdrawal signs after high-dose therapy, and more subjects required drug treatment for withdrawal signs.[138]

Neuromuscular blocking agents, such as pancuronium bromide or succinylcholine chloride or other curare-like drugs, block nerve transmission at the neuromuscular end plate by preventing the action of acetylcholine. These drugs are typically used to block ventilatory effort and activity in mechanically ventilated infants. Paralyzing agents do not provide any sedation or analgesic effect, nor do they blunt the stress response induced by pain, handling, or stressful environment. Rather, neuromuscular blocking agents affect only skeletal muscle activity. Pain is difficult to assess in the infant who has received neuromuscular blocking agents since the ability to evidence pain cues through motor activity is hindered. Pancuronium bromide may elevate blood pressure with implications for changes in CBF and IVH and PVH.[158]

Effects of Drug Exposure In Utero

The fetus is a passive recipient of all drugs entering the mother's system. Drug use in pregnancy is common. From laxatives and antacids to cocaine and heroin, all of these substances are chemicals that may have an effect on the fetus and newborn. Medications are not "approved" for use in pregnancy; rather, medications are "presumed safe" for use in pregnancy. Some classes of drugs are more significant to CNS development and function after birth than are others. Drugs known to produce significant CNS effects are ethanol, narcotics, and cocaine. Since these classes of drugs affect the integrity and organization of the CNS, alterations in neurobehavioral organization are frequently observed and provide a basis for nursing care.[58]

Neonatal Abstinence Syndrome

Neonatal abstinence syndrome refers to particular withdrawal behaviors observed in neonates exposed to dependency-producing drugs in utero.[181] These drugs include ethanol, barbiturates, and all narcotics. The fetus is not immune from developing chemical dependency. After birth the neonate who has been exposed to narcotics in utero exhibits withdrawal symptoms. These infants are often small for gestational age.[189] The timing and severity of withdrawal are based on the type of drug, the mother's drug dosage, the length of time since the mother's last dose, the duration of exposure, the neonate's degree of immaturity, and the neonate's general health status.[56, 189] Symptoms usually appear within 72 hours after birth but can be seen as late as 2 to 4 weeks of age.[56] The neonate's withdrawal responses may last from 6 days to 8 weeks.[56] At birth the drug supply is removed, leading to withdrawal symptoms, called neonatal abstinence syndrome (Table 12–16).

The responses to drug withdrawal are similar to those in the adult, but because of the nature of neurologic organization, the implications are more severe in neonates. Neonatal abstinence syndrome includes both physiologic and behavioral responses. The Finnegan Scale[56] has been developed to aid observation and measurement of the responses to neonatal abstinence (Fig. 12–13). Interventions are initiated based on the severity of withdrawal as assessed by the Finnegan Scale. Withdrawal may be treated pharmacologically with paregoric, diazepam, tincture of opium, or phenobarbital.

Cocaine

Cocaine is a central and peripheral stimulant that produces its effects by preventing the reuptake of norepinephrine, resulting in increased levels of norepinephrine at the neuronal junction.[25] The actions of cocaine are similar to those of amphetamines, causing intense sympathetic nervous system activity. Cocaine produces vasoconstriction, tachycardia, and elevation of blood pressure in addition to a sense of excitement and euphoria. Cocaine is lipid-soluble, easily crossing the placenta and, in the fetus, produces increased motor activity and tachycardia; cocaine crosses the fetal blood–brain barrier.[166]

Because cocaine is a potent vasoconstrictor, blood flow to the placenta is reduced and associated with a high incidence of abruptio placentae (see Chapter 2). Blood flow to the fetus through the placenta is also curtailed. The resultant placental ischemia has been attributed as the cause of low birth weight, decreased body length, and smaller head circumference found among infants of cocaine-abusing mothers. Cocaine also increases uterine irritability and results in contractions. Fig. 12–14 summarizes the impact of cocaine on the mother, fetus, and neonate.

After birth cocaine does not produce withdrawal behaviors, per se, but its effect appears to be related to an alteration of neurobehavioral organization that probably results from its direct influence on the developing brain. In addition, cocaine may cause cerebral infarcts. Neonates exposed in utero to cocaine are irritable, tremulous, and difficult to soothe and have rapid respiratory and heart rates; these infants exhibit excessive motor activity, altered sleep–wake patterns, poor feeding and feeding intolerance, and diarrhea.[25, 166] Testing using the BNBAS has demonstrated poor neurobehavioral organization, particularly in the area of social interaction.[27] Cocaine-exposed infants have been reported to have an increased risk of sudden infant death syndrome (SIDS), although this finding has been challenged by subsequent studies.[25, 168a] The half-life of cocaine is longer in the fetus and neonate than in the adult since the enzyme systems governing the drug's metabolism are not mature, and cocaine may persist in the neonate for several days after birth. Cocaine passes easily into breast milk; active use of cocaine by a lactating mother may produce severe reactions and possibly death in the neonate.[26] Cocaine has been found in breast milk as late as 36 hours after maternal use.[26]

MATURATIONAL CHANGES DURING INFANCY AND CHILDHOOD

Brain growth and maturation continue after birth into childhood and adolescence, with

TABLE 12–16
Signs of Neonatal Abstinence Syndrome

W	=	Wakefulness
I	=	Irritability
T	=	Tremulousness, Temperature instability, Tachypnea
H	=	Hyperactivity, High-pitched cry, Hyperacusia, Hyperreflexia, Hypertonus
D	=	Diarrhea, Diaphoresis, Disorganized suck
R	=	Rub marks, Respiratory distress, Rhinorrhea
A	=	Apnea, Autonomic dysfunction
W	=	Weight loss
A	=	Alkalosis (respiratory)
L	=	Lacrimation

From Torrence, C.R. & Horn, K.H. (1989). Appraisal and caregiving for the drug addicted infant. *Neonatal Network, 8,* 54.

	Signs and Symptoms	Score	AM	PM	Comments
Central Nervous System Disturbances	Excessive High Pitched Cry Continuous High Pitched Cry	2 3			Daily Weight:
	Sleeps < 1 Hour After Feeding Sleeps < 2 Hours After Feeding Sleeps < 3 Hours After Feeding	3 2 1			
	Hyperactive Moro Reflex Markedly Hyperactive Moro Reflex	2 3			
	Mild Tremors Disturbed Moderate-Severe Tremors Disturbed	1 2			
	Mild Tremors Undisturbed Moderate-Severe Tremors Undisturbed	3 4			
	Increased Muscle Tone	2			
	Excoriation (Specify Area:_____	1			
	Myoclonic Jerks	3			
	Generalized Convulsions	5			
Metabolic/Vasomotor/Respiratory Disturbances	Sweating	1			
	Fever < 101 (99–100.8°F./37.2–38.2°C) Fever > 101 (38.4°C. and Higher)	1 2			
	Frequent Yawning (3> 3–4 times/interval)	1			
	Mottling	1			
	Nasal Stuffiness	2			
	Sneezing (> 3–4 times/interval)	1			
	Nasal Flaring	2			
	Respiratory Rate > 60/Min. Respiratory Rate > 60/Min. with Retractions	1 2			
Gastrointestinal Disturbances	Excessive Sucking	1			
	Poor Feeding	2			
	Regurgitation Projectile Vomiting	2 3			
	Loose Stools Watery Stools	2 3			
	TOTAL SCORE INITIALS OF SCORER				

FIGURE 12–13. Finnegan scoring system assessing neonatal abstinence syndrome (From Finnegan, L.P. (1985). Neonatal abstinence. In N. Nelson (Ed.), *Current therapy in neonatal-perinatal medicine* (p. 265). Toronto: BC Decker.)

some processes continuing to mature into adulthood. The neonatal period and early infancy are periods of increased vulnerability to insults because of the rapid brain growth during this period. The brain reaches 90% of adult weight by 2 years because of increases in nerve fibers and development of nerve tracts. Myelinization continues through late adolescence and early adulthood. Nociceptive receptor density gradually decreases to adult levels by 2 years.[11] The cerebellar growth spurt begins later (about 30 weeks' gestation) and ends earlier (about 1 year)

than other areas and thus is particularly vulnerable to nutritional and other insults during infancy.

The cranial bones are not fully fused until 16 to 18 months of age. With increasing gestational age conduction rates increase. The speed of transmission becomes similar to adults by 3 to 4 years of age.[189] Electrical responses after stimulation become like those observed in the adult at 8 months.[171] By 8 months of age the six EEG patterns observed in the mature brain are found in the EEG of the infant.[143] The Moro reflex disappears by

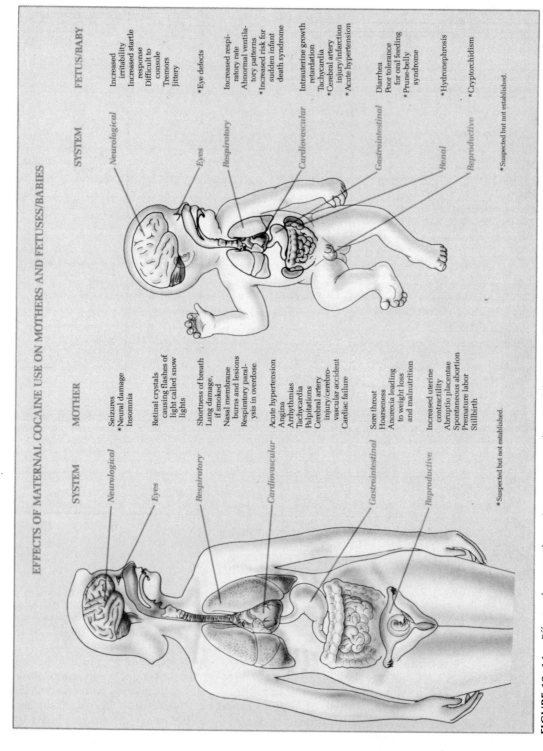

EFFECTS OF MATERNAL COCAINE USE ON MOTHERS AND FETUSES/BABIES

SYSTEM	MOTHER
Neurological	Seizures *Neural damage Insomnia
Eyes	Retinal crystals causing flashes of light called snow lights
Respiratory	Shortness of breath Lung damage, if smoked Nasal membrane burns and lesions Respiratory paral- ysis in overdose
Cardiovascular	Acute hypertension Angina Arrhythmias Tachycardia Palpitations Cerebral artery injury/cerebro- vascular accident Cardiac failure
Gastrointestinal	Sore throat Hoarseness Anorexia leading to weight loss and malnutrition
Reproductive	Increased uterine contractility Abruptio placentae Spontaneous abortion Premature labor Stillbirth

*Suspected but not established.

SYSTEM	FETUS/BABY
Neurological	Increased irritability Increased startle response Difficult to console Tremors Jittery
Eyes	*Eye defects
Respiratory	Increased respi- ratory rate Abnormal ventila- tory patterns *Increased risk for sudden infant death syndrome
Cardiovascular	Intrauterine growth retardation Tachycardia *Cerebral artery injury/infarction *Acute hypertension
Gastrointestinal	Diarrhea Poor tolerance for oral feeding *Prune-belly syndrome
Renal	*Hydronephrosis
Reproductive	*Cryptorchidism

*Suspected but not established.

FIGURE 12–14. Effects of maternal cocaine use on mothers and fetuses, and infants. (From Smith, J. (1988). The dangers of prenatal cocaine use. *MCN, 13,* 175. By permission of Network Graphics.)

6, palmar grasp by 2, and tonic neck reflex by 7 months of age.

Sensory abilities are similar to that of the adult at approximately 2 years of age. Visual acuity is adult-like at 6 months of age. Depth perception matures sometime after 3 months of age. Color vision is present to some degree by 2 months of age and increases at 3 months.[76] By 4 to 5 months visual–motor neuroconnections begin to develop, although the prehensile stage is not reached until 6 to 7 months. By 5 to 6 months visual impulses begin to be retained (memory), with recognition of familiar and strange objects and faces.

As the infant develops, total sleep time (the total number of hours spent asleep) per day decreases to about 12 hours by the 1st year. Sleep cycles increase in length, reaching the adult length in roughly the late school-age years. The infant is increasingly capable of chaining together two or more sleep cycles, leading to increased duration of sleep periods.[85] Sleep first exhibits longer periods and then gradually becomes consolidated into the night-time hours. The percentage of sleep time spent in active sleep decreases and the percentage of time in quiet sleep increases.[85] The reduction in active sleep is paralleled by an increase in wakefulness.[29] By the 1st year 30 to 40% of sleep time is active sleep. This proportion becomes adult-like in the early teen years.

SUMMARY

Transition from intrauterine to extrauterine life involves numerous changes in the nervous system as the infant adapts to his or her new environment and caregivers. The term newborn has the ability to receive and process information and respond in ways suited to neonatal development. These abilities are less well developed in the preterm infant. In the past 2 decades our knowledge of response

---

TABLE 12–17
Summary of Recommendations for Clinical Practice Related to the Neuromuscular and Sensory Systems During Pregnancy

Know the major stages for development of the neuromuscular and sensory systems (pp. 549–551).
Provide parent counseling and teaching regarding development of CNS defects (pp. 531–548, Table 12–8).
Recognize stages of CNS development and vulnerabilities in preterm infants (pp. 546–548, Table 12–8).
Recognize processes of fetal neurosensory development (pp. 549–553).
Recognize the sensorimotor capabilities of term infant and provide appropriate interventions (pp. 552–553, 555–557).
Recognize the sensorimotor capabilities of preterm infant and provide appropriate interventions (pp. 549–551, 555–557).
Promote neurosensory adaptations during transition to extrauterine life (pp. 551–553).
Protect term and preterm infants from overstimulation (pp. 549–555).
Recognize implications of differences in CBF and autoregulation within the neonate (pp. 553–555).
Implement interventions to prevent or minimize changes in oxygenation and intracranial pressure (pp. 554–555, 566–567).
Position term and preterm infants to enhance motor development (pp. 550–551, 557–558).
Assess reflexes, motor tone, and sensory capabilities (pp. 551–560, Tables 12–9, 12–10, and 12–11).
Recognize normal and abnormal neonatal reflex responses (pp. 557–560, Table 12–9).
Recognize different states and their implications (pp. 560–564, Table 12–11).
Interact with infants appropriate to their state (pp. 560–564, Table 12–11).
Promote state modulation in term and preterm infants (pp. 563–564).
Promote neurobehavioral organization in term and preterm infants (pp. 564–565).
Recognize stress, stability, engagement, and disengagement cues and respond appropriately (pp. 564–565, Table 12–12).
Modify the neonatal intensive care unit environment to reduce sensory overload (pp. 563–566).
Teach parents to recognize infant states, stress, stability, engagement, disengagement cues, and sensorimotor capabilities (pp. 560–566, Tables 12–11 and 12–12).
Recognize factors that may increase the risk of PVH and IVH (pp. 554–555, 566–567).
Implement interventions to reduce the risk of PVH and IVH (pp. 566–567).
Recognize signs of seizure activity (pp. 568–569, Table 12–13).
Differentiate between seizures and jitteriness (pp. 568–569, Table 12–14).
Recognize consequences of pain in the neonate (pp. 569–570).
Assess infants for signs of pain (p. 570, Table 12–15).
Use pharmacologic and nonpharmacologic interventions to treat neonatal pain (pp. 570–572).
Recognize factors influencing pharmacokinetics of analgesics, narcotics and neuromuscular blocking agents in neonates (pp. 570–572).
Assess infants for signs of intrauterine drug exposure from maternal substance abuse (pp. 572–574, Table 12–6, Figs. 12–13 and 12–14).

Page numbers in parentheses following each recommendation refer to pages in the text where the rationale for that intervention is discussed.

patterns, interactive abilities, and cues used by term and preterm infants to communicate with caregivers has expanded dramatically. An understanding of the level of maturation and organization of these systems in the neonate is critical for providing appropriate environments, promoting neurobehavioral organization, and influencing parent teaching. Recommendations for clinical practice related to the neuromuscular and sensory systems in the neonate are summarized in Table 12–17.

REFERENCES

1. Alahuta, S., et al. (1990). Visceral pain during caesarean section under spinal and epidural anesthesia with bupivacaine. *Acta Anaesthesiol Scand, 34,* 95.
2. Allen, M.C. & Capute, A.J. (1990). Tone and reflex development before term. *Pediatrics, 85,* 393.
3. Als, H. (1986). A synactive model of neonatal organization: framework for the assessment of neurobehavioral development in the premature infant and for support of infants and parents in the neonatal intensive care unit. *Phys Occup Ther Pediatr, 6,* 3.
4. Als, H. & Gibes, R. (1985). Neonatal Individualized Developmental Care and Assessment Program, Children's Hospital and Brigham & Womens' Hospital, Boston, MA.
5. Als, H., Lester, B.M., & Brazelton, T.B. (1979). Dynamics of the behavioral organization of the premature infant: A theoretical perspective. In T.M. Field (Ed.), *Infants born at risk: Behavior and development* (pp. 173–192). New York: SP Medical and Scientific Books.
6. Als, H., et al. (1982). Toward a research instrument for the assessment of preterm infants' behavior (APIB). In H.B. Fitzgerald, B.M. Lester, & M.W. Yogman (Eds.), *Theory and research in behavioral pediatrics* (Vol. 1, pp. 35–63). New York: Plenum Press.
7. Als, H., et al. (1986). Individualized behavioral and environmental care for the very low birth weight preterm infant at high risk for bronchopulmonary dysplasia: Neonatal intensive care unit and developmental outcome. *Pediatrics, 78,* 1123.
8. American Academy of Pediatrics Committee on Drugs. (1979). Anticonvulsants and pregnancy. *Pediatrics, 63,* 331.
9. Amiel-Tison, C. (1977). Evaluation of the neuromuscular system of the infant. In A. Rudolph (Ed.), *Pediatrics* (pp. 155–164). New York: Appleton-Century-Crofts.
10. Aminoff, M.J. (1989). Neurologic disorders. In R.K. Creasy & R. Resnik (Eds.), *Maternal-fetal medicine: Principles and practice* (2nd ed., pp. 1073–1109). Philadelphia: WB Saunders.
11. Anand, K.J.S., Phil, D., & Hickey, P.R. (1987). Pain and its effects in the human neonate and fetus. *N Engl J Med, 317,* 1321.
12. Avasthi, P., Sethi, P., & Mithal, S. (1976). Effect of pregnancy and labor on intraocular pressure. *Int Surg, 6,* 82.
13. Ballinger, C.B., et al. (1979). Emotional disturbance following childbirth and the excretion of cyclic AMP. *Psychol Med, 9,* 293.
14. Barb, S.A. & Lemons, P.K. (1989). The premature infants: Toward improving neurodevelopmental outcomes. *Neonatal Network, 7,* 7.
15. Bellur, S. (1985). Diseases of the striated muscles in pregnancy. In N. Gleicher (Ed.), *Principles of medical therapy in pregnancy* (pp. 932–937). New York: Plenum Press.
16. Bellur, S. (1985). Neurologic disorders in pregnancy. In N. Gleicher (Ed.), *Principles of medical therapy in pregnancy* (pp. 916–931). New York: Plenum Press.
17. Birk, K. & Rudick, R. (1986). Pregnancy and multiple sclerosis. *Arch Neurol, 43,* 719.
18. Blackburn, S. (1983). Fostering behavioral development of high-risk infants. *J Obstet Gynecol Neonatal Nurs, 12*(Suppl), 76s.
18a. Blackburn, S.T. & VandenBerg, K.A. (in press). Assessment and management of neonatal neurobehavioral development. In C. Kenner, L.P. Gunderson, & A. Bruegemeyer (Eds.), *Comprehensive neonatal nursing care.* Philadelphia: WB Saunders.
19. Boetez, M.I. & Lambert, B. (1977). Folate deficiency and restless legs syndrome in pregnancy. *N Engl J Med, 297,* 670.
20. Borsellino, A. (1980). Neuronal death in embryonic development: A model for selective cell competition and dominance. *Dev Neurosci, 9,* 495.
21. Branchey, M. & Petre-Quadens, O. (1968). A comparative study of sleep parameters during pregnancy. *Acta Neurol Belg, 68* 453.
22. Brazelton, T.B. (1973). Neonatal behavioral assessment scale. *Clin Dev Med, 50,* 1.
23. Brazelton, T.B. (1984). Neonatal behavioral assessment scale. (2nd ed) *Clin Dev Med, 88,* 1.
24. Briggs, G.G., Freeman, R.K., & Yaffe, S.J. (1986). *Drugs and lactation.* Baltimore: Williams & Wilkins.
25. Chasnoff, I.J. (1987). Perinatal effects of cocaine. *Contemp Obstet/Gynecol, 29,* 163.
26. Chasnoff, I.J., Lewis, D.E., & Squires, L. (1987). Cocaine intoxification in a breast-fed infant. *Pediatrics, 80,* 836.
27. Chasnoff, I.J., et al. (1985). Cocaine use in pregnancy. *N Engl J Med, 313,* 666.
28. Chaudhuri, P. & Wallenburg, N.C.S. (1980). Brain tumors and pregnancy. *Eur J Obstet Gynecol Reprod Biol, 11,* 109.
29. Coons, S. (1987). Development of sleep and wakefulness during the first 6 months of life. In C. Guilleminault (Ed.), *Sleep and its disorders in children* (pp. 17–27). New York: Raven Press.
30. Coons, S. & Guilleminault, C. (1984). Development of consolidated sleep and wakeful periods in relation to the day/night cycle in infancy. *Dev Med Child Neurol, 26,* 169.
31. Crepel, F. (1980). Electrophysiological correlates of brain development. *Dev Neurosci, 9,* 155.
32. Crook, C.K. (1978). Taste perception in the newborn infant. *Infant Behav Dev, 1,* 52.
33. Crook, C.K. & Lipsitt, L.P. (1976). Neonatal nutritive sucking: Effects of taste stimulation upon sucking rhythm and heart rate. *Child Dev, 47,* 518.
34. Cullen, J.A. & Carella, D.M. (1988). Periventricular intraventricular hemorrhage: Nursing implications. *Crit Care Nurs, 8* 72.
35. D'Apolito, K. (1984). The neonate's response to pain. *MCN, 9,* 256.
36. Dale, J.C. (1986). A multidimensional study of

infants' responses to painful stimuli. *Pediatr Nurs*, *12*, 27.

37. Dalessio, D.J. (1990). Epilepsy in pregnancy. In N.M. Nelson (Ed.), *Current therapy in neonatal-perinatal medicine—2* (pp. 54–58). Toronto: BC Decker.

38. Dalessio, D.J. (1985). Seizure disorders and pregnancy. *N Engl J Med, 312*, 559.

39. DeCasper, A.J. & Fifer, W.P. (1980). Of human bonding: newborns prefer their mother's voices. *Science, 208*, 1174.

40. Diamond, M.C. (1984). Cortical change in response to environmental enrichment and impoverishment. In *The many facets of touch* (pp. 22–29). Johnson & Johnson Pediatric Round Table 10. Skillman, NJ: Johnson & Johnson.

41. Dobbing, J. (1975). Human brain development and its vulnerability. In *Biologic and clinical aspects of brain development* (pp. 1–12). Mead Johnson Symposium on Perinatal and Developmental Medicine, No. 6. Evansville, IN: Mead Johnson.

42. Dobbing, J. & Sands, J. (1970). Timing of neuroblast multiplication in developing human brain. *Nature, 226*, 639.

43. Dommisse, J. (1990). Phenytoin Na and magnesium sulfate in the management of eclampsia. *Br J Obstet Gynaecol, 97*, 104.

44. Donaldson, J.O. (1978). *Neurology of pregnancy*. Philadelphia: WB Saunders.

45. Donaldson, J.O. (1981). Stroke. *Clin Obstet Gynecol, 24*, 825.

46. Donaldson, J.O. (1986). Does magnesium sulfate treat eclamptic convulsions? *Clin Neuropharmacol, 9*, 37.

47. Donaldson, J.O. (1988). Neurologic complications. In G.N. Burrow & T.F. Ferris (Eds.), *Medical complications during pregnancy* (pp. 485–498). Philadelphia: WB Saunders.

48. Dreyfus-Brisac, C. (1968). Sleep ontogenesis in early human prematurity from 24 to 27 weeks of conceptional age. *Dev Psychobiol, 1*, 162.

49. Dreyfus-Brisac, C. (1975). Neurophysiological studies in human premature and full-term newborns. *Biol Psychol, 10*, 485.

50. Drury, M.I., et al. (1983). Pregnancy in the diabetic patient. *Obstet Gynecol, 62*, 279.

51. Duncan, T.E. (1974). Krukenberg spindles in pregnancy. *Ophthalmology, 91*, 355.

52. Ekborn, K.A. (1960). Restless legs syndrome. *Neurology, 10*, 868.

53. Ellingson, R.J. (1972). Development of wakefulness-sleep cycles and associated EEG patterns in mammals. In C.D. Clemente, D.P. Purpura, & F.E. Mayer (Eds.), *Sleep and the maturing nervous system* (pp. 165–174). New York: Academic Press.

54. Fennell, D.F. & Ringel, S.P. (1987). Myasthenia gravis and pregnancy. *Obstet Gynecol Surv, 41*, 414.

55. Ferris, T.F. (1988). Toxemia and hypertension. In G.N. Burrow & T.F. Ferris (Eds.), *Medical complications during pregnancy* (pp. 1–33). Philadelphia: WB Saunders.

56. Finnegan, L.P. (1985). Neonatal abstinence. In N. Nelson (Ed.), *Current therapy in neonatal-perinatal medicine* (pp. 262–270). Toronto: BC Decker.

57. Fisher, S. (1989). Obstetrical analgesia and anesthesia. In W.R. Cohen, D.B. Acker, & E. Friedman (Eds.), *Management of labor* (2nd ed., pp. 77–130). Rockville, MD: Aspen.

58. Flandermeyer, A.A. (1987). A comparison of the effects of heroin and cocaine abuse upon the neonate. *Neonatal Network, 6*, 42.

59. Franck, L.S. (1987). A national survey of the assessment and treatment of pain and agitation in the neonatal intensive care unit. *J Obstet Gynecol Neonatal Nurs, 16*, 387.

60. Franck, L.S. (1986). A new method to quantitatively describe pain behavior in infants. *Nurs Res, 35*, 28.

61. Freeman, L.N. (1985). Neurosis and psychiatric diseases. In N. Gleicher (Ed.), *Principles of medical therapy in pregnancy* (pp. 897–906). New York: Plenum Press.

62. Friedman, A.P. & Merritt, H.H. (1959). *Headache—Prognosis and treatment*. Philadelphia: FA Davis.

63. Gerhardt, K.J. (1989). Characteristics of the fetal sheep sound environment. *Semin Perinatol, 13*, 362.

64. Gianoulakis, C. & Chretien, M. (1985). Endorphins in fetomaternal physiology. In N. Gleicher (Ed.), *Principles of medical therapy in pregnancy* (pp. 162–172). New York: Plenum Press.

65. Gilles, F.J., Shankle, W., & Dooling, E.C. (1983). Myelinated tracts: Growth patterns. In F.H. Gilles, A. Leviton, & E.C. Dooling (Eds.), *The developing human brain: Growth and epidemiologic neuropathology* (pp. 117–138). Boston: John Wright

66. Giwa-Osagie, O.F., Newton, J.R., & Larcher, V. (1981). Obstetrical performance of patients with myasthenia gravis. *Int J Obstet Gynecol, 19*, 267.

67. Gleiss, J. & Stuttgen, G. (1970). Morphologic and functional development of the skin. In U. Stave (Ed.), *Physiology of the perinatal period* (Vol. 2, pp. 889–906). New York: Appleton-Century-Crofts.

68. Goldstein, G.W. (1981). Special features of the brain microcirculation: Role in brain edema formation. In *Perinatal brain insult* (pp. 43–48). Mead Johnson Symposium on Perinatal and Developmental Medicine, No. 17. Evansville, IN: Mead Johnson.

69. Goldstein, G.W. & Donn, S.M. (1984). Periventricular and intraventricular hemorrhages. In H.B. Sarnat (Ed.), *Topics in neonatal neurology* (pp. 83–108). New York: Grune & Stratton.

70. Gorga, D., Stern, F.M., & Ross, G. (1985). Trends in neuromotor behavior of preterm and fullterm infants in the first year of life. *Dev Med Child Neurol, 27*, 756.

71. Gorski, P.A., Lewkowicz, D.J., & Huntington, L. (1987). Advances in neonatal and infant behavioral assessment: Toward a comprehensive evaluation of early patterns of development. *Dev Behav Pediatr, 8*, 39.

72. Gunderson, L.P. & Kenner, C. (1987). Neonatal stress: Physiologic adaptation and nursing implications. *Neonatal Network, 6*, 37.

73. Guttman, L. (1976). *Spinal cord injuries* (2nd ed.). Oxford: Blackwell Scientific Publications.

74. Hack, M. (1983). The sensorimotor development of the preterm infant. In A.A. Fanaroff & R.J. Martin (Eds.), *Behrman's neonatal-perinatal medicine* (pp. 328–345). St. Louis: CV Mosby.

75. Hagne, I. (1972). Development of the EEG in normal infants during the first year of life. *Acta Paediatr Scand*, (Suppl 232), 1.

76. Haith, M.M. (1986). Sensory and perceptual processes in early infancy. *J Pediatr, 109*, 158.

77. Hammer, M., Larsson, L., & Tegler, L. (1981). Calcium treatment of leg cramps in pregnancy. *Acta Obstet Gynecol Scand, 60*, 345.

78. Harris, B. (1980). Maternity blues. *Br J Psych, 136,* 520.

79. Harrison, L. (1985). Effects of early supplemental stimulation programs for premature infants: Review of the literature. *Matern Child Nurs J, 14,* 69.

80. Hawkins, J.W. & Gorvine, B. (1985). *Postpartum nursing.* New York: Springer.

81. Hess, L.M. (1990). Cues NICU nurses use as indicating pain in the intubated infant. Unpublished thesis, University of Washington, Seattle, WA.

82. Hill, J.H. & Applebaum, E.L. (1985). Otolaryngology: Head and neck problems in pregnancy. In N. Gleicher (Ed.), *Principles of medical therapy in pregnancy* (pp. 875–881). New York: Plenum Press.

83. Hilsinger, R.L., Adour, K.K., & Doty, H.E. (1975). Idiopathic facial paralysis, pregnancy and the menstrual cycle. *Ann Otol Rhinol Laryngol, 84,* 433.

84. Hopkins, A. & Wray, S. (1967). The effect of pregnancy on dystrophia myotonia. *Neurology, 17,* 166.

85. Hoppenbrouwers, T. (1987). Sleep in infants. In C. Guilleminault (Ed.), *Sleep and its disorders in children* (pp. 1–15). New York: Raven Press.

86. Hoppenbrouwers, T., et al. (1988). Sleep and waking states in infancy: Normative studies. *Sleep, 11,* 387.

87. Horven, I. & Gjonnaess, H. (1974). Corneal indentation pulse and intraocular pressure in pregnancy. *Arch Ophthalmol, 91,* 92.

88. Howard, J.H., et al. (1976). A neurologic comparison of pre-term and full-term infants at term conceptional age. *J Pediatr, 88,* 995.

89. Izard, C.E. & Buechler, S. (1979). Emotion expression and personality integration in infancy. In C.E. Izard (Ed.), *Emotions in personality and psychopathology* (pp. 445–472). New York: Plenum Press.

90. Jaffee R, et al. (1986). Myonic dystrophy and pregnancy: A review. *Obstet Gynecol Surv, 41,* 272.

91. Janz, D. (1982). Antiepileptic drugs and pregnancy: Altered utilization patterns and teratogenesis. *Epilepsia, 23* (Suppl 1), S53.

92. Janz, D., et al. (Eds.). (1982). *Epilepsy, pregnancy and the child.* New York: Raven Press.

92a. Jimenez, S.L.M. (1983). Application of the body's natural pain relief mechanisms to reduce discomfort in labor and delivery. NAACOG Update Series, *1(1),* 1.

92b. Jones, L.C. (1990). Postpartum emotional disorders. *ICEA Review, 14*(4), 21.

93. Kaneko, S., et al. (1982). The problems of antiepileptic medication in the neonatal period: Is breastfeeding advisable. In D. Janz, et al. (Eds.), *Epilepsy, pregnancy and the child.* New York: Raven Press.

94. Karacan, I., et al. (1968). Characteristics of sleep patterns during late pregnancy and the postpartum periods. *Am J Obstet Gynecol, 10,* 579.

95. Karacan, I., et al. (1969). Some implications for the sleep pattern for post partum emotional disorder. *Br J Psych, 115,* 929.

96. Kass, M.A. & Sears, M.L. (1977). Hormonal regulation of intraocular pressure. *Surv Ophthalmol, 22,* 153.

97. Keefe, M. (1988). The impact of infant rooming-in on maternal sleep at night. *J Obstet Gynecol Neonatal Nurs, 17,* 122.

98. Killien, M. & Lentz, M. (1985). Sleep patterns and adequacy during the postpartum period. *Commun Nurs Res, 18,* 56.

99. King, C.R. & Chow, S. (1985). Dermatomyositis and pregnancy. *Obstet Gynecol, 66,* 589.

100. Knight, A.H. & Rhind, E.G. (1975). Epilepsy and pregnancy: A study of 153 patients. *Epilepsia, 16,* 99.

101. Kooner, K.S. & Zimmerman, T.J. (1988). Antiglaucoma therapy during pregnancy. *Ann Ophthalmol, 166,* 208.

102. Korn-Lubetzki, I., et al. (1984). Activity of multiple sclerosis during pregnancy and puerperium. *Ann Neurol, 16,* 229.

103. Kovnar, E. & Volpe, J.J. (1982). Current concepts in neonatal neurology. 2. Periventricular-intraventricular hemorrhage. *Perinatol Neonatol, 6,* 81.

104. Landesman, R., Douglas, R.G., & Holze, E. (1954). The bulbar conjunctival vascular bed in the toxemia of pregnancy. *Am J Obstet Gynecol, 68,* 170.

105. Landesman, R., et al. (1953). The bulbar conjunctival vascular bed in normal pregnancy. *Am J Obstet Gynecol, 65,* 876.

106. Lary, S., et al. (1985). Hearing threshold in preterm and term infants by auditory brainstem response. *J Pediatr, 107,* 593.

107. Lawhon, G. (1986). Management of stress in premature infants. In D.J. Angelini, C.M. Whelan-Knapp, & R.M. Gibes (Eds.), *Perinatal/neonatal nursing* (pp. 319–328). Boston: Blackwell Scientific.

108. Lawrence, R.A. (1989). *Breastfeeding: A guide for the medical profession* (3rd ed.). St. Louis: CV Mosby.

109. Lawson, W. & Biller, H.F. (1985). Ear, nose and throat disorders in pregnancy. In S.H. Cherry, R.L. Berkowitz, & N.G. Kase (Eds.), *Rovinsky and Guttmacher's medical, surgical, and gynecologic complications of pregnancy* (3rd ed., pp. 496–500). Baltimore: Williams & Wilkins.

110. Lee, R.V., McComb, L.E., & Mezzardi, F.C. (1990). Pregnant patients, painful legs: The obstetrician's dilemma. *Obstet Gynecol Surv, 45,* 290.

111. Leners, D. (1989). Vestibular stimulation. In M. Craft & J. Denehy (Eds.), *Nursing interventions for infants and children* (pp. 274–284). Philadelphia: WB Saunders.

111a. Lentz, M.J. & Killien, M.G. (1991). Are you sleeping? Sleep patterns during postpartum hospitalization. *J Perinatal Neonatal Nurs, 4*(4), 30.

112. Lott, J.W. (1989). Developmental care of the preterm infant. *Neonatal Network, 7,* 21.

113. Lynn, A.M. & Slattery, J.T. (1987). Morphine pharmacokinetics in early infancy. *Anesthesiology, 66,* 136.

114. Macfarlane, J.A. (1975). Olfaction in the development of social preferences in the human neonate. In *Parent-infant interaction* (pp. 103–117). CIBA Foundation Symposium 33. Amsterdam: Elsevier.

115. Mantle, M.J., Greenwood, R.M., & Currey, H.L.F. (1977). Backache in pregnancy. *Rheumatol Rehabil, 16,* 95.

116. Marchette, L., Main, R., & Redick, E. (1989). Pain reduction during neonatal circumcision. *Pediatr Nurs, 15,* 207.

117. Massey, E.W. (1977). Migraine during pregnancy. *Obstet Gynecol Surv, 32,* 693.

118. Massey, E.W. (1978). Carpal tunnel syndrome in pregnancy. *Obstet Gynecol Surv, 33,* 145.

119. Massey, E.W. & Cefalo, R.C. (1979). Neuropathies of pregnancy, *Obstet Gynecol Surv, 34,* 489.

120. Maymon, R. & Fejin, M. (1990). Intracranial hemorrhage during pregnancy and puerperium. *Obstet Gynecol Surv, 45,* 157.

121. McGregor, J.A. & Meeuwsen, J. (1985). Autonomic hyperreflexia: A mortal danger for spinal-cord damaged women in labor. *Am J Obstet Gynecol, 151,* 330.

123. Melvin, J.L., Burnett, C.N., & Johnson, E.W. (1969). Median nerve conduction in pregnancy. *Arch Phys Med, 50,* 75.

124. Millodot, M. (1977). The influence of pregnancy on the sensitivity of the cornea. *Br J Ophthalmol, 58,* 752.

125. Melzack, R. & Wall, P.D. (1983). *The challenge of pain.* New York: Basic Books.

126. Mogil, L.G. & Friedman, A.H. (1985). Ocular complications of pregnancy. In S.H. Cherry, R.L. Berkowitz, & N.G. Kase (Eds.), *Rovinsky and Guttmacher's medical, surgical, and gynecologic complications of pregnancy* (3rd ed., pp. 476–493). Baltimore: Williams & Wilkins.

127. Moloney, J.B.M. & Drury, M.I. (1982). The effect of pregnancy on the natural course of diabetic retinopathy. *Am J Ophthalmol, 93,* 745.

128. Moore, K.L. (1982). *The developing human: Clinically oriented embryology* (3rd ed.) Philadelphia: WB Saunders.

129. Moore, M.L. (1983). *Realities in childbearing* (2nd ed.). Philadelphia: WB Saunders.

130. Movshon, J.A. & Van Sluyters, R.C. (1981). Visual neural development. *Annu Rev Psychol, 32,* 477.

131. Namba, T., Brown, S.B., & Grob, D. (1970). Neonatal myasthenia gravis: Report of two cases and a review of the literature. *Pediatrics, 45,* 488.

132. Nau, H., et al. (1982). Anticonvulsants during pregnancy and lactation-transplacental, maternal and neonatal pharmacokinetics. *Clin Pharmacokinet, 7,* 508.

133. Nausieda, P.A., et al. (1979). Chorea induced by oral contraceptives. *Neurology, 29,* 1605.

134. NCAST Learning Resource Manual (1987). Nursing Child Assessment Satellite Training. University of Washington Child Development and Mental Retardation Center, Seattle, WA.

135. Nelson, K.B. & Ellenberg, J.H. (1982). Maternal seizure disorder, outcome of pregnancy, and neurologic abnormalities in children. *Neurology, 32,* 1247.

136. Niebyl, J.R., et al. (1979). Carbamazepine levels in pregnancy and lactation. *Obstet Gynecol, 53,* 139.

137. Nijhuis, J.G. (1986). Behavioral states: Concomitants, clinical implications and the assessment of the condition of the nervous system. *Eur J Obstet Gynecol Reprod Biol, 21,* 301.

138. Norton, S.J. (1988). Aftereffects of morphine and fentanyl analgesia: A retrospective study. *Neonatal Network, 7,* 25.

139. Nowlis, G.H. & Kesson, W. (1976). Human newborns differentiate concentrations of sucrose and glucose. *Science, 191,* 865.

140. O'Connell, J.E.A. (1960). Lumbar disc protrusions in pregnancy. *J Neurol Neurosurg Psych, 23,* 138.

141. Omar, S.Y., et al. (1985). Blood pressure responses to care procedures in ventilated preterm infants. *Acta Paediatr Scand, 74,* 920.

142. Owens, M.E. (1984). Pain in infancy: Conceptual and methodological issues. *Pain, 20,* 213.

143. Parmelee, A.H. & Stern, E. (1972). Development of states in infants. In C.D. Clemente, D.P. Purpura, & F.E. Mayer (Eds.), *Sleep and the maturing nervous system* (pp. 199–219). New York: Academic Press.

144. Porter, F. (1989). Pain in the newborn. *Clin Perinatol, 16,* 549.

145. Parmelee, A.H. & Sigman, M.D. (1983). Perinatal brain development and behavior. In P.H. Mussen (Ed.), *Handbook of child psychology; Vol II. Infancy and developmental psychobiology* (4th ed.). New York: John Wiley & Sons.

146. Patterson, R.M. (1989). Seizure disorders in pregnancy. *Med Clin North Am, 73,* 661.

147. Pearson, M.F. (1957). Neuralgia paresthetica: With reference to its occupance in pregnancy. *J Obstet Gynaecol Br Comm, 64,* 427.

148. Phillips, C.I. & Gore, S.M. (1985). Ocular hypotensive effect of late pregnancy with and without high blood pressure. *Br J Ophthalmol, 69,* 117.

149. Plauche, W.C. (1983). Myasthenia gravis in pregnancy: An update. *Clin Obstet Gynecol, 26,* 592.

150. Pritchard, J.A. (1980). Management of preeclampsia and eclampsia. *Kidney Int, 18,* 259.

151. Purpura, D.P. (1975). Neuronal migration and dendritic differentiation: Normal and aberrant development of human cerebral cortex. *Biologic and clinical aspects of brain development* (pp. 13–27). Mead Johnson Symposium on Perinatal and Developmental Medicine, No. 6. Evansville, IN: Mead Johnson.

152. Purves, D. & Lichtman, J.W. (1980). Elimination of synapses in the developing nervous system. *Science, 210,* 153.

153. Riss, B. & Riss, P. (1981). Corneal sensitivity in pregnancy. *Ophthalmology, 183,* 57.

154. Robertson, D.N.S. (1972). Pregnancy and labour in the paraplegic. *Paraplegia, 10,* 209.

155. Robertson, I.G. (1986). Epilepsy in pregnancy. *Clin Obstet Gynaecol, 13,* 365.

156. Robinson, J.L., Hall, C.S., & Sedzimir, C.B. (1974). Arteriovenous malformations, aneurysms and pregnancy. *J Neurosurg, 4,* 63.

157. Roscow, C., et al. (1984). Hemodynamics and histamine release during induction with sufentanil or fentanyl. *Anesthesiology, 60,* 489.

158. Runkle, B. & Bancalari, E. (1984). Acute cardiopulmonary effects of pancuronium bromide in mechanically ventilated newborn infants. *J Pediatr, 99,* 614.

159. Schnachner, S.M. & Reynolds, A.C. (1982). Horner's syndrome during lumbar epidural analgesia. *Obstet Gynecol, 59,* 315.

160. Schnidt, D., et al. (1983). Changes of seizure frequency in pregnant epileptic women. *J Neurol Neurosurg Psych, 46,* 751.

161. Serup, L. (1986). Influence of pregnancy on diabetic retinopathy. *Acta Endocrinol, 112,* 122.

162. Shapiro, C. (1989). Pain in the neonate: Assessment and intervention. *Neonatal Network, 8,* 7.

163. Shapiro, S., et al. (1976). Anticonvulsant and parental epilepsy in the development of birth defects. *Lancet, 1,* 272.

164. Sibai, B.M. (1990). Magnesium sulfate is the ideal anti-convulsant in pre-eclampsia. *Am J Obstet Gynecol, 162,* 1141.

165. Siesjo, B.K. & Blennow, G. (1980). The effects of hypoxia, hypoglycemia, and epileptic seizures on brain development. *Dev Neurosci, 9,* 241.

166. Smith, J. (1988). The dangers of prenatal cocaine use. *MCN, 13,* 174.

167. Somerville, B.W. (1972). A study of migraine in pregnancy. *Neurology, 22,* 824.

168. Seidel, B.D. & Meadow, S.R. (1972). Maternal

epilepsy and abnormalities of the fetus and new-born. *Lancet, 2,* 839.

168a. Srinivasan, G. (1991). Infants of drug-dependent mothers. In Yeh, T.H. (Ed.), *Neonatal therapeutics* (2nd ed., pp 32–39). St. Louis: CV Mosby.

169. Srinivasan, K. (1983). Cerebral venous and arterial thrombosis in pregnancy and puerperium. A study of 135 patients. *Angiology, 34,* 731.

170. Srinivasan, K., et al. (1982). Maternal anticonvulsant therapy and hemorrhagic disease of the newborn. *Obstet Gynecol, 59,* 250.

171. Starr, A., et al. (1977). Development of auditory function in newborn infants revealed by auditory brainstem potentials. *Pediatrics, 60,* 831.

172. Stein, G.S. (1981). Headaches in the first postpartum week and their relationship to migraines. *Headache, 21,* 201.

173. Steinbrook, A.R., et al. (1982). Dissociation of plasma and cerebrospinal fluid beta-endorphin-like immunoreactivity levels during pregnancy and parturition. *Anesth Analg, 61,* 893.

174. Sterman, M.B. (1972). The basic rest-activity cycle and sleep: Developmental considerations in man and cats. In C.D. Clemente, D.P. Purpura, & F.E. Mayer (Eds.), *Sleep and the maturing nervous system* (pp. 175–197). New York: Academic Press.

175. Strauss, R.G. & Bernstein, R. (1974). Folic acid and dilantin antagonism in pregnancy. *Obstet Gynecol, 44,* 345.

175a. Strickler, S.M., et al. (1985). Genetic predisposition to phenytoin-induced birth defects. *Lancet, 2,* 746.

176. Sunderland, S. (1968). *Nerves and nerve injuries.* Edinburgh: Churchill Livingstone.

177. Taylor, H.J. (1985). Choice of analgesia and anaesthesia during labour and delivery. *Clin Invest Med, 8,* 345.

178. Teich, S.A. (1985). Common disturbances of vision and ocular movement and surgery of the eye in the pregnant patient. In N. Gleicher (Ed.), *Principles of medical therapy in pregnancy* (pp. 861–874). New York: Plenum Press.

179. Thompson, D.S., et al. (1986). The effects of pregnancy in multiple sclerosis: A retrospective study. *Neurology, 36,* 1097.

180. Torrence, C.R. (1985). Neonatal seizures: Part II. Recognition, treatment, and prognosis. *Neonatal Network, 4*(2), 21.

181. Torrence, C.R. & Horns, K.H. (1989). Appraisal and caregiving for the drug addicted infant. *Neonatal Network, 8,* 49.

182. Touwen, B.C.L. (1980). The preterm infant in the extrauterine environment. Implications for neurology. *Early Hum Dev, 4*(3), 287.

183. Trange, J.M., Kluza, R.B., & Kearns, G.L. (1984). Pharmacokinetics for pediatric nurses. *Pediatr Nurs, 10,* 267.

184. Vannucci, R.C. & Hernandez, M.J. (1981). Perinatal cerebral blood flow. *Perinatal brain insult* (pp. 17–29). Mead Johnson Symposium on Perinatal and Developmental Medicine, No. 17. Evansville, IN: Mead Johnson.

185. VandenBerg, K.A. (1990). Behaviorally supportive care for the extremely premature infant. In L.P. Gunderson & C. Kenner (Eds.), *Care of the 24–25 week gestational age infant (small baby protocol)* (pp. 129–157). Petaluma, CA: Neonatal Network.

186. Vert, P. & Deblay, M.F. (1982). Hemorrhagic disease in infants of epileptic mothers. In D. Janz, et al. (Eds.), *Epilepsy, pregnancy and the child.* New York: Raven Press.

187. Villar, M.A. & Sibai, B.M. (1988). Eclampsia. *Obstet Gynecol Clin North Am, 15,* 355.

188. Visser, G.H.A., et al. (1987). Fetal behavior at 30 to 32 weeks gestation. *Pediatr Res, 22,* 655.

189. Volpe, J.J. (1987). *Neurology of the newborn* (2nd ed.). Philadelphia: WB Saunders.

190. Webb, D., et al. (1978). Myotonia dystrophia: Obstetric complications. *Am J Obstet Gynecol, 132,* 265.

191. Weinreb, R.M., Lu, A., & Key, T. (1987). Maternal ocular adaptations during pregnancy. *Obstet Gynecol Surv, 42,* 471.

192. Wiebers, D.O. (1985). Ischemic cerebrovascular complications of pregnancy. *Arch Neurol, 42,* 1106.

193. Wigglesworth, J.S. (1981). Brain development and the structural basis of perinatal brain damage. *Perinatal brain insult* (pp. 3–10). Mead Johnson Symposium on Perinatal and Developmental Medicine, No. 17. Evansville, IN: Mead Johnson.

194. Wolff, P.H. (1966). The causes, controls, and organization of behavior in the neonate. *Psychol Issues, 5,* Monogr 17, 1.

195. Yahr, M.D., Gudesblatt, M. & Cohen, J.A. (1985). Neurological complications of pregnancy. In S.H. Cherry, R.L. Berkowitz, & N.G. Kase (Eds.), *Rovinsky and Guttmacher's medical, surgical, and gynecologic complications of pregnancy* (3rd ed., pp. 434–446). Baltimore: Williams & Wilkins.

196. Yerby, M.S. (1987). Problems and management of the pregnant woman with epilepsy. *Epilepsia, 28*(Suppl), S29.

197. Young, B.K. & Kirshenbaum, N.W. (1987). Neurologic disorders in pregnancy. In C.J. Pauerstein (Ed.), *Clinical obstetrics.* New York: John Wiley & Sons.

Adaptations in Metabolic Processes in the Pregnant Woman, Fetus, and Neonate

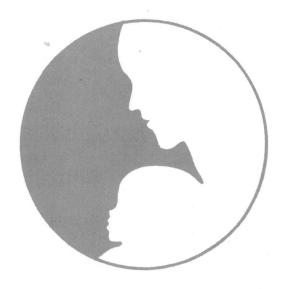

CHAPTER 13

Carbohydrate, Fat, and Protein Metabolism

Maternal Physiologic Adaptations
  The Antepartum Period
    Carbohydrate Metabolism
    Protein Metabolism
    Fat Metabolism
    Insulin
    Absorptive versus Postabsorptive States
    Effects of Placental Hormones
  The Intrapartum Period
  The Postpartum Period
Clinical Implications for the Pregnant Woman and Her Fetus
  Pregnancy as a State of Facilitated Anabolism
  Pregnancy as a State of "Accelerated Starvation"
  Pregnancy as a Diabetogenic State
  Effects of Metabolic Changes on the Glucose Tolerance Test

  Maternal-Fetal Relationships
  The Pregnant Diabetic Woman
Fetal Development of Carbohydrate, Fat, and Protein Metabolism
Neonatal Physiology
  Transitional Events
  Carbohydrate Metabolism
  Fat Metabolism
  Protein Metabolism
Clinical Implications for Neonatal Care
  Neonatal Hypoglycemia
  Neonatal Hyperglycemia
Maturational Changes During Infancy and Childhood

Metabolism comes from the Greek word meaning "to change." It is essentially the totality of chemical reactions within a living organism.[98] Cahill, as cited by Hare, identified four principles that underlie and guide metabolic functions in humans:[50]

1. Plasma glucose must be maintained within normal limits.
2. An optimal source of glycogen must be maintained as an emergency fuel.
3. An optimal supply of protein must be

maintained for use in enzymatic mechanisms of metabolism as well as muscular mobility. Excess protein is converted to fat and the nitrogen released is excreted in urine.

4. Protein must be conserved when it is scarce and stored fat used in time of caloric need.[50, p.2]

Metabolic processes in the neonate and pregnant woman are closely linked with and mediated by the function of various endocrine glands. Major alterations in metabolic processes arise during pregnancy. These changes are essential for the mother to provide adequate nutrients to support fetal growth and development. Maternal metabolic changes also alter the course of pregnancy in women with chronic disorders such as diabetes mellitus. After birth, major changes occur in both the sources of nutrients and the use of substrates by the neonate. Limitations in metabolic processes and related endocrine function during this period can compromise extrauterine adaptations and health. This chapter examines alterations in carbohydrate, fat, and protein metabolism and related endocrinology during pregnancy and in the fetus and neonate.

MATERNAL PHYSIOLOGIC ADAPTATIONS

Metabolic adaptations during pregnancy are directed toward

1. Ensuring satisfactory growth and development of the fetus;
2. Providing the fetus with adequate stores of energy and substrates needed for transition to extrauterine life;
3. Meeting maternal needs to cope with the increased physiologic demands of pregnancy;
4. Providing energy and substrate stores for the demands of pregnancy, labor and lactation.[6]

The first two demands listed above are in competition with the third and fourth demands. As a result, alterations in maternal metabolic processes can significantly affect maternal and fetal health status.

Pregnancy involves a "coordinated series of physiologic adjustments which act in concert to preserve maternal homeostasis while at the same time providing for fetal growth and development."[50, p.259] Pregnancy is primarily an anabolic state in which food intake and appetite are increased, activity is decreased, approximately 3.5 kg of fat is deposited, and 900 g of new protein is synthesized (by the mother, fetus, and placenta). The overall energy cost of reproduction is estimated at 75,000 to 84,000 kcal.[6, 65] Anabolic aspects are most prominent during the first half of pregnancy when accumulation of maternal fat and increased blood volume lead to maternal weight gain. During the second

half the woman's metabolic status becomes more catabolic as stored fat is used, insulin resistance increases, and serum glucose falls (Fig. 13–1). During this phase, weight gain is primarily due to the growing fetus and placenta.[65]

The Antepartum Period

Pregnancy is associated with major changes in metabolic processes and endocrine function. Hare characterizes pregnancy as a metabolic "tug of war" between the mother and the fetus.[50] The fetus and placenta influence maternal metabolic alterations since these tissues become an additional site for metabolism of maternal hormones as well as a new site for hormonal biosynthesis. Many of these changes are aimed at providing substances (especially glucose and amino acids) for the growth and development of the fetus. As the conceptus grows, it alters maternal fuel economy.

Metabolic processes during pregnancy are influenced by human placental lactogen (hPL), estrogen, and progesterone, which alter glucose utilization and insulin action. These changes contribute to the diabetogenic effects of pregnancy, stimulate alterations in

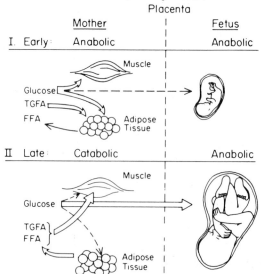

FIGURE 13–1. Fuel disposition in pregnancy during early (I) and late (II) gestation. (From Knopp, R.H., Childs, M.T., & Warth, M.R. (1979). Dietary management of the pregnant diabetic. In M. Winick (Ed.), *Nutritional management of genetic disorders* (p. 129). New York: Wiley-Interscience.)

lipid and protein metabolism, and increase the availability of glucose and amino acid for transfer to the fetus while providing an alternative energy substrate (free fatty acids) to meet maternal needs and maintain homeostasis.

Carbohydrate Metabolism

Baird notes that the literature regarding carbohydrate metabolism during pregnancy is vast, confused, and contradictory.[6] Blood glucose levels in pregnancy are generally 10 to 20% lower than in nonpregnant women. In addition, during the overnight fasting period maternal plasma glucose values fall to levels 15 to 20 mg/dl lower than in nonpregnant women.[124] This decrease in glucose leads to lower insulin levels during the postabsorptive state and a tendency toward ketosis.

As pregnancy progresses, peripheral glucose use by the mother decreases because of increasing insulin resistance. This reduces maternal glucose utilization and makes glucose more readily available to the fetus. The mechanisms underlying the insulin resistance of pregnancy are not completely understood. Insulin resistance is believed to be due to a decrease in sensitivity of tissue cell receptors that results from the insulin antagonism effects of hPL, progesterone, and cortisol. The insulin antagonism is partially modulated by beta-cell hyperplasia and hypertrophy with increased insulin availability after feeding. Pregnancy is also characterized by greater oscillations in insulin and glucagon levels.[50] A reduction in the extraction of insulin by the liver may contribute to peripheral hyperinsulinemia. Variations in hepatic insulin binding may contribute to alterations in the ratio of insulin to glucagon.[6]

Progesterone augments insulin secretion, decreases peripheral insulin effectiveness, and increases insulin levels after a meal. Estrogen increases the level of plasma cortisol (an insulin antagonist), stimulates beta-cell hyperplasia (and thus insulin production), and enhances peripheral glucose utilization. Increased levels of both bound and free cortisol decrease hepatic glycogen stores and increase hepatic glucose production. These changes further increase glucose availability for the fetus.[55]

Human placental lactogen is a single-chain polypeptide that is similar to human growth hormone. hPL levels correlate with fetal and placental weight and are higher in multiple

pregnancy. Levels higher than 4 µg/ml in the third trimester are considered abnormal.[128] hPL increases synthesis and availability of lipids. Lipids can be used by the mother as an alternative fuel, enhancing availability and transfer of glucose and amino acids to the fetus. A mild form of the metabolic changes seen during pregnancy can be induced by giving hPL to nonpregnant women. There is no consistent relationship between hPL levels and insulin requirements in the pregnant diabetic, however.

Protein Metabolism

Decreased serum amino acid and serum protein levels are found in pregnancy (see Chapter 5). This decrease is related to increased placental uptake, increased insulin levels, hepatic diversion of amino acids for gluconeogenesis, and transfer of amino acids to the fetus for use in glucose formation. Maternal plasma levels of amino acids such as alanine, glycine, and serine are reduced because of placental transfer of amino acids. Plasma alanine levels are lower because alanine is a key precursor for glucose formation (gluconeogenesis) by the fetal liver.

Alterations in protein metabolism during pregnancy seem to have a biphasic pattern in animals, and possibly in humans.[91] During the first half of gestation protein storage increases; during the second half, maternal protein use is more economic and some of the stored protein is broken down to use as an alternate energy source and for transfer to the fetus.[82, 83, 84] The early changes may be mediated by decreased activity of hepatic enzymes involved in amino acid deamination and urea synthesis.[91]

Fat Metabolism

Pregnancy results in alteration of every aspect of lipid metabolism.[124] Lipid metabolism in pregnancy is characterized by two phases and is analogous to the patterns of change in carbohydrate and protein metabolism.[6, 20, 64, 124] During the first two trimesters triglyceride synthesis and fat storage increase. Promotion of lipogenesis and suppression of lipolysis in this anabolic storage phase are mediated by the progressive increase in insulin and enhanced by progesterone and cortisol.[6, 63, 124] During this period ketogenesis is increased after fasting, suggesting enhanced fat utilization.[91]

The third trimester is characterized by a balance between lipogenesis and lipolysis. The increased lipolysis is probably primarily due to rising hPL levels. Accelerated ketogenesis in the liver is a consequence of increased oxidation of free fatty acids for energy, which increases the risk of maternal ketosis. The fat mobilization is associated with increased glucose and amino acid uptake by the fetus. Thus, fats are probably serving as alternative maternal energy substrates that allow the mother to conserve glucose for the fetus and her central nervous system during the second half of gestation.[6, 91, 124]

The two phases of lipid metabolism during pregnancy are reflected in changes in maternal serum free fatty acid concentrations as well as plasma triglyceride, cholesterol, and phospholipid levels (Fig. 13–2A). Maternal plasma free fatty acid levels are not significantly elevated until after about 30 weeks' gestation (Fig. 13–2B). The minimal change in free fatty acids during the first part of pregnancy is probably due to increased fat storage and augmented fat utilization. As maternal fat stores are mobilized, serum levels of free fatty acids increase and peak at term. Since elevations in free fatty acids are due to catabolism of stored triglycerides (into free fatty acid and glycerol), changes in free fatty acids are mirrored by changes in glycerol (Fig. 13–2B).[6, 91, 124] Hypertriglyceridemia during the third trimester is due to increases in very-low-density lipoproteins (VLDLs).[55]

Changes in lipid metabolism are accompanied by functional and morphologic changes in the adipocytes (Fig. 13–3).[124] Hypertrophy of these cells accommodates the increased fat storage during the first two thirds of pregnancy. In the last trimester maximal glucose transport, glucose oxidation, and lipogenesis within the adipocytes decrease.[54] The number of insulin receptors on the adipocytes increases in the first part of pregnancy and returns to nonpregnant levels by term.[6] Since responsiveness of adipose tissue to insulin is not diminished as much as that of other tissues, these changes in the adipocytes facilitate fat storage. After a meal, maternal fat stores are replenished by increased glucose uptake, incorporation of glucose into glycerol, and esterification of fatty acids by adipocytes.[6]

Insulin

Insulin levels and responsiveness of tissues to insulin change dramatically during pregnancy. Actions of insulin are summarized in Table 13–1. Maternal insulin levels increase twofold by the third trimester.[50] Increased insulin secretion ensures adequate maternal protein synthesis in the face of increasing resistance of peripheral tissues to the effects of insulin.[91] Tissue resistance is most prominent in liver, adipose, and muscle cells.[124]

Insulin antagonism is mediated by the increasing levels of placental hormones (especially estrogens, progesterone, and hPL), to a lesser extent by prolactin and cortisol, and is minimally affected by changes in blood glucose levels. In late pregnancy, although basal insulin levels are elevated, maternal blood glucose values are similar to nonpregnant levels.[6] Increased insulin secretion after a meal (in response to the higher blood glucose) offsets the contrainsulin effects of the placental hormones. As a result these effects are most noticeable in the postabsorptive state.[50] If the pregnant woman is not able to elevate her insulin secretion to overcome the increasing pregnancy-induced insulin resistance, metabolic abnormalities such as gestational diabetes may develop or existing metabolic problems such as diabetes will be aggravated.

Alterations in insulin production and responsiveness are critical in integrating changes in carbohydrate and fat metabolism throughout the course of pregnancy. Baird summarizes these interactions as follows: During early pregnancy increased insulin in response to glucose, minimal changes in insulin sensitivity, and increased number of insulin receptors on the adipocytes result in normal or slightly enhanced carbohydrate tolerance. The increased hepatic synthesis and secretion of triglycerides during this period, along with a normal or slightly elevated removal of triglycerides from the circulation, lead to a net storage of fat. During late pregnancy the elevated plasma insulin, decrease in numbers of adipocyte insulin receptors to nonpregnant levels, and increasing insulin resistance result in reduced assimilation of glucose and triglycerides by maternal tissues, greater transfer of these substances to the fetus, and increased lipolysis. The net result is a decrease in maternal blood glucose, increased glucose turnover, and greater maternal reliance on lipid catabolism for energy.[6] Changes in lipid, carbohydrate, and protein metabolism are summarized in Table 13–2.

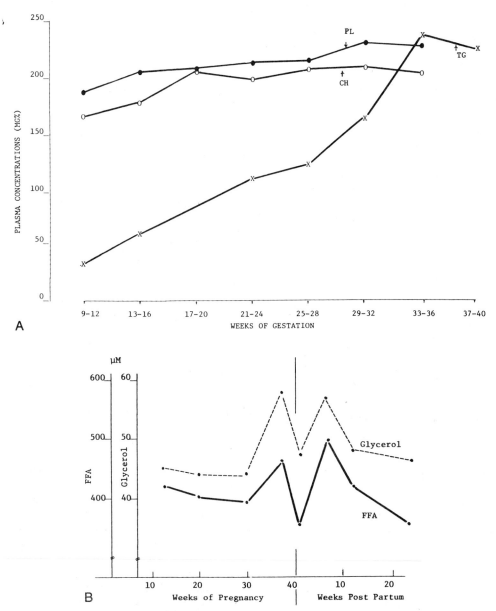

FIGURE 13–2.   Changes in plasma lipid concentrations during pregnancy. *A*, Changes in triglyceride (TG) concentrations during pregnancy with a progressive rise in phospholipid (PL) and cholesterol (CH). *B*, Plasma free fatty acid (FFA) and serum glycerol concentrations in normal women during pregnancy. Changes in FFA and glycerol concentrations parallel each other. Lipolysis is more rapid in the last trimester and early in the postpartum period with a transient reduction at term. (From Kalkhoff, R.K., Kissebah, A.H., & Kim, H.J. (1979). Carbohydrate and lipid metabolism during normal pregnancy: Relationship to gestational hormone action. In I.R. Merkatz & P.A.J. Adams (Eds.), *The diabetic pregnancy: A perinatal perspective* (pp. 11–13). New York: Grune & Stratton.)

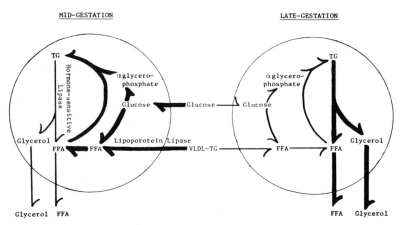

FIGURE 13–3. Changes in adipocyctes during pregnancy. The thick arrows represent the predominant metabolic activity. During the first half of pregnancy lipogenesis predominates with a net lipolysis in late gestation. (From Kalkhoff, R.K., Kissebah, A.H., & Kim, H.J. (1979). Carbohydrate and lipid metabolism during normal pregnancy: Relationship to gestational hormone action. In I.R. Merkatz & P.A.J. Adams (Eds.), *The diabetic pregnancy: A perinatal perspective* (p. 17). New York: Grune & Stratton.)

Absorptive versus Postabsorptive States

In addition to phasic changes in metabolic processes throughout the course of pregnancy, metabolism of amino acids, carbohydrates, and fats also varies on a daily basis depending on whether the mother is in the absorptive (fed) or postabsorptive state (Fig. 13–4). As a result of these changes pregnancy has been characterized as a period of both "accelerated starvation" and "facilitated anabolism."[36, 39] These periods are described in the section on Clinical Implications for the Pregnant Woman and Her Fetus.

THE ABSORPTIVE STATE

During the absorptive (fed) state, ingested nutrients (amino acid, glucose, triglyceride) are entering the blood from the gastrointestinal tract (see Chapter 9) and must be oxidized for energy, used for protein synthesis, or stored. The average meal takes about 4 hours for complete absorption. In this state anabolism exceeds catabolism and glucose is the major energy source. Small amounts of amino acid and fat are converted into energy or used to resynthesize body proteins or for structural fat. Most of the amino acid and fat and any extra carbohydrate are transformed into adipose tissue; carbohydrate is also stored as glycogen.[124]

The absorptive state during pregnancy (Fig. 13–4A) is characterized by relative hyperinsulinemia (related to decreased insulin sensitivity), hyperglycemia (due to failure of liver glucose uptake), and hypertriglyceridemia and lipogenesis (more glucose is converted to triglyceride for storage).[22, 121, 128] Maternal blood glucose levels may rise transiently to 130 to 140 mg/dl.[29] Gluconeogenesis and circulating free fatty acids are decreased. The hyperinsulinemic response is

TABLE 13–1
Metabolic Effects of Insulin and Glucagon

HORMONE	METABOLIC ACTIONS
Insulin	Acts in the liver to
	Increase glycogen synthesis from carbohydrate (glycogenesis) or fat and protein (glyconeogenesis)
	Decrease formation of glucose from fats and protein (gluconeogenesis)
	Increase protein synthesis
	Acts in muscle to
	Increase glucose uptake
	Increase glycogen and protein synthesis
	Retard proteolysis
	Acts in adipose cells to
	Increase glucose uptake
	Increase conversion of carbohydrate to fat
	Decrease lipolysis
	Increase uptake of free fatty acids
Glucagon	Acts in the liver to
	Decrease glycogen synthesis and increase conversion of glycogen to glucose (glycogenolysis)
	Increase uptake of amino acids
	Increase conversion of alanine to glucose
	Increase ketogenesis
	Acts in adipose tissue to
	Increase lipolysis

Compiled from Vander, A., et al. (1985). *Human physiology.* New York: McGraw-Hill and Guyton, A.C. (1987). *Textbook of medical physiology* (7th ed.). Philadelphia: WB Saunders.

TABLE 13–2
Maternal Metabolic Processes During Pregnancy: Relationship Between Hormonal and Metabolic Changes

HORMONAL CHANGE	EFFECT	METABOLIC CHANGE
Increased hPL	Diabetogenic Decreased glucose tolerance	Facilitated anabolism during feeding *and*
Increased prolactin	Insulin resistance	Accelerated starvation during fasting ↓
Increased bound and free cortisol	Decreased hepatic glycogen stores Increased hepatic glucose production	Ensures glucose and amino acids to fetus
Increased estrogen, progesterone, and insulin during early pregnancy	Increased fat synthesis Fat cell hypertrophy Inhibition of lipolysis	Anabolic fat storage during early pregnancy
Increased hPL in late pregnancy	Lipolysis	Catabolic fat mobilization in late pregnancy

Adapted from Hollingsworth, D.R. & Moore, T.R. (1989). Diabetes and pregnancy. In R.K. Creasy & R. Resnik (Eds.), *Maternal-fetal medicine: Principles and practice* (2nd ed., pp. 932, 935). Philadelphia: WB Saunders.

most marked during the third trimester because of hypertrophy and hyperplasia of islet beta cells. These cells become more responsive to alterations in blood glucose and amino acid levels.[124] Under the influence of placental hormones, resistance of the liver and peripheral tissues to insulin is reduced by as much as 60 to 80%.[85, 121] Even with increased production of insulin, however, overall glucose levels are maintained, although at a relatively lower level than in the nonpregnant woman because of the counterbalancing effects of estrogen, progesterone, and hPL.

THE POSTABSORPTIVE STATE

In the postabsorptive (fasting) state energy must be supplied by body stores. Most energy is produced by catabolism of fat. In this state fat and protein synthesis are decreased and catabolism exceeds anabolism. Plasma glucose levels are maintained during the postabsorptive state by use of alternate sources of glucose and glucose-sparing or fat-utilization reactions.[124] In the postabsorptive state the central nervous system continues to use glucose while other organs and tissues become glucose sparing, depending on fat as the primary energy source. Fatty acids are liberated by breakdown of triglycerides by the Krebs cycle, with production of ketone bodies that can produce ketoacidosis if allowed to accumulate.

Maternal responses during the fasting or postabsorptive state are exaggerations of normal postabsorptive responses, especially during the first half of pregnancy. These responses are influenced by (1) continuous placental uptake of glucose and amino acids from the maternal circulation; (2) decreased peripheral utilization of glucose as plasma concentrations of ketones and free fatty acids

increase; (3) decreased renal absorption of glucose; and (4) decreased hepatic glucose production. Thus, the postabsorptive state in pregnancy is characterized by relative hypoglycemia (due to the fetal siphon, increased renal losses, and decreased liver production), hyperketonuria (as an alternative energy source), hypoalaninemia (due to placental transfer for use in fetal glucose production), and hypoinsulinemia (Fig. 13–4B).[22, 121]

During the first half of pregnancy, glucose metabolism in the fasting postabsorptive state is an exaggeration of normal responses and leads to lower plasma glucose, blood glucose, and insulin levels. During the second half of pregnancy, effectiveness of insulin in translocating glucose into cells is reduced.[22] Since insulin is the ultimate arbitrator of both the absorptive and postabsorptive states, alterations in insulin secretion alter substrate availability to the mother and fetus.[50] The insulin antagonism in pregnancy is progressive, paralleling the growth of the fetoplacental unit, and disappears immediately after delivery. Placental hormones are probably major factors in producing this insulin antagonism.

Effects of Placental Hormones

The phasic changes in carbohydrate, lipid, and protein metabolism during pregnancy are probably due to the interplay of placental hormones, especially estrogen, progesterone, and hPL. During the first half of pregnancy, metabolism is affected primarily by estrogens and progesterone. In late pregnancy the influences of increasing concentrations of hPL become more prominent. Maternal metabolic changes are also influenced by prolactin and cortisol.[7]

Estrogen stimulates islet beta-cell hyper-

Fed State

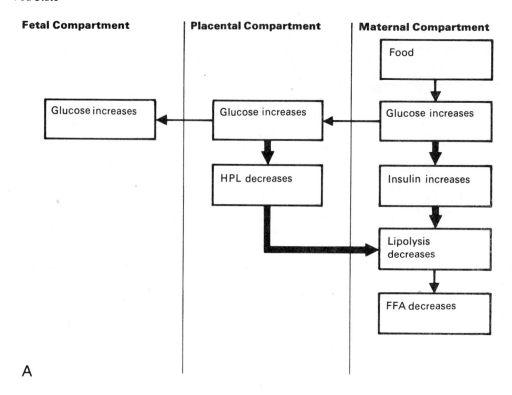

A

Fasting State

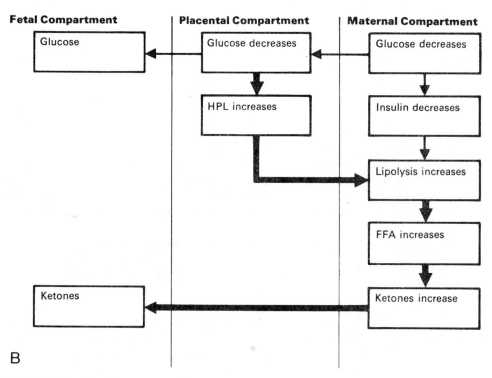

B

FIGURE 13–4. The absorptive and nonabsorptive states during pregnancy. *A*, Absorptive or fed state. *B*, Postabsorptive or fasting state. (From Speroff, L., Glass, R.H., & Kase, N.G. (1989). *Clinical gynecologic endocrinology and fertility* (4th ed., pp. 333–334). Baltimore: Williams & Wilkins.)

plasia and insulin secretion, enhances glucose utilization in peripheral tissues, and increases plasma cortisol, an insulin antagonist. As a result, particularly in the first half of gestation, estrogen decreases fasting glucose levels, improves glucose tolerance, and increases glycogen storage.[7, 22] Progesterone augments insulin secretion, increases fasting plasma insulin concentrations, and diminishes peripheral insulin effectiveness. Cortisol mediates these changes by inhibiting glucose uptake and oxidation, increasing liver glucose production, and possibly augmenting glucagon secretion.[7, 58, 149]

Human placental lactogen, a polypeptide hormone produced by the syncytiotrophoblast (see Chapter 2), is the most potent insulin antagonist of the placental hormones. This hormone is secreted primarily into the maternal circulation, with levels increasing markedly after 20 weeks. Since effects of hPL are similar to those of growth hormone, it has been called the "growth hormone" of the second half of pregnancy.[7] hPL action increases availability of maternal glucose and amino acids to the fetus. Other effects of hPL include diminished tissue response to insulin; lipolysis, which increases plasma free fatty acids; enhanced nitrogen retention; decreased urinary potassium excretion; and increased calcium excretion. The major effect is sparing of maternal carbohydrate (glucose) by providing alternative energy sources such as free fatty acids (Fig. 13–5).[58, 91]

The Intrapartum Period

The processes of parturition are dependent on an available supply of glucose and triglycerides as energy sources. In addition, essential fatty acids are important as precursors of prostaglandins (arachidonic acid is a derivative of essential fatty acid), which are critical to the onset of labor. These relationships are described in Chapter 3.

During labor and delivery maternal glucose consumption increases markedly to produce the energy required by the uterus and skeletal muscles.[42, 50, 57] As a result maternal insulin requirements fall. Oxytocin may augment or supplant insulin during this period. In animals, oxytocin has been demonstrated to act similarly to insulin, that is, oxytocin stimulates glucose oxidation, lipogenesis, glycogen synthesis, and protein formation.[48, 50]

The Postpartum Period

With removal of the placenta, concentrations of placental hormones such as hPL, estrogens, and progesterone fall rapidly within hours after delivery (see Chapter 4).[89, 149] The postpartum woman is in a state of relative hypopituitarism with blunted production of gonadotropins and growth hormone.[21, 50] This hypopituitarism may result from the feedback effects of elevated hPL and prolactin levels during pregnancy on the pituitary gland. hPL is similar to growth hormone, and its disappearance with removal of the placenta leaves the woman without its contrainsulin effects during a period of relative deficiency of growth hormone.[50]

Plasma free fatty acids fall during the first postpartal week then increase to late pregnancy levels by 6 weeks, followed by a decrease to nonpregnant levels by 3 to 6 months (see Fig. 13–2B).[6] The initial decrease during the 1st week coincides with the fall in hPL. The increasing levels of fatty acids from 1 to 6 weeks post partum may reflect maternal use of other nutrients for milk production.[124] Maternal plasma amino acid levels return to nonpregnant values of approximately 4.3 mg/dl (versus pregnant values of 3.5 mg/dl) by several days after birth.[91]

CLINICAL IMPLICATIONS FOR THE PREGNANT WOMAN AND HER FETUS

The metabolic adaptations of pregnancy safeguard against variations in maternal caloric intake through decreased activity (assumed but not well documented), increased metabolic efficiency, and changes in the metabolism of carbohydrates, fats, and proteins.[6, 91] These metabolic changes occur in a phasic pattern, probably programmed by placental hormones, that spreads the energy costs and protein requirements of pregnancy over the entire 9 months of gestation. In early pregnancy energy is conserved (facilitated anabolism) followed by later redirection of energy (glucose) to the fetus ("accelerated starvation"), whereas throughout pregnancy the mother uses protein more economically to provide adequate amino acids for development of the fetal brain and other organs.[6, 50]

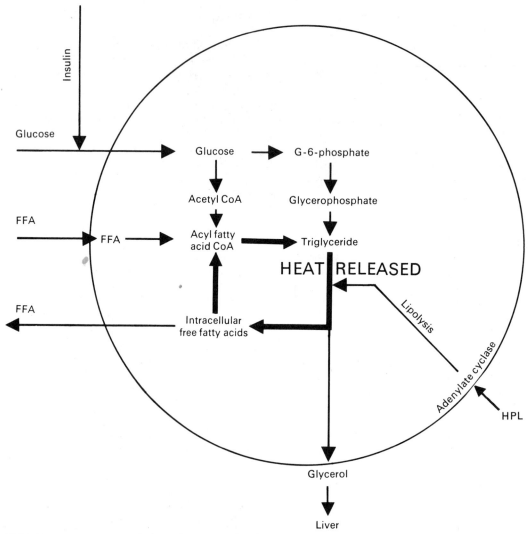

FIGURE 13–5. Fat metabolism during pregnancy and the actions of insulin and human placental lactogen (hPL). CoA, coenzyme A; FFA, free fatty acid. (From Speroff, L., Glass, R.H., & Kase, N.G. (1989). *Clinical gynecologic endocrinology and fertility* (4th ed., p. 332). Baltimore: Williams & Wilkins.)

Pregnancy has also been characterized as a diabetogenic state.[66] This state is reflected in the elevated blood glucose levels in association with increasing insulin resistance. These states are described in this section along with the basis for alterations in the glucose tolerance test and the effects of the normal metabolic changes of pregnancy on the diabetic woman and her fetus.

Pregnancy as a State of Facilitated Anabolism

Pregnancy has been called a state of facilitated anabolism to describe metabolic alterations that conserve energy during early preg-

nancy and help offset the accelerated starvation (described below).[39] After a meal the pregnant woman has higher glucose, insulin, and triglyceride levels and suppression of glycogen. These changes increase glucose availability for transport to the fetus, increase availability of an alternate energy source (triglycerides) for maternal needs, and provide less stimulus for maternal gluconeogenesis, glycogenolysis, and ketogenesis.[50]

Pregnancy as a State of "Accelerated Starvation"

During the postabsorptive state, when glucose is not being continuously supplied from the gastrointestinal tract, plasma glucose levels fall. The magnitude of the decline is greater in pregnant than nonpregnant women and is associated with a more rapid conversion to fat metabolism. This response is an exaggeration of the changes normally seen in the postabsorptive (fasting) state in nonpregnant women and similar to changes that occur during starvation ketosis. This state is characterized by lower fasting glucose and amino acid levels, increased blood glucose levels after eating, and increased plasma free fatty acids, triglycerides, ketones, and insulin secretion in response to glucose.[7, 22, 36, 96]

Maternal metabolic changes associated with this state of "accelerated starvation" include increased lipolysis due to hPL with increased free fatty acids, which increases ketogenesis in the liver and liver gluconeogenic potential. These changes would normally raise blood glucose levels, but in the pregnant woman the fasting glucose level tends to be lower because of the limited availability of substrate for gluconeogenesis. For example, as early as 15 weeks' gestation, maternal glucose levels after a 12- to 14-hour overnight fast are 15 to 20 mg lower than levels in nonpregnant women. The decrease in glucose during the overnight "fasting" period is especially prominent during the second and third trimesters.[6, 22, 124] Hypoalaninemia also develops because maternal protein stores can provide only limited substrate, which is insufficient to meet both maternal and fetal amino acid needs.[36, 50]

Thus, the accelerated starvation of pregnancy is characterized by hypoglycemia, hypoalaninemia, hyperketonemia, and increased levels of free fatty acids (see Fig. 13–4B) after a normal overnight (12- to 16-hour) fast.[33] These changes are similar to those seen in insulin-dependent diabetics with ketoacidosis except that a diabetic woman would be hyperglycemic rather than hypoglycemic. This disparity is due to differences in tissue sensitivity to insulin.[50]

Metabolic changes characteristic of this state are primarily due to hPL, which promotes lipolysis to increase free fatty acid levels and opposes insulin action, thus increasing glucose availability to the fetus. Other factors influencing this response include increased glucose utilization by the fetus ("the fetal siphon") and mother, along with an increase in the volume of distribution for glucose (i.e., hemodilution).[22]

Drainage of glucose and amino acids by the fetus may lead to increased maternal appetite and a feeling of faintness sometimes experienced during early pregnancy. Pregnant women may experience more rapid development of ketosis and fasting hypoglycemia after food deprivation or in the postabsorptive state. With greater maternal reliance on fat utilization during pregnancy, production of ketone bodies and risks of abnormalities such as acidosis are increased. Ketones readily cross the placenta and have been associated with neurologic deficits in infants. Although all studies have not confirmed this finding, dieting and caloric restrictions during pregnancy should be considered potentially dangerous to both the mother and fetus.[46]

Pregnancy as a Diabetogenic State

The diabetogenic effects of pregnancy are reflected by alterations in the glucose tolerance test, with higher glucose values after a meal reflecting an acquired resistance to insulin.[124] The alterations in carbohydrate metabolism are most evident during late pregnancy in the absorptive state (see Fig. 13–4A). When the woman is in this state and glucose is being added to the plasma, her blood glucose levels do not drop as rapidly as usual, even in the face of higher circulating insulin levels. This response results from decreased maternal sensitivity to insulin due to the action of hormones such as hPL, progesterone, and cortisol. Secretion of these hormones increases during the second half of pregnancy, therefore diabetogenic effects are most prominent during this period. Insulin resistance is somewhat compensated by increased plasma insulin concentrations.[2, 22]

The changes in insulin sensitivity tend to protect the fetus if the mother is fasting by keeping glucose in the blood and thus available for placental transfer. hPL decreases insulin effectiveness (and thus movement of glucose out of the blood into cells) by decreasing tissue sensitivity and mobilizes free fatty acids and amino acids. The result is an increase in available glucose and amino acid for transfer to the fetus and increased free fatty acids for maternal energy.

Effects of Metabolic Changes on the Glucose Tolerance Test

The alterations in carbohydrate metabolism in the absorptive state during pregnancy result in an elevated blood glucose response to a carbohydrate load. This progressive decrease in glucose tolerance is reflected in the criteria for an abnormal glucose tolerance test (GTT) in pregnancy. These changes are most marked in the second and third trimesters.[17, 85, 124]

As can be seen from values in Table 13–3, the initial fasting blood glucose value is lower because of decreased glucose utilization and increased fat utilization by the mother (making increased glucose available to the fetus) and the subsequent effects of the fetal siphon. Blood glucose levels tend to remain high after ingestion of carbohydrates for a longer period of time secondary to insulin antagonism and decreased insulin sensitivity. Normally the magnitude of the increase in blood glucose after a carbohydrate feeding is a refection of failure in glucose uptake by the liver. During pregnancy the increased glucose response in the face of increased endogenous insulin confirms the relative insensitivity and resistance of the liver (as well as peripheral tissues such as muscle and adipose tissue) to insulin.[22, 55]

Maternal-Fetal Relationships

Growth and development of the fetus is dependent on the availability of a constant supply of glucose from the mother for energy and protein synthesis. The fetus also requires transfer of amino acids and lipids for synthesis of new tissues. The fetus must develop adequate stores of these substances to meet the demands of the intrapartum period and transition to extrauterine life. Placental transfer of selected nutrients and hormones is summarized in Figure 13–6. Fetal requirements for substrates involved in carbohydrate, fat, and protein metabolism are discussed in the next section.

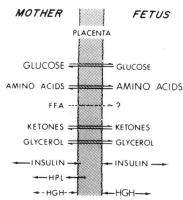

FIGURE 13–6. The interrelationships between maternal and fetal fuels and hormones. (From Freinkel, N. & Metzger, B.E. (1979). Pregnancy as a tissue culture experience: The critical implications of maternal metabolism for fetal development. *Pregnancy, metabolism, diabetes and the fetus: Ciba Foundation Symposium No. 63* (p. 4). Amsterdam: Excerpta Medica.)

Alterations in maternal metabolic processes or in placental transfer of essential nutrients reduce or increase the availability of specific substrates and can be both an advantage and a potential disadvantage to the fetus (Table 13–4). For example, since fetal energy requirements are met almost exclusively by glucose, the diabetogenic state increases availability of glucose in maternal plasma for placental transfer by reducing efficiency of maternal glucose storage. If the usual metabolic changes of pregnancy or placental function is altered, however, variations in fetal growth, such as occur in the infant of a diabetic mother or infant with intrauterine growth retardation, may develop.

Maternal glucose infusions during the intrapartum period can lead to a fetal hyperglycemia that stimulates insulin and inhibits glucagon secretion. This may delay gluconeo-

TABLE 13–3
Criteria for an Abnormal 3-hour 100-g Glucose Tolerance Test (GTT) in a Pregnant Woman

TIME	NONPREGNANT STATE (mg/dl)	PREGNANT* (WHOLE BLOOD) (mg/dl)	PREGNANT* (PLASMA)† (mg/dl)
Fasting	110	90	105
1 hour	180	165	190
2 hours	120	145	165
3 hours	110	125	145

*Upper limits of normal.
†Plasma values modified by National Diabetes Data Group.
Compiled from National Diabetes Data Group. (1979). Classification and diagnosis of diabetes mellitus and other categories of glucose intolerance. *Diabetes, 28*, 1039, and O'Sullivan, J.B. & Mahan, C.M. (1964). Criteria for the oral glucose tolerance tests in pregnancy. *Diabetes, 13*, 278.

TABLE 13–4
Potential Advantages and Disadvantages to the Fetus of Alterations in Maternal Metabolism
During Pregnancy

PARAMETER	POTENTIAL ADVANTAGES	POTENTIAL DISADVANTAGES
Diabetogenic effects	Increased availability of glucose for the fetus since the mother stores glucose less readily	Increased tendency to maternal and subsequent fetal hyperglycemia with increased risk of fetal hyperinsulinemia and macrosomia
Accelerated starvation		May lead to maternal ketosis; ketones cross the placenta and have been associated with impaired neurologic development by some investigators
Increased availability of free fatty acids	Free fatty acids are not transferred to the fetus in significant amounts and serve as an alternate maternal energy source, especially during the postabsorptive state, conserving maternal glucose for transfer to the fetus	Ketones from metabolism of free fatty acids are probably transferred to the fetus when maternal glucose levels are reduced (as an alternate fetal energy source) and have been associated with neurologic deficits by some investigators

genesis after birth and increase the risk of neonatal hypoglycemia.[59, 73, 107]

The Pregnant Diabetic Woman

The metabolic changes during pregnancy contribute to alterations in insulin requirements in insulin-dependent pregnant diabetic women. Since the metabolic changes in pregnancy normally lead to increased insulin availability by the end of pregnancy, it is not surprising that pregnant diabetic women experience an increase in insulin requirements by this time.[22, 50, 55]

The classification system for diabetes proposed by the National Diabetes Data Group consists of type I (insulin dependent), type II (noninsulin dependent), type III (gestational diabetes), and type IV (secondary diabetes).[85] Hare identifies three levels of insulin deficit in pregnancy:[50]

1. Women with mild gestational diabetes (type III) whose primary alteration is an abnormal glucose tolerance test. These women essentially have a disorder of underutilization of glucose characterized by a normal fasting glucose, but elevated glucose levels after being given a glucose load.

2. Women with moderate to severe gestational diabetes (type III) who have an increased fasting glucose, indicating an overproduction of glucose.

3. Women with type I diabetes who have little or no available endogenous insulin. These women cannot achieve the usual balance between the accelerated starvation and the facilitated anabolism characteristic of pregnancy since homeostasis is dependent on

the availability of additional insulin to promote facilitated anabolism.

Gestational diabetes is defined as the onset or first recognition of carbohydrate intolerance in pregnancy.[85] These women have decreased numbers of insulin receptors and decreased binding of insulin to target cells, which, along with a relative deficiency of circulating insulin, result in a progressive alteration in glucose tolerance.[29]

Pregnant insulin-dependent diabetic women often experience decreased insulin requirements during the first half of pregnancy because of increased glucose siphoning by the fetus, which decreases maternal blood glucose levels. Maternal food intake may also decrease during this period because of the nausea and vomiting of pregnancy. Since circulating glucose levels are reduced, maternal insulin requirements are also lowered. As pregnancy progresses, the diabetogenic actions of increasing amounts of placental hormones and the increasing insulin insensitivity outweigh the effects of the fetal siphon. Thus, maternal insulin requirements increase during the second half of gestation to levels 2 to 3 times higher than prepregnancy values.[22, 50, 55]

The diabetic woman may have little or no insulin requirement during labor, probably because of an increase in energy needs, and thus glucose utilization, and the presence of oxytocin, with its insulin-like effects.[42, 57] After delivery and removal of the placenta, levels of estrogens, progesterone, and hPL fall rapidly. This quickly reverses the insulin insensitivity of pregnancy. Maternal insulin requirements usually fall rapidly to prepregnancy levels or even below (due to a rebound phenomenon). Oxytocin may also contribute to these changes. As a result, the insulin-dependent diabetic woman may need little or no exogenous insulin the first few days after delivery. Insulin requirements generally return to prepregnancy levels by 4 to 6 weeks post partum.[46] These changes are summarized in Figure 13–7.

Levels of glycosylated hemoglobin and other glycosylated proteins are useful in monitoring glucose concentrations over time and in genetic counseling and have been used to evaluate fetal and maternal risks for complications in a pregnancy complicated by maternal diabetes.[7, 15, 80, 97, 124, 127] Glycosylated hemoglobin is formed slowly over the life span of the red blood cell and represents an overall measure of glycemia. The parameters used most frequently are hemoglobin A_{1c} (the most abundant component of hemoglobin A) and total amounts of hemoglobin A. Levels of glycosylated hemoglobin A reflect ambient glucose concentrations over the previous 4 to 6 weeks and have been used to monitor maternal glycemic control on a monthly basis.[124] Hemoglobin A_{1c} is higher in preg-

nant diabetics than in other pregnant women, but lower than in nonpregnant diabetics.[15, 124]

Hemoglobin A_{1c} is not as useful as an independent measure of glycemic control in pregnancy, since these levels may not be a good predictor of capillary blood glucose levels in the woman.[66a, 66b] The use of verified glucose data (i.e., a glucose reflectance meter with memory capability) collected by the pregnant woman (using protocols for self-monitoring of blood glucose) has been shown to provide more reliable data.[66a]

Fetus of a Diabetic Mother

Maternal metabolic abnormalities, particularly hyperglycemia during the period of embryonic organogenesis (3 to 8 weeks), have been associated with an increased risk of congenital anomalies (Fig. 13–8).[7, 43, 76, 124] The incidence of anomalies ranges from 3% in infants of women with good glycemic control to up to 22% in women with poor control.[76] Rigid glycemic control before conception and during early pregnancy has been associated with a reduction in the frequency of congenital anomalies.[41, 61a, 66a, 77a, 79] Thus,

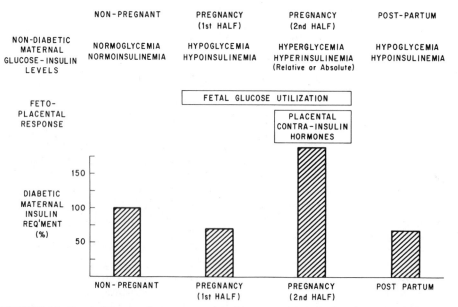

FIGURE 13–7. Influence of pregnancy on glucose and insulin levels in nondiabetic women and on insulin requirements in diabetic women. The prepregnancy insulin dose is shown as 100%. The insulin requirement may decline in the first half of pregnancy and in the puerperium and is increased in the second half of pregnancy. (From Tyson, J.E. & Felig, P. (1971). Medical aspects of diabetes in pregnancy. *Med Clin North Am, 55,* 953.)

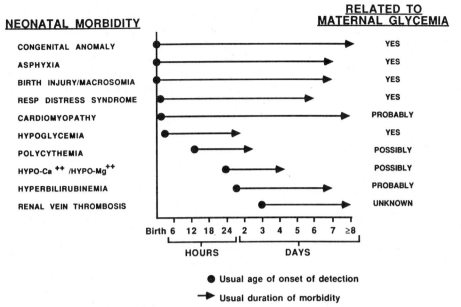

NEONATAL MORBIDITY

**RELATED TO
MATERNAL GLYCEMIA**

CONGENITAL ANOMALY	YES
ASPHYXIA	YES
BIRTH INJURY/MACROSOMIA	YES
RESP DISTRESS SYNDROME	YES
CARDIOMYOPATHY	PROBABLY
HYPOGLYCEMIA	YES
POLYCYTHEMIA	POSSIBLY
HYPO-Ca ++ /HYPO-Mg++	POSSIBLY
HYPERBILIRUBINEMIA	PROBABLY
RENAL VEIN THROMBOSIS	UNKNOWN

Birth 6 12 18 24 2 3 4 5 6 7 ≥8

HOURS   DAYS

● Usual age of onset of detection

➤ Usual duration of morbidity

FIGURE 13–8. Relationship of fetal and neonatal morbidities in the infant of a diabetic mother to maternal blood glucose control. (From Merkatz, I.R. & Adams, P.A.J. (Eds.). (1979). *The diabetic pregnancy: A perinatal perspective* (p. 197). New York: Grune & Stratton.)

preconceptual counseling and control are critical for improving pregnancy outcome in a diabetic mother.

Although the exact basis for development of macrosomia and other problems in the fetus of a diabetic woman has not been completely determined, this phenomenon is generally thought to arise from increased fetal production of insulin in response to fetal hyperglycemia (Fig. 13–9).[7, 38, 41, 52, 75, 81, 124] Since maternal insulin does not cross the placenta (see Fig. 13–6), fetal hyperinsulinemia arises as a response to increased placental transfer of substrates, particularly glucose. Thus, maternal hyperglycemia in diabetic women results in fetal hyperglycemia and subsequent hyperplasia of the fetal islet cells, with increased production of insulin, enhanced glycogen synthesis, lipogenesis, and increased protein synthesis.[23, 29] Increased levels of other substances ("mixed nutrients"), particularly amino acids and fatty acids, may also be important in the development of fetal macrosomia.[23, 94, 123]

Levels of endogenous insulin are correlated with the development of macrosomia.[7] Insulin is the major fetal growth hormone, therefore fetal hyperinsulinemia leads to increased body fat and organ size. The major organs affected are the heart, lungs, liver, spleen, thymus, and adrenal gland. The brain and kidney are not affected. The organo-

megaly probably arises from increased protein synthesis.[7, 33, 81] Stringent maternal glucose control, especially during the third trimester, when fetal growth peaks, reduces the risk of macrosomia.[12, 29, 99]

Maternal diabetes also alters lipid metabolism and transfer of fatty acids to the fetus. In diabetic women transfer of fatty acids to the fetus is increased, as is the amount of triglyceride stored in the placenta. These changes are secondary to alterations in several factors that influence fatty acid transfer, including maternal and fetal blood flow and concentrations of serum proteins and placental fatty acid–binding protein.[18]

The placenta is also affected, especially in women whose diabetes is poorly controlled, with increased peripheral and capillary surface area and intervillous space volume.[29, 75] These changes may result from the increased glucose load and abnormal metabolic environment with fetal hyperinsulinemia (fetal "growth" hormone), or as a compensatory mechanism to increase oxygen delivery. The fetus of a diabetic mother shows increases in metabolic rate and oxygen consumption owing to metabolism of excessive glucose and other substrates.[75]

SUMMARY

Maternal adaptations during pregnancy alter the woman's metabolic processes. These

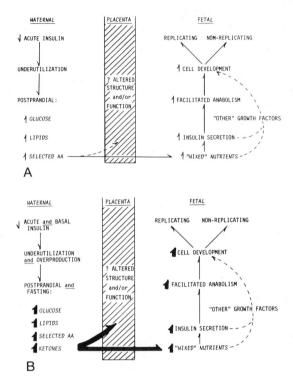

FIGURE 13–9. *A,* Fetal development in mild gestational diabetes (maternal underutilization only). *B,* Fetal development in more severe diabetes in pregnancy (maternal underutilizaiton and overproduction). (From Freinkel, N. & Metzger, B.E. (1979). Pregnancy as a tissue culture experience: The critical implications of maternal metabolism for fetal development. *Pregnancy, metabolism, diabetes and the fetus: Ciba Foundation Symposium No. 63* (pp. 10–11). Amsterdam: Excerpta Medica.)

changes are critical for protection of the mother and promote her ability to adapt to pregnancy. Maternal adaptations are essential to ensure that the fetus obtains an adequate supply of nutrients to support growth and development. Alterations in metabolic processes in the mother also interact with the course of disorders such as diabetes mellitus. Through an understanding of the normal metabolic changes during pregnancy, the nurse gains greater understanding of the alterations seen in the pregnant diabetic, her fetus, and newborn. Implications for clinical practice are summarized in Table 13–5.

FETAL DEVELOPMENT OF CARBOHYDRATE, FAT, AND PROTEIN METABOLISM

Fetal metabolic processes are dominated by anabolism and governed primarily by glucose with little oxidation of fat. The fetus must produce energy and maintain oxidative phosphorylation in the face of a low-oxygen environment. Although energy is produced in the fetus under aerobic conditions, the fetus has a greater capacity for anaerobic metabolism and is efficient in using lactate.[56, 123] Oxygen consumption in the fetus is 8 ml/kg/min. Glucose contributes more than half of the substrate for oxygen consumption.[125]

The fetal caloric requirement has been estimated to average 90 to 100 kcal/kg/day.[109] Almost all of the fetal fuel requirements are met by metabolism of glucose, lactate, and amino acids (especially alanine).[8] The fetus also uses these substrates as major precursors for storage of fuels such as fatty acids and glycogen. The stored fuels are critical energy sources during the intrapartum period and transition to extrauterine life. By term, the fetus has increased its weight 175-fold, protein content 400-fold, and fat content 5000-fold.[130]

Carbohydrate Metabolism

The fetus, who has been described as a "glucose-dependent parasite," uses glucose from the mother as the major substrate for energy production.[60, 65, 125] Fetal glucose utilization rates (6 mg/kg/min) are higher than in neonates (4.2 mg/kg/min) or adults (2 to 3 mg/kg/min).[23, 32, 92] The placenta has a high facility for glucose uptake and transport. Approximately two thirds of maternal glucose entering the uteroplacental circulation is used by the uterus and placenta to meet their energy needs.[106]

Under basal, nonstressed conditions, the fetal glucose pool is in equilibrium with the maternal pool and almost all fetal glucose is of maternal origin.[121] Fetal glucose levels are generally 10 to 20 mg/dl less than maternal levels and increase slightly toward the end of gestation.[7, 22, 60, 124] This gradient favors transfer of glucose across the placenta from the mother through carrier-mediated facilitated diffusion (Fig. 13–10). The levels at which these carriers become saturated is significantly above the usual maternal blood glucose level, which promotes a constant supply of glucose to the fetus.[65] There is no net transfer of insulin or glucagon to the fetus.[23]

Fetal glucose utilization is independent of maternal glucose availability. The mother meets this demand by an increasing reliance on fat metabolism for her own fuel needs. If

TABLE 13–5
Summary of Recommendations for Clinical Practice Related to Changes in Carbohydrate, Protein, and Fat Metabolism: Pregnant Woman

Recognize usual changes in carbohydrate, protein, and fat metabolism during pregnancy (pp. 584–591, Table 13–2).
Assess and monitor maternal nutrition in terms of carbohydrate, protein, and fat intake (pp. 585–591).
Counsel women regarding nutrient and energy requirements to meet maternal and fetal needs during pregnancy (pp. 584–595, 597–606, Figs. 13–10 and 13–12).
Monitor maternal glucose and ketone status (pp. 588–589, 592–595, 598–599)
Monitor fetal growth (pp. 594–595, 600–603, Figs. 13–6, 13–10, and 13–12).
Understand implications of changes in the absorptive and postabsorptive states for the pregnant woman and fetus (pp. 588–591, Figure 13–4).
Monitor maternal energy status during intrapartum period (p. 591).
Counsel women regarding changes in appetite and weight during pregnancy (pp. 585, 591–593, Chapter 9).
Counsel women regarding risks of dieting and caloric restriction during pregnancy (p. 593, 600–601, Chapter 9).
Know usual parameters for the glucose tolerance test during pregnancy (pp. 593–594, Table 13–3).
Recognize the effects of metabolic changes on insulin requirements of diabetic women during the prenatal, intrapartum, and postpartum periods (pp. 595–596, Fig. 13–7).
Evaluate and monitor metabolic and insulin status in the pregnant diabetic woman (pp. 595–597, Fig. 13–7).
Counsel diabetic women regarding the effects of diabetes on pregnancy and the fetus and of pregnancy on diabetes (pp. 596–597, Fig. 13–8, Table 13–9).
Counsel diabetic women regarding prepregnancy strategies to optimize maternal and fetal outcomes (pp. 596–597).
Recognize the potential effects of diabetes on the fetus and newborn (pp. 596–597, 607–608, Fig. 13–8, Table 13–9).

Page numbers in parentheses following each recommendation refer to the page(s) in the text where the rationale for that intervention is discussed.

the maternal system is not able to meet the fetal demand for gluconeogenic precursors, hypoglycemia can result. Since fetal blood glucose levels are 70 to 80% of maternal values, maternal hypoglycemia leads to even lower fetal blood glucose levels.[22]

Glucose is also needed by the fetus for protein synthesis, as a precursor for fat synthesis, for conversion to glycogen for storage, and as the primary substrate for oxidative metabolism. Most of the transferred glucose is oxidized to CO_2 and H_2O by the Krebs cycle and oxidative phosphorylation.

The fetus has an active capacity for anaerobic metabolism, which has a greater role in fetal metabolic processes than it does in adults.[126] The fetus has increased amounts of glycolytic isoenzymes such as hexokinase, glu-

PLACENTAL TRANSFER OF MATERNAL NUTRIENTS

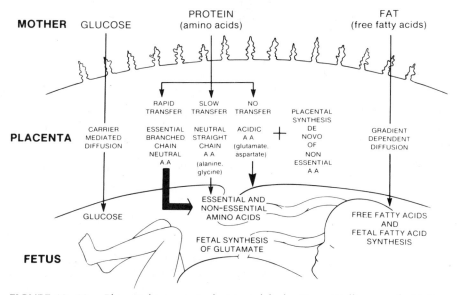

FIGURE 13–10. Placental transport of maternal fuels. (From Hollingsworth, D.B. (1983). Alterations of maternal metabolism in normal and diabetic pregnancies in insulin-dependent, noninsulin-dependent, and gestational diabetes. *Am J Obstet Gynecol, 146,* 420.)

cose-6-phosphate dehydrogenase (G6PD), and pyruvate dehydrogenase, which favor anaerobic glycolysis (Fig. 13–11).[56, 60, 125, 126] Fetal and placental tissues actively metabolize glucose to lactate. The greater amount of lactate generated by the fetus serves as an important nutrient.[8, 123] Lactate rather than glucose may be the major precursor of fetal hepatic glycogen and fatty acid synthesis.[9, 60] Under aerobic conditions, the fetus is a net consumer of lactate. The placenta produces large amounts of lactate and ammonia, which may help in regulating metabolic activities in the fetal hepatocytes.[8]

Glycogen synthesis is greater than glycogenolysis in the fetus. Glycogen synthetase can be found in the liver from the 8th week.[60] Deposition of hepatic glycogen during the perinatal period is regulated by glucocorticoids and insulin. Glucocorticoids may induce glycogen synthetase, which is then activated by insulin.[31] Fetal cells are believed to have increased insulin receptors, greater receptor affinity for glucose, and delayed maturation of hepatic glucagon receptors. These changes promote storage of glucose as glycogen and fat.

Glycogen is stored in fetal tissues from 9 weeks' gestation on and increases significantly during the third trimester. Until 20 to 24 weeks the fetal liver is the main glycogen storehouse; after that time glycogen is stored in heart and skeletal muscle. Compared with adults, the term fetus has 2 to 3 times more liver glycogen, 3 to 5 times more skeletal muscle glycogen, and 10 times more cardiac muscle glycogen stores.[91] The placenta has enzymes for gluconeogenesis and glycolysis and also accumulates glycogen, with greatest storage at 8 to 10 weeks' gestation.

Insulin is present in fetal islet tissue from about 9 to 11 weeks' gestation and can be found in plasma by 13 weeks' gestation. Insulin levels are dependent on fetal glucose levels. Insulin production is stimulated by increasing glucose and amino acid concentrations, especially after 20 weeks.[44, 67] Fetal glucose metabolism is relatively independent of the insulin–glucagon regulatory mechanisms seen after birth, however. Acute changes in glucose concentrations leading to hypo- or hyperglycemia do not significantly alter fetal insulin or glucagon secretion. Secretion of these hormones is markedly al-

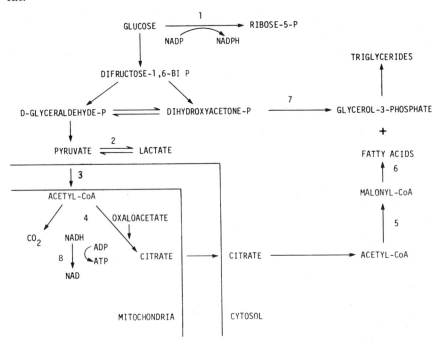

FIGURE 13–11. Major metabolic fates of glucose: *1*, Glucose-6-phosphate dehydrogenase. *2*, Lactate dehydrogenase. *3*, Pyruvate dehydrogenase. *4*, Citric acid cycle. *5*, Acetyl-CoA carboxykinase. *6*, De novo synthesis of fatty acids. *7*, Glycerol-3-phosphate dehydrogenase. *8*, Oxidative phosphorylation. (From Kimura, R.E. & Warshaw, J.B. (1983). Metabolism during development. In J.B. Warshaw (Ed.), *The biological basis of reproductive and developmental medicine* (p. 340). New York: Elsevier Biomedical.)

tered by chronic changes such as long-term hyperglycemia in a diabetic woman, which augments insulin secretion and suppresses glucagon, or by chronic maternal malnutrition, which depresses insulin and stimulates release of fetal glucagon.[121] Since insulin is a fetal growth hormone, fetal hyperinsulinemic states are associated with fetal and neonatal macrosomia.[52, 78]

Glucagon is found in fetal plasma by 15 weeks' gestation and reaches peak concentrations at 24 to 26 weeks. In comparison with adults, the number of fetal hepatic glucagon receptors is decreased and insulin receptors are increased. The fetal liver, erythrocyte, monocyte, and lung have an increased affinity for insulin. These attributes promote insulin-mediated anabolic processes such as glycogen formation and decrease glucagon-mediated catabolism.[121]

The fetal liver receives the highest net flux of maternal glucose because it is the first organ system encountered by blood returning from the placenta (see Chapter 6). Hepatic enzyme systems in the fetus have reduced activity to promote glycogen storage. Thus, enzymes for glycogenesis (carbohydrate to glycogen) are increased, whereas enzymes for glycolysis (carbohydrate to pyruvate and lactate) and gluconeogenesis (fat and protein to glucose) are present but decreased (Fig. 13–11). For example, glucose-6-phosphatase, an enzyme involved in gluconeogenesis and inhibited by glucose and amino acids, is at 20 to 50% of adult levels at mid-gestation.[60] These relationships are maintained until birth, when decreased glucose availability and onset of high-fat feedings stimulate decreases in glycogenolytic enzymes.[122, 126]

Fat Metabolism

Fetal fat content increases during gestation from 0.5% of body weight in early gestation to approximately 3.5% by 28 weeks and 16% at term.[129] This increase is due to transfer of fatty acids from the mother and active lipogenesis in the fetal liver and other tissues. Lipogenesis is primarily through the fatty acid synthetase pathway, which is highly active in the fetus.[18, 61, 126] Free fatty acids cross the placenta from mother to fetus in limited amounts by diffusion with a net flux of unesterified fatty acids to the fetus.[7, 60] These fatty acids are derived primarily from maternal circulating free fatty acids or cleavage of maternal triglycerides by lipoprotein lipase (Fig. 13–12).[91] The maternal diet is reflected in the fatty acid content of fetal tissues.[18, 60]

Since transport of fatty acids is primarily controlled by maternal concentrations, increased maternal levels are associated with increased transfer and fetal storage.[51] Other factors influencing free fatty acid transfer include serum albumin level, fatty acid chain length, uteroplacental and umbilical blood flow, and binding affinity.[18] The essential fatty acids, linoleic and alpha-linolenic acids, cannot be synthesized by the fetus and must be transported across the placenta. These substances can be desaturated by the fetus to form other fatty acids. Transfer of essential fatty acids increases in late pregnancy.[120]

Increased fat deposition during the third trimester is associated with increasing fetal weight and decreased serum triglycerides because these are used in fat deposition.[30] Most (80%) of the fetal fat accretion during this period is due to de novo synthesis from acetyl coenzyme A (CoA) (Fig. 13–13A) with formation of palmitic acid, especially in the brain and liver.[61, 120]

Fetal lipid metabolism is characterized by early development of mechanisms for lipogenesis with decreased lipolytic activity throughout gestation, except in the liver.[91, 125] Fetal fatty acid synthesis occurs through lipogenesis and desaturation of essential fatty acids. Lipogenesis is dependent on substrate availability. Lipogenic precursors include glucose, lactate, and ketone bodies; the latter two are the most important.[60, 61]

The rate of synthesis is primarily controlled by the ratio of plasma insulin-to-glucagon levels. Insulin stimulates and glucagon inhibits fatty acid synthesis. The action of glucagon is mediated by cyclic adenosine monophosphate (cAMP), which inhibits acetyl CoA enzymes.[61] The high insulin-to-glucagon ratio in the fetus promotes fatty acid synthesis. Lipogenesis is increased by glucose, fatty acids, and T_4 (see Chapter 16) and reduced by catecholamines.[60, 120] The fetal liver and brain contain enzymes for ketone oxidation as an alternative energy substrate.[7, 104] Lipolytic activity becomes active after delivery, when the infant can no longer rely on a constant glucose supply from the mother and must cope with relatively high fat intake.

By 15 weeks the fetus has developed enzymes to convert acetate or citrate to fatty acid and thus the potential to use fat as an

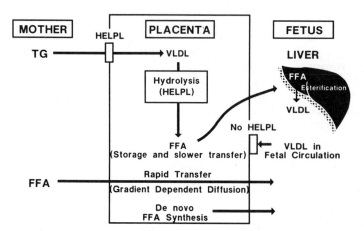

FIGURE 13–12. Mechanisms by which maternal free fatty acids and triglycerides give rise to free fatty acids in the fetal circulation (TG, triglycerides; FFA, free fatty acids; HELPL, heparin-elutable lipoprotein lipase; VLDL, very-low-density lipoprotein). (From Hollingsworth, D.B. & Moore, T.R. (1989). Diabetes and pregnancy. In R.K. Creasy & R. Resnik (Eds.), *Maternal-fetal medicine: Principles and practice* (p. 934). Philadelphia: WB Saunders.)

alternative source of energy.[91] Blood lipid and free fatty acid levels are relatively stable after about 26 weeks but remain low until after delivery.[125] The limited amounts of free fatty acids that cross the placenta are used by the fetus in organ development; synthesis of pulmonary surfactant, phospholipids, bile, and serum lipoprotein; formation of cell membranes; and as second messenger precursors. Fatty acids needed by developing neuronal and glial cells and in formation of the myelin sheath are synthesized within the brain.[126]

Activity of the pentose phosphate intermediary metabolic pathway is also high in the fetus. Activity of this pathway is associated with cell proliferation and an increased requirement for ribose phosphate precursors

of nucleic acids and provision of nicotinamide-adenine dinucleotide (NADH) for synthesis of long-chain fatty acids.[126]

Amino Acid Metabolism

At least 10 amino acids are essential for the fetus, including those essential for adults plus cysteine and histidine, with a dependency on arginine and tyrosine. Because of the relative inactivity of hepatic enzymes such as cystathionase and phenylalanine hydroxylase, the fetus cannot synthesize tyrosine and cysteine from phenylalanine and methionine.[49] The fetus uses amino acids for protein synthesis or oxidation since organ development involves continuous remodeling (breakdown and resynthesis) of tissue.

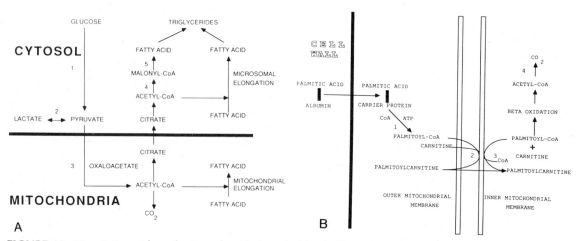

FIGURE 13–13. Fatty acid synthesis and oxidation. *A*, Metabolic pathways involved in fatty acid synthesis: *1*, glycolysis; *2*, lactate dehydrogenase; *3*, pyruvate dehydrogenase; *4*, acetyl-CoA carboxylase; *5*, fatty acid synthase complex. *B*, Metabolic pathways involved in fatty acid oxidation: *1*, palmitoyl-CoA synthetase; *2*, carnitine palmitoyl transferase I; *3*, carnitine palmitoyl transferase II; *4*, citric acid cycle. (From Kimura, R.E. (1989). Fatty acid metabolism in the fetus. *Semin Perinatol, 13*, 202.)

There is a net flux of most amino acids from the mother to the fetus (see Fig. 13–10).[65] Since concentrations of most amino acids are higher in fetal than maternal blood, amino acids are actively transported across the placenta. Fetal-to-maternal amino acid nitrogen ratios average 1.03 to 3.0 with a net active transfer of nitrogen to the fetus of 54 nmol/day and a total accumulation of about 400 g of protein by term.[6, 65, 91]

Levels of most amino acids remain higher in fetal than in maternal blood until near term, when fetal blood amino acid levels, particularly those of nonessential amino acids, fall. Levels of gluconeogenetic amino acids such as alanine are the only ones that remain elevated in late gestation. In the third trimester alanine is the most common amino acid transferred across the placenta; transfer of glutamine, glycine, and serine also remains high.[91, 125] The urea cycle is decreased or absent until mid-gestation.[65]

Until about 26 weeks' gestation most of the increase in fetal weight is due to accumulation of protein; after that time weight gain is due to fat accumulation. During the last weeks before term, fetal uptake of nitrogenous compounds falls and fetal nitrogen levels decrease because of the increased deposition of fat.[91]

NEONATAL PHYSIOLOGY

Neonates must develop a homeostatic balance between energy requirements and the supply of substrates as they move from the constant glucose supply of fetal life to the normal intermittent variations in the availability of glucose and other fuels that characterize the absorptive and postabsorptive states. The development of this homeostasis is dependent on substrate availability and maturation of hormonal, neuronal, and enzymatic systems and influenced by gestational age, health status, and intake.[23] Alterations in metabolic substrates and hormones in the fetus and neonate are summarized in Table 13–6.

Transitional Events

Metabolic transition is characterized by a shift from the anabolic-dominant fetal state to the catabolic state of the neonate. This transition is influenced by genetic, environmental, and endocrine factors as well as by major alterations in energy metabolism within the mitochondria.[8, 126] The ability of the fetus to use glucose anaerobically and to readily metabolize lactate may be important in maintaining homeostasis during the stresses of labor and delivery. The fetus prepares for this transition during the last weeks of gestation by increasing fuel storage in the form of glycogen and lipids. Glycogen is critical in order to maintain glucose homeostasis immediately after birth, whereas the fat stores, through lipolysis of fatty acids and ketone bodies, serve as an alternate energy source.[86] Postnatal changes in metabolism involve the transition from the almost exclusive reliance on glucose for energy production in the fetus to markedly increased use of fatty acid oxidation and ketone body use for energy production in the neonate.[8, 91]

Carbohydrate Metabolism

Birth results in the loss of the maternal glucose source. As a result, neonatal blood glucose normally falls, reaching a nadir at 2 to 6 hours after birth (Fig. 13–14). These values generally stabilize at levels of 50 to 60 mg/dl during the first few hours after birth. The basis for the fall in blood glucose is summarized in Table 13–7.

The newborn responds to the decrease in blood glucose in several ways. The rapid glycogenolysis (liberation of glucose from glycogen) after birth is stimulated by falling insulin levels and sluggish insulin (due to the decreased blood glucose with removal of the placenta), increased serum glucagon, stimulation of the sympathetic nervous system and catecholamine release, and increases in hepatic cAMP.[13] Since insulin promotes transfer of glucose out of the blood into cells, the lowered levels decrease transfer and elevate blood glucose levels. Glucagon stimulates conversion of glycogen into glucose, also raising blood glucose levels.[110]

Hepatic glycogen stores decrease markedly during this period. An estimated 90% of liver and 50 to 80% of muscle glycogen are used within the first 24 hours after birth.[1] After depletion of glycogen stores, the newborn responds by mobilizing fat stores with release of free fatty acids. This response is stimulated by the catecholamine release associated with cooling at birth (see Chapter 17). Catecholamines tend to stimulate glucagon, suppress insulin, and augment growth hormone secretion.[121] Production of glucose

TABLE 13–6
Alterations in Metabolic Substrates and Hormones in the Fetus and Neonate

	FETUS	NEWBORN
Hormone concentration		
Insulin	Low	Low
Glucagon	Low	High
Epinephrine	Low	High
Hormone receptors		
Insulin Density	High	Decrease
Affinity	High normal	Decrease
Structure	Normal	Normal
Functional kinase	Present	Present
Glucagon Density	Low	Rapid increase
Structure	?	Normal
Functional linkage to cAMP	Absent to low	Rapid increase
Epinephrine β-Receptor	Present	Present
Functional linkage	Present	Present
Liver enzymes		
Phosphorylase	Low	High
PEPCK	Low	High
Source of nutrients	Mother	Endogenous
Endogenous glucose production	Minimal	Highly active
Lipolysis/ketogenesis	Minimal	Highly active
	Anabolic	Catabolic

From Sperling, M.A. (1988). Glucose homeostasis after birth. In C.T. Jones (Ed.), *Research in perinatal medicine (VII). Fetal and neonatal development* (p. 464). Ithaca, NY: Perinatology Press.

from amino acids, especially alanine, increases and accounts for 4 to 10% of the glucose used for energy in term infants. Glycogen stores remain low for several days before rising.

Gluconeogenic enzyme activity develops after birth. From late fetal life to 3 days after birth blood glucose regulation is glucose dominant. As a result, gluconeogenesis is diminished during this period. After this period blood glucose regulation becomes insulin dominant (the adult pattern).[125] The

increased gluconeogenesis after birth is regulated by changes in the serum insulin-to-glucagon ratio, catecholamine secretion, fatty acid oxidation, and activation of hepatic enzyme systems.[60]

Increased secretion of catecholamines at birth, stimulated by postbirth cooling, increases glucagon secretion and reverses the fetal insulin-to-glucagon ratio. Increased glucagon concentrations and norepinephrine are important in subsequent activation of the hepatic gluconeogenic enzymes.[74] The predominant enzymes activated during this period are hepatic glycogen phosphorylase, G6PD, and phosphoenolpyruvate carboxykinase (PEPCK). Hepatic glycogen phospho-

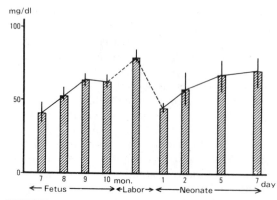

FIGURE 13–14. Blood glucose concentrations during the perinatal period. (From Takeda, Y. (1988). Metabolic adjustment in perinatal period. In G.H. Wiknjosastro, W.H. Prakoso, & K. Maeda (Eds.), *Perinatology* (p. 138). Amsterdam: Elsevier.)

TABLE 13–7
Basis for Changes in Glucose Levels in the First Few Hours After Birth

CHARACTERISTIC	BASIS
Immature liver enzyme systems	Promotes glucose storage rather than release
Larger brain in proportion to body size	Obligatory glucose user
Increased red blood cell volume	Obligatory glucose user
Decreased liver response to glucagon	Limits release of glucose from glycogen stores
Increased energy needs	Increased metabolic and motor activity with birth

rylase is activated by norepinephrine and glucagon and stimulates glycogenolysis. G6PD activity increases markedly after birth, increasing hepatic release of glucose. This is probably due to surges of glucagon and cAMP, which help to shift the activity of the liver from glycogen to glucose production. PEPCK is the rate-limiting enzyme for gluconeogenesis. PEPCK is inhibited by insulin. With changes in the insulin-to-glucagon ratio after birth, this enzyme increases about 20-fold, thus increasing gluconeogenesis.[60] Concentrations of these enzymes continue to increase over the first 2 weeks after birth in both term and preterm infants.[72]

The resumption of a carbohydrate source, that is, feeding, generally stabilizes the infant's glucose concentration, and most neonates achieve a steady state in their glucose concentrations by about 5 days.[125] The first enteral feeding immediately increases blood glucose levels. This increase is accompanied by an increase in plasma insulin levels in term infants and development of cyclic changes in insulin and blood glucose levels.[4, 5] In preterm infants the initial feeding is not accompanied by similar hormonal changes and the cyclic responses in insulin and blood glucose take 2 to 3 days to develop, probably longer in VLBW infants.[11] Enteral feeding stimulates production of digestive hormones and secretion of peptides critical for induction of gastrointestinal tract maturation and development of the enteroinsular axis. These changes lead to additional modifications of hepatic metabolism (see Chapter 9).[110]

Fat Metabolism

The inability of the fetus to oxidize fatty acids is rapidly reversed at birth because of changes in the functional ability of enzymes such as carnitine palmitoyltransferase (see Fig. 13–13).[126] During this period the levels of glucose and free fatty acids are mirror images of each other.[125] Lipolysis increases quickly after birth, reaching a maximum within a few hours.[13, 86, 126] This increase is reflected in changes in plasma free fatty acid levels, which rise rapidly beginning 4 to 6 hours after birth and reach adult levels by 24 hours. At this time two thirds of the infant's energy is produced from oxidation of fat.[91, 125]

Fat is the major form of stored calories in the newborn and the preferred energy source for tissues such as the heart and ad-renal cortex, which have high energy demands.[60] After birth mobilization of fatty acids from these stores is reflected in the rise in serum levels over the first few hours. This process is initiated by the increase in catecholamines and glucagon, resulting in increased cAMP followed by an increase in protein kinases, phosphorylation, and activation of adipose tissue lipase with release of fatty acids.[60]

The transition from glucose to fatty acid oxidation after birth is reflected in the fall of the respiratory quotient from 1.0 to 0.7 by 3 days.[103] This indicates that the infant has moved from obtaining nearly two thirds of its energy from oxidation of glycogen immediately after birth, to deriving most of its energy from fat metabolism by 3 days (and probably by 24 hours) of age.[91] This transition reflects increasing dependence on oxidative metabolism and is associated with an increase in the number of mitochondria and enzymes of the Krebs cycle and changes in blood free fatty acid levels. The neonate's brain may use free fatty acids, along with branched-chain amino acids and ketones, as additional energy sources.[60, 126]

The increase in fatty acid oxidation and ketogenesis after birth is related to increased enzyme activity, especially carnitine palmitoyltransferase (see Fig. 13–13), which reaches adult values by 30 days.[60, 125] Carnitine activity enhances fatty acid oxidation. Concentrations of carnitine are high in human milk for 2 to 3 days after delivery.[26] Another factor influencing this change is alteration in the insulin-to-glucagon ratio with increased glucagon. This increases the availability of substrates such as acetyl CoA and carnitine for fatty acid oxidation in the mitochondria.[61]

Protein Metabolism

Serum amino acid levels are higher during the first few weeks of life.[70] Urinary amino acids are elevated immediately after birth, with excretion of 8.8 mg/day in preterm and 7.6 mg/day in term infants versus 2.5 mg/day in older children.[124] The average body nitrogen content at birth is 2%.[70]

The newborn has a limited capacity to synthesize protein, primarily because of the relative inactivity of several hepatic enzymes (see Chapter 9).[49] This limitation is especially marked in preterm infants, whose capacity to use excess amino acid is reduced. Preterm infants who receive excess protein or an un-balanced amino acid intake are at risk for hyperammonemia, azotemia, metabolic acidosis, and altered plasma amino acid profiles. The latter changes are associated with altered protein synthesis and growth, central nervous system function, and bile acid uptake. The ability to metabolize excess amino acids may also be altered in the newborn depending on maturity of enzyme systems in the liver and skeletal muscle and activity of the urea cycle to eliminate nitrogen.[60]

CLINICAL IMPLICATIONS FOR NEONATAL CARE

The newborn's transitional state in relation to glucose homeostasis can result in problems even for healthy newborns as they attempt to provide adequate energy for maintenance and growth. Alterations in metabolic processes in the newborn can result in clinical problems, most notably hypoglycemia. The status of metabolic function in the newborn also influences nutritional needs (see Chapter 9).

Neonatal Hypoglycemia

The neonate may develop hypoglycemia if glycogen stores are insufficient to provide fuel during transition and until production of energy by fat oxidation is adequate or if the infant fails to adequately mobilize available glycogen stores.[126] Until recently hypoglycemia during the first 72 hours after birth was defined as a whole blood glucose value less than 35 mg/dl (term) or 25 mg/dl (preterm) or plasma glucose concentrations less than 40 mg/dl (term) or 30 mg/dl (preterm), with lower limits for normal values of 40 mg/dl (whole blood) and 45 mg/dl (plasma) after 72 hours.[74] These levels are controversial and have been abandoned by many clinicians, who instead believe that the lowest acceptable whole blood glucose for both term and preterm infants is 40 mg/dl. A recent panel concluded that the ". . . rational definition of hypoglycemia is clearly not a specific value but a continuum of falling blood glucose values, creating thresholds for neurologic dysfunction, which may vary from one cause of hypoglycemia or clinical circumstance to another."[21, p.836] They recommended that the concept of "cutoff" blood glucose values be discarded and the focus be on promoting normoglycemia for all infants with prompt intervention for values less than 40 mg/dl.

Clinical signs of hypoglycemia include tremors, jitteriness, irregular respirations, hypotonia, apnea, cyanosis, poor feeding, high-pitched cry, hypothermia, and seizures. Since hypoglycemic infants may be symptomatic or asymptomatic and signs of hypoglycemia are often nonspecific, careful monitoring of infants at risk for development of hypoglycemia is critical. Multiple factors influence the outcome of infants with hypoglycemia including severity and duration of the episode, cerebral blood flow and central nervous system glucose levels, rates of glucose uptake, maturity, availability of alternative substrates, response to intervention, and type of clinical manifestation.[21] Infants with symptomatic hypoglycemia and seizures have been reported to have a high incidence of later neurologic impairment.[35, 53] Most infants with asymptomatic hypoglycemia were reported to have generally good outcomes in earlier studies but this finding has also been challenged.[21] Most studies on the outcome of infants with hypoglycemia have significant methodologic limitations and there have been no controlled prospective studies.

Monitoring of blood glucose values is also an issue. Glucose oxidase reagent sticks are difficult to use in newborns because these sticks are dependent on the hematocrit, have great variance, and lack reproducibility, especially at levels less than 50 mg/dl.[19, 21] Glucose reflectance meters are also reported to be unreliable in evaluation of capillary blood glucose concentrations in high-risk neonates (i.e., hematocrits over 55% tend to reduce readings; hematocrits below 35% tend to result in falsely high readings).[19, 68]

Neonatal hypoglycemia can arise from an inadequate supply of glucose, alterations in endocrine regulation, or increased glucose regulation.[74] Preterm and small for gestational age (SGA) infants tend to develop hypoglycemia because of insufficient glycogen and fat stores and a decreased rate of gluconeogenesis. Infants of diabetic mothers usually have sufficient stores, however, but glycogenolysis is prevented by their high insulin levels and inability to secrete glucagon despite falling blood glucose levels.[126] Infants at risk for neonatal hypoglycemia and associated mechanisms are summarized in Table 13–8.

The Low Birth Weight Infant

Hypoglycemia is a common problem of low birth weight infants, including both appro-

TABLE 13–8
Causes and Time Course of Neonatal Hypoglycemia

MECHANISM	CLINICAL SETTING	EXPECTED DURATION
Decreased substrate availability	Intrauterine growth retardation	Transient
	Prematurity	Transient
	Glycogen storage disease	Prolonged
	Inborn errors of metabolism	Prolonged
Endocrine disturbances: hyperinsulinemia	Infant of a diabetic mother	Transient
	Beckwith-Wiedemann syndrome	Prolonged
	Erythroblastosis fetalis	Transient
	Exchange transfusion	Transient
	Islet cell dysplasia	Prolonged
	Maternal β-sympathomimetics	Transient
	Improperly placed umbilical artery catheter	Transient
Other endocrine disorders	Hypopituitarism	Prolonged
	Hypothyroidism	Prolonged
	Adrenal insufficiency	Prolonged
Increased utilization	Perinatal asphyxia	Transient
	Hypothermia	Transient
Miscellaneous or multiple factors	Sepsis	Transient
	Congenital heart disease	Transient
	CNS abnormalities	Prolonged

From Merenstein, G.B. & Gardner, S.L. (1989). *Handbook of neonatal intensive care* (2nd ed., p. 229). St. Louis: CV Mosby.

priate for gestational age (AGA) preterm infants and infants with intrauterine growth retardation. AGA preterm infants usually develop hypoglycemia secondary to inadequate intake or decreased hepatic glucose production. These infants have decreased glycogen and fat stores, since accumulation of these stores occurs during the third trimester, and immature hepatic function with low levels of gluconeogenic and glycogenolytic enzymes. Preterm infants may also have altered metabolic demands from tachypnea, respiratory distress syndrome, hypoxia, hypothermia, or other events that increase glucose use. Infants of mothers treated with β-sympathomimetics for preterm labor may develop hypoglycemia secondary to hyperinsulinemia. These agents rapidly cross the placenta and stimulate beta receptors on the fetal pancreas with subsequent insulin release and altered glucose, homeostasis in the fetus and newborn.

SGA infants are at risk for hypoglycemia primarily because of alterations in hepatic glucose production and increased glucose utilization.[74] These infants may have reduced glycogen stores owing to altered placental transport of substrates during fetal life. SGA infants have increased energy demands owing to their greater brain-to-body mass size, increased metabolic rate, and a tendency toward polycythemia. Since the brain and red blood cells are obligatory glucose users, these factors can markedly increase glucose needs even in nonstressed infants. Glucose utilization may be further increased by chronic or acute perinatal hypoxia. Secretion of hepatic gluconeogenic enzymes, especially PEPCK, is impaired in SGA infants, further limiting their ability to increase glucose production to meet metabolic demands.

The Infant of a Diabetic Mother

Although improved preconceptual care and careful metabolic control of pregnant diabetic women have reduced the incidence of significant macrosomia and improved perinatal mortality, these infants continue to be at risk for a variety of health problems. The cause of these problems relates to fetal and neonatal responses to maternal metabolic alterations and consequences to the neonate of cessation of placental transfer of substrates after birth (see Table 13–9 and Figs. 13–8 and 13–9). Many infants of diabetic mothers are large for gestational age, lethargic, poor feeders, and at risk for the problems listed in Table 13–9. Infants born to mothers with vascular involvement are usually SGA, however, with more mature liver enzyme systems and lungs owing to the effects of intrauterine stress. This group of infants is at particular risk for problems associated with chronic hypoxia such as perinatal asphyxia and polycythemia.

A prominent problem seen in these infants is hypoglycemia. Hyperinsulinemia and a

TABLE 13–9
Pathophysiology of Morbidity and Mortality of the Infant of a Diabetic Mother

PROBLEM	PATHOPHYSIOLOGY
Fetal demise	Acute placental failure?
	Hyperglycemia–lactic acidosis–hypoxia
Macrosomia	Hyperinsulinism
Respiratory distress syndrome	Insulin antagonism of cortisol
	Variant surfactant biochemical pathways
Transient tachypnea of the newborn	Cesarean section
Hypoglycemia	↓ Glucose and fat mobilization
Polycythemia	Erythropoietic "macrosomia"?
	Mild fetal hypoxia?
	↓ O_2 delivery to fetus—HbA_{1c}
Hypocalcemia	↓ Neonatal parathyroid hormone
	↑ Calcitonin
Hyperbilirubinemia	↑ Erythropoietic mass
	↑ Bilirubin production
	Immature hepatic conjugation?
	Oxytocin induction
Congenital malformations	Hyperglycemia?
	Genetic linkage?
	Insulin as teratogen?
	Vascular accident?
Renal vein thrombosis	Polycythemia
	Dehydration?
Neonatal small left colon syndrome	Immature GI motility?
Cardiomyopathy	Reversible septal hypertrophy
	↑ Glycogen
	↑ Muscle
Family psychological stress	High-risk pregnancy
	Fear of diabetes in infant

From Kliegman, R. M. & Wald, M. K. (1986). Problems in metabolic adaptation: Glucose, calcium and magnesium. In M. H. Klaus & A. A. Fanaroff (Eds.), *Care of the high risk neonate* (3rd ed., p. 225). Philadelphia: WB Saunders; as adapted from Kliegman, R.M. & Fanaroff, A.A. (1989). Developmental metabolism and nutrition. In G.A. Gregory (Ed.), *Pediatric anesthesia* (Vol. 1, 2nd ed.). New York: Churchill Livingstone.

blunted glucagon response, aggravated by decreased hepatic responsiveness to glucose, are responsible for the hypoglycemia (see p. 597).[7, 126] Levels of epinephrine and norepinephrine are also elevated, suggesting that hypoglycemia in these infants may also be related to adrenal medullary exhaustion.[3, 23, 122]

The Infant with Perinatal Asphyxia

Hypoxia and asphyxia alter glucose production and utilization with an increase in glycogenolysis to meet the increased metabolic and energy demands. Since oxygen availability is compromised, the infant switches from aerobic to anaerobic glycolysis. Anaerobic metabolism is less efficient than aerobic metabolism, producing a net increase of only two molecules of adenosine triphosphate (ATP) per molecule of glucose oxidized (versus 36 molecules of ATP per glucose molecule under aerobic conditions). These changes rapidly deplete glucose (glycogen) reserves, with decreased energy production that may be inadequate to maintain normal cell biologic processes and accumulation of

lactic acid.[126] Hypoxic-ischemic damage to the liver may further impair glucose production and delay the postnatal increase in gluconeogenesis.[74]

Since the fetus normally produces large amounts of lactate, intermediary pathways to metabolize lactate are relatively mature and efficient in the fetus and the newborn. As a result, metabolic acidosis with birth and perinatal asphyxia, if it is not severe enough to overwhelm these pathways or associated with postnatal alterations in oxygenation, is often readily reversed without administration of sodium bicarbonate.[8] Even with moderate to severe perinatal asphyxia this ability is probably an advantage.

The ability of the infant to mobilize fat stores may be impaired in hypoxia. During hypoxia release of catecholamines and fatty acids is impaired and oxidation of fats inhibited.[126] These changes impair the ability of the infant to generate the energy necessary for normal cell functions and to meet the increased demands of the hypoxic states. The infant of a diabetic woman may be further compromised, since although this infant has adequate (or excessive) fat stores, the concomitant hyperinsulinemia and reduced glucagon secretion result in inadequate lipolysis.[10, 11]

Neonatal Hyperglycemia

Neonatal hyperglycemia is a blood glucose level greater than 125 mg/dl (whole blood) or 145 to 150 mg/dl (plasma). Hyperglycemia occurs less frequently than hypoglycemia, but has the potential for significant alterations in neurodevelopmental outcome.[21, 74] Hyperglycemia is seen predominantly in preterm infants, especially those weighing less than 1000 g and receiving parenteral glucose infusions. Hyperglycemia is negatively correlated with birth weight and positively correlated with the rate of glucose infusion.[69] Markedly increased blood glucose levels can lead to osmotic changes and fluid shifts within the central nervous system (with a risk of intraventricular hemorrhage) and to glycosuria (with increased fluid and electrolyte loses and subsequent dehydration).

Neonatal hyperglycemia is believed to arise primarily from an inability of the infant to suppress endogenous glucose production while receiving a glucose infusion.[62] Stressed infants seem to be at particular risk for hyperglycemia becasue of the simultaneous increase in catecholamine release (as a stress response), which further increases glucose levels by inhibiting insulin release and glucose utilization.[24, 25] Other infants at risk for hyperglycemia include infants treated with methylxanthines for apnea or with lipid infusions given at rates greater than 0.25 g/kg/hour, infants with sepsis or after surgery, and term newborns with severe growth retardation who develop a transient neonatal diabetes. The latter disorder may be due to partial insulin insensitivity and the effects of stress on glucose homeostasis.[25, 74]

MATURATIONAL CHANGES DURING INFANCY AND CHILDHOOD

Energy and calorie requirements per unit of body weight remain higher in children than in adults because of their higher metabolic rate and growth needs. The relative requirement for carbohydrates is similar for children and adults. For infants, generally not more than 40% of the total calories should be carbohydrates; for children and adults this value is 40 to 60%.[70]

Serum amino acid levels decrease and urinary excretion increases until early childhood. Total body protein increases and reaches adult proportions (3%) by 4 years. Retention of nitrogen decreases during this time to adult values (11 mg/kg/day).[70] Diet alters the fatty acid composition of adipose tissue during periods of rapid weight gain in the 1st year of life and possibly the composition of structural lipids. This may affect functional ability of tissues and structures.[127]

SUMMARY

Growth "is an accretion of materials brought together in a synergism involving anabolism and catabolism."[65, p.169] Growth involves increases in cell size and in the complexity of cells, tissues, and organs. Alterations in

---

TABLE 13–10
Summary of Recommendations for Clinical Practice Related to Carbohydrate, Protein, and Fat Metabolism: Neonate

Know usual changes in carbohydrate, protein, and fat metabolism during the fetal and neonatal periods (pp. 598–606, Table 13–6).
Monitor neonates for alterations in metabolic processes (pp. 598–606).
Monitor newborn glucose status during transition and in the early neonatal period (pp. 603–605, Table 13–7).
Initiate early enteral feeding as appropriate (pp. 603–605, Table 13–7).
Monitor neonates for signs of excessive and inadequate intake of carbohydrates, protein, and fat (pp. 603–605).
Recognize infants at risk for hypoglycemia (pp. 606–609, Table 13–8).
Know clinical signs of hypoglycemia (p. 606).
Assess and monitor infants at risk for neonatal hypoglycemia (pp. 606–609, Table 13–8).
Recognize infants at risk for hyperglycemia (p. 609).
Assess and monitor infants at risk for hyperglycemia (p. 609).
Monitor infants at risk for hyperglycemia for alterations in fluid and electrolyte balance (p. 609).
Recognize and monitor for problems for which the infant of a diabetic mother is at increased risk (pp. 596–597, 607–608, Fig. 13–8, Table 13–9).

Page numbers in parentheses following each recommendation refer to page(s) in the text where the rationale for that intervention is discussed.

growth during the perinatal period arise from maternal, fetal, or placental factors that alter the availability, accretion, or use of substrates or nutrients. When this occurs the fetus or neonate may be unable to adapt to environmental stress and is at increased risk for morbidity and mortality.[65] Implications for clinical practice are summarized in Table 13–10.

REFERENCES

1. Allen, D., Kornhauser, D., & Schwartz, R. (1966). Glucose homeostasis in the newborn puppy. *Am J Dis Child, 112,* 343.
2. Anast, C.S. & David. L'. (1983). The physiology of calcium in the human neonate. In M.F. Holick, C.S. Anast, & T.K. Gray (Eds.), *Perinatal calcium and phosphorus metabolism* (pp. 363–383). Amsterdam: Elsevier.
3. Artal, R., et al. (1982). Sympatho-adrenal activity in infants of diabetic mothers. *Am J Obstet Gynecol, 142,* 436.
4. Aynsley-Green, A., et al. (1977). Endocrine and metabolic responses in the human newborn to the first feed of breast milk. *Arch Dis Child, 52,* 291.
5. Aynsley-Green, A. (1985). Metabolic and endocrine interrelations in the human fetus and neonate. *Am J Clin Nutr, 41,* 399.
6. Baird, J.D. (1986). Some aspects of the metabolic and hormonal adaptation to pregnancy. *Acta Endocrinol, 112* (Suppl. 277), 11.
7. Barss, V. (1989). Diabetes and pregnancy. *Med Clin North Am, 73,* 685.
8. Battaglia, F. (1982). New facts about fetal and placental metabolism. *Contemp OB/GYN, 19,* 189.
9. Battaglia, F.C. & Meschia, G. (1981). Foetal and placental metabolism: Their interrelationship and impact upon maternal metabolism. *Proc Nutr Soc, 40,* 99.
10. Baum, D. (1969). The inhibition of norepinephrine stimulated lipolysis by acute hypoxia. *J Pharmacol Exper Ther, 169,* 87.
11. Baum, D., Anthony, C.L., & Stowers, C. (1971). Impairment of cold stimulated lipolysis by acute hypoxia. *Am J Dis Child, 121,* 115.
12. Berk, M.A. et al. (1989). Macrosomia in infants of insulin-dependent diabetic mothers. *Pediatrics, 83,* 1029.
13. Blazquez, E., et al. (1974). Neonatal changes in the concentration of rat cyclic AMP and serum glucose, FFA, insulin, pancreatic glucagon and total glucagon in man and the rat. *J Lab Clin Med, 83,* 957.
14. Bloom, S.R. & Johnston, D.I. (1972). Failure of glucagon release in infants of diabetic mothers. *Br J Med, 25,* 453.
15. Brownlee, M., Vlassara, H., & Cerami, A. (1984). Nonenzymatic glycosylation and the pathogenesis of diabetic complications. *Ann Intern Med, 101,* 527.
16. Cahill, G.F. (1971). Physiology of insulin in man. *Diabetes, 20,* 785.
17. Carpenter, M.W. & Coustan, D.R. (1982). Criteria for screening tests for gestational diabetes. *Am J Obstet Gynecol, 144,* 768.
18. Coleman, R.A. (1989). The role of the placenta in lipid metabolism and transport. *Semin Perinatol, 13,* 180.
19. Conrad, P.D., et al. (1989). Clinical application of a new glucose analyzer in the neonatal intensive care unit: Comparison with other methods. *J Pediatr, 114,* 281.
20. Cooney, G.J. & Newsholme, E.A. (1982). The maximum capacity of glycolysis in brown adipose tissue and its relationship to control of the blood glucose concentration. *FEBS Letters, 148,* 198.
21. Cornblath, M., et al. (1990). Hypoglycemia in infancy: The need for a rational definition. *Pediatrics, 85,* 834.
22. Coustan, D.R. & Felig, P. (1988). Diabetes Mellitus. In G.N. Burrow & T.F. Ferris (Eds.), *Medical complications during pregnancy* (3rd ed., pp. 34–64). Philadelphia: WB Saunders.
23. Cowett, R.M. (1986). Metabolism in the fetus and infant of the diabetic mother. *Infant of the diabetic mother: Report of the 93rd Ross conference on pediatric research* (pp. 26–32). Columbus, OH: Ross Laboratories.
24. Cowett, R.M., Oh, W., & Schwartz, R. (1983). Persistent glucose production during glucose infusion in the neonate. *J Clin Invest, 71,* 467.
25. Cowett, R.M., et al. (1988). Ontogeny of glucose homeostasis in low birth weight infants. *J Pediatr, 112,* 462.
26. Curry, E. & Warshaw, J.B. (1978). Higher serum carnitine levels and ketogenesis in breast fed as compared to formula fed infants. *Pediatr Res, 12,* 504.
27. DeLucchi, C., et al. (1987). Effects of dietary nucleotides on the fatty acid composition of erythrocyte membrane lipids in term infants. *J Pediatr Gastroenterol, 6,* 568.
28. Desci, T., Molnar, D., & Klujber L. (1990). Lipid levels in VLBW preterm infants. *Acta Paediatr Scand, 29,* 577.
29. Dickson, J.E. & Palmer, S.P. (1990). Gestational diabetes: Pathophysiology and diagnosis. *Semin Perinatol, 14,* 2.
30. Economides D.L., et al. (1990). Hypertriglyceridemia and hypoxemia in SGA fetuses. *Am J Obstet Gynecol, 162,* 382.
31. Eisen, H.J., Goldfine, D., & Glinsman, W. (1973). Regulation of hepatic glycogen synthesis during fetal development: Role of hydrocortisone, insulin and insulin receptors. *Proc Natl Acad Sci USA, 70,* 3454.
32. Felig, P. (1973). Maternal and fetal fuel homeostasis in human pregnancy. *Am J Clin Nutr, 26,* 998.
33. Felig, P. & Lynch, V. (1970). Starvation in human pregnancy: Hypoglycemia, hypoinsulinemia, and hyperketonemia. *Science, 170,* 990.
34. Fisher, P.M., Sutherland, H.W., & Bewsher, P.D. (1980). Insulin response to glucose infusion in normal human pregnancy. *Diabetologia, 19,* 15.
35. Fluge, G. (1975). Neurological findings at follow-up in neonatal hypoglycemia. *Acta Paediatr Scand, 64,* 629.
36. Freinkel, N. (1965). Effects of the conceptus on maternal metabolism in pregnancy. In B.S. Leibel & G.A. Wrenshall (Eds.), *On the nature and treatment of diabetes* (pp. 679–691). Amsterdam: Excerpta Medica.
37. Freinkel, N. (1980). Of pregnancy and progeny. *Diabetes, 29,* 1023.
38. Freinkel, N. & Metzger, B.E. (1979). Pregnancy as a tissue culture experience: The critical implications of maternal metabolism for fetal develop-

ment. In *Pregnancy, metabolism, diabetes and the fetus: Ciba foundation symposium No. 63* (pp. 3–23). Amsterdam: Excerpta Medica.

39. Freinkel, N., et al. (1974). Facilitated anabolism in late pregnancy. In W.J. Malaise & J. Pirart (Eds.), *Proceedings of the VIIIth congress of the international diabetes foundation* (pp. 474–488). Amsterdam: Excerpta Medica.

40. Freinkel, N., et al. (1972). "Accelerated starvation" and mechanisms for the conservation of maternal nitrogen during pregnancy. *Isr J Med Sci, 8*, 426.

41. Fuhrman, K., Reiner, H., & Semmler, K. (1983). Prevention of congenital malformations in infants of insulin-dependent diabetic mother. *Diabetes Care, 6*, 219.

42. Golde, S.H., et al. (1982). Insulin requirements during labor: A reappraisal. *Am J Obstet Gynecol, 144*, 556.

43. Goldman, J.A., et al. (1986). Pregnancy outcome in patients with insulin-dependent diabetes mellitus with preconceptual diabetic control: A comparative study. *Am J Obstet Gynecol, 155*, 293.

44. Grasso, S., et al. (1968). Serum insulin response to glucose and amino acids in premature infants. *Lancet, 2*, 755.

45. Grasso S., et al. (1990) Glucose and insulin secretion in low birth weight preterm infants. *Acta Paediatr Scand, 79*, 280.

46. Gross, T.L. & Kazzi, G.M. (1985). Effects of maternal malnutrition and obesity on pregnancy outcome. In N. Gleicher (Ed.), *Principles of medical therapy in pregnancy* (pp. 332–351). New York: Plenum Press.

47. Guyton, A.C. (1987). *Textbook of medical physiology* (7th ed.). Philadelphia: WB Saunders.

48. Hanif, K., et al. (1982). Oxytocin action: Mechanisms for insulin-like activity in isolated rat adipocytes. *Mol Pharmacol, 22*, 381.

49. Hanning, R.M. & Zlotkin, S.H. (1989). Amino acid and protein needs of the neonate: Effects of excess and deficiency. *Semin Perinatol, 13*, 131.

50. Hare, J.W. (1989). *Diabetes complicating pregnancy: The Joslin Clinic method*. New York: Alan R. Liss.

51. Hendrickse, W., Stammers, J.P., & Hull, D. (1989). The transfer of free fatty acids across the human placenta. *Br J Obstet Gynaecol, 92*, 945.

52. Hill, D.E. (1978). Effect of insulin on fetal growth. *Semin Perinatol, 2*, 319.

53. Hirabayashi, S., Kitakara, O., & Hishidi, T. (1980). Computed tomography in perinatal hypoxic and hypoglycemic encephalopathy with emphasis on follow-up studies. *J Comput Asstist Tomogr, 4*, 451.

54. Hjollund, E., et al. (1986). Impaired insulin receptor binding and postbinding defects of adipocytes from normal and diabetic pregnant women. *Diabetes, 35*, 598.

55. Hollingsworth, D.B. & Moore, T.R. (1989). Diabetes and pregnancy. In R.K. Creasey & R. Resnik (Eds.), *Maternal-fetal medicine: Principles and practice* (pp. 925–988). Philadelphia: WB Saunders.

56. Hommes, F.A. & Wilmink, O.W. (1968). Developmental changes of glycolytic enzymes in rat brain, liver and skeletal muscle. *Biol Neonate, 12*, 181.

57. Jovanovic, L. & Peterson, C.M. (1983). Insulin and glucose requirements during the first stage of labor in insulin-dependent diabetic women. *Am J Med, 75*, 607.

58. Kalkhoff, R.K., Kissebah, A.H., & Kim, H.J. (1979). Carbohydrate and lipid metabolism during normal pregnancy: Relationship to gestational hormone action. In I.R. Merkatz & P.A.J. Adams (Eds.), *The Diabetic pregnancy: A perinatal perspective* (pp. 3–21). New York: Grune & Stratton.

59. Kenepp N.S., et al. (1980). Fetal and neonatal hazards of maternal hydration with 5% dextrose before caesarean section. *Lancet, 1*, 1150.

60. Kimura, R.E. & Warshaw, J.B. (1983). Metabolism during development. In J.B. Warshaw (Ed.), *The biological basis of reproductive and developmental medicine* (pp. 337–364). New York: Elsevier Biomedical.

61. Kimura, R.E. (1989). Fatty acid metabolism in the fetus. *Semin Perinatol, 13*, 202–210.

61a. Kitzmiller, J.L., et al. (1991). Preconception care of the diabetic: Glycemic control prevents congenital anomalies. *JAMA, 265*, 731.

62. Kliegman, R.M. & Wald, M.K. (1986). Problems in metabolic adaptation: Glucose, calcium and magnesium. In M.H. Klaus & A.A. Fanaroff (Eds.), *Care of the high risk neonate* (3rd ed., pp. 220–238). Philadelphia: WB Saunders.

63. Knoop, R.H., Herrrera, E., & Freinkel, N. (1970). Carbohydrate metabolism in pregnancy. VII: Metabolism of adipose tissue isolated from fed and fasted pregnant rats during late gestation. *J Clin Invest, 49*, 1438.

64. Knoop, R.H., et al. (1973). Two phases of adipose tissue metabolism in pregnancy: Maternal adaptations for fetal growth. *Endocrinology, 92*, 984.

65. Kretchmer, N., Schumacher, L.B., & Silliman, K. (1989). Biological factors affecting intrauterine growth. *Semin Perinatol, 13*, 169.

66. Kyle, G.C. (1963). Diabetes and pregnancy: Pregnancy as a diabetogenic event. *Ann Intern Med, 59* (Suppl. 3), 1.

66a. Langer, O. (1990). Critical issues in diabetes and pregnancy: Early identification, metabolic control, and prevention of adverse outcome. In I.R. Merkatz & J.E. Thompson (Eds.), *New perspectives on prenatal care* (pp. 445–459). New York: Elsevier.

66b. Langer, O. & Mazze, R.S. (1986). The relationship between glycosylated hemoglobin and verified self-monitored blood glucose among pregnant and non-pregnant women with diabetes. *Practical Diabetes, 4*, 32.

67. Like, A. & Orci, L. (1972). Embryogenesis of the human pancreatic islets: A light and electron microscopic study. *Diabetes, 21*, 511.

68. Lin, H.C., et al. (1989). Accuracy and reliability of glucose reflectance meters in the high-risk neonate. *J Pediatr, 115*, 998.

69. Louik, C., et al. (1985). Risk factors for neonatal hyperglycemia associated with 10% dextrose infusion. *Am J Dis Child, 139*, 783.

70. Lowrey, G. (1986). *Growth and development of children*. Chicago: Yearbook.

71. Lucas, A. & Bloom, S.R. (1978). Metabolic and endocrine events at the time of the first feed of human milk in preterm and term infants. *Arch Dis Child, 53*, 731.

72. Marsac, C., et al. (1976). Development of gluconeogenic enzymes in the liver of human newborns. *Biol Neonate, 28*, 317.

73. Mediola, J., Grylack, L.J., & Scanlon, J.W. (1982). Effect of intrapartum glucose infusion on the normal fetus and newborn. *Anesth Analg, 61*, 32.

74. Merenstein, G.B. & Gardner, S.L. (1989). *Handbook of neonatal care* (2nd ed.). St. Louis: CV Mosby.

75. Meyer, B.A. & Palmer S.A. (1990). Pregestational diabetes. *Semin Perinatol, 14,* 12.

76. Miller, E., et al. (1981). Elevated maternal hemoglobin A1c in early pregnancy and major congenital anomalies in infants of diabetic mothers. *N Engl J Med, 304,* 1331.

77. Milley, J.R. (1989). Fetal protein metabolism. *Semin Perinatol, 13,* 192.

77a. Mills, J.L., et al. (1988). Lack of relation of increased malformation rates in infants of diabetic mothers to glycemic control during organogenesis. *N Engl J Med, 318,* 672.

78. Milner, R.D.G. & Hill, D.J. (1984). Fetal growth control: The role of insulin and related peptides. *Clin Endocrinol, 21,* 415.

79. Miodovinik, M., et al. (1988). Major malformations in infants of IDDM women: Vasculopathy and early first-trimester poor glycemic control. *Diabetes Care, 11,* 713.

80. Morris, M.A., Grandis, A.S., & Litton, J.C. (1986). Longitudinal assessment of glycosylated blood protein concentrations in normal pregnancy and gestational diabetes. *Diabetes Care, 9,* 107.

81. Naeye, R.L. (1965). Infants of diabetic mothers: A qualitative, morphologic study. *Pediatrics, 35,* 980.

82. Naismith, D.J. (1980). Maternal nutrition and the outcome of pregnancy: A critical appraisal. *Proc Nutr Soc, 39,* 1.

83. Naismith, D.J. (1981). Diet during pregnancy: A rationale for prescription. In J. Dobbing (Ed.), *Maternal nutrition in pregnancy: Eating for two?* (pp. 21–40). New York: Academic Press.

84. Naismith, D.J. & Morgan, B.L.G. (1976). The biphasic nature of protein metabolism during pregnancy in the rat. *Br J Nutr, 36,* 563.

85. National Diabetes Data Group. (1979). Classification and diagnosis of diabetes mellitus and other categories of glucose intolerance. *Diabetes, 28,* 1039.

86. Novak, M., et al. (1965). Release of free fatty acids from adipose tissue obtained from newborn infants. *J Lipid Res, 6,* 91.

87. Novak, M. & Monkus, E. (1972). Metabolism of subcutaneous adipose tissue in the immediate postnatal period of human newborns: I. Developmental changes in lipolysis and glycogen content. *Pediatr Res, 6,* 73.

88. O'Sullivan, J.B. & Mahan, C.M. (1964). Criteria for the oral glucose tolerance tests in pregnancy. *Diabetes, 13,* 278.

89. Osathanondh, R. & Tuchinsky, D. (1980). Placental polypeptide hormones. In D. Tulchinsky & K. Ryan (Eds.), *Maternal-fetal endocrinology* (pp. 17–42). Philadelphia: WB Saunders.

90. Oski, F.A. & Komazaw, M. (1975). Metabolism of the erythrocytes of the newborn infant. In F.A. Oski, R.F. Jaffee, & P.A. Miescher (Eds.), *Current problems in pediatric hematology.* New York: Grune & Stratton.

91. Page, E.W., Villee, C.A., & Villee, D.B. (1981). *Human reproduction: Essentials of reproductive and perinatal medicine* (3rd ed.). Philadelphia: WB Saunders.

92. Page, E.W. (1969). Human fetal nutrition and growth. *Am J Obstet Gynecol, 104,* 378.

93. Paterson, P., et al. (1967). Maternal and foetal ketone concentration in plasma and urine. *Lancet, 1,* 862.

94. Pedersen, J. (1977). *The pregnant diabetic and her newborn: Problems and management.* Baltimore: Williams & Wilkins.

95. Peevy, K.J., Landow, S.A., & Gross, S.J. (1980). Hyperbilirubinemia in infants of diabetic mothers. *Pediatrics, 66,* 417.

96. Phelps, R.L., Metzger, B.E., & Freinkel, N. (1981). Carbohydrate metabolism in pregnancy, XVII. Diurnal profiles of plasma glucose, insulin, free fatty acids, triglycerides, cholesterol and individual amino acids in late normal pregnancy. *Am J Obstet Gynecol, 140,* 730.

97. Phelps, R.L., et al. (1983). Biphasic changes in hemoglobin A1c concentration during normal human pregnancy. *Am J Obstet Gynecol, 147,* 651.

98. Pitkin, R.M. (1983). Human maternal-fetal calcium homeostasis. In M.F. Holick, C.S. Anast, & T.K. Gray (Eds.), *Perinatal calcium and phosphorus metabolism* (pp. 259–279). Amsterdam: Elsevier.

99. Reece, E.A., et al. (1990). A longitudinal study comparing growth in diabetic pregnancies with growth in normal gestations: I. Fetal weight. *Obstet Gynecol Rev, 45,* 160.

100. Rudolph A. (1977). *Pediatrics* (pp. 176–177). New York: Appleton-Century-Crofts.

101. Sanders, T.A.B. & Naismith, D.J. (1979). A comparison of the influence of breast feeding and bottle feeding on the fatty acid composition of erythrocytes. *Br J Nutr, 4,* 619.

102. Schwartz, H.C., et al. (1976). Effects of pregnancy on hemoglobin A1c in normal, gestational diabetic, and diabetic women. *Diabetes, 25,* 1118.

103. Senterre, J. & Karlberg, P. (1970). Respiratory quotient and metabolic rate in normal fullterm and small for date newborn infants. *Acta Paediatr Scand, 59,* 653.

104. Shamburgh, G.E., Mrozak, S.C., & Freinkel, N. (1977). Fetal fuels. I: Utilization of ketones by isolated tissues at various stages of maturation and maternal nutrition during late gestation. *Metabolism, 26,* 623.

105. Shenolikar, I.S. (1970). Absorption of dietary calcium in pregnancy. *Am J Clin Nutr, 23,* 63.

106. Simmons, M.A., Battaglia, F.C., & Meschia, G. (1979). Placental transfer of glucose. *J Dev Physiol, 1,* 227.

107. Singhi, S. (1988). Effect of maternal intrapartum glucose therapy on neonatal blood glucose levels and neurobehavioral status of hypoglycemic term newborns. *J Perinat Med, 16,*217.

108. Skouby, S.O., et al. (1990). Mechanisms of action of oral contraceptives on CHO metabolism at the cellular level. *Am J Obstet Gynecol, 163,* 343.

109. Sparks, J.W., Girard, J.R., & Battaglia, F.C. (1980). An estimate of the caloric requirements of the human fetus. *Biol Neonate, 38,* 13.

110. Sperling, M.A. (1982) Integration of fuel homeostasis by insulin and glucagon in the newborn. *Monogr Pediatr, 16,* 39.

111. Sperling, M.A. (1988). Glucose homeostasis after birth. In C.T. Jones (Ed.), *Research in perinatal medicine (VII). Fetal and neonatal development* (pp. 458–467). Ithaca, NY: Perinatology Press.

112. Stern, L., Ramos, A., & Leduc, J. (1968). Urinary catecholamine excretion in infants of diabetic mothers. *Pediatrics, 42,* 598.

113. Susa, J.B., McCormick, K.L., & Widness, J.A. (1979). Chronic hyper-insulinemia in the fetal rhesus monkey. *Diabetes, 28,* 1058.

114. Swislocki, A. & Kraemer, F.B. (1989). Maternal

metabolism in diabetes mellitus: Pathophysiology of diabetes in pregnancy. In S.A. Brody & K. Ueland (Eds.), *Endocrine disorders in pregnancy* (pp. 247–272). Norwalk, CT: Appleton & Lange.

115. Takeda, Y. (1988). Metabolic adjustment in perinatal period. In G.H. Wiknjosastro, W.H. Prakoso, & K. Maeda (Eds.), *Perinatology* (pp. 135–143). Amsterdam: Elsevier.

116. Thomas, C.R. & Lowy, C. (1982). The clearance and placental transfer of free fatty acids and triglycerides in the pregnant guinea pig. *J Dev Physiol, 4,* 163.

117. Tlinen, K., Rairo, K., & Teramo, K. (1981). Hemoglobin A1c predicts the prenatal outcome in insulin-dependent pregnancies. *Br J Obstet Gynecol, 88,* 961.

118. Tsang, R.C. et al. (1976). Hypomagnesemia in infants of diabetic mothers: Perinatal studies. *J Pediatr, 89,* 115.

119. Tulchinsky, D. & Ryan, K. (1980). *Maternal-fetal endocrinology.* Philadelphia: WB Saunders.

120. Uauy, R., Treen, M., & Hoffman, D.R. (1989). Essential fatty acid metabolism and requirements during development. *Semin Perinatol, 13,* 118.

121. Vander, A., Sherman, J., & Luciano, D. (1985). *Human physiology: The mechanism of body function.* New York: McGraw-Hill.

122. Vernon, R.G. & Walker, D.G. (1968). Adaptive behavior of some enzymes involved in glucose utilization and formation in rat liver during the weaning period. *Biochem J, 106,* 331.

123. Villee, C.A. & Hagerman, D. (1958). Effect of oxygen deprivation on the metabolism of fetal and adult tissues. *Am J Physiol, 144,* 457.

124. Waisman, H.A. & Kerr, G.R. (1965). Amino acid and protein metabolism in the developing fetus and newborn infant. *Pediatr Clin North Am, 12,* 551.

125. Warshaw, J.B. (1972). Cellular energy metabolism during fetal development: IV. Fatty acid activation, acetyl transfer and fatty acid oxidation during development of the chick and rat. *Dev Biol, 28,* 537.

126. Warshaw, J.B. & Maniscalco, W.M. (1978). Perinatal adaptations in carbohydrate and lipid metabolism. In L. Stern, W. Oh, & B. Friis-Hansen (Eds.), *Intensive care of the newborn II* (pp. 251–260). New York: Masson.

127. Warshaw, J.B. & Terry, M.L. (1976). Cellular energy metabolism during fetal development: VI. Fatty acid oxidation by developing brain. *Dev Biol, 52,* 161.

128. Weiss, P.A.M. (1988). *Gestational diabetes.* New York: Springer-Verlag.

129. Widdowson, E. (1950). Chemical composition of newly born mammals. *Nature, 166,* 626.

130. Widdowson, E.M. (1981). The demands of the fetal and maternal tissues for nutrients, and the bearing of these on the needs of the mother to "eat for two." In J. Dobbing (Ed.), *Maternal nutrition in pregnancy—eating for two?* (pp. 1–19). London: Academic Press.

131. Widness, J.A., et al. (1981). Increased erythropoiesis and elevated erythropoietin in infants born to diabetic mothers and in hyperinsulinemic rhesus fetuses. *J Clin Invest, 67,* 637.

132. Zlotkin, S.H. & Anderson, G.H. (1982). The development of cystathionase activity during the first year of life. *Pediatr Res, 16,* 65.

CHAPTER 14

Calcium and Phosphorus Metabolism

Maternal Physiologic Adaptations
    The Antepartum Period
    The Intrapartum Period
    The Postpartum Period
Clinical Implications For The Pregnant Woman And Her Fetus
    Maternal Calcium and Phosphorus Needs
    Leg Cramps
    Hypertension and Calcium
    Magnesium Sulfate Therapy
    Women on Heparin Therapy
    Maternal-Fetal Interactions
Development Of Calcium And Phosphorus Metabolism in the Fetus
    Anatomic Development
    Functional Development
Neonatal Physiology
    Transitional Events
    Calcium

    Phosphorus
    Parathyroid Hormone
    Vitamin D
    Calcitonin
    Magnesium
Clinical Implications for Neonatal Care
    Nutritional Needs
    Bone Mineralization
    Neonatal Hypocalcemia
    Alterations in Magnesium
    Neonatal Rickets
    Neonatal Hypercalcemia
Maturational Changes During Infancy and Childhood

Calcium and phosphorus are critical in cardiovascular, nervous, hemostatic, and muscular processes and in the function of many hormones and enzyme systems. Maternal calcium metabolism is altered to enhance transport of this mineral to the fetus, who needs adequate calcium and phosphorus for growth and development, especially for bone mineralization for normal skeletal growth. After birth the neonate loses the placental supply of calcium and must quickly establish homeostasis of this system to avoid metabolic derangements. This chapter discusses alterations in these substances and related hormones during pregnancy and the neonatal period.

MATERNAL PHYSIOLOGIC ADAPTATIONS

Calcium and phosphorus metabolism are altered during pregnancy with an increase in

614

the amount and efficiency of intestinal calcium absorption.[39] The increased absorption is mediated by increased parathyroid hormone (PTH) and vitamin D.[71] Calcium accumulation by term totals 25 to 30 g.[72] Most of the calcium is used for fetal bone formation and mineralization.

The Antepartum Period

Maternal calcium, phosphorus, and magnesium levels fall during pregnancy. These changes are associated with increased production of PTH, calcitonin, and vitamin D under the influence of hormones such as estrogen and human placental lactogen (hPL). Calcium homeostasis during pregnancy is interrelated with changes in extracellular fluid volume, renal function, and fetal needs.

Calcium

Maternal serum calcium levels fall progressively beginning soon after fertilization and decrease by an average of 1.0 to 1.5 mg/dl. Calcium reaches its lowest levels at 28 to 32 weeks, followed by a plateau or slight rise to term (Fig. 14–1A).[71–73, 112] Serum calcium levels during pregnancy average 9 to 10 mg/dl, a decrease of 5 to 6%.[72] Most investigators report a slight, nonsignificant decrease in ionized calcium.[71, 72, 74, 102]

The question of whether there is a net increase in calcium storage in the maternal skeleton during pregnancy (in preparation for lactation) or net bone loss of calcium is controversial and data conflict.[71] The rate of bone turnover is increased.[74] When recommended dietary calcium intake during pregnancy is maintained, however, there does not appear to be a large change in maternal skeletal mass or bone density, probably because the fetal calcium accumulation of 30 g represents only a small proportion of maternal skeletal stores.[74, 121] In addition, any increase in bone reabsorption of calcium (due to hPL) is counteracted by an estrogen-induced decrease in reabsorption. Estrogen-increased PTH enhances intestinal calcium absorption, reduces urinary calcium losses, and stabilizes bone turnover.[71] Low vitamin D intake during pregnancy, combined with decreased exposure to sunlight, is associated with osteomalacia.[44, 93]

The decrease in serum calcium is primarily related to and parallels the fall in serum proteins, especially albumin, with a decrease in both total and bound calcium (Fig. 14–1A).[71] Other factors that contribute to alterations in serum calcium include increased plasma volume and hemodilution, increased urinary calcium excretion, and fetal transfer (primarily in the third trimester).[50, 71, 74, 95]

Urinary calcium excretion is reported to rise in early pregnancy (because of the increased glomerular filtration rate), but falls near term.[72, 74, 121] Since normally nearly 100% of urine calcium is conserved, this mechanism is probably not of major importance. After 36 weeks urinary calcium excretion decreases by about 35%, increasing calcium availability by 50 mg/day. Since fetal needs at this point are approximately 350 mg/day, however, other maternal calcium sources (i.e., dietary sources or the maternal skeleton) are essential.[43, 68, 72, 110, 121] Increased urinary excretion of calcium has been reported in women with good dietary calcium intake who are given calcium supplements.[32]

Phosphorus and Magnesium

Serum inorganic phosphate levels fall slightly and progressively until approximately 30 weeks' gestation, then rise slightly to levels near nonpregnant levels by term.[71, 74] Serum magnesium changes in a similar manner, paralleling ionized calcium. These changes are related to hemodilution and decreased serum albumin.[24, 74]

Parathyroid Hormone

Most investigators report that PTH production increases during pregnancy because of parathyroid gland hyperplasia. The cause of this change is unknown but it may be due to estrogen and hPL or a secondary response to changes in serum calcium or other parameters.[71] Even the relatively slight decrease in serum calcium during pregnancy stimulates increased PTH and, over time, hypertrophy of the parathyroids. Increased PTH favors bone release of calcium (Table 14–1) and increased maternal serum calcium levels (and thus increased availability of calcium for fetal transfer) and counteracts factors that decrease calcium in maternal extracellular fluid. PTH levels are reported to rise gradually and progressively during pregnancy, leading to a 30 to 50% increase by term (Fig. 14–1B).[74]

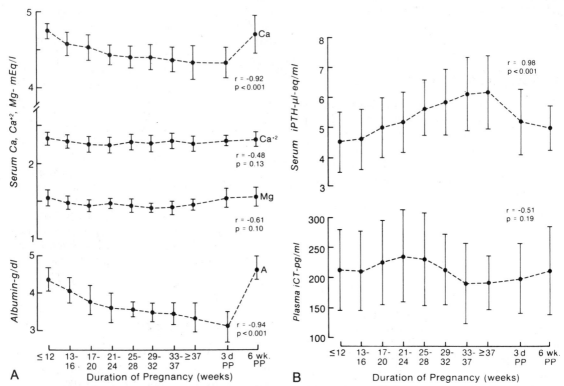

FIGURE 14–1.   Serum calcium, ionized calcium, and albumin concentrations (*A*) and serum parathyroid hormone and calcitonin concentrations (*B*) during pregnancy. (From Pitkin, R.M., et al. (1979). Calcium metabolism in pregnancy: A longitudinal study. *Am J Obstet Gynecol, 133*, 781.)

TABLE 14–1
Summary of Hormonal Actions Controlling Calcium and Phosphorus Levels

HORMONE	BONE	INTESTINE	KIDNEY
Parathyroid hormone	Increased calcium release		Increased calcium reabsorption
	Increased phosphorus release		Decreased phosphorus reabsorption
Calcitonin	Decreased calcium release	May inhibit calcium and phosphorus reabsorption	Increased calcium excretion
	Decreased phosphorus release		Increased phosphorus excretion
Vitamin D	Increased calcium release	Increased calcium absorption	Increased calcium reabsorption
		Increased phosphorus absorption	Increased phosphorus reabsorption

Some researchers, however, report that PTH levels are within normal limits until the third trimester, then progressively increase, whereas others have found that PTH does not show any significant changes.[21, 25, 71] There is little correlation between maternal serum calcium and PTH levels.

Vitamin D

Levels of 1,25-dihydroxyvitamin D [1,25-$(OH)_2D$] increase by 10 weeks' gestation but usually remain within normal limits until 24 to 36 weeks. Then they rise above nonpregnant levels to 70 to 100 pg/ml.[5, 54, 76, 117] Serum 25-hydroxyvitamin D [25(OH)D] levels do not change significantly during pregnancy.[74] The first trimester increase in intestinal absorption of calcium is probably mediated by prolactin rather than 1,25$(OH)_2D$.[33] The increase in 1,25$(OH)_2D$ after 34 to 36 weeks has been associated with an increase in a vitamin D–binding protein and bound vitamin D. Intestinal absorption of vitamin D is enhanced throughout gestation.[32]

These changes are influenced by the lower maternal serum calcium level and mediated by increased PTH activity, which increases renal formation of 1,25$(OH)_2D$ (Fig. 14–2). Other hormones that may also influence these changes include prolactin, hPL, growth hormone, and estrogens.[8, 35, 96] Elevated vitamin D is necessary to maintain normocalcemia, adequate intestinal absorption of calcium, and normal fetal bone metabolism (Table 14–1).[39] Daily requirements increase several times over by term.[33]

Calcitonin

Calcitonin levels are also reported to increase during pregnancy (see Fig. 14–1B), although there is controversy regarding the pattern of change.[28, 71, 101, 117] The increase is stimulated by increased serum calcium and influenced by estrogen and hPL. Increased calcitonin inhibits calcium and phosphorus release from the bones, counteracting the action of PTH (Table 14–1). This helps to conserve the maternal skeleton while simultaneously permitting the intestinal and renal actions of PTH to provide the additional calcium needed by the fetus.[104]

The Intrapartum Period

Calcium is essential for activation of myosin light chain kinase in smooth muscle and thus

---

Calcium and Phosphorus Homeostasis

PTH and vitamin D are the major hormones involved in calcium homeostasis. Calcitonin also influences calcium, but appears to be less important. Actions of PTH and intestinal absorption of vitamin D are enhanced by magnesium. Hormonal regulation of calcium metabolism is summarized in Figure 14–2. Calcium and phosphorus are absorbed in the small intestine under the influence of 1,25$(OH)_2D$, which stimulates a calcium-binding protein. PTH mobilizes calcium and phosphorus in bone by stimulating osteolysis. This process is vitamin D dependent and releases calcium and phosphorus into extracellular fluid (ECF). In the kidneys, PTH inhibits proximal tubular reabsorption of PO_4, leading to increased urinary loss and decreased ECF levels. PTH increases distal tubular reabsorption of Ca^{2+} to conserve calcium by decreasing renal excretion. Thus, PTH increases the release of both calcium and phosphorus from the bones, increasing ECF levels. Since concentrations of Ca^{2+} and PO_4 in ECF are closely tied to each other (i.e., $[Ca^{2+}] \times [PO_4]$ is a constant of solubility), if ECF PO_4 levels increase, further release of calcium from the bones would normally be impaired to keep the total concentration of calcium and phosphorus constant. If the kidneys increase PO_4 excretion, however, extracellular phosphorus decreases and more calcium is released from bone. The net result is increased ECF and serum calcium and decreased phosphorus. Decreased serum PO_4 occurs because the phosphaturic actions of PTH exceed serum phosphate–elevating activities. Release of PTH is regulated by concentrations of serum calcium. Even small changes in serum ionized calcium stimulate PTH release.

Vitamin D also enhances PTH action to increase calcium release from bone and tubular reabsorption of these minerals (see Fig. 14–2). Vitamin D can be produced endogenously in the epidermal layer of skin by ultraviolet light irradiation of 7-dehydrocholesterol to D_3 (cholecalciferol) or ingested as D_2 (ergocalciferol) or D_3. Ingested vitamin D requires bile salts for intestinal absorption. Vitamin D is converted to 25(OH)D (major circulating metabolite) in the liver. In the kidneys 25(OH)D is hydroxylated to 1,25$(OH)_2D$ (see Fig. 14–2). Regulation of vitamin D is through negative feedback from serum 25(OH)D levels.

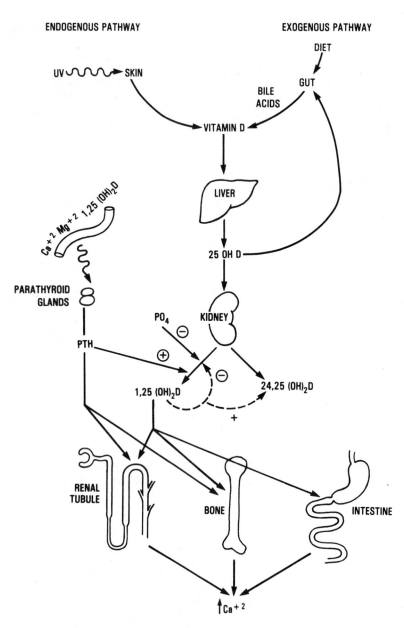

FIGURE 14–2. Hormonal regulation of serum calcium. (From Zaloga, G.P. & Eil, C. (1989). Diseases of the parathyroid glands and nephrolithiasis during pregnancy. In S.A. Brody & K. Ueland (Eds.), *Endocrine disorders in pregnancy* (p. 233). Norwalk, CT: Appleton & Lange.)

myometrial contraction. Without calcium, much of which comes from extracellular sources, myometrial contraction does not occur. The role of calcium in uterine contraction is discussed in Chapter 3.

The Postpartum Period

Serum calcium, PTH, and calcitonin gradually return to prepregnant values by 6 weeks post partum (see Fig. 14–1).[72] Hyperplasia of the parathyroid glands continues during lactation to meet the increased need for maternal calcium for milk production.[38] Lactation physiology is discussed in Chapter 4.

CLINICAL IMPLICATIONS FOR THE PREGNANT WOMAN AND HER FETUS

Changes in calcium and phosphorus metabolism are essential to provide adequate substrate for fetal growth and development and to simultaneously ensure maternal homeostasis. To support these changes maternal calcium and phosphorus intake must increase during pregnancy and lactation. This section considers these needs as well as implications of alterations in calcium, phosphorus, and magnesium in relation to disorders such as leg cramps and pregnancy-induced hypertension (PIH).

Maternal Calcium and Phosphorus Needs

During pregnancy an additional 400 mg/day of both calcium and phosphorus is recommended, especially during the second and third trimesters. This results in a total calcium intake of 1200 mg/day in the pregnant woman (or 1600 mg/day in the pregnant adolescent).[82, 120] Supplementation may be needed by pregnant adolescents with low dietary intakes (<600 mg/day). Current evidence does not suggest that pregnant women over age 35 have special needs for calcium supplementation nor that depletion of maternal stores over multiple pregnancies increases the risk of osteoporosis in later life.[29] The increased calcium and phosphorus needs during lactation are discussed in Chapter 4.

Vitamin D intake is critical in maintaining calcium homeostasis. Vitamin D intakes of 400 IU (10 μg)/day are recommended in pregnancy. Vitamin D helps ameliorate fluctuations in the calcium-to-phosphorus ratio and enhances calcium absorption. Alterations in calcium and bone metabolism, including increased risk of maternal osteomalacia and neonatal hypocalcemia, tend to occur primarily in women who have diets that are low in both calcium and vitamin D.[82] Supplementation is recommended for women with low dietary intakes and those who live in northern latitudes during the winter, where sunlight exposure is minimal.

Milk is an excellent source of calcium, vitamin D, and phosphorus. Alternatives for women who are lactose intolerant (see Chapter 9) include cheese, yogurt, lactose-free milks, sardines, whole or enriched grains, and green leafy vegetables. Calcium absorption is altered by other substances. Lactose increases calcium absorption, possibly by decreasing luminal pH or through chelate formation. Excessive fats, phosphate, phytates (found in many vegetables), or oxalates interfere with calcium absorption by forming insoluble calcium salts within the intestinal lumen. High sodium concentrations may also decrease calcium absorption by interfering with active transport mechanisms.[14, 121]

Adequate intake of phosphorus is as important as that of calcium since these two minerals exist in a constant of solubility in the blood (see box on p. 617). Excess dietary phosphorus binds calcium in the intestine, limiting absorption; excess blood phosphorus leads to increased urinary excretion of calcium. Therefore, it is essential for the pregnant and lactating woman's diet to be balanced in regard to these substances. Foods such as processed meats, snack foods, and cola drinks have high phosphorus but low calcium levels.[120]

Leg Cramps

Sudden tonic or clonic contraction of the gastrocnemius muscles and occasionally the thigh and gluteal muscles is experienced by over 25% of pregnant women. These cramps are felt most frequently at night or on awakening and are most common after 24 weeks' gestation.[27]

Cramps may be associated with increased neuromuscular irritability due to decreased serum ionized calcium levels combined with increased serum inorganic phosphate levels.[67, 71] The incidence of leg cramps is not correlated with ionized calcium levels, however.[36] Some women who drink more than 1 quart of milk per day report relief from leg cramps after a decrease in milk intake.[27] Muscular irritability in pregnancy also arises from the lowered calcium levels and mild alkalosis caused by changes in the respiratory system (see Chapter 7).[120] Interventions have included reducing milk intake (although milk is rich in calcium, it also contains large amounts of phosphate), supplementation with nonphosphate calcium salts, or use of aluminum hydroxide antacids to promote formation of insoluble aluminum phosphate salts in the gut, thus reducing absorption of phosphorus.[71] Treatment with oral calcium versus a placebo has not been reported to significantly reduce the incidence of leg cramps.[40] Thus the specific basis for leg cramps in pregnant women remains unclear.

Hypertension and Calcium

Women with acute and chronic hypertension during pregnancy tend to have lower serum calcium and higher magnesium levels.[78, 113] The incidence of PIH has been reported to vary inversely with calcium intake.[4, 53] The interrelationships between calcium homeostasis and PIH are still unclear, as are the implications for management.

Magnesium Sulfate Therapy

Magnesium sulfate is used as a tocolytic (see Chapter 3) and in management of PIH. Magnesium sulfate therapy elevates serum magnesium levels. This slows transmission of nerve impulses at neuromuscular junctions and in the cardiac conduction system, decreases central nervous system irritability, and decreases smooth muscle contractility. Thus this drug has an anticonvulsant effect but little effect on blood pressure. Magnesium sulfate therapy is associated with decreased uterine contractility, depressed respirations, altered cardiac conduction, electrocardiographic changes, and depression of deep tendon reflexes.[79] Magnesium sulfate increases urinary calcium excretion, decreasing serum levels.[71]

Intravenous infusions of magnesium sulfate increase serum magnesium by 150% and decrease serum calcium by about 16%.[17] Significant maternal hypocalcemia is rare because of increased PTH levels during pregnancy. Deep tendon reflexes should be monitored in these women because loss of these reflexes signifies a dangerously high magnesium level. The converse, that brisk deep tendon reflexes signify inadequate magnesium dosage, is not true, however.[79] Infants born to these women tend to have elevated magnesium levels and lower calcium levels for the first 48 hours.[17, 19, 60] These infants usually do not develop hypocalcemia.[72]

Women on Heparin Therapy

Women on long-term heparin therapy for thromboembolism during pregnancy may occasionally develop heparin-induced osteopenia.[72] Heparin inhibits 1-alpha-hydroxylation of 25(OH)D, decreasing levels of 1,25(OH)$_2$D, altering calcium homeostasis, and increasing bone calcium absorption.[1] Calcium status should be monitored carefully in women receiving this therapy.

Maternal-Fetal Interactions

Maternal-placental-fetal calcium metabolism is interrelated (Fig. 14–3). Calcium is believed to be actively transported across the placenta, mediated by vitamin D and a placental calcium-binding protein.[72, 111] Calcium transport increases from 50 mg/day (20 weeks) to 350 mg/day (range, 120 to 150 mg/kg/day) at term.[118] Peak accretion occurs at 34 to 36 weeks' gestation.

Fetal serum calcium (10 to 11 mg/dl) is about 1 mg/dl above maternal values. The higher fetal values are primarily due to increased ionic calcium.[77] Fetal calcium accretion increases during pregnancy from 100 mg (4 months) to 28 to 30 g at term.[11, 33, 50a] About two thirds of fetal calcium deposits are amassed during the third trimester, coinciding with bone development.

Approximately 30% of fetal calcium deposits are taken directly from the maternal skeleton; the rest are from maternal dietary calcium.[39, 43] Thus fetal calcium accumulation is mediated by increased maternal absorption of calcium. Fetal phosphorus and magnesium levels are also higher than maternal levels and these minerals are actively transported across the placenta.[71] Magnesium is transported to the fetus in increasing amounts after the 5th month.[20] Fetal magnesium levels depend on adequate placental function and maternal stores. Placental insufficiency and inadequate nutritional intake increase the risk of neonatal hypomagnesemia.[91]

Placental transport of 1,25(OH)$_2$D is low.[72, 97] The placenta is a source of this metabolite and contains 1,25(OH)$_2$D receptors and enzymes such as 1-hydroxylase.[34, 121] The fetus is dependent on maternal 25(OH)D, which is transported across the placenta (Fig. 14–3) since fetal hepatic enzyme processes are limited. Maternal vitamin D deficiency is associated with an increased incidence and severity of neonatal hypocalcemia.[16, 59] PTH and calcitonin do not appear to cross the placenta.[23, 71] Implications of these changes are summarized in Table 14–2.

SUMMARY

Calcium and phosphorus are essential minerals for many body processes and growth. Alterations in metabolic processes related to these elements during pregnancy can alter maternal, fetal, and infant health status. Health can be promoted by careful assessment and monitoring of maternal and fetal status and initiation of appropriate interventions. Recommendations for clinical practice related to calcium and phosphorus metabolism during pregnancy are summarized in Table 14–3.

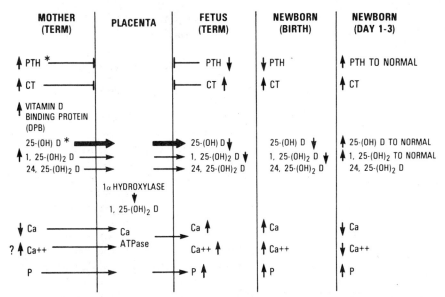

FIGURE 14–3. Interrelationships between maternal, placental, fetal, and newborn infant parathyroid hormone, calcitonin, and vitamin D. PTH, parathyroid hormone; CT, calcitonin; 25-(OH) D, 25-hydroxyvitamin D; 1, 25-(OH)$_2$ D, 1,25-dihydroxyvitamin D; 24, 25-(OH)$_2$ D, 24,25-dihydroxyvitamin D; Ca, calcium; Ca^{++}, ionized calcium; P, phosphorus; ATPase, adenosine triphosphatase. *Data in the literature are conflicting. (From Hollingsworth, D.R. (1989). Endocrine disorders of pregnancy. In R.K. Creasy & R. Resnik (Eds.), *Maternal-fetal medicine: Principles and practice* (2nd ed., p. 1015). Philadelphia: WB Saunders.)

DEVELOPMENT OF CALCIUM AND PHOSPHORUS METABOLISM IN THE FETUS

Anatomic Development

Calcium and phosphorus metabolism are regulated by a variety of hormones, including PTH, vitamin D, and calcitonin. This section reviews development of the parathyroid glands; development of the thyroid glands (calcitonin) is discussed in Chapter 16. Since calcium and phosphorus are critical for bone mineralization processes, skeletal growth is also considered.

Parathyroid Glands

Many structures of the head and neck, including the maxillary process, mandibular arch, several muscles of the jaw, hyoid and ear bones, thyroid, and cricoid cartilage, develop from the branchial or pharyngeal arches. These are bars of mesenchymal tissue separated by pharyngeal clefts. The pharyngeal pouches are outpouchings along the lateral walls of the pharyngeal gut (Fig. 14–4). Structures that develop from these pouches include the palatine tonsil, thymus, primitive tympanic cavity, and (from the third and fourth pouches) the parathyroid glands.

TABLE 14–2
Potential Advantages and Disadvantages to the Fetus of Alterations in Maternal Calcium and Phosphorus Metabolism During Pregnancy

PARAMETER	POTENTIAL ADVANTAGES	POTENTIAL DISADVANTAGES
Increased PTH	Favors bone release of calcium and higher maternal serum calcium levels, thus, more calcium is available for fetal transfer	
Increased calcitonin		Inhibits release of calcium and phosphorus from maternal bone (and thus availability to fetus), but counteracts elevated PTH to help protect maternal system

TABLE 14–3
Summary of Recommendations for Clinical Practice Related to Changes in Calcium and Phosphorus Metabolism: Pregnant Woman

Recognize usual changes in calcium and phosphorus metabolism during pregnancy (pp. 615–617).

Assess and monitor maternal nutrition in terms of calcium, phosphorus, and vitamin D intake (pp. 615–617, 619).

Counsel women regarding calcium, phosphorus, and vitamin D requirements to meet maternal and fetal needs during pregnancy (pp. 615–617, 619).

Monitor fetal growth (pp. 619, 622–623).

Know usual parameters for serum calcium during pregnancy (p. 615).

Evaluate diet of women complaining of leg cramps (p. 619).

Counsel women regarding leg cramps and appropriate interventions (p. 619).

Monitor calcium and magnesium status and deep tendon reflexes in women receiving magnesium sulfate therapy (pp. 619–620).

Page numbers in parentheses following each recommendation refer to pages in the text where the rationale for that intervention is discussed.

The inferior parathyroid glands differentiate from the dorsal part of the third pharyngeal pouch during the 5th week. The ventral portion of this pouch forms the thymus. These parathyroid glands initially migrate caudally and medially with the thymus, later separating and attaching to the dorsal surface of the thyroid. The superior parathyroid glands develop from the fourth pouch

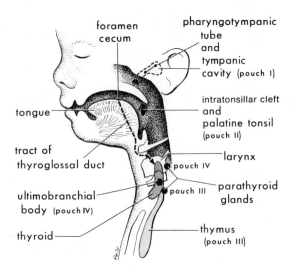

FIGURE 14–4. Schematic sagittal section of the head and neck of a 20-week-old fetus showing the adult derivatives of the pharyngeal pouches and descent of the thyroid gland. (From Moore, K. (1989). *The developing human* (4th ed., p. 179). Philadelphia: WB Saunders.)

and attach to the dorsal side of the caudally migrating thyroid gland.[64, 83]

Skeletal Development and Growth

Skeletal growth occurs in two phases. During fetal life a cartilage anlage (primordium) is formed that is later replaced by bone. Bone formation also occurs by differentiation of mesenchyme directly into bone cells. Later, linear growth depends on cartilaginous growth in the endochondral ossification centers at the epiphyses; appositional growth of the skeleton depends on laying down of new bone by bone-forming cells with subsequent remodeling (reabsorption of existing bone followed by formation of new bone).[26] Bone formation and remodeling is a cyclic process that occurs continuously throughout life. During growth bone formation is greater than remodeling. Once maximal growth is achieved, the skeletal mass is stable for 10 to 15 years and remodeling and bone formation occur at the same rate. With aging remodeling is greater than bone formation, with a gradual loss of bone mass. Excessive differences between bone formation and remodeling can lead to osteoporosis and compromised skeletal integrity.[26, 41] Stress, such as subjecting bone to heavy loads or that occurs with exercise, stimulates osteoblastic deposition of new bone, leading to thickening of bones.[38]

Skeletal development begins in early embryonic life and continues into postnatal life. Bone consists primarily of organic matrix and bone salts. Compact bone is 30% organic matrix and 70% bone salts; newer bone has more organic matrix. The organic matrix is composed primarily of collagen fibers that give the bone its tensile strength. The rest of the matrix is ground substance, consisting of extracellular fluid and proteoglycans, which may assist in controlling deposition of calcium salts. Crystalline bone salts (hydroxyapatites) give bone compressional strength and consist primarily of calcium and phosphorus with small deposits of sodium, potassium, magnesium, and carbonate salts.[38]

Bone is formed by either intramembranous or endochondral ossification. With intramembranous ossification, the mesenchyme condenses to form a collagenous membrane in which some cells differentiate into osteoblasts. Osteoblasts produce a collagenous material and ground substance to fill the extracellular spaces. The collagen polymerizes to form collagen fibers and the tissue becomes osteoid and similar to cartilage.[38] Osteoblasts later secrete alkaline phosphatase, which leads to deposition of calcium salts in the form of calcium hydroxyapatite crystals, with gradual conversion of the osteoid to bone. Some osteoblasts are trapped within lacunae in the bone matrix to form osteocytes. The bone matrix grows in all directions as spicules and ossification centers are established.

The osteoblasts deposit spongy bone first, followed by plates of compact bone (periosteal ossification). Spongy bones are filled with fibrous and cellular mesenchymal derivatives that later differentiate into elements characteristic of red bone marrow (reticular tissue, fat cells, sinusoids, and developing blood cells). Bone growth is accompanied by remodeling in which much of the original matrix is reabsorbed by osteoclasts simultaneously with formation of new bone by osteoblasts. During this process the osteoclasts project villi that secrete proteolytic enzymes to dissolve the organic matrix and citric, lactic, and other acids that cause solution of bone salts.[38]

The long bones form by endochondral ossification in which the condensed mesenchymal cells give rise to hyaline cartilage models that are shaped like the eventual bone. This cartilage is eroded locally and destroyed as bone is formed. Endochondral ossification involves the progressive destruction of cartilage, deposition of calcium salts, and formation of a central area of spongy bone (that will develop a red marrow matrix) surrounded by compact bone. This process begins in the middle of the bone shaft and progresses toward the epiphysis. At birth the long bones consist of central ossification centers and bony shafts with cartilaginous ends. Secondary areas of ossification later appear in the epiphyses.[26, 64, 103]

Bone growth is mediated by a variety of regulating hormones and mediating substances including calcium-regulating hormones (PTH, vitamin D, calcitonin); systemic growth-regulating hormones (growth hormone, insulin, glucocorticoids, thyroid hormones, sex steroids); circulating growth factors (somatomedin, insulin-like growth factor, epidermal growth factor, platelet-derived growth factor, fibroblast growth factor); and local factors (osteoclast activity factor, cartilage-derived growth factor).[26] Many factors, including growth hormone, thyroid hor-

mones, cortisol, and estrogen, do not seem to be as important in regulating bone development in the fetus as in older individuals.

Functional Development

Fetal calcium requirements are met by transport of calcium across the placenta (see Fig. 14–3). From 28 weeks' gestation to term bone mineralization increases fourfold and fetal calcium acquisition ranges from 120 to 150 mg/kg/day.[51] In contrast, calcium accretion immediately after birth ranges from 15 mg/kg on day 1 to 45 mg/kg on day 3.[20] Phosphate levels peak at mid-gestation (15 mg/dl) then decrease to 5.5 to 7 mg/dl by term.[118]

Vitamin D, PTH, and calcitonin levels are altered in the fetus, although there is much contradictory evidence as to the rate and pattern of change.[71] The fetus is reported to have lower PTH levels. The parathyroid gland contains PTH by 10 to 12 weeks and actively secretes PTH by 25 to 26 weeks in response to decreased extracellular fluid calcium.[12, 56] The fetal parathyroid is less responsive to decreased serum calcium, perhaps because of suppression of the parathyroid by the relative fetal hypercalcemia or placental PTH production.[75]

Calcitonin-containing cells appear in the thyroid at about 14 weeks' gestation and secrete immunoreactive calcitonin from 28 weeks.[91] Calcitonin levels are high in the fetus, with increasing concentrations during the third trimester that promote calcium storage in the bones. 25(OH)D is transferred from the mother since fetal liver processes for vitamin D metabolism are limited. Renal 1-alpha-hydroxylation to form $1,25(OH)_2D$ occurs in the fetal kidneys and probably in the placenta and decidua.[116] The fetus needs to store vitamin D to cope with the relatively high calcium requirements of the early postbirth period.[6]

NEONATAL PHYSIOLOGY

The newborn is hypercalcemic and hyperphosphatemic when compared with the mother.[71] The infant must quickly move from the intrauterine dependence on maternal calcium sources and placental hormones to independent extrauterine control of calcium and phosphorus metabolism and homeostasis with reliance on oral intake and bone stores.

Failure to do so may lead to hypocalcemia and other metabolic abnormalities.

Transitional Events

At birth maternal supplies of calcium and other minerals are no longer available to the infant. Total and ionized calcium levels are higher in cord blood than in maternal serum; PTH is decreased and calcitonin is normal or increased.[23, 71, 77] Cord blood magnesium levels are slightly increased and related to maternal levels, whereas phosphorus levels are markedly increased.[25, 51, 88, 119] Maternal serum 25(OH)D levels at term correlate with cord blood levels, although cord blood values are 20 to 30% lower; 1,25(OH)$_2$D levels are about half maternal values.[25,119] Cord blood levels of calcium, PTH, magnesium, and phosphorus in relation to maternal values are illustrated in Figure 14–5.

Calcium

The relative hypercalcemia at birth is followed by a physiologic hypocalcemia over the next 24 to 48 hours as calcium falls (Fig. 14–5) to levels lower than those found in older infants and about 1 mg/dl lower than birth values.[14, 72] Term infant calcium values increase by 5 to 10 days after birth.[23] Serum calcium levels in the first 3 days correlate with gestational age.[14] In term infants values average 8 to 9 mg/dl (total), with a range of 8 to 11, and 3.5 to 4 mg/dl (ionized) calcium; values are lower in preterm infants.[50a, 51, 65]

Intestinal absorption of calcium is correlated with both gestational and postbirth age, but the major factor in determining absorption is postnatal age.[45] Immature intestinal function or decreased intake may limit calcium absorption. Renal calcium excretion is relatively efficient in both term and preterm infants, although increased renal sodium losses in very low birth weight (VLBW) infants may also increase calcium loss.[14] Renal calcium excretion increases with gestational and postbirth age, ranging from 60 to 88 mg/day during the first 2 weeks to 180 mg/day by 3 to 12 weeks in the term infant and from less than 8 to 80 mg/day to 120 mg/day by 2 weeks of age in the preterm infant.[21]

Phosphorus

Phosphorus levels may decrease slightly during the first 1 to 2 days after birth but remain higher than those of adults (4–7.1 versus 2.7–4 mg/dl) (Fig. 14–5).[72] Endogenous stores of calcium are released after birth leading to elevated serum phosphorus in the first 3 days. Renal excretion of phosphorus is delayed because of decreased glomerular filtration rate and increased tubular reabsorption of phosphorus. Increased energy demands during birth with conversion of adenosine triphosphate (ATP) to adenosine diphosphate (ADP) lead to additional phosphorus release. Delayed feeding further elevates phosphorus levels because of tissue catabolism. Levels are lower in small for gestational age infants and correlate with the degree of growth retardation.[65]

Parathyroid Hormone

As serum calcium levels decrease over the first few days after birth, PTH levels gradually increase (Fig. 14–5).[23] Although the neonatal parathyroid can respond to a hypocalcemic stimulus by increasing PTH output, in many infants the parathyroid glands remain functionally immature for 2 to 3 days after birth.[14] These glands respond less readily to decreased serum calcium leading to a "functional hypoparathyroidism." This state is observed more frequently in VLBW infants and infants of diabetic mothers. Renal responsiveness to PTH is also decreased during the first 48 hours.[21] Neonatal parathyroid gland responsiveness is dependent on gestational and postnatal age.[14] By 3 to 4 days of age, the preterm infant's parathyroid gland generally responds effectively to calcium.[51] PTH levels do not appear to change with oral administration of calcium supplements, but intravenous bolus administration of calcium (i.e., with an exchange transfusion) can suppress parathyroid function.[14]

Vitamin D

Plasma concentrations of 25(OH)D in term infants correlate with maternal serum values.[23] With elimination of 25(OH)D from maternal sources after birth, the neonate must metabolize and hydroxylate vitamin D (see Fig. 14–2). Term infants are able to effectively metabolize vitamin D in the liver and kidneys. The kidneys can convert 25(OH)D to 1,25(OH)$_2$D by 28 to 32 weeks.[21, 105] Vitamin D metabolism remains limited in the preterm infant because 25-hydroxylation by the liver does not occur at

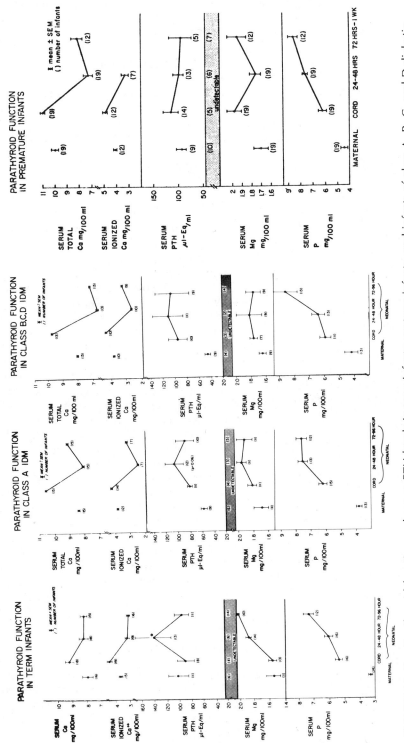

FIGURE 14–5. Parathyroid function and serum PTH levels in term infants, preterm infants, and infants of class A, B, C, and D diabetic mothers. In term infants, decrease in serum calcium (total and ionized) is associated with significant increase in serum PTH at 24 hours of age. In infants of class A diabetic mothers, the increase of PTH is equivocal. In infants of insulin-dependent (class B, C, D) diabetic mothers, there is no significant increase in serum PTH values in spite of marked decrease in serum calcium. Similarly, in preterm infants there is no significant increase in serum PTH values. (From Tsang, R.C., et al. (1975). Parathyroid function in infants of diabetic mothers. J Pediatr, 86, 401; and Tsang, R.C., et al. (1973). Neonatal parathyroid function: Role of gestational age and postnatal age. J Pediatr, 83, 731.

625

significant rates until 36 to 38 weeks' gestation.[97] Absorption of exogenous vitamin D may be limited because of immature fat absorption. Serum 25(OH)D and 1,25(OH)$_2$D levels increase during the first 24 to 48 hours, probably because of decreased serum calcium or increased PTH. This helps to maintain calcium levels within physiologic limits by stimulating bone and intestinal reabsorption.[91, 100]

Calcitonin

Calcitonin levels may be normal or slightly elevated at birth, followed by a surge that is reported to peak anywhere from 2 to 5 to 13 to 24 hours of age, then reach a plateau.[14, 23] The elevated calcitonin may be accompanied by an increase in plasma glucagon, a hypocalcemic agent.[14] After about 36 hours calcitonin levels gradually fall, but they remain elevated for 1 to 2 weeks in term infants.[23, 47, 85] Calcitonin levels are negatively correlated with gestational age. Levels in VLBW infants may exceed 1000 pg/ml (versus <100 pg/ml in adults).[85] Calcitonin is also higher in infants with asphyxia.[51]

Increased calcitonin may protect the infant against excessive bone reabsorption and promote mineralization during a period of active bone growth and in the face of increased PTH and 1,25(OH)$_2$D.[14, 45, 97] High calcitonin levels may contribute to the lower serum calcium levels and increased risk of hypocalcemia seen in preterm infants.[22] Calcitonin levels remain high in preterm infants for a longer period of time, slowly decreasing over the first 2 to 3 months to reach normal levels by about 40 weeks' postconceptual age.[45] Oral calcium supplementation does not stimulate (and may decrease) calcitonin secretion, although early oral supplementation decreases the postdelivery calcitonin surge. Intravenous calcium does not appear to affect calcitonin levels.[14, 45, 87]

Magnesium

Serum magnesium levels increase initially after birth (see Fig. 14–5), then fall to levels similar to those in adults (range, 1.5 to 2.8 mg/dl) by 2 weeks.[14] Urinary excretion of magnesium may be low for the first few days after birth.

CLINICAL IMPLICATIONS FOR NEONATAL CARE

Bone mineralization and synthesis of new tissues continue after birth and are dependent on adequate substrate. Alterations in calcium and phosphorus metabolism in the neonatal period have implications for nutritional needs of term and preterm infants and are critical in ensuring adequate postnatal growth and development. In addition, these alterations may increase the risk for disorders such as hypocalcemia in certain groups of infants. This section examines postnatal nutritional needs related to calcium and phosphorus metabolism and the demands of bone mineralization and the basis for common disorders.

Nutritional Needs

Daily enteric requirements for calcium are approximately 60 mg of elemental calcium per kilogram per day in term infants and may range up to 200 mg/kg/day in preterm infants. Phosphorus requirements are 40 mg/kg/day in term and 100 to 120 mg/kg/day in preterm infants; the requirement for magnesium is approximately 6 to 8 mg/kg/day.[20] A calcium-to-phosphorus ratio of 2:1 is thought to be ideal for human infants.[20]

The ratio of calcium to phosphorus can have a significant impact on mineral homeostasis. Hyperphosphatemia may lead to hypocalcemia by blunting the responsiveness of the bone to PTH and vitamin D. Conversely, low serum phosphorus levels can lead to reduction of calcium entry into bone, bone demineralization, and hypercalcemia.[20] Infant formulas have higher phosphorus and lower ionized calcium concentrations than does human milk.[98] The calcium-to-phosphorus ratio of 1.3:1 found in some formulas may result in an excessive phosphorus load for some infants. Many commercial formulas currently have ratios that more closely approximate those of human milk.[97] Nutritional needs are discussed further in Chapter 9.

Infants Fed Human Milk

Levels of calcium are lower in human milk than in cow's milk formulas. Human milk averages 24 to 35 mg/dl of calcium and 11 to 16 mg/dl of phosphorus.[20, 84] The 2:1 ratio of calcium to phosphorus promotes calcium-phosphorus homeostasis. The efficiency of intestinal calcium absorption is increased with human milk feedings (80% versus 44%).[42] Vitamin D supplementation of infants fed human milk increases 25(OH)D levels with no difference in $1,25(OH)_2D$ values.[97] Calcium and phosphorus levels of human milk are not adequate for very low birth weight infants, and supplementation is recommended (see Chapter 9).

Calcium Intake in Preterm Infants

Preterm infants may have difficulty maintaining an adequate calcium intake because of increased growth needs and a low intake. Calcium levels in mature breast milk and standard formulas are significantly below daily intrauterine calcium accretion rates in the third trimester.[14] As a result, bone mineralization is reduced in infants fed these substances.[45] If supplementation is used for preterm infants fed human milk, calcium-to-phosphorus ratios should not be greater than 2:1 to prevent hyperphosphatemia.[84]

Preterm formulas, which average 140 mg/kg/day of calcium and 75 mg/kg/day of phosphorus, come closer to duplicating intrauterine calcium accretion rates during the last trimester (120 to 150 mg/kg/day).[118] Vitamin D levels are increased in these formulas to enhance intestinal calcium absorption. Medium-chain triglycerides (MCTs) are also added to increase fat absorption and thus absorption of vitamin D and calcium.[94]

Bone Mineralization

VLBW infants have been reported to have decreased postnatal bone mineralization and a significant delay in completing bone development in comparison with intrauterine rates (Fig. 14–6).[62] Low birth weight infants given a calcium and phosphorus intake similar to intrauterine accretion rates mineralize their bones at rates similar to those of the fetus.[94, 99] These infants tend to have more stable calcium, phosphorus, magnesium, PTH, and 25(OH)D concentrations with a lower than expected calcitonin level. This suggests that the major problem in bone mineralization for the preterm infant is a lack of calcium and phosphorus.[14, 63, 97] Mineralization can also be altered in preterm infants by decreased absorption of fat-soluble vitamin K, an important factor in osteoclast formation.[45] As a result, preterm infants are at increased risk for both rickets and osteopenia (demineralization of the bone with or without signs of rickets).[97] Mineralization may also be delayed in small for gestational age infants.

Neonatal Hypocalcemia

The serum calcium level below which an infant is considered to be hypocalcemic varies in the literature from 7.0 to 8.5 mg/dl.[23, 50a, 51, 72] Most sources use a lower limit of 7 in preterm and 7.8 in term infants.[20] Ideally determination of hypocalcemia should be based on the ionized calcium fraction (<4.4 mg/dl), since this is the biologically active form.[20] These determinations are becoming increasingly accurate even with small amounts of blood. Calcium levels can be altered by hypoproteinemia or acid–base changes. Serum calcium is either ionized (physiologically active form) or undissociated and bound to protein or complexed to anions. Since these two forms of serum calcium are in equilibrium, hypoproteinemia lowers serum calcium levels. This equilibrium is influenced by acid–base status. Acidosis increases the movement of calcium from bone and decreases the amount of protein-bound calcium. As a result levels of ionized calcium increase. Opposite effects are seen during alkalosis.[20]

Infants at greatest risk for hypocalcemia are preterm infants, those born to diabetic mothers, or those born after perinatal asphyxia.[66, 107, 109] Possible pathogenic mechanisms are discussed below and summarized in Table 14–4. Hypocalcemia due to decreased ionized calcium may occur after exchange transfusion (see Chapter 15), with renal dysfunction, after furosemide therapy, or with magnesium deficiency.[51] Hypocalcemia with a decrease in ionized calcium but without a decrease in total calcium can occur with alkalosis, after exchange transfusion with citrated blood, or with elevated serum free fatty acids after lipid infusion.[20]

The usual physiologic course involves a decrease in serum calcium (<7 to 8 mg/dl) to a nadir at 24 to 48 hours of age in term and slightly earlier in preterm infants. This is associated with a concomitant increase in phosphorus levels (>8 mg/dl). Magnesium levels may be normal or low (<1.5 mg/dl). Infants can be asymptomatic or symptomatic. Symptoms may include tremors, twitching, hyperexcitability, irritability, high-pitched cry, laryngospasm, tachycardia, apnea, and, rarely, seizures.

Hypocalcemia in the Preterm Infant

Hypocalcemia is seen frequently in preterm infants with serum calcium levels lower than

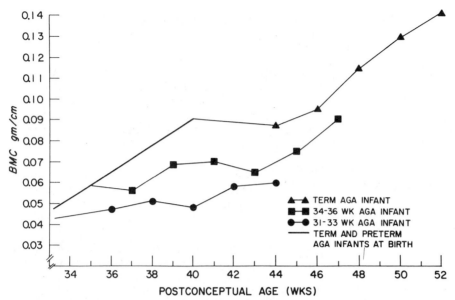

FIGURE 14–6.   Bone mineralization after birth in preterm infants fed standard proprietary formulas. The rate of bone mineralization is slower than that seen in the fetus. (From Minton, S.D., et al. (1979). Bone mineral content in term and preterm appropriate-for-gestational-age infants. *J Pediatr, 95,* 1037; as redrawn in Koo, W.W.K. & Tsang, R.C. (1987). Calcium and magnesium homeostasis in the newborn. In G.B. Avery (Ed.), *Neonatology: Pathophysiology and management of the newborn* (3rd ed., p. 717). Philadelphia: JB Lippincott.)

7 mg/dl (total) or 3 to 3.5 mg/dl (ionized) reported in 30 to 40%.[51] These infants are often asymptomatic. The hypocalcemia usually occurs early (beginning by 12 to 24 hours after birth) with a spontaneous return to normal values in untreated infants by 5 to 10 days.[2] Possible causes include lack of available calcium due to decreased early intake, decreased PTH response to move calcium out of the bones, immature absorption, interference with calcium metabolism by acidosis, increased calcitonin levels, decreased vitamin D intake and absorption, and $1,25(OH)_2D$ in very low birth weight infants.[20, 53, 61, 91]

Hypocalcemia in preterm infants may not be due to parathyroid immaturity per se since PTH increases as serum calcium decreases in these infants.[23] By 24 hours of age most preterm infants have elevated PTH levels that are sustained for 2 to 3 days, falling with correction of the hypocalcemia.[2] There may be an imbalance between calcium needs and PTH production, however, with increased calcium needs due to growth and a decreased supply.[91] The preterm infant also has a limited renal response to PTH during the first 48 hours.[57]

A refractory response to PTH or alterations in calcitonin may be important in the cause of this disorder.[23, 78, 91] The preterm infant has a marked elevation of calcitonin at 2 to 5 hours that reaches a plateau at 12 to 24 hours. Serum calcium values are negatively correlated with calcitonin at 12 to 24 hours of age, possibly impeding resolution of the hypocalcemia.[2, 23] Alterations in vitamin D metabolism or availability may also impede resolution. Hyperphosphatemia has also been observed by some investigators, along with an occasional transient decrease in magnesium at 24 to 48 hours.[107] The decrease in magnesium can be prevented by calcium, suggesting that hypomagnesemia is a consequence and not a cause of this hypocalcemia.[23]

Hypocalcemia in the Infant of a Diabetic Mother

Hypocalcemia occurs in about 50% of infants of insulin-dependent diabetic women.[53, 61] This form of hypocalcemia tends to appear within the first 24 hours of age and to be more severe and last longer than hypocalcemia seen in preterm infants.[23] The decrease in calcium level is directly correlated with the severity of the maternal diabetes.[61]

Cord blood of these infants contains decreased total and ionic calcium and PTH (see Fig. 14–5). The cause of this form of hypocalcemia may be related to suppression of the fetal parathyroid by maternal hypomag-

TABLE 14–4

TABLE 14–4
Possible Pathogenic Mechanisms in Early Neonatal Hypocalcemia

CLINICAL PARAMETER	POSSIBLE PATHOGENIC MECHANISMS
Prematurity	Decreased calcium and phosphorus intake
	Decreased PTH responsiveness altering ability to move calcium out of bone
	Increased calcitonin
	Immature absorption
	Immature renal function with decreased phosphorus excretion
	Decreased vitamin D intake and absorption
	Interference with calcium metabolism by acidosis
	Increased needs
Infant of a diabetic mother	Prematurity (see above)
	Transient hypoparathyroidism due to fetal parathyroid suppression by maternal hyperparathyroidism
Perinatal asphyxia	Increased tissue breakdown with phosphorus release
	Effects of pH and bicarbonate on protein binding of calcium and levels of ionized calcium
	Impaired parathyroid function
	Increased calcitonin

nesemia or by the relative maternal hyperparathyroidism seen in many diabetic women. The metabolic disorders in the diabetic woman are believed to be caused by increased urinary losses and lead to chronic fetal hypomagnesemia and decreased PTH secretion.[20] This results in a transient neonatal hypoparathyroidism.[66, 108] The pregnant diabetic woman has lower magnesium levels and a failure of the usual increase in PTH, although serum total and ionic calcium values are often within normal limits for pregnancy.[18] This disorder may be related to immaturity since it is seen more frequently in infants who are also immature. Since these infants are often hypomagnesemic also, magnesium therapy may be needed to correct both the hypocalcemia and hypomagnesemia.[72]

Hypocalcemia and Perinatal Asphyxia

With birth asphyxia there is increased tissue breakdown with release of phosphorus as well as accelerated conversion of ATP to ADP (to meet the increased energy demands) with subsequent phosphorus release. Administration of bicarbonate increases pH, which alters protein binding and decreases ionized cal-

cium.[91] Alkalosis from bicarbonate therapy reduces the flux of calcium from bone and reduces serum ionized calcium.[20] Birth asphyxia is also associated with an impairment of parathyroid function, increased calcitonin levels, and decreased serum levels of magnesium and phosphorus.[23, 51, 61] Administration of vitamin D has been reported to prevent development of hypocalcemia in many of these infants.[69]

Late Neonatal Hypocalcemia

Late hypocalcemia is seen infrequently and primarily in formula-fed term infants at 3 to 30 days of age.[51, 91] Late hypocalcemia may be asymptomatic, but is associated with tetany. Symptoms range from mild tremors to seizures.[23]

These infants demonstrate hypoparathyroidism in the face of decreased serum calcium and a reduction in efficient parathyroid activity that extends the usual postnatal decrease in calcium beyond 72 hours. The cause of persistent hypoparathyroidism is unknown. These changes may be aggravated by other factors such as vitamin D deficiency or high phosphorus loads from cow's milk formulas.[23, 53, 91] Late hypocalcemia was seen more often in the past when higher phosphate formulas (with calcium-to-phosphorus ratios of 1.3 to 1.4) were more common. The disorder is uncommon with current formulas and essentially nonexistent in breast-fed infants (human milk has a calcium-to-phosphorus ratio of 2.3). Late hypocalcemia is occasionally seen in preterm infants secondary to immature renal function, transient parathyroid dysfunction, or altered responsiveness to $1,25(OH)_2D$.[51]

Alterations in Magnesium

Hypomagnesemia in the neonate (<1.5 mg/dl) occurs most often in infants who are small for gestational age, preterm, or born to diabetic women. Less frequent causes of neonatal hypomagnesemia include decreased intake due to malabsorption or short bowel syndrome, increased losses with frequent exchange transfusions or diuretic use, maternal hyperparathyroidism, neonatal hypoparathyroidism, and hyperphosphatemia from cow's milk formula.[14] Hypocalcemia and hypomagnesemia usually occur simultaneously and symptoms are similar. Magnesium plays an important role in bone–serum calcium homeostasis and intestinal absorption of calcium (see Fig. 14–2). Decreased magnesium leads to decreased PTH secretion with subsequent reduction in calcium levels.

Hypermagnesemia (>2.5 mg/dl) is most often associated with administration of magnesium sulfate to the mother for treatment of PIH or preterm labor prevention. This can lead to elevated neonatal magnesium levels during the first 48 hours and respiratory depression, hypotonia, flaccidity, ileus, and poor feeding (magnesium has a curare-like effect). These infants have lower calcium levels, although they are not necessarily hypocalcemic. Hypermagnesemia may be treated with calcium, which increases magnesium excretion.[51, 91]

Neonatal Rickets

Rickets occurs because of a deficiency of calcium or phosphorus in extracellular fluid, usually associated with inadequate vitamin D to ensure adequate intestinal absorption of these minerals (Table 14–5). This results in increased secretion of PTH, which stimulates osteoclastic breakdown and absorption of bone. Additional calcium is then available to maintain serum levels and prevent hypocalcemia. After a time the bone weakens and becomes stressed. Osteoblast activity is stimulated to replace the absorbed bone, leading to production of large amounts of osteoid (organic bone matrix) that never becomes completely calcified because of lack of calcium and phosphorus.

In preterm infants rickets develops from inadequate intake of calcium or phosphorus over an extended period of time during which the infant is growing rapidly.[10, 55] In preterm infants rickets is associated with increased levels of $1,25(OH)_2D$, a finding consistent with inadequate calcium and phosphorus.[14] The 2nd month of life seems to be an especially vulnerable period for development of rickets in VLBW infants. Rickets may be treated by providing a supplemental elemental calcium intake of 100 mg/kg/day, phosphorus intake of 50 mg/kg/day, and 400 IU vitamin D/day (provided a calcium- and phosphorus-fortified formula is not already being used).[50a] Infants on total parenteral nutrition, with chronic health problems such as bronchopulmonary dysplasia, or on long-term diuretic therapy have higher mineral requirements and are at greater risk to develop

TABLE 14–5
Factors Predisposing Infants to Rickets of Prematurity

Prematurity
  Decreased stores of calcium and phosphorus
Bronchopulmonary dysplasia (BPD)
  Decreased intake of calcium and phosphorus secondary to fluid restriction and low content of calcium and phosphorus in hyperalimentation solutions
  Prolonged total parenteral nutrition (TPN)
    Direct bone toxicity (vitamin D, aluminum?)
    Hypercalciuria
    Cholestatic jaundice (vitamin D malabsorption)
  Furosemide therapy; hypercalciuria
  Increased serum 1,25-dihydroxyvitamin D (bone resorption?)
Prolonged TPN without BPD
  Decreased intake of calcium and phosphorus
  Inadvertent omission of calcium and vitamin D from solutions
  Direct bone toxicity (vitamin D, aluminum?)
  Hypercalciuria
  Cholestatic jaundice (vitamin D malabsorption)
Smallness for gestational age
  Placental insufficiency with decreased stores of calcium and phosphorus at birth
Soy formula feeding
  Decreased absorption of calcium and phosphorus
Human milk feeding
  Decreased intake of calcium and phosphorus
  Hypercalciuria secondary to inadequate intake of phosphorus
  Increased serum 1,25-dihydroxyvitamin D (bone resorption?)

From Greer, F.R. & Tsang, R.C. (1986). Calcium and vitamin D metabolism in term and low-birthweight infants. *Perinatology-Neonatology*, 9, 14.

rickets. Acidosis increases urinary calcium losses and interferes with synthesis of $1,25(OH)_2D$.[45] Factors predisposing to rickets are summarized in Table 14–5.

Rickets has been reported in breast-fed infants (Table 14–5), but in most cases appears to be related more to lack of ultraviolet (sunlight) exposure of the mother than nutritional deficiencies per se. The greatest risks to the infant seem to occur if the mother's diet is deficient in vitamin D and she also does not get enough sun exposure.[97]

Neonatal Hypercalcemia

Hypercalcemia is much less common than hypocalcemia in the neonate and is generally defined as a serum calcium level over 10.5 to 11.0 mg/dl, or ionized calcium over 5.0 to 5.8 mg/dl.[3, 50a] Infants may be asymptomatic or symptomatic (hypotonia, poor feeding, lethargy, vomiting, seizures, polyuria, and hypertension). Neurologic manifestations arise from the effects of calcium on nerve cells and cerebral ischemia. Polyuria is due to interference with the action of argininevasopressin on the collecting ducts and can lead to dehydration. Hypertension is related to the vasoconstrictive effects of calcium and subsequent increased activity of the renin–angiotensin system.[3] Hypercalcemia may be idiopathic, iatrogenic, or due to hypervitaminosis (vitamins A or D) or underlying metabolic or genetic disorders.

MATURATIONAL CHANGES DURING INFANCY AND CHILDHOOD

Age-related changes in calcium and phosphorus and their regulating hormones reflect needs of the infant and child to maintain calcium stability while providing for skeletal growth. Phosphorus levels decrease during the 1st year. With increasing exposure to ultraviolet light, 25(OH)D levels increase during this same period. Levels of $1,25(OH)_2D$ are higher than adult values

TABLE 14–6
Summary of Recommendations for Clinical Practice Related Calcium and Phosphorus Metabolism: Neonate

Know usual changes in calcium, phosphorus, and magnesium metabolism during the neonatal period (pp. 624–626).

Monitor newborn calcium, phosphorus, and magnesium status during transition and in the early neonatal period (pp. 624–631).

Recognize factors that influence bone mineralization and growth (pp. 622–623, 627).

Initiate early enteral feeding as appropriate (pp. 623–624).

Monitor nutritional intake of calcium, phosphorus, and vitamin D in infants (pp. 624–630).

Monitor neonates for signs of excessive and inadequate intake of calcium, phosphorus, and magnesium (pp. 627–631).

Recognize infants at risk for hypocalcemia (pp. 627–629, Table 14–4).

Know clinical signs of hypocalcemia (p. 627).

Assess and monitor infants at risk for hypocalcemia (pp. 627–629).

Recognize infants at risk for hypo- and hypermagnesemia (pp. 629–630).

Know clinical signs of hypo- and hypermagnesemia (pp. 629–630).

Assess and monitor infants at risk for hypo- and hypermagnesemia (pp. 629–630).

Recognize and monitor infants at risk for late neonatal hypocalcemia (pp. 630–631).

Recognize and monitor infants at risk for neonatal rickets (p. 630, Table 14–5).

Page numbers in parentheses following each recommendation refer to pages in the text where the rationale for that intervention is discussed.

for the 1st year.[89] Levels of this biologically active metabolite may remain even higher in preterm infants for up to 3 months, perhaps to compensate for immature calcium absorption.[84] Levels of $1,25(OH)_2D$ tend to be elevated during periods of growth.[80]

From 3 weeks to 6 months serum calcium values in breast-fed infants gradually increase, leading to a transient physiologic hypercalcemia. This increase may be related to decreased phosphorus intake due to the lower levels of phosphorus in human milk.[37, 91, 97] Serum calcium levels do not change significantly in formula-fed infants from birth to 18 months. Serum calcium levels gradually decrease from 6 to 20 years.[98]

Infants on standard formulas experience a progressive fall in serum PTH during the neonatal period that reaches a nadir at about 3 months, at which time bone mineralization increases.[63] This is analogous to the lowered PTH levels seen in utero and may promote extrauterine bone development.[14] By 2 to 4 months the renal response to exogenous PTH is similar to that seen in adults.[52]

SUMMARY

Calcium and phosphorus are essential minerals for many body processes and normal growth and development. Alterations in metabolic processes related to these elements can significantly alter the infant's health status. Many of these problems can be prevented and normal growth and development promoted by careful assessment and monitoring of neonatal nutritional status and initiation of appropriate interventions. Recommendations for clinical practice related to calcium and phosphorus metabolism are summarized in Table 14–6.

REFERENCES

1. Aarskog, D., et al. (1984). Heparin-induced inhibition of 1,25-dihydroxyvitamin D formation. *Am J Obstet Gynecol, 148*, 1141.
2. Anast, C.S. & Dirksen, H. (1978). Studies related to the pathogenesis of neonatal hypocalcemia. In D.H. Copp & R.V. Talmage (Eds.), *Endocrinology of calcium metabolism*. Amsterdam: Excerpta Medica.
3. Anast, C.S. & David. L. (1983). The physiology of calcium in the human neonate. In M.F. Holick, C.S. Anast, & T.K. Gray (Eds.), *Perinatal calcium and phosphorus metabolism* (pp. 363–383). Amsterdam: Elsevier.
4. Belizan, J.M. & Villar, J. (1980). The relationship

between calcium intake and edema, proteinuria, and hypertension-gestosis: A hypothesis. *Am J Clin Nutr, 33*, 2202.

5. Bouillon, R., et al. (1981). Influence of vitamin D binding protein on the serum concentration of 1,25-dihydroxyvitamin D. *J Clin Invest, 67*, 589.

6. Bouillon, R. (1983). Vitamin D metabolites in human pregnancy. In M.L. Holick, C.S. Anast, & T.K. Gray (Eds.), *Perinatal calcium and phosphorus metabolism* (pp. 291–300). Amsterdam: Elsevier.

7. Bouillon, R. & Van Assche, F.A. (1982). Perinatal vitamin D metabolism. *Dev Pharmacol Ther, 4*(Suppl.), 38.

8. Brown, D.J., Spanos, E., & MacIntyre, I. (1980). Role of pituitary hormones in regulating renal vitamin D metabolism in man. *Br Med J, 280*, 277.

9. Bruns, E. (1983). Vitamin D action during pregnancy: The induction of calcium binding protein in intestine, placenta and yolk sac. In M.F. Holick, C.S. Anast, & T.K. Gray (Eds.), *Perinatal calcium and phosphorus metabolism* (pp. 183–196). Amsterdam: Elsevier.

10. Campbell, D.E. & Fleischman, A.R. (1988). Rickets of prematurity: Controversies in causation and prevention. *Clin Perinatol, 15*, 879.

11. Care, A.W.C. (1980). Calcium homeostasis in the fetus. *J Dev Physiol, 2*, 85.

12. Care, A.D. & Ross, R. (1984). Fetal calcium homeostasis. *J Dev, 6*, 59.

13. Chan, G.M., et al. (1982). Growth and bone mineralization of normal breast-fed infants and effects of lactation on maternal bone mineral status. *Am J Clin Nutr, 36*, 438.

14. Chan, G.M., Venkataraman, P., & Tsang, R.C. The physiology of calcium in the human neonate. In M.F. Holick, C.S. Anast, & T.K. Gray (Eds.), *Perinatal calcium and phosphorus metabolism* (pp. 331–349). Amsterdam: Elsevier.

15. Clemens, T.L. & Holick, M.F. (1983). Recent advances in the hormonal regulation of calcium and phosphorus in adult animals and humans. In M.F. Holick, C.S. Anast, & T.K. Gray (Eds.), *Perinatal calcium and phosphorus metabolism* (pp. 1–24). Amsterdam: Elsevier.

16. Cockburn, F., et al. (1980). Maternal vitamin D intake and mineral metabolism in mothers and their newborn infants. *Br Med J, 281*, 11.

17. Cruikshank, D.P., et al. (1979). Effects of magnesium sulfate on perinatal calcium metabolism; I. Maternal and fetal responses. *Am J Obstet Gynecol, 134*, 243.

18. Cruikshank, D.P., et al. (1980). Altered maternal calcium homeostasis in diabetic pregnancy. *J Clin Endocrinol Metab, 50*, 264.

19. Cruishank, D.P., et al. (1981). Urinary magnesium, calcium and phosphate excretion duirng magnesium sulfate infusion. *Obstet Gynecol, 58*, 430.

20. Cruz, M.L. & Tsang, R.C. (1991). Disorders of calcium and magnesium homeostasis. In T.F. Yeh (Ed.), *Neonatal therapeutics* (2nd ed., pp. 253–271). St. Louis: Mosby–Year Book.

21. Cushard, W.G., et al. (1972). Physiologic hyperparathyroidism in pregnancy. *J Clin Endocrinol, 34*, 767.

22. David, L., et al. (1981). Serum immunoreactive calcitonin in low birth weight infants. Description of early changes, effect of intravenous calcium, relationship with early changes in serum calcium, phosphorus, magnesium, parathyroid hormone, and gastrin levels. *Pediatr Res, 15*, 803.

23. David, L., et al. (1983). The physiology of calcium in the human neonate. In M.F. Holick, C.S. Anast, & T.K. Gray (Eds.), *Perinatal calcium and phosphorus metabolism* (pp. 351–361). Amsterdam: Elsevier.

24. De Jorge, F.B., et al. (1965). Magnesium concentration in the blood serum of normal pregnant women. *Obstet Gynecol, 25*, 253.

25. Devlin, E.E., et al. (1982). Control of vitamin D metabolism in preterm infants: Feto-maternal relationships. *Am J Dis Child, 57*, 754.

26. Disousa, S.M. & Mundy, G.R. (1983). Hormonal regulation of fetal skeletal growth and development. In M.F. Holick, C.S. Anast, & T.K. Gray (Eds.), *Perinatal calcium and phosphorus metabolism* (pp. 233–257). Amsterdam: Elsevier.

27. Donaldson, J.O. (1988). Neurologic complications. In G.N. Burrow & T.F. Ferris (Eds.), *Medical complications during pregnancy* (pp. 485–498). Philadelphia: WB Saunders.

28. Drake, T.S., Kaplan, R.A., & Lewis, T.A. (1979). The physiologic hyperparathyroidism of pregnancy: Is it primary or secondary. *Obstet Gynecol, 53*, 746.

29. Duggin, G.G., et al. (1974). Calcium balance in pregnancy. *Lancet, 2*, 926.

30. Edidin, D.V., et al. (1980). Resurgence of nutritional rickets associated with breast feeding and special dietary practices. *Pediatrics, 65*, 232.

31. Forbes, G.B. (1976). Calcium accumulation by the human fetus. *Pediatrics, 57*, 976.

32. Gertner, J.M., et al. (1986). Pregnancy as a state of physiologic absorptive hypercalciuria. *Am J Med, 81*, 451.

33. Gray, T.K. (1983). Vitamin D and human pregnancy. In M.F. Holick, C.S. Anast, & T.K. Gray (Eds.), *Perinatal calcium and phosphorus metabolism* (pp. 281–290). Amsterdam: Elsevier.

34. Gray, T.K., Lesaer, G.F., & Lorene, R.S. (1979). Evidence for extra-renal 1-alpha-hydroxylation of 25OHD3 in pregnancy. *Science, 204*, 1311.

35. Gray, T.K., Lowe, W., & Lester, G.E. (1981). Vitamin D and pregnancy: The maternal-fetal metabolism of vitamin D. *Endocrinol Rev, 2*, 264.

36. Greer, F.R., et al. (1981). Bone mineral content and serum 25-hydroxyvitamin D concentration in breast-fed infants with and without supplemental vitamin D. *J Pediatr, 98*, 696.

37. Greer, F.R., et al. (1982). Increasing serum calcium and magnesium concentrations in breast-fed infants: Longitudinal studies of minerals in human milk and sera of nursing mothers and their infants. *J Pediatr, 100*, 59.

38. Guyton, A.C. (1987). *Textbook of medical physiology* (7th ed., pp. 605–618). Philadelphia: WB Saunders.

39. Halloran, B.P. & DeLuca, H.F. (1983). Vitamin D: Its role in pregnancy and lactation. In M.F. Holick, C.S. Anast, & T.K. Gray (Eds.), *Perinatal calcium and phosphorus metabolism* (pp. 103–129). Amsterdam: Elsevier.

40. Hammar, M., et al. (1987). Calcium and magnesium status in pregnant women: A comparison between treatment with calcium and vitamin C in pregnant women with leg cramps. *Int J Vitam Nutr Res, 57*, 179.

41. Harris, W.H. & Heaney, R.P. (1969). Skeletal renewal and metabolic bone disease. *N Engl J Med, 280*, 1460.

42. Harrison, H.E. & Harrison, H.C. (1974). Calcium. *Biomembranes, 4B*, 793.

43. Hearney, R.P. & Skillman, T.G. (1971). Calcium metabolism in normal human pregnancy. *J Clin Endocrinol, 33*, 661.

44. Heckman, J.Z., et al. (1979). Plasma 25-hydroxy-vitamin D in pregnant Asian women and their babies. *Lancet, 2*, 546.

45. Hillman, L.S., et al. (1977). Serial measurements of serum calcium, magnesium, parathyroid hormone, calcitonin and 25-dihydroxyvitamin D in premature and term infants during the first week of life. *Pediatr Res, 11*, 739.

46. Hillman, L.S. & Blethen, S.L. (1981). Serum somatomedin-C concentrations (SMC) in preterm infants. *Pediatr Res, 15*, 509.

47. Hillman, L.S. (1983). Mineralization and late mineral homeostasis in infants: Role of mineral and vitamin D sufficiency and other factors. In M.F. Holick, C.S. Anast, & T.K. Gray (Eds.), *Perinatal calcium and phosphorus metabolism* (pp. 301–329). Amsterdam: Elsevier.

48. Hirata, T. & Brady, J. (1977). *Newborn intensive care: Chemical aspects* (pp. 92–103). Springfield, IL: Charles C Thomas.

49. Hollingsworth, D.R. (1989). Endocrine disorders of pregnancy. In R.K. Creasy & R. Resnik (Eds.), *Maternal-fetal medicine: Principles and practice* (pp. 989–1031). Philadelphia: WB Saunders.

50. Howarth, A.T., Morgan, D.B., & Payne, R.B. (1977). Urinary excretion of calcium in late pregnancy and its relation to creatinine clearance. *Am J Obstet Gynecol, 129*, 499.

50a. Itani, O. & Tsang, M.B.B.S. (1991). Calcium, phosphorus, and magnesium in the newborn: Pathophysiology and management. In W.W. Hay (Ed.), *Neonatal nutrition and metabolism* (pp. 171–202). St. Louis: CV Mosby.

51. Kleigman, R.M. & Wald, M.K. (1986). Problems in metabolic adaptation: Glucose, calcium and magnesium. In M.H. Klaus & A.A. Fanaroff (Eds.), *Care of the high risk neonate* (3rd ed., pp. 220–238). Philadelphia: WB Saunders.

52. Kodama, S., et al. (1975). Etiologic analysis of neonatal hypocalcemia. Relationship with reactivity to parathyroid hormone. *Kobe J Med Science, 21*, 69.

53. Koo, W.W.K. & Tsang, R.C. (1987). Calcium and magnesium homeostasis in the newborn. In G.B. Avery (Ed.), *Neonatology: Pathophysiology and management of the newborn* (pp. 710–723). Philadelphia: JB Lippincott.

54. Kumar, R., et al. (1979). Elevated 1,25-dihydroxy-vitamin D plasma levels in normal human pregnancy and lactation. *J Clin Invest, 63*, 342.

55. Laing, I.A., et al. (1985). Rickets of prematurity: Calcium and phosphorus supplementation. *J Pediatr, 106*, 265.

56. Leroyer-Alizon, E., et al. (1981). Immunocytological evidence for parathyroid hormone in human parathyroid glands. *J Clin Endocrinol Metab, 52*, 513.

57. Linarelli, L.G., Bobik, C., & Bobik, J. (1973). Urinary cAMP and renal responsiveness to parathormone in premature hypocalcemic infants. *Pediatr Res, 7*, 329.

58. Mallet, E., et al. (1978). Neonatal parathyroid secretion and renal receptor maturation in premature infants. *Biol Neonate, 33*, 304.

59. Marya, R.K., et al. (1981). Effects of vitamin D supplementation in pregnancy. *Gynecol Obstet Invest, 12*, 155.

60. McGuinness, G.A., et al. (1980). Effects of magnesium sulfate treatment on perinatal calcium metabolism; II. Neonatal responses. *Obstet Gynecol, 56*, 595.

61. Mimouni, F. & Tsang, R.C. (1987). Disorders of calcium and magnesium metabolism. In A.A. Fanaroff & R.J. Martin (Eds.), *Neonatal-perinatal medicine: Diseases of the fetus and infant* (pp. 1077–1092). St. Louis: CV Mosby.

62. Minton, S.D., Steichen, J.J., & Tsang, R.C. (1979). Bone mineral content in term and preterm appropriate-for-gestational-age infants. *J Pediatr, 95*, 1037.

63. Minton, S.D., Steichen, J.J., & Tsang, R.C. (1983). Decreased bone mineral content in SGA compared with AGA infants: Normal serum 25-hydroxyvitamin D and decreasing parathyroid hormones in SGA and AGA infants. *Pediatrics, 71*, 383.

64. Moore, K. (1989). *The developing human: Clinically oriented embryology*. Philadelphia: WB Saunders.

65. Nelson, N. et al. (1989). Plasma ionized calcium, phosphate and magnesium in preterm and SGA infants. *Acta Paediatr Scand, 78*, 351.

66. Noguchi, A., Eren, M., & Tsang, R.C. (1980). Parathyroid hormone in hypocalcemic and normocalcemic infants of diabetic mothers. *J Pediatr, 97*, 112.

67. Page, E.W., Villee, C.A., & Villee, D.B. (1981). *Human reproduction: Essentials of reproductive and perinatal medicine* (3rd ed.). Philadelphia: WB Saunders.

68. Page, E.W. & Page, E.P. (1953). Leg cramps in pregnancy: Etiology and treatment. *Obstet Gynecol, 1*, 94.

69. Petersen, S., Christensen, N.C., & Fogh-Andersen, N. (1981). Effect on serum calcium of 1-hydroxy-vitamin D3 supplementation in infants of low birthweight, infants with perinatal asphyxia, and infants of diabetic mothers. *Acta Paediatr Scand, 70*, 897.

70. Pitkin, R.M. (1975). Calcium metabolism in pregnancy: A review. *Am J Obstet Gynecol, 121*, 724.

71. Pitkin, R.M. (1983). Human maternal-fetal calcium homeostasis. In M.F. Holick, C.S. Anast, & T.K. Gray (Eds.), *Perinatal calcium and phosphorus metabolism* (pp. 259–279). Amsterdam: Elsevier.

72. Pitkin, R.M. (1985). Calcium metabolism in pregnancy and the perinatal period: A review. *Am J Obstet Gynecol, 151*, 99.

73. Pitkin, R.M. & Gebhardt, M.P. (1977). Serum calcium concentrations in human pregnancy. *Am J Obstet Gynecol, 127*, 775.

74. Pitkin, R.M., et al. (1979). Calcium metabolism in pregnancy: A longitudinal study. *Am J Obstet Gynecol, 133*, 781.

75. Pitkin, R.A., et al. (1980). Fetal calcitropic hormones and neonatal calcium homeostasis. *Pediatrics, 66*, 77.

76. Reddy, G.S., et al. (1983). Regulation of vitamin D metabolism in normal human pregnancy. *J Clin Med, 56*, 363.

77. Reitz, R.E., et al. (1977). Calcium, magnesium, phosphorus and parathyroid hormone interrelationships in pregnancy and newborn infants. *Obstet Gynecol, 50,* 701.

78. Richards, S.R., Nelson, D.M., & Zuspan, F.P. (1984). Calcium levels in normal and hypertensive patients. *Am J Obstet Gynecol, 149,* 168.

79. Roberts, J.M. (1989). Pregnancy-related hypertension. In R.K. Creasy & R. Resnik (Eds.), *Maternal-fetal medicine: Principles and practice* (pp. 777–823). Philadelphia: WB Saunders.

80. Rosen, J.F. & Chesney, R.W. (1983). Circulating calcitriol concentrations in health and disease. *J Pediatr, 103,* 1.

81. Rosli, A. & Fanconi, A. (1973). Neonatal hypocalcemia. "Early type" in low birth weight newborns. *Helv Paediatr Acta, 28,* 443.

82. Rush, D., Johnstone, F.D., & King, J.C. (1988). Nutrition and pregnancy. In G.N. Burrow & T.F. Ferris (Eds.), *Medical complications during pregnancy* (pp. 117–135). Philadelphia: WB Saunders.

83. Sadler, T.W. (1985). *Langman's medical embryology* (5th ed.). Baltimore: Williams & Wilkins.

84. Salle, B.L., et al. (1987). Vitamin D metabolism in preterm infants. *Biol Neonate, 52* (Suppl.), 119.

85. Salle, B.L., et al. (1982). Early oral administration of vitamin D and its metabolites in premature neonates. Effect on mineral homeostasis. *Pediatr Res, 16,* 75.

86. Salle, B., et al. (1986). Effects of calcium and phosphorus supplementation on calcium retention and fat absorption in preterm infants fed pooled human milk. *J Pediatr Gastroenterol Nutr, 5,* 638.

87. Sann, L., et al. (1980). Effect of early calcium supplementation on serum calcium and immunoreactive calcitonin in preterm infants. *Arch Dis Child, 55,* 611.

88. Schauberger, C.W. & Pitkin, R.M. (1980). Maternal-perinatal calcium relationships. *Obstet Gynecol, 53,* 74.

89. Schilling, R., et al. (1990). High total and free 1,25-dihydroxyvitamin D concentrations in the serum of preterm infants. *Acta Paediatr Scand, 79,* 36.

90. Senterre, J. & Salle, B. (1982). Calcium and phosphorus economy of the preterm infant and its interaction with vitamin D and its metabolites. *Acta Paediatr Scand, 296,* 85.

91. Senterre, J. & Salle, B. (1987). Calcium, phosphorus, magnesium and vitamin D. In L. Stern & P. Vert (Eds.), *Neonatal medicine* (pp. 831–848). New York: Masson.

92. Senterre, J., et al. (1983). Effects of vitamin D and phosphorus supplementation on calcium retention in preterm infants fed banked human milk. *J Pediatr, 103,* 305.

93. Sersnius, F., Elidrissy, A., & Dandona, P. (1984). Vitamin D nutrition in pregnant women at term and in newly born babies in Saudi Arabia. *J Clin Pathol, 37,* 444.

94. Shaw, J.C.L. (1976). Evidence for defective skeletal mineralization in low-birthweight infants: The absorption of calcium and fat. *Pediatrics, 57,* 16.

95. Shenolikar, I.S. (1970). Absorption of dietary calcium in pregnancy. *Am J Clin Nutr, 23,* 63.

96. Simpson, A.A., et al. (1973). Changes in the concentrations of prolactin and adrenocorticosteroids in rat plasma during pregnancy and lactation. *J Endocrinol, 58,* 675.

97. Specker, B.L. & Tsang, R.C. (1986). Vitamin D in infancy and childhood: Factors determining vitamin D status. *Adv Pediatr, 33,* 1.

98. Specker, B.L., et al. (1985). Reduction of serum ionized calcium and elevation of serum phosphorus in cow milk formula-fed infants compared to breast-fed infants in the first six months of life. *Pediatr Res, 19,* 233A.

99. Steichen, J.J., et al. (1980). Osteopenia of prematurity: The cause and possible treatment. *J Pediatr, 96,* 528.

100. Steichen, J.J., et al. (1980). Vitamin D homeostasis in the perinatal period: 1,25-dihydroxyvitamin D in maternal, cord and neonatal blood. *N Engl J Med, 302,* 315.

101. Stevenson, J.C., et al. (1979). A physiological role for calcitonin: Protection of the maternal skeleton. *Lancet, 2,* 769.

102. Tan, C.M., Raman, A., & Sinnathyray, T.A. (1979). Serum ionic calcium levels during pregnancy. *Br J Obstet Gynaecol, 79,* 694.

103. Tassinari, M.S. & Holtrop, M.E. (1983). Development of the fetal skeleton: Factors determining normal and abnormal growth. In M.F. Holick, C.S. Anast, & T.K. Gray (Eds.), *Perinatal calcium and phosphorus metabolism* (pp. 197–231). Amsterdam: Elsevier.

104. Taylor, T.G., Lewis, P.E., & Balderstone, O. (1975). Role of calcitonin in protecting the skeleton during pregnancy and lactation. *J Endocrinol, 66,* 297.

105. Tsang, R.C. (1983). The quandary of vitamin D in the newborn. *Lancet, 1,* 1370.

106. Tsang, R.C., et al. (1972). Hypocalcemia in infants of diabetic mothers. *J Pediatr, 80,* 384.

107. Tsang, R.C., et al. (1973). Possible pathogenic factors in neonatal hypocalcemia of prematurity. *J Pediatr, 82,* 423.

108. Tsang, R.C., et al. (1976). Hypomagnesemia in infants of diabetic mothers. *J Pediatr, 89,* 115.

109. Tsang, R.C., et al. (1974). Neonatal hypocalcemia in infants with birth asphyxia. *J Pediatr, 84,* 428.

110. Tulchinsky, D. & Ryan, K. (1980). *Maternal-fetal endocrinology.* Philadelphia: WB Saunders.

111. Umeki, S., Nagao, S., & Nozawa, Y. (1981). The purification and identification of calmodulin from human placenta. *Biochem Biophys Acta, 674,* 319.

112. Vander, A., Sherman, J., & Luciano, D. (1985). *Human physiology: The mechanism of body function* (pp. 71–98, 393–395, 440–457). New York: McGraw-Hill.

113. Varner, M.W., Cruikshank, D.P., & Pitkin, R.A. (1983). Calcium metabolism in the hypertensive mother, fetus and newborn. *Am J Obstet Gynecol, 147,* 762.

114. Venkataraman, P.S., et al. (1983). Profound neonatal hypocalcemia in very low birth weight infants with unresponsive parathyroid glands refractory to 1,25-dihydroxyvitamin D3. *Pediatr Res, 17,* 340A.

115. Villar, J., Belizan, J.M., & Fisher, P.J. (1983). Epidemiologic observations on the relationship between calcium intake and eclampsia. *Int J Obstet Gynecol, 21,* 271.

116. Weisman, Y., et al. (1979). 1,25-dihydroxyvitamin

D3 and 24,25-dihydroxyvitamin D in vitro synthesis by human decidua and placenta. *Nature, 281,* 317.

117. Whitehead, M., et al. (1981). Interrelationships of calcium-regulating hormones during normal pregnancy. *Br Med J, 3,* 10.

118. Widdowson, E.M. & Dickerson, J.T. (1961). Chemical composition of the body. In C.L. Comar & F. Bronner (Eds.), *Mineral metabolism* (Vol. 2). New York: Academic Press.

119. Wieland, P., et al. (1980). Perinatal parathyroid hormone, vitamin D metabolites and calcitonin in man. *Am J Perinatol, 239,* E388.

120. Worthington-Roberts, B.S., Vermeersch, J., & Williams, S.R. (1989). *Nutrition during pregnancy and lactation.* St. Louis: CV Mosby.

121. Zaloga, G.P. & Eil, C. (1989). Diseases of the parathyroid glands and nephrolithiasis during pregnancy. In S.A. Brody & K. Ueland (Eds.), *Endocrine disorders in pregnancy* (pp. 231–246). Norwalk, CT: Appleton & Lange.

CHAPTER 15

Bilirubin Metabolism

Maternal Physiologic Adaptations
Clinical Implications for the Pregnant Woman and
    Her Fetus
Development of Bilirubin Metabolism in the Fetus
Neonatal Physiology
    Transitional Events
    Bilirubin Production in the Neonate
    Physiologic Jaundice
Clinical Implications for Neonatal Care
    Neonatal Hyperbilirubinemia
    Measurement of Serum Bilirubin

Management of Neonatal Hyperbilirubinemia
    Pharmacologic Agents
    Exchange Transfusion
    Phototherapy
Breast-Feeding and Neonatal Jaundice
Competition for Albumin Binding
Bilirubin Encephalopathy
Maturational Changes During Infancy and
Childhood

Physiologic jaundice is a common problem in term and preterm infants during the 1st week after birth. For most of these infants this phenomenon is mild and resolves without treatment. A small group of infants develop neonatal hyperbilirubinemia, however, which may herald underlying disorders such as hemolytic disease of the newborn or sepsis. When any infant develops significant hyperbilirubinemia, concerns arise about possible sequelae in the form of bilirubin encephalopathy. This chapter focuses on bilirubin metabolism and its pattern in the fetus and neonate along with issues related to neonatal hyperbilirubinemia and its management. Maternal adaptations are discussed only briefly, since bilirubin metabolism is not normally significantly altered in pregnancy. Bilirubin

synthesis, transport, and metabolism are summarized in Figure 15–1 and the boxes on pages 638 and 639.

MATERNAL PHYSIOLOGIC ADAPTATIONS

Alterations in the liver and hepatic function during pregnancy are described in Chapter 9. Bilirubin metabolism is not significantly altered in the pregnant woman, with bilirubin levels generally reported to be similar to those in nonpregnant women with upper limits of 0.4 mg/dl for total and 0.2 mg/dl for direct values.[7, 11] Fallon reports that slight increases in serum bilirubin levels may be seen in approximately 5% of healthy preg-

636

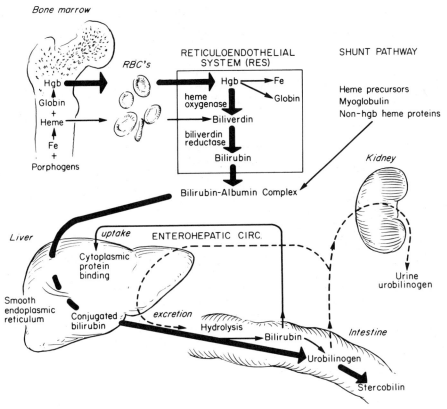

FIGURE 15–1. Bilirubin synthesis, transport, and metabolism. (From Gartner, L.M. & Hollander, M. (1972). Disorders of bilirubin metabolism. In N.S. Assali (Ed.), *Pathophysiology of gestation.* (Vol. 2, p. 457.) New York: Academic Press.)

nant women, possibly secondary to hormonal influences.[55]

CLINICAL IMPLICATIONS FOR THE PREGNANT WOMAN AND HER FETUS

The major difference between fetal and adult handling of bilirubin is that the fetus uses the placenta rather than the intestines as the major elimination pathway. Most of the bilirubin produced by the fetus remains in the indirect state, a form that can be readily cleared by the placenta. The indirect fetal bilirubin eliminated across the placenta is conjugated and excreted by the maternal liver. Even with severe hemolysis, infants are rarely born jaundiced since the placenta efficiently clears excess fetal indirect bilirubin. These infants may have an accumulation of direct bilirubin and are often severely anemic. In addition the maternal system effi-

ciently handles the fetal bilirubin load and has sufficient reserve so maternal hyperbilirubinemia secondary to fetal hemolysis is rare.[7] Immunologic aspects of hemolytic disorders secondary to blood group incompatibility are discussed in Chapter 10.

Maternal Hyperbilirubinemia

The effects of excessive maternal bilirubin production on the fetus depend on whether the woman has direct or indirect hyperbilirubinemia. Direct (conjugated) bilirubin is not transferred across the placenta in either direction.[55] Therefore the fetus of a woman with direct hyperbilirubinemia and jaundice secondary to hepatitis or other functional liver disorders does not have an elevated direct bilirubin level. Indirect (unconjugated) bilirubin can be transferred across the placenta in both directions, however. Cord bilirubin levels of mothers and newborns are similar.[38] Isolated indirect hyperbilirubinemia is rare in adults; however, several cases

Bilirubin Synthesis, Transport, and Metabolism

Bilirubin is an end-product of hemoglobin catabolism. Hemoglobin is broken down into heme iron–porphyrin complex and globin in the reticuloendothelial system (see Fig. 15–1). The iron is released and stored. Heme is further degraded by macrophages to carbon monoxide and biliverdin under the influence of microsomal heme oxygenase. Biliverdin is catabolized to indirect (unconjugated) bilirubin (IXa) by action of nicotinamide adenine dinucleotide phosphate (NADPH)-dependent biliverdin reductase. Most of the heme comes from catabolism of senescent RBCs and ineffective erythropoiesis (each gram of hemoglobin produces 34 to 35 mg of unconjugated bilirubin). Some bilirubin also comes from catabolism of nonhemoglobin heme proteins and free heme in the liver. Indirect bilirubin is orange-yellow, fat soluble, and not readily excreted in bile or urine. Indirect bilirubin is transported in plasma, bound to albumin (1 g albumin binds 8.5 to 10 mg of bilirubin) with a small amount of free bilirubin, to the liver for metabolism and excretion. Direct (conjugated) bilirubin is a water-soluble complex that has been metabolized by the liver to form bilirubin monoglucuronides or diglucuronides (see Fig. 15–2). Direct bilirubin is excreted through the biliary tree into the intestines and forms a major component of bile and feces; small amounts may also be excreted through the kidneys (increases with elevated direct bilirubin).[1, 9–11, 20, 23, 25, 29, 139]

In the intestines conjugated bilirubin is further catabolized by intestinal bacterial flora into urobilinogen and stercobilinogen, which are further oxidized to urobilin or stercobilin. These latter substances have a characteristic orange color that contributes to the color of feces. Direct bilirubin is unstable and can by hydrolyzed by the relatively alkaline environment of the duodenum and jejunum or by specific enzymes such as β-glucuronidase back into indirect bilirubin. Some urobilinogen is deconjugated in the small intestine by β-glucuronidase, absorbed across the intestinal mucosa, and returned to the circulation and portal venous system through enterohepatic circulation (see Fig. 15–1). Recirculated bilirubin eventually is reconjugated by the liver.[1, 12–15, 17, 20, 28, 34]

of elevated indirect bilirubin levels in cord blood have been reported in infants of women with end-stage cirrhosis.[11, 55, 179] Maisels questions whether this increase resulted from maternal-to-fetal transfer or if the elevated maternal bilirubin levels prevented the normal fetal-to-maternal transfer.[105]

DEVELOPMENT OF BILIRUBIN METABOLISM IN THE FETUS

Since the placenta transfers only unconjugated (indirect) bilirubin, fetal bilirubin must remain in this state.[7, 31] This is facilitated by immaturity of the liver and intestine, decreased hepatic blood flow from shunting of blood away from the liver by the ductus venosus, and increased recirculation of bilirubin by the enterohepatic shunt. Hepatic uptake is reduced by very low levels of ligandin (Y carrier protein).[155] Conjugation of indirect bilirubin by the fetal liver is reduced because of immaturity of uridine diphosphoglucuronyl (UDP-glucuronyl) transferase and other liver enzyme systems and decreased hepatocyte uptake and excretion of bilirubin (Fig. 15–2). UDP-glucuronyl transferase can be detected by 16 weeks' gestation.[56, 86] Activity of this enzyme remains low in the fetus (Fig. 15–3) and is 0.1% of adult activity at 17 to 30 weeks, increasing to 1% by term.[86]

The elevated concentrations of β-glucuronide in the fetal small intestine lead to increased deconjugation of direct bilirubin with recirculation to the blood for removal by the placenta. Limited intestinal motility also promotes intestinal reabsorption of bilirubin by lengthening the time available for β-glucuronide to act.

Indirect bilirubin can be found in the amniotic fluid beginning at about 12 weeks' gestation. Amniotic fluid bilirubin levels initially rise, then decrease with increasing gestational age and essentially disappear by about 36 weeks. This pattern has been plotted on graphs used to monitor and manage the fetus in pregnancies complicated by Rh sensitization and other blood group incompatibilities.

The mechanism by which bilirubin reaches amniotic fluid is uncertain. Bilirubin may be transferred directly across placental tissue from the mother or across the amnion or umbilical cord from fetal blood vessels.[86, 105]

Bilirubin Transport and Conjugation by Hepatocytes

Cell membranes of hepatocytes have receptor sites for bilirubin. Bilirubin is also removed from albumin and transported into the hepatocyte by two intracellular carrier proteins (Y and Z) that bind organic anions (see Fig. 15–2). Protein Y (ligandin) is the major intracellular carrier protein for bilirubin. Protein Z is used when levels of bilirubin are high. Indirect bilirubin is conjugated in the smooth endoplasmic reticulum of the liver to form bilirubin monoglucuronide or diglucuronide. The major conjugation pathway involves action of the enzyme UDP-glucuronyl transferase. There are at least four forms of this liver enzyme including a bilirubin-specific form. Other forms are involved in conjugation of various drugs and hormones and may provide alternative methods for bilirubin conjugation in the immature liver.

Conjugation of each bilirubin molecule involves a two-step process and two molecules of UDP-glucuronic acid (see Fig. 15–2). In the first step the bilirubin is converted to a monoglucuronide. About two thirds of the monoglucuronides are conjugated to form diglucuronides. The glucuronyl-conjugating system is dependent on adequate supplies of glucose and oxygen for proper functioning. Most conjugated bilirubin passes into the intestines in bile and is excreted in feces. A small amount is reabsorbed in the colon and subsequently excreted in urine. The excretion of bilirubin into the biliary tree is by carrier-mediated active transport. These carriers may become saturated at high bilirubin levels. This is a rate-limiting step in clearance of bilirubin from the blood. If these carriers become saturated (as occurs with hepatocellular disorders such as hepatitis), direct hyperbilirubinemia develops.[1, 12–15, 17, 20, 28, 34]

The lipid-soluble indirect bilirubin may enter the amniotic fluid dissolved in phospholipids in tracheobronchial secretions. In animal studies serum bilirubin concentrations correlate with concentrations of bilirubin in tracheal fluid.[112] Failure of amniotic fluid bilirubin levels to decrease during gestation is associated with hemolytic disease or disorders that interfere with the normal production and turnover of amniotic fluid, such as high intestinal obstruction or anencephaly with decreased fetal swallowing (see Chapter 2).

NEONATAL PHYSIOLOGY

Before birth bilirubin clearance is handled efficiently by the placenta and mother. After birth the liver of the newborn must assume full responsibility for bilirubin metabolism. Immaturity of liver and intestinal processes for metabolism, conjugation, and excretion can result in physiologic jaundice and interact with other factors to increase the risk of neonatal hyperbilirubinemia.

Transitional Events

Cord blood bilirubin levels are normally less than 2 mg/dl and average 1.7 to 1.8 ± 0.7 mg/dl.[105] With clamping of the umbilical cord, blood flow and pressure in the venous circulation decrease, the ductus venosus constricts, and flow of relatively unoxygenated blood to the liver increases. Persistent or fluctuating patency of the ductus venosus, which occurs in some immature or ill infants, results in shunting of portal blood past the liver sinusoidal circulation, reducing the amount of blood perfusing the liver, and may interfere with normal clearance of bilirubin from the plasma.[30, 105, 155]

At birth the intestines may contain up to 200 g of meconium, which may be comprised of up to 175 mg of bilirubin. About half of this is unconjugated bilirubin and equals 5 to 10 times the daily bilirubin production rate in the term neonate. Any delay in passage of meconium through the intestinal tract increases the likelihood that conjugated bilirubin will be deconjugated (see box, p. 638) and returned to the circulation.

Studies have postulated important roles for bilirubin as an antioxidant and oxygen scavenger.[113] Highly reactive metabolites of oxygen (free radicals) are a by-product of oxidative phosphorylation. Cellular enzymes normally scavenge for and destroy these radicals before they can interfere with cell metabolic functions and destroy cell lipid membranes. Stocker and associates suggest that bilirubin may be a more potent antioxidant scavenger of peroxyl radicals than vitamin E (see Chapter 5) and may suppress oxidation of linoleic acid in cell membranes.[161] Bilirubin may help protect the fetus in moving from the lower oxygenation of the intrauterine environment to the extrauterine environment. Bilirubin has also been suggested to have a protective role in prevention of reti-

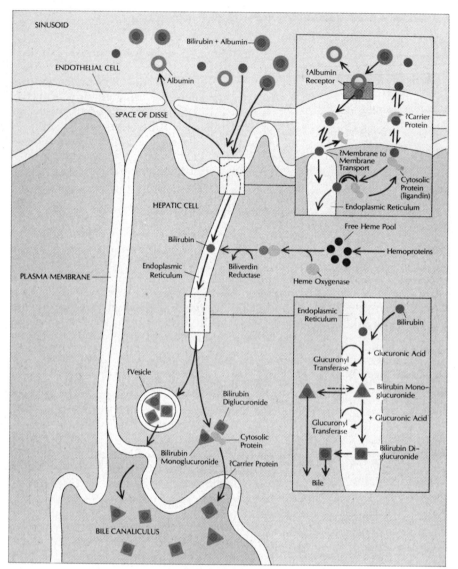

FIGURE 15–2. Transport and conjugation of bilirubin by the hepatocyte. The upper box illustrates bilirubin uptake by the hepatocyte by two proposed mechanisms: membrane-to-membrane transport or a carrier protein. The lower box illustrates proposed mechanisms for conjugation of bilirubin. (From Gollan, J.L. & Knapp, A.B. (1985). Bilirubin metabolism and congenital jaundice. *Hosp Pract, 20*(2), 87.)

nopathy of prematurity, again because of its activity in scavenging and detoxifying oxygen radicals.[15]

Bilirubin Production in the Neonate

Usual destruction of circulating red blood cells (RBCs) accounts for about 75% of the bilirubin produced in the healthy term newborn.[105] Catabolism of nonhemoglobin heme, ineffective erythropoiesis, and enterohepatic recirculation (enterohepatic shunt) account for 21 to 25% of the bilirubin produced in

the term and 30% in the preterm infant.[16, 91, 105] In newborns the amount of nonhemoglobin heme is increased by heme from the large pool of hematopoietic tissue that ceases to function after birth.[61] Bilirubin produced by catabolism of nonhemoglobin heme and immature RBCs is sometimes referred to as "early" bilirubin.[4]

The newborn produces up to 8.5 to 10 mg/kg/day of bilirubin (which is about twice as much as adults).[5, 105] Bilirubin production is inversely correlated with gestational age and remains higher (per kilogram) for 3 to 6 weeks.[5] Increased bilirubin production in

FIGURE 15–3. Developmental pattern of hepatic bilirubin UDP-glucuronyl transferase activity from fetal life to adulthood. (From Kawade, N. & Onishi, S. (1981). The prenatal and postnatal development of UDP-glucuronyl transferase activity towards bilirubin and the effect of premature birth on this activity in the human liver. *Biochem J*, 196, 257.)

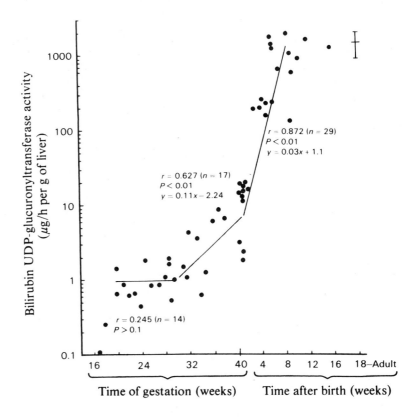

$r = 0.872 (n = 29)$
$P < 0.01$
$y = 0.03x + 1.1$

$r = 0.627 (n = 17)$
$P < 0.01$
$y = 0.11x - 2.24$

$r = 0.245 (n = 14)$
$P > 0.1$

Time of gestation (weeks)   Time after birth (weeks)

the newborn is due to a greater circulating RBC volume per kilogram (and subsequent breakdown of senescent cells), decreased RBC life span (70 to 90 versus 120 days), increased numbers of immature or fragile cells, and an increase in early bilirubin.[105]

Levels of unbound bilirubin are also higher in the newborn, and more so in the preterm infant, because of lower albumin concentrations, decreased albumin-binding capacity, and decreased affinity of albumin for bilirubin.[28, 32, 61, 142] The reasons for these alterations are unclear. There may be a maturational defect in albumin structure, or endogenous metabolic products produced during periods of stress or abnormal metabolism may block or interfere with albumin-binding sites.[31]

Physiologic Jaundice

Physiologic jaundice in the newborn is seen in 45 to 60% of term and up to 80% of preterm infants during the first days after birth.[61, 105] Visible jaundice usually appears as the bilirubin level reaches 5 to 7 mg/dl.[105, 155] Up to 90% of term infants develop bilirubin levels over 2 mg/dl in the 1st week.[105]

Patterns of Physiologic Jaundice

The usual pattern of bilirubin change is a two-phase process. During phase I bilirubin levels increase to around 6 mg/dl by the 3rd day, then gradually fall to 2 to 3 mg/dl by day 5 (Table 15–1). During phase II bilirubin remains relatively stable for several days, then gradually decreases to less than 1 mg/dl by 11 to 12 days (Fig. 15–4). In preterm infants, bilirubin follows a similar pattern, but peak concentrations are higher and rise over a longer period of time. Phase II is also altered and bilirubin levels may not fall to less than 1 mg/dl until the end of the 1st month.[105] In preterm infants mean peak concentrations reach 10 to 12 mg/dl by 5 days, then gradually fall over several weeks.[61]

Causes of Physiologic Jaundice

Physiologic jaundice is probably not caused by a single factor, but rather reflects a combination of factors related to the newborn's physiologic maturity (Table 15–2). The increased levels of circulating indirect bilirubin in the newborn are due to the combination of increased bilirubin availability and decreased clearance from the plasma. Gartner

TABLE 15–1
Clinical Parameters Associated with Jaundice in Term and Breast-fed Infants

PARAMETERS	PHYSIOLOGIC JAUNDICE IN TERM INFANTS	BREAST-FEEDING JAUNDICE	
		Early Onset	Late Onset
Age at onset (days)	1–3	3–4	4–5
Age at peak level (day)	3–4	4.5	10–15
Peak level (mg/dl)	6–12	12–20	10–30
Age when level normal (wk)	1.5–2	—	3–12
Incidence	50%	25%	2–30%

From Lascari, A.D. (1986). "Early" breast-feeding jaundice: Clinical significance. *J Pediatr, 108,* 157.

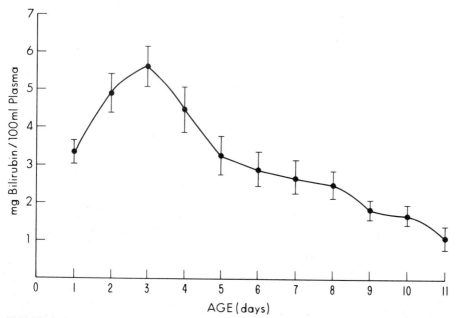

FIGURE 15–4. Changes in mean total bilirubin concentrations in 29 normal term human newborns after birth. Vertical bars represent one SE of the mean. (From Gartner, L.M., et al. (1977). Development of bilirubin transport and metabolism in the newborn rhesus monkey. *J Pediatr, 90,* 518.)

TABLE 15–2
Factors Associated with the Pathogenesis of Physiologic Jaundice

Increased bilirubin availability	Increased bilirubin production	Increased RBC
		Decreased RBC life span
		Increased early bilirubin
	Increased recirculation through the enterohepatic shunt	Increased β-glucuronidase activity
		Absent bacterial flora
		Delayed passage of meconium
Decreased clearance of bilirubin	Decreased clearance from plasma	Deficiency of carrier proteins
	Decreased hepatic metabolism	Decreased UDP-glucuronyl transferase activity

and Lee suggest that phase I bilirubin elevations are primarily due to a sixfold increase in bilirubin load, decreased bilirubin-specific hepatic UDP-glucuronyl transferase activity (see Fig. 15–3), and increased enterohepatic circulation.[61] Phase II elevations are primarily due to increased reabsorption of bilirubin by the enterohepatic shunt (see Fig. 15–1) and increased bilirubin production. Table 15–3 lists factors associated with increased bilirubin levels in newborns.

Increased bilirubin availability results from greater production (with more RBCs per kilogram), decreased RBC life span, and greater early bilirubin. Active recirculation of bilirubin by the enterohepatic shunt also raises serum indirect bilirubin levels (see box on p. 638 and Fig. 15–1). Increased recirculation of bilirubin is promoted by absent bacterial flora (which normally further metabolizes direct bilirubin for excretion in feces) and high levels of β-glucuronidase activity (which deconjugates direct bilirubin) and decreased intestinal motility.[138]

The longer direct bilirubin remains in the small intestine, the greater the likelihood it will be deconjugated. Thus, infants who are fed before 4 hours of age (versus after 24 hours) or fed more frequently and infants with meconium staining or early passage of meconium tend to have a lower incidence of physiologic jaundice.[13, 33, 39, 128, 129, 145, 186] Bottle-fed infants tend to excrete more bilirubin in their meconium during the first 3 days

after birth than breast-fed infants. Among breast-fed infants, levels tend to be lower in those who defecate more frequently.[45] Infants with delayed passage of meconium, meconium ileus, or intestinal obstructions are more likely to develop physiologic jaundice. Recirculated bilirubin puts an additional load on an already stressed and functionally immature liver.

Decreased clearance of bilirubin from the plasma and metabolism by the liver are impaired in the newborn because of deficient Y-acceptor intracellular carrier proteins (ligandin), reduced UDP-glucuronyl transferase activity, and diminished excretion by a liver overloaded with bilirubin. Levels of Y carrier proteins reach adult values by 5 days of age.

UDP-glucuronyl transferase activity is minimal during the first 24 hours after birth. Activity is lower in preterm than term infants; however, increases in activity after birth are related more to postbirth age than to gestational age. Activity of this enzyme increases rapidly after the first 24 hours but does not reach adult levels for 6 to 12 weeks (see Fig. 15–3).[86] Hypoglycemia or hypoxemia may interfere with bilirubin conjugation. Decreased liver perfusion due to persistent patency of the ductus venosus may also impede clearance of bilirubin from plasma, particularly in preterm infants.[30, 105, 155] Hypoxemia further alters blood flow to the liver and hepatocyte function. The ability

TABLE 15–3
Epidemiologic Factors Associated with the Development of Neonatal Jaundice

EFFECT ON SERUM BILIRUBIN LEVELS	FACTOR	SPECIFIC PARAMETERS
Increase	Race	Oriental, Greek, Native American
	Maternal	Diabetes, hypertension, first trimester bleeding, decreased plasma zinc level
	Drugs administered to mother	Diazepam, oxytocin (?), epidural anesthesia
	Labor and delivery	Premature rupture of membranes, forceps delivery, breech delivery, vacuum extraction
	Infant	Low birth weight, prematurity, male sex, infection, breast-feeding, increased weight loss after delivery, caloric deprivation, decreased fluid intake, delayed meconium passage, delayed cord clamping, low serum magnesium and zinc, increased cord bilirubin level
Decrease	Race	Black
	Maternal	Smoking
	Drugs administered to mother	Phenobarbital, meperidine, reserpine, aspirin, chloral hydrate, heroin, phenytoin, antipyrine, alcohol
No association	Maternal	Parity
	Drugs administered to mother	β-adrenergic agents
	Labor and delivery	Fetal distress, low Apgar scores

Modified from Maisels, M.J. (1987). Neonatal jaundice. In G.B. Avery (Ed.), *Neonatology, pathophysiology and management of the newborn* (p. 545). Philadelphia: JB Lippincott.

of the newborn's liver to excrete conjugated bilirubin may also be decreased. This may be critical in disorders with large bilirubin loads (e.g., severe erythroblastosis fetalis) and accounts for the direct hyperbilirubinemia in these infants.[105]

The preterm infant is more likely to develop physiologic jaundice and hyperbilirubinemia than the term infant. All of the factors described above that contribute to physiologic jaundice in the term infant are magnified in the preterm infant. In addition, RBC life span is related to gestational age and may be only 40 days in the very low birth weight infant. These infants often have a low caloric intake initially and slower intestinal transit time. The major factor contributing to the increased risk in the preterm infant is believed to be decreased UDP-glucuronyl transferase activity (see Fig. 15–3).[117]

CLINICAL IMPLICATIONS FOR NEONATAL CARE

Alteration in bilirubin metabolism is a relatively common event during the 1st week after birth. Physiologic jaundice, described above, occurs in 45 to 60% of term and up to 80% of preterm infants. Some of these infants also develop pathologic jaundice or hyperbilirubinemia. The risk of this disorder is increased in breast-fed infants and preterm infants. Neonatal hyperbilirubinemia is of concern because of its association with bilirubin encephalopathy or kernicterus, especially in immature or ill infants. This section addresses these issues and discusses the basis for phototherapy and other methods of managing hyperbilirubinemia.

Neonatal Hyperbilirubinemia

Neonatal hyperbilirubinemia or pathologic jaundice is usually defined as jaundice within the first 24 hours after birth or persistence of visible jaundice after 1 week of age in term infants (2 weeks in preterm infants), or bilirubin values that exceed any of the following parameters: (1) rise in total bilirubin over 5 mg/dl per day; (2) total bilirubin over 12.9 mg/dl in a term infant or over 15 mg/dl in a preterm infant; or (3) direct bilirubin over 1.5 to 2.0 mg/dl.[105] Maisels and Gifford suggest that for breast-fed infants the upper limit might more appropriately be 15 mg/

dl.[109] Bilirubin levels over 12.9 mg/dl are reported in approximately 6% and over 15 mg/dl in 3% of term infants.[31, 110] Jaundice associated with other abnormal findings such as feeding problems, irritability, hepatosplenomegaly, acidosis, or metabolic abnormalities is also of concern. A specific pathologic cause for hyperbilirubinemia is identified in only about 30% of term infants with bilirubin levels over 12.9 mg/dl.[105]

Neonatal hyperbilirubinemia is due to increased production or decreased hepatic clearance (Table 15–4) of bilirubin and occurs more frequently in immature infants. Significant hyperbilirubinemia within the first 36 hours after birth is usually due to increased production (primarily from hemolysis), since hepatic clearance is rarely altered enough during this period to produce bilirubin values over 10 mg/dl.[61, 105] An increase in the hemoglobin destruction rate by 1% leads to a fourfold increase in the bilirubin production rate.

Direct or conjugated hyperbilirubinemia (obstructive jaundice), common in adults with jaundice, is rare in the neonate. Elevations of direct bilirubin involve cholestasis and are associated with alterations in hepatic function and interference with excretion of bilirubin into bile or obstruction of bile flow in the biliary tree. In neonates this can occur with hepatitis, severe erythroblastosis, sepsis, biliary atresia, and inborn errors of metabolism including galactosemia, α_1-antitrypsin deficiency, tyrosinemia, and cystic fibrosis. Prolonged use of parenteral alimentation is also associated with conjugated hyperbilirubinemia.[120]

Measurement of Serum Bilirubin

Serum bilirubin levels are measured by laboratory and transcutaneous methods. Clinical estimations of serum bilirubin levels by the cephalopedal progression of jaundice are correlated with serum bilirubin concentrations.[20, 190] These observations only approximate actual serum bilirubin values, so laboratory assessments are also necessary. Laboratory methods involve measurement of total and direct bilirubin and calculation of indirect values. These measurements are often unreliable with wide interlaboratory variability and are influenced by hemoglobin and lipid concentrations and methods of specimen handling.[151, 153] Newer techniques, such as measurement in whole blood rather

TABLE 15-4
Causes of Neonatal Indirect Hyperbilirubinemia

BASIS	CAUSES
Increased Production of Bilirubin	
Increased hemoglobin destruction	Fetomaternal blood group incompatibility (Rh, ABO)
	Congenital RBC abnormalities
	Congenital enzyme deficiencies (G6PD, galactosemia)
	Enclosed hemorrhage (cephalhematoma, bruising)
	Sepsis
Increased amount of hemoglobin	Polycythemia (maternal-fetal or twin-twin transfusion, SGA)
	Delayed cord clamping
Increased enterohepatic circulation	Delayed passage of meconium, meconium ileus or plug
	Fasting or delayed initiation of feeding
	Intestinal atresia or stenoses
Altered Hepatic Clearance of Bilirubin	
Alteration in glucuronyl transferase production or activity	Immaturity
	Metabolic/endocrine disorders (Criglar-Najjar disease, hypothyroidism, disorders of amino acid metabolism)
Alteration in hepatic function and perfusion (and thus conjugating ability)	Asphyxia, hypoxia, hypothermia, hypoglycemia
	Sepsis (also causes inflammation)
	Drugs and hormones (novobiocin, pregnanediol)
Hepatic obstruction (associated with direct hyperbilirubinemia)	Congenital anomalies (biliary atresia, cystic fibrosis)
	Biliary stasis (hepatitis, sepsis)
	Excessive bilirubin load (often seen with severe hemolysis)

G6PD, glucose-6-phosphate dehydrogenase; RBC, red blood cell; SGA, small for gestational age.

than serum using a hematofluorometer and direct photometric measurement of bilirubin after it is complexed with an anionic polymeric mordant layer, may improve reliability.[105]

Alternatives to laboratory measurement are reference devices to assess color (icterometer) and transcutaneous measurements.[153] Transcutaneous bilirubinometry is most appropriate for screening and monitoring healthy term infants with physiologic jaundice because it avoids repeated heel sticks.[152, 189, 190] Maisels and Conrad reported a mean 95% confidence interval of 3.1 mg/dl (range, 1.96 to 3.72) in infants with bilirubin levels between 3.7 and 12.7 mg/dl.[106] This is similar to intervals reported for laboratory measurements.[105, 152]

Transcutaneous measurements provide a quantification of skin color by an arbitrary "bilirubin index." This index is obtained by measuring color as a function of light wavelength over the visible portion of the light spectrum.[105, 152] These instruments are placed over the infant's skin, and pressure is applied to blanch the skin. Light is reflected through the skin to the subcutaneous tissues and back into the instruments through fiberoptic filaments. The intensity of the yellow skin coloration is calculated within the spectrophotometric module.

Transcutaneous bilirubin is linearly related to laboratory measurements of total serum bilirubin.[47, 62, 106, 154, 169] These measurements are affected by gestation, skin color differences, and birth weight, so different standards must be used.[62, 70, 76, 152, 190] Transcutaneous measurements are also altered by phototherapy. Variations may be reduced by covering the area of the skin used for measurement by an opaque patch.[76, 105, 136, 169, 170] Other factors altering the reliability of transcutaneous bilirubin measurements include interoperator differences, using an angle other than 90 degrees between the instrument and the skin surface, the presence of unevaporated isopropyl alcohol on the probe, and exchange transfusion.[105, 152]

Management of Neonatal Hyperbilirubinemia

Various techniques have been used to manage neonates with indirect hyperbilirubinemia. Strategies have included prevention, use of pharmacologic agents, exchange transfusion, and phototherapy. Prevention has focused on early initiation of feedings and frequent breast-feedings to decrease enterohepatic shunting, promote establishment of normal bacterial flora, and stimulate intestinal activity.[13, 39, 128, 129, 145] Specific pharmacologic agents have been used to prevent hyperbilirubinemia or reduce bilirubin levels.

Pharmacologic Agents

Pharmacologic agents have been used in the management of hyperbilirubinemia to stimulate the activity of hepatic enzymes and carrier proteins, to interfere with heme degradation, or to bind bilirubin in the intestines to decrease enterohepatic reabsorption. Inert nonabsorbable substances such as charcoal and agar have been tried for the latter purpose with equivocal results and are not recommended.[87, 171]

Phenobarbital has been demonstrated to be effective in stimulating activity and concentrations of hepatic glucuronyl transferase and Y carrier proteins and may increase the number of bilirubin-binding sites.[99, 105, 180, 184] Postbirth use of phenobarbital is controversial and generally not recommended. Several days of therapy may be required before a significant change is seen, which makes postbirth use undesirable since phototherapy is effective much earlier.[170, 171] Phenobarbital has been used primarily with Rh incompatibility to reduce the number of exchange transfusions.[170] Phenobarbital is effective if given to both the pregnant woman (for at least 3 and preferably 10 days before delivery) and the newborn. Combined antenatal (over 3 days) and postnatal therapy (3 to 5 days) seems to be most effective.

Phenobarbital administration after birth results in a greater reduction in bilirubin levels in term than preterm neonates. Preterm infants at 32 weeks' gestation or less require higher doses or a longer period of treatment (at least 3 to 5 days) to effectively reduce bilirubin levels.[99] Long-term effects of this therapy are unclear.[171]

Recently prevention of hyperbilirubinemia with the use of metalloprotoporphyrins has been investigated. These substances are synthetic heme analogues. Protoporphyrin has been shown to be an effective inhibitor of heme oxygenase, the enzyme necessary for catabolism of heme to biliverdin (see Fig. 15–1) and the rate-limiting step in formation of bilirubin.[49] In animal and a few human studies, tin-protoporphyrin in particular has significantly decreased serum bilirubin levels.[37, 48, 85, 177, 178] Use with human infants in conjunction with phototherapy has been associated with phototoxic side effects such as erythema. These agents are still experimental and dosage, route of administration, safety, and clinical effectiveness have not been established.

Exchange Transfusion

Exchange transfusions are used in the management of indirect hyperbilirubinemia and hemolytic disease of the newborn. An exchange transfusion removes antibody-coated blood cells and bilirubin and helps to correct the anemia associated with hemolytic disease. A two-volume exchange replaces 85% of the circulating RBC volume and reduces the bilirubin by approximately 50%.[91] This rebounds up to 70 to 80% of previous values over the next hours as bilirubin diffuses into the vascular space from extravascular tissues. The frequency of exchange transfusions has been significantly reduced with the availability of Rho(D) immune globulin (see Chapter 10).

The type of blood used for the exchange can increase the risk of side effects. For example, citrate-phosphate-dextrose (CPD) blood may increase serum glucose, potassium, and sodium and decrease pH, chloride, and bicarbonate levels. This may lead to electrolyte abnormalities or acidosis. Elevated glucose during the exchange stimulates sulin secretion that results in rebound hypoglycemia after the exchange. These preparations may bind ionic calcium and magnesium, decreasing ionized calcium and increasing the risk of hypocalcemia. Calcium is sometimes given during an exchange transfusion to prevent hypocalcemia, although some authors have not reported an increase in the incidence of this disorder or a significant change in serum ionized calcium values when calcium is not given routinely.[105]

Blood more than 4 to 5 days old may have a decreased ability to transport oxygen. Potassium levels increase with the length of storage and may be significantly elevated in blood stored over 4 days.[6] Heparinized blood is associated with decreased glucose and transiently increased concentrations of nonesterified fatty acids. Free fatty acids compete with bilirubin for albumin-binding sites, increasing concentrations of unbound bilirubin.

Phototherapy

Phototherapy was first introduced in 1958 and has been used extensively and effectively in treating neonatal indirect hyperbilirubinemia since the late 1960s.[40,46,121] Phototherapy appears to be most effective in the first 24 to 48 hours of usage.[23]

PHYSICS OF PHOTOTHERAPY
Light reduces bilirubin by photoisomerization and photo-oxidation (Fig. 15–5). Indirect bilirubin (IXa) is composed of four pyr-

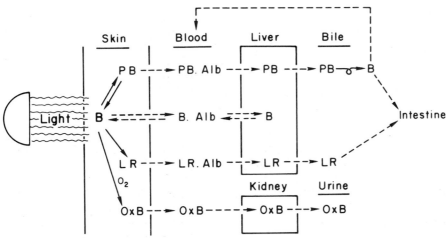

FIGURE 15–5. Mechanisms of action for phototherapy. (Chemical reactions are illustrated by solid arrows; transport processes by dotted arrows.) B, bilirubin (Z,Z isomer); PB, photobilirubin (E,E and E,Z isomers); LR, lumirubin (E and Z isomers); O x B, bilirubin oxidation products; Alb, albumin. (From McDonagh, A.F. & Lightner, D.A. (1985). "Like a shriveled blood orange": Bilirubin, jaundice and phototherapy. *Pediatrics, 75,* 452. Reproduced by permission of *Pediatrics.*)

role rings. Photoisomerization involves conversion of poorly soluble indirect bilirubin into water-soluble configurational (rearrangement of chemical groups in the molecule) or structural (rearrangement of the atoms) photoisomers (i.e., photobilirubin or lumirubin). These photoisomers can be excreted into bile without conjugation. Formation of configurational isomers, which are unstable and readily excreted in bile, is rapid, but these isomers are excreted slowly with a serum half-life of 12 to 21 hours.[52, 117] Lumirubin, a structural nonreversible isomer, is formed at a slower rate but excreted more rapidly with a serum half-life of 2 hours. Lumirubin is probably the major pathway through which bilirubin is eliminated during phototherapy.[54] Excretion of these isomers increases bile flow, which may stimulate intestinal activity and more rapid removal of bilirubin. As a result phototherapy is often more effective in infants being fed and less effective in infants who are NPO or infants with bowel obstruction.

Photo-oxidation probably has a minor role in elimination of bilirubin with phototherapy.[52] In this process the bilirubin molecule absorbs light energy from the phototherapy lights. Some of this energy is transferred to oxygen, leading to the formation of a highly reactive oxygen molecule (singlet oxygen). This molecule aids in oxidation and breakdown of bilirubin into water-soluble breakdown products such as monopyrroles and dipyrroles that are excreted primarily in urine.[117] Decomposition of bilirubin under phototherapy occurs primarily in the skin.[185]

SIDE EFFECTS OF PHOTOTHERAPY

Many concerns have been raised about the safety of phototherapy and possible short-term and long-term effects. Short-term concerns have focused on complications of photoisomerization and photo-oxidation; long-term concerns focus on irradiation damage, retinal damage, and neurodevelopmental issues.[61] Studies done in vitro and in animals have demonstrated adverse effects of phototherapy, including altered cell growth, damage to cell membranes, breaks in deoxyribonucleic acid (DNA), and alterations in hormonal and enzyme release.[10, 114, 115, 118, 158, 186] Investigations have generally failed to demonstrate any significant problems with phototherapy usage in human infants and side effects are usually transient.[148] These transient effects include thermal and metabolic changes, increased insensible water loss, altered physiologic function and weight gain, skin and ocular effects, behavioral alterations, and hormonal changes (Table 15–5).[186]

There are also a variety of psychobehavioral concerns associated with the use of phototherapy, including the potential impact of isolation and the lack of usual sensory experiences, behavioral and activity changes (including lethargy, irritability, and altered feeding behavior), and alterations in state organization and biologic rhythms as well as effects of parental stress (Table 15–5).[88, 122, 133, 134, 165] These concerns may alter parental perceptions of their infant and parent–infant interactions.

INTERMITTENT VERSUS CONTINUOUS PHOTOTHERAPY

An issue in caring for infants under phototherapy is whether to turn off the "lights" or remove the infant from under them during feeding and other caregiving. The benefits to both the infant and the parents of removing the eye shields and holding the infant during feeding seem to outweigh concerns regarding the effectiveness of bilirubin reduction.[155] Intermittent phototherapy has been shown to be effective in some studies, although other studies demonstrate increased effectiveness for continuous treatment.[97, 111, 185, 187] The most rapid catabolism of bilirubin appears to take place within the first few hours after the start of each phototherapy period. The irradiance, area of skin exposed, and initial effects of phototherapy on bilirubin in the skin seem to have more influence than whether the infant is removed for short periods of feeding or holding.[31]

EQUIPMENT ISSUES

Effective phototherapy requires sufficient illumination over an adequate area of exposed skin at a sufficiently short distance to produce the desired effect of light on bilirubin molecules.[155] Various types and configurations of light have been used with little consensus on which are best. In terms of phototherapy equipment, the irradiance of the light source (radiant power per unit area) within the therapeutic wavelength of maximum light absorbance by the bilirubin molecule (425 to 550 nm), not the intensity (i.e., illumination or brightness), determines effectiveness.[116] There is a significant linear relationship between the amount of irradiance received by

the infant and the decrease in serum bilirubin levels over a 24-hour period.[162]

The effective range for irradiance is 1 to 3 mW/cm² in the 425- to 475-nm waveband.[117] The minimum irradiance can usually be provided by 8 daylight fluorescent bulbs. Since units vary in effectiveness and light emission may decrease over time, however, irradiance levels should be monitored using the instructions in equipment manuals or unit protocol. Phototherapy units attached to radiant warmers have been reported to provide reduced and potentially ineffective irradiance because of insufficient number of bulbs and increased distance.[12] Increasing the amount of skin exposed to direct light can produce similar effects with less irradiance.

Woven fiberoptic pads (Wallaby system) have become available as an alternative method of providing phototherapy. Halogen light beams are transmitted through a cord of fiberoptic filaments to a flexible pad that is placed beneath or wrapped around the infant. These pads remain at room temperature and deliver light within the 425- to 475-nm wavelength.[52, 190] Initial reports using this equipment with term infants suggest that it is effective in reducing bilirubin levels and may be associated with fewer side effects.[58a, 120a]

For phototherapy to be effective, light photons must penetrate the skin and be absorbed by bilirubin molecules. Only certain wavelengths are absorbed by bilirubin; longer waves penetrate deeper into the skin.[52] Light wavelengths in the blue-green spectrum (425 to 550 nm) are most effective in reducing bilirubin levels. Green, daylight white, blue, and special blue (super blue) fluorescent bulbs have been used. Special blue (narrow spectrum) bulbs appear to be more effective than regular blue or daylight white bulbs. Difficulty in determining infant skin color and side effects in staff such as nausea and headaches have been reported with the use of blue bulbs. Green lights have been reported to be less effective than special blue bulbs by many but not all investigators.[1, 109, 160, 183, 188] Green light may be less effective in producing photoisomers.

Cashore identified several issues to consider in choosing a light source: What is the cost of the light bulb? How long will it maintain its irradiance? What is the energy output of the light source in the 425- to 475-nm wavelength (wavelength at which bilirubin

TABLE 15–5
Side Effects of Phototherapy

SIDE EFFECT	SPECIFIC CHANGES	IMPLICATIONS
Thermal and other metabolic changes	Increased environmental and body temperature Increased oxygen consumption Increased respiratory rate Increased skin blood flow	Influenced by maturity, caloric intake (energy to respond to thermal changes), adequacy of heat dissipation from phototherapy unit, distance of unit from infant and incubator hood (space for air flow, radiant heat loss), use of servocontrol
Fluid status	Increased peripheral blood flow	Increase fluid loss May alter uptake of IM medications
	Increased insensible water loss	Due to increases in evaporative water loss, metabolic rate, and possibly respiratory rate Influenced by environment (air flow, humidity, temperature); characteristics of phototherapy unit (heat dissipation, distance from infant); ambient temperature alteration; infant alterations in skin and core temperature, HR, RR, metabolic rate, caloric intake; type of bed (increased with radiant warmer and incubator)
Gastrointestinal function	Increased number, frequency of stools Watery, greenish-brown stools Decreased time for intestinal transit Decreased absorption; retention of nitrogen, water, electrolytes Altered lactose activity, riboflavin	May be related to increased bile flow, which stimulates GI activity Increases stool water loss Increases stool water loss and risk of dehydration Temporary lactose intolerance with decreased lactase at epithelial brush border and increased frequency and water content of stools
Altered activity	Lethargy or irritability Decreased eagerness to feed	May impact on parent–infant interaction May alter fluid and caloric intake
Altered weight gain	Decreased initially but generally catches up in 2 to 4 weeks	Due to poor feeding and increased GI losses
Ocular effects	Not documented in humans, but continued concerns about effects of light versus effects of eye patches	Lack of appropriate sensory input and stimulation Eye patches increase risk of infection, corneal abrasion, increased ICP (if too tight)
Skin changes	Tanning	Due to induction of melanin synthesis or dispersion by UV light
	Rashes	Due to injury to skin mast cells with release of histamine; erythema from UV light
	Burns	From excessive exposure to short-wave emissions from fluorescent light
	Bronze baby syndrome	Due to decreased hepatic excretion of bilirubin photodegradation by-products (especially in infants with elevated direct bilirubin)
Hormonal changes	Alterations in serum gonadotropins (increased LH and FSH)	Significance unclear May also affect circadian rhythms (unclear)
Hematologic changes	Increased rate of platelet turnover	May be a problem in infants with low platelets and sepsis
	Injury to circulating RBC with decreased potassium and increased ATP activity	May lead to hemolysis, increased energy needs
Psychobehavioral concerns	Isolation/lack of usual sensory experiences including visual deprivation	Impact can be mediated by provision of appropriate nursing care
	Alteration in state organization and neurobehavioral organization	May interfere with parent–infant interaction and increase parental stress

ATP, adenosine triphosphate; FSH, follicle-stimulating hormone; GI, gastrointestinal; HR, heart rate; ICP, intracranial pressure; IM, intramuscular; LH, luteinizing hormone; RBC, red blood cell; RR, respiratory rate; UV, ultraviolet.

maximally absorbs light)? Do the lights interfere with the ability of the staff to diagnose cyanosis?[27] Considerations regarding phototherapy equipment are summarized in Table 15–6.

Breast-Feeding and Neonatal Jaundice

Older studies tended to demonstrate no difference in bilirubin levels between breast-fed and bottle-fed infants.[14, 20, 41, 108, 160] Recent investigations with larger sample sizes have shown clear differences in patterns of bilirubin production between these groups of infants.[7, 80, 84, 105, 109, 128, 147, 150] Breast-fed infants are significantly more likely to develop hyperbilirubinemia than bottle-fed infants. The increased incidence of hyperbilirubinemia in the United States over the past 25 years has been attributed to the increase in breast-feeding.[109] Approximately 80% of infants with hyperbilirubinemia for which no specific cause can be found are breast-fed.[108]

Two forms of neonatal jaundice are seen in breast-fed infants: early and late onset (see Table 15–1). The early form (also referred to as breast–feeding–related jaundice) is believed to be related to the process of feeding, the late form to attributes of breast milk that interfere with normal conjugation and excretion.[50] Breast-fed infants have significantly higher bilirubin levels at 3 to 4 days of age (mean difference of 1.6 mg/dl), and greater numbers of these infants have bilirubin values over 12 mg/dl (12.1% versus 3.6%).[109] This pattern generally does not require any treatment. Although the cause of this form of jaundice is unknown, it is believed to be related to inadequate caloric or fluid intake and decreased frequency of feedings.[96] This may increase enterohepatic reabsorption of bilirubin.

Breast-fed infants also develop a late-onset, prolonged hyperbilirubinemia. This syndrome is seen in approximately 1 in 100 to 200 breast-fed infants.[50, 61] Late-onset jaundice is characterized by increasing bilirubin levels from day 4 on, peaking at 10 to 30 mg/dl by 10 to 15 days, followed by a slow decrease in bilirubin values to normal limits over the next 3 to 12 weeks. If breast-feeding is interrupted for 48 hours, bilirubin levels fall rapidly, followed by a slight increase (1 to 3 mg/dl) with resumption of nursing.[61] These infants do not have any signs of hemolysis or abnormal liver function.

The cause of late-onset jaundice in breast-fed infants is unknown but has been attributed to the presence of 3-α-20-β-pregnanediol in breast milk (which may interfere with UDP-glucuronyl transferase activity or release of conjugated bilirubin from the hepatocyte); increased breast milk lipoprotein lipase activity with subsequent release of free fatty acids in the intestines; inhibition of conjugation by the increased amounts of unsaturated fatty acids such as palmitic, stearic, oleic, and linoleic acid found in breast milk; or β-glucuronidase or other factors in breast

TABLE 15–6
Equipment Considerations with Phototherapy

PARAMETER	CONSIDERATIONS
Energy output	Irradiance of light source, not light intensity (i.e., illumination or brightness), determines effectiveness
Irradiance levels	Effective range: 4 to 9 μW/cm²/nm
Distance of light from infant	Amount of radiant energy delivered to infant is related to distance (increasing distance decreases irradiance, i.e., a twofold increase in distance produces a fourfold decrease in irradiance); generally lights should be 40 to 50 cm above infant
Wavelength	Bilirubin absorbs light maximally over wavelengths of 425 to 475 nm (450 to 470 nm may be safest and most effective)
Ultraviolet irradiation	Reduced by placing a Plexiglas shield (¼″ thick) between light source and infant
Electrical hazards	Phototherapy units should be checked regularly for grounding and electrical leakage
Effectiveness	Light emission may decrease over time, therefore monitor energy levels (irradiance) in the effective wavelength range and replace bulbs as recommended by the manufacturer
Thermal hazards	Reduce risk for overheating or hyperthermia by monitoring of infant thermal status and maintaining a space of about 2″ between the incubator hood and lamp cover to allow free flow of air Risk of overheating is increased in infants in radiant warmers with three-sided lights since these prevent radiant heat loss
Alteration in blood samples	Phototherapy off while blood for bilirubin values is drawn

milk that may increase enterohepatic shunting.[3, 20, 59, 61, 65, 73, 74, 105, 137, 139, 140] Inhibition of conjugation by the increased amounts of free fatty acids that are released in the duodenum of breast-fed infants may occur as these fatty acids are absorbed into the circulation. When fatty acids reach the liver, they may inhibit glucuronyl transferase activity or saturate the hepatic protein carrier system.[44, 122] In vitro levels of free fatty acids are increased in milk stored over 3 to 5 days or frozen.[123, 124]

Prevention of Early-Onset Jaundice in Breast-fed Infants

Early-onset jaundice may be prevented or reduced by early initiation of breast-feeding, increasing frequency of feeding, and early passage of meconium (colostrum acts as a laxative). Infants fed in the first 1 to 3 hours after birth pass meconium sooner than infants fed after 4 hours.[13] Feeding stimulates the gastrocolonic reflex, increases intestinal motility, and stimulates meconium passage. This removes conjugated bilirubin from the small intestine, thus reducing the likelihood that this bilirubin will be recirculated by the enterohepatic shunt.

A critical factor in reducing the risk of jaundice in breast-fed infants seems to be enhancing breast milk intake. Bilirubin levels in these infants tend to correlate negatively with breast milk intake, that is, as intake decreases, bilirubin levels tend to rise. Supplemental feedings with dextrose and water have been found to decrease breast milk intake and increase bilirubin levels in these infants by 4 to 6 days of age.[93, 98, 124] Supplementation with dextrose and water feedings may satiate the infant but lead to inadequate caloric intake; caloric deprivation increases bilirubin levels.[128] Use of supplementation was also associated with a significant decrease in the number of infants still breast-feeding at 3 months.[78] Use of any form of supplementation can alter intake of breast milk and establishment of the mother's milk supply (see Chapter 4). A linear relationship between the number of feedings per day and bilirubin levels has been reported.[44, 45] Bilirubin levels were lowest in infants who were breast-fed more than eight times in 24 hours during the first 3 days after birth. Increasing the frequency of feedings may stimulate gut motility and decrease intestinal absorption of bilirubin.[44, 127]

Management of Jaundice in Breast-fed Infants

Management of jaundice in breast-fed infants is often problematic. Multiple issues and concerns, including maternal desire to breast-feed, advantages of breast-feeding to both mother and infant, effects on maternal-infant interaction, parental stress with the potential for bilirubin toxicity, and legal implications related to "safe" (and possibly artificial) bilirubin values, must be balanced.[20, 61] Maisels notes that no cases of overt bilirubin encephalopathy have been documented in healthy term infants, but also acknowledges that no studies have been done.[105] He recommends that if bilirubin levels reach 16 to 17 mg/dl in an otherwise healthy term infant, breast-feeding be interrupted for 48 hours and the infant fed formula. Although this is difficult, he suggests that interruption of breast-feeding at this point may prevent the need for phototherapy and its associated side effects and reduce the number of heel sticks. Amato and associates report no difference in the time needed to reduce bilirubin levels with jaundice managed by discontinuing breast-feeding versus the use of phototherapy and continued nursing.[2]

Lawrence emphasizes a more proactive approach, focusing on prevention and modifying factors, particularly inadequate frequency of feeding, that are associated with early-onset jaundice in breast-fed infants (Table 15–7).[98] Interruption of breast-feeding must be accompanied by strong parental

TABLE 15–7
Management Outline for Early Jaundice While Breast-feeding

1. Monitor all infants for initial stooling. Consider stimulating stooling if no stool in 24 hours.
2. Initiate breast-feeding early and frequently. Frequent short feeding more effective than infrequent prolonged feeding, although total time may be the same.
3. Discourage water, dextrose water, or formula substitutes.
4. Monitor weight, voidings, stooling in association with breast-feeding pattern.
5. When bilirubin level approaches 15 mg/dl, augment feeds, stimulate breast milk production with pumping, and use phototherapy if this aggressive tack fails.
6. There is no evidence that early jaundice is associated with an "abnormality" of the breast milk, therefore withdrawing breast milk as a trial is only indicated if jaundice persists longer than 6 days or rises above 15 mg/dl or the mother has a history of a previously affected infant.

Modified from Lawrence, R.A. (1989). *Breastfeeding: A guide for the medical profession* (3rd ed., p. 357). St. Louis: CV Mosby.

emotional support and facilitation of breast pumping or manual expression of milk. Elander and Lindberg measured maternal stress with urinary cortisol levels.[50] They found that separating the mother and infant for phototherapy increased both maternal stress and the likelihood that she would stop breast-feeding.

Competition for Albumin Binding

Most indirect bilirubin is transported in plasma bound to albumin (1 g albumin binds 8.5 to 10 mg of bilirubin).[90, 125] Two terms used to describe albumin binding are capacity and affinity. Each molecule of albumin has a certain number of binding sites available (the binding capacity). The tightness by which bilirubin is bound to sites available for binding is the affinity.

The binding sites may be primary (tight or high affinity) or secondary (weak affinity). Each albumin molecule is believed to have one primary binding site and one or more secondary sites. If the primary site is saturated, there is a rapid increase in loosely bound or free bilirubin.[105] Unbound bilirubin can leave the vascular system and enter the brain and other organs. Various techniques have been developed to measure albumin binding of bilirubin but none of them are acceptable for widespread clinical management in terms of either application or interpretation.[31, 61, 105]

Bilirubin bound to secondary sites is easily displaced by competing substances. Drugs such as sulfonamides, salicylate, furosemide, certain x-ray contrast substances, and sodium benzoate (a preservative used in multiple injection vials for drugs such as diazepam and plasma expanders) may displace bilirubin.[18, 22, 31] The actions of many drugs used in neonates in competing with bilirubin for binding sites have not been well studied. Oxytocin use for labor induction has also been reported to increase the risk of subsequent hyperbilirubinemia in the neonate.[25, 26, 83, 156] In several of these studies the oxytocin-induced groups contained less mature infants and if maturity was controlled for, differences were minimal or nonexistent.[33, 94, 105]

Albumin binding of bilirubin can be altered by pathologic events. Plasma free fatty acids compete with bilirubin for albumin-binding sites.[130] Hypothermia increases metabolism and catabolism of fatty acids, which

may displace bilirubin from albumin. Concerns have been raised about risks with the use of emulsified lipid solutions (e.g., Intralipid) in neonates.[157, 166] Spear and associates reported that doses below 1 g/kg every 15 hours had no significant effect on bilirubin levels, but at higher levels, increased doses were correlated with increased levels of free fatty acids and decreased binding of bilirubin, especially in preterm infants.[157] The amount of unbound indirect bilirubin may also be increased if there is more bilirubin than available albumin because of excess production of bilirubin or decreased albumin (e.g., with malnourishment). Acidosis decreases the affinity of albumin for bilirubin, thus increasing levels of unbound bilirubin.[32, 92, 105]

Bilirubin Encephalopathy

Development of bilirubin encephalopathy, commonly called kernicterus, is a concern for any infant with elevated bilirubin levels. Bilirubin encephalopathy involves permanent brain damage secondary to deposition of bilirubin in brain cells, with yellow staining and neuronal necrosis. Although the specific toxic effect is uncertain, acidic forms of bilirubin act as mitochondrial poisons that uncouple oxidative phosphorylation in the mitochondria, interfering with cellular respiration, blocking adenosine triphosphate (ATP) production, inhibiting cellular enzymes, and altering water and electrolyte transport.[19, 29, 31, 105, 131, 183, 191] Areas of the brain most often affected include the basal ganglia, hippocampal cortex, and subthalamic cerebellar nuclei. Some infants (30 to 50%) also have extraneural lesions, primarily in the renal tubular cells and gastrointestinal system.[61, 71]

Early signs of bilirubin encephalopathy include progressive lethargy, poor feeding, vomiting, temperature instability, hypotonia, and a high-pitched cry.[79] Many infants, particularly those born prematurely, are asymptomatic in the neonatal period. Later signs include ataxia, opisthotonos, deafness, seizures, and, less frequently, mental retardation.[31, 61, 117] These so-called "classic" findings of kernicterus are rarely seen today. Bilirubin encephalopathy has been implicated in the minimal brain damage, hearing loss, and learning problems found in follow-up of preterm infants, however.[71] Serum bilirubin levels have also been correlated with sensorineural hearing impairment, especially in low

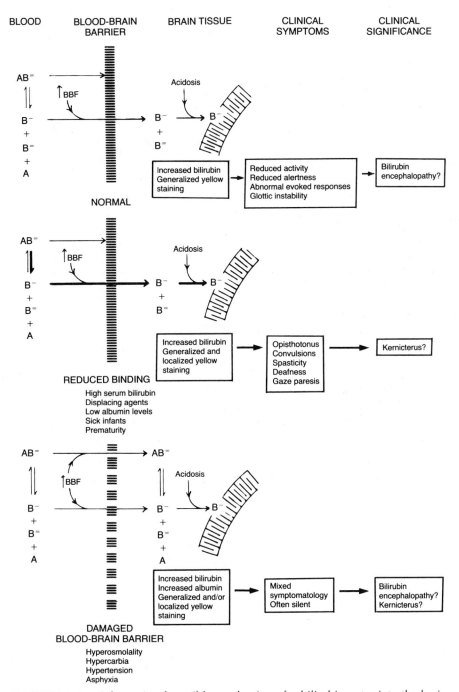

FIGURE 15–6. Schematic of possible mechanisms for bilirubin entry into the brain and binding to neuronal cell membranes. The different factors affecting this process are also indicated. A, albumin; AB=, albumin–bilirubin complex; B⁻, bilirubin monoanion; B=, bilirubin dianion; BBF, brain blood flow. (From Bratlid, D. (1990). How bilirubin gets into the brain. *Clin Perinatol, 17,* 460.)

birth weight infants.[42] The neurotoxic effects of bilirubin are exacerbated by other pathologic conditions such as hypoxia, asphyxia, and hypercapnia.[165]

Current theories regarding the mechanisms by which bilirubin passes into neural tissue include the free bilirubin theory and opening of the blood–brain barrier hypothesis.[17, 117] For many years bilirubin encephalopathy was believed to be caused by passage of unbound indirect bilirubin across the blood–brain barrier (free bilirubin theory) with deposition of this fat-soluble form of bilirubin in the basal ganglia and other areas of the brain with a high lipid content. Some bilirubin does cross into the brain, but is not considered harmful.[17] More recently a hypothesis was proposed suggesting that reversible alterations ("opening") in the blood–brain barrier (caused by infection, dehydration, hyperosmolality, or hypoxemia) allow entry of albumin-bound bilirubin as well (Fig. 15–6).[16, 31]

The critical level of bilirubin beyond which brain damage occurs is not certain. Indications for exchange transfusion have used bilirubin levels of 20 mg/dl in term infants (and 15 mg/dl or lower in preterm infants) as critical levels for many years. Bilirubin levels of 20 mg/dl are used as an upper level for exchange transfusion for legal reasons ("vigintiphobia").[181] Most studies report no adverse effects of elevated bilirubin levels in healthy term infants.[121, 123, 146, 171] Lower (less than 20 mg/dl) bilirubin values are not "safe" for all infants, since pathologic changes associated with bilirubin encephalopathy have clearly been demonstrated on autopsy at much lower values.[28, 105, 141] Factors associated with the greatest risk for developing kernicterus at lower bilirubin levels are prematurity, respiratory distress syndrome, hypoxia, and acidosis.[31, 92] Maximum serum total bilirubin levels have been correlated with neurodevelopmental outcome in preterm infants.[172] Newer techniques to assess risks of hyperbilirubinemia include brain stem auditory evoked response and cry analysis.[175, 176]

MATURATIONAL CHANGES DURING INFANCY AND CHILDHOOD

The bilirubin load tends to remain higher in infants for 3 to 6 weeks after birth. Bilirubin-specific UDP-glucuronyl transferase activity increases to adult values by 6 to 12 weeks of age (see Fig. 15–3).[86]

SUMMARY

Alterations in bilirubin metabolism that occur with birth result in one of the more frequent problems seen in the neonate, physiologic jaundice. These changes also interact with pathologic factors in the development of hyperbilirubinemia. Hyperbilirubinemia is of concern because it may be a sign of underlying pathologic processes, such as hemolysis or sepsis, and may lead to adverse conse-

TABLE 15–8
Summary of Recommendations for Clinical Practice Related to Bilirubin Metabolism: Neonate

---

Know substances and pathophysiologic events that may compete with bilirubin for albumin-binding sites and monitor status of exposed infants (p. 652).

Know usual cord blood values for serum bilirubin (p. 639).

Know usual patterns for serum bilirubin in the term and preterm neonate, and breast-fed infants (pp. 640–644, 650–652, Table 15–1, Figure 15–4).

Recognize infants at risk for physiologic jaundice (pp. 641–644, Tables 15–2 and 15–3).

Monitor fluid intake and stooling patterns (pp. 641–644).

Assess and monitor infants at risk for physiologic jaundice (pp. 641–644).

Recognize infants at risk for hyperbilirubinemia (pp. 644–645, Table 15–4).

Assess and monitor infants at risk for hyperbilirubinemia (pp. 644–645, Table 15–4).

Know methods of monitoring serum bilirubin levels and factors that can alter accuracy of measurement (pp. 644–645).

Monitor infants during and after exchange transfusion for alterations in fluid, electrolyte, and acid–base status (p. 646).

Recognize and monitor for physiologic and psychobehavioral side effects associated with phototherapy (pp. 647–648, Table 15–5).

Provide a safe environment for the infant under phototherapy (pp. 647–649, Tables 15–5 and 15–6).

Counsel and support the family of a jaundiced infant (pp. 647–648, 651–652, Table 15–5).

Monitor breast-fed infants for early and late hyperbilirubinemia (pp. 650–652).

Institute interventions to prevent early-onset jaundice in breast-fed infants (pp. 651–652, Table 15–7).

Counsel and support parents of a jaundiced breast-fed infant (pp. 651–652).

Recognize infants at risk for bilirubin encephalopathy (pp. 652–653).

Monitor for signs of bilirubin encephalopathy (pp. 652–653).

Page numbers in parentheses following each intervention refer to page(s) in the text where the rationale for that intervention is discussed.

quences, namely kernicterus. Therefore it is essential for caregivers to appreciate the processes involved in bilirubin metabolism and its maturation to understand the basis for physiologic jaundice and hyperbilirubinemia and to recognize infants at risk for these disorders. Clinical recommendations are summarized in Table 15–8.

REFERENCES

1. Amanuliah, A. (1976). Neonatal jaundice. *Am J Dis Child, 130,* 1274.
2. Amato, M., Howald, H., & van Murah, G. (1985). Interruption of breastfeeding versus phototherapy as treatment of hyperbilirubinemia in full term infants. *Helv Paediatr Acta, 40,* 127.
3. Arias, I., et al. (1964). Prolonged neonatal unconjugated hyperbilirubinemia associated with breastfeeding and a steroid pregnane–3α, 20β-diol in maternal milk that inhibits glucuronide formation in vitro. *J Clin Invest, 43,* 2037.
4. Arias, I.M. (1968). Formation of bile pigment. In *Handbook of Physiology* (Section 7, p. 2347). Washington, D.C.: American Physiological Society.
5. Bartoletti, A.L., et al. (1979). Pulmonary excretion of carbon monoxide in the human infant as an index of bilirubin production. I. Effects of gestational age and postnatal age and some common neonatal abnormalities. *J Pediatr, 94,* 952.
6. Batton, D.G., Maisels, M.J., & Schulman, G. (1983). Serum potassium changes following packed red cell transfusion in newborn infants. *Transfusion, 23,* 163.
7. Bergstein, N.A.M. (1973). *Liver and pregnancy.* Amsterdam: Excerpta Medica.
8. Berk, P.D., et al. (1974). Comparison of plasma bilirubin turnover and carbon monoxide production in man. *J Lab Clin Med, 83,* 29.
9. Bernstein, R.B., et al. (1969). Bilirubin metabolism in the fetus. *J Clin Invest, 48,* 1678.
10. Bhatia, J., Mims, L.C., & Rosel, R.A. (1980). The effect of phototherapy on animo acid solutions containing multivitamins. *J Pediatr, 96,* 284.
11. Blanco, J.D. (1987). Gastrointestinal problems and jaundice. In C.J. Pauerstein (Ed.), *Clinical Obstetrics* (pp. 703–716). New York: John Wiley & Sons.
12. Bonta, B.W. & Warshaw, J.B. (1976). Importance of radiant flux in the treatment of hyperbilirubinemia: Failure of overhead phototherapy units in intensive care units. *Pediatrics, 57,* 502.
13. Boyer, D.B. & Vidyasagar, D. (1987). Serum indirect bilirubin levels and meconium passage in early fed normal newborns. *Nurs Res, 36,* 174.
14. Boylan, P. (1976). Oxytocin and neonatal jaundice. *Br Med J, 3,* 564.
15. Bracci, R., et al. (1988). Neonatal hyperbilirubinemia: Evidence for a role of the erythrocyte enzyme activities involved in the detoxification of oxygen radicals. *Acta Paediatr Scand, 77,* 349.
16. Bratlid, D. (1985). The importance of blood-brain barrier function on bilirubin transfer from plasma to brain: An animal study. In L. Stern, M. Xanthou, & B. Friis-Hansen (Eds.), *Physiologic foundations of perinatal care* (pp. 136–147). New York: Praeger.
17. Bratlid, D. (1990). How bilirubin gets into the brain. *Clin Perinatol, 17,* 449.
18. Broderson, R. (1978). Free bilirubin in blood plasma of the newborn: Effects of albumin, fatty acids, pH, displacing drugs, and phototherapy. In L Stern, W. Oh, & B. Friis-Hansen (Eds.), *Intensive care of the newborn, II* (pp. 331–345). New York: Masson Publishing.
19. Brodersen, R. & Robertson A. (1983). Chemistry of bilirubin and its interaction with albumin. In *Hyperbilirubinemia in the newborn, report of the 85th Ross Conference on pediatric research* (pp. 91–101). Columbus, OH: Ross Laboratories.
20. Brooten, D., et al. (1985). Breast-milk jaundice. *J Obstet Gynecol Neonatal Nurs, 13,* 220.
21. Brown, A. (1976). Bilirubin metabolism in fetus and newborn. In C.A. Smith & N.M. Nelson (Eds.), *The physiology of the newborn infant* (pp. 312–353). Springfield, IL: Charles C Thomas.
22. Brown, A.K., Kim, M.H., & Bryla, D. (1983). Report on the NIH Cooperative Study of Phototherapy: Efficacy of phototherapy in controlling hyperbilirubinemia and preventing kernicterus. In *Hyperbilirubinemia in the newborn, report of the 85th Ross Conference on pediatric research* (pp. 55–63). Columbus, OH: Ross Laboratories.
23. Brown, A.K., et al.(1985). Efficacy of phototherapy in prevention and management of neonatal hyperbilirubinemia. *Pediatrics 75*(Suppl.), 393.
24. Brown, W.R., Grodsky, G.M., & Carbone, J.V. (1965). Intracellular distribution of tritiated bilirubin during hepatic uptake and excretion. *Am J Physiol, 207,* 1237.
25. Buchan, P.C. (1979). Pathogenesis of neonatal hyperbilirubinemia after induction of labour with oxytocin. *Br Med J, 2,* 1255.
26. Calder, A.A., et al. (1974). Increased bilirubin levels in neonates after induction of labour by intravenous prostaglandin E2 or oxytocin. *Lancet, 2,* 1339.
27. Cashore, W.J. (1983). Neonatal hyperbilirubinemia. In R.A. Polin & F.D. Burg (Eds.), *Workbook in practical neonatology* (p. 80). Philadelphia: WB Saunders.
28. Cashore, W.J. & Oh, W. (1982). Unbound bilirubin and kernicterus in low birthweight infants. *Pediatrics, 69,* 481.
29. Cashore, W.J. (1990). The neurotoxicity of bilirubin. *Clin Perinatol, 17,* 437.
30. Cashore, W.J. & Stern, L. (1984). The management of hyperbilirubinemia. *Clin Perinatol, 11,* 339.
31. Cashore, W.J. & Stern, L. (1987). Neonatal hyperbilirubinemia. In L. Stern & P. Vert (Eds.), *Neonatal medicine* (pp. 791–808). New York: Masson.
32. Cashore, W.J., et al. (1977). Influence of gestational age and clinical status on bilirubin-binding capacity in newborn infants. *Am J Dis Child, 131,* 898.
33. Clarkson, J.E., et al. (1984). Jaundice in full term healthy neonates—A population study. *Aust Paediatr J, 20,* 303.
34. Cohen, A.N. & Ostrow, J.D. (1980). New concepts in phototherapy: Photoisomerization of bilirubin IX alpha and potential toxic effects of light. *Pediatrics, 65,* 740.
35. Cole, A. & Hargreaves, T. (1972). Conjugation inhibitors and early neonatal hyperbilirubinemia. *Am J Dis Child, 47,* 415.
36. Connolly, A.M. & Volpe, J.J. (1990). Clinical features of bilirubin encephalopathy. *Clin Perinatol, 17,* 371.
37. Cornelius, C.E. & Rogers, P.A. (1984). Prevention

of neonatal hyperbilirubinemia in rhesus monkeys by tin-protoporphyrin. *Pediatr Res, 18,* 728.

38. Cotton, D.B., Brock, B.J., & Schifrin, B.S. (1981). Cirrhosis and fetal hyperbilirubinemia. *Obstet Gynecol, 57,* 25s.

39. Cottrell, B.H. & Anderson, G.C. (1984). Rectal or axillary temperature measurement: Effect on plasma bilirubin level and intestinal transit of meconium. *J Pediatr Gastroenterol Nutr, 3,* 734.

40. Cremer, R.J., Perryman, P.W., & Richards, D.H. (1958). Influence of light on the hyperbilirubinemia of infants. *Lancet, 1,* 1094.

41. Dahms, B.B., et al. (1973). Breast feeding and serum bilirubin values during the first four days of life. *J Pediatr, 83,* 1049.

42. de Vries, L.S., et al. (1987). Relationship of serum bilirubin levels and hearing impairment in newborn infants. *Early Human Dev, 15,* 269.

43. De Carvalho, M., Holl, M., & Harvey, D. (1981). Effects of water supplementation on physiological jaundice in breastfed babies. *Am J Dis Child, 56,* 568.

44. De Carvalho, M., Klaus, M., & Merkatz, R.B. (1982). Frequency of breast-feeding and serum bilirubin concentration. *Am J Dis Child, 136,* 737.

45. De Carvalho, M., Robertson, S., & Klaus, M. (1985). Fecal bilirubin excretion and serum bilirubin concentrations in breast-fed and bottle-fed infants. *J Pediatr, 107,* 786.

46. Dobbs R.H. & Cremer, R.J. (1975). Phototherapy (looking back). *Arch Dis Child, 50,* 833.

47. Douville, P., Masson, M., & Forest, J. (1983). Diagnostic value of sequential readings with a Minolta transcutaneous bilirubinometer in normal and low-birthweight infants. *Clin Chem, 29,* 740.

48. Drummond, G.S. & Kappas, A. (1982). Chemoprevention of neonatal jaundice: Potency of tin-protoporphyrin in an animal model. *Science, 217,* 1250.

49. Drummond, G.S. & Kappas, A. (1981). Prevention of neonatal hyperbilirubinemia by tin-protoporphyrin IX, a potent competitive inhibitor of heme oxidation. *Proc Natl Acad Sci, 78,* 6466.

50. Elander, G. & Lindberg, T. (1986). Hospital routines in infants with hyperbilirubinemia influence the duration of breastfeeding. *Acta Paediatr Scand, 75,* 708.

51. Ennever, J.F. (1988). Phototherapy for neonatal jaundice. *Photochem Photobiol, 47,* 871.

52. Ennever, J.F. (1990). Blue light, green light, white light, more light: Treatment of neonatal jaundice. *Clin Perinatol, 17,* 467.

53. Ennever, J.F., McDonagh, A.F., & Speck, W.T. (1983). Phototherapy for neonatal jaundice: Optimal wavelengths of light. *J Pediatr, 103,* 295.

54. Ennever, J.F., et al. (1987). Rapid clearance of structural isomer of bilirubin during phototherapy. *J Clin Invest, 79,* 1671.

55. Fallon, H.J. (1988). Liver diseases. In G.N. Burrow & T.F. Ferris (Eds.), *Medical complications during pregnancy* (3rd ed., pp. 318–344). Philadelphia: WB Saunders.

56. Felsher, B.F., et al. (1978). Reduced hepatic bilirubin uridine diphosphate glucuronyl transferase and uridine diphosphate glucose dehydrogenase activity in the human fetus. *Pediatr Res, 12,* 838.

57. Fleischner, G.M. & Arias, I.M. (1976). Structure and function of ligandin and Z protein in the liver: A progressive report. In H. Popper & F. Schaffner

(Eds.), *Progress in Liver Disease.* New York: Grune & Stratton.

58. Foerder, B. (1987). Neonatal jaundice: Effects on development to age two years. *Commun Nurs Res, 20,* 38.

58a. Gale, R., et al. (1990). A randomized, controlled application of the Wallaby phototherapy system compared with standard phototherapy. *J Perinatol, 10,* 239.

59. Gartner, L.M. (1983). Breast milk jaundice. In *Hyperbilirubinemia in the newborn, report of the 85th Ross Conference on pediatric research* (pp. 75–91). Columbus, OH: Ross Laboratories.

60. Gartner, L.M. & Arias, I.M. (1969). Formation, transport, metabolism and excretion of bilirubin. *N Engl J Med, 280,* 1339.

61. Gartner, L.M. & Lee, K-S. (1978). Unconjugated hyperbilirubinemia. In A.A. Fanaroff & R.J. Martin (Eds.), *Neonatal-perinatal medicine, Diseases of the fetus and infant* (pp. 946–965). St. Louis: CV Mosby.

62. Goldman, S.L., Penalver, A., & Penaranda, R. (1982). Jaundice meter: Evaluation of new guidelines. *J Pediatr, 101,* 253.

63. Gollan, J.L. & Knapp, A.B. (1985). Bilirubin metabolism and congenital jaundice. *Hosp Pract, 20*(2), 83.

64. Goodlin, R. & Lloyd, D. (1968). Fetal tracheal excretion of bilirubin. *Biol Neonate, 12,* 1.

65. Gourley, G.R. & Arend, R.A. (1986). Beta-glucuronidase and hyperbilirubinemia in breast-fed and formula-fed babies. *Lancet, 22,* 644.

66. Grodsky, G.M., et al. (1970). The effect of age on rate of development of hepatic carriers for bilirubin: A possible explanation for physiologic jaundice and hyperbilirubinemia in the newborn. *Metabolism, 19,* 246.

67. Gutcher, G. (1981). Breast milk jaundice: An evolving tale. *Wis Med J, 80,* 26.

68. Guyton, A.C. (1987). *Textbook of medical physiology* (7th ed.). Philadelphia: WB Saunders.

69. Hammerman, C., et al. (1981). Comparative measurements of phototherapy: A practical guide. *Pediatrics, 67,* 368.

70. Hanneman, R.E., et al. (1982). Evaluation of the Minolta bilirubin meter as a screening device in white and black infants. *Pediatrics, 69,* 107.

71. Hansen, T.W.R. & Bratlid, D. (1986). Bilirubin and brain toxicity. *Acta Paediatr Scand, 75,* 513.

72. Hargreaves, T. (1970). Breast milk jaundice. *Br Med J, 3,* 647.

73. Hargreaves, T. (1973). Effect of fatty acids on bilirubin conjugation. *Am J Dis Child, 48,* 446.

74. Hargreaves, T. & Piper, R.F. (1971). Breast milk jaundice: Effect of inhibitory breast milk on 3α,20β-pregnanediol on glucuronyl transferase. *Am J Dis Child, 46,* 145.

75. Hegyi, T. (1986). Transcutaneous bilirubinometry in the newborn: State of the art. *J Clin Monitoring, 2,* 53.

76. Hegyi, T., Hiatt, I.M., & Indyk, L. (1982). Transcutaneous bilirubinometry: I. Correlations in term infants. *J Pediatr, 98,* 454.

77. Heirwegh, K.P.M. & Brown, S.B. (1982). *Bilirubin, Vol. 2: Metabolism.* Boca Raton, FL: CRC Press.

78. Herrera, H.A. (1984). Supplemented versus unsupplemented breastfeeding. *Perinatol Neonatol, 8*(3), 70.

79. Hung K.-L. (1989). Auditory brainstem responses

in patients with neonatal hyperbilirubinemia and bilirubin encephalopathy. *Brain Dev, 11,* 297.

80. Indyk. L. (1976). Physical aspects of phototherapy. In D. Bergsma & S.H. Blondheim (Eds.), *Bilirubin metabolism in the newborn* (Vol. 2). New York: Elsevier.

81. Ives, N.K., et al. (1988). The effects of bilirubin on brain energy metabolism during normoxia and hypoxia: An in vitro study using 31P nuclear magnetic resonance spectroscopy. *Pediatr Res, 23,* 569.

82. Jacques, S.G., Wessling, C., & Larson, E. (1985). Phototherapy in neonates. *Neonatal Network, 3*(4), 50.

83. Jeffaries, M.J. (1977). A multifactorial survey of neonatal jaundice. *Br J Obstet Gynaecol, 84,* 452.

84. Johnson, C.A., Lieberman, B., & Hassanein, R.E. (1985). The relationship of breastfeeding to third-day bilirubin levels. *J Fam Pract, 20,* 147.

85. Kappas, A., et al. (1988). Sn-Protoporphyrin use in the management of hyperbilirubinemia in term newborns with direct Coombs-positive ABO incompatibility. *Pediatrics, 81,* 485.

86. Kawade, N. & Onishi, S. (1981). The prenatal and postnatal development of UDP-glucuronyl transferase activity towards bilirubin and the effect of premature birth on this activity in the human liver. *Biochem J, 196,* 257.

87. Kemper, K., Horowitz, R.I., & McCarthy, P. (1988). Decreased neonatal serum bilirubin with plain agar: A meta-analysis. *Pediatrics, 82,* 631.

88. Kemper, K., Forsyth, B., & McCarthy, P. (1989). Jaundice, terminating breast feeding, and the vulnerable child. *Pediatrics, 84,* 773.

89. Kivlahan, C. & James, E.J.P. (1984). The natural history of neonatal jaundice. *Pediatrics, 74,* 364.

90. Klatskin, G. & Bungards, L. (1956). Bilirubin-protein linkage and their relationship to the Van den Berg reaction. *J Clin Invest, 35,* 537.

91. Korones, S.B. (1986). *High-risk newborn infants: The basis for intensive nursing care* (4th ed.). St. Louis: CV Mosby.

92. Kozuki, K., et al. (1979). Increase in bilirubin binding to albumin with correction of neonatal acidosis. *Acta Paediatr Scand, 68,* 213.

93. Kuhr, M. & Paneth, N. (1982). Feeding practices and early neonatal jaundice. *J Pediatr Gastroenterol Nutr, 1,* 485.

94. Lange, A.P., et al. (1982). Neonatal jaundice after labour induced or stimulated by prostaglandin E2 or oxytocin. *Lancet, 1,* 991.

95. Lanzkowsky, P. (1975). The jaundiced newborn: Causes and importance. Paper presented at the Symposium in Hematologic Diseases in Children, NY City Department of Health, Bureau of Health. Mead Johnson Publication No. L-B13–4–78.

96. Lascari, A.D. (1986). "Early" breast-feeding jaundice: Clinical significance. *J Pediatr, 108,* 156.

97. Lau, S.P. & Fung, K.P. (1984). Serum bilirubin kinetics in intermittent phototherapy of physiological jaundice. *Am J Dis Child, 59,* 892.

98. Lawrence, R.A. (1989). *Breastfeeding: A guide for the medical profession.* St. Louis: CV Mosby.

99. Lee, K., Moscioni, A.D., & Choi, J. (1991). Jaundice. In T.H. Yeh (Ed.), *Neonatal therapeutics* (2nd ed., pp. 352–363). St. Louis: Mosby–Year Book.

100. Levi, A.J., Gatmaitan, Z., & Arias, I.M. (1969). Two hepatic cytoplasmic protein fractions, Y and Z, and their possible role in the hepatic uptake of bilirubin, sulfobromophthalein and other anions. *J Clin Invest, 48,* 2156.

101. Linn, S., et al. (1985). Epidemiology of neonatal hyperbilirubinemia. *Pediatrics, 75,* 770.

102. Lucey, J.F. (1989). Bilirubin and brain damage—A real mess. *Pediatrics, 69,* 381.

103. Maisels, M.J. (1972). Bilirubin: On understanding and influencing its metabolism in the newborn infant. *Pediatr Clin North Am, 19,* 447.

104. Maisels, M.J. (1983). Clinical studies of the sequelae of hyperbilirubinemia. In *Hyperbilirubinemia in the newborn, report of the 85th Ross Conference on pediatric research* (pp. 26–38). Columbus, OH: Ross Laboratories.

105. Maisels, M.J. (1987). Neonatal jaundice. In G.B. Avery (Ed.), *Neonatology, pathophysiology and management of the newborn* (pp. 534–629). Philadelphia: JB Lippincott.

106. Maisels, M.J. & Conrad, S. (1982). Transcutaneous bilirubin measurements in full term infants. *Pediatrics, 70,* 464.

107. Maisels, M.J. & D'Arcangelo, M.R. (1983). Breast feeding and jaundice in the first six weeks of life. *Pediatr Res, 17,* 324A.

108. Maisels, M.J. & Gifford, K. (1983). Neonatal jaundice in full-term infants: Role of breastfeeding and other causes. *Am J Dis Child, 137,* 561.

109. Maisels, M.J. & Gifford, K.L. (1986). Normal serum bilirubin levels in the newborn and the influence of breastfeeding. *Pediatrics, 78,* 837.

110. Maisels, M.J., et al. (1988). Jaundice in the healthy newborn infant: A new approach to an old problem. *Pediatrics, 81,* 505.

111. Maurer, H.M., et al. (1973). Control trial comparing agar, intermittent phototherapy, and continuous phototherapy for reducing neonatal hyperbilirubinemia. *J Pediatr, 82,* 73.

112. McDonagh, A.F. & Lightner, D.A. (1985). "Like a shriveled blood orange"—Bilirubin, jaundice and phototherapy. *Pediatrics, 75,* 443.

113. McDonagh, A.F. (1990). Is bilirubin good for you? *Clin Perinatol, 17,* 359.

114. Messner, K.H. (1978). Light toxicity to newborn retina. *Pediatr Res, 12,* 530.

115. Messner, K.H., Maisels, M.J., & Leure du Pree, A.E. (1978). Phototoxicity to the newborn primate retina. *Invest Ophthalmol, 17,* 178.

116. Modi, N. & Keay, A.J. (1983). Phototherapy for neonatal hyperbilirubinemia: The importance of dose. *Am J Dis Child, 58,* 406.

117. Modi, N. (1989). Jaundice. In D. Harvey, R.W.I. Cooke, & G.A. Levitt (Eds.), *The baby under 1000 g* (pp. 120–133). Kent, England: Wright.

118. Montichone, R.E. & Schneider, E.L. (1979). Induction of sister chromatid exchanges in human cells by fluorescent light. *Mutation Res, 59,* 215.

119. Morales, W.S. & Koerten, J. (1986). Prevention of intraventricular hemorrhage in very low birth weight infants by maternally administered phenobarbital. *Obstet Gynecol, 68,* 295.

120. Morecki, R., Gartner, L.M., & Lee, K-S. (1978). Conjugated hyperbilirubinemia. In A.A. Fanaroff & R.J. Martin (Eds.), *Neonatal-perinatal medicine, diseases of the fetus and infant* (pp. 966–980). St. Louis: CV Mosby.

120a. Murphy, M.R. & Oellrich, R.G. (1990). A new method of phototherapy: Nursing perspectives. *J Perinatol, 10,* 249.

121. National Institute of Child Health and Human

Development. (1985). Randomized controlled trial of phototherapy for neonatal hyperbilirubinemia. *Pediatrics, 75,* 365.

122. Nelson, C.A. & Horowitz, F.D. (1982). The short-term behavioral sequelae of neonatal jaundice treated with phototherapy. *Infant Behavior Dev, 5,* 289.

123. Newman, T.B. & Maisels, M.J. (1990). Does hyperbilirubinemia damage the brain of healthy full-term infants. *Clin Perinatol, 17,* 331.

124. Nicoll, A., Ginsburg, G., & Tripp, J.H. (1982). Supplementary feeding and jaundice in newborns. *Acta Paediatr Scand, 71,* 759.

125. Odell, G.B. (1959). The dissociation of bilirubin from albumin and its clinical implications. *J Pediatr, 55,* 268.

126. Onishi, S., et al. (1986). Wavelength-dependence of the relative rate constants for the main geometric and structural photoisomerization of bilirubin IXa bound to human serum albumin. *Biochem J, 109,* 119.

127. Osborn, L.M. (1986). Management of neonatal jaundice. *Nurse Pract, 11,* 41.

128. Osborn, L.M., Reiff, M.I., & Bolus, R. (1984). Jaundice in the full-term neonate. *Pediatrics, 73,* 520.

129. Ostler, C.W. & Anderson-Shanklin, G.C. (1979). Initial feeding time of new-born infants: Effect upon first meconium passage and serum indirect bilirubin levels. *Q Pediatr Bull, 5,* 63.

130. Ostrea, M., et al. (1983). Influence of free fatty acids and glucose infusion on serum bilirubin and bilirubin binding to albumin. *J Pediatr, 102,* 426.

131. Palmer, C. & Smith M. (1990). Assessing the risk of kernicterus using nuclear magnetic resonance. *Clin Perinatol, 17,* 307.

132. Palmer, D.C. & Drew, J.H. (1983). Jaundice: A 10-year review of 41,000 live born infants. *Aust Pediatr J, 19,* 86.

133. Paludetto, R. (1983). The behavior of jaundiced infants treated with phototherapy. *Early Human Dev, 8,* 259.

134. Park, T.S., et al. (1976). Effect of phototherapy and nursery light on neonatal biorhythms. *Pediatr Res, 10,* 429.

135. Pasnick, M. & Lucey, J.F. (1976). Riboflavin and bilirubin response during phototherapy. *Pediatr Res, 10,* 854.

136. Pasnick, M. & Lucey, J.F. (1982). Transcutaneous bilirubinometry can be used duirng phototherapy (abstract). *Pediatr Res, 16,* 302A.

137. Poland, R.L. (1981). Breast milk jaundice. *J Pediatr, 99,* 86.

138. Poland, R.D. & Odell, G.B. (1971). Physiologic jaundice: The enterohepatic circulation of bilirubin. *N Engl J Med, 284,* 1.

139. Poland, R. & Schultz, G. (1980). High milk lipase activity associated with breast milk jaundice. *Pediatr Res, 14,* 1328.

140. Poland, R.L., Schultz, G.E., & Garg, G. (1980). High milk lipase activity associated with breast milk jaundice. *Pediatr Res, 14,* 1328.

141. Ritter, D.A., et al. (1982). A prospective study of free bilirubin and other high-risk factors in the development of kernicterus in premature infants. *Pediatrics, 69,* 260.

142. Robinson, R.J. & Rapoport, S.I. (1987). Binding effect of albumin on uptake of bilirubin by the brain. *Pediatrics, 79,* 553.

143. Romagnoli, C., et al. (1988). Phototherapy for hyperbilirubinemia in preterm infants: Green versus blue or white light. *J Pediatr, 112,* 476.

144. Rosenfeld, W., Twist, P., & Concepcion, L. (1989). A new device for phototherapy. *Pediatr Res, 25,* 227A.

145. Rosta, J., Makol, Z., & Kertesz, A. (1968). Delayed meconium passage and hyperbilirubinemia. *Lancet, 73,* 515.

146. Rubin, R.A., et al. (1979). Neonatal bilirubin levels related to cognitive development at ages 4 through 7 years. *J Pediatr, 94,* 601.

147. Saigal, S., et al. (1982). Serum bilirubin levels in breast- and formula-fed infants in the first five days of life. *Can Med Assn J, 127,* 985.

148. Scheidt, P.C., et al. (1990). Phototherapy for neonatal hyperbilirubinemia: Six year followup of the NICHD clinical trial. *Pediatrics, 85,* 455.

149. Schmid, R. & McDonagh, A.F. (1979). Formation and metabolism of bile pigments in vivo. In D. Dolphin (Ed.), *The porphyrin* (Vol. 6). New York: Academic Press.

150. Schneider, A.P. (1986). Breast milk jaundice in the newborn. *JAMA, 255,* 3270.

151. Schreiner, R.L. & Glick, M.R. (1982). Interlaboratory bilirubin variability. *Pediatrics, 69,* 277.

152. Schumacher, R.E. (1990). Noninvasive measurements of bilirubin in the newborn. *Clin Perinatol, 17,* 417.

153. Schumacher R.E., Thornberry, J.M., & Gutcher, G.R. (1985). Transcutaneous bilirubinometry: A comparison of old and new methods. *Pediatrics, 76,* 10.

154. Sheridan-Pereira, M. & Gorman, W. (1982). Transcutaneous bilirubinometry: An evaluation. *Am J Dis Child, 57,* 708.

155. Sisson, T.R.C. (1978). Bilirubin metabolism. In U. Stave (Ed.), *Perinatal physiology* (pp. 523–546). New York: Plenum Press.

156. Sivasuriya, M., et al. (1978). Neonatal serum bilirubin levels in spontaneous and induced labor. *Br J Obstet Gynecol, 85,* 619.

157. Spear, M.L., et al. (1985). The effect of 15-hour fat infusions of varying dosage on bilirubin binding to albumin. *J Parenter Enteral Nutr, 9,* 144.

158. Speck, W.T. & Rosenkranz, H.S. (1979). Intracellular deoxyribonucleaic acid-modifying activity of phototherapy lights. *Pediatr Res, 10,* 553.

159. Speck, W.T. (1979). Effect of phototherapy on fertilization and embryonic development. *Pediatr Res, 13,* 506.

160. Stiehm, E.R. & Ryan, J. (1965). Breast milk jaundice. *Arch Dis Child, 109,* 212.

161. Stocker, R., et al. (1987). Bilirubin is an antioxidant of possible physiologic importance. *Science, 235,* 1043.

162. Tan, K.L. (1989). Efficacy of fluorescent daylight, blue and green lamps in the management of non-hemolytic hyperbilirubinemia. *J Pediatr, 114,* 132.

163. Tan, K.L. (1982). The pattern of bilirubin response to phototherapy for neonatal hyperbilirubinemia. *Pediatr Res, 16,* 670.

164. Tan, K.L. (1982). Transcutaneous bilirubinometry in full term Chinese and Malay infants. *Acta Paediatr Scand, 71,* 593.

165. Telzrow, R.W., et al. (1980). The behavior of jaundiced infants under phototherapy. *Dev Med Child Neurol, 22,* 317.

166. Thaler, M.M. & Pelger, A. (1977). Influence of

intravenous nutrients on bilirubin transport. III. Emulsified fat infusion. *Pediatr Res, 11,* 171.

167. Tolentino, T., et al. (1982). Transcutaneous bilirubinometry: Correlations during phototherapy. *Pediatr Res, 16,* 312A.

168. Trolle, D. (1968). Decreased total serum bilirubin concentration in newborn infants after phenobarbitone treatment. *Lancet, 2,* 705.

169. Tudehope, D.I. & Chang, A. (1982). Multiple site readings from a transcutaneous bilirubinometer. *Aust Pediatr J, 18,* 102.

170. Valaes, T., et al. (1980). Effectiveness and safety of prenatal phenobarbital for the prevention of neonatal jaundice. *Pediatr Res, 14,* 947.

171. Valaes, T.N. & Harvey-Wilkes, K. (1990). Pharmacologic approaches in the prevention and treatment of neonatal hyperbilirubinemia. *Clin Perinatol, 17,* 245.

172. Van de Bor, M., et al. (1989). Hyperbilirubinemia in preterm infants and neurodevelopmental outcome at 2 years of age: Results of a national collaborative study. *Pediatrics, 83,* 915.

173. Vecchi, C., et al. (1986). Phototherapy for neonatal jaundice: Clinical equivalence of fluorescent green and "special" blue lamps. *J Pediatr, 108,* 452.

174. Vogl, T.P., et al. (1978). Intermittent phototherapy in the treatment of jaundice in the premature infant. *J Pediatr, 92,* 627.

175. Vohr, B.R. (1989). Behavioral changes correlated with cry characteristics and brainstem auditory evoked response (BAER) in term infants with moderate hyperbilirubinemia. *Pediatr Res, 25,* 19A.

176. Vohr, B. (1990). New approaches to assessing the risks of hyperbilirubinemia. *Clin Perinatol, 17,* 293.

177. Vreman, H.J. & Stevenson, D.K. (1990). Metalloporphyrin-enhanced photodegradation of bilirubin in vitro. *Am J Dis Child, 144,* 590.

178. Vreman, H.J., et al. (1988). Effects of oral administration of tin and zinc protoporphyrin on neonatal and adult rat tissue heme oxygenase activity. *J Pediatr Gastroenterol Nutr, 7,* 902.

179. Waffarn, F., et al. (1982). Fetal exposure to maternal hyperbilirubinemia. *Am J Dis Child, 136,* 416.

180. Wallin, A. & Boreus, L.O. (1984). Phenobarbital prophylaxis for hyperbilirubinemia in preterm infants: A control study of bilirubin disappearance and infant behavior. *Acta Paediatr Scand, 73,* 488.

181. Watchko, J.F. & Oski, F.A. (1983). Bilirubin 20 mg/dl: Vigintiphobia. *Pediatrics, 71,* 660.

182. Watson, C. J., Campbell, M., & Lowrey, P.T. (1958). Preferential reduction of conjugated bilirubin to urobilinogen by normal fecal flora. *Proc Soc Exp Biol Med, 98,* 707.

183. Wennberg, R.P., Pal, N., & Bessman, S.P. (1986). Effects of blood-brain barrier disruption and bilirubin on cerebral metabolism. *Pediatr Res, 20,* 469A.

184. Wolkoff, A.W., et al. (1978). Hepatic accumulation and intracellular binding of conjugated bilirubin. *J Clin Invest, 61,* 142.

185. Wu, P.Y.K. (1981). Phototherapy update: Factors effecting efficiency of phototherapy. *Perinatol Neonatol, 5(5),* 45.

186. Wu, P.Y.K. (1982). Phototherapy: In vivo side effects. *Perinatol Neonatol, 6(2),* 21.

187. Wu, P.Y.K., et al. (1974). Effect of phototherapy in preterm infants on growth in the neonatal period. *J Pediatr, 85,* 563.

188. Wu, P.Y.K., et al. (1983). Metabolic aspects of phototherapy. *Pediatrics, 75(Suppl.),* 427.

189. Yamauchi, Y. & Yamanouchi, I. (1989). Transcutaneous bilirubinometry. *Acta Paediatr Scand, 78,* 844.

190. Yamauchi, Y. & Yamanouchi, I. (1990). Clinical application of transcutaneous bilirubin measurement. Early prediction of hyperbilirubinemia. *Acta Paediatr Scand, 79,* 385.

191. Zetterstrom, R. & Ernster, L. (1956). Bilirubin, an uncoupler of oxidative phosphorylation in isolated mitochondria. *Nature, 178,* 1335.

CHAPTER 16

Thyroid Function

Maternal Physiologic Adaptations
  The Antepartum Period
  The Intrapartum Period
  The Postpartum Period
Clinical Implications for the Pregnant Woman and Her Fetus
  Thyroid Function Tests During Pregnancy
  Thyroid Function and Nausea and Vomiting of
    Pregnancy
  The Pregnant Woman with Hyperthyroidism
  The Pregnant Woman with Hypothyroidism
  Postpartum Thyroid Disorders
  Breast-Feeding in Women with Thyroid
    Disorders

  Use of Radioiodine and Iodides
  Effects of Thyroid and Antithyroid Agents on the
    Fetus
Development of Thyroid Function in the Fetus
  Anatomic Development
  Functional Development
Neonatal Physiology
Clinical Implications for Neonatal Care
  Thyroid Function and Thermoregulation
  Transient Hypothyroidism in the Preterm Infant
  Neonatal Hyperthyroidism
  Neonatal Hypothyroidism
**Maturational Changes During Infancy and
  Childhood**

Thyroid hormones play a critical role in body functions such as metabolism and are necessary for development of the central nervous system (CNS) and other growth processes. Thyroid function is linked with reproductive function. Disorders of the thyroid are associated with infertility, alterations in normal changes at puberty, and complications of pregnancy. Concentrations of thyroid hormones are altered in healthy pregnant women and neonates. In the neonate the marked changes in thyroid function that occur with birth are interrelated with thermal regulation. This chapter examines changes in the thyroid and its hormones during pregnancy, development of thyroid function in the fetus and neonate, and implications for the mother, fetus, and neonate. Figures

16–1 and 16–2 review thyroid hormone metabolism.

MATERNAL PHYSIOLOGIC ADAPTATIONS

Significant alterations in concentrations of thyroid hormones (thyroxine [T_4] and triiodothyronine [T_3]) and thyroxine-binding globulin (TBG) occur during pregnancy. These changes are influenced by hormones, particularly estrogen and human chorionic gonadotropin (hCG), and alterations in liver and kidney function. These changes are important in supporting the altered carbohydrate, protein, and lipid metabolism of pregnancy (see Chapter 13).

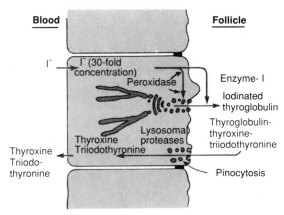

Blood   **Follicle**

FIGURE 16–1. Thyroid cellular mechanisms for iodine transport and thyroxine (T_4) and triiodothyronine (T_3) formation and release into the blood. Iodide is actively transported into the thyroid cell, stored, and oxidized. Oxidized iodide is bound to tyrosine to form iodotyrosines. These substances are held within the thyroglobulin and used to form T_4 and T_3. T_4 and T_3 are stored in the thyroid, bound to thyroglobulin. Under the influence of thyroid stimulating hormone (TSH), T_4 and a small amount of T_3 are cleaved from thyroglobulin and secreted. In peripheral tissue, T_4 is deiodinated to T_3 (70 to 80% of T_3 in tissues is derived from this process). Released iodine is reconcentrated by the thyroid or excreted by the kidneys. T_4 can also be metabolized to reverse T_3 (rT_3), which is an inactive compound. T_3 and rT_3 are in a reciprocal relationship. Nearly all of the thyroid hormones circulate in plasma bound to proteins, including thyroxine-binding globulin or TBG (major carrier), thyroxine-binding prealbumin (TBPA), or albumin. Changing levels of TBG, such as occurs during pregnancy, alter serum thyroxine levels without changing thyroid status. The small amounts of free T_3 and T_4 in the blood form the physiologically active fraction. (From Guyton, A. C. [1991]. *Textbook of medical physiology* [8th ed., p. 832]. Philadelphia: WB Saunders.)

The Antepartum Period

Adaptations during pregnancy related to thyroid physiology mimic hyperthyroidism. The pregnant woman can be described as being in a state of euthyroid hyperthyroxinemia, however, since thyroid function per se does not change during pregnancy. This state is associated with periods of increased estrogen (pregnancy, oral contraceptives, or estrogen replacement therapy), liver dysfunction, and use of drugs (heroin and methadone).[77]

Under the influence of estrogen, hepatic synthesis of TBG increases 50 to 100% beginning in the first trimester.[5, 27, 29, 39, 112] The ability of TBG to bind thyroxine doubles during this period; thyroxine-bind-

ing prealbumin (TBPA)–binding capacity decreases.[12, 94] These changes increase serum TBG levels, decrease the percent of T_4 bound to prealbumin, and increase total T_4 and T_3 (Table 16–1). Concentrations of free T_3 and T_4 remain within normal physiologic limits, however.[64, 75, 77]

Resin T_3 uptake (RT_3U) decreases during pregnancy. RT_3U measures TBG-binding capacity, quantifies the number of unbound sites, and approximates the amount of free T_4. Although T_4-binding sites and binding capacity increase in pregnancy, the number of binding sites exceeds nonpregnant levels

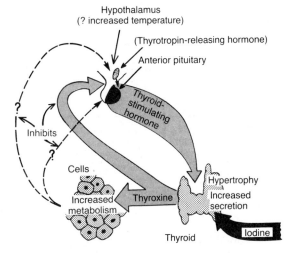

FIGURE 16–2. Regulation of thyroid hormone secetion. Thyroid stimulating hormone (TSH) acts through receptors on the thyroid cell membrane to activate adenyl cyclase. This stimulates formation of cyclic adenosine monophosphate (cAMP), which activates cellular systems to alter thyroid processes. TSH secretion is stimulated by thyrotropin releasing hormone or factor (TRH). TRH is secreted primarily by paraventricular nuclei of the hypothalamus and released into the hypothalamic–pituitary portal system. TRH binds to receptors on the plasma membrane of thyrotropic cells within the anterior pituitary to activate synthesis and secretion of TSH. Secretion of thyroid hormones decreases the responsiveness of the pituitary to TRH. Secretion of TSH is also influenced by both circulating levels of free thyroid hormone and intrapituitary T_3 levels via negative feedback to the pituitary gland; that is, increased free thyroid hormone levels decrease secretion of TSH by the pituitary and vice versa. Circulating T_4 regulates TSH primarily through intrapituitary deiodination of T_4 to T_3. The pituitary–thyroid axis is controlled in turn by the hypothalamus and TRH. TSH is inhibited by excess circulating thyroid hormone. (From Guyton, A. C. [1991]. *Textbook of medical physiology* [8th ed., p. 838]. Philadelphia: WB Saunders.)

TABLE 16–1
**Thyroid Function Tests in Nonpregnant and Pregnant Women and Those Taking Oral Contraceptives
Containing Estrogens***

TEST	METHOD	NORMAL NONPREGNANT	PREGNANCY OR ORAL CONTRACEPTIVES	COMMENT
Thyroid-stimulating hormone "sensitive TSH" (μU/ml)	RIA	<2	No changes	↑ in primary hypothyroidism
Thyroxine T_4 (μg/100 ml)	RIA	4.5–12.5	↑ 2–4 μg/dl	↑ normal range secondary to ↑ TBG levels
Triiodothyronine T_3 (ng/100 ml)	RIA	90–190	↑ 25–50 ng/dl	↑ normal range with ↑ TBG levels
RT_3U (%)	Resin T_3 uptake	25–35	↓ to 20–25	Indirect test of protein binding (Not a measurement of T_3)
Free thyroxine FT_4 (ng/100 ml)	Equilibrium dialysis	1.4 ± 0.16	No change	Helpful in evaluating function in women who are pregnant or on oral contraceptives
Free T_4 or Free T_3	Index†			
Thyroid autoantibodies			May be positive in subacute and Hashimoto's thyroiditis and Graves' disease	
Thyroglobulin	Hemagglut	None		
Microsomal (MSA)	Hemagglut	None		
[131]I (%)	Uptake of ^{131}I or ^{125}I by thyroid gland	10–25% at 24 hr	*Contraindicated in pregnancy*	
[125]I (%)				
TSH receptor antibodies measured by (TRAb)‡				

*Normal values must be determined for each laboratory in which the test is performed.

†Calculation based on the product of the in vitro resin uptake value of T_3 or T_4 and the serum total T_4 concentration. This is not a thyroid test or measurement.

‡Because of proliferation of methods for detecting TSH receptor antibodies characteristic of Graves' disease, the present terminology is suggested to replace terms such as long-acting thyroid stimulator (LATS) and TSH-displacing activity (TDA). (The normal values on this table and nomenclature are those adopted in 1987 by the American Thyroid Association Committee on Nomenclature.)

TBG, thyroid-binding globulin.

From Hollingsworth, D.R. (1989). Endocrine disorders of pregnancy. In R.K. Creasy & R. Resnik (Eds.), *Maternal-fetal medicine: principles and practice* (2nd ed., p. 1001). Philadelphia: WB Saunders.

and available T_4. The increased number of unbound sites is reflected by decreased RT_3U.[12, 64]

T_3 and T_4 peak at 10 to 15 weeks' gestation (Fig. 16–3).[39, 55] The increased T_3 and T_4 may be related to increased thyroid-stimulating hormone (TSH) bioactivity stimulated by hCG, which peaks at about the same time. hCG has a mild TSH-like activity (the alpha subunits of hCG and TSH are similar) that increases secretion of T_4. Levels of T_3 are elevated because of increased available T_4 for deiodination to T_3 in peripheral tissue rather than increased T_3 production. Elevated T_3 and T_4 suppress endogenous TSH secretion by the anterior pituitary (see Fig. 16–2).[39, 55]

The increased T_4 and T_3 stimulate increased serum protein-bound iodine (PBI).[55, 75, 77] Since circulating levels of free thyroid hormone are not significantly altered, increased PBI does not reflect maternal hyperthyroidism.[5] Thyroid iodine uptake increases because of a decrease in the total body iodine pool. This pool is altered because of increased renal iodide clearance secondary to the increased glomerular filtration rate (see

Chapter 8) and placental transfer of iodine to the fetus.[1, 5, 74]

For many years thyroid enlargement was believed to be a normal finding during pregnancy due to increased thyroid activity in response to elevated renal iodide losses. Changes in thyroid size are currently minimal or nonexistent among most pregnant women in North America because of diets that are relatively high in iodine.[12, 17, 27] Therefore, moderate to marked thyroid enlargement in these women cannot be considered normal and requires further evaluation.

Changes in Basal Metabolic Rate

The basal metabolic rate (BMR) increases during pregnancy by 20 to 25% beginning at 4 months. This does not reflect an actual change of this magnitude since 70 to 80% of the increase can be accounted for by the increased surface area of the mother and fetus and the remainder by increased maternal work.[5, 12, 15, 16]

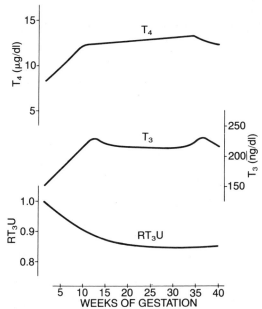

FIGURE 16–3. Changes in thyroid hormones (T$_3$ and T$_4$) and T$_3$ resin uptake (RT$_3$U) during pregnancy. The early increase in serum T$_4$ and T$_3$ is due to estrogen-stimulated increase in hepatic production of TBG. Serum TBG, T$_4$, and T$_3$ peak or plateau by 10 to 15 weeks' gestation. The decrease in RT$_3$U reflects the increase in TBG-binding sites. (From Harada, A., et al. (1979). Comparison of thyroid stimulators and thyroid hormone concentrations in the sera of pregnant women. J Clin Endocrinol Metab, *48*, 793; as redrawn by Fisher, D. A. [1983]. Maternal-fetal thyroid function. *Clin Perinatol, 10*, 617.)

The Intrapartum Period

Levels of total and free T$_3$ increase during labor.[5] This change probably reflects the energy demands of labor on the maternal system. T$_3$ and T$_4$ have similar functions, but T$_3$ is 3 to 5 times more active. T$_3$ and T$_4$ increase intracellular enzymes (increased cellular metabolism), the number and activity of mitochondria (to provide energy for cellular enzyme systems), and Na-K adenosine triphosphatase (ATPase) (because of the increased energy use).[53, 113]

The Postpartum Period

After delivery and with decreased estrogen, hepatic synthesis of TBG decreases, as does the increased renal excretion of iodine. As a result, the metabolic alterations in thyroid processes gradually reverse, but may persist for up to 6 to 12 weeks.[56] Thyrotropin-releasing hormone (TRH) is a (minor) stimulus of prolactin release and has been used to induce relactation.[71] Transient disorders in thyroid function are seen in some postpartum women.

Thyroid hormones are secreted in breast milk. Levels are low initially, then rise to mean levels of 4.3 μg/dl, equivalent to approximately 40 to 50 μg of T$_4$ per day.[114] Breast milk T$_4$ and T$_3$ have been reported to delay the development of hypothyroidism in some infants.[85, 103, 107] These hormones may also mask clinical symptoms and impede the diagnosis of congenital hypothyroidism.[114]

CLINICAL IMPLICATIONS FOR THE PREGNANT WOMAN AND HER FETUS

Thyroid disorders are more common in women and are not uncommon in pregnant women. Diagnosis of thyroid dysfunction during pregnancy may be more difficult since symptoms of several thyroid disorders mimic some of the usual physiologic changes of pregnancy and radioactive iodine tests cannot be used because of fetal risks. Implications of alterations in thyroid function and changes in laboratory tests during pregnancy are discussed in this section along with disorders of thyroid function unique to the postpartum period.

Thyroid Function Tests During Pregnancy

Changes in TBG and thyroid hormones during pregnancy alter parameters for many tests used to assess thyroid status (Table 16–1). These alterations must be considered when evaluating thyroid function in pregnant and postpartum women.

Thyroid Function and Nausea and Vomiting of Pregnancy

Nausea and vomiting in early pregnancy have been linked to alterations in T$_4$, TSH, and hCG (which has TSH-like activity). Morning sickness severity has been correlated with increased free T$_4$ and decreased TSH, with values returning to normal (for the pregnant woman) as the nausea and vomiting resolve.[12, 83] These findings may lead to or be a consequence of emesis during early pregnancy.

Hyperemesis gravidarum in women without any history or evidence of thyroid dysfunction has also been associated with increased free T$_4$ and decreased TSH. These findings are similar to the euthyroid sick syndrome seen with severe illness. T_4 levels in women with hyperemesis return to usual values in 1 to 4 weeks with or without treatment with antithyroid drugs.[5, 9, 30]

The Pregnant Woman with Hyperthyroidism

The diagnosis of hyperthyroidism during pregnancy may be difficult since many of the signs and symptoms associated with this disorder are often seen normally during pregnancy. Findings common to hyperthyroidism and certain stages of pregnancy include fatigue, heat intolerance, warm skin, emotional lability, increased appetite, sweating, breathlessness, ankle edema, full pulse, and increased pulse pressure.[15, 25, 64, 77] Increased free T_3 and total T_4 (over 15 µg/dl) and increased or high-normal RT_3U are seen with hyperthyroidism. Alterations in thyroid function tests during pregnancy (Table 16–1) must be considered when interpreting test results. For example, since RT_3U is decreased in pregnancy, values in the nonpregnant range suggest hyperthyroidism.

Hyperthyroidism in pregnant women in North America is usually due to either an autoimmune disorder or an unknown cause; it is rarely due to goiter. The risk of goiter during pregnancy is attributed to increased avidity of the thyroid for iodine in response to increased renal loss and placental transport. In most women these losses are compensated by a high dietary iodine intake.

Hyperthyroidism in pregnant women is almost always due to Graves' disease.[77] Graves' disease is an autoimmune disorder in which a group of thyroid-stimulating antigens (TSIs) attach to and activate TSH receptors on the thyroid follicular cells. This leads to increased production of thyroid hormones and the clinical finding of hyperthyroidism.

Women with mild hyperthyroidism generally do well during pregnancy since increased serum TBG offsets the increased secretion of thyroid hormones. Women with Graves' disease often improve during pregnancy, with remission and occasionally complete resolution seen in some women during the third trimester.[12, 77, 84, 97] This improvement is related to changes in the immune system (see Chapter 10) that lower TSI levels and to decreased thyroid hormone production. Relapse or exacerbation generally occurs within several weeks of delivery as the immune system alterations and production of TBG return to prepregnancy levels.[77] Hyperthyroidism is treated with antithyroid drugs or surgery. Propylthiouracil (PTU) effects must be monitored carefully, particularly during the third trimester in women with Graves' disease, when remission can lead to decreased thyroid hormone production and decreased requirements for PTU.[2]

Pregnant women with hyperthyroidism will usually require a caloric intake that is higher than that usually recommended during pregnancy to compensate for their increased metabolic rate. These women are also at risk for fluid loss and dehydration as the result of the diarrhea and tachycardia that often accompany hyperthyroidism.[112a]

Pregnancy complicated by hyperthyroidism, particularly if this disorder is poorly controlled, is associated with intrauterine growth retardation and preterm labor. Treatment of preterm labor with beta agonists (see Chapter 3) is contraindicated since these agents can aggravate symptoms related to alterations in sympathetic nervous system function in hyperthyroidism and precipitate a thyroid storm.[25] Transplacental passage of TSIs can lead to a transient neonatal hyperthyroidism (see Chapter 10).

Pregnant women may also develop a transient subacute thyroiditis that often occurs in association with viral infections. The inflammation and destruction of thyroid tissue lead to release of stored thyroid hormone into serum and a transient hyperthyroxinemia. As the disorder resolves, the woman may develop hypothyroidism since the released thyroid hormones are used up before the thyroid gland can produce an adequate new supply. If treatment is initiated, β-blockers such as propranolol are required rather than antithyroid drugs that block thyroid hormone production, since with subacute thyroiditis the thyroid is not making hormones.[64]

Trophoblastic disorders such as a molar pregnancy occasionally cause biochemical and sometimes clinical findings of hyperthyroidism because of the high levels of hCG secreted by the trophoblastic mass. Biochemical hyperthyroidism has been reported to occur with hCG levels over 100,000 mIU/ml, with clinical findings of hyperthyroidism seen with hCG levels over 300,000 mIU/ml.[77]

The Pregnant Woman with Hypothyroidism

Hypothyroidism in pregnant women is usually secondary to autoimmune disorders (after surgical removal or ablation of the thyroid with ^{131}I for Graves' disease and idiopathic myxedema) or Hashimoto's thyroiditis.[12,64] Women with untreated hypothyroidism have a high incidence of infertility.[112a] The diagnosis of hypothyroidism during pregnancy may be missed since some of the signs and symptoms associated with this disorder, such as fatigue, weight gain, constipation, and amenorrhea, are also seen normally during pregnancy.[15, 25, 77, 112a]

In the absence of severe iodine deficiency or exposure to teratogenic drugs, fetal development often proceeds normally because the fetal thyroid is not dependent on maternal hormones for development.[12, 17] Pregnancy in women with hypothyroidism may be complicated by an increased risk of fetal loss or prolonged pregnancy, however, possibly owing to compromised placental blood flow or the inability of the thyroid gland to meet the metabolic demands of pregnancy.[25, 112a] Weight gain patterns must be carefully monitored in the woman with hypothyroidism.[112a] These women may also have difficulty with fatigue and constipation during pregnancy.

Postpartum Thyroid Disorders

The postpartum period is associated with a transient postpartum thyroiditis or hypothyroidism. Physiologic alterations and experiences of pregnancy can mask clinical findings of hypo- or hyperthyroidism. As a result, these disorders may first become apparent in the postpartum period.[17]

Postpartum thyroiditis is a transient, mild form of hyperthyroidism seen in 3 to 6% of postpartum women.[80] This disorder generally appears 6 to 8 weeks after delivery. It is characterized by weeks or months (average, 2 to 3 months) of mild hyperthyroidism, followed by weeks or months of hypothyroidism, and finally a return to normal thyroid function in about 90% of these women.[12, 17, 64, 77] Biochemical abnormalities include elevated free T_4, suppression of TSH, presence of microsomal antibodies, and a low ^{131}I uptake.[12, 77] Postpartum thyroiditis may be misdiagnosed as postpartum depression and often recurs with subsequent deliveries.[17, 119] Transient hypothyroidism is also seen occasionally during the postpartum period. Findings include fatigue, weight gain, low free T_4, and elevated TSH levels, and elevated

antimicrosomal and antithyroglobulin antibody titers.[17]

Breast-Feeding in Women with Thyroid Disorders

Breast-feeding is generally not contraindicated in women with hypothyroidism since thyroid hormones cross in only small amounts and the infant should receive a dose no higher than that from a euthyroid woman.[22, 71] Breast-feeding in women with hyperthyroidism is controversial, primarily because of passage of antithyroid medications in breast milk.[25, 26, 71, 77] PTU is excreted in breast milk in relatively small amounts (0.025 to 0.077% of the maternal dose).[71] Most sources suggest that breast-feeding is probably not routinely contraindicated in women on PTU who are carefully monitored, but that each women needs to weigh the risks and benefits and the infant must be carefully monitored. PTU is preferred over methimazole (Tapazole), which crosses in much higher amounts.[5] Propranolol and thiouracil cross in significant amounts and are generally contraindicated in breast-feeding women.[71, 104]

The mammary glands actively take up, concentrate, and secrete iodine in breast milk. Thus, breast-feeding is interrupted if the woman requires thyroid uptake studies or scans involving use of ^{123}I or [131]I. McDougall recommends that breast-feeding not be resumed unless the dose of radioactivity in the milk is below 1 rad of exposure to the infant's thyroid.[77]

Use of Radioiodine and Iodides

Iodine is actively transported across the placenta and taken up by the fetal thyroid (Fig. 16–4). Avidity (affinity) of the fetal thyroid for iodine is 20 to 50 times greater than that of the mother. Administration of any form of iodine to pregnant women results in significantly higher concentrations per weight in fetal tissues and can lead to development of a goiter.[12] Fetal risks of radioactive substances include thyroid damage, microcephaly, intrauterine growth retardation, mental retardation, later malignancy, and death. As a result, radioiodine has been contraindicated during pregnancy.

The use of nonradioactive iodides has also been reported to result in fetal goiter with

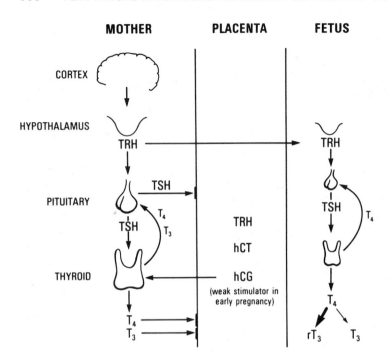

FIGURE 16–4. Maternal, placental, and fetal thyroid relationships. Placental hCG is a weak stimulator of the maternal thyroid during the first trimester. Maternal TRH crosses the placenta, whereas TSH does not; placental transfer of T_4 and T_3 is minimal. Therefore fetal thyroid function is independent of maternal influences. TRH, thyrotropin releasing hormone; TSH, thyroid stimulating hormone; T_4, thyroxine; T_3, triiodothyronine; hCT, human chorionic thyrotropin; hCG, human chorionic gonadotropin; rT_3 reverse triiodothyronine. (From Hollingsworth, D. R. [1989]. Endocrine disorders of pregnancy. In R. K. Creasy & R. Resnik [Eds.], *Maternal-fetal medicine: Principles and practice* [2nd ed., p. 998]. Philadelphia: WB Saunders.)

tracheal obstruction, hypothyroidism, and fetal death.[48, 56] Iodides are found in betadine-containing vaginal suppositories and douches, saturated solution of potassium iodide (SSKI), iodinized medications for asthmatics, and some contrast materials.[56, 93, 97, 103] The incidence of drug-induced fetal goiter is 1 in 10,000 and is seen primarily with daily iodide doses over 12 µg.[7, 12, 18]

McDougall suggested that radioiodine uptake studies using small doses of ^{123}I (10 to 20 µCi) during early pregnancy may be warranted if it can be demonstrated that treatment of the woman would be altered or to differentiate between Graves' disease and subacute (silent) thyroiditis.[77] This distinction is critical since subacute thyroiditis does not respond to standard pharmacologic regimens used in hyperthyroidism, and requires the use of β-blocking agents. Since fetal thyroid uptake and concentration of iodide are minimal before 10 to 12 weeks of gestation, the risks of a small dose of radiation with ^{123}I at this time may be small. Use of even the small doses suggested by McDougall is controversial.

All women should have a pregnancy test before radioactive iodine studies. If these studies are done in a woman who is later found to be pregnant, however, the risks are minimal since the dose of ^{123}I used is generally low.[12] The use of ^{131}I for definitive diagnosis and therapy of Graves' disease is associated with increased pregnancy loss and destruction of the fetal thyroid; thus, this agent is not used during pregnancy.

Effects of Thyroid and Antithyroid Agents on the Fetus

Transplacental passage of thyroid and antithyroid agents (Fig. 16–4) is of interest in terms of the potential for intrauterine treatment of fetal thyroid disorders and possible adverse effects. The drugs used most frequently to treat hyperthyroidism are antithyroid agents, primarily PTU and methimazole (Tapazole), and β-blockers such as propranolol. Antithyroid drugs block production of thyroid hormones by blocking iodination of tyrosine. The antithyroid drug of choice in pregnancy is PTU since it blocks conversion of T_4 to T_3 as well as inhibits production of thyroid hormones.[12]

PTU crosses the placenta and can block synthesis of thyroid hormones by the fetus. The incidence of hypothyroidism in exposed infants is 1 in 100. The lower hormone levels stimulate increased TSH production, which can lead to goiter and tracheal obstruction. Infants of mothers treated with PTU may have decreased T_4 and increased TSH levels after birth. These values are generally within normal neonatal limits by 4 to 5 days of age and later development is usually normal.[13, 19, 113] Propranolol is generally not indicated for long-term treatment of pregnant women with hyperthyroidism. This drug crosses the placenta and has been associated with fetal growth retardation and impaired response to anoxia and neonatal hypoglycemia and bradycardia.[12, 104]

Intrauterine treatment of fetal disorders is an area of intense investigation. Fetal hyperthyroidism, which is most often secondary to transfer of TSIs across the placenta from the mother with Graves' disease, can be treated by giving medication to the mother since antithyroid agents are readily transferred across the placenta. Treatment of fetal hypothyroidism with maternal medication is not possible since the placenta is essentially impermeable to T_4, T_3, and TSH.[77, 95] Treatment by weekly intra-amniotic injections of T_4 is being investigated.[113]

SUMMARY

Changes in thyroid function can alter reproductive processes. The pregnant woman is in a state of euthyroid hyperthyroxinemia because of an increased availability of TBG. As a result, parameters for thyroid function tests are altered. These changes must be considered when evaluating thyroid function during pregnancy. Thyroid disorders are not uncommon in pregnant women. Knowledge of the effects of these disorders and their treatment is important to optimize fetal and neonatal outcome. Clinical recommendations related to thyroid function during pregnancy are summarized in Table 16–2.

DEVELOPMENT OF THYROID FUNCTION IN THE FETUS

As a result of the relative impermeability of the placenta to maternal TSH, T_4, and T_3, the fetal hypothalamic–pituitary–thyroid axis develops and functions independent of maternal influences (Fig. 16–4).[34, 60, 99] Maternal TRH does cross the placenta but does not seem to have a major influence on fetal pituitary or thyroid function.[25] Lack of significant transfer of T_3 and T_4 may be due to the presence in the placenta of alpha iodothyronine, which increases levels of the inactive reverse T_3, or to deiodinase enzymes, which deiodinate (degrade) T_3 and T_4 into inactive products.[99, 100] Increased T_4 transfer

TABLE 16–2
Summary of Recommendations for Clinical Practice Related to Changes in Thyroid Function: Pregnant Woman

Recognize usual changes in thyroid metabolism during pregnancy (pp. 660–662).

Assess and monitor maternal nutrition in terms of iodine intake (pp. 660–662, 664).

Monitor fetal growth in women with normal and abnormal thyroid function (pp. 664–665, 667).

Know usual parameters for thyroid function tests during pregnancy (p. 663, Table 16–1).

Recognize signs and symptoms of thyroid dysfunction and similarities with certain pregnancy-related findings (pp. 664–665).

Counsel women with hyper- and hypothyroidism regarding the effects of their disorder on pregnancy and the fetus and of pregnancy on the thyroid disorder (pp. 664–665).

Monitor medication levels and requirements in the pregnant woman with hyperthyroidism (pp. 664–666).

Avoid use of beta agonists in hyperthyroid women (p. 664).

Know fetal and neonatal risks of maternal iodide and radioactive iodine administration (pp. 665–666).

Avoid use of iodides and radioactive iodine in pregnant women (pp. 665–666).

Know fetal and neonatal risks associated with use of thyroid and antithyroid agents (pp. 666–667).

Recognize and monitor for transient postpartum thyroid disorders (p. 665).

Counsel women with hypo- and hyperthyroidism regarding breast-feeding considerations (p. 665).

Page numbers in parentheses following each recommendation refer to the pages in the text where the rationale for that intervention is discussed.

has been reported in late gestation with fetuses with severe congenital hypothyroidism.[118] The placenta is permeable to commonly used antithyroid drugs (PTU and methimazole) and β-blockers (propranolol and iodine).[77, 95] Placental permeability to TSIs can lead to development of transient neonatal hyperthyroidism in infants of women with Graves' disease (see Chapter 10).

Anatomic Development

The hypothalamus and anterior pituitary glands develop simultaneously but independently of each other. As a result, growth of the thyrotropic cells within the anterior pituitary is not dependent on the presence of the hypothalamus. For example, anencephalic infants do not have a hypothalamus but have TSH cells with their anterior pituitary glands.[99]

The hypothalamus develops during the 12th week from the ventral portion of the diencephalon. Hypothalamic nuclei and supraoptic track fibers develop by 12 to 14 weeks with maturation of the hypothalamic neurons by 30 to 35 weeks.[50, 99] The anterior pituitary arises from the anterior wall of Rathke's pouch, an offshoot of the oral cavity; the posterior pituitary and stalk develop from the infundibulum, a thickening on the floor of the diencephalon.[108] The anterior pituitary can be seen by 4 weeks and is independent of the oral cavity by 12 weeks. During the 5th week the primitive anterior pituitary becomes connected with the infundibulum. Cellular differentiation within the anterior pituitary gland begins at 7 to 8 weeks, with appearance of thyrotrophic cells at 12 to 13 weeks. A marked increase in TSH-secreting cell volume occurs by 23 weeks.[99]

Thyroid Gland

The thyroid gland develops during the first 12 weeks of gestation. The thyroid begins as an epithelial thickening at the base of the tongue. As the primordial gland migrates down the trachea it becomes bilobular with a small median isthmus. The thyroid initially descends in front of the pharyngeal gut. Later the thyroid descends in front of the hyoid bone and larynx to reach its final position in front of the trachea by 7 weeks.[108]

Functional Development

Maturation of thyroid function is interrelated with that of the hypothalamic–pituitary–thyroid axis. This process can be divided into three overlapping phases: embryogenesis (Phase I), hypothalamic maturation (Phase II), and maturation of thyroid system function (Phase III).[32, 34, 39, 61, 99] During the first phase (10 to 12 weeks) the thyroid gland develops morphologically, accumulates and concentrates iodine, and begins to synthesize and secrete iodothyronines. T_4 can be detected in fetal serum at 9 to 12 weeks. TSH can be detected in the pituitary by 10 to 12 weeks and in fetal serum by 11 to 18 weeks.[38, 52, 60, 99] Thyroxine-binding proteins can be found from 12 weeks.[85]

Hypothalamic function matures during Phase II (from 4 to 5 until about 35 weeks). TRH, gonadotropin-releasing hormone (GnRH), and somatostatin are detected in the hypothalamus by 10 to 12 weeks by radioimmunoassay and in fetal blood in the third trimester.[50, 99]

Phase III lasts from mid-gestation until term or 1 month after birth if transitional changes are considered. This stage involves increasing maturation and integration of thyroid system function. Fetal thyroid function remains at basal levels until mid-gestation, even though the capacity to secrete TSH and other hormones develops earlier.[39] After about 22 weeks TSH, T_4, and reverse T_3 (rT_3) rise rapidly.[38, 50, 113, 120] Changes in fetal concentrations of thyroid hormones are summarized in Figure 16–5. At term, T_4 levels are similar to or slightly higher than maternal values.[71] TBG parallels T_4 and reaches term values at mid-gestation.[85]

TSH has been detected in amniotic fluid by 16 to 19 weeks, although the usefulness of this hormone for evaluating fetal thyroid function is unclear.[57, 67, 68, 96, 99, 123] Some success in using amniotic fluid iodothyronine levels for prenatal diagnosis of hypothyroidism has been reported.[62] Amniotic fluid T_4 levels peak at 25 to 30 weeks, then decrease; T_3 levels increase slowly throughout pregnancy.[62]

Serum T_3 levels remain low until 30 weeks, then increase slightly, never approaching maternal values.[27, 38, 99] T_3 levels remain low because the fetus is unable to convert T_4 to T_3 peripherally, possibly because of incomplete enzyme systems.[12]

A greater proportion of T_4 is converted to rT_3 in the fetus than in the adult. Serum rT_3 levels rise early in the third trimester, then gradually increase until term to values greater than those in adults (Fig. 16–5). The elevated serum rT_3 levels in the fetus are believed to be due to increased beta-ring iodothyronine monodeiodinase activity.[20, 32, 39, 60] This increases conversion of T_4 to the biologically inactive rT_3 rather than to biologically active T_3 and may be a way the fetus counteracts high T_4 levels and maintains metabolic homeostasis.[113]

Thyroid maturation in Phase III is related to progressive increases in hypothalamic TRH secretion, TRH responsiveness by the pituitary (the fetus responds to TRH similarly to adults by 26 to 28 weeks), sensitivity of the thyroid to TSH, and maturation of feedback mechanisms.[39, 60, 61] Since the fetal pituitary gland develops independent of hypothalamic control until late in gestation, circulating TRH is also derived from extra-hypothalamic sources such as the placenta.[27]

NEONATAL PHYSIOLOGY

Thyroid hormones are needed for lung development and surfactant production, bone

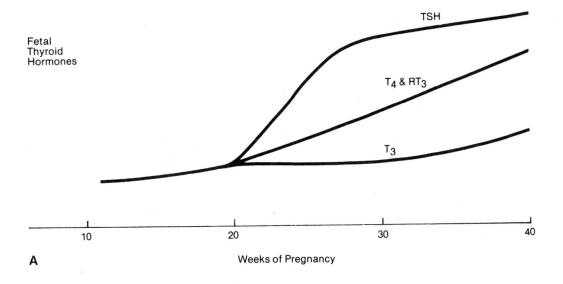

Fetal
Thyroid
Hormones

TSH

T4 & RT3

T3

A

Weeks of Pregnancy

10 20 30 40

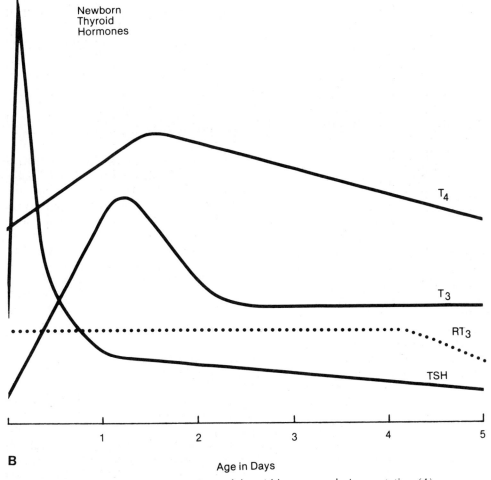

Newborn
Thyroid
Hormones

T4

T3

RT3

TSH

B

Age in Days

1 2 3 4 5

FIGURE 16–5. Changes in concentrations of thyroid hormones during gestation *(A)* and at birth *(B)*. TSH, thyroid stimulating hormone; T_4, thyroxine; T_3, triiodothyronine; rT_3, reverse triiodothyronine. (From Speroff, L., Glass, R. H., & Kase, N. G. [1989]. *Clinical gynecologic endocrinology and fertility* [4th ed., pp. 340–341]. Baltimore: Williams & Wilkins.)

growth, and CNS maturation. Intra-amniotic injections of T_4 may accelerate lung maturation in immature infants.[98] Within the CNS these hormones are critical for dendritic arborization, synaptogenesis, and cerebellar cell migration and growth (see Chapter 12).[33, 53] Effects on bone growth and CNS development continue into early childhood.

The newborn is in a state of relative hyperthyroidism because of marked changes in thyroid function with birth. TSH levels increase rapidly after birth (Fig. 16–5). Exposure of the newborn to the cooler extrauterine environment is believed to stimulate skin thermal receptors, release of TRH by the hypothalamus, and TSH release by the pituitary gland. The TSH surge may also be related to cutting of the umbilical cord, since this surge has been reported to occur even if cooling is prevented.[106] TSH increases from 9 to 10 μU/ml at birth to peak values of 85 to 100 μU/ml by 15 to 60 (mean, 30) minutes after birth.[24, 42, 60, 99] TSH rapidly decreases to 50% of peak values by 2 hours and to 20% by 24 hours, followed by a progressive decrease over the next 2 to 3 days to levels similar to cord blood values (Fig. 16–5).[24, 42, 85] During the 1st week periodic oscillations in serum TSH have been reported, possibly reflecting establishment of a new equilibrium in the negative feedback exerted by thyroid hormone on the anterior pituitary.[99]

The TSH surge leads to a rapid increase in T_4 and T_3 secretion (Fig. 16–5). T_4, T_3, and rT_3 levels are correlated with gestational age and birth weight.[38] Cord blood levels of total and free T_4 in term infants are similar to adult values.[37, 85] Newborn T_4 levels are usually 10 to 20% less than maternal values.[85] T_4 levels peak at 24 to 48 hours after birth (Fig. 16–5), then slowly decrease over the next few weeks.[45, 113]

Cord blood T_3 values average 45 to 50 ng/dl (30 to 50% of maternal values).[40] The newborn quickly changes from a state of T_3 deficiency to T_3 excess. T_3 levels increase rapidly with birth and peak at 24 hours at approximately 300 ng/ml (values exceeding those in adults) in most infants, then gradually fall.[38, 60] T_3 increases more than T_4 since some T_4 is converted to T_3 by the liver and peripheral tissues.[27] The increase in T_3 may be related to early cutting of the umbilical cord that augments increased liver blood flow and conversion of T_3 to T_4.[113] T_3 and T_4 levels gradually fall to high-normal adult values by 4 to 6 weeks.[85]

Levels of rT_3 remain high for 3 to 5 days (Fig. 16–5), then gradually decrease to adult values by 2 weeks.[85, 113] TBG tends to be high because of transplacental passage of estrogens that stimulate its production. TBG-binding capacity in the infant is higher than in the pregnant woman and about 1.5 times that of the adult.[85] Radioactive iodine uptake by the thyroid is higher in the newborn because of increased avidity of the neonatal thyroid for iodine. Values for parameters related to thyroid function in the neonate are summarized in Table 16–3.

The TSH surge is seen in term, preterm, and small for gestational age (SGA) infants and seems unrelated to type of delivery.[42, 105] Thyroid hormones in preterm infants follow patterns similar to those in term infants, but may take longer to reach stable values.[85] T_4 and T_3 levels are lower and rT_3 levels higher in preterm and SGA infants than in term infants.[45] Some ill preterm infants develop a characteristic syndrome with elevated TSH and low T_4 levels without other evidence of hypothyroidism.[21, 32, 60]

CLINICAL IMPLICATIONS FOR NEONATAL CARE

Alterations in thyroid function influence the transition to extrauterine life. Thyroid function is closely linked to thermoregulation and production of heat from brown adipose tissue. Alterations in health status from immaturity or acute illness can result in transient thyroid dysfunction. Screening for hypothyroidism and recognition of hyper- and hypothyroidism have important ramifications for the infant's future growth and development. This section examines implications of these events.

Thyroid Function and Thermoregulation

Thyroid function and neonatal temperature regulation are interrelated (see Chapter 17). T_3 and T_4 increase basal metabolic rate and heat production, whereas T_4 and norepinephrine stimulate metabolism of brown adipose tissue (BAT). T_4 potentiates the effects of catecholamines to increase oxygen consumption (and metabolic rate) and increases BAT lipolysis. Within 6 hours of birth the term neonate can respond to cold stress by

TABLE 16–3
Normal Range for T_4, T_3, RT_3U, TBG, and TSH in Infancy and Childhood*

AGE	TOTAL T_4 (μg/dl)		TOTAL T_3 (ng/dl)		T_3 RESIN UPTAKE (%)		TBG (mg/dl)		TSH (μU/ml)	
	Mean	Range†	Mean	Range†	Mean	Range†	Mean	Range†	Mean	Range†
Cord blood	10.2	7.4–13.0	45	15–75	0.90	0.75–1.05	5.6	—	9.0	<2.5–17.4
1 to 3 days	17.2	11.8–22.6	124	32–216	1.15	0.90–1.40	5.0	—	8.0	<2.5–13.3
1 to 2 weeks	13.2	9.8–16.6	—	—	1.00	0.85–1.15	—	—	—	—
2 to 4 weeks	11.0	7.0–15.0	160	160–240	0.95	0.80–1.15	—	—	4.0	0.6–10.0
1 to 4 months	10.3	7.2–14.4	163	117–209	0.90	0.75–1.05	—	—	<2.5	<2.5
4 to 12 months	11.0	7.8–16.5	176	110–280	0.98	0.88–1.12	4.4	3.1–5.6	2.1	0.6–6.3
1 to 5 years	10.5	7.3–15.0	168	105–269	0.99	0.88–1.12	4.2	2.9–5.4	2.0	0.6–6.3
5 to 10 years	9.3	6.4–13.3	150	94–241	1.00	0.88–1.12	3.8	2.5–5.0	2.0	0.6–6.3
10 to 15 years	8.1	5.6–11.7	113	83–213	1.01	0.88–1.12	3.3	2.1–4.6	1.9	0.6–6.3
Adult	8.4	4.3–12.5	125	70–204	1.01	0.85–1.14	3.5	2.1–5.5	1.8	0.2–7.6

*T_4, T_3, TSH, and TBG are measured by radioimmunoassay; T_4 results measured by competitive protein binding are 15% lower.
†Range equals ±2 S.D. from mean value.
From La Franchi, S.H. (1979). Hypothyroidism. *Pediatr Clin North Am, 26,* 33.

increasing his or her metabolic rate 100%; by 6 to 9 days this increase may be 170%. The preterm infant responds similarly to cold stress, although at a slower rate and lower percentage increase (40%).[10]

Transient Hypothyroidism in the Preterm Infant

In healthy preterm infants cord blood T_4 levels range from 5.5 to 6 μg/dl, increasing to 7 to 9 μg/dl by 21 to 28 days and reaching values similar to term infants by 4 to 6 weeks.[32, 63] As a result, preterm infants are more likely to have below normal values on thyroid screening tests compared with term infants. The prevalence of these alterations is 1 in 6000.[85]

Ill or stressed preterm infants, usually those with respiratory distress syndrome, may develop a transient hypothyroxinemia, often without other signs of hypothyroidism, characterized by lower serum T_4 and TSH levels than those seen in nonstressed infants of similar gestational ages and TBG values in the low to normal range.[23, 63, 116] T_3 levels are also lower because of persistence of increased deiodination of the inner thyronine ring with abnormally high levels of rT_3 (similar to the fetus) and an inability to convert T_4 to T_3.[21, 60]

The incidence of transient hypothyroidism varies depending on the values used as lower limits for normal, with an overall reported incidence of 25% in infants younger than 36 weeks' gestation.[54] Thyroid function tends to return to normal as the infant recovers from the underlying illness, with achievement of stable serum T_4 values by 6 to 7 weeks.[85] At 1 year intellectual development is similar to infants without transient hypothyroidism.[54]

The cause of transient hypothyroidism in preterm infants is unclear. These findings might be due to inadequate enteral feeding, since malnutrition results in similar alterations; delayed maturation of the hypothalamic–pituitary–thyroid axis; or may be a physiologic response to preterm birth or respiratory distress. This disorder is similar to the euthyroid sick syndrome seen in severely ill adults and children.[21, 32]

The decision of whether to treat healthy or ill preterm infants with transient hypothyroidism is controversial.[45, 85] Exogenous TRH significantly increases serum T_4 and TSH levels.[32, 54] Use of T_4 for thyroid hormone replacement does not result in significant differences in the age at which serum T_4 values normalize or in infant growth parameters, however.[21] Erenberg identifies several theoretical disadvantages to T_3 or T_4 therapy in these infants.[32] Early use of thyroid drugs alters development of the thyroid and adrenal axes in animal models. Administration of exogenous iodothyronines to neonates has been associated with decreased deoxyribonucleic acid (DNA) content and cellular proliferation in the brain. Many infants with transient hypothyroidism also have respiratory problems and are receiving oxygen therapy. Thyroid replacement may be a disadvantage if tissue oxygenation is marginal, since thyroid hormones increase oxygen consumption.[32]

Neonatal Hyperthyroidism

Neonatal hyperthyroidism is rare and is usually associated with transplacental passage of maternal TSIs (see Chapter 10) in women with Graves' disease. TSI levels correlate positively with development of neonatal hyperthyroidism. The incidence of neonatal effects is 1 in 70.[78] Although this disorder is usually transient, mortality rates of up to 20 to 25% have been reported, usually due to respiratory obstruction, difficult delivery due to the enlarged thyroid, or high-output cardiac failure secondary to tachycardia (heart rates greater than 200 beats/min).[72] T_4 and free T_4 levels are increased but they are also increased in the normal newborn.

Clinical findings such as low birth weight, irritability, hunger, tachycardia, diarrhea, sweating, and arrhythmias may be present at birth. If the mother is on antithyroid medication, manifestations may be delayed for 2 to 10 days.[72] These infants have an advanced bone age and occasionally craniosynostosis. Clinical effects, although transient, may last for 1 to 5 months.[25] If this disorder is recognized before birth, the fetus may be treated with propylthiouracil through the mother.

Neonatal Hypothyroidism

The most common cause of congenital hypothyroidism in North America is thyroid dysgenesis, with an incidence of 1 in 4000 live births.[32, 60] Hypothyroidism and cretinism secondary to endemic goiter are rare in North America. Infants with intrauterine hypothyroidism generally do not experience significant impairment of somatic or brain growth. Since neither maternal T_3 nor T_4 crosses the placenta, this is due to some unknown factor or factors that substitute for fetal T_4 supplies until birth.[60]

Most infants appear normal at birth with clinical signs apparent in fewer than 30%. Common findings such as a large fontanel, hypotonia, macroglossia, and umbilical hernia may not develop for several weeks or months.[85, 86, 99] By the time these findings are apparent, significant neurologic damage has already occurred, since inadequate thyroid hormone during fetal life and early infancy alters CNS development. The exact mechanism of injury is not well understood, but the degree of neurologic abnormality correlates with the duration and severity of the hypothyroidism.[88]

Newborn Screening for Hypothyroidism

Diagnosis and treatment of congenital hypothyroidism before 1 to 3 months of age are associated with an increased likelihood of normal mental development.[87,121] Therefore, routine screening of newborns for hypothyroidism has been implemented in many countries. Screening involves evaluating T_4 (more common in North America) or TSH (more common in Europe) levels. Infants with congenital hypothyroidism have decreased T_4 levels because of the thyroidal dysgenesis and elevated TSH levels. TSH levels are elevated since the low T_4 level does not provide the usual negative feedback inhibition of the anterior pituitary. Infants with a positive diagnosis are treated with thyroid hormone replacement therapy to normalize serum T_4 levels.[17]

Screenings for hypothyroidism and phenylketonuria (PKU) are done concurrently at 2 to 5 days of age. Specimens taken immediately after birth are avoided because of the usual TSH surge. If T_4 values fall into the lowest percentile (usually the third), TSH values are measured. If these are elevated, the infant is recalled for further evaluation.[85, 86] This test has a high selectivity and low (1 to 2%) recall rate.[85]

MATURATIONAL CHANGES DURING INFANCY AND CHILDHOOD

Thyroid function gradually changes during infancy and childhood (Table 16–3). The ability of the infant to convert T_4 to T_3 matures over the 1st month.[40] Twenty-four–hour ^{131}I uptake by the thyroid at 1 month is similar to adult values.[85] During childhood TSH levels tend to remain higher than those found in adults.[70] Maturation of negative feedback control of TSH secretion occurs by 2 months.[40, 99] The T_4 turnover rate is higher in infants and children, accounting for the increased requirement of children for thyroid hormone per unit weight.[85] TBG levels gradually fall over the first few years. Thyroid hormones fall to high adult values by 4 to 6 weeks, but do not reach mean adult values until puberty.[85]

SUMMARY

Normal thyroid function in the fetus and infant is essential for development of the CNS and other systems. Thyroid function

TABLE 16–4
Summary of Recommendations for Clinical Practice Related to Thyroid Function: Neonate

Know usual changes in thyroid function during the neonatal period (pp. 668–670, Fig. 16–5).

Recognize normal parameters related to thyroid function in the neonate (pp. 669–670, Table 16–3).

Recognize and monitor for transient hypothyroidism in the preterm infant (p. 661).

Recognize signs of and monitor for transient hyperthyroidism in infants of mothers with Grave's disease (pp. 664, 671–672).

Recognize clinical signs of hypothyroidism in infants (p. 672).

Screen newborns for congenital hypothyroidism (pp. 671–672).

Monitor growth and neurologic status in infants with congenital hypothyroidism (p. 672).

Page numbers in parentheses following each recommendation refer to the pages in the text where the rationale for that intervention is discussed.

is interrelated with thermoregulation and changes dramatically at birth. Newborns normally have a relative hyperthyroidism, but immaturity or illness can lead to transient hypothyroidism. Screening for congenital hypothyroidism is a part of routine newborn care in most of North America. Use of this screening is essential for early identification and reduction of mental retardation in these infants. Table 16–4 summarizes clinical recommendations related to neonatal thyroid function.

REFERENCES

1. Aboul-Khair, S.A., et al. (1964). The physiological changes in thyroid function during pregnancy. *Clin Science, 27*, 195.
2. Amino, N., et al. (1978). Changes of serum antithyroid antibodies during and after pregnancy in autoimmune thyroid diseases. *Clin Exp Immunol, 31*, 30.
3. Amino, N., et al. (1982). High prevalence of transient post-partum thyrotoxicosis and hypothyroidism. *N Engl J Med, 306*, 849.
4. Banerji, A. & Prasad, C. (1982). The postnatal development of the pituitary thyrotropin-releasing hormone receptor in male and female rats. *Endocrinol, 110*, 663.
5. Becker, R.A. (1987). Thyroid disease in pregnancy. In C.J. Pauerstein (Ed.), *Clinical obstetrics* (pp. 717–730). New York: John Wiley & Sons.
6. Bernal, J. & Pekonen, F. (1984). Ontogenesis of the nuclear 3, 5, 3'-triiodothyronine receptor activity in the human fetal brain. *Endocrinology, 114*, 677.
7. Black, J.A. (1963). Neonatal goiter and mental deficiency: The role of iodides taken during pregnancy. *Am J Dis Child, 38*, 526.
8. Bode, H.H., Vonjonack, K., & Crawford, J.T. (1977). Mitigation of cretinism by breast feeding. *Pediatr Res, 11*, 423.
9. Bouillon, R., et al. (1982). Thyroid function in patients with hyperemesis gravidarum. *Am J Obstet Gynecol, 143*, 922.
10. Bruck, K. (1961). Temperature regulation in the newborn infant. *Biologia Neonatorum, 3*, 65.
11. Burr, W.A., et al. (1977). Concentration of thyroxine-binding globulin: Value of a direct assay. *Br Med J, 1*, 485.
12. Burrow, G.N., Klastskin, E.H., & Genel, M. (1978). Intellectual development in children whose mothers received propylthiouracil during pregnancy. *Yale J Biol Med, 51*, 151.
13. Burrow, G.N., et al. (1968). Children exposed in utero to propylthiouracil: Subsequent intellectual and physical development. *Am J Dis Child, 116*, 161.
14. Burrow, G.N. (1978). Maternal-fetal considerations in hyperthyroidism. *Clin Endocrinol Metabol, 7*, 115.
15. Burrow, G.N. (1989). Thyroid diseases. In G.N. Burrow & T.F. Ferris (Eds.), *Medical complications during pregnancy* (pp. 224–253). Philadelphia: WB Saunders.
16. Burwell, C.S. (1954). Circulatory adjustments to pregnancy. *Bull Johns Hopkins Hosp, 95*, 115.
17. Camargo, C. A. (1989). Hypothyroidism and goiter during pregnancy. In S.A. Brody & K. Ueland (Eds.), *Endocrine disorders in pregnancy* (pp. 165–176). Norwalk, CT: Appleton & Lange.
18. Carswell, F., Kerr, M.M., & Hutchison, J.H. (1970). Congenital goitre and hypothyroidism produced by maternal ingestion of iodides. *Lancet, 1*, 1241.
19. Cheron, R.G., et al. (1981). Neonatal thyroid function after propylthiouracil therapy for maternal Graves'disease. *N Engl J Med, 304*, 525.
20. Chopra, I.J. & Crandall, B.F. (1975). Thyroid hormones and thyrotropin in amniotic fluid. *N Engl J Med, 293*, 740.
21. Chowdry, P., et al. (1981). The nature of hypothyroxinemia in sick preterm infants. *Pediatr Res,* Suppl, 505.
22. Crooks, J., et al. (1987). Comparative incidence of goitre in pregnancy in Ireland and Scotland. *Lancet, 2*, 625.
23. Cuestas, R.A. & Engel, R.R. (1979). Thyroid function in preterm infants with respiratory distress syndrome. *J Pediatr, 94*, 643.
24. Czernichow, P., et al. (1971). Thyroid function studied in paired maternal cord sera and subsequential observations of thyrotropic-hormone release during the first 72 hours of life. *Pediatr Res, 5*, 53.
25. Decherney, A. & Naftolin, F. (1980). The structural and functional development of neuroendocrine tissue in the human fetus. *Clin Obstet Gynecol, 23*, 749.
26. DeGroot, L.J., Robertson, M., & Rue, P.A. (1977). Tri-iodothyronine receptors during maturation. *Endocrinology, 100*, 1511.
27. Dowling, J.T. (1961). Effects of pregnancy on iodine metabolism in a primate. *J Clin Endocrinol Metab, 21*, 779.
28. Dowling, J.T., Frenkel, N., & Ingbar, S.H. (1960). The effect of estrogens upon the peripheral metabolism of thyroxine. *J Clin Invest, 39*, 1119.
29. Dowling, J.T., Frenkel, N., & Ingbar, S.H. (1974). Thyroxine-binding by sera of pregnant women, newborn infants, and women with spontaneous abortion. *J Clin Invest, 53*, 1263.
30. Dozeman, R., et al. (1983). Hyperthyroidism ap-

pearing as hyperemesis gravidarum. *Arch Int Med*, *143*, 2202.

31. Erenberg, A. (1978). The effect of perinatal factors on cord thyroxine concentrations. *Early Hum Devel*, *2*, 283.

32. Erenberg, A. (1982). Thyroid function in the preterm infant. *Pediatr Clin North Am*, *29*, 1205.

33. Ferreiro, B., et al. (1988). Estimation of nuclear thyroid hormone receptor saturation in human fetal brain and lung during early gestation. *J Clin Endocrinol Metab*, *67*, 853.

34. Fisher, D.A., Lehman, H., & Lackey, C. (1964). Placental transport of thyroxine. *J Clin Endocrinol Metab*, *24*, 339.

35. Fisher, D.A., Oddie, T.H., & Burroughs, J.C. (1962). Thyroidal radioiodine uptake rate measurement in infants. *Am J Dis Child*, *103*, 738.

36. Fisher, D.A. & Klein, A.H. (1980). The ontogenesis of thyroid function and its relationship to neonatal thermogenesis. In D. Tulchinsky & K. Ryan (Eds.), *Maternal-fetal endocrinology* (pp. 281–293). Philadelphia: WB Saunders.

37. Fisher, D.A., et al. (1969). Thyroid function in the term fetus. *Pediatrics*, *44*, 526.

38. Fisher, D.A., et al. (1977). Ontogenesis of hypothalamic-pituitary-thyroid function and metabolism in man, sheep and rat. *Recent Prog Horm Res*, *33*, 59.

39. Fisher, D.A. (1983). Maternal-fetal thyroid function in pregnancy. *Clin Perinatol*, *10*, 615.

40. Fisher, D.A. & Klein, A.H. (1981). Thyroid development and disorders of thyroid function in the newborn. *N Engl J Med*, *304*, 702.

41. Fisher, D.A. (1985). Control of thyroid hormone production in the fetus. In E.D. Albrecht & G.J. Pepe (Eds.), *Research in perinatal medicine (IV)* (pp. 55–69). Ithaca, NY: Perinatology Press.

42. Fisher, D.A. & Odell, W.D. (1969). Acute release of thyrotropin in the newborn. *J Clin Invest*, *48*, 1670.

43. Fisher, D.A., et al. (1970). Thyroid function in the preterm fetus. *Pediatrics*, *45*, 208.

44. Fisher, D.A. (1986). The unique endocrine milieu of the fetus. *J Clin Invest*, *78*, 603.

45. Forest, M.G. (1987). Endocrine disorders in the newborn. Problems related to thyroid and adrenal disorders in the neonatal period. In L. Stern & P. Vert (Eds.), *Neonatal medicine* (pp. 863–873). Chicago: Year Book Medical Publishers.

46. Fukuchi, M., et al. (1970). Thyrotropin in human fetal pituitaries. *J Clin Endocrinol Metab*, *31*, 565.

47. Furth, E.D. (1983). Thyroid and parathyroid hormone function in pregnancy. In F. Fuchs & A. Klopper (Eds.), *Endocrinology of pregnancy* (pp. 176–190). Philadelphia: Harper & Row.

48. Galina, M.P., Avnet, N.L., & Einhorn, A. (1962). Iodides during pregnancy. An apparent cause of neonatal death. *N Engl J Med*, *267*, 1124.

49. Gibson, M. & Tulchinsky, D. (1980). The maternal thyroid. In D. Tulchinsky & K. Ryan (Eds.), *Maternal-fetal endocrinology* (pp. 115–128). Philadelphia: WB Saunders.

50. Gluckman, P.D., et al. (1981). The neuroendocrine regulation and function of growth hormone and prolactin in the mammalian fetus. *Endocrinol Rev*, *2*, 363.

51. Grasso, S., et al. (1980). Thyroid-pituitary function in eight anencephalic infants. *Acta Endocrinol*, *93*, 396.

52. Greenberg, A.H., et al. (1970). Observations on

the maturation of thyroid function in early fetal life. *J Clin Invest*, *49*, 1790.

53. Guyton, A.C. (1987). *Textbook of medical physiology* (7th ed.). Philadelphia: WB Saunders.

54. Hadeed, A.J., et al. (1981). Significance of transient postnatal hypothyroxinemia in premature infants with and without respiratory distress syndrome. *Pediatrics*, *68*, 494.

55. Harada, A., et al. (1979). Comparison of thyroid stimulators and thyroid hormone concentrations in the sera of pregnant woman. *J Clin Endocrinol Metab*, *48*, 793.

56. Hollingsworth, D.R. & Alexander, N.M. (1983). Amniotic fluid concentrations of iodothyronines and thyrotropin do not reliably predict fetal thyroid status in pregnancies complicated by maternal thyroid disorders or anencephaly. *J Clin Endocrinol Metab*, *57*, 349.

57. Hollingsworth, D.R. (1989). Endocrine disorders of pregnancy. In R.K. Creasy & R. Resnik (Eds.), *Maternal-fetal medicine: Principles and practice* (pp. 989–1031). Philadelphia: WB Saunders.

58. Ingbar, S.H. (1972). Autoregulation of the thyroid: Response to iodide excess and depletion. *Mayo Clin Proc*, *47*, 814.

59. Kampmann, J.P., et al. (1980). Propylthiouracil in human milk: Revision of a dogma. *Lancet*, *1*, 736.

60. Kaplan, S.A. (1983). Ontogenesis of hormone action: Insulin, adrenal corticoids, thyroid hormones and growth hormone. In J.B. Warshaw (Ed.), *The biological basis of reproductive and developmental medicine* (pp. 291–305). New York: Elsevier Biomedical.

61. Klein, A.H., et al. (1982). Developmental changes in pituitary-thyroid function in the human fetus and newborn. *Early Hum Devel*, *6*, 321.

62. Klein, A.H., et al. (1980). Amniotic fluid thyroid hormone concentrations during human gestation. *Am J Obstet Gynecol*, *136*, 626.

63. Klien, A.H., et al. (1979). Thyroid hormone and thyrotropin responses to parturition in premature infants with and without the respiratory distress syndrome. *Pediatrics*, *63*, 380.

64. Kohler, P.O. (1987). Thyroid function and reproduction. In D.H. Riddick (Ed.), *Reproductive physiology in clinical practice* (pp. 171–187). New York: Thieme Medical Publishers.

65. Koivusalo, F. (1981). Evidence of thyrotropin releasing hormone activity in autopsy pancreata from newborns. *J Clin Endocrinol Metab*, *53*, 734.

66. Koshimizu, T., et al. (1985). Peripheral plasma concentrations of somatostatin-like immunoreactivity in human newborns and infants. *J Clin Endocrinol Metab*, *61*, 78.

67. Kourides, I.A., et al. (1984). Antepartum diagnosis of goitrous hypothyroidism by fetal ultrasonography and amniotic fluid thyrotropin concentrations. *J Clin Endocrinol Metab*, *59*, 1016.

68. Kourides, I.A., Heath, C., & Ginsberg-Fellner, F. (1982). Measurement of thyroid stimulating hormone in human amniotic fluid. *J Clin Endocrinol Metab*, *54*, 635.

69. LaFranchi, S.H. (1979). Hypothyroidism. *Pediatr Clin North Am*, *26*, 33.

70. LaFranchi, S.H. (1982). Disorders of the thyroid: Hypothyroidism. In S.A. Kaplan (Ed.), *Clinical pediatric and adolescent endocrinology*. Philadelphia: WB Saunders.

71. Lawrence, R.A. (1989). Breastfeeding and medical disease. *Med Clin North Am, 73*, 583.

72. Levy, R.P., et al. (1980). The myth of goiter in pregnancy. *Am J Obstet Gynecol, 137*, 701.

73. Lightner, E.S., et al. (1977). Intra-amniotic injection of thyroxine (T4) to a human fetus: Evidence for conversion of T4 to reverse T3. *Am J Obstet Gynecol, 127*, 487–490.

74. London, W.T., Money, W.L., & Rawson, R.W. (1964). Placental transfer of ^{131}I labelled iodide in the guinea pig. *J Endocrinol, 28*, 247.

75. Malkasian, G.D. & Mayberry, W.E. (1970). Serum total and free thyroxine and thyrotropin in normal and pregnant women, neonates and women receiving progesterone. *Am J Obstet Gynecol, 108*, 1236.

76. McDougall, I.R. & Bayer, M.F. (1986). Should a woman taking propylthiouracil breast feed? *Clin Nucl Med, 11*, 249.

77. McDougall, I.R. (1989). Hyperthyroidism and maternal-fetal thyroid hormone metabolism. In S.A. Brody & K. Ueland (Eds.), *Endocrine disorders in pregnancy* (pp. 151–163). Norwalk, CT: Appleton & Lange.

78. McKenzie, J.M. & Zakaraija, M. (1978). Pathogenesis of neonatal Graves' disease. *J Endocrinol Invest, 2*, 182.

79. Mestman, J.H. (1977). A practical approach to thyroid function tests. *Contemp OB/GYN, 9*, 28.

80. Mitchell, M.L., et al. (1982). Pitfalls in screening for neonatal hypothyroidism. *Pediatrics, 70*, 16.

81. Miyamoto, J. (1984). Prolactin and thyrotropin responses to thyrotropin-releasing hormone during the peripartal period. *Obstet Gynecol, 63*, 639.

82. Momotani, N., et al. (1986). Antithyroid drug therapy for Graves' disease during pregnancy: Optimal regimen for fetal thyroid status. *N Engl J Med, 315*, 24.

83. Mon, M., et al. (1988). Morning sickness and thyroid function in normal pregnancy. *Obstet Gynecol, 72*, 355–359.

84. Montoro, M. & Mestman, J.H. (1981). Graves' disease and pregnancy. *N Engl J Med, 305*, 48.

85. Morishima, A. (1987). Thyroid disorders. In A.A. Fanaroff & R.J. Martin (Eds.), *Neonatal-perinatal medicine-diseases of the fetus and infant* (pp. 1093–1114). St. Louis: CV Mosby.

86. Moshand, T. & Bongiovanni, A.M. (1987). Endocrine disorders in the newborn. In G.B. Avery (Ed.), *Neonatology-pathophysiology and management of the newborn* (pp. 1274–1297). Philadelphia: JB Lippincott.

87. New England Congenital Hypothyroidism Collaborative. (1981). Effects of neonatal screening for hypothyroidism: Prevention of mental retardation by treatment before clinical manifestations. *Lancet, 2*, 1095.

88. New England Congenital Hypothyroidism Collaborative. (1985). Neonatal hypothyroidism screening: Status of patients at 6 years of age. *J Pediatr, 107*, 915.

89. Oddie, T.H., et al. (1979). Comparison of T4, T3, rT3 and TSH concentrations in cord blood and serum of infants up to 3 months of age. *Early Hum Develop, 3*, 239.

90. Oddie, T.H., et al. (1977). Thyroid function at birth in infants of 30 to 45 weeks gestation. *J Pediatr, 90*, 803.

91. Penny, R., et al. (1984). Cord serum thyroid stimulating hormone and thyroglobulin levels decline with increasing birth weight in newborns. *J Clin Endocrinol Metab, 59*, 979.

92. Pezzino, V., et al. (1982). Role of thyrotropin-releasing hormone in the development of pituitary-thyroid axis in four anencephalic infants. *Acta Endocrinol, 101*, 538.

93. Prager, E.M. & Gardiner, R.E. (1979). Iatrogenic hypothyroidism from topical iodine containing medications. *West J Med, 130*, 553.

94. Robin, N.L., et al. (1969). Parameters of thyroid function in maternal and cord serum at term pregnancy. *J Clin Endocrinol Metab, 29*, 1276.

95. Robinson, P.L., O'Mullane, N.M., & Alderman, B. (1979). Prenatal treatment of fetal thyrotoxicosis. *Br Med J, 1*, 383.

96. Robuschi, G., et al. (1985). Amniotic fluid thyrotropin (TSH) does not reflect elevated fetal serum TSH following maternal administration of thyrotropin releasing hormone. *J Perinatal Med, 13*, 219.

97. Rodesch, F., et al. (1976). Adverse effect of amniofetography on fetal thyroid function. *Am J Obstet Gynecol, 123*, 723.

98. Romaguera J., et al. (1990). Responsiveness of the L-S ratio of the amniotic fluid to intra-amniotic administration of thyroxine. *Acta Obstet Gynecol Scand, 69*, 119.

99. Roti, E. (1988). Regulation of thyroid-stimulating hormone (TSH) secretion in the fetus and neonate. *J Endocrinol Invest, 11*, 145.

100. Rovet, J.F. (1990). Does breast-feeding protect the hypothyroid infants whose condition is diagnosed by newborn screening? *Am J Dis Child, 144*, 319.

101. Roti, E., et al. (1982). Ontogenesis of placental inner ring thyroxine deiodinase and amniotic fluid 3,3',5-triiodothyronine concentration in the rat. *Endocrinology, 111*, 959.

102. Roti, E., Gnudi, A., & Braverman, L.E. (1983). The placental transport, synthesis and metabolism of hormones and drugs which affect thyroid function. *Endocrinol Rev, 4*, 131.

103. Roti, E., et al. (1981). Human cord blood concentrations of thyrotropin, thyroglobulin and iodothyronines after maternal administration of thyrotropin releasing hormone. *J Clin Endocrinol Metab, 53*, 813.

104. Rubin, P.C. (1981). Current concepts: Beta-blockers in pregnancy. *N Engl J Med, 305*, 1323.

105. Sack, J., Fisher, D.A., & Wang, C.C. (1976). Serum thyrotropin, prolactin and growth hormone levels during the early neonatal period in the human infant. *J Pediatr, 89*, 298.

106. Sack, J., et al. (1976). Umbilical cord cutting triggers hypertriiodothyroninemia and nonshivering thermogenesis in the newborn lamb. *Pediatr Res, 10*, 169.

107. Sack, J., et al. (1977). Thyroxine concentrations in human milk. *J Clin Endocrinol Metab, 45*, 171.

108. Sadler, T.W. (1985). *Langman's medical embryology* (5th ed., pp. 353–355). Baltimore: Williams & Wilkins.

109. Schenker, J.G., et al. (1975). Prolactin in normal pregnancy: Relationship of maternal, fetal and amniotic fluid levels. *Am J Obstetr Gynecol, 123*, 834.

110. Senior, B. & Chernoff, H.L. (1971). Iodide goiter in the newborn. *Pediatrics, 47*, 510.

111. Sherwin, J.R. (1982). Development of the regulatory mechanisms in the thyroid: Failure of iodide to suppress iodide transport activity. *Proc Soc Exp Biol Med, 169*, 458.

112. Skjoldebrand, L., et al. (1982). Thyroid associated components in serum during normal pregnancy. *Acta Endocrinol, 100,* 504.

112a. Smith, J.E. (1990). Pregnancy complicated by thyroid disease. *J Nurs Midwifery, 35,* 143.

113. Speroff, L., Glass, R.H. & Kase, N.G. (1989). *Clinical gynecologic endocrinology and infertility* (4th ed.). Baltimore: Williams & Wilkins.

114. Tulchinsky, D. (1980). The postpartum period. In D. Tulchinsky & K. Ryan (Eds.), *Maternal-fetal endocrinology* (pp. 144–166). Philadelphia: WB Saunders.

115. Tyson, J.E. (1980). Changing role of placental lactogen and prolactin in human gestation. *Clin Obstet Gynecol, 23,* 737.

116. Uhrmann, S., et al. (1978). Thyroid function in the preterm infant: A longitudinal assessment. *J Pediatr, 92,* 968.

117. Uhrmann, S., et al. (1981). Frequency of transient hypothyroxinaemia in low birthweight infants: Potential pitfall for neonatal screening programmes. *Arch Dis Child, 56,* 214.

118. Vulsma, T., et al. (1989). Maternal-fetal transfer of thyroxine in congenital hypothyroidism due to a total organification defect or thyroid agenesis. *N Engl J Med, 321,* 13.

119. Walfish, P.G. & Chan, J.Y.C. (1985). Post-partum hyperthyroidism. *J Clin Endocrinol Metab, 14,* 417.

120. Wilson, D.M., et al. (1982). Serum free thyroxine values in term, premature and sick infants. *J Pediatr, 101,* 113.

121. Wolter R., et al. (1979). Neurophysiological study in treated thyroid dysgenesis. *Acta Paed Scand Suppl, 277,* 41.

122 Yamamoto, T., et al. (1979). Longitudinal study of serum thyroid hormones, chorionic gonadotropin and thyrotropin during and after normal pregnancy. *Clin Endocrinol, 10,* 459.

123 Yoshida, K., et al. (1986). Measurement of TSH in human amniotic fluid diagnosis of fetal thyroid abnormality in utero. *Clin Endocrinol, 25,* 313.

CHAPTER 17

Thermoregulation

Maternal Physiologic Adaptations
    The Antepartum Period
    The Intrapartum and Postpartum Periods
Clinical Implications for the Pregnant Woman and Her Fetus
    Fetal Thermoregulation
    Maternal Hyperthermia and Fever
Neonatal Physiology
    Transitional Events
    Heat Transfer
    Heat Production and Conservation
    Heat Dissipation and Loss

Clinical Implications for Neonatal Care
    Neutral Thermal Environment
    Prevention of Heat Loss and Excessive Heat Gain
    Equipment Considerations
    Neonatal Hypothermia and Cold Stress
    Hyperthermia in the Neonate
Maturational Changes During Infancy and Childhood

Thermoregulation is the balance between heat production and heat loss involved in maintaining thermal equilibrium. Heat is produced by the body as a by-product of metabolic processes and muscular activity; thus a major function of the thermoregulatory system is dissipation of this heat.[25] The thermoregulatory system must also respond appropriately to alterations in environmental temperature to preserve thermal equilibrium. Maintenance of thermal stability is particularly critical in the newborn since exposure to cold environments and lowered body temperatures are closely correlated with survival, especially in very low birth weight (VLBW) infants. Maternal temperature changes are also important in relation to fetal well-being and the potential adverse consequences of maternal hyperthermia. Regulation of body temperature is summarized in Fig. 17–1.

MATERNAL PHYSIOLOGIC ADAPTATIONS

Hormonal and metabolic alterations during pregnancy result in changes in maternal temperature. These changes are transient and may cause discomfort but are generally not associated with significant physiologic alterations.

The Antepartum Period

The amount of heat generated increases 30 to 35% during pregnancy because of the thermogenic effects of progesterone and alterations in maternal metabolism and basal metabolic rate (BMR) (see Chapter 16).[91] As a result, many pregnant women develop an increased tolerance for cooler weather and decreased tolerance for heat. The additional heat is dissipated by peripheral vasodilation

Body Temperature Regulation

Regulation of temperature depends on the ability to (1) sense temperature changes in the external environment by skin receptors; (2) regulate heat production by increasing or decreasing metabolic rate; (3) conserve or dissipate heat (by sweating or altering skin blood flow); and (4) coordinate sensory input about environmental changes with appropriate body-temperature regulating responses.[116] Thermoregulation involves a "multiple-input system" controlled by the anterior and posterior portions of the hypothalamus. The anterior hypothalamus is temperature-sensitive and controls heat loss mechanisms. The preoptic nucleus of the anterior hypothalamus is the site of the set-point or threshold temperature. The set-point is a mechanism through which heat production and loss are regulated to maintain the core temperature within a narrow range.[67] The posterior hypothalamus, the central controller of responses (heat production or dissipation) to cold or heat stimuli, receives input from central and peripheral receptors (skin, abdomen, spinal cord, hypothalamic preoptic nuclei, internal organs). With cold stress the thermoregulatory center acts to conserve heat (through cutaneous vasoconstriction and abolition of sweating) or increase heat production (through voluntary skeletal muscle activity, shivering, or nonshivering thermogenesis). This center dissipates heat by activation of sweat glands to increase evaporative loss, peripheral vasodilation, and respiration.

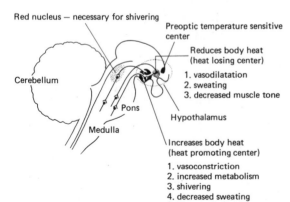

FIGURE 17–1. Regulation of body temperature. (From Guyton, A.C. (1974). *Function of the human body* (4th ed., p. 404). Philadelphia: WB Saunders).

with a four- to sevenfold increase in cutaneous blood flow and increased activity of the sweat glands. Cutaneous vasodilation leads to skin warmth. The maternal temperature usually increases by 0.5°C (0.3°F).

The Intrapartum and Postpartum Periods

Maternal temperature is monitored closely during the intrapartum period since elevations may indicate infection or dehydration. A transient postpartum chill is often experienced about 15 minutes after birth of the infant or delivery of the placenta. The cause of this chill is unknown and various causes have been proposed. This phenomenon may represent muscular exhaustion or result from disequilibrium between the internal and external thermal gradients secondary to muscular exertion during labor and delivery, sudden changes in intra-abdominal pressure with emptying of the uterus, or small amniotic fluid emboli.

Transient maternal temperature elevations up to 38°C (100.4°F) occur in up to 6.5% of vaginally-delivered women during the first 24 hours after delivery. In most women this resolves spontaneously and is secondary to noninfectious causes such as dehydration or a transient bacterial endometritis.[38, 113] Maternal fever in the postpartum period may be a sign of puerperal infection, mastitis, endometritis, or urinary tract infection, although these infections are usually the cause of fever after 24 hours. Any temperature elevation merits close monitoring, especially with increasingly early discharge.[102]

CLINICAL IMPLICATIONS FOR THE PREGNANT WOMAN AND HER FETUS

Fetal Thermoregulation

Since fetal temperature is linked to maternal temperature and the maternal-fetal thermal gradient, the fetus cannot control its temperature independently. Under normal resting conditions, the temperature of the fetus is approximately 0.5°C (0.9°F) higher than that of the mother, or about 37.6 to 37.8°C (99.7 to 100.0°F). Fetal heat dissipation is influenced by fetal and placental metabolic activity, thermal diffusion capacity of heat exchange sites within the placenta, and rates of blood flow in the placental and intervillous spaces.[3]

Heat generated by fetal metabolism is dissipated by the amniotic fluid or the placenta to maternal blood in the intervillous spaces. Transfer of heat is facilitated by the maternal-fetal temperature gradient. If the mother has an elevated temperature (from exercise, illness, or exposure to hot environments such as a sauna), this gradient may be reduced or reversed, leading to an increase in the fetal temperature. Changes in fetal temperature lag behind maternal changes since the amniotic fluid provides some insulation.[70]

Maternal Hyperthermia and Fever

There has been concern in recent years about the effects of elevated maternal temperature on the fetus. Maternal fever has three potential effects on the fetus: hypoxia secondary to maternal and fetal tachycardia and altered hemodynamics; teratogenesis; and preterm labor either from the fever per se, underlying infection, or associated hemodynamic alterations.[47] Maternal hyperthermia increases maternal oxygen consumption and shifts the oxygen-hemoglobin dissociation curve to the right. Although this latter change increases the oxygen supply to the placenta, fetal oxygen uptake becomes more difficult because of the altered thermal gradient.[57]

Research regarding adverse fetal effects has focused on three causes of maternal temperature elevations: fever secondary to illness, exercise, and the use of saunas or hot tubs. Many of these studies have been retrospective and suggestive but inconclusive. Maternal exercise (see Chapter 6) is associated with increased heat production and temperature that may alter the maternal-fetal thermal gradient and fetal heat dissipation. In addition uterine blood flow decreases during exercise, further altering the ability of the mother to dissipate fetal heat.[57, 70] The ability of the mother to dissipate the heat generated by exercise may improve as pregnancy progresses.[27]

Elevated maternal temperature secondary to illness-induced fever during early pregnancy, especially around the time of neural tube closure (22 to 28 days), has been associated with increased risk of anencephaly, microcephaly, and other central nervous system disorders; alterations in growth; cleft lip; and facial dysmorphogenesis in humans.[81, 89, 104] Whether these disorders are primarily due to the elevated temperature, the underlying infection, or a combination of these events is unclear. Several studies have reported similar patterns of defects in infants born to women whose extended heat exposure was secondary to sauna or hot tub use, suggesting that an elevated temperature may be the critical factor.[89, 104]

SUMMARY

Alterations in thermal status during pregnancy increase the risk of alterations in fetal health and development. Ongoing assessment and monitoring of thermal status in the pregnant woman and neonate and initiation of appropriate interventions to maintain thermal stability can prevent or minimize these risks. Clinical recommendations related to these processes include

1. Counsel pregnant women regarding basis for heat intolerance during pregnancy and intervention strategies.
2. Monitor maternal temperature during the intrapartum and postpartum periods.
3. Evaluate women with elevated temperatures for signs of infection
4. Counsel pregnant women to avoid activities that may lead to hyperthermia.

NEONATAL PHYSIOLOGY

Thermoregulation is a critical physiologic function in the neonate that is closely linked to the infant's survival and health status. An understanding of transitional events and neonatal physiologic adaptations is essential for provision of an appropriate environment to maintain thermal stability. Heat losses are greater, more rapid, and can easily exceed heat production in both term and preterm neonates if they are left unclothed in an environment comfortable for an adult. This is because of the infant's larger surface area–to–body mass ratio, decreased insulating subcutaneous fat, increased skin permeability to water, and small radius of curvature of exchange surfaces.[31]

Transitional Events

With birth the fetus moves from the warm intrauterine environment to the colder extrauterine environment. The newborn loses heat rapidly after birth, especially through evaporative losses. Although stimulation of cutaneous thermal receptors is a stimulus for initiation of respiration (see Chapter 7), significant heat loss must be prevented to reduce mortality and morbidity. Interventions in the delivery room to reduce evaporative and other losses support transition, reduce cold stress, and have been associated with a higher PO_2 at 1 hour of age.[87] An effective way to conserve heat after birth in the healthy term infant is to wrap the infant in a warm, dry towel and either give him or her to the mother for skin–to–skin contact or place him or her in a prewarmed incubator.[29, 31] Other interventions are listed in Table 17–1.

The infant's temperature may fall 2 to 3°C after birth, triggering cold-induced metabolic responses and heat production.[25] Term newborns can increase their metabolic rate by 100% by 15 to 30 minutes after birth and 170% at 1 week.[4, 23, 25] This response is delayed in larger preterm infants, who do not approximate term values until 2 to 3 weeks of age; further delay is seen in VLBW infants.[23] Thermal transition at birth is interrelated with thyroid function (see Chapter 16).

Heat Transfer

The usual rectal temperature for a newborn is 36.5 to 37.0°C (97.6 to 98.6°F); skin temperature is 36.0 to 36.5°C (97.1 to 97.8°F). Heat transfer involves two interrelated processes, the internal and external gradients. The internal gradient involves transfer of heat from within the body to the surface and relies primarily on blood flow within an extensive capillary and venous plexus. Efficiency of heat conduction is influenced by tissue insulation (subcutaneous fat) and convective movement of heat through blood. Heat conduction can be altered by vasomotor control processes mediated by the sympathetic nervous system that change skin blood flow with peripheral vasoconstriction to conserve heat and vasodilation to eliminate heat. Heat transfer through the internal gradient is increased in neonates because of their thinner layer of subcutaneous fat (i.e., less insulation) and a larger surface-to-volume ratio, especially in preterm infants. The subcutaneous layer of insulating fat accounts for only 16% of body fat in infants compared with 30 to 35% in adults.[32] The body mass of the neonate is about 5% of adult mass, whereas the surface area is 15%. [108] In term infants the surface-to-volume ratio may be three times, and in preterm infants five times, greater than that of adults.[25]

The external gradient involves transfer of heat from the body surface to the environment. The rate of heat loss is directly proportional to the magnitude of the difference between skin temperature and the environmental temperature and can be expressed as: heat loss = h (skin temperature − environmental temperature) × (surface area).[25,86] In this equation h equals the thermal transfer coefficient (the rate at which heat leaves the body surface) and is influenced by body size, tissue conductance, skin blood flow, and vasoactivity.[86] Heat loss per unit of body mass is inversely proportional to body size.[25] The mechanisms by which heat is transferred from the body surface are conduction, convection, radiation, and evaporation.

Heat transfer by the external gradient is also increased in the neonate because of increased surface area and an increased thermal transfer coefficient.[86] In terms of heat loss, the amount of exposed surface area is most critical, thus an infant who is not in an incubator or radiant warmer will lose less heat if he or she is diapered or swaddled. Factors that increase the thermal transfer coefficient (and thus heat loss) such as decreased skin thickness and altered conductance are present in the neonate. The threshold for heat production in the newborn is more closely linked to skin temperature than in the adult. As a result, cold responses, especially in preterm infants, are related primarily to skin rather than core temperatures changes.[80]

Heat Production and Conservation

Heat production is a result of metabolic processes that generate energy by oxidative metabolism of glucose, fats, and proteins. The amount of metabolic heat produced varies with activity, feeding (calorigenic or specific dynamic action), and environmental temperature.[25] Organs that generate the greatest amount of metabolic energy are the brain,

TABLE 17–1
Prevention of Heat Loss and Overheating in the Neonate

MECHANISMS	SOURCES OF HEAT LOSS / OVERHEATING	INTERVENTIONS
Conduction	Cool mattress, blanket, scale, table, x-ray plate, or clothing	Place warm blankets on scales, x-ray plates, other surfaces in contact with the infant Warm blankets and clothing before use Preheat incubators, radiant warmers, heat shields
	Heating pads, hot water bottles, chemical bags	Avoid placing infant on any surface or object that is warmer than the infant (see Table 17–3)
Convection	Cool room, corridors, or outside air	Maintain room temperature at levels adequate to provide a safe thermal environment for infant (72 to 76°F) Transport infants in enclosed, warmed incubators through internal hallways and between external environments (e.g., ambulance to nursery) Open incubator portholes only when necessary and for brief periods Use plastic sleeves on portholes Swaddle with warm blankets (unless under radiant warmer) or stretch transparent plastic across infant between radiant warmer side guards; use caps with adequate insulation quality or hooded blankets
	Convective air flow incubator	Monitor incubator temperature to avoid temperatures warmer than infant's body temperature
	Drafts from air vents, windows, doors, heaters, fans, air conditioners	Place infants away from air vents, drafts, and other sources of moving air particles Use side guards on radiant warmers to decrease cross current air flow across infant; stretch transparent plastic across infant between radiant warmer side guards
	Cold oxygen flow (especially near facial thermal receptors)	Warm oxygen and monitor temperature inside oxygen hood
Evaporation	Wet body surface and hair in delivery room or with bathing	Dry infant, especially head, immediately after birth with a warm blanket or towel Use caps with adequate insulation quality or hooded blankets Replace wet blankets with dry, warm ones and place in warm environment Delay initial bath until temperature has stabilized then give sponge bath Bathe in warm, draft-free environment and place on warmed towels and dry immediately; bathe under a radiant warmer
	Application of lotions, solutions, wet packs, or soaks to infant	Prewarm solutions and soaks; maintain warmth during use Avoid overheating solutions and soaks
	Water loss from lungs	Warm and humidify oxygen
	Increased insensible water loss in VLBW or ill infants	Increased incubator humidity levels may be necessary, especially in dry climates or with VLBW infants
Radiation	Placement near cold or hot external windows or walls, placement in direct sunlight	Place incubators, cribs, and radiant warmers away from external walls and windows, direct sunlight Use thermal shades on external windows Line incubator with aluminum foil
	Cold incubator walls	Use double-walled incubators or heat shields or cover with plastic film Prewarm incubators, radiant warmers, heat shields
	Heat lamps	Avoid use whenever possible; if used, monitor temperature every 10 to 15 minutes to avoid burns (Table 17–3)

heart, and liver. To maintain a constant body temperature, heat production must equal heat loss from the body surface over a given time. Basal heat production to maintain this stability is generated by body metabolic processes. In the event of cold stress, heat above basal needs can be generated by physical or chemical mechanisms.

Physical methods include involuntary (shivering) and voluntary muscular activity. Shivering is the most important mechanism for the generation of additional heat in adults. The neonate uses physical methods (shivering and increased muscular activity) to some extent to generate additional heat. Shivering is not as important in the neonate as in the adult, however, and is primarily seen as a late event associated with decreased spinal cord temperature after prolonged cold exposure. The cervical spinal region is protected from cold stress and preferentially receives heat generated by nonshivering thermogenesis (NST) through metabolism of brown adipose tissue (BAT) in the intrascapular area. If NST is blocked or unable to generate adequate heat to compensate for severe or prolonged cold stress, the temperature of the spinal cord eventually decreases.[25]

Infants produce some heat by increasing muscular activity with restlessness, hyperactivity, or crying. Infants may try to conserve heat by postural changes such as flexion that reduce the surface area and heat loss through the internal gradient. The ability to produce heat by physical methods can be markedly reduced or obliterated with the use of anesthetics, muscle relaxants, or sedatives and in infants who are tightly restrained or brain-damaged.[5, 25, 28, 32, 86, 99, 103, 107, 108]

Heat can be generated by chemical or nonshivering thermogenesis through increased metabolic rate and, in neonates, BAT metabolism. Both infants and adults can generate heat by increasing their metabolic rate above basal levels. An adult can increase heat production by 10 to 15% by NST; the neonate can have an increase of 100% or more.[46] NST is mediated by epinephrine in the adult and by norepinephrine in the neonate.[107] This results in activation of an adipose tissue lipase and splitting of triglycerides into glycerol and nonesterified fatty acids (NEFA), which are oxidized to produce heat, esterified to form triglycerides, or released into the circulation.[33, 92, 107]

NST is the major mechanism through which the infant produces heat above basal needs. Increasing the metabolic rate may lead to further problems in immature or compromised neonates since any increase in metabolic rate increases oxygen consumption. Stressed infants may be unable to provide enough oxygen; oxygen debt with lactic acidosis from anaerobic metabolism and finally exhaustion can result.

Thermal receptors in the skin are important mediators of the hypothalamic thermal center's response to temperature changes or cold stress. Stimulation of these receptors initially leads to heat-conserving responses with peripheral vasoconstriction. This may lead to acrocyanosis in the neonate. In the infant, thermal receptors are most prominent and sensitive over the trigeminal area of the face.[80] For example, cooling the face of an infant who is normothermic causes a responsive rise in metabolic rate. Conversely, warming the facial skin (i.e., use of warmed oxygen in an oxygen hood) when an infant is cold may suppress the usual increase in metabolic rate and other heat-generating mechanisms and can be dangerous.[86]

Brown Adipose Tissue Metabolism

The neonate relies primarily on brown adipose tissue (BAT) metabolism for nonshivering thermogenesis. Large amounts of BAT are found in human and animal newborns, hibernators, and in adult animals after cold acclimatization.[59, 105] Small amounts of BAT remain in the human adult and can be found around the kidneys and possibly the great vessels. In the adult, BAT produces minimal energy. In the term newborn BAT accounts for 2 to 7% of the infant's weight.[24, 25] The major function of BAT is heat production. BAT is found in the midscapular region, nape of the neck, around the neck muscles extending under the clavicles into the axillae, in the mediastinum, and around the trachea, esophagus, heart, lungs, liver, intercostal and mammary arteries, abdominal aorta, kidneys, and adrenal glands.[6, 32, 79] The total amount of heat produced by BAT metabolism in the neonate is unknown, but it may account for nearly 100% of the infant's needs.

BAT cells begin to differentiate at 26 to 30 weeks' gestation and continue developing until 3 to 5 weeks after birth. BAT stores increase up to 150% during this time and account for one tenth of the adipose tissue in term infants.[107, 132] BAT stores are lower in preterm and minimal in VLBW infants.

BAT is markedly different in appearance and composition from white adipose tissue (Table 17–2).[6, 25, 32, 79, 89, 103] These characteristics promote rapid metabolism, heat production, and heat transfer to the peripheral circulation. The lipolysis rate in BAT is three times higher than in white adipose tissue.[33]

BAT metabolism is controlled by the sympathetic nervous system and hormonal mediators (Fig. 17–2). Changes in temperature are transmitted from peripheral cutaneous receptors to the posterior hypothalamus (see Fig. 17–1). The sympathetic nervous system is stimulated to release norepinephrine within BAT stores and to stimulate catecholamine release from the adrenal medulla. Catecholamines stimulate glycogenolysis to provide glucose for thermoregulatory metabolic processes. The thyroid gland is also stimulated by the pituitary release of thyroid stimulating hormone to produce thyroxine (T_4). Thyroxine enhances the effect of norepinephrine on the BAT cells and may also act directly on BAT.[25, 32, 36, 55, 66, 90]

Heat production within the BAT cell has been proposed to occur by several mechanisms. Davis summarizes four possible mechanisms (see Fig. 17–2).[32] The first two mechanisms involve activation by norepinephrine of adenyl cyclase on the BAT cell membrane. Adenyl cyclase catalyzes conversion of adenosine triphosphate (ATP) to cyclic adenosine monophosphate (cAMP), which activates a

TABLE 17–2
Characteristics of Brown Adipose Tissue and Their Significance

CHARACTERISTIC	SIGNIFICANCE
Many small fat vacuoles	Large fat-to-cytoplasm ratio enhancing the rapidity of fat use
Many mitochondria	Production of energy (ATP) for rapid metabolic turnover and heat production
Glycogen stores	Source of glucose for production of ATP and energy
Abundant blood supply	Brings nutrients to cell and transports heat produced to other areas of the body
Abundant sympathetic nerve supply	Metabolism of BAT is mediated by norepinephrine

Compiled from references 24, 25, 32, 33, 59, 79, and 105.

lipase that breaks triglycerides into glycerol and fatty acids. Activity of adenyl cyclase is enhanced by thyroxine. Heat is produced by either reformation of triglycerides (reaction 1 on Fig. 17–2) or oxidation of the fatty acids to acetyl coenzyme A (CoA) followed by resynthesis of the fatty acids (reaction 2 on Fig. 17–2). Heat may also be produced by stimulation or disruption of the sodium pump by norepinephrine or thyroxine. This leads to activation of ATP, with a release of energy to run the pump and restore equilibrium and a loss of excess energy as heat (reaction 3 on Fig. 17–2). Finally, interference with the process of oxidative phosphorylation within the mitochondria by norepinephrine, thyroxine, or fatty acids (reaction 4 on Fig. 17–2) could result in loss of the excess energy produced by these reactions as heat. This energy is normally recycled to reform ATP from adenosine diphosphate (ADP).[32, 36, 55, 56, 66]

Production of heat from BAT metabolism involves breakdown of triglycerides into glycerol and nonesterified fatty acids (NEFA). Approximately 30% of the NEFA are oxidized with formation of energy and metabolic heat.[33] Since oxidation of NEFA is dependent on the availability of oxygen, glucose, and ATP, the ability of the neonate to generate heat can be altered by pathologic events such as hypoxia, acidosis, and hypoglycemia.

Heat Dissipation and Loss

The neonate can dissipate heat by peripheral vasodilation or by sweating. As the infant's core temperature rises above 37.3°C, cutaneous blood flow and skin thermal conductance increase along with heat loss through the external gradient.[112, 114]

Sweating increases evaporative loss. Each milliliter of water evaporated results in 0.58 cal of heat loss.[86] Term infants can increase evaporative losses up to 100%, but are less effective at sweating than adults.[49] Although the density of sweat glands is six times greater in the neonate, the capacity of these glands is only about one third of adult values.[40] Sweat appears first on the infant's forehead, generally beginning after 35 to 40 minutes of exposure to an ambient temperature above 37°C. By 70 to 75 minutes, evaporative water losses increase four times. In the term small for gestational age (SGA) infant, the onset of sweating is slower (55 to 60 minutes) but

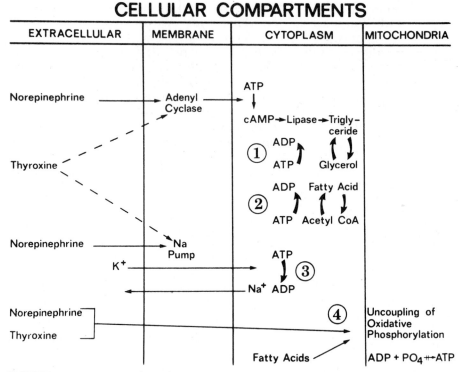

FIGURE 17–2. Proposed mechanisms of heat production in brown adipose tissue. See text for description. (From Davis, V. (1980). The structure and function of brown adipose tissue in the neonate. *J Obstet Gynecol Neonatal Nurs*, 9, 368.)

evaporative losses increase more rapidly to five times basal levels.[112]

Sweating is also altered in infants with central nervous system dysfunction and in preterm infants. In preterm newborns over 30 weeks' gestation the onset of sweating is delayed. SGA infants demonstrate thermoregulatory potential similar to that in infants of comparable gestations but are limited by their body size. In preterm infants, the maximal rate of sweating is less than that of either term or SGA infants.[112] Sweating is minimal or nonexistent in infants of less than 30 weeks' gestation because of inadequate development of sweat glands.[40] Even without large numbers of functional sweat glands, these infants have significant transepidermal water and heat losses (see Chapter 11).[49, 114] These losses are significantly increased in infants cared for in a radiant warmer or receiving phototherapy. Neonates also lose heat by radiation, conduction, and convection (discussed in the next section).

CLINICAL IMPLICATIONS FOR NEONATAL CARE

Prevention of cold stress and hypothermia is critical for the intact survival of the neonate.

Lowered body temperatures are inversely correlated with survival, especially in VLBW infants.[15, 26, 35, 41, 88, 91] Exposure to cool environments and subsequent cold stress often result in physiologic changes that significantly alter the infant's health status. Major components of neonatal care include maintenance of infant thermoregulatory processes, provision of an appropriate thermal environment, and prevention of heat loss, hypothermia, and cold stress.

Neutral Thermal Environment

Body temperature and oxygen consumption are closely related. As the body temperature falls, the amount of oxygen needed for survival increases rapidly. Oxygen consumption is minimal in two thermal regions: the neutral thermal environment and with severe hypothermia (Fig. 17–3). The neutral thermal environment (thermoneutrality) is an idealized setting defined as a range of ambient temperatures within which the metabolic rate is minimal and thermoregulation is achieved by basal nonevaporative physical processes alone.[21, 25, 31, 96, 107] Within this range the person is in thermal equilibrium with the environment. Since all newborns lose fluid through their skin continuously, evaporative loss is always present. Thus, Darnell proposes the following clinical definition of thermoneutrality for infants: ". . . that environment (usually a range of air temperatures in an incubator or abdominal skin temperature under a radiant warmer) in which the infant, when quiet or asleep, is not required to increase heat production above 'resting' levels to maintain body temperature."[31, p. 21] Figure 17–3 illustrates the relationships between thermoneutrality, body temperature, and metabolism.

In the thermoneutral state an infant is neither gaining nor losing heat, oxygen consumption is minimal, and the core-to-skin temperature gradient is small. A normal skin or core temperature does not necessarily mean that the infant is in a thermal neutral zone since an infant may be maintaining that temperature by increasing metabolic rate and BAT metabolism.

Thermoneutrality is generally achieved at environmental temperatures of 25 to 30°C in the adult, at 32 to 34°C in the term infant, and at higher temperatures in VLBW infants.[25, 107] Thus environmental conditions that do not tax an adult may require increased metabolic work by the neonate. Guidelines for determining neutral thermal zones for infants of varying ages and weights are available.[50, 64, 85, 86, 77, 100] These guidelines were developed for healthy infants at set environmental conditions and must be used in conjunction with evaluation of the temperature of the incubator walls and external environment, humidity, air velocity, health status and activity level, and, especially in the first week, gestational age.[96] These guidelines are not appropriate for extremely low birth weight infants.[73] These infants require higher neutral temperatures because of increased evaporative losses.[47, 94] Hey and Katz provide a formula for increasing ambient temperature if incubator wall and air temperatures are unequal: operative temperature for T (neutral) = 0.4 T (air) + 0.6 T (wall).[50]

Preterm infants cared for in environments outside the thermoneutral zone do not grow as well as infants with similar caloric intakes cared for in a thermoneutral environment.[44] VLBW infants may respond to temperatures outside the thermoneutral zone by a change in body temperature unaccompanied by an increase in oxygen consumption. Data indicate that there may not be a thermoneutral range for extremely preterm infants. The very high transepidermal water losses in these infants seem to be the major factor in determining their appropriate thermal environment.[73] Sauer and associates proposed a redefinition of the neutral thermal environment for VLBW infants as "the ambient temperature at which the core temperature of the infant at rest is between 36.7 and 37.3°C and the core and mean skin temperatures are changing less than 0.2 and 0.3°C/hour respectively."[96, p. 19]

Prevention of Heat Loss and Excessive Heat Gain

The four mechanisms by which heat is transferred to and from the body surface are conduction, convection, radiation, and evaporation. Examples of each mechanism in the neonate and appropriate interventions are listed in Table 17–1.

Conduction

Conduction involves transfer of heat from the body core to the surface through body tissue and from the body surface to objects in contact with the body (mattress, clothing,

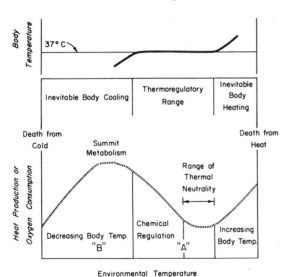

FIGURE 17–3. Effects of environmental temperature on oxygen consumption and body temperature. (From Klaus, M.H., Fanaroff, A.A., & Martin, R.J. (1986). The physical environment. In M.H. Klaus & A.A. Fanaroff (Eds.), *Care of the high-risk neonate.* (3rd. ed., p. 99). Philadelphia: WB Saunders.)

scales). The rate at which heat is transferred is directly proportional to the size of the temperature gradient.[11] Conductive loss can be minimized through insulation such as blankets or clothing or through skin-to-skin contact and is increased by placing the infant on conductive surfaces such as metal.[42] The 1-inch foam rubber mattress used in most incubators and radiant warmers has a low conductivity. Room temperature blankets and mattresses can be associated with significant heat loss, especially in the preterm infant, and must be warmed before use.[68, 120]

Heat can also be transferred from an object to the infant through conduction. Thus, if an infant is placed on a heated pad or hot water bottle that is warmer than the infant, hyperthermia or burns can develop (Table 17–3). Heat is also conducted to the surrounding stable air (boundary layer) in direct contact with the infant's body. This form of heat loss is minimal unless the air around the infant is moving such that the warmed air is constantly being replaced with cooler air, leading to convective losses.[46]

Convection

With convective losses, heat is dissipated from the interior of the body to the skin surface through the blood, conducted from the body surface to surrounding air (boundary layer), and carried away by diffusion to moving air particles (drafts, colder room or outside air) at the skin surface. Natural or passive convection involves movement of heat molecules into the boundary layer and then gradually away from the infant. Forced convection occurs when a mass of air is physically moving over the infant, conveying heat away from the body.[11, 69] Transfer is dependent on ambient temperature, air flow velocity, and relative humidity (which determines the air's thermal density). In low birth weight infants, convective losses are increased by the shorter radius of curvature of the body surface.[114] Heat can be lost by convective means through transfer of warmed inspired air to colder exterior air (or unheated oxygen) through exhalation. Convective losses are increased at higher air-flow velocities.[69] This is known as the wind-chill factor and may also be induced by incubator air circulation or gas flow into an oxygen hood. Environments with higher air temperatures and minimal air circulation

TABLE 17–3
Guidelines to Prevent Thermal Injury to the VLBW Neonate

Heat lamps should be avoided because of the increased potential for burns, unless strict measures are taken to measure the actual temperature of the exposed skin every 10 to 15 minutes during use.

Whenever heating pads are used, the pre-set temperature should never exceed 40°C. The infant's position should be changed frequently (possibly every 30 minutes at first) to prevent overexposure of the delicate skin surface to the heat.

Whenever transcutaneous heated electrodes are used, the lowest possible temperature should be used (under 44°C). Creative methods of securing the electrode should also be attempted to avoid adhesive use, such as wrapping the electrode with an elastic wrap around an extremity. Always observe the extremity carefully for changes in perfusion. A report from England recommends applying the electrode to the skin after a 1 to 2 second spray of Op-Site. If the adhesive disc is used, try dabbing the exterior adhesive with the loose fibers from a cotton swab to prevent the adhesive from adhering to the adjacent skin.

Pulse oximetry has been demonstrated to be an effective alternative to transcutaneous monitoring, since adhesive use is minimal and heat is not involved.

Before heelstick labwork, the heel should be prewarmed, but care should be taken to avoid temperatures over 40°C, especially when the foot is wrapped in plastic, which retains heat. The maximum temperature of chemical hot packs should be measured before routine use. Additionally, to avoid skin breakdown on the ankles or heels from routine heelsticks, labwork should be reduced to the absolute minimum.

Warmed ambient humidity is effective in maintaining thermoregulation and reducing insensible water loss and therefore maintaining skin integrity. The temperature should be constantly monitored so as not to exceed 40°C, and the humidity hose (if used) should be directed away from the baby. Warm aerosolized sterile water should be used. The combination of high humidity and denuded skin may predispose the infant to secondary infection, and therefore should be used cautiously.

From Malloy, M.B. (1989). High risk skin and high tech care: Skin care of the very low birthweight neonate. NAACOG Update Series, Vol.6, Lesson 8, p 5. Princeton, NJ: CPEC. (The NAACOG Update Series is a program sponsored by NAACOG and published by CPEC, Inc.)

can reduce convective loss by up to two thirds.[107]

Convective heat losses can be minimized by swaddling or using caps on infants in cribs, warming oxygen, and placing infants away from drafts or air vents (see Table 17–1). Warming of oxygen used in oxygen hoods is essential because of the sensitivity of the thermal receptors in the trigeminal area. If the infant's environment is well heated below the neck but cool around the face, the infant will react as if cold stressed. This can lead to metabolic alterations and hyperthermia.[86] If the infant's face is warmer than the body, apnea may result.

Evaporation

Evaporative heat loss occurs as moisture on the body surface or respiratory tract mucosa vaporizes. These losses depend on air speed and relative humidity.[47, 84, 119] Evaporative loss is the major source of heat loss immediately after delivery or during bathing, accounting for up to 25% of the total heat loss.[108] A wet newborn in the delivery room loses heat and lowers his or her skin temperature at a rate of 0.3°C/min (0.5°F/min) and rectal temperature by 0.1°C/min (0.2°F/min). This change is equivalent to a temperature loss of 3°C (5°F) over 10 minutes and represents a heat loss of at least 100 cal/lb/min.[103]

Evaporative losses are correlated with gestational age. In immature infants higher evaporative loss due to poor skin resistance to water passage from a lack of skin keratinization (see Chapter 11), constitutes a significant portion of overall heat loss (Fig. 17–4).[54] In these infants evaporative losses in the first days exceed all other sources of heat loss and often exceed heat production.[12, 69, 123] VLBW infants may lose up to 120 ml/kg/day through skin water loss. This represents a loss of 72 kcal/kg/day, a significant portion of the infant's total caloric intake.[37] Evaporative insensible water losses increase with activity, tachypnea, under radiant warmers, or with phototherapy (see Chapter 8).

Evaporative losses may be minimized by drying infants immediately after delivery or bathing; the use of sponge baths; warming

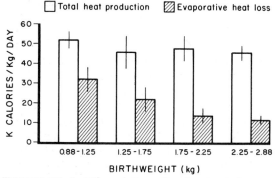

FIGURE 17–4. The relative role of evaporative heat loss at different birth weights. (From Klaus, M.H., Fanaroff, A.A., & Martin, R.J. (1986). The physical environment In M.H. Klaus & A.A. Fanaroff (Eds.), *Care of the high-risk neonate* (3rd ed., p. 99) Philadelphia: WB Saunders.)

soaks and solutions; and warming and humidifying oxygen (see Table 17–1). In term and preterm infants the evaporative heat loss is inversely proportional to the partial pressure of water vapor.[69, 97] Increasing relative humidity reduces evaporative losses; at a relative humidity of 100% evaporative loss is nonexistent.[111, 114] Incubator humidity levels may need to be increased to reduce evaporative losses in VLBW infants. These infants may have subnormal temperatures in spite of incubator temperatures above their body temperatures. The elevated air temperature reduces convective and radiant losses but does little to reduce the extremely high transepidermal evaporative loss in these infants.[73] Evaporative water losses in infants under radiant warmers can be reduced by stretching a layer of plastic wrap across the infant between the side guards of the radiant warmer.[11, 12, 13, 39] Hey and Scopes estimate that increasing the humidity of the VLBW infant by 50% is similar to increasing the ambient temperature 1.5°C.[54]

Radiation

The major form of heat loss in infants in incubators is radiation. Radiation involves the transfer of radiant energy from the body surface (through absorbance and emission of infrared rays) to surrounding cooler or warmer surfaces (walls, windows, heat lamps, light bulbs) not in contact with the infant. The rate of transfer depends on the temperature gradient, surface absorption, and geometry (the amount and angle of the infant's surface area facing the object).[11, 69] Radiant heat losses are independent of ambient temperature and other heat loss mechanisms.[107] Regulating incubator temperature only does not prevent heat loss by radiation. Thus, infants can get cold in a room containing air warmer than the infant if the walls and windows are cold.[33] Infants in warm incubators can be cold stressed if they radiate body heat to cooler incubator walls or cooler windows and walls. The amount of radiant loss is related to the temperatures of the window and walls rather than the temperature of the air in the incubator. Conversely, a baby in a cool incubator can get overheated if the incubator walls or room windows or walls are too hot.[33]

Incubators tend to act as greenhouses by trapping heat. The acrylic walls of the incubator are opaque to infrared rays. The walls allow short light waves to enter the incubator and subsequently the infant's body. The infant converts the short waves to heat and re-emits them as longer infrared rays. Since these rays cannot escape from the incubator, they heat the incubator and then the infant ("greenhouse effect"). Infants in incubators can become hyperthermic even if they are not subjected to obvious heating and without a change in incubator temperature.[33, 107] Radiant heat losses can be reduced by placing vulnerable infants away from the cooler exterior walls and windows, and by the use of thermal shades and heat shields or double-walled incubators (see Table 17–1). Overheating of infants by radiation can be prevented by placing infants away from windows and walls that are warmer than the infant and by avoiding or carefully monitoring the use of heat lamps.

Equipment Considerations

A major consideration in monitoring thermal status and promoting thermal stability in the neonate involves issues related to the various types of equipment that are currently available. Temperature can be monitored by rectal, skin, or axillary measurements and by manual or servocontrol methods. High-risk neonates are generally cared for in either convectively heated incubators or open radiantly heated beds. Each of these pieces of equipment and methods has inherent advantages and disadvantages. Unfortunately there are few good controlled studies that provide data to address most of these issues.

Monitoring Body Temperature

In the neonate, body temperature is monitored clinically by rectal, skin, or axillary methods. Rectal temperature provides an approximation of core temperature. The reading varies depending on the depth of insertion, with greatest variation found in the first 4 to 5 cm. The reading is higher as the depth of insertion increases. For example, increasing the depth of insertion from 1 to 5 cm may result in a variation in temperature of up to 1.5°C.[86] Disadvantages of rectal temperatures include trauma, perforation, and cross-contamination with repeated insertions.[54]

Axillary temperatures are noninvasive and approximate core temperature. Although axillary and rectal temperatures are correlated in neonates, reported mean differences have ranged from −0.05°C (axillary higher) to +0.55°C (rectal higher).[14, 58, 77, 98] The optimal length of time to obtain an accurate assessment of temperature with axillary measurement using a mercury glass thermometer carefully placed in the axilla was reported as 5 minutes in one study.[77] Recommendations in clinical texts vary from 90 seconds to 11 minutes.[109]

In a cold environment, core temperature may not indicate thermal stability. In a cold-stressed infant, the core temperature may be within normal limits because the infant has successfully compensated by increasing chemical thermogenesis. By the time the rectal temperature falls, the infant may be significantly compromised and difficult to rewarm.[86] Skin temperature measurement is frequently used with preterm and other neonates at risk for thermoregulatory problems. Skin temperature changes provide an early indication of cold or heat stress (Fig. 17–5). Thermocouplers or thermistors must be carefully placed since skin temperature can vary widely. Appropriate sites include the skin surface over the liver or between the umbilicus and pubis. The probe should not be placed over areas of BAT, poorly vasoreactive areas such as extremities and body prominences, or excoriated areas. Disadvantages of skin temperature include accidental displacement of the probe, risk of skin irritation, and misleading values with rapid temperature changes.[54]

Servocontrol

Servocontrol methods have been used with increasing frequency to maintain an infant's temperature within specified ranges. The temperature from either a skin or rectal probe (not currently recommended) is electronically monitored and used to control heater output decisions in either a convectively heated incubator or radiant warmer. Considerations related to use of skin probes were discussed above. Risks of servocontrol include hyperthermia if the probe becomes detached or is left in the manual mode and failure to detect early signs of sepsis since alterations in body temperature are masked.

Servocontrol is less effective in immature infants because of their higher evaporative water losses. The servocontrol system is based

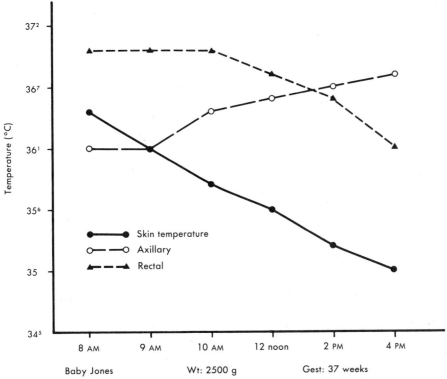

FIGURE 17–5. Temperature measurement at various sites during cold stress. In an environment that is less than thermal neutral, cold stress begins as skin temperature decreases (9 A.M.) because of vasoconstriction of the skin. Axillary temperature increases (10 A.M.) as infant burns brown adipose tissue to keep warm; rectal temperature is unchanged since core temperature is maintained. At noon the infant is still cold stressed (decreased skin temperature); axillary temperature is up as infant continues to compensate (burns brown adipose tissue); rectal temperature is still in normal range. From 2 to 4 P.M., the skin temperature reflects severe cold stress; the axilla is warm but the baby is cold; rectal temperature (core temperature) falls as body decompensates (severe cold stress). (From Merenstein, G.B. & Gardner, S.L. (1989). *Handbook of neonatal intensive care* (2nd ed., p. 115). St. Louis: CV Mosby.)

on the assumption that the temperature of the skin under the probe represents that of the surrounding skin; however, attaching the probe to the skin reduces evaporative losses at the site where temperature is being monitored. Thus, the servocontrol system may record skin temperatures that are higher than that of the rest of the infant's body and fail to keep the infant warm.[54, 86] Increasing humidity may reduce these differences.[86]

Incubators and Radiant Warmers

Preterm and other high-risk infants are usually cared for in closed convectively warmed incubators or open radiant warmers. There is no consistent evidence supporting either as more effective in reducing morbidity or mor-

tality and each has advantages and disadvantages.

INFANT INCUBATORS

The standard single- or double-walled convective incubator operates by circulation of warmed air. Air entering the incubator is filtered, providing a barrier against airborne pathogenic organisms from the environment. Air leaving the incubator is not filtered, so personnel or infants in open warmers and cribs are not protected from airborne organisms in the incubator air.

Up to 60 to 70% of total heat loss in infants cared for in convectively heated incubators is radiation.[114, 123] Since plexiglass is relatively opaque to radiant waves, infants radiate their body heat primarily to the inner side of the incubator wall. In a single-walled incubator, the temperature of this wall is midway between the incubator and room air temperatures. Since in most nurseries room air is considerably cooler than incubator air, this can lead to significant radiant heat loss, particularly in immature infants.

Radiant losses can be reduced by the use of double-walled incubators or heat shields.[75, 126] These devices place a second layer of plexiglass between the infant and the outer incubator wall. The infant radiates heat to the inner wall or shield, which is surrounded on both sides by warmed incubator air.[51] Heat shields should have closed ends to prevent a wind-tunnel effect, which further increases convective losses. Radiant losses in infants in incubators can also be reduced by increasing the ambient temperature of the room and placing the infant away from windows or exterior walls (see Table 17–1). Further alterations in radiant losses occur when incubators are covered with blankets or quilts to reduce light and noise levels.[118] Owing to extremely high transepidermal evaporative losses, VLBW infants may have subnormal temperatures in spite of incubator temperatures above their body temperatures and the use of heat shields and double-walled incubators.[5]

A major disadvantage of convective incubators is temperature fluctuations that occur with opening and closing of the portholes or hood. When the portholes are open the temperature of the air in the incubator falls rapidly and recovers slowly. Temperature changes with opening of the portholes can be reduced by the use of plastic sleeves. Laminar flow incubators minimize these fluctuations.

RADIANT WARMERS

Radiant warmers maintain the infant's temperature by a servocontrol system. These warmers are convenient to use, allow direct access to the infant, decrease radiant losses, and eliminate temperature fluctuations with opening of the portholes. Evaporative and convective losses are increased, however, with a risk of dehydration.[10, 123] Radiant warmers may also be associated with an increase in oxygen consumption.[51, 74] Other disadvantages of radiant warmers include those associated with servocontrol.

Insensible water loss in infants in radiant warmers is increased 50 to 200%.[22, 46, 61, 78, 124, 125] These losses may counteract the reduc-

tion in radiant losses in VLBW infants. Hey and Scopes note that although it may be possible to compensate for variations in evaporative and convective heat losses, the increased evaporative water losses are more difficult to manage.[54]

Convective losses can be reduced by using the sides on the warming bed or by stretching a layer of plastic wrap across the infant between the radiant warmer's side guards or on a special frame.[11, 12, 13, 39] Plastic wrap does not block radiant heat waves as does Plexiglass; thus, heat shields are not recommended for use with radiant warmers. Plastic wrap also reduces insensible water loss; plastic shields do not have a similar effect.[12, 13, 19]

Use of Head Coverings and Other Clothing

In the neonate the head accounts for one fifth of the total body surface area. Brain heat production is estimated to account for 55% of total metabolic heat production in the newborn.[93] Thus, the neonate's head accounts for a significant proportion of total heat loss. Head coverings are often used to reduce heat loss from this area. Head coverings or caps made of stockinette, which is a poor insulator, are relatively ineffective in reducing heat losses.[45, 93, 110] More effective materials include caps made of insulated fabrics or wool, lined with Gamgee, or insulated with a plastic liner. These head coverings have been found to significantly decrease heat loss after delivery and in neonates cared for in cribs and incubators.[20, 45, 76, 92, 93, 95, 110] Head coverings and clothing interfere with radiant heat loss and gain and are not appropriate for infants under radiant warmers.

Neonatal Hypothermia and Cold Stress

Alterations in health status or maturity can compromise the ability of the newborn to efficiently and effectively regulate heat production and respond to cold stress. Infants at risk and the basis for this risk are summarized in Table 17–4.

Signs of hypothermia are often absent or nonspecific in neonates. Clinical findings may include lethargy, restlessness, pallor, cool skin, tachypnea, grunting, poor feeding, or decreased weight gain.[86, 107, 116] The initial

TABLE 17–4
Infants at Risk for Problems in Thermoregulation

INFANT CATEGORY	BASIS FOR RISK
Preterm infants	Decreased subcutaneous fat for insulation
	Decreased BAT and ability to mobilize norepinephrine and fat
	Large surface area to weight ratio
	Inadequate caloric intake
	Inability to effectively increase oxygen consumption
	Increased open resting posture with less flexion
	Immature thermal regulatory mechanisms
	Increased evaporative water losses and higher body water content
Infants with neurologic problems	Alterations in hypothalamic control of body temperature
Infants with endocrine problems	Impairment of BAT metabolism due to inadequate catecholamines, thyroxine, or other hormones
Hypoglycemic infants	Decreased substrate for energy and ATP production in BAT
	Decreased metabolic response to cold stress
Infants with cardiorespiratory problems	Inability to increase oxygen consumption or minute ventilation further
	Inability to increase metabolic rate and reduce metabolic response to cold
	Impairment of BAT metabolism by hypoxia (impaired with P_{O_2} of 45 to 55 torr, essentially ceases at values below 30 torr) [99]
	Inadequate caloric intake to meet metabolic demands
	Increased risk of metabolic acidosis
	Increased temperature losses through evaporation of water from lungs
Infants with nutritional problems	Inadequate caloric intake to meet increased metabolic demands
Infants with electrolyte imbalances	Alterations in Na and K may lead to Na pump failure interfering with BAT metabolism
Infants with congenital anomalies such as meningomyelocele, omphalocele, gastroschisis	Increased surface area for heat loss
	Increased evaporative losses
Small for gestational age infants	Decreased subcutaneous fat for insulation
	Increased surface area for weight
	Higher basal metabolic rate and energy demands
Sedated infants or maternal intrapartal analgesia	Limited physical activity to generate heat
	Maternal diazepam (over 30 mg within 15 minutes of delivery) or meperidine (200 to 400 mg within 3 to 5 hours of delivery) administration associated with decreased newborn temperature for up to 20 hours [5, 28]

Compiled from references 5, 25, 28, 32, 86, 99, 103, 107, and 108.

temperature decrease is peripheral with stimulation of cutaneous receptors and initiation of nonshivering thermogenesis. If the heat generated by this method is insufficient, the core (rectal) temperature will drop.

The hypothermic or cold-stressed neonate tries to compensate by conserving heat and increasing heat production. These compensatory mechanisms can lead to physiologic alterations that may set off a series of adverse metabolic events (Fig. 17–6). If uninterrupted, this chain of events can result in hypoxemia, metabolic acidosis, glycogen depletion, hypoglycemia, and altered surfactant production. Physiologic effects of hypothermia and their consequences are summarized in Table 17–5.

Prevention of hypothermia and cold stress is a major component of neonatal health care. Strategies include careful monitoring of all infants, especially those at increased risk for hypothermia; decreasing heat losses by preventing evaporative, convective, conductive, and radiative losses; reducing the frequency and duration of cold exposure; and monitoring both infant and environmental temperatures.

Rewarming the Hypothermic Infant

The goal of rewarming a hypothermic infant in an incubator is to provide an environment in which the infant's temperature can increase through heat generated by the infant's internal mechanism while reducing sources of heat loss.[86] A radiant warmer may be more effective than an incubator for some infants, since it heats the baby, whereas an incubator reduces heat loss. Specific approaches to rewarming are controversial, since both slow and rapid rewarming have inherent limitations. Slow rewarming prolongs the hypothermia and pathologic consequences of cold

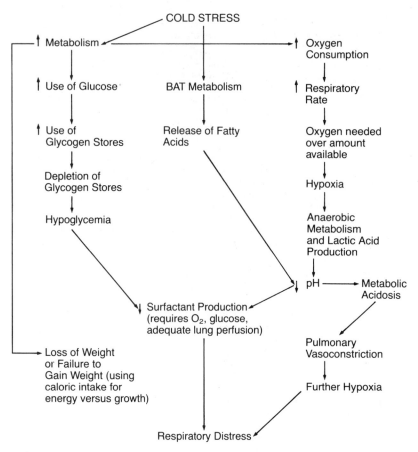

FIGURE 17–6. Physiologic consequences of cold stress.

stress. Rapid rewarming has been associated with heat-induced apnea and decreased blood pressure and shock due to rapid vasodilation with shunting and pooling of blood.[30, 86, 87, 107]

Perlstein recommends the following strategy for rewarming based on the principle of producing heat gain from the environment while eliminating further heat loss from the infant[86]:

1. Warm incubator air over the infant to 36°C, and simultaneously increase the humidity to reduce evaporative losses and decrease radiant losses with a heat shield.
2. Monitor with simultaneous skin and rectal temperatures (skin temperature should not be more than 1° warmer than rectal temperature).
3. If the temperature ceases to decrease or begins to slowly rise, maintain the infant and continue to monitor.
4. If the infant's temperature continues to fall, raise the incubator temperature to 37°C, evaluate for missed sources of heat loss, and check that the humidity is greater than 70%.

5. If the infant's temperature is still falling 15 minutes later, raise the incubator temperature to 38°C and add a radiant warmer over the incubator to increase the external wall temperature.
6. If the infant becomes apneic or shocky, slow the rate of rewarming.[86]

Hyperthermia in the Neonate

Although discussions regarding alterations in neonatal thermoregulation often focus primarily on hypothermia, the neonate is also at risk for hyperthermia. Hyperthermia increases metabolic demands, so even a slight increase in temperature can result in a significant increase in oxygen consumption, especially in preterm infants.[1] Other consequences of hyperthermia include increased heart, respiratory, and metabolic rates; increased insensible water loss (IWL); dehydration; peripheral vasodilation with a risk of decreased blood pressure; alteration in weight gain; and the risk of hypoxia and metabolic acidosis.[108] Neonatal hyperthermia

TABLE 17–5
Consequences of Neonatal Hypothermia

PHYSIOLOGIC EFFECT	PHYSIOLOGIC CONSEQUENCE
Peripheral vasoconstriction	Increased internal (core to skin) gradient and tissue insulation
	Persistent vasoconstriction can lead to reduced tissue perfusion and metabolism with accumulation of ketone bodies and development of metabolic acidosis
Increased metabolic rate	Increased oxygen consumption by increasing minute ventilation and respiratory rate
	Risk of hypoxia and respiratory failure in infants unable to increase oxygen intake (e.g., infant with respiratory distress syndrome or other respiratory problems, VLBW)
Increased requirements for oxygen, glucose, and calories	Exhaustion of supplies with subsequent development of hypoglycemia, hypoxia, aggravation of respiratory distress syndrome, or weight loss
Increased production of ketone bodies and accumulation of lactic acid from anaerobic metabolism	Metabolic acidosis with subsequent pulmonary vasoconstriction with further reduction in pulmonary perfusion
	Risk of hypoxia and altered surfactant synthesis
Norepinephrine release	Increased pulmonary vascular resistance with altered ventilation perfusion relationships and increased right-to-left shunting through the patent ductus arteriosus
	Risk of hypoxia and altered surfactant synthesis
Elevation in plasma nonesterified fatty acids	Alteration in glucose–to–fatty acid relationship with fall in blood glucose
	Risk of hypoglycemia and altered surfactant synthesis
	Competition with bilirubin for albumin binding sites with risk of bilirubin encephalopathy
Dissociation of albumin and bilirubin due to acidosis	Increased indirect (unbound) bilirubin
	Risk of bilirubin encephalopathy

Compiled from references 25, 32, 103, and 107.

(>37.5°C) is primarily due to overheating and less often to hypermetabolism. Hyperthermia also results from dehydration, drugs, or alterations in hypothalamic control mechanisms secondary to birth trauma.

Overheating due to increased environmental temperatures or radiant gains from exposure to sunlight or heat lamps is associated with peripheral vasodilation, a "flushed" appearance especially prominent in extremities, warm extremities, increased activity, irritability, increased IWL, and sweating in older preterm or term infants. Skin temperatures are higher than core temperatures.[86] Infants, particularly VLBW infants, are at risk for thermal injury from environmental sources (see Table 17–3)

The neonate is more vulnerable to overheating than are older individuals. At environmental temperatures above the neutral thermal zone, thermal equilibrium is reestablished by increasing evaporative losses.[25] The adult responds by increasing skin water losses and sweating. The neonate's initial response is to increase respiratory water loss (tachypnea). Infants over 30 weeks' gestation can sweat if the environmental temperature exceeds their threshold.[40,49]

Hyperthermia secondary to hypermetabolism can result from sepsis, cardiac problems, drug withdrawal, or other metabolic alterations. Clinical signs include peripheral vasoconstriction, pale, cool extremities, and a core body temperature that is higher than skin temperature.[86] Regardless of the cause, hyperthermia can lead to heat stroke, dehydration, and brain damage.

MATURATIONAL CHANGES DURING INFANCY AND CHILDHOOD

With increasing age nonshivering thermogenesis becomes less prominent and the infant begins to rely more on physical methods of heat generation such as activity and shivering.[25] Brown adipose tissue gradually disappears within the 1st year of life. This change is correlated with the switch in the major thermoregulatory mechanism from nonshivering thermogenesis to shivering.[107] Sweating becomes more efficient as a method of heat dissipation. The threshold body temperature for sweating decreases and maximal sweat production increases.[114]

TABLE 17–6
Summary of Recommendations for Clinical Practice Related to Thermoregulation: Neonate

Know mechanisms of heat production and dissipation in the neonate (pp. 680–688).

Initiate interventions to conserve body heat and reduce neonatal heat loss during transition (p. 680, Table 17–1).

Recognize usual values for neonatal temperature (p. 680).

Avoid overheating or cooling the trigeminal area of the neonate's face (pp. 682, 686).

Recognize and monitor for events that increase heat loss by conduction, convection, evaporation, and radiation (pp. 685–688, Table 17–1).

Institute interventions to reduce heat loss in the term and preterm infant by conduction, convection, evaporation, and radiation (pp. 685–688, Table 17–1).

Provide the term and preterm neonate with an appropriate thermal environment (pp. 684–688).

Know methods for monitoring thermal status and their advantages and limitations (pp. 688–689).

Understand differences between and implications of core versus skin temperature (pp. 680, 688).

Know advantages and limitations of different types of infant incubators and radiant warmers (pp. 689–690).

Use infant incubators and radiant warmers appropriately to maintain neonatal thermal status and reduce heat loss (pp. 689–690).

Monitor insensible water loss in infants cared for in radiant warmers (p. 690).

Use head coverings made of appropriate materials to reduce heat loss in infants in incubators and cribs (p. 690).

Recognize infants at risk for hypothermia and cold stress (pp. 690–691, Table 17–4).

Monitor neonates for signs of hypothermia and cold stress (pp. 690–691).

Monitor hypothermic or cold-stressed infants for adverse physiologic effects (pp. 690–691, Table 17–5, Figure 17–6).

Monitor infants during rewarming (pp. 691–692).

Recognize infants at risk for hyperthermia and thermal injury (pp. 692–693, Table 17–3).

Monitor neonates for signs of hyperthermia (p. 692).

Monitor hyperthermic infants for adverse physiologic effects (pp. 692–693).

Implement interventions to prevent thermal injury (Table 17–3).

Page numbers in parentheses following each recommendation refer to the page(s) in the text where the rationale for that intervention is discussed.

Higher rectal temperatures predominate in infants. Average temperatures at 18 months of age are 37.7°C (99.8°F), with marked daily variations seen in some children.[14] Body temperatures gradually decrease from 2 years to puberty, stabilizing at 13 to 14 years in girls and 16 to 17 in boys.[58]

SUMMARY

Thermal stability is one of the most critical processes during the transition to extrauter-ine life. Thermoregulation is essential for survival and has priority over most other metabolic demands. The infant who does not achieve thermal stability after birth or who is cold stressed in the neonatal period is more likely to experience health problems, poor growth, and increased morbidity and mortality. Ongoing assessment and monitoring of thermal status in the neonate and initiation of appropriate interventions to maintain thermal stability can prevent or minimize these risks. Clinical recommendations related to neonatal thermoregulation are summarized in Table 17–6.

REFERENCES

1. Adams, F.H., et al. (1964). Temperature regulation in premature infants. *Pediatrics, 33,* 487.
2. Adamsons, K. (1959). Breathing and the thermal environment in rabbits. *J Physiol, 146,* 144.
3. Adamsons, K. (1966). The role of thermal factors in fetal and neonatal life. *Pediatr Clin North Am, 13,* 599.
4. Adamsons, K., Gandy, G.M., & James, L.S. (1965). The influence of thermal factors upon oxygen consumption of the newborn human infant. *J Pediatr, 66,* 495.
5. Adamsons, K. & Towell, M.E. (1965). Thermal homeostasis in the fetus and newborn. *Anesthesiology, 4,* 531.
6. Aherne, W. & Hull, D. (1964). The site of heat production in the newborn infant. *Proc R Soc Med, 57,* 1172.
7. American Academy of Pediatrics and American College of Obstetricians and Gynecologists (1988). *Guidelines for perinatal care* (2nd ed.). Elk Grove, IL: AAP and Washington, DC: ACOG.
8. Artal, R. & Wiswell, R. (1986). *Exercise in pregnancy.* Baltimore: Williams & Wilkins.
9. Atkins, E. (1970). Fever. In C. MacBryde & R.S. Blacklow (Eds.), *Signs and symptoms* (5th ed., 451–475). Philadelphia: JB Lippincott.
10. Baumgart, S. (1985). Partitioning of heat losses and heat gains in premature newborn infants under radiant warmers. *Pediatrics, 75,* 89.
11. Baumgart, S. (1987). Current concepts and clinical strategies for managing low-birth-weight infants under radiant warmers. *Med Instrum, 21,* 23.
12. Baumgart, S., Fox, W.W., & Polin, R.A. (1982). Physiologic implications of two different heat shields for infants under radiant warmers. *J Pediatr, 100,* 787.
13. Baumgart, S., et al. (1981). Effect of heat shielding on convection and evaporation, and radiant heat transfer in the premature infant. *J Pediatr, 97,* 948.
14. Bayley, N. & Stolz, H.R. (1937). Maturational changes in rectal temperatures of 61 infants from 1 to 36 months. *Child Dev, 8,* 195.
15. Beautow, K.C. & Klein, S.W. (1964). Effect of maintenance of normal skin temperature on survival of infants of low birth weight. *Pediatrics, 34,* 163.
16. Belgaumkar, T.K. & Scott, K.E. (1975). Effects of low humidity on small premature infants in servo

control incubators. II. Increased severity of apnea. *Biol Neonate, 26,* 348.

17. Bell, E.F. (1983). Infant incubators and radiant warmers. *Early Hum Develop, 8,* 351.
18. Bell, E.F. & Rios, G.R. (1983). Air versus skin temperature servo control of infant incubators. *J Pediatr, 103,* 954.
19. Bell, E.F., Weinstein, M.R., & Oh, W. (1980). Heat balance in premature infants: Comparative effects of convectively heated incubator and radiant warmer with and without plastic shields. *J Pediatr, 96,* 460.
20. Besch, N.J., et al. (1971). The transparent baby bag: A shield against heat loss. *N Engl J Med, 284,* 121.
21. Bligh, J. & Johnson, K.G. (1973). Glossary of terms for thermal physiology. *J Appl Physiol, 35,* 941.
22. Brengelmann, G.L. (1983). Circulatory adjustments to exercise and heat stress. *Ann Rev Physiol, 45,* 191.
23. Bruck, K. (1961). Temperature regulation in the newborn infant. *Biol Neonate, 3,* 65.
24. Bruck, K. (1970). Non-shivering thermogenesis and brown adipose tissue in relation to age, and their integration in the thermoregulatory system. In O. Lindberg (Ed.), *Brown adipose tissue* (pp. 117–154). New York: Elsevier.
25. Bruck, K. (1978). Heat production and temperature regulation. In U. Stave (Ed.), *Perinatal physiology* (pp. 455–492). New York: Plenum Press.
26. Budin, P. (1907). *The nursling: The feeding and hygiene of premature and full-term infants.* New York: Imperial.
27. Clapp, J., Wesley, M., & Sleamaker, R. (1987). Thermoregulatory and metabolic responses to jogging prior to and during pregnancy. *Med Sci Sports Exerc, 19,* 124.
28. Cree, J.E., Meyer, J., & Hailey, D.M. (1973). Diazepam in labour: Its metabolism and effect on the clinical condition and thermogenesis of the newborn. *Br Med J, 4,* 251.
29. Dahm, L.S. & James, L.S. (1972). Newborn temperature and calculated heat loss in the delivery room. *J Physiol, 49,* 504.
30. Daily, W.J.R., Klaus, M., & Meyer, H.B.P. (1969). Apnea in premature infants: Monitoring, incidence, heart rate changes and an effect of environmental temperature. *Pediatrics, 43,* 510.
31. Darnell, R.A. (1987). The thermophysiology of the newborn infant. *Med Instrum, 21,* 16.
32. Davis, V. (1980). The structure and function of brown adipose tissue in the neonate. *J Obstet Gynecol Neonatal Nurs, 9,* 368.
33. Dawkins, M.J. & Hull, D. (1964). Brown adipose tissue and the response of newborn rabbits to cold. *J Physiol, 172,* 216.
34. Dawkins, M.J.R. & Scopes, J.W. (1965). Non-shivering thermogenesis and brown adipose tissue in the human newborn infant. *Nature, 206,* 201.
35. Day, R.L., et al. (1964). Body temperature and survival of premature infants. *Pediatrics, 34,* 171.
36. Edelman, I.S. (1974). Thyroid thermogenesis. *N Engl J Med, 290,* 1303.
37. Fanaroff, A.A., et al. (1972). Insensible water loss in low birth weight infants. *Pediatrics, 50,* 236.
38. Filker, R. & Monif, G.R.G. (1979). The significance of temperature during the first 24 hours postpartum. *Obstet Gynecol, 53,* 358.
39. Fitch, C.W. & Korones, S.B. (1984). Heat shield reduces water loss. *Arch Dis Child, 59,* 886.
40. Foster, K.G., Hey, E.N., & Katz, G. (1969). The response of the sweat glands of the newborn baby to thermal stimuli and to intradermal acetylcholine. *J Physiol, 203,* 13.
41. Gandy, G.M., et al. (1964). Thermal environment and acid base homeostasis in human infants during the first few hours of life. *J Clin Invest, 43,* 751.
42. Gardner, S. (1979). The mother as an incubator after delivery. *J Obstet Gynecol Neonatal Nurs, 8,* 174.
43. Gibbs, R.S. (1987). Fever and infections. In C. J. Pauerstein (Ed.), *Clinical obstetrics* (pp. 751–770). New York: John Wiley & Sons.
44. Glass, L., Silverman, W.A., & Sinclair, J.C. (1968). Effect of the thermal environment on cold resistance and growth of small infants after the first week of life. *Pediatrics, 41,* 1033.
45. Greer, P.S. (1988). Head coverings for newborns under radiant warmers. *J Obstet Gynecol Neonatal Nurs, 17,* 265.
46. Guyton, A.C. (1991). *Textbook of medical physiology* (8th ed.). Philadelphia: WB Saunders.
47. Hammarlund, K., et al. (1980). Transepidermal water loss in newborn infants versus evaporation from the skin and heat exchange during the first hours of life. *Acta Paediatr Scand, 69,* 385.
48. Hensel, H. (1974). Thermoreceptors. *Ann Rev Physiol, 36,* 233.
49. Hey, E.N. & Katz, G. (1969). Evaporative water loss in the new-born baby. *J Physiol, 200,* 605.
50. Hey, E.N. & Katz, G. (1970). The optimal thermal environment for naked babies. *Arch Dis Child, 45,* 328.
51. Hey, E.N. & Mount, L.E. (1966). Temperature control in incubators. *Lancet, 2,* 202.
52. Hey, E.N. & Mount, L.E. (1967). Heat losses from babies in incubators. *Arch Dis Child, 42,* 75.
53. Hey, E.N. & O'Connell, B. (1970). Oxygen consumption and heat balance in the cot-nursed baby. *Arch Dis Child, 45,* 335.
54. Hey, E. & Scopes, J.W. (1987). Thermoregulation in the newborn. In G.B. Avery (Ed.), *Neonatology-Pathophysiology and management of the newborn* (pp. 201–211). Philadelphia: JB Lippincott.
55. Himms-Hagen, J. (1976). Cellular thermogenesis. *Ann Rev Physiol, 38,* 315.
56. Horwitz, B.A. (1973). Quabain-sensitive component of brown fat thermogenesis. *Am J Physiol, 224,* 352.
57. Huch, R. & Erkkola, R. (1990). Pregnancy and exercise—exercise and pregnancy. A short review. *Br J Obstet Gynaecol, 97,* 208.
58. Iliff, A. & Lee, V.A. (1952). Pulse rate, respiratory rate and body temperature of children between two months and 18 years of age. *Child Dev, 23,* 238.
59. Johannson, B. (1959). Brown fat: A review. *Metabolism, 8,* 221.
60. Jones, R., et al. (1985). Thermoregulation during aerobic exercise in pregnancy. *Obstet Gynecol, 65,* 340.
61. Jones, R.W., Rocheforst, M.J., & Baum, J.D. (1976). Increased insensible water loss in newborn infants nursed under radiant heaters. *Br Med J, 2,* 1347.
62. Karlberg, P. (1949). The significance of the depth of insertion of the thermometer for recording rectal temperatures. *Acta Paediatr Scand, 38,* 359.

63. Kaunitz, A.M., et al. (1985). Causes of maternal mortality in the United States. *Obstet Gynecol, 65,* 605.

64. Klaus, M.H., Fanaroff, A.A., & Martin, R.J. (1986). The physical environment. In M.H. Klaus & A.A. Fanaroff (Eds.), *Care of the high risk infant* (pp. 96–112). Philadelphia: WB Saunders.

65. Kornienko, I.A. & Gokhblit, I.I. (1980). Age differences of temperature regulation in children age 5–12 years. *Human Physiol, 6,* 443.

66. Krishna, G., et al. (1968). Effects of thyroid hormones on adenyl cyclase in adipose tissue and on free fatty acid mobilization. *Proc Natl Acad Sci (USA), 59,* 884.

67. Kruse, J. (1988). Fever in children. *Am Fam Physician, 37,* 127.

68. LeBlanc, M.H. (1984). Evaluation of two devices for improving thermal control of premature infants in transport. *Crit Care Med, 12,* 3.

69. LeBlanc, M.H. (1987). The physics of thermal exchange between infants and their environment. *Med Instrum, 21,* 11.

70. Lotering, F.K. & Longo, L.D. (1984). Exercise and pregnancy: How much is too much? *Contemp Obstet Gynecol, 23,* 63.

71. Main, S.W. & Baumgart, S. (1987). Optimal thermal management for low birth weight infants nursed under high-powered radiant warmers. *Pediatrics, 79,* 47.

72. Malloy, M.B. (1989). High risk skin and high tech care: Skin care of the very low birthweight neonate. NAACOG Update Series (Vol. 6, Lesson 8, pp. 1–8). Princeton, NJ: Continuing Professional Education Center.

73. Marks, K.H. (1987). Incubators. *Med Instrum, 21,* 29.

74. Marks, K.H., Gunther, C., & Rossi, J.A. (1980). Oxygen consumption and insensible water loss in premature infants under radiant heater. *Pediatrics, 66,* 228.

75. Marks, K.H., et al. (1980). Oxygen consumption and temperature control of premature infants in a double-wall incubator. *Pediatrics, 68,* 93.

76. Marks, K.M., et al. (1985). Thermal head wrap for infants. *J Pediatr, 107,* 956.

77. Mayfield, S.R., et al. (1984). Temperature measurement in term and preterm neonates. *J Pediatr, 104,* 271.

78. Merenstein, G.B. (1970). Rectal perforation by thermometer. *Lancet, 1,* 1007.

79. Merklin, R.J. (1974). Growth and distribution of human fetal brown fat. *Anat Rec, 178,* 537.

80. Mestyan, J., et al. (1964). Surface temperature versus deep body temperature and the metabolic response to cold of hypothermic premature infants. *Biol Neonate, 1,* 230.

81. Miller, P., Smith, D.W., & Shepherd, T.H. (1978). Maternal hyperthermia as a possible cause of anencephaly. *Lancet, 1,* 519.

82. Motil, K.J., Blackburn, M.G., & Pleasure, J.R. (1974). The effects of four different radiant warmer temperature set points used for rewarming neonates. *J Pediatr, 85,* 546.

83. Nicholls, D.G. & Locke, R.M. (1984). Thermogenic mechanisms in brown fat. *Physiol Rev, 64,* 1.

84. Okken, A., et al. (1982). Effects of forced convection of heated air on insensible water loss and heat loss in preterm infants in incubators. *J Pediatr, 101,* 108.

85. Oliver, T.K. (1965). Temperature regulation and heat production in the newborn. *Pediatr Clin North Am, 12,* 765.

86. Perlstein, P.H. (1987). Physical environment. In A.A. Fanaroff & R.J. Martin (Eds.), *Neonatal-perinatal medicine—Diseases of the fetus and infant* (pp. 398–416). St. Louis: CV Mosby.

87. Perlstein, P.H., Edwards, N.K., & Sutherland, J.M. (1970). Apnea in premature infants and incubator-air-temperature changes. *N Engl J Med, 282,* 461.

88. Perlstein, P.H., et al. (1976). Computer-assisted newborn intensive care. *Pediatrics, 57,* 494.

89. Pleet, H.B., et al. (1980). Patterns of malformations resulting from the teratogenic effects of first trimester hyperthermia. *Pediatr Res, 14,* 587.

90. Polk, D.H., et al. (1987). Effect of fetal thyroidectomy on newborn thermogenesis in lambs. *Pediatr Res, 21,* 453.

91. Prichard, J.A., MacDonald, P.C., & Gant, N.F. (1985). *Williams obstetrics* (17th ed.). Norwalk, CT: Appleton-Century-Crofts.

92. Rizak, M. (1964). Activation of epinephrine-sensitive lipolytic activity from adipose tissue by adenosine 3,5 phosphate. *J Biol Chem, 239,* 392.

93. Rowe, M.E., Weinberg, G., & Andrew, W. (1983). Reduction of neonatal heat loss by an insulated head cover. *J Pediatr Surg, 18,* 909.

94. Rutter, N. & Hull, D. (1979). Water loss from the skin of term and preterm babies. *Arch Dis Child, 58,* 858.

95. Rutter, N., Brown, S.M., & Hull, D. (1977). Variations in resting oxygen consumption of small babies. *Arch Dis Child, 53,* 850.

96. Sauer, P.J.J., Dane, H.J., & Visser, H.K.A. (1984). New standards for neutral thermal environment of healthy very low birthweight infants in week one of life. *Arch Dis Child, 59,* 18.

97. Sauer, P.J.J., Dane, H.J., & Visser, H.K.A. (1984). Influences of variations in ambient humidity on insensible water loss and thermoneutral environment of low birth weight infants. *Acta Paediatr Scand, 73,* 615.

98. Schiffman, R.F. (1982). Temperature monitoring in the neonate: A comparison of axillary and rectal temperatures. *Nurs Res, 31,* 274.

99. Scopes, J.W. (1966). Metabolic rate and temperature control in the human baby. *Br Med Bull, 22,* 88.

100. Scopes, J.W. & Ahmed, J. (1966). Range of critical temperatures in sick and premature newborn infants. *Arch Dis Child, 41,* 417.

101. Silverman, W.A., Fértig, J.W., & Berger, A.D. (1958). The influence of the thermal environment upon survival of newly born premature infants. *Pediatrics, 22,* 876.

102. Simpson, M.L., et al. (1988). Bacterial infections during pregnancy. In G.N. Burrows & T.F. Ferris (Eds.), *Medical complications during pregnancy* (pp. 345–371). Philadelphia: WB Saunders.

103. Sinclair, J. (1976). Metabolic rate and temperature control. In C.A. Smith & N.N. Nelson (Eds.), *The Physiology of the newborn infant* (4th ed.). Springfield, IL: Charles C Thomas.

104. Smith, D.W., Clarren, S.K., & Harvey, M.A. (1978). Hyperthermia as a possible teratogenic agent. *J Pediatr, 92,* 878.

105. Smith, R.E. & Horwitz, B.A. (1969). Brown fat and thermogenesis. *Physiol Rev, 49,* 330.

106. Stern, L. (1977). Thermoregulation in the new-

born. Physiologic and clinical consequences. *Acta Paediatr Belg, 30*, 3.

107. Stern, L. (1979). Clinical aspects of thermoregulation in the newborn. *Contemp Obstet Gynecol, 13*, 109.

108. Streeter, N.S. (1986). *High-risk neonatal care* (pp. 87–106). Rockville, MD: Aspen.

109. Stephen, S.B. & Sexton, P.R. (1987). Neonatal axillary temperatures: Increases in readings over time. *Neonatal Network, 5*(6), 25.

110. Strothers, S.J.K. (1981). Head insulation and heat loss in the newborn. *Arch Dis Child, 56*, 530.

111. Sulyok, E., Jequier, E., & Ryser, G. (1982). Effect of relative humidity on the thermal balance of the newborn infant. *Biol Neonate, 21*, 210.

112. Sulyok, E., Jequier, E., & Prod'hom, L.S. (1973). Thermal balance of the newborn infant in a heat gaining environment. *Pediatr Res, 7*, 888.

113. Sweet, R.L. & Gibbs, R.S. (1985). *Infectious diseases of the female genital tract* (pp. 277–290). Baltimore: Williams & Wilkins.

114. Swyer, P.R. (1987). Thermoregulation in the newborn. In L. Stern & P. Vert (Eds.), *Neonatal medicine* (pp. 773–790). New York: Masson Publishing.

115. Templeman, M.C. & Bell, E.F. (1986). Head insulation for premature infants in servocontrolled incubators and radiant warmers. *Am J Dis Child, 140*, 940.

116. TePas, K.E. (1988). *Thermoregulation in newborns.* White Plains: March of Dimes Birth Defects Foundation.

117. Thomas, K. (1986). The influence of air temperature on the respiratory responses of preterm infants. Unpublished doctoral dissertation, University of Washington, Seattle, WA.

118. Thomas, K. (1990). Personal communication.

119. Thompson, M.H., Strothers, J.K., & McLellan, N.J. (1984). Weight and water loss in the neonate in natural and forced convection. *Arch Dis Child, 59*, 951.

120. Topper, W.H. & Stewart, T.P. (1984). Thermal support for the very-low-birth weight infant: Role of supplemental conductive heat. *J Pediatr, 105*, 810.

121. Torrance, J.T. (1968). Temperature readings of premature infants. *Nurs Res, 17*, 312.

122. Vaughans, B. (1990). Early maternal-infant contact and neonatal thermoregulation. *Neonatal Network, 8(5)*, 19.

123. Wheldon, A.E. & Rutter, N. (1982). The heat balance of small babies nursed in incubators and under radiant warmers. *Early Hum Develop, 6*, 131.

124. Williams, P.R. & Oh, W. (1974). Effects of radiant warmer on insensible water loss in newborn infants. *Am J Dis Child, 128*, 511.

125. Wu, P.Y.K. & Hodgman, J.E. (1974). Insensible water losses in pre-term infants: Changes with postnatal development and non-ionizing radiant energy. *Pediatrics, 54*, 704.

126. Yeh, T.F., et al. (1980). Oxygen consumption and insensible water loss in premature infants in single- versus double-walled incubators. *J Pediatr, 97*, 967.

127. Znamenacek, K. & Pribylowa, H. (1964). Some parameters of respiratory metabolism in the first three days after birth. *Acta Paediatr Scand, 53*, 241.

Index

Note: Page numbers in italics refer to illustrations;
page numbers followed by t refer to tables.

A

ABO incompatability, 462–464, *463*
Abortion, spontaneous, 48–49
Abruptio placentae, 93
Absorption, in gastrointestinal tract, *381*
  of carbohydrates in neonate, physiologic limitations
    of, 413t, 414–415
  of fats in neonate, physiologic limitations of, 413t,
    415–416
  of proteins in neonate, physiologic limitations of,
    412–414, 413t
  transepidermal, in neonate, 512, 513t–514t, 514
Absorptive state, of pregnancy, carbohydrate, fat and
  protein metabolism in, 588–589, *590*
Accelerated starvation, pregnancy as state of, 592–593
Accidental capillary breaks, placental transport by, 79t,
  81
Acid-base balance, in antepartum period, 266t, 266–
  267
  in intrapartum period, 267–269
Acid-base homeostasis, in neonate, 363
Acidosis, metabolic, late, in neonate, 369–370
Acquired immunodeficiency syndrome (AIDS). See also
  Human immunodeficiency virus (HIV).
  perinatal, 451–452
Actin, in myometrial cells, 111, *112*
Acyanotic congenital heart disease, management of,
  252
Adhesives, neonatal skin and, 511–512
Adipocytes, in pregnancy, 586, *588*
Adipose tissue, fetal development of, 505
Adrenal gland, in fetal endocrinology, 20
β-Adrenergic agonists, in labor inhibition, 127–128
Adrenocorticotropic hormone (ACTH), breast
  development and, 142t
Aerobic capacity, in antepartum period, exercise and,
  272
Afterload, in antepartum period, 206
  in functional development of fetal cardiovascular sys-
    tem, 239
Air flow, in antepartum period, 265–266
Airway resistance, increased, in neonate, respiratory
  risk and, 309
Airways, development of, in persistent pulmonary
  hypertension, 323t

Albumin, binding of bilirubin by, competition for, 652
Allergies, development of, 486
Allogenic fetoplacental units, nonrejection of,
  mechanisms of, 448t
Allograft, definition of, 441t
Alveolar-capillary membrane, in neonatal physiology,
  305–309
Amino acids, metabolism of, 583–610. See also
  Protein(s), metabolism of.
Aminoglycosides, toxicity of, in pregnant woman, fetus,
  and neonate, 454t–455t
Amniocentesis, genetic, in fetal status assessment, 89
Amnion, 82–83
Amniotic cavity, development of, in placentation, 65,
  67
Amniotic fluid, 83–84
  analysis of, in fetal status assessment, 89, 90t
  composition of, 84
  disposition of, 83–84, *85*
  in fetal development, 506–507
  in protection of fetus from infection, 464
  production of, 83–84, *85*
  turnover of, 83
  volume of, 83
    alterations in, 91–92
Ampicillin toxicity, in pregnant woman, fetus and
  neonate, 454t–455t
Anabolism, facilitated, pregnancy as state of, 592
Analgesics, for neonatal pain, 570–571
Androgens, in female reproductive processes, 25
Anemia, in pregnancy, megaloblastic, 173
  severe, 172–174
  sickle cell, 173–174
  physiologic, of infancy, 193–195
  vitamin E deficiency, in preterm infant, 190–191
Anencephaly, 542–543
Anesthesia, balanced, without epinephrine for cesarean
  section, hemodynamic changes from, 217
  epidural, without epinephrine for cesarean section,
    hemodynamic changes from, 217
  for cesarean section, cardiovascular system and, 217
  inhalation, respiratory effects of, 275–276
Aneuploidy, 7
Angiomas, spider, in pregnancy, 495–496
Angiotensin II, impaired response to, in pregnancy-
  induced hypertension, 351–352

Angiotensin II *(Continued)*
in pregnancy, 344
Angiotensinogen levels, in pregnancy, 343
Anomalies, gastrointestinal, 399t
in fetus of diabetic mother, 596–597
of central nervous system, 542–546
of foregut development, *401*
of hindgut, 405
of midgut, 404
of renal system, developmental basis for, 357
Anoxia, brain edema and hemorrhage related to, *566*
Antepartum period. See also *Pregnancy.*
ABO incompatibility in, 462–464, *463*
antibiotic use in, 452–455
arrhythmias in, 212
asthma in, 272–274
autoimmune disease in, 458
back pain in, 529
blood cellular components in, 162–165
blood pressure in, 206–207
blood volume changes in, 160–162, 202–203
brain tumor in, 536, 538
calcium and phosphorus metabolism in, 615, *616,*
616t, 617
carbohydrate metabolism in, 584–585
cardiac disease in, 218–222. See also *Heart, disease of,*
in pregnancy.
cardiac output in, 203–205
cardiovascular system in, 202–210
changes in, clinical implications for pregnant
woman and fetus from, 212–228
functional, 202–208
physical, 208–210
cell-mediated immunity in, 440
cerebral vascular disorders in, 538
chronic neurologic disorders in, 531–535
coagulation factor changes in, 166–167
complement system in, 444
connective tissue changes in, 494–495
constipation in, 391–392
cutaneous tissue changes in, 496–497
dependent edema in, 346–348
drug absorption and metabolism in, 397
dyspnea in, 270
echocardiographic changes in, 210
effects of altered maternal nutrition on, 394–395
electrocardiographic changes in, 210
epilepsy in, 531–535
exercise in, cardiovascular system and, 213–217
respiratory system and, 271–272
fat metabolism in, 584–586, *592*
gastrointestinal system in, 380–385
changes in, clinical implications for pregnant
woman and fetus and, 389–396, 397
nursing recommendations for, 391t, 398t
disorders of, 395–396
hair growth in, 497
headache in, 530–531
heart rate in, 205–206
heart sounds in, 209–210
heartburn in, 390–391
HELLP syndrome in, 227–228, 457–458
hematologic changes in, 495–496
hemodynamic changes in, 202–208
hemorrhoids in, 392
hemostasis in, 166–167
host defense mechanisms in, 440
changes in, implications for pregnant woman and
fetus and, 446–464, 465t

Antepartum period *(Continued)*
humoral immunity in, 440, 444
immune system in, 440, 444
immunization in, 455–456
integumentary system in, 492–497
liver disease in, 396–397
liver function tests in, 386t–387t
malignancy in, 456
management of renal function during, 350–352
maternal infection in, HIV, 451–452
preterm labor and, 450–451
risk of, 449–450
maternal tolerance of fetus in, 446–449
mucous membrane changes in, 496–497
musculoskeletal changes in, 524
musculoskeletal discomforts in, 529–530
nails in, 497
nausea and vomiting in, 392–393
neuromuscular system in, 523–524
nocturia in, 346
nutritional requirements in, 389–390
ocular adaptations in, 528–529
ocular changes in, 523–524
otolaryngeal changes in, 524
oxygen consumption in, 208
paresthesias in, 529
peripheral neuropathies in, 535–536, 537t
pigmentation alterations in, 492–494
plasma components in, 164t–165t, 165–166
plasma volume changes in, 160–162
platelets in, 162t–163t, 164–165
pregnancy-induced hypertension in, 222–227, 538
immunologic aspects of, 456–457
pregnancy-induced immune states in, 457–458
protection of fetus from infection in, 464
protein metabolism in, 584–585
pruritus in, 497
red blood cells in, 162t–163t, 162–164
regional blood flow in, 207–208
renal disease in, 352–354
renal system in, 337–345
arginine vasopressin and, 344–345
changes in, clinical implications for pregnant
woman and fetus and, 346–354, 347t, 355t
in glomerular filtration, 339, 341
in renal hemodynamics, 339
in tubular function, 341–342
structural, 337–339, 338t
fluid and electrolyte homeostasis and, 342
regulation of osmolarity and, 344
renin-angiotensin-aldosterone system and, 342–
344
sodium homeostasis and, 342
volume homeostasis and, 344
respiratory infection in, 271
respiratory system in, 263–267
changes in, clinical implications for pregnant
woman and fetus from, 270–276
Rho(D) isoimmunization in, 459–462, *461–462*
risk of urinary tract infection in, 348
secretory gland changes in, 497
sleep in, 524
smoking in, 274–275
spinal cord transection in, 536
spinal cord tumor in, 536, 538
stroke volume in, 206
supine hypotensive syndrome of pregnancy in, 213
systemic vascular resistance in, 207
thermoregulation in, 677–678

Antepartum period *(Continued)*
  thyroid function in, 660–663
    tests of, 663
  transplacental passage of maternal antibodies in, 458–459
  upper respiratory capillary engorgement in, 270–271
  urinary frequency in, 346
  vascular changes in, 495–496
  white blood cells in, 162t–163t, 164
Antibiotics, toxicity of, in pregnant woman, fetus, and neonate, 454t–455t
  use of, in neonate, 480–481
  used in pregnancy, 452–455
Antibody(ies), blocking, definition of, 441t
    in protection of fetus from rejection, 447–449
  definition of, 441t
  maternal, transplacental passage of, 458–459
Antibody-mediated immunity, definition of, 441t
  in neonate, 470–471
  in pregnancy, 440, 444
Anticonvulsant drugs, metabolism of, pregnancy and, 533t
Antidiuretic hormone, in pregnancy, 344–345
Antigen, definition of, 441t
Antioxidant protective mechanisms, 286t
Antioxidants, oxygen, in functional development of fetal respiratory system, 285
Antithyroid agents, fetal effects of, 666–667
Anus, imperforate, fetal development of, 405
Aorta, coarctation of, management of, 252–253
Aortic arches, fetal development of, 236
Aortocaval compression, in pregnancy, 213, *214*
Apneustic center, in respiratory control in neonate, 294
Appendages, epidermal, fetal development of, 505–506
Appendicitis, acute, in pregnancy, 395
Arachidonic acid, metabolism of, prostaglandin formation and, *115*, 116
Arginine vasopressin (AVP), in pregnancy, 344–345
  in renal system regulation in neonate, 365
Arrector pili muscle, fetal development of, 506
Arrhythmias, in pregnancy, 212
Artery(ies), fetal development of, 236
  intra-acinar, development of, in persistent pulmonary hypertension, 323t
  pulmonary, prenatal development of, 278–279
Artificial insemination, donor, 45–46
Asphyxia, intrauterine, 311–313
    management of, 313
    risk factors for, 312
  perinatal, 312
    hypocalcemia and, 629
    hypoglycemia in infant with, 608–609
    resuscitation for, 314–315
Aspirin, low dose, for pregnancy-induced hypertension, 226
Asthma, in antepartum period, 272–274
Atrial septal defect (ASD), in pregnancy, 220
Atrioventricular (AV) node, fetal development of, 234–235
Atrioventricular canal, septation of, in fetus, 231
Atrioventricular valves, fetal development of, 235
Atrium, septation of, in fetus, 231, *232–233*
Autoimmune disease, pregnant woman with, 458
Automatic walking reflex, 560t
Autonomic nervous system, fetal development of, 548–549

Autonomic regulation, in transition to extrauterine life, 552
Autonomic stress syndrome, in labor in paralyzed mother, 536
Autoregulation, cerebral, 554–555
Autosomal inheritance, 9–10

B

Babinski reflex, 558
Bacterial infections, immune responses of neonate to, 474–477
Bacteriocidal activity, altered, in neonate, 469
Baroreceptors, in regulation of fetal circulation, 243
Barrier methods, of contraception, 32
Basal metabolic rate (BMR) changes, in antepartum period, 662
Baseline heart rate, in fetal circulation regulation, 244–245
Battledore placenta, 94
Bell's palsy, in pregnancy and lactation, 537t
Bilirubin, albumin binding of, competition for, 652
  conjugation of, by hepatocytes, 639, *640*
  entry into brain, mechanisms of, *653*
  metabolism of, 636–655, *637*
    changes in, clinical implications for neonatal care and, 644–654
      clinical implications for pregnant woman and fetus and, 637–638
      maturational, during infancy and childhood, 654
    fetal development of, 638–639
    in maternal physiologic adaptations, 636–637
    in neonatal physiology, 639–644
      transitional events in, 639–640
  production of, in neonate, 640–641
  serum, measurement of, in neonate, 644–645
  synthesis of, *637*, 638
  total concentrations of, in neonate, *642*
  transport of, *637*, 638
    by hepatocytes, 639, *640*
Bilirubin encephalopathy, 652–654
Biochemical changes, in respiratory system in pregnancy, 263–264
Biochemical evaluation, of placental function, 88–89
Bladder, exstrophy of, 357
  hypertonic, post partum, 348
  neonatal, 365
  tone of, decreased, in pregnancy, 338–339
Blastocyst, early implantation of, *47*
Blastomeres, 43
Blocking antibody(ies), definition of, 441t
  in protection of fetus from rejection, 447–449
Blood, flow of, cerebral, local control of, 554–555
  in extremities in antepartum period, 208
  mammary, in antepartum period, 207
  pulmonary, in neonatal physiology, 300–301
  pulmonary vascular, in antepartum period, 208
  regional, in antepartum period, 207–208
  renal, in antepartum period, 208
    in fetus, 357
  uterine, in antepartum period, 207–208
  transfusions of, in neonate, 189–190
  volume of, changes in, in antepartum period, 160–162, 171
    in postpartum period, 169–170
      following vaginal and cesarean birth, *170*
    in antepartum period, 202–203
    in neonate, 181–182

Blood (*Continued*)
    in postpartum period, 212
    in pregnancy-induced hypertension, 224–225
Blood-brain barrier, in neonate, 553–554
Blood cells, formation of, in fetus, 176–178
    red, in antepartum period, 162t–163t, 162–164
    white, in antepartum period, 162t–163t, 164
Blood gases, fetal, in functional development of fetal
        respiratory system, 287
    maternal exercise and, 272
        normal, 288t
    maternal, exercise and, 271
Blood pressure, in antepartum period, 206–207
    in intrapartum period, 211
    in twin pregnancy, 218
Blood vessels, changes in, in pregnancy, 495–496
    fetal development of, 235–237
    pulmonary, prenatal development of, 278–279
Blues, postpartum, 527–528
Body composition of neonate, renal system and, 359
Body temperature, neonatal, monitoring, equipment
        for, 688
    regulation of, 677–694. See also *Thermoregulation.*
Bone mineralization, postnatal, calcium and
        phosphorus intake and, 627, *628*
Bradycardia, fetal, 244–245
    from maternal exercise, 216
Brain, bilirubin entry into, mechanisms of, *653*
    blood flow in, local control of, 554–555
    defects in, 542t–543t
    development of, 542t–543t
    edema of, anoxia and hemorrhage related to, *566*
    maturation of, sleep-wake states related to, 561–562
    neonatal, circulation in, 553–555
    tumor of, pregnancy in woman with, 536, 538
    vesicles of, embryonic development of, *544*
Brain barriers, in neonate, 553–554
Breast(s), blood flow in, in antepartum period, 207
    development of, hormonal contributions to, 142t–
        143t
    postpartum changes in, involution of, 138–139
    structure of, 141–142
Breast-feeding. See also *Lactation.*
    drugs contraindicated in, 152t
    in epileptic women, 535
    in women with thyroid disorders, 665
    neonatal jaundice and, 650–652
    neuropathies associated with, 537t
Breathing movements, fetal, in functional development
        of fetal respiratory system, 288–289
    maternal exercise and, 272
Bromocriptine, breast-feeding and, 152t
Bronchopulmonary dysplasia (BPD), hyperoxia and,
        308–309
    in newborn, 318–321
        factors affecting development of, *319*
        nursing care in, 320–321
        pathogenesis of, 318–320
        risk factors for, 318t
        treatment of, 320
    management of, 249–250
Brown adipose tissue (BAT), metabolism of, in heat
        production by neonate, 682–683, *684*
Bulbus cordis, fetal development of, 234
Bulk flow, placental transport by, 79t, 81
Bundle of His, fetal development of, 234–235

C

Café au lait spots, in neonate, 493t
Calcitonin, calcium levels and, in antepartum period,
    617
    in control of calcium and phosphorus levels, 616t
    levels of, in neonate, 626
    maternal-placental-fetal-neonatal interrelationships
        of, *621*
Calcium, absorption of, in neonate, 46
    antagonists of, in labor inhibition, 127
    for hypermagnesemia in neonate, 630
    homeostasis of, 617
    hypertension and, 619
    in milk, 148–149
    intake of, in preterm infants, 627
    levels of, hormonal actions controlling, 616t
        in neonate, 624
    maternal needs for, 619
    metabolism of, 614–631
        changes in, clinical implications for neonatal care,
            626–631
            clinical implications for pregnant woman and fe-
                tus and, 618–620
            fetal effects of, 621t
            maturational, during infancy and childhood, 631
        fetal development of, 621–623
        in antepartum period, 615
        in maternal physiologic adaptations, 614–618
        in neonatal physiology, 623–626
        maternal-fetal interactions and, 620, *621*
    myometrial contraction and, 117
    neonatal requirements for, 421
Calmodulin, myometrial contraction and, 117
Calories, neonatal requirements for, 417
    renal solute load and, for neonate, 422
Capacitation, 43
Capillary breaks, accidental, placental transport by, 79t,
    81
Capillary hemangiomas, in pregnancy, 496
Carbohydrate(s), absorption and digestion of, in
        neonate, physiologic limitations of, 413t, 414–415
    digestion of, *381*
    metabolism of, 583–610
        changes in, clinical implications for pregnant
            woman and fetus and, 591–598
            clinical implications for neonatal care, 606–609
            glucose tolerance test and, 593–594, 594t
            maturational, during infancy and childhood, 609
        fetal development of, 598–601
        in antepartum period, 584–585
        in intrapartum period, 591
        in maternal physiologic adaptations, 584–591
        in neonatal physiology, 603–605
        in postpartum period, 591
        maternal-fetal relationships and, 594–595, 595t
    neonatal requirements for, 420
    synthesis and release of, in milk, 150
Carbon dioxide, effects of ventilation-perfusion
        mismatching on, 304
    transfer of, in functional development of fetal respi-
        ratory system, 288
Carbon dioxide pressure, arterial, in antepartum
        period, 266–267
    in intrapartum period, 268–269
Cardiac output, in antepartum period, 203–205
    in intrapartum period, 210–211
    in transition, 241–242
    in twin pregnancy, 218

Cardinal veins, fetal development of, 237
Cardiovascular system, 201–254
  changes in, clinical implications of, for neonatal care, 246–253. See also specific disorder.
    for pregnant woman and fetus, 212–228
      maturational, 253–254
      physical, in antepartum period, 208–210
  conversion to extrauterine life, 291–292
  development of, timetable of, 54t, 57, *58*
  fetal development of, 228–240
    anatomic, 229–237
    blood vessels in, 235–237
    bulbus cordis in, 234
    cardiac valves in, 234
    conducting system in, 234–235
    functional, 237–240
      afterload in, 239
      Frank-Starling relationship in, 238–239
      inotropy in, 239–240
    primitive heart development in, 229–231
    septation of heart in, 231–234
    truncus arteriosus in, 234
  functional, contractile properties in, 238
    stress-strain relationship in, 237–238
  functions of, 201
  in antepartum period, 202–210
  in intrapartum period, 210–211
  in maternal physiologic adaptation, 202–212
  in neonatal physiology, 240–246. See also *Heart, physiology of.*
    cardiac physiology in, 242–246
    transitional events in, 240–242
  in postpartum period, 211–212
  twins and, 217–218
Caregiving environment, risks posed to neuromuscular and sensory development by, 565–574
Carpal tunnel syndrome, transient, in pregnancy and lactation, 537t
Catecholamines, in fetal circulation regulation, 244
  in functional development of fetal respiratory system, 284
  maternal exercise and, 215, 216
Caudal anesthesia, cardiac output and, 210–211, 217
Cavernous hemangioma, in neonate, 493t
Cell-mediated immunity, definition of, 441t
  in neonate, 471
  in pregnancy, 440
Cells, adhesion of, in morphogenesis, 51
  death of, programmed, in morphogenesis, 50
  differentiation of, in morphogenesis, 50
  division of, 5–6
  migration of, in morphogenesis, 50–51
  proliferation of, differential, in morphogenesis, 50
  recognition of, in morphogenesis, 51
  shape changes in, in morphogenesis, 50
  size changes in, in morphogenesis, 50
Central nervous system, anomalies of, 542–546
  function in preeclampsia, 226
Cephalosporin toxicity, in pregnant woman, fetus and neonate, 454t–455t
Cerebral autoregulation, 554–555
Cerebral vascular disorders, in pregnancy, 538
Cervix, development of, *16*, 17
  dilatation of, 122
  in pregnancy, 120–122
  involution of, postpartum, 138
  ripening of, 121–122
    control of, 125–126
  structure of, 120–121

Cesarean delivery, blood volume and hematocrit after, *170*
  hemodynamic changes and, 211
Chadwick's sign, of pregnancy, 38
Chemoreceptors, in fetal circulation regulation, 243–244
  in respiratory control in neonate, 292–293
Chemotaxis, altered, in neonate, 468
  definition of, 441t
Chest wall, compliance of, in postpartum period, 270
  muscles of, in respiratory pump, 295
  reflexes from, in respiratory control in neonate, 293
Childhood, maturational changes during, of bilirubin metabolism, 654
  of calcium and phosphorus metabolism, 631
  of cardiovascular system, 253–254
  of gastrointestinal system, 429–431
  of hematologic and hemostatic systems, 195–197
  of host defense mechanisms, 482–486
  of integumentary system, 516–517
  of metabolic processes, 609
  of neuromuscular and sensory systems, 572–573, 575
  of renal system, 371–373
  of respiratory system, 324–327
  of thermoregulation, 693
  of thyroid function, 672
Chimerism, 98
Chloasma, in pregnancy, 492, 494
Chloramphenicol, toxicity of, in pregnant woman, fetus, and neonate, 454t–455t
Cholecystitis, in pregnancy, 396
Cholelithiasis, in pregnancy, 396
Cholestasis, intrahepatic, in pregnancy, 397
Chorea gravidarum, 530
Chorion, 82–83
Chorionic gonadotropin, human, 75
Chorionic villus sampling (CVS), in fetal status assessment, 89–91
Chorionic villus(i), development of, in placentation, 67–68
Chromosomes, 3–4
  abnormalities of, age and, 24
  breaks in, teratogenesis by, 62
  deletions of, 8
  duplication of, 8
  inversion of, 8
  nondisjunction of, teratogenesis by, 62
  number of, changes in, genetic diseases from, 7
  structure of, changes in, genetic diseases from, 7–8
  translocation of, 8
Cimetidine, breast-feeding and, 152t
Circulation, fetal, 240
  regulation of, 243–246
    baseline heart rate in, 244–245
    beat-to-beat variability in, 245–246
    humoral, 244
    neural, 243–244
  fetal-placental, 72
  in neonatal brain, 553–555
  maternal uteroplacental, 72–74
  placental, 71–74
    at term, *68*
Circumarginate placenta, 94
Circumvallate placenta, 94
Cleavage of zygote, 45
Clemastine, breast-feeding and, 152t
Climacteric, in female, 27–28
  in male, 29

Clindamycin toxicity, in pregnant woman, fetus, and neonate, 454t–455t
Clitoris, development of, 18
Closing capacity in neonate, 299–300
Clothing, in neonatal body temperature maintenance, 690
Clotting factors. See *Coagulation factors.*
Coagulation, in labor, delivery, and postpartum period, *170*
  in neonate, 184–186
  physiology of, pregnancy and, *168*
Coagulation factors, 167t
  in antepartum period, 166–167
  in intrapartum period, 167, 169
  in preterm, term, and older infants, 187t
Coagulopathies, consumptive, in pregnancy, 175
Coarctation of aorta, management of, 252–253
Cocaine, in-utero exposure to, effects of, 572, *574*
Codominance, 4
Cold stress, neonatal, 690–692
  physiologic consequences of, *692*
Collagen instability, in neonate, 510
Complement, definition of, 441t
Complement system, in neonate, 471–472, *472*
  in pregnancy, 444
Compliance, lung, 297
  rib cage, in respiratory pump, 295–296
Conception, 40–45
  cleavage in, 45
  clinical implications related to, 45–49
  fertilization in, 43–45
  ovarian function in, 40–42
  sperm transport in, 42–43
  zygote transport in, 45
Conducting system of heart, fetal development of, 235
Conduction, heat loss in neonate by, preventing, 681t, 685–686
Connective tissue changes, in pregnancy, 494–495
Constipation, in pregnancy, 391–392
  nursing recommendations for, 391t
Consumptive coagulopathies, in pregnancy, 175
Contraception, 31–33
Contraceptive implants, 33
Contraceptives, oral, 32
Contractile properties, in functional development of fetal cardiovascular system, 238
Contraction(s), myometrial, 117–120
  cellular mechanisms controlling, *118*
  coordination of, 119–120
  uterine, coordination of, 119–120
  in pregnancy, 113–117
  physiologic events during, 120
Contraction stress test (CST), in fetal heart rate evaluation, 89
Convection, heat loss in neonate by, preventing, 681t, 686
Copper, neonatal requirements for, 422
Cordocentesis, in fetal status assessment, 91
Corpus luteum, in conception, 42
Corticosteroids, for skin disorders in pregnancy, 499
Countercurrent multiplier system, in neonatal water balance, 363, *364*
Cradle cap, in neonate, 493t
Cramps, leg, in pregnancy, calcium levels and, 619
Creatinine clearance, 24-hour, in GRF measurement, 350
Crossed extension reflex, 560t
Cutaneous innervation, fetal development of, 505

Cutaneous tissue alterations, in pregnancy, 496–497
Cutis marmorata, in pregnancy, 495
Cyanosis, in respiratory distress syndrome, 317
Cyanotic congenital heart disease, management of, 251–252
Cyclic adenosine monophosphate (cAMP), myometrial contraction and, 117–118
Cyclophosphamide, breast-feeding and, 152t
Cytotoxic T cell, definition of, 441t
Cytotrophoblast, migratory, 73

D

Dead space ventilation, in neonate, 299
Decidua, in placental development, 65, *66*
  layers of, changes in, with embryonal and fetal growth, *66*
Dehydration, in neonate, 428–429
  risk of, in neonate, 369
Deletions, of chromosomes, 8
Delivery. See also *Intrapartum period; Labor.*
  cesarean, blood volume and hematocrit after, *170*
    hemodynamic changes and, 211
  in woman with spinal cord transsection, 536
  vaginal, blood volume and hematocrit after, *170*
Dendrites, growth of, 548
Dense protein bodies, in myometrial cells, 111, 113
Deoxyribonucleic acid (DNA), function of, 4
  replication of, 5
  structure of, 4–5
Dependent edema, in pregnancy, 346–348
Depression, postpartum, 528
Dermatitis, of pregnancy, papular, 500t–501t
Dermatoses, associated with pregnancy, 498, 500t–501t
Dermis, cohesion between epidermis and, in neonate, 510
  fetal development of, 504–505
  structural components of, *503*
Desensitization, to β-adrenergic agents in labor inhibition, 128
Developmental defect, pathogenesis of, 63t
Diabetic mother, 595–597
  fetus of, 596–597
  glycosuria in pregnancy and, 351
  infant of, hypocalcemia in, 628–629
    hypoglycemia in, 607–608
    pathophysiology of morbidity and mortality of, 608t
Diabetogenic state, pregnancy as, 593
Diaphragm, in respiratory pump, 294–295
Diarrhea, in neonate, 428–429·
Diffusing capacity, in antepartum period, 266
Diffusion, across alveolar-capillary membrane, 305–306
  placental transport by, facilitated, 79t, 80–81
    factors influencing, 84–85
    simple, 78–80, 79t
Digestion, of carbohydrates in neonate, physiologic limitations of, 413t, 414–415
  of fats in neonate, physiologic limitations of, 413t, 415–416
  of proteins in neonate, physiologic limitations of, 412–414, 413t
  summary of, *381*
Digestive system, development of, timetable of, 54t, *57*
2,3–Diphosphoglycerate (2,3–DPG), in neonate, 183
Disseminated intravascular coagulation (DIC), in pregnancy, 175
  infant at risk for, 192

Disseminated intravascular coagulation (DIC) *(Continued)*
 pathophysiology of, *176*
Diuretics, pregnancy and, 352
Dizygotic (DZ) twins, 98, *99*
DNA (deoxyribonucleic acid), function of, 4
 replication of, 5
 structure of, 4–5
Dominant inheritance, autosomal, 9–10
 X-linked, 9
Donor artificial insemination, 45–46
Drug(s), absorption and metabolism of, in neonate, 429
 in pregnancy, 397
 distribution of, in fetus, factors influencing, 87t
 fetal effects of, 86
 for neonatal hyperbilirubinemia, 645–646
 in breast milk, 151–152
 in-utero exposure to, effects of, 571–572, *574*
 renal effects of, in neonate, 372t
 renal handling of, in neonate, 370
Ductus arteriosus, closure of, in transition, 241
 patent, management of, 250
Duncan's mechanism, of placental separation, 71
Duodenum, fetal development of, 401–402
Duplication, of chromosomes, 8
Dyspnea, in antepartum period, 270
Dystocia, 128
 reasons for, 129t

E

Ecchymoses, in neonate, 493t
Eccrine gland, increased activity of, in pregnancy,
 nursing intervention for, 495t
Echocardiographic changes, in antepartum period, 210
Eclampsia, 538
Ectopic pregnancy, 64
Edema, cerebral, anoxia and hemorrhage related to,
 566
 dependent, in pregnancy, 346–348
 fetal, management of, 247–249
 nonpitting, in pregnancy, 496
 nursing interventions for, 495t
Eisenmenger's syndrome, in pregnancy, 221
Ejaculatory duct, development of, 17
Elastic recoil, of chest wall in respiratory pump, 295
Elastin, instability of, in neonate, 510
Electrical activity, in fetus, 548
Electrocardiographic changes, in antepartum period,
 210
Electrolytes, fluids and. See *Fluid(s) and electrolytes.*
 imbalances of, in neonate, 369
 neonatal requirements for, 422
 serum, in antepartum period, 164t, 165
Embryo, brain of, folding of, *544*
 brain vesicle development in, *544*
 development of, 49–55
 clinical implications related to, 60–63
 critical periods of, 60–61
 morphogenesis in, 49–51
 organogenesis in, 51, 53t–54t
 overview of, 51–55
 folding of, in morphogenesis, 51
 neuromuscular system development in, 539, 541–
 546
 sensory system development in, 539, 541–546
 stages of hematopoiesis in, *177*
Embryonic development, of reproductive system, 10–18
Encephaloceles, 543

Encephalopathy, bilirubin, 652–654
 hypoxic-ishemic brain injury in neonate from, 567–
 568
Endocrine changes, postpartum, 139–141
Endocrinology, fetal, 18, 20
 of female reproductive processes, 24–25
 of male reproductive processes, 28–29
 placental, 75–78
Endocytosis, in placental transport, 79t, 81
Endogenous inhibitors, of prostaglandin synthase
 (EIPS), 116
Endometrial cycle, 26–27
Endometrium, in placental development, 64–65
Endorphins, in intrapartum period, 526–527
 in neonate, 569
Endothelial lining, of vessels, fetal development of,
 235–236
Endotracheal tube (ETT), in neonate, nursing
 interventions for, 311
 placement of, in resuscitation of neonate, 315
Endovascular migratory cytotrophoblast, 73
Energy sources, altered, teratogenesis by, 62–63
Engorgement of breasts, postpartum, 138–139
Enteral feeding, initiation of, 410
Environment, caregiving, risks posed to neuromuscular
 and sensory development by, 565–574
 neutral thermal, in neonatal care, 684–685
 thermal, of neonate, integumentary system and,
 509–510
Environment, intrauterine, 59–60
Enzyme(s), gastrointestinal, 382t
 inhibition of, teratogenesis by, 63
Epidermal appendages, fetal development of, 505–506
Epidermis, cohesion between dermis and, in neonate,
 510
 fetal development of, 501–504
 structural components of, *503*
Epididymis, development of, 15, *16*, 17
Epidural anesthesia, without epinephrine for cesarean
 section, hemodynamic changes from, 217
Epilepsy, breast feeding and, 535
 effects of, on fetus and neonate, 534–535
 on pregnancy, 534
 effects of pregnancy on, 531–533
 pregnant woman with, 531–535
Episiotomies, 138
Epispadias, 22
Epulis formation, in pregnancy, 382
Ergotamine, breast-feeding and, 152t
Erythema, palmar, in pregnancy, 496
Erythema toxicum, in neonate, 493t
Erythromycin estolate, toxicity of, in pregnant woman,
 fetus, and neonate, 454t–455t
Erythropoietin, in neonate, 183
Esophagus, fetal development of, 399, 401
 in pregnancy, 383–384
 motility of, in neonate, 411
Estradiol, in conception, 40
 production of, in pregnancy, 77–78
Estriol production, in pregnancy, 78
Estrogen(s), breast development and, 142t
 effects on carbohydrate, fat, and protein metabolism,
 591
 in female reproductive processes, 25
 in initiation of labor, 114
 postpartum levels of, 139–140
 production of, in pregnancy, 71–78
Estrone production, in pregnancy, 77–78
Ethanol, in labor inhibition, 127

Evaporation, heat loss in neonate by, preventing, 681t, 687

Exchange transfusions, for neonatal hyperbilirubinemia, 646

Exercise, in antepartum period, cardiovascular system and, 213–217
respiratory system and, 271–272

Exstrophy, of bladder, 357

Extremity(ies), blood flow in, in antepartum period, 208

Eye(s), adaptations of, in pregnancy, 528–529
changes in, in antepartum period, 523–524
hyperoxia and, effects of, 308–309

F

Facilitated anabolism, pregnancy as state of, 592

Facilitated diffusion, placental transport by, 79t, 80–81

Fallopian tubes, development of, 17

Fat(s), concentrations of, in pregnancy, *587*
digestion and absorption of, in neonate, physiologic limitations of, 413t, 415–416
digestion of, *381*
metabolism of, 583–610
changes in, clinical implications for pregnant woman and fetus, 591–598
maturational, during infancy and childhood, 609
fetal development of, 601–602
in antepartum period, 584–586, *592*
in intrapartum period, 591
in maternal physiologic adaptations, 584–591
in neonatal physiology, 605
in postpartum period, 591
maternal-fetal relationships and, 594–595, 595t
neonatal requirements for, 420
serum, in antepartum period, 164t, 166
synthesis and release of, in milk, 149–150

Fatty acids, in fetal metabolism, 601–602

Fatty liver, of pregnancy, 396–397

Feeding, enteral, initiation of, 410
for infants, method of, considerations related to, 425–427
with health problems, 423–425

Female, reproductive processes in, 24–28

Fenoterol, in labor inhibition, 127–128

Fentanyl, for neonatal pain, 571

Ferritin, serum, in antepartum period, 164t, 166
in neonate, 183–184

Fertility, problems with, 30–31

Fertilization, 43–45
diagrammatic summary of, *46*
in vitro, 46–47

Fetal blood gases, in functional development of fetal respiratory system, 287–288
maternal exercise and, 272
normal, 288t

Fetal development, of reproductive system, 10–18

Fetal distress, from maternal exercise, 216

Fetal heart rate (FHR), antepartum surveillance of, 89

Fetal state patterns, 551

Fetal stress response, management of, 246–247

Fetus, activity of, maternal exercise and, 272
asphyxia in, 311–313. *See also* Asphyxia, intrauterine.
bilirubin metabolism development in, 638–639
blood cell formation in, 176–178
breathing movements of, in functional development of fetal respiratory system, 288–289
maternal exercise and, 272

Fetus *(Continued)*
calcium metabolism development in, 621–623
carbohydrate metabolism development in, 598–501
cardiovascular system development in, 228–237. See also *Cardiovascular system, fetal development of.*
circulation in, 240
regulation of, 243–246
development of, clinical implications related to, 60–63
overview of, 56–59, *58–59*
development of host defense mechanisms in, 464–467, 466t
drug distribution in, factors influencing, 87t
drug effects on, 86
edema in, management of, 247–249
effects of anticonvulsants on, 534
effects of antithyroid agents on, 666–667
effects of epilepsy on, 534
effects of maternal cocaine use on, *574*
effects of maternal exercise on, 215–216
endocrinology of, 18, 20
fat metabolism development in, 601–602
gastrointestinal system in, development of, 397–408. See also *Gastrointestinal (GI) system, fetal, development of.*
in amniotic fluid production and exchange, 84
growth of, 172, 406
retardation of, 406–408
hematologic system development in, 176–186
hemoglobin formation in, 178–179, *179*
hemostatic system development in, 179
hepatic system development in, 402
integumentary system development in, 499–507
iron requirements of, 172
lungs of, maturity of, assessment of, 284–285
maternal hyperthermia and fever and, 679
maternal tolerance of, immune system in, 446–449
metabolic substrate and hormone alterations in, 604t
movements of, 550–551
neurodevelopment in, 546–548
neuromuscular system development in, 546–549
nutritional needs of, 390
of diabetic mother, 596–597
oxygen content of, 240–241
oxygenation of, 172
phosphorus metabolism development in, 621–623
protection from infection, 464
protein metabolism development in, 602–603
renal system development in, 354–358. See also *Renal system, fetal development of.*
respiratory system of, development of, 276–289. See also *Respiratory system, fetal development of.*
in amniotic fluid production and exchange, 84
sensory system development in, 546–549
skin of, in amniotic fluid production and exchange, 84
stages of hematopoiesis in, *177*
status of, assessment of, placental function in, 88–89
thermoregulation in, 678–679
toxicity of antibotics for, 454t–455t
urinary tract of, in amniotic fluid production and exchange, 84

Fever, maternal, fetus and, 679

Fibrinolysis, in neonate, 186

Fibrinolytic activity, in fetus, 179
in labor, delivery, and postpartum period, *170*
in postpartum period, 171

Fibromata molle, in pregnancy, 496–497

Fibronectin, definition of, 441t

Fibronectin *(Continued)*
  in neonate, 469
  maturation and, 482
Fick diffusion equation, in placental transport, 79
Finnegan scoring system, for neonatal abstinence
    syndrome, *573*
Fluid(s), amniotic. See *Amniotic fluid.*
  and electrolytes, balance of, in neonate, management
      of, 365–370
    estimating needs of, in neonate, 367
    homeostasis of, 336–374. See also *Kidney(s).*
    , in pregnancy, 342
      maternal-fetal, 354
  distribution of, in antepartum period, 203
  intake of, in labor, 393–394
  lung, composition of, 286t
    in functional development of fetal respiratory sys-
        tem, 285–287
  needs for, in labor, 349–350
Folate, neonatal requirements for, 421
Follicle, maturation of, in conception, 40–41
Follicle-stimulating hormone (FSH), in conception, 40
  in female reproductive processes, 25
  in follicle maturation, 41
  in male reproductive processes, 28
Follicular phase, of ovarian cycle, 26
Folliculostatin, in female reproductive processes, 25
Food(s), allergies to, development of, 486
  intake of, in labor, 393–394
  solid, introduction of, 429, 431
Footdrop, postpartum, 537t
Foregut, fetal development of, 399–402
Formula, composition of, 418t
  infant fed with, hypocalcemia and, 629
Frank-Starling relationship, in functional development
    of fetal cardiovascular system, 238–239
FSH. See *Follicle-stimulating hormone (FSH).*
Functional residual capacity (FRC), in neonate, 299–
    300

G

Galactopoiesis, 146
Gallbladder, fetal development of, 402
  in pregnancy, 385
Gallstones, in pregnancy, 396
Gamete intrafallopian transfer (GIFT), 47–48
Gametes, abnormal development of, 24
Gametogenesis, 23–24
Gap junction formation, in coordination of uterine
    contractions, 119–120
Gastroesophageal reflux (GER), in neonate, 427–428
Gastrointestinal (GI) system, 379–431
  anomalies of, 399t
  changes in, clinical implications for neonatal care,
      417–431
    implications for pregnant woman and fetus, 389–
        396, 397
    maturational, during infancy and childhood, 429,
        431
  disorders of, in pregnancy, 395–396
  drug absorption by, in pregnancy, 397
  enzymes of, 382t
  fetal, development of, 397–408
    anatomic, 398–405
    developmental markers in, 406t
    functional, 405–408
    in amniotic fluid production and exchange, 84

Gastrointestinal (GI) system *(Continued)*
  function of, maturation of, 409
  in antepartum period, 380–385
  in intrapartum period, 388
  in maternal physiologic adaptations, 380–385
  in neonatal physiology, 408–416
    functional and anatomic limitations in, 410–412
    physiologic limitations in, 412–416
    transitional events in, 408–410
  in postpartum period, 388–389
Gastroschisis, fetal development of, 404
Gate control theory, of pain, 525–526, *526*
Gene(s), 3–4
  mutation of, teratogenesis by, 62
  structure of, 4–5
Genetic diseases, causes of, 6–10
  inheritance of, autosomal, 9–10
    sex-linked, 8–9
  transmission of, 6–10
Genetic mechanisms/principles, 3–6
Genital ducts, development of, 15–17
Genitalia, external, development of, 17–18, *19*
Genitourinary system, development of, timetable of,
    53t, *57, 59*
Genotype, 4
Germ cells, meiosis in, 6, *7*
Germinal matrix, bleeding in, injury from, 567
Gestation, postdate, placental function and, 88
Gestational age, infant state parameters by, 561t
Gestational trophoblastic disease, 95
Gingivitis, in pregnancy, 380–382
Gland(s), parathyroid, fetal development of, 621
  sebaceous, fetal development of, 506
  secretory, alterations in, in pregnancy, 497
  sweat, fetal development of, 506
Globulin concentrations, in antepartum period, 164t,
    165
Glomerular filtration, *340*
Glomerular filtration rate (GFR), in antepartum
    period, 208
  in fetus, 357
  in neonate, 360–361
  in pregnancy, 339–341
  physiologic and pathophysiologic changes in, 347t
Glucagon, fatty acid synthesis and, 601
  metabolic effects of, 588t
  metabolism of, fetal development of, 601
Glucocorticoids, in functional development of fetal
    respiratory system, 282–283
Glucose, levels of, in first hours after birth, 604t
  in perinatal period, *604*
  metabolic rates of, *600*
  metabolism of, fetal development of, 598–600
  renal handling of, in neonate, 362
Glucose tolerance test, effect of metabolic changes on,
    593–594, 594t
Glycogen metabolism, fetal development of, 600
Glycosuria, in pregnancy, 350–351
Gold salts, breast-feeding and, 152t
Gonadotropin(s), chorionic, human, 75
  pituitary, in female reproductive processes, 25
  postpartum levels of, 140–141
Gonadotropin-releasing hormone (GnRH), in female
    reproductive processes, 24
  in male reproductive processes, 28
Gonads, agenesis of, 21
  development of, 11–15
    indifferent stage in, 12–13, *14*
    in fetal endocrinology, 20

Goodell's sign, of pregnancy, 38
Graves' disease, in pregnancy, 664
    transplacental transfer of maternal antibodies in, 459
Growth, fetal, 406
        retardation of, 406–408
    hair, alterations in, in pregnancy, 497
    influences of, on hematologic parameters in neonate, 187–188
    skeletal, 622–623
Growth hormone, breast development and, 142t
    human, plasma concentrations of, during nursing, 147
Grunting, in respiratory distress syndrome, 317
Gut, host defense mechanisms of, in neonate, 472–474, 473t

H

Hair, fetal development of, 505–506
    growth of, alterations in, in pregnancy, 497
    loss of, post partum, 497–498
Head, coverings for, in neonatal body temperature maintenance, 690
Headache, in pregnancy, 530–531
Hearing, sense of, development of, 549–550
Heart, congenital malformations of, management of, 251–253
    disease of, congenital, acyanotic, management of, 252–253
        cyanotic, management of, 251–252
        in pregnancy, 218–222
            atrial septal defect as, 222
            Eisenmenger's syndrome as, 221
            left-to-right shunts as, 220
            Marfan's syndrome as, 221–222
            mitral regurgitation as, 219
            mitral stenosis as, 219
            mitral valve prolapse as, 219–220
            nursing care for, 222
            obstructive lesions as, 219
            patent ductus arteriosus as, 220–221
            pulmonary artery hypertension as, 221
            right-to-left shunts as, 221
            tetralogy of Fallot as, 221
            ventricular septal defect as, 220
    massage of, external, in resuscitation of neonate, 315
    physiology of, in neonate, 242–246
        central mechanism in, 243
        metabolic rate and, 242–243
        oxygen transport and, 242–243
        regulation of fetal circulation and, 243–246
    primitive, development of, in fetus, 229–231
    problems of, infants with, feeding of, 424–425
    rate of, baseline, in fetal circulation regulation, 244–245
        beat-to-beat variability in, in fetal circulation regulation, 245–246
        in antepartum period, 205–206
        in intrapartum period, 211
        in postpartum period, 212
    septation of, in fetus, 231
    valves of, fetal development of, 235
Heart sounds, in antepartum period, 209–210
Heartburn, in pregnancy, 390–391
    nursing recommendations for, 391
Heat, conservation of, by neonate, 680
    dissipation of, by neonate, 683–684
    excessive, in neonate, preventing, 681t

Heat (Continued)
    gain of, by neonate, excessive, prevention of, 685–688
    loss of, by neonate, 683–684
        excessive, prevention of, 685–688
        preventing, 681t
    production of, by neonate, 680, 682–683, 684
    transfer of, in neonate, 680
Hegar's sign, of pregnancy, 38
HELLP syndrome, 227–228, 457–458
Helper T cell, definition of, 441t
Hemangiomas, capillary, in pregnancy, 496
    in neonate, 493t
Hematocrit, following vaginal and cesarean birth, 170
    in antepartum period, 163–164
    in neonate, 183
    in postpartum period, 212
Hematologic changes, in pregnancy, 495–496
Hematologic parameters, in childhood, 195–196
    in infancy, 195–196
    in intrapartum period, 167
    in neonate, 181–184
        factors influencing, 186–188
        growth infuences on, 187–188
        hemolysis detection and, 188
        iatrogenic losses and, 187
        site of sampling and, 186–187
    in postpartum period, 170–171
Hematologic system(s), 159–197
    fetal development of, 176–186
    in antepartum period, 160–167
    in intrapartum period, 167–169
    in postpartum period, 169–171
Hematopoiesis, stages of, in embryo and fetus, 177
Hemodynamic changes, from cesarean section, 217
    in antepartum period, in cardiovascular system, 202–208
        in renal system, 339
    in intrapartum period, 210–211, 217
    in postpartum period, 211–212
Hemoglobin, catabolism of, bilirubin from, 638
    fetal, in neonate, 182–183
    formation of, in fetus, 178–179
    in antepartum period, 163
    levels of, in neonate, 182–183
    in postpartum period, 170
Hemoglobin-oxygen affinity, alterations in, in childhood, 196–197
    in infancy, 196–197
    in neonate, 188
Hemoglobinopathy, infant with, 191–192
Hemolysis detection, in neonate, 188
Hemorrhage, anoxia and brain edema related to, 566
    intraventricular, brain injury in neonate from, 566–567
    periventricular, brain injury in neonate from, 566–567
Hemorrhagic disease of newborn (HDN), vitamin K and, 188–189
Hemorrhoids, in pregnancy, 392
    nursing recommendations for, 391t
Hemostasis, altered, infant at risk for, 192–193
    changes in, in antepartum period, 166–167
        in neonate, 184–186
    in intrapartum period, 167
    in postpartum period, 171
Hemostatic factors, in preterm, term, and older infants, 187t
Hemostatic system, development of, in fetus, 179

Heparin therapy, in pregnancy, calcium levels and, 620
Hepatitis B virus (HBV) infection, immune response of neonate to, 477–479
Hepatocytes, bilirubin transport and conjugation by, 639, *640*
Hering-Breuer reflex, 293
Hermaphroditism, 21
Hernia, umbilical, fetal development of, 404
Herpes gestationis, 500t–501t
Herpes simplex virus (HSV) infection, immune response of neonate to, 477
Hexoprenaline, in labor inhibition, 127–128
Hindgut, fetal development of, 404
Hirsutism, in pregnancy, 497
Hormonal factors, influence on host defense mechanisms in pregnancy and, 444
Hormone(s), contributing to breast development, 142–143t
  in regulation of renal system in neonate, 365
  parathyroid. See *Parathyroid hormone (PTH)*.
  placental, effects of, on carbohydrates, fat, and protein metabolism, 591
  thyroid, in functional development of fetal respiratory system, 283–284
Host defense factors, maturation of, 482–483
Host defense mechanisms, 439–486. See also *Immune system; Immunity*.
  disturbances of, clinical implications for neonatal care and, 474–482
  fetal development of, 464–467, 466t
  gut, in neonate, 472–474
  in neonatal physiology, 467–474
    alterations in specific immune responses in, 470–472
    gut, alterations in, 472–474
    primary alterations in, 468–470
    transitional events in, 467–468
  in pregnancy, alterations in, 443t
  maturational changes in, in infancy and childhood, 482–486
  primary, in pregnancy, 440
Host defense responses, primary, definition of, 441t
  secondary, definition of, 441t
  tertiary, definition of, 441t
Human chorionic gonadotropin (hCG), 75
Human immunodeficiency virus (HIV), infection of neonate by, 479–480
  perinatal infection with, 451–452
  replication of, *451*
Human placental lactogen (hPL), 75–76
  breast development and, 142t
Humoral-mediated immunity, definition of, 441t
  in neonate, 470–471
  in pregnancy, 440, 444
Humoral regulation, of fetal circulation, 244
Hydatidiform mole, 95
Hydration status of neonate, measurement of, 370
Hydronephrosis, physiologic, in pregnancy, 337
Hydrops fetalis, management of, 247–249
Hydroureter, physiologic, in pregnancy, 337–338
Hyperbilirubinemia, maternal, 637–638
  neonatal, 644
    exchange transfusion for, 646
    indirect, causes of, 645t
    management of, 645–650
    pharmacologic agents for, 645–646
    phototherapy for, 646–650
Hypercalcemia, at birth, 624
  neonatal, 630–631

Hypercoagulable state, of pregnancy, 166–167
Hyperemesis gravidarum, 393
  thyroid function and, 663
Hyperglycemia, neonatal, 609
Hypermagnesemia, neonatal, 630
Hypernatremia, neonatal, 369
Hyperoxia, cellular, consequences of, 308–309
Hyperpigmentation, in pregnancy, 492
  nursing intervention for, 495t
Hypertension, calcium and, 619
  essential, women with, renal system in, 352
  pregnancy-induced. See *Pregnancy-induced hypertension (PIH)*.
  pulmonary artery, in pregnancy, 221
  renal system and, 351, *352*
Hyperthermia, fetal effects of, 213–215
  maternal, fetus and, 679
  neonatal, 692–693
Hyperthyroidism, in pregnancy, 664
  neonatal, 671–672
Hyperventilation, in intrapartum period, 268–269
Hyperviscosity, neonatal, 191, *192*
Hypervolemia, in antepartum period, 162
  of pregnancy, 171
Hypocalcemia, neonatal, 624
  calcium and phosphorus intake and, 627–629
  in infant of diabetic mother, 628–629
  in preterm infant, 627–628
  late, 629
  perinatal asphyxia and, 629
Hypogammaglobulinemia, physiologic, 483–484
Hypoglycemia, in infant with perinatal asphyxia, 608–609
  neonatal, causes of, 607t
    clinical implications of, 606–609
    in infant of diabetic mother, 607–608
    in low-birth-weight infant, 606–607
    time course of, 607t
Hypomagnesemia, neonatal, 629–630
Hyponatremia, neonatal, 369
Hypospadias, 22
Hypotension, from supine position in pregnancy, 213
Hypothalamic hormones, in female reproductive processes, 24
Hypothalamic-pituitary-thyroid axis, thyroid function and, 668
Hypothermia, neonatal, 692–693
  consequences of, 693t
Hypothermic infant, rewarming, 691–692
Hypothyroidism, in pregnancy, 664–665
  neonatal, 672
  transient, in preterm infant, 671
Hypoxia, causes of, 308
  cellular, consequences of, 306–307
    systemic manifestations of, 307–308
  fetal, smoking and, 274–275
  injury from, vulnerability of neuromuscular and sensory systems to, 565–568
Hypoxic-ischemic encephalopathy, brain injury in neonate from, 567–568

I

Immune responses, altered, in neonate, 470–472
  of neonate, to bacterial infections, 474–477
    to viral infections, 477–480
Immune states, pregnancy-induced, 457–458

Immune system, 439–486, *442–443*. See also *Host defense mechanisms; Immunity.*
  changes in, clinical implications of, for neonatal care, 474–482
    for pregnant woman and fetus, 446–464
    maturational, during infancy and childhood, 482–486
      allergy development and, 486
      immunizations and, 484–486
      physiologic hypogammaglobulinemia and, 483–484
  fetal development of, 464–467
  in antepartum period, 440, 444
  in intrapartum period, 444
  in maternal physiologic adaptations, 440–446
  in neonatal physiology, 467–474
  in postpartum period, 444–446
Immunity, active, definition of, 441t
  antibody-mediated, definition of, 441t
    in neonate, 470–471
    in pregnancy, 440, 444
  cell-mediated, definition of, 441t
    in neonate, 471
    in pregnancy, 440
  humoral-mediated, definition of, 441t
    in neonate, 470–471
    in pregnancy, 440, 444
  passive, definition of, 441t
Immunization(s), 484–486
  for hepatitis B virus infection, 478–479
  pregnant woman and, 455–456
Immunoglobulin(s), definition of, 441t
  levels of, in fetus, newborn, and infant, 470, *471*
Immunologic aspects of pregnancy-induced hypertension, 456–457
Immunologic functions, of placenta, 78
Immunologic properties of human milk, 445t, 445–446
Immunoprophylaxis for group B *Streptococcus* infection, 482
Immunotherapy for neonatal sepsis, 481–482, 483t
Imperforate anus, fetal development of, 405
Impetigo herpetiformis, 500t–501t
Implantation, of blastocyst, early, *47*
  processes in, 63–64
Impulse conduction, in fetus, 548
  in transition to extrauterine life, 553
In vitro fertilization (IVF), 46–47
Incubators, in neonatal body temperature maintenance, 689–690
Independent movement, placental transport by, 79t, 81
Induction, in morphogenesis, 50
Infancy, maturational changes during, of bilirubin metabolism, 654
  of calcium and phosphorus metabolism, 631
  of cardiovascular system, 253–254
  of gastrointestinal system, 429–431
  of hematologic and hemostatic systems, 195–197
  of host defense mechanisms, 482–486
  of integumentary system, 516–517
  of metabolic processes, 609
  of neuromuscular and sensory systems, 572–573, 575
  of renal system, 371–373
  of respiratory system, 324–327
  of thermoregulation, 693
  of thyroid function, 672
Infant(s), at risk for altered hemostasis, 192–193
  effects of maternal cocaine use on, *574*
  hematologic parameters in, 195–196

Infant(s) *(Continued)*
  low-birth-weight, hypoglycemia in, 606–607
  maturational changes in gastrointestinal system in, 429, 431
  of diabetic mother. See *Diabetic mother, infant of.*
  older, coagulation factors in, 187t
    hemostatic factors in, 187t
  pain reception in, 569
  pain responses in, 570t
  postmature, integumentary system in, 515
  preterm. See *Preterm infant(s).*
  receiving phototherapy, integumentary system in, 515–516
  small-for-gestational-age. See *Small-for-gestational-age (SGA) infant(s).*
  very-low-birth-weight. See *Very-low-birth-weight (VLBW) infant(s).*
  with health problems, feeding of, 423–425
  with hemoglobinopathy, 191–192
Infant state(s), chart of, 562t–563t
  definition of, 560–561
  development of, 562–563
  modulation of, 563–564
  parameters of, by gestational age, 561t
Infection(s), bacterial, immune responses of neonate to, 474–477
  hepatitis B virus, immune response of neonate to, 477–479
  herpes simplex virus, immune response of neonate to, 477
  HIV, in neonate, 479–480
  inability of neonate to localize, 469–470
  maternal, preterm labor and, 450–451
    risk of, immune system and, 449–450
  neonatal, diagnosis of, 480
    protection from, skin in, 512
  protection of fetus from, 464
  respiratory, in antepartum period, 271
  viral, immune responses of neonate in, 477–480
Infectious processes, risk of specific, in neonate, 474–480
Infertility, 30–31
Inhalation anesthesia, respiratory effects of, 275–276
Inheritance, autosomal, 9–10
  mendelian principles of, 6, 8t
  modes of, 4
  sex-linked, 8–9
  X-linked, 8–9
  Y-linked, 9
Innervation, cutaneous, fetal development of, 505
Inotropy, in functional development of fetal cardiovascular system, 239–240
Insemination, artificial, donor, 45–46
Insulin, fat metabolism in pregnancy and, *592*
  fatty acid synthesis and, 601
  in antepartum period, 586
  in functional development of fetal respiratory system, 284
  metabolic effects of, 588t
  metabolism of, fetal development of, 600–601
Integumentary system, 491–517
  changes in, clinical implications of, for neonatal care, 511–516
    for pregnant woman and fetus, 498–499
    maturational, during infancy and childhood, 516–517
  components of, 491
  fetal development of, 499–507
    anatomic, 500–506
    functional, 506–507

Integumentary system *(Continued)*
  in antepartum period, 492–497
  in maternal physiologic processes, 492–498
  in neonatal physiology, 508–511
    barrier properties and, 508
    cohesion between epidermis and dermis in, 510
    collagen and elastin instability and, 510
    permeability and, 508
    protective mechanisms in, 510–511
    thermal environment and, 509–510
    transepidermal water loss and, 508–509
  in postpartum period, 497–498
  transitional events and, 507–508
Interleukin-2, definition of, 441t
Intersexuality, classification of, 21t
Interstitial migratory cytotrophoblast, 73
Intestines, atresia of, fetal development of, 404
  in pregnancy, 384–385
  motility of, in neonate, 411–412
  stenosis of, fetal development of, 404
  surface area of, in neonate, 412
Intrapartum period. See also *Delivery; Labor.*
  calcium metabolism in, 617–618
  carbohydrate metabolism in, 591
  cardiovascular system in, 210–211, 217
  fat metabolism in, 591
  fluid intake in, 393–394
  fluid needs in, 349–350
  food intake in, 393–394
  gastrointestinal system in, 388
  hematologic parameters in, 167
  hemostatic changes in, 167, 169
  hepatic system in, 388
  immune system in, 444
  neuromuscular system in, 524–527
  phosphorus metabolism in, 617–618
  pregnancy-induced hypertension management during, 226–227
  protein metabolism in, 591
  renal system in, 345
  respiratory system in, 267–269
  sensory system in, 524–527
  thermoregulation in, 678
  thyroid function in, 663
Intrauterine devices (IUDs), 32
Intrauterine environment, 59–60
Intrauterine growth retardation, 406–408
Intrauterine transfusions, for fetus of Rho(D)-immunized woman, 460
Intravenous fluid administration, in labor, conditions associated with, 349t
Intraventricular hemorrhage (IVH), brain injury in neonate from, 566–567
Inversion, of chromosomes, 8
Iodides, use of, in pregnancy, 665–667
Iron, absorption of, in neonate, 416
  balance of, postnatal, changes in, *196*
  in neonate, 183–184
  requirements for, in pregnancy, 171–172
    of fetus, 172
    of neonate, 421–422
  supplemental, for physiologic anemia of infancy, 195
Isoimmunization, ABO, 462–464, *463*
  Rho(D), 459–462, *461–462*
Isoniazid toxicity, in pregnant woman, fetus and neonate, 454t–455t
Isoxsuprine, in labor inhibition, 127–128

J

Jaundice, in breast-fed infants, 650–652
  management of, 651t, 651–652
  prevention of, 651
  physiologic, 641–644
    causes of, 641, 642t, 643
    clinical parameters of, 642
    development of, epidemiologic factors associated with, 643t
    patterns of, 641
Junctional nevi, in neonate, 493t

K

Kernicterus, 652–654
Kidney(s). See also *Renal system.*
  agenesis of, 357
  blood flow in, in antepartum period, 208
  changes in, clinical implications for pregnant woman and fetus, 346–354, 347t
  disease of, pregnancy and, 352–354
  effects of pharmacologic agents on, in neonate, 372t
  embryology of, *356*
  fetal, development of, 354–357
    in amniotic fluid production and exchange, 84
  function of, in neonate, during illness, 370–371
    measurement of, 370
    values for assessing, 371t
    in preeclampsia, 226, 227
    in pregnancy, effects of position on, 346–348
      laboratory values associated with, 340t
      measurement of, 350–352
    maturational changes during infancy and childhood in, 371, 373
  handling by, of glucose in neonate, 362
    of pharmacologic agents in neonate, 370
    of solutes in neonate, 362–363
  hypertension and, 351, *352*
  in antepartum period, 337–345
  in intrapartum period, 345
  in maternal physiologic adaptation, 337–346
  in postpartum period, 345–346
  polycystic, 357
  solute load on, calories and, for neonate, 422
  transplantation of, pregnancy following, 353–354
Killer T cell, definition of, 441t

L

Labia majora, development of, 18
Labia minora, development of, 18
Labor. See also *Delivery; Intrapartum period.*
  dysfunctional, 128
  flood and fluid intake in, 393–394
  fluid needs in, 349–350
  hormonal control of, *114*
  in woman with spinal cord transection, 536
  induction of, pharmacologic agents in, 126
  inhibition of, pharmacologic agents in, 126–128
  initiation of, 113
    estrogen in, 114
    oxytocin in, 116
    progesterone in, 114
    prostaglandins in, 114–116
    relaxin in, 117

Labor *(Continued)*
   maternal position during, physiologic processes and, 122–123
   pain and discomfort during, 524–526
   pharmacology of, physiologic processes and, 124–128
   postterm, 28–130
   preterm, 124
     factors associated with, 125t
     infection and, 450–451
   second stage of, maternal pushing efforts during, physiologic processes and, 123–124
Lactacting women, prolactin patterns in, 146
Lactation, galactopoiesis in, 146
   hormonal preparation of breast for, in pregnancy, *144*
   lactogenesis in, 143–146
   mammogenesis in, 142–143
   nutrition during, 151
   peripheral neuropathies in, 537t
   physiology of, 141–152
   resumption of, menstruation and ovulation and, 140–141
Lactogen, human placental, 75–76
   breast development and, 142t
   effects on carbohydrate, fat, and protein metabolism, 591
   fat metabolism in pregnancy and, *592*
Lactogenesis, 143–146
Lactose, synthesis and release of, in milk, 150
Large-for-gestational-age (LGA) infants, maternal obesity and, 394–395
Large intestines, in pregnancy, 384–385
Lecithin-to-sphingomyelin (L/S) ratio, in fetal lung maturity assessment, 284–285
Left-to-right shunts, in pregnancy, 220–221
Leg cramps, in pregnancy, calcium levels and, 619
Let-down reflex, 146
LH. *See Luteinizing hormone (LH).*
Lincomycin toxicity, in pregnant woman, fetus and neonate, 454t–455t
Linea alba, 492
Lipids. See *Fat(s).*
Liver, disease of, in pregnancy, 396–397
   drug absorption and metabolism by, in pregnancy, 397
   fatty, of pregnancy, 396–397
   fetal development of, 402
   function of, in neonate, 416
     in pregnancy, tests of, 386t–387t
     post partum, tests of, 386t–387t
   in pregnancy, 385–386
Lochia, postpartum, 137–138
Low-birth-weight (LBW) infant, hypoglycemia in, 606–607
Lower esophageal sphincter (LES), function of, in neonate, 411
   in pregnancy, 383–384
Lung(s), blood flow in, in antepartum period, 208
   in neonatal physiology, abnormal distribution of, 300
     normal, 300
   blood vessels of, prenatal development of, 278–279
   compliance of, 297
   fetal, maturity of, assessment of, 284–285
   fluid in, composition of, 286t
     in functional development of fetal respiratory system, 285–287
   function of, in antepartum period, 265–267

Lung(s) *(Continued)*
   prenatal growth of, 277–278
   reflexes of, in respiratory control in neonate, 293–294
   resistance of, 297–298
   vascular bed of, excessive muscularization of, in persistent pulmonary hypertension, 322–323
     maladaptation of, in persistent pulmonary hypertension, 322
     underdevelopment of, in persistent pulmonary hypertension, 323–324
   ventilation-perfusion of, ideal, *303*
   zones of, *301*
Lung volumes, in antepartum period, *264*, 264–265, 265t
   in infant and adult, *296*
   in neonate, 299–300
Lupus erythematosus, systemic, pregnant woman with, 458
Luteal phase, of ovarian cycle, 26
Luteinizing hormone (LH), in female reproductive processes, 25
   in follicle maturation, 41
   in male reproductive processes, 28
   in ovulation, 42
Lymphokine, definition of, 441t

M

Macrosomia, in fetus of diabetic mother, 597
Magnesium, alterations in, in neonate, calcium and, 630
   levels of, in neonate, 626
   metabolism of, in antepartum period, 615
   neonatal requirements for, 421
Magnesium sulfate, in labor inhibition, 127
   therapy with, in pregnancy, calcium levels and, 620
Major histocompatibility complex (MHC), definition of, 441t
Male, reproductive processes in, 28–29
Malignancy, pregnancy and, 456
Malrotation, fetal development of, 404
Mammary glands, development of, hormonal contributions to, 142t–143t
   postpartum change in, 138–139
   structure of, 141–142
Mammogenesis, 142–143
Marfan's syndrome, in pregnancy, 221–222
Marginate placenta, 94
Maternal physiologic adaptations, bilirubin metabolism in, 636–637
   calcium metabolism in, 614–618
   carbohydrate metabolism in, 584–591
   cardiovascular system in, 202–212
   fat metabolism in, 584–591
   gastrointestinal system in, 380–385
   hematologic and hemostatic systems in, 160–171
   hepatic system in, 385–386
   immune system in, 440–446
   integumentary system in, 492–498
   neuromuscular system in, 523–528
   phosphorus metabolism in, 614–618
   protein metabolism in, 584–591
   renal system in, 337–346
   respiratory system in, 263–270
   sensory system in, 523–528
   thermoregulation in, 677–678
   thyroid function in, 660–663

Maturation, of respiratory system, 324–325
Maturational changes, during infancy and childhood,
 in bilirubin metabolism, 654
 in calcium metabolism, 631
 in carbohydrate metabolism, 609
 in cardiovascular system, 253–254
 in fat metabolism, 609
 in gastrointestinal system, 429–431
 in host defense mechanisms, 482–486
 in integumentary system, 516
 in neuromuscular system, 575–576
 in phosphorus metabolism, 631
 in protein metabolism, 609
 in renal system, 371, 373
 in sensory system, 575–576
 in thermoregulation, 693
 in thyroid function, 672
Maturity, differential, in morphogenesis, 51
Mechanoreceptors, of lung airways in respiratory
 control in neonate, 293
Meconium, passage of, 410
Meconium aspiration syndrome, 321–322
Medullary center, in respiratory control in neonate,
 294
Meiosis, in germ cells, 6, 7
Melasma, in pregnancy, 492, 494
 nursing interventions for, 495t
Membranes, characteristics of, altered, teratogenesis by,
 63
 fetal, appearance of, alterations in, 86–88
 in amniotic fluid production and exchange, 83–84
Memory cell, definition of, 441t
Menarche, 25–26
Mendelian diseases, 6
Meningomyelocele, 545–546, 546
Menstrual cycle, 26–27
 ovarian cycle correlated with, 28
Menstrual phase, of endometrial cycle, 27
Menstruation, resumption of, postpartum, 140–141
Meralgia paresthesia, in pregnancy and lactation, 537t
Mesonephric duct, in male genital duct development,
 15, 16, 17
Metabolic acidosis, late, in neonate, 369–370
Metabolic rate, of neonate, 242–243
Metabolism, of anticonvulsant drugs, pregnancy and,
 533t
 of bilirubin, 636–655. See also *Bilirubin, metabolism of.*
 of carbohydrates, 583–610. See also *Carbohydrate(s),
  metabolism of.*
 of drugs, in neonate, 429
  in pregnancy, 397
 of fat, 583–610. See also *Fat(s), metabolism of.*
 of protein, 583–610. See also *Protein(s), metabolism of.*
 placental, 74–75
Methimazole, breast-feeding and, 152t
Methotrexate, breast-feeding and, 152t
Metronidazole toxicity, in pregnant woman, fetus and
 neonate, 454t–455t
Midgut, congenital anomalies of, 404
 fetal development of, 402–404
Migraine headaches, in pregnancy, 531
Migratory cytotrophoblast, 73
Milia, in neonate, 493t
Miliaria, in neonate, 493t
Milk, human, composition of, 147–151, 418t
 drugs in, 151–152
 for neonate, 422–423
 immunologic properties of, 445t, 445–446
 infants fed with, calcium homeostasis and, 626–627

Milk *(Continued)*
 preterm versus term, 151
 production of, 146–151
  functional unit of, 144
  initiation of, 143, 145–146
 transfer of antibiotics in, 454–455, 455t
Mineralization, of bone, postnatal, calcium and
 phosphorus intake and, 627, 628
Minerals, in milk, 148–149
 neonatal requirements for, 420, 421–422
Mitosis, in somatic cells, 5–6, 7
 interference with, teratogenesis by, 62
Mitral valve, fetal development of, 234
 prolapse of (MVP), in pregnancy, 219–220
 regurgitation in, in pregnancy, 219
 stenosis of, in pregnancy, 219
Mongolian spots, in neonate, 493t
Monosomy, 7
Monozygotic (MZ) twins, 95–96
 development and placentation of, 96, 97
Moro reflex, 558–559, 560t
Morphine, for neonatal pain, 571
Morphogenesis, principles of, 49–51
Mortality, perinatal, weight gain in pregnancy and, 387
Mother, effects of cocaine use on, 574
 infection in, risk of, immune system and, 449–450
 tolerance of fetus by, immune system and, 446–449
 toxicity of antibiotics for, 454t–455t
Motility, esophageal, in neonate, 411
 intestinal, in neonate, 411–412
Motor abilities, fetal development of, 550–551
Motor function, in transition to extrauterine life, 552
 neonatal, 557–560
Mouth, in pregnancy, 380, 382–383
Mucous membranes, alterations in, in pregnancy, 496–
 497
Multiple sclerosis, implications for mother and infant,
 532t
Muscle(s), arrector pili, fetal development of, 506
 chest wall, in respiratory pump, 295
 development of, in neonate, 557
 rib cage, in respiratory pump, 295
Muscle tone, active, by gestational age, 559
 fetal development of, 550
 passive, by gestational age, posture and, 558
Musculoskeletal changes, in antepartum period, 524
Musculoskeletal discomforts, in pregnancy, 529–530
Mutations, genetic, diseases from, 6–10
Myasthenia gravis, implications for mother and infant,
 532t
Myelinization, in fetus, 547–548
Myocardial contractility, in neonate, 242
Myometrium, 111–113. See also *Uterus.*
 cells of, structure of, 111, 112, 113
 changes in, in pregnancy, 113
 contractility of, hormonal control of, 114
 contraction of, 117–120
  cellular mechanisms controlling, 118
  coordination of, 119–120
 structure of, 110
Myosin filaments, in myometrial cells, 111, 112
Myosin light chain kinase (MLK), in myocardial
 contraction, 117–118
Myotonic dystrophy, implications for mother and
 infant, 532t

N

Nails, alterations in, in pregnancy, 497
Narcotics, for neonatal pain, 570–571

Nausea and vomiting, in pregnancy, 392–393
  causes of, 392t
  nursing recommendations for, 391t
  thyroid function and, 663–664
Necrotizing enterocolitis (NEC), in neonate, 428
Neonatal abstinence syndrome, 571–572, 572t
  Finnegan scoring system for, *573*
Neonate, adaptation of, after birth, placental
    transfusion and, 181t
  antibiotic use in, 480–481
  asphyxia in, 312
  at risk for altered hemostasis, 192–193
  bilirubin production in, 640–641
  blood transfusions in, 189–190
  blood volume changes in, 181–182
  cardiovascular conversion in, 291–292
  care of, clinical implications for, of bilirubin metabo-
    lism, 644–654
    of calcium metabolism, 626–631
    of carbohydrate metabolism, 606–609
    of cardiovascular disorders, 246–253
    of host defense mechanism alterations, 474–482
    of integumentary system, 511–516
    of renal system disorders, 365–371
    of respiratory disorders, 309–324
    of thyroid function, 670–672
  coagulation factors in, 187t
  coagulation in, 184–186
  cold stress in, 690–692
  control of respiration in, 292–294
  dehydration and diarrhea in, 428–429
  2,3–diphosphoglycerate changes in, 183
  drug absorption and metabolism in, 429
  effects of anticonvulsants on, 534
  effects of epilepsy on, 534
  effects of in-utero drug exposure on, 571–572, *574*
  erythropoietin in, 183
  extremely immature, integumentary system in, 514–
    515
  feeding methods for, considerations on, 425–427
  fibrinolysis in, 186
  fluid and electrolyte balance in, management of,
    365–370
  growth of, 417
  heat loss/overheating in, preventing, 681t
  hematocrit in, 183
  hematologic parameters in, 181–184
  hemoglobin development in, *179*
  hemoglobin levels in, 182–183
  hemoglobin-oxygen affinity alterations in, 188
  hemorrhagic disease of, vitamin K and, 188–189
  hemostasis in, 184–186
  hemostatic factors in, 187t
  HIV infection in, 479–480
  hyperbilirubinemia in, 644, 645–650. See also *Hyper-
    bilirubinemia, neonatal.*
  hypercalcemia in, 630–631
  hyperthermia in, 692–693
  hyperthyroidism in, 671–672
  hyperviscosity in, 191, *192*
  hypocalcemia in, 627–629
  hypoglycemia in, 606–607. See also *Hypoglycemia,
    neonatal.*
  hypothermia in, 692–693
    consequences of, 693t
  hypothyroidism in, 672
  immune responses of, to bacterial infections, 474–
    477
    to viral infections, 477–480

Neonate *(Continued)*
  immunotherapy for sepsis in, 481–482, 483t
  infection in, diagnosis of, 480
  iron in, 183–184
  liver function in, 416
  maturational changes in gastrointestinal system in,
    429
  measurement of renal function and hydration status
    in, 370
  metabolic substrate and hormone alterations in, 604t
  necrotizing enterocolitis in, 428
  nutritional requirements of, 417–423
  nutritional status of, monitoring, 427
  pain in, 568–572. See also *Pain, neonatal.*
  physiologic anemia in, 193–195
  physiology of, 179–180
    bilirubin metabolism in, 639–644
    calcium metabolism in, 623–626
    carbohydrate metabolism in, 603–605
    cardiovascular system in, 240–246. See also *Cardio-
      vascular system in neonatal physiology.*
    fat metabolism in, 605
    gastrointestinal system in, 408–416. See also *Gas-
      trointestinal (GI) system in neonatal physiology.*
    hematologic and hemostatic systems in, 180–186
    host defense mechanisms in, 467–474. See also
      Host defense mechanisms in neonatal physiology.
    integumentary system in, 508–511
    neuromuscular system in, 551–565
    phosphorus metabolism in, 623–626
    protein metabolism in, 605–606
    renal system in, 358–365. See also *Renal system in
      neonatal physiology.*
    respiratory system in, 289–309. See also *Respiratory
      system in neonatal physiology.*
    sensory system in, 551–565. See also *Sensory system
      in neonatal physiology.*
    thermoregulation in, 679–684. See also *Thermoreg-
      ulation in neonatal physiology.*
    thyroid function in, 668, *669*, 670
  platelets in, 184
  polycythemia in, 191, *192*
  preterm. See also *Preterm infant(s).*
  red blood cells in, 182
  reflexes in, 557–560
  regurgitation and reflux in, 427–428
  renal function during illness in, 370–371
  renal handling of pharmacologic agents in, 37(
  respiratory conversion in, 289–291
  respiratory risk in, factors increasing, 309–310
  respiratory stability in, nursing interventions to pro-
    mote, 310–311
  reticulocytes in, 183
  rickets in, 630
  screening for hypothyroidism in, 672
  seizures in, 568t, 568
  sensory function in, 555–557
  serum ferritin in, 183–184
  thermal status of, monitoring equipment for, 688–
    690
  toxicity of antibiotics for, 454t–455t
  transepidermal absorption in, 512, 513t–514t, 514
  transitional events in, 180–181
  very-low-birth-weight. See *Very-low-birth-weight
    (VLBW) infant(s).*
  white blood cells in, 184
Nervous system, autonomic, fetal development of,
    548–549
  development of, timetable of, 53t, *56, 58*

Nervous system *(Continued)*
  peripheral, fetal development of, 549
Neural connections, in transition to extrauterine life, 553
Neural crest, derivatives of, *545*
Neural plate, embryonic formation of, 539, *541*
Neural regulation, of fetal circulation, 243–244
Neural tube, closure of, failure of, anomalies from, 542
  embryonic formation of, 539, *541*, 541–542
Neurobehavioral cues, infant, 565t
Neurobehavioral organization, 564–565
Neurodevelopment, fetal, 546–548
Neurologic disorder, chronic, pregnant woman with, 531–535
Neuromuscular blocking agents, for neonatal pain, 570–571
Neuromuscular system, 522–576
  changes in, clinical implications of, for mother and infant, 532–533t
    for neonatal care, 565–574
    for pregnant woman and fetus, 528–538, 540t
    maturational, during infancy and childhood, 575–576
  effects of drug exposure in-utero on, 572–573, *574*
  embryonic development, 539, 541–546
  fetal development of, 546–551
    anatomic, 546–549
    functional, 549–551
  in antepartum period, 523–524
  in intrapartum period, 524–527
  in maternal physiologic adaptations, 523–528
  in neonatal physiology, 551–564
    circulation in brain and, 553–555
    conduction of impulses and, 553
    motor function in, 557–560
    neural connections and, 553
    neurobehavioral organization in, 564
    sensory function and, 555–557
    sleep-wake pattern in, 553, 560–564
    transitional events in, 551–553
  in postpartum period, 527–528
  neonatal pain and, 569–572
  neonatal seizures and, 568–569
  vulnerability of, to hypoxic and pressure-related injury, 566–568
Neurons, migration of, fetal, 547
  proliferation of, fetal, 546–547
Neuropathy(ies), peripheral, in pregnancy, 535–536, 537t
Neutral thermal environment, in neonatal care, 684–685
Nevus(i), junctional, in neonate, 493t
  spider, in pregnancy, 495–496
    nursing interventions for, 495t
Nevus flammeus, in neonate, 493t
Nitrofurantoin toxicity, in pregnant woman, fetus and neonate, 454t–455t
NK cells, definition of, 441t
Nocturia, in pregnancy, 346
Nondisjunction, 24
Nonshivering thermogenesis (NST), in heat production by neonate, 682
Nonstress testing (NST), in fetal heart rate evaluation, 89
Norplant, 33
Nucleic acid, integrity and function of, altered, teratogenesis by, 62
Nutrition, during postpartum period and lactation, 151

Nutrition *(Continued)*
  inadequate, in reproductive cycle, consequences of, 394t
  maternal, altered, effects of, 394–395
  parenteral, total, solutions for, components of, 423, 424t
Nutritional needs, of fetus, 390
  of neonate, for calcium, 626–627
    for phosphorus, 626–627
Nutritional requirements, of full and preterm infants, 417–423
  of pregnancy, 389–390
Nutritional status, of neonate, monitoring of, 427

O

Obesity, maternal, 394–395
Obstructive lesions, of heart in pregnancy, 219–220
Oligohydramnios, 91–92
Omphalocele, fetal development of, 404
Oocyte, in follicle maturation, 40–41
  in ovulation, 42
Oogenesis, 23–24
Open-glottis pushing, in second stage of labor, 123–124
Opsonization, definition of, 441t
Oral contraceptives, 32
  estrogen-containing, thyroid function tests and, 662t
  lactation and, 152
Orciprenaline, in labor inhibition, 127–128
Organogenesis, 51, 53t–54t, *56–57*
  period of, sensitivity teratogens in, 61
Osmolar imbalance, teratogenesis by, 63
Osmolarity, regulation of, in pregnancy, 344
Otolaryngeal changes, in antepartum period, 524
Ovarian cycle, 26
  diagrammatic summary of, *46*
  menstrual cycle correlated with, *28*
Ovary(ies), development of, 13, *14*, 15
  function of, in conception, 40–42
  hormones of, in female reproductive processes, 25
Overhydration, risk of, in neonate, 368–369
Ovulation, 26
  in conception, 42
  resumption of, postpartum, 140–141
Ovulatory phase, of ovarian cycle, 26
Oxygen, effects of ventilation-perfusion mismatching on, 304
Oxygen antioxidants, in functional development of fetal respiratory system, 285
Oxygen consumption, in antepartum period, 208
  exercise and, 272
  in neonatal physiology, 306
Oxygen content, of fetus, 240–241
Oxygen-hemoglobin affinity, alterations in, in childhood, 196–197
  in infancy, 196–197
  in neonate, 188
Oxygen-hemoglobin dissociation curve, in antepartum period, 267
  in neonatal physiology, 306, *307*
Oxygen transfer, in functional development of fetal respiratory system, 287
Oxygen transport, in neonate, 242–243
Oxygenation, fetal, 172
Oxytocin, breast development and, 142t
  in initiation of labor, 116
  in labor induction, 126

Oxytocin *(Continued)*
in let-down reflex, 146
postpartum levels of, 141
Oxytocin challenge test (OCT), in fetal heart rate
evaluation, 89

P

Pacemaker, of cardiac muscle, fetal development of,
234
Pacemaker potential, in coordination of uterine
contractions, 119
Pain, gate control theory of, 525–526, *526*
in labor, 524–526
endorphins and, 526–527
physiologic changes secondary to, *525*
neonatal, 568–572
assessment of, 570
consequences of, 569
management of, 570–571
reception of, 569
responses to, 570t
postpartum, 527
Palmar erythema, in pregnancy, 496
Palmar grasp reflex, 559, 560t
Pancreas, fetal development of, 402
in pregnancy, 385
Pancreatitis, in pregnancy, 396
Pancuronium bromide, for neonatal pain, 571–572
Papular dermatitis, of pregnancy, 500t–501t
Paramesonephric duct, in female genital duct
development, *16*, 17
Parathyroid glands, fetal development of, 621
Parathyroid hormone (PTH), calcium and phosphorus
homeostasis and, 617
calcium levels and, in antepartum period, 615, *616*,
616t, 617
in control of calcium and phosphorus levels, 616t
levels of, in neonate, 624, *625*
maternal-placental-fetal-neonatal interrelationships
of, *621*
Paresthesia(s), in antepartum period, 529
meralgia, in pregnancy and lactation, 537t
Partial thromboplastin time (PTT), in neonate, 185–
186
Parturition, physiologic processes of, clinical
implications of, 122–130
dystocia and, 128
maternal position during labor and, 122–123
maternal pushing efforts during second stage and,
123–124
pharmacology of labor and, 124–128
postterm labor and, 128–130
preterm labor and, 124
physiology of, 113–122
Passive immunity, definition of, 441t
Patent ductus arteriosus (PDA), in pregnancy, 220–221
management of, 250
Penicillin toxicity, in pregnant woman, fetus and
neonate, 454t–455t
Penis, development of, 18, *19*
in hypospadias, 22
Peptic ulcer, in pregnancy, 395–396
Perception, tactile, in neonate, 511
Percutaneous umbilical blood sampling (PUBS), in fetal
status assessment, 91
Perfusion, in neonatal physiology, 300–301

Perfusion *(Continued)*
matching of ventilation to, 301–305. See also *Ventila-
tion-perfusion matching.*
skin, in antepartum period, 208
Perinatal asphyxia, 312
hypocalcemia and, 629
hypoglycemia in infant with, 608–609
Perinatal HIV infection, 451–452
Perinatal mortality, weight gain in pregnancy and, *387*
Perinatal nutrition, 379–431. See also *Gastrointestinal
(GI) system; Nutrition.*
Perinatal pharmacology, 86
Peripheral nervous system, fetal development of, 549
Peripheral neuropathies, in pregnancy, 535–536, 537t
Periventricular hemorrhage (PVH), brain injury in
neonate from, 566–567
Periventricular leukomalacia (PVL), brain injury in
neonate from, 567
Permeability, of fetal skin, 507
Persistent pulmonary hypertension (PPHN), in
newborn, 322–324
Petechiae, in neonate, 493t
Phagocytosis, altered, in neonate, 468–469
Pharmacologic agents. See *Drug(s).*
Pharmacologic treatment, of skin disorders in
pregnancy, 498–499
Pharmacology, of labor, physiologic processes and,
124–128
perinatal, 86
Pharyngeal gut, fetal development of, 398–399, *400*
Phenindione, breast-feeding and, 152t
Phenobarbital, for neonatal hyperbilirubinemia, 646
Phenotype, 4
Phosphatidylcholine (PC), in pulmonary surfactant, 279
synthesis of, 280–282, *281*, *282*
Phosphatidylglycerol (PG), in pulmonary surfactant,
279, 280
synthesis of, 281, *281*
Phospholipids, biosynthesis of, *281*, 281–282
gestational alterations in, 282, *283*
Phosphorus, homeostasis of, 617
levels of, hormonal actions controlling, 616t
in neonate, 624
maternal needs for, 619
metabolism of, 614–631
changes in, clinical implications for pregnant
woman and fetus and, 618–620
fetal effects of, 621t
fetal development of, 621–623
in antepartum period, 615, 616t, 617, 625
in maternal physiologic adaptations, 614–618
in neonatal physiology, 623–626
neonatal requirements for, 421
renal handling of, in neonate, 362, 363
Phototherapy, for neonatal hyperbilirubinemia, 646–
650
equipment for, 648, 650, 650t
intermittent versus continuous, 648
mechanisms of action of, *647*
physics of, 646–647
side effects of, 647–648, *649*
infants receiving, integumentary system in, 515–516
Physiologic anemia of infancy, 193–195
Physiologic hypogammaglobulinemia, 483–484
Pigmentary demarcation lines, in pregnancy, 494
Pigmentation, alterations of, in pregnancy, 492
Pinocytosis, in placental transport, 79t, 81
Pituitary gland, gonadotropins of, in female
reproductive processes, 25

Pituitary gland (*Continued*)
  in fetal endocrinology, 18, 20
Pituitary gonadotropin, postpartum levels of, 140–141
Placenta, 63–81
  abnormalities of, 92–94
  appearance of, alterations in, 86–88
  circulation in, 71–74
    at term, *68*
  development of, 63–71
  function of, 74–81
    endocrinologic, 75–78
    evaluation of, 88–89
    immunologic, 78
    metabolic, 74–75
    postdate gestation and, 88
  growth of, 68–70
  implantation of, abnormalities of, 92–94
  in amniotic fluid production and exchange, 83–84
  in multiple pregnancy, 95–96, 98, *100*, 101
  perfusion of, in pregnancy-induced hypertension,
    226
  physiology of, clinical implications related to, 84–95
  separation of, 70–71
    abnormalities of, 92–94
  smoking and, 274–275
  structure of, 71
    at term, *68*
  transport across, 78–81
    active, 79t, 81
    by accidental capillary breaks, 79t, 81
    by bulk flow, 79t, 81
    by facilitated diffusion, 79t, 80–81
    by independent movement, 79t, 81
    by simple diffusion, 78–80, 79t
    by solvent drag, 79t, 81
    endocytosis in, 79t, 81
    of maternal fuels, *599*
    of substances, clinical implications of, 84–86
    pinocytosis in, 79t, 81
Placenta accreta, 93–94
Placenta increta, 93
Placenta percreta, 93–94
Placenta previa, 92–93
Placental hormones, effects of, on carbohydrate, fat
    and protein metabolism, 589, 591
Placental lactogen, human, 75–76
  breast development and, 142t
  effects on carbohydrate, fat, and protein metabolism,
    591
  fat metabolism in pregnancy and, *592*
Placental transfusion, effects of, on neonatal adaptation
    after birth, 181t
Placentation, 65, 67–68
  abnormalities of, 94
  of dizygotic twins, 98, *99*
  of monozygotic twins, 96, *97*
Plasma, components of, in antepartum period, 164t–
    165t, 165–166
  volume of, in antepartum period, 160–162, 171, 203
Plasma cell, definition of, 441t
Platelets, activity of, in labor, delivery, and postpartum
    period, *170*
  development of, in fetus, 178
  in antepartum period, 162t–163t, 164–165
  in neonate, 184
Pleural pressure, in neonate, 299
Pneumotaxic center, in respiratory control in neonate,
    294
Polycystic kidneys, 357

Polycythemia, neonatal, 191, *192*
Polyhydramnios, 91
Polymorphonuclear neutrophils (PMNs), altered, in
    neonate, 468
Polyploidy, 7
Position, maternal, in labor, physiologic processes and,
    122–123
  renal function in pregnancy and, 346–348
Postabsorptive state, of pregnancy, carbohydrate, fat
    and protein metabolism in, 589, *590*
Postmature infants, integumentary system in, 515
Postmaturity syndrome, 129–130
Postpartum foot drop, 537t
Postpartum period, 136–153
  blood volume changes in, 169–170
  blues in, 527–528
  calcium metabolism in, 618
  carbohydrate metabolism in, 591
  cardiovascular system in, 211–212
  discomfort in, 527
  endocrine changes in, 139–141
  fat metabolism in, 591
  gastrointestinal system in, 388–389
  hematologic parameters in, 170–171
  hemostasis in, 171
  hepatic system in, 388–389
  immune system in, 444–446
  inability to void in, 348
  integumentary system in, 497–498
  involution in, of breasts, 138–139
    of cervix, 138
    of uterus, 137–138
    of vagina, 138
  lactation in, 141–152. See also *Lactation.*
  neuromuscular system in, 527–528
  neuropathies in, 537t
  nutrition during, 151
  phosphorus metabolism in, 618
  protein metabolism in, 591
  renal system in, 345–346
  respiratory system in, 269–270
  sensory system in, 527–528
  sexual function and activity in, 139
  sleep in, 527
  thermoregulation in, 678
  thyroid disorders in, 665
  thyroid function in, 663
Potassium, renal handling of, in neonate, 362
Preeclampsia, complications of, 223–224
  diagnosis of, 222–223
  prediction of, 224
  proteinuric, risk in twin pregnancy, 218
  severe, HELLP syndrome and, 227–228
Pregnancy, 36–63. See also *Antepartum period.*
  as diabetogenic state, 593
  as state of accelerated starvation, 592–593
  as state of facilitated anabolism, 592
  blood cellular components in, 162t–163t, 162–165
  cervix in, 120–122
  coagulation in, *168*
  consumptive coagulopathies in, 175
  ectopic, 64
  effects of, on epilepsy, 531, 533
  effects of epilepsy on, 534
  first trimester of, 37–38
  hypercoagulable state of, 166–167
  hypervolemia of, 171
  immune states induced by, 457–458
  iron requirements in, 171–172

Pregnancy *(Continued)*
  location of uterus in, *39*
  loss of, recurrent, 48–49
  megaloblastic anemia in, 173
  multiple, 95–101. See also *Twin(s).*
  plasma components in, 164t–165t, 165–166
  second trimester of, 38
  severe anemia of, 172–174
  sickle cell anemia in, 173–174
  supine hypotensive syndrome of, 213
  β-thalassemia in, 174
  third trimester of, 39–40
  thromboembolism and, 174–175
  uterus in, 113
    growth of, 110–111
Pregnancy-induced hypertension (PIH), 74, 222–227
  blood volume in, 161
  cerebral manifestations of, 538
  immunologic aspects of, 457–458
  intrapartum management of, 226–227
  plasma volume in, 161
  platelet aggregation in, 164
  prenatal therapy of, 226
  renal system in, 351–352
Prematurity, rickets of, factors predisposing to, 630t
  urinary tract infection and, 348
Prenatal period, 36–63. See also *Antepartum period;*
  Pregnancy.
Prenatal testing, timeline for, *90*
Preoxygenation, in suctioning of endotracheal tube,
  311
Pressure-related injury, to neuromuscular and sensory
  systems, 565–568
Preterm infant(s), calcium intake in, 627
  coagulation factors in, 187t
  feeding of, 423–424
  hemostatic factors in, 187t
  human milk for, 422–423
  hypocalcemia in, 627–628
  intestinal motility in, 412
  nutritional requirements of, 417–423, 419t
  respiratory stability in, nursing interventions to pro-
    mote, 310–311
  sensory modalities in, 556
  sodium balance in, 361–362
  sodium requirements of, 367–368
  sucking and swallowing in, 411
  transfusion of, 190
  transient hypothyroidism in, 671
  vitamin E and, 190–191
Preterm labor, 224
  factors associated with, 125t
  infection and, 450–451
Progesterone, breast development and, 142t
  effects on carbohydrate, fat, and protein metabolism,
    591
  in female reproductive processes, 25
  in initiation of labor, 114
  in labor inhibition, 127
  postpartum levels of, 139–140
  production of, in pregnancy, 76–77
  respiratory changes in pregnancy from, 263–264
Prolactin, breast development and, 142t
  in female reproductive processes, 25
  in milk production, 144–145
  pattern of, in lactating women, 146
  plasma concentrations of, during nursing, *147*
  postpartum levels of, 141

Prolactin-inhibiting factor (PIF), breast development
  and, 142t
Proliferative phase, of endometrial cycle, 26–27
Propranolol, fetal effects of, 666–667
Propylthiouracil (PTU), fetal effects of, 666
  for hyperthyroidism in pregnancy, 664
Prostaglandin(s), in initiation of labor, 114–116
  in labor induction, 126
  respiratory changes in pregnancy from, 264
  synthesis of, abnormal, in pregnancy-induced hyper-
    tension, 224, 225
  to enhance cervical ripening, 125
Prostaglandin A1, for pregnancy-induced
  hypertension, 226
Prostaglandin synthetase inhibitors, in labor inhibition,
  127
Protective mechanisms, of skin in neonate, 510–511
Protein(s), absorption of, in neonate, physiologic
  limitations of, 412–414, 413t
  digestion of, *381*
    in neonate, physiologic limitations of, 412–414,
      413t
  metabolism of, 583–610
    changes in, clinical implications for pregnant
      woman and fetus and, 591–598
      maturational, during infancy and childhood, 609
    fetal development of, 602–603
    in antepartum period, 584–586
    in intrapartum period, 591
    in maternal physiologic adaptations, 584–591
    in neonatal physiology, 605–606
    in postpartum period, 591
    maternal-fetal relationships and, 594–595, 595t
  neonatal requirements for, 419–420
  plasma, total, in antepartum period, 164t, 165
  synthesis and release of, in milk, 150–151
Proteinuria, in pregnancy, 341
Prurigo gestationis of Besnier, 500t–501t
Pruritic urticarial papules and plaques of pregnancy
  (PUPPP), 500t–501t
Pruritus, in pregnancy, 497
  nursing interventions for, 495t
Pruritus gravidarum, 500t–501t
Pseudohermaphroditism, 21–22
Ptyalism, in pregnancy, 382–383
Puberty, in female, 25–26
  in male, 29
Pulmonary artery hypertension, in pregnancy, 221
Pulmonary hypertension, persistent, in newborn, 322–
  324
Pulmonary vascular blood flow, in antepartum period,
  208
Pulmonary vascular resistance (PVR), in transition to
  extrauterine life, 241
Purkinje fibers, fetal development of, 234

R

Radiant warmers, in neonatal body temperature
  maintenance, 690
Radiation, heat loss in neonate by, preventing, 681t,
  687–688
Radioiodine, use of, in pregnancy, 665–667
Recessive inheritance, autosomal, 10
  X-linked, 8–9
Red blood cell volume, in antepartum period, 202–203
Red blood cells (RBCs), development of, in fetus, 178
  in antepartum period, 162t–163t, 162–164

Red blood cells (RBCs) (*Continued*)
    in neonate, 182
Reflex(es), chest wall, in respiratory control in neonate, 293
    lung, in respiratory control in neonate, 293–294
    neonatal, 557–560
Reflux, gastroesophageal, in neonate, 427–428
Regurgitation, in neonate, 427–428
    mitral, in pregnancy, 219
Relaxin, in initiation of labor, 117
Renal blood flow (RBF), in fetus, 357
    in neonate, 360–361
Renal plasma flow (RPF), physiologic and pathophysiologic changes in, 347t
Renal system, 336–374. See also *Fluid(s) and electrolytes, homeostasis of; Kidney(s).*
    anomalies of, developmental basis for, 357
    changes in, clinical implications of, for neonatal care, 365–371
        for pregnant woman and fetus, 346–354, 347t, 355t
        maturational, during infancy and childhood, 371, 373
    fetal development of, 354–358
        anatomic, 354–357
        anomalies in, 357
        functional, 357–358
    hypertension and, 351, *352*
    in antepartum period, 337–345
    in maternal physiologic adaptation, 337–346
    in neonatal physiology, 358–365
        bladder in, 365
        body composition in, 359
        glomerular filtration rate and, 360–361
        hormonal regulation in, 365
        renal blood flow and, 360–361
        transitional events in, 359
        tubular function and, 361–363
        urine output in, 359–360
        water balance and, 363–364
    in postpartum period, 345–346
Renin-angiotensin-aldosterone system, in neonate, 365
    in pregnancy, 342–344, *343*
Renin-angiotensin system, in fetal circulation regulation, 244
    in fetus, 358
Reproduction, biologic basis for, 3–33
    physiologic basis for, 3–33
    processes of, 24–29
        female, 24–28
        male, 28–29
Reproductive organs, involution of, postpartum, 137–139
Reproductive system, anomalies of, 20–23
    embryonic/fetal development of, 10–18
Respiration, control of, in neonate, 292–294
    maternal, exercise and, 271
    tissue, in neonatal physiology, 306–307
Respiratory capillary engorgement, upper, in antepartum period, 270–271
Respiratory distress syndrome (RDS), in newborn, 316–318
    clinical symptoms of, 317
    pathogenesis of, 316–317
    treatment of, 317–318
    L/S ratio in prediction of, 285
Respiratory infection, in antepartum period, 271
Respiratory pump, in neonatal physiology, 294–296
Respiratory system, 262–326

Respiratory system (*Continued*)
    changes in, clinical implications of, for neonatal care, 309–324. See also *specific disorder.*
        for pregnant woman and fetus, 270–276
    conversion to extrauterine life, 289–291
    development of, timetable of, 53t, *57, 58*
    fetal, in amniotic fluid production and exchange, 84
    fetal development of, 276–289
        anatomic, 277–279
        functional, 279–289
            assessment of fetal lung maturity in, 284–285
            carbon dioxide transfer in, 287–288
            catecholamines in, 284
            fetal blood gases in, 287
            fetal breathing movements in, 288–289
            glucocorticoids in, 282–283
            insulin in, 284
            lung fluid in, 285–287
            normal fetal blood gases in, 288
            oxygen antioxidants in, 285
            oxygen transfer in, 287
            thyroid hormones in, 283–284
    in antepartum period, 263–267
        biochemical changes in, 263–264
        lung function changes in, 265–267
        lung volumes in, *264,* 264–265, 265t
        mechanical changes in, 263
    in intrapartum period, 267–269
    in maternal physiologic adaptation, 263–270
    in neonatal physiology, 289–309
        alveolar-capillary membrane in, 305–309
        control of respiration in, 292–294
        lung volumes in, 299–300
        mechanical properties in, 297–299
        perfusion in, 300–301
        respiratory pump in, 294–296
        transitional events in, 289–292
        ventilation in, 299
        ventilation-perfusion matching in, 301–305
    in postpartum period, 269–270
    maturation of, during infancy and childhood, 324–325
    problems of, infants with, feeding of, 424
Response, to traction reflex, 560t
Restless leg syndrome, in pregnancy, 529–530
Resuscitation, of newborn, 314–315
Reticulocytes, in neonate, 183
Retinopathy, of prematurity, 308–309
Retractions, in neonate, physiologic basis for, 310
    in respiratory distress syndrome, 317
Rewarming hypothermic infant, 691–692
RhIG, in prevention of Rho(D) isoimmunization, 460–462
Rho(D) isoimmunization, 459–462, *461–462*
Rib cage, compliance of, in respiratory pump, 295–297
    muscles of, in respiratory pump, 295
Ribonucleic acid (RNA), function of, 4
    structure of, 4
Rickets, neonatal, 630
    of prematurity, factors predisposing to, 630t
Right-to-left shunts, in pregnancy, 221
Ritodrine, in labor inhibition, 127–128
RNA (ribonucleic acid), function of, 4
    structure of, 4
Roll-over test, to predict preeclampsia, 224
Rooting reflex, 559–560

S

Salbutamol, in labor inhibition, 127–128
Salivation, excessive, in pregnancy, 382–383
Salmon patch hemangioma, in neonate, 493t
Schultze's mechanism, of placental separation, 71
Sebaceous glands, fetal development of, 506
Secretory glands, alterations in, in pregnancy, 497
Secretory phase, of endometrial cycle, 27
Seizures, neonatal, 568t, 568
    jitteriness differentiated from, 569t
Semen abnormalities, etiology of, 31t
Semilunar valves, fetal development of, 234
Seminal vesicle, development of, *16*, 17
Sense organs, development of, timetable of, 54t, *56*, *58*
Sensory abilities, fetal development of, 549–550
Sensory experiences, during birth, 552
Sensory function, in transition to extrauterine life,
        552–553
    neonatal, 555–557
Sensory modalities, neonatal, 556
Sensory processing, neonatal, 556–557
Sensory system, 522–576
    changes in, clinical implications of, for neonatal care,
            565–574
        for pregnant woman and fetus, 528–529, 540t
        maturational, during infancy and childhood, 575–
            576
    development of specific systems in, 548–549
    embryonic development of, 539, 541–546
    fetal development of, 546–551
        anatomic, 546–549
        functional, 549–551
    fetal neurodevelopment and, 546–548
    in antepartum period, 523–524
    in intrapartum period, 524–527
    in maternal physiologic adaptations, 523–528
    in neonatal physiology, 551–565
        neural connections and, 553
        sensory function and, 555–557
        transitional events in, 551–553
    in postpartum period, 527–528
Septation, of heart in fetus, 231–234
Serum factors, influence on host defense mechanisms
        in pregnancy on, 444
Servocontrol methods, of neonatal thermoregulation,
        688–689
Sex-linked inheritance, 8–9
Sexual function/activity, postpartum, 139
Shivering, in heat production by neonate, 682
Short bowel syndrome, infants with, feeding of, 425
Shunting, in newborn lung, 303
Skeletal system, development of, growth and, 622–623
    timetable of, 54t, *59*
Skin, 491–517. See also *Integumentary system.*
    appearance of, by gestational age, 508t
    barrier properties of, in neonate, 508
    disorders of, pharmacologic treatment of, during
            pregnancy, 498–499
        preexisting, effects of pregnancy on, 498
    fetal, in amniotic fluid production and exchange, 84
    neonatal, care of, 511
        in protection from infection, 512
        variations in, 493t
    perfusion of, in antepartum period, 208
    permeability of, in neonate, 508
    protective mechanisms of, in neonate, 510–511
Sleep, in antepartum period, 524
    in postpartum period, 527

Sleep-wake patterns, fetal, 551
    in neonate, 560–564
    in transition to extrauterine life, 553
    related to brain maturation, 561–562
Sleep-wake states, 562t–563t
Small-for-gestational-age (SGA) infant(s), cell-mediated
        immunity in, 471
    fetal hemoglobin concentrations in, 182
    perinatal adaptive problems of, 40lt
    risk of thrombosis in, 193
Small intestines, in pregnancy, 384–385
Smell, sense of, development of, 549
Smoking, in antepartum period, 274–275
Smooth muscle, contraction and relaxation of,
        mechanisms of, *112*
Sodium, balance of, in preterm infants, 361–362
    excretion of, physiologic and pathophysiologic
            changes in, 347t
    homeostasis of, in pregnancy, 342
    requirements of preterm infants for, 367–368
    tubular handling of, in neonate, 361
Solvent drag, placental transport by, 79t, 81
Somatic cells, mitosis in, 5–6, *7*
Somatic pain, in labor, 525
Somatomammotropin, human chorionic, 75–76
Sperm, abnormalities of, infertility from, 30
    production of, 29
    transport of, in conception, 42–43
Spermatogenesis, 23
Spider nevi, in pregnancy, 495–496
    nursing interventions for, 495t
Spina bifida, 543
    types of, *546*
Spina bifida cystica, 545, *546*
Spina bifida occulta, 543, 545, *546*
Spinal cord, transection of, pregnancy in woman with,
        536
    tumor of, pregnancy in woman with, 536, 538
Starvation, accelerated, pregnancy as state of, 592–593
Stenosis, mitral, in pregnancy, 219
Steroidogenesis, in pregnancy, 76–78
Stomach, emptying of, in neonate, 411
    fetal development of, 401
    in pregnancy, 384
Strawberry hemangioma, in neonate, 493t
Streptococcus, group B (GBS), immune response to, in
        neonate, 474–477, *476*
Stress, cold, neonatal, 690–692
    physiologic consequences of, *692*
Stress-strain relationship, in functional development of
        fetal cardiovascular system, 237–238
Striae gravidarum, 494–495
    in pregnancy, nursing intervention for, 495t
Stroke volume, in antepartum period, 206
    in intrapartum period, 211
    in postpartum period, 212
Subarachnoid block, for cesarean section,
        hemodynamic changes from, 217
Subcutaneous tissue, structural components of, *503*
Succenturiate placenta, 94
Sucking, maturation of, 410–411
Sucking reflex, 559–560, 560t
Suckling, neuroendocrine reflexes initiated by, *145*
    prolactin release and, 144–145
Suctioning, of endotracheal tube, sighing after, 311
    two-person, 311
Sulfonamide toxicity, in pregnant woman, fetus and
        neonate, 454t–455t
Supine hypotensive syndrome, of pregnancy, 213

Supine pressor test, to predict preeclampsia, 224
Suppressor T cell, definition of, 441t
Supraventricular tachycardia, hydrops fetalis from, 248
Surfactant, composition of, 279, *280*
    exogenous replacement of, for bronchopulmonary dysplasia, 320
    in fetal lung development, 279–282
    inadequate, respiratory distress syndrome and, 317
Swallowing, by fetus, 405
    maturation of, 410–411
Sweat glands, fetal development of, 506
Sweating, heat dissipation by, in neonate, 683–684
Systemic lupus erythematosus (SLE), pregnant woman with, 458
Systemic vascular resistance (SVR), in antepartum period, 207
    in transition to extrauterine life, 241

T

T cell(s), cytotoxic, definition of, 441t
    in cell-mediated immunity, 471
    killer, definition of, 441t
    suppressor, definition of, 441t
Tachycardia, fetal, 244
    supraventricular, hydrops fetalis from, 248
Tachypnea, in neonate, physiologic basis for, 310
    transient, in newborn, 315–316
Tactile perception, in neonate, 511
Taste, sense of, development of, 549
Teratogenesis, mechanisms of, 62–63
    principles of, 61–63
Terbutaline, in labor inhibition, 127–128
Testes, development of, 13, *14*, 18
Testosterone, in male reproductive processes, 28–29
Tetracycline toxicity, in pregnant woman, fetus, and neonate, 454t–455t
Tetralogy of Fallot, in pregnancy, 221
β-Thalassemia, in pregnancy, 174
Thermal environment, neutral, in neonatal care, 684–685
    of neonate, integumentary system and, 509–510
Thermogenesis, nonshivering, in heat production by neonate, 682
Thermoregulation, 677–694
    changes in, clinical implications of, for neonatal care, 684–693
        for pregnant woman and fetus, 678–679
        maturational, during infancy and childhood, 693
    fetal, 678–679
    in maternal physiologic adaptations, 677–678
    in neonatal physiology, 679–684
        heat dissipation and loss in, 683–684
        heat production and conservation in, 680, 682–683
        heat transfer in, 680
        in transitional events, 680
    in neonate, thyroid function and, 670–672
    infants at risk for problems in, 691t
Thiouracil, breast-feeding and, 152t
Thrombocytopenia, in pregnancy-induced hypertension, 226
Thromboembolism, pregnancy and, 174
Thrombosis, in neonate, 193
Thyroid function, 660–673
    changes in, clinical implications of, for neonatal care, 670–672
        for pregnant woman and fetus, 663–667

Thyroid function *(Continued)*
        maturational, during infancy and childhood, 672
    fetal development of, 667–668
    in maternal physiologic adaptations, 660–663
    in neonatal physiology, 668, *669*, 670
    in neonate, thermoregulation and, 670–672
    nausea and vomiting of pregnancy and, 663–664
    tests of, during pregnancy, 663
        estrogen-containing oral contraceptives and, 662t
Thyroid gland, disorders of, breast-feeding in women with, 665
        postpartum, 665
    fetal development of, 668
    function of, 660–673. See also *Thyroid function.*
Thyroid hormones, concentration of, changes in, in gestation and birth, *669*
    in functional development of fetal respiratory system, 283–284
    secretion of, regulation of, *661*
Thyroiditis, postpartum, 665
Thyrotropin-releasing hormone, breast development and, 142t
Thyroxine (T4), 660. See also *Thyroid hormones.*
    breast development and, 142t
    in functional development of fetal respiratory system, 283
Time constants, in respiratory system, 298–299
Tissue(s), respiration of, in neonatal physiology, 306–307
    subcutaneous, structural components of, *503*
Tonic neck reflex, 559
Total anomalous pulmonary venous return, management of, 251–252
Total blood volume (TBV), in antepartum period, 202–203
Total parenteral nutrition (TPN), solutions for, components of, 423, 424t
Touch, sense of, development of, 549
Trace elements, neonatal requirements for, 420, 422
Transepidermal absorption, in neonate, 512, 513t–514t, 514
Transfusion(s), blood, in neonate, 189–190
    exchange, for neonatal hyperbilirubinemia, 646
    intrauterine, for fetus of Rho(D)-immunized woman, 460
    placental, effects of, on neonatal adaptation after birth, 181t
Transient tachypnea in newborn, 315–316
Transitional events, bilirubin metabolism in, 639–640
    calcium and phosphorus metabolism in, 624
    cardiovascular system in, 240–242
    gastrointestinal system in, 408–412
    hematologic and hemostatic systems in, 180–181
    host defense mechanisms in, 467–468
    integumentary system in, 507–508
    metabolic processes in, 603
    neuromuscular and sensory systems in, 551–553
    renal system in, 359
    respiratory system in, 289–292
    thermoregulation in, 680
Translocation, of chromosomes, 8
Transplacental passage, of maternal antibodies, 458–459
Transplant, renal, pregnancy following, 353–354
Transpulmonary pressure–to–lung volume curve, 299, *300*
Traumatic neuropathies, in pregnancy and lactation, 537t
Tricuspid valve, atresia of, management of, 252

Tricuspid valve (*Continued*)
fetal development in, 234
Triiodothyronine (T3), 660
in functional development of fetal respiratory system, 283
Trimethoprim toxicity, in pregnant woman, fetus, and neonate, 454t–455t
Trisomy, 7
Trophoblastic disease, gestational, 95
Truncus arteriosus, fetal development of, 234
management of, 252
Tubular functions, *340*
alterations in, in pregnancy, *341*, 341–342
in neonate, 361–363
Turner's syndrome, 22
Twin(s), cardiovascular system and, 217–218
dizygotic, 95–96, 98
incidence of, 95
monozygotic, 95–96
perinatal mortality in, 96
placental abnormalities in, 98, *100*, 101
Twin-to-twin transfusion syndrome, 98, 101

U

Ulcer, peptic, in pregnancy, 395–396
Umbilical blood sampling, in fetal status assessment, 91
Umbilical cord, 81–82
abnormalities of, 94
clamping of, 180–181
in amniotic fluid production and exchange, 84
Umbilical hernia, fetal development of, 404
Umbilical vein, fetal development of, 237
Undernutrition, in pregnancy, 394
Uric acid, renal handling of, in neonate, 362
Uridine diphosphoglucuronyl (UDP-glucuronyl) transferase activity, development of, *641*, 643–644
Urinary frequency, in pregnancy, 346
Urinary tract, fetal, development of, 357
in amniotic fluid production and exchange, 84
infection of (UTI), risk of, in pregnancy, 348
Urine, output of, in neonate, 359–360
water loss in, in neonate, 366–367
Uropathy, obstructive, 357
Uterovaginal malformation, 23
Uterus. See also *Myometrium.*
blood flow in, in antepartum period, 207–208
contraction of, coordination of, 119–120
physiologic events during, 120
development of, *16*, 17
growth of, 110–111
involution of, postpartum, 137–138
location of, in pregnancy, *39*
physiology of, 109–111
structure of, 110

V

Vagina, development of, *16*, 17
involution of, postpartum, 138
Valsalva pushing, in second stage of labor, 123, *124*
Valves, cardiac, fetal development of, 235
Varicosities, in pregnancy, 496
nursing intervention for, 495t
Vas deferens, development of, 17
Vascular anastomoses, placental, in multiple gestations, 98, *100*

Vasopressin, arginine, in pregnancy, 344–345
in renal system regulation in neonate, 365
in fetal circulation regulation, 244
Vein(s), fetal development of, 236–237
pulmonary, prenatal development of, 278–279
Velamentous insertion, of umbilical cord, 94
Ventilation, in antepartum period, 265
in intrapartum period, 268–269
in neonate, 299
in resuscitation of neonate, 315
wasted, in newborn lung, 303
Ventilation-perfusion, lung, ideal, *303*
Ventilation-perfusion matching, developmental differences in, 304–305
in neonatal physiology, 301–305
Ventilation-perfusion mismatching, effect on carbon dioxide, 304
effect on oxygen, 304
Ventilation-perfusion ratios, 301–305
Ventricles, septation of, in fetus, 231, *234*, 235
Ventricular septal defects (VSDs), in pregnancy, 220
management of, 253
Vernix caseosa, 507
Very-low-birth-weight (VLBW) infant(s), altered hemostasis in, 193
bone mineralization in, 627
feeding of, 424
iatrogenic blood losses in, 187
integumentary system in, 514–515
thermal injury prevention in, 686t
Vestibular sense, development of, 549
Villi, development of, in placentation, 65, 67–68
Viral infections, immune responses of neonate to, 477–480
Virchow's triad, predisposing to thromboembolic disorder, 174
Visceral pain, in labor, 524–525
Vision, sense of, development of, 550
Vitamin(s), absorption of, in neonate, 416
in milk, 148, 149t
neonatal requirements for, 420–421
Vitamin A, neonatal requirements for, 420–421
Vitamin C, neonatal requirements for, 421
Vitamin D, calcium levels and, in antepartum period, 617
in control of calcium and phosphorus levels, 616t
levels of, in neonate, 624, 626
maternal-placental-fetal-neonatal interrelationships of, *621*
neonatal requirements for, 421
Vitamin E, for bronchopulmonary dysplasia, 320
neonatal requirements for, 421
preterm infant and, 190–191
Vitamin K, hemorrhagic disease of newborn and, 188–189
Vitelline veins, fetal development of, 236–237
Voiding, postpartum problems with, 348
Volume homeostasis in pregnancy, 344
Vomiting, nausea and, in pregnancy, 392–393
causes of, 392t
nursing recommendations for, 391t
thyroid function and, 663–664

W

Warmers, radiant, in neonatal body temperature maintenance, 690
Water, loss of, in urine, in neonate, 366–367

Water (*Continued*)
    insensible, in neonate, 366, 367t
    transepidermal, in neonate, 508–509
Water balance, in neonate, 363–364
Weight gain, in pregnancy, 386, 388
    perinatal mortality and, *387*
    recommended ranges of, 388t
White blood cells (WBCs), development of, in fetus,
    178
    in antepartum period, 162t–163t, 164
    in neonate, 184

X

X-linked inheritance, 8–9

Y

Y-linked inheritance, 9
Yolk sac, formation of, 51, *52*

Z

Zinc, neonatal requirements for, 422
Zygote, cleavage of, 45
    transport of, 45

ISBN 0-7216-2936-9

90038